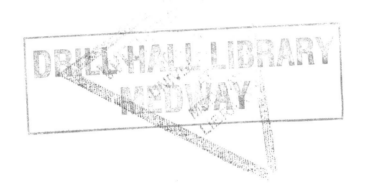

Giles R. Scuderi · Alfred J. Tria

Editors

Minimally Invasive Surgery
in Orthopedics

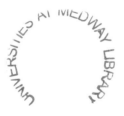

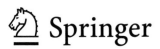

Springer

Editors

Giles R. Scuderi, MD, FACS
Director
Insall Scott Kelly Institute for Orthopaedics and Sports Medicine
Attending Orthopedic Surgeon
North Shore-LIJ Health System
Assistant Clinical Professor of Orthopedic Surgery
Albert Einstein College of Medicine
New York, NY
USA
grscudri@aol.com

Alfred J. Tria, MD
Clinical Professor of Orthopaedic Surgery
Institute for Advanced Orthopaedic Study
The Orthopaedic Center of New Jersey
Clinical Professor
Department of Orthopedic Surgery
Robert Wood Johnson Medical School
Piscataway, NJ
USA
atriajrmd@aol.com

ISBN 978-0-387-76607-2   e-ISBN 978-0-387-76608-9
DOI 10.1007/978-0-387-76608-9
Springer New York Dordrecht Heidelberg London

Library of Congress Control Number: 2009933884

Springer is part of Springer Science+Business Media (www.springer.com)

Preface

Minimally invasive surgery has evolved as an alternative to the traditional approaches in orthopedic surgery and has gathered a great deal of attention. Many surgeons are now performing all types of procedures through smaller surgical fields. Along with changes in the surgical technique, there have been rapid advances in computer navigation and robotics as tools to enhance the surgeon's vision in the limited operative fields. With these new techniques and technologies, we must ensure that these procedures are performed safely and effectively with predictable clinical outcomes. This book has been expanded from our previous publications to include spine and foot and ankle surgery, along with updated sections on knee arthroplasty, hip arthroplasty, and upper extremity surgery. The clinical information and surgical techniques, along with tips and pearls, provided by experts in the field allows the reader to grasp a comprehensive understanding of the nuances of MIS. It is our intention that this text will be a valuable reference for all orthopedic surgeons.

New York, NY Giles R. Scuderi, MD
Piscataway, NJ Alfred J. Tria, MD

Contents

Contributors

Kenneth Accousti, MD Shoulder Fellow, Mount Sinai Medical Center, New York, NY, USA

Jamal Ahmad, MD Assistant Professor, Department of Orthopaedic Surgery, Rothman Institute and Thomas Jefferson University Hospital, Philadelphia, PA, USA

Rodney K. Alan, MD Attending Surgeon, Department of Surgery, Saint Peters University Hospital, New Brunswick, NJ, USA

David W. Altchek, MD Professor, Department of Orthopaedic Surgery, Weill Medical College of Cornell University, New York, NY, USA
Co-Chief, Sports Medicine and Shoulder Service, Hospital for Special Surgery, New York, NY, USA

B. Sonny Bal, MD, MBA Associate Professor, Department of Orthopaedic Surgery, University of Missouri-Columbia, Columbia, MO, USA

John-Erik Bell, MD Assistant Professor, Shoulder, Elbow, and Sports Medicine, Department of Orthopaedic Surgery, Dartmouth-Hitchcock Medical Center, One Medical Center Drive, Lebanon, NH

Richard A. Berger, MD Assistant Professor, Department of Orthopaedic Surgery, Rush-Presbyterian-St. Luke's Medical Center, Chicago, IL, USA

Gregory C. Berlet, MD Chief Foot and Ankle Ohio State University, Orthopaedic Foot and Ankle Center, Columbus, Ohio

Roberto Bevoni, MD Staff, Rizzoli Orthopedic Institute, University of Bologna, Via GC Pupilli 1, 40136 Bologna, Italy

Eddie Bibbiani, MD Attending Surgeon, Centro Chirurgia Protesica, Istituto Ortopedico "R. Galeazzi," 20161 Via R. Galeazzi 4, Milano, Italy

Louis U. Bigliani, MD Frank E. Stinchfield Professor and Chairman, Department of Orthopaedic Surgery, New York-Presbyterian Hospital, Columbia University Medical Center, New York, NY, USA

Theodore A. Blaine, MD Associate Professor, Department of Orthopaedic Surgery, Brown Alpert Medical School, Providence, RI, USA
Rhode Island Hospital and the Miriam Hospitals, Providence, RI, USA

Peter Bonutti, MD Founder and CEO, Bonutti Clinic, Effingham, IL, USA
Associate Clinical Professor, Department of Orthopaedics, University of Arkansas, Little Rock, AK, USA

Matteo Cadossi, MD Staff, Rizzoli Orthopedic Institute, University of Bologna, Bologna, Italy

James B. Carr, MD Private Practice, Lewis Gale Orthopedics, Salem, VA, USA
Associate Clinical Professor, Department of Orthopedics, University of South Carolina,
Columbia, SC, USA

Dominic S. Carreira, MD Private Practice, Broward Health Orthopedics, Fort Lauderdale,
FL, USA

Filippo Casella, MD Attending Surgeon, Department of Orthopaedic and Traumatology,
S. Spirito in Sassia Hospital, Rome, Italy

Nicolò Castelnuovo, MD Attending Surgeon, Centro Chirurgia Protesica, Istituto
Ortopedico "R. Galeazzi," 20161 Via R. Galeazzi 4, Milano, Italy

Louis W. Catalano III, MD Assistant Clinical Professor, Department of Orthopaedic
Surgery, Columbia College of Physicians and Surgeons, New York, NY, USA
Attending Hand Surgeon, C.V. Starr Hand Surgery Center, St. Luke's – Roosevelt Hospital
Center, New York, NY, USA

Michael P. Clare, MD Director of Fellowship Education, Division of Foot & Ankle
Surgery, The Florida Orthopaedic Institute, Tampa, FL, USA

J. Chris Coetzee, MD, FRCSC Attending Physician, Fairview University Medical Center,
Minneapolis, MN, USA
Surgeon, Minnesota Sports Medicine and Twin Cities Orthopedics, Eden Prairie, MN, USA

Frances Cuomo, MD Chief, Division of Shoulder and Elbow Surgery, Department of
Orthopedics and Sports Medicine, Beth Israel Medical Center, Phillips Ambulatory Care
Center, New York, NY, USA

F. d'Amario, MD Attending Surgeon, Centro Chirurgia Protesica, Istituto Ortopedico
"R. Galeazzi," Milano, Italy

Phani K. Dantuluri, MD Assistant Clinical Professor, Department of Orthopaedics,
Thomas Jefferson University Hospital, Jefferson Medical College, The Philadelphia Hand
Center, Philadelphia, PA, USA

P. A. J. de Leeuw, MD Department of Orthopaedic Surgery, Academic Medical Centre,
University of Amsterdam, Amsterdam, The Netherlands

Christopher W. DiGiovanni, MD Associate Professor and Chief, Division of Foot and
Ankle, Department of Orthopedic Surgery, Brown University Medical School, Rhode Island
Hospital, Providence, RI, USA

Christopher C. Dodson, MD Fellow, Sports Medicine and Shoulder Service, Hospital for
Special Surgery, New York, NY, USA

Lawrence D. Dorr, MD Director, Dorr Arthritis Institute, Los Angeles, CA, USA

Xavier Duralde, MD Private Practice, Peachtree Orthopaedic Clinic, Atlanta, GA, USA

Sara L. Edwards, MD Fellow, Department of Orthopedic Surgery, New York-Presbyterian
Hospital, Columbia University Medical Center, New York, NY, USA

Kurt M. Eichholz, MD Assistant Professor, Department of Neurological Surgery,
Vanderbilt University, Nashville, TN, USA

Francesco Falez, MD Chief, Department of Orthopaedic and Traumatology, S. Spirito in
Sassia Hospital, Rome, Italy

Richard G. Fessler, MD, PhD Professor, Department of Neurosurgery, Feinberg School of
Medicine, Northwestern University, Chicago, IL, USA

Evan L. Flatow, MD Lasker Professor and Chair, Peter & Leni May Department of Orthopaedic Surgery, Mount Sinai Medical Center, New York, NY, USA

Kyle Fox, PA-C Physician Assistant, Milwaukee Neurological Institute, Milwaukee, WI, USA

W. Anthony Frisella, MD, MA Fellow, Shoulder and Elbow Service, Department of Orthopedics and Sports Medicine, Beth Israel Medical Center, Phillips Ambulatory Care Center, New York, NY, USA

Andrew A. Freiberg, MD Arthroplasty Service Chief, Department of Orthopedic Surgery, Massachusetts General Hospital, Yawkey Center For Outpatient Care, Boston, MA, USA

Leesa M. Galatz, MD Associate Professor, Program Director, Shoulder & Elbow Fellowship, Department of Orthopaedic Surgery, Washington University School of Medicine, St. Louis, MO, USA

Sandro Giannini, MD Director, School of Orthopaedics at Instituto Ortopedico Rizzoli, Bologna University, Bologna, Italy

Steven Z. Glickel, MD Associate Clinical Professor of Orthopaedic Surgery, Columbia College of Physicians and Surgeons, New York, NY, USA
Director, Hand Service, C.V. Starr Hand Surgery Center, St. Luke's – Roosevelt Hospital Center, New York, NY, USA

Steven B. Haas, MD, MPH Chief of Knee Service, Department of Orthopedic Surgery, Hospital for Special Surgery, New York, NY, USA
Associate Professor, Weill Medical College of Cornell University, New York, NY, USA

Richard H. Hallock, MD CEO, The Orthopedic Institute of Pennsylvania, Camp Hill, PA, USA

Sanaz Hariri, MD Arthroplasty Fellow, Department of Orthopedics, Massachusetts General Hospital, Boston, MA, USA

Jodi F. Hartman, MS President, Orthopaedic Research & Reporting, Ltd., Gahanna, OH, USA

Mark A. Hartzband, MD Director, Joint Replacement Service, Department of Orthopedics, Hackensack University Medical Center, Hackensack, NJ, USA
Hartzband Center for Hip and Knee Replacement, Paramus, NJ, USA

Michael R. Hausman, MD Professor, Department of Orthopaedics, Mount Sinai School of Medicine, New York, NY, USA

Peter F. Heeckt, MD Chief Medical Officer, Smith & Nephew, Inc., Memphis, TN, USA

Jonathon Herald, MD Department of Orthopaedics, Mount Sinai School of Medicine, New York, NY, USA AAD Hertzband

John E. Herzenberg, MD, FRCSC Director, International Center for Limb Lengthening Director, Pediatric Orthopedics, Sinai Hospital of Baltimore, Baltimore, MD, USA

Beat Hintermann, MD Associate Professor, Chairman, Department of Orthopedic Surgery, University of Basel, Basel, Switzerland

Jim C. Hsu, MD Private Practice, The Sports Medicine Clinic, Seattle, WA, USA

Juha Jaakkola, MD Staff Physician, Southeastern Orthopedic Center, Savannah, GA, USA

Anish R. Kadakia, MD Clinical Lecturer, Department of Orthopedic Surgery, University of Michigan, Ann Arbor, MI, USA

Gregg R. Klein, MD Attending Physician, Department of Orthopedics, Hackensack University Medical Center, Hackensack, NJ, USA
Hartzband Center for Hip and Knee Replacement, Paramus, NJ, USA

Martin Knight, MD, FRCS, MBBS Hon Senior Lecturer, The University of Manchester, Manchester, UK
Hon Senior Lecturer, The University of Central Lancashire, Preston, UK
Medical Director, The Spinal Foundation, Sunnyside, Congleton, Cheshire, UK

Mohanjit Kochhar, MD Attending Surgeon, North Middlesex University Hospital, London, UK

Raymond A. Klug, MD Assistant Professor, Department of Orthopaedics, Mount Sinai School of Medicine, New York, NY, USA

Bradley M. Lamm, DPM Head of Food and Ankle Surgery, International Center for Limb Lengthening, Rubin Institute for Advanced Orthopedics, Sinai Hospital of Baltimore, Baltimore, MD, USA

Richard L. Lebow, MD Fellow, Department of Neurological Surgery, Vanderbilt University Medical Center, Nashville, TN, USA

Edward W. Lee, MD Attending Surgeon, The CORE Institute, Phoenix, AZ, USA

Max C. Lee, MD Private Practice, Milwaukee Neurological Institute, Milwaukee, WI, USA

Steve K. Lee, MD Associate Chief, Division of Hand Surgery, Department of Orthopaedic Surgery, The NYU Hospital for Joint Diseases, New York, NY, USA
Assistant Professor, Department of Orthopaedic Surgery, The New York University School of Medicine, New York, NY, USA
Co-Chief, Hand Surgery Service, Bellevue Hospital Center, New York, NY, USA

Baron S. Lonner, MD Director, Scoliosis Associates, New York, NY, USA
Assistant Professor of Orthopaedic Surgery at New York University Medical School, New York, NY, USA

Jess H. Lonner, MD Director, Knee Replacement Surgery, Director, Orthopaedic Research, Booth Bartolozzi Balderston Orthopaedics, Pennsylvania Hospital, Philadelphia, PA, USA

Samuel J. Macdessi, MBBS (Hons), FRACS Staff, Sydney Knee Specialists, Edgecliff, Australia

Nicola Maffulli, MD, MS, PhD, FRCS(Orth) Centre Lead and Professor of Sports and Exercise Medicine, Consultant Trauma and Orthopaedic Surgeon, Queen Mary University of London, Centre for Sports and Exercise Medicine, Barts and the London School of Medicine and Destistry, London, UK

Brian Magovern, MD Attending Physician, Shoulder Service, Harbor-UCLA Medical Center Private Practice, Orthopaedic Institute, Torrance, CA, USA

Sabine Mai, MD Attending Orthopaedic Surgeon, Kassel Orthopaedic Center, Kassel, Germany

Aamer Malik, MD Orthopedics Fellow, Adult Joint Reconstruction, Hospital for Special Surgery, New York, NY, USA

Mary Ann Manitta, RN Clinical Nurse, Department of Orthopedics, Hospital for Special Surgery, New York, NY, USA

David R. Marker, BS Research Trainee/Medical Student, Rubin Institute for Advanced Orthopaedics, Center for Joint Preservation and Replacement, Sinai Hospital of Baltimore, Baltimore, MD, USA

Guido Marra, MD Assistant Professor, Chief, Section of Shoulder and Elbow Surgery, Loyola University Medical Center, Maywood, IL, USA

Joel Matta, MD Founder and Director, Hip and Pelvis Institute, St. John's Health, Santa Monica, CA, USA

Peter B. Maurus, MD Orthopaedic Surgeon, Steindler Orthopedic Clinic, Iowa City, IA, USA

Michael A. Mont, MD Director, Rubin Institute for Advanced Orthopaedics, Center for Joint Preservation and Reconstruction, Sinai Hospital of Baltimore, Baltimore, MD, USA

Griffin R. Myers, MD The Boston Consulting Group, Chicago, IL, USA

Mark S. Myerson, MD Director, Foot and Ankle Institute, Mercy Medical Center, Baltimore, MD, USA

James A. Nunley, MD Chairman, Division of Orthopaedic Surgery, Department of Surgery, Duke University Medical Center, Durham, NC, USA

Alfred T. Ogden, MD Department of Neurological Surgery, Northwestern Memorial Hospital, Chicago, IL, USA

John E. O'Toole, MD Assistant Professor, Department of Neurosurgery, Rush University Medical Center, Chicago, IL, USA

Geert I. Pagenstert, MD Attending Physician, Department of Orthopaedic Surgery, University of Basel, Basel, Switzerland

Mark W. Pagnano, MD Associate Professor, Department of Orthopedic Surgery, Mayo Clinic College of Medicine, Mayo Clinic, Rochester, MN, USA

Dror Paley, MD, FRCSC Director, Paley Advanced Limb Lengthening Institute, St. Mary's Hospital, West Palm Beach, FL, USA

Bradford O. Parsons, MD Assistant Professor, Department of Orthopaedics, Mount Sinai School of Medicine, New York, NY, USA

Milan M. Patel, MD Fellow, C.V. Starr Hand Surgery Center, St. Luke's – Roosevelt Hospital Center, New York, NY, USA

Fernando A. Pena, MD Assistant Professor, Department of Orthopaedic Surgery, University of Minnesota, Minneapolis, MN, USA

Steven M. Raikin, MD Director, Foot and Ankle Service, Assistant Professor, Department of Orthopaedic Surgery, Rothman Institute and Thomas Jefferson University Hospital, Philadelphia, PA, USA

Matthew L. Ramsey, MD Private Practice, Rothman Institute, Philadelphia, PA, USA

John A. Repicci, DDS, MD Private Practice, Joint Reconstruction Orthopedic Center, Buffalo, NY, USA

Martinus Richter, MD Professor, II Chirurgische Klinik, Unfallchirurgie, Orthopädie und Fußchirurgie, Klinikum Coburg, Coburg, Germany

Sergio Romagnoli, MD Attending Surgeon, Centro Chirurgia Protesica, Istituto Ortopedico "R. Galeazzi," Milano, Italy

Michael M. Romash, MD Private Practice, Orthopedic Foot and Ankle Center of Hampton Roads, Chesapeake Regional Medical Center, Chesapeake, VA, USA

Aaron G. Rosenberg, MD Professor, Department of Orthopaedic Surgery, Rush Medical College, Rush-Presbyterian-St. Luke's Medical Center, Chicago, IL, USA

S. Robert Rozbruch, MD Director and Chief, Limb Lengthening and Deformity Service, Hospital for Special Surgery, New York, NY, USA
Associate Professor of Clinical Orthopaedic Surgery, Weill Medical College of Cornell University, New York, NY, USA

Paul L. Saenger, MD Private Practice, Blue Ridge Bone & Joint Clinic, PA, Asheville, NC, USA

Jonathan R. Saluta, MD Private Practice, Los Angeles Orthopaedic Center, Los Angeles, CA, USA

Roy W. Sanders, MD Director, Orthopaedic Trauma Service, Tampa General Hospital, The Florida Orthopaedic Institute, Tampa, FL, USA

Nicholas Savva, MBBS, BMedSci, FRCS (Tr & Orth) Staff, Foot and Ankle Surgery, Brisbane Private Hospital, Brisbane, Australia

Murali K. Sayana, MB, ChB, AFRCSI, FRCS Senior Specialist Registrar, Department of Trauma & Orthoapedics, Royal College of Surgeons in Ireland, Dublin, Ireland

Terry Saxby, MBBS, FRACS Staff, Foot and Ankle Surgery, Brisbane Private Hospital, Brisbane, Australia

Amol Saxena, DPM, FACFAS Section Chief, Podiatric Surgery, Department of Sports Medicine, Palo Alto Medical Foundation, Palo Alto, CA, USA

Pierce Scranton, MD Associate Clinical Professor, Department of Orthopedics, University of Washington, Seattle, WA, USA

Giles R. Scuderi, MD, FACS Director, Insall Scott Kelly Institute for Orthopaedics and Sports Medicine, New York, NY, USA
Attending Orthopedic Surgeon, North Shore-LIJ Health System, Great Neck, NY, USA
Assistant Clinical Professor of Orthopedic Surgery, Albert Einstein College of Medicine, New York, NY, USA

Thorsten M. Seyler, MD Fellow, Rubin Institute for Advanced Orthopaedics, Center for Joint Preservation and Replacement, Sinai Hospital of Baltimore, Baltimore, MD, USA

Steven L. Shapiro, MD Director, Savannah Orthopaedic Foot and Ankle Center, Savannah, GA, USA

Werner Siebert, MD Professor of Orthopaedic Surgery and Chairman, Kassel Orthopaedic Center, Kassel, Germany

James B. Stiehl, MD Clinical Associate Professor, Department of Orthopaedic Surgery, Medical College of Wisconsin, Milwaukee, WI, USA

A.C. Stroïnk, MD Department of Orthopaedic Surgery, Academic Medical Center, University of Amsterdam, Amsterdam, The Netherlands

C. Christopher Stroud, MD Attending Physician, Department of Surgery, William Beaumont Hospital-Troy, Troy, MI, USA

S. David Stulberg, MD Clinical Professor, Department of Orthopaedic Surgery, Feinberg School of Medicine, Northwestern University, Chicago, IL, USA

Steven J. Thornton, MD Fellow, Department of Orthopaedic Surgery, Hospital for Special Surgery, New York, NY, USA

Alfred J. Tria, Jr., MD Clinical Professor of Orthopaedic Surgery, Institute for Advanced Orthopaedic Study, The Orthopaedic Center of New Jersey, Somerset, NJ, USA
Clinical Professor, Department of Orthopedic Surgery, Robert Wood Johnson Medical School, Piscataway, NJ, USA

Slif D. Ulrich, MD Fellow, Center for Joint Preservation and Reconstruction, Rubin Institute for Advanced Orthopedics, Sinai Hospital of Baltimore, Baltimore, MD, USA

Victor Valderrabano, MD, PhD Associate Professor, Department of Orthopaedics, University Hospital, University of Basel, Basel, Switzerland

C.N. van Dijk, MD, PhD Department of Orthopaedic Surgery, Academic Medical Centre, University of Amsterdam, Amsterdam, The Netherlands

Francesca Vannini, MD, PhD Assistant Professor, Department of Orthopaedics and Traumatology, Rizzoli Orthopedic Institute, University of Bologna, Bologna, Italy

Francesco Verde, MD Attending Surgeon, Centro Chirurgia Protesica, Istituto Ortopedico "R. Galeazzi," Milano, Italy

Mordechai Vigler, MD Chief of Hand Surgery, Department of Orthopaedic Surgery, Rabin Medical Center, Hasharon Hospital, Tel-Aviv University, Sackler School of Medicine, Petach-Tikva, Israel

Stephen M. Walsh, MD, FRCSC Fellow, Department of Orthopaedic Surgery, Rush Medical College, Rush-Presbyterian-St. Luke's Medical Center, Chicago, IL, USA

Zhinian Wan, MD Director of Research, Dorr Arthritis Institute, Los Angeles, CA, USA

Jonathan Young, MB, ChB, MRCS (Edin) Specialist Registrar, Department of Orthopaedics and Trauma, University Hospitals Coventry and Warwickshire, Coventry, UK

Christopher M. Zarro, MD Private Practice, Spine Care and Rehabilitation Inc., Roseland, NJ, USA

Section I
The Upper Extremities

Chapter 1
What Is Minimally Invasive Surgery and How Do You Learn It?

Aaron G. Rosenberg

Innovation in surgery is not new and should not be unexpected. As an example, the history of total joint replacement has demonstrated continuous evolution, and the relatively high complication rates associated with early prostheses and techniques eventually led to the improvement of implants and refinement of the surgical procedures. Gradual adoption of these improvements and their eventual diffusion into the surgical community led to improved success and increased rates of implantation.[1] Increased surgical experience was eventually accompanied by more rapid surgical performance and then by the development of standardized hospitalization protocols, which eventually led to more rapid rehabilitation and return to function. These benefits are well accepted and can be seen as helping contribute to the establishment of a more "consumer driven" and medical practice.

Most surgeons would agree that as experience guides the surgeon to more accurate incision placement, more precise dissection, and more skillful mobilization of structure, the need for *wide* exposure diminishes. Indeed, less invasiveness appears to be a hallmark of experience gained with a given procedure. From a historical perspective, this appears to be true of total hip replacement. The operation as initially described by Charnley required trochanteric osteotomy. The osteotomy served several purposes: generous exposure, access to the intramedullary canal for proper component placement and cement pressurization, and the ability of the surgeon to "tension" the abductors to improve stability. However, over time, it became apparent that trochanteric nonunion and retained trochanteric hardware could be problematic. In attempts to minimize these problems, some worked to develop improved techniques for trochanteric fixation. However, others went in a different direction, eventually demonstrating that the operation could be performed quite adequately without osteotomy. Many purists complained that this was not the Charnley operation, and that the *benefits* of trochanteric osteotomy were lost. Yet the eventual acceptance of the nonosteotomy approaches by almost all surgeons performing primary total hip arthroplasty (THA) in the vast majority of circumstances would attest to the fact that osteotomy was not required to achieve the result that had come to be expected.

These developments led to the popularity of the posterior approach to the hip for THA. Initially the gluteus maximus tendon insertion into the posterolateral femur was routinely taken down to obtain adequate exposure of the acetabulum. Indeed, the generous exposure provided by this release was needed to adequately control acetabular component position, to reduce bleeding for cement interdigitation, and to allow pressurization of acetabular cement. However, this generous exposure was associated with a higher dislocation rate than was seen with the trochanteric osteotomy technique. But with the advent of improved component design (offset) and better understanding of component positioning, as well as the introduction of cementless techniques, less exposure was needed in the majority of cases. Eventually, careful closure of the posterior structures also led to a significant reduction in the dislocation rate.[2] Seen in this example is a finding typically noted in the close examination of most evolutionary processes: initial benefits are obtained at some expense in the form of new or different complications or alterations in the complication rate. Further modifications are then required to overcome the new problems that arise from the adaptation of the innovation. The study of the factors that lead to the adoption (and alterations) of innovations has been extensively studied by Rogers and is well described in his landmark work, *The Diffusion of Innovation*.[3]

The trend to *less* or minimally invasive procedures has been noted in other specialties[4] and perhaps can be seen most dramatically in the field of interventional radiology.[5]

It would be fair to say that almost all surgical techniques improve over time by leading to less invasive approaches, which are frequently adopted only reluctantly by the surgical community. For skeptics it is instructive to review the career of Dr. Kurt Semm.[6] His reports of surgical techniques were shouted down at professional meetings and his lectures were greeted with "laughter, derision, and suspicion." He was forbidden to publish by his dean, and his first papers submitted were rejected because they were "unethical." The President

A.G. Rosenberg
Department of Orthopaedic Surgery, Rush Medical College,
1725 West Harrison Street, Suite 1063, Chicago, IL 60612, USA

G.R. Scuderi and A.J. Tria (eds.), *Minimally Invasive Surgery in Orthopedics*,
DOI 10.1007/978-0-387-76608-9_1, © Springer Science+Business Media, LLC 2010

of the German Surgical Society demanded that his license be revoked and he be barred from practice. His associates at the University of Kiel asked him to have psychological testing because his ideas were considered so radical. Despite this opprobrium, he invented 80 patented surgical devices, published more than 1,000 scientific papers, and developed dozens of new techniques. His obituary in the *The British Medical Journal* hailed him as "the father of laparoscopic surgery." Who today would choose a standard open cholecystectomy over the benefits of the laparoscopic approach?

Hip replacement is currently being performed by a variety of minimalist modifications of the standard hip approaches as well as by nontraditional approaches. Knee replacement is similarly being attempted through shorter incisions with various arthrotomy approaches. The proponents of all call them *minimally invasive*, but this term has really become a catchall, and has no specificity or agreed upon meaning.

The purported benefits of these techniques include earlier, more rapid, and more complete recovery of function, less perioperative bleeding, and improved cosmesis. There has been, to date, few data by other than those proponents of specific techniques to substantiate any of these potential benefits. Of course, these purported benefits must be weighed against their potential to change the nature and/or incidence of complications that may arise secondary to the modifications of these approaches.

There is general consensus that adoption of new techniques initially results in a greater incidence of complications. This is the so-called learning curve,[7,8] well known to all surgeons learning a new procedure. Whether this learning curve is extended or contracted has been shown to depend on both individual as well as the systemic features of the operation.[9]

It should therefore come as little surprise that, in the hands of those initially reporting these modified procedures (and presumably who have developed their expertise gradually and over considerable time), the complication rates are comparable to those found in the standard approaches, while others report a higher complication rate.[10–14] There has been insufficient time for the scientific evidence to accumulate in sufficient volume to clarify the specific benefits and risks of these modifications in the hands of specialist surgeons, let alone the generalist who performs these procedures.

Clearly, the modern era's communications technologies, coupled with more sophisticated marketing techniques, have dramatically influenced the speed with which new techniques are recognized, popularized, and thus demanded by an easily influenced public. However, continued accumulation of data through the performance of appropriate studies will eventually determine the most appropriate role for these techniques in the orthopedic surgeon's armamentarium.[15] Prior to that occurrence, what is the surgeon to do?

A purely prescriptive approach is prohibited by the multifactorial nature of the surgical endeavor. The vast majority of surgeons who perform THA on a regular basis have already modified their operative approaches to incorporate less invasive techniques. Each surgeon has an individual tolerance for and willingness to undergo the struggles involved in learning a new procedure, differing levels of commitment to the change required for the performance of the technique, as well as a varying ability to tolerate the potential complications encountered while on the so-called learning curve. Unfortunately, the removal of standard visual, auditory, and tactile feedback cues during the performance of these "less" invasive procedures may require the development of alternate cues, which may not be readily available, well established, or assimilated.[11] Thus, the overall complication rate may rise while familiarization with these cues (and the appropriate response to them) matures or while alternate methods of incorporating similar or comparable information is developed. As attempts are made to limit the invasiveness of surgical procedures, surgeons must be prepared to cultivate and take advantage of nontraditional sensory feedback and other alternate visualization methods to direct their efforts. As these evolve, it can be expected that surgical intervention will continue to become less invasive.

The ultimate question implied in the title of this chapter, that is, how to learn a minimally invasive surgery (MIS) technique, can only be answered by first understanding the current methods of surgical training and their relationship to the practice requirements of standard orthopedic procedures. Only then can we evaluate the way these methods relate specifically to the requirements of MIS and so answer the question: do the specific surgical requirements of the MIS procedure require an alteration in the manner in which we train surgeons? An additional implied assumption is the perception, which appears to be correct but has not yet been rigorously established, that the performance of minimally invasive procedures in the training environment substantially alters the educational experience for the learning surgeon. A series of linked questions is raised that deserves inquiry: (1) What are the performance requirements for MIS surgery? (2) Do they differ substantially from that of routine non-MIS surgery (begging the question of whether we really understand these!)? (3) What are the relationships between surgical training methods and patient outcomes and do we understand these relationships sufficiently well to proceed to alter them in a meaningful fashion? (4) Does the routine adoption of MIS surgical procedures alter the current teaching environment in a way that is deleterious to the learning surgeon? (5) To what extent do the answers to the proceeding questions demand the development of new methods for surgical teaching as regards the MIS procedures? And, finally, (6) What form might this take?

The old adage "It takes 1 year to teach someone how to operate, 5 years to teach them when to operate, and a lifetime to learn when not to operate." seems to make the point that, in the surgeon's repertoire, it is the psychomotor skills that are the easiest and most readily taught. The implication is that the psychomotor skills required in the operating room are substantively different (and easier to teach) than the cognitive skills required. But this is clearly simplistic. Surgical performance is based on a continuous feedback loop of psychomotor performance intimately coupled with cognitive function. It is the continuous and ongoing making of decisions (albeit almost always at a subconscious level for the experienced) in the midst of physical performance that influences the quality of the surgical intervention.

To what extent the development of these cognitive and motor skills, and their interaction, governs the eventual outcome is a complex problem that has not yet been fully investigated and remains poorly understood. It has been said, "Many more surgeons have done a video analysis of their golf swing than have evaluated their operative performance." While there are few studies that have effectively evaluated real-time surgical performance characteristics in a meaningful way, even more fundamentally and unfortunately, there is little research in the realm of surgical education that would help us determine the specific performance requirements for most surgical procedures in general and of less invasive procedures in particular. Additionally, there are few data on the pedagogical aspects of surgical procedure training for either minimally or maximally invasive procedures. A recent comprehensive review of expert performance indicates that there has been more attention directed to the study of musicians, athletes, pilots, and military commanders than to surgeons.[16] Clearly, however, advances in surgical technology and technique has led to a renewed interest in these issues.

While the performance of arthroscopic procedures has resulted in a premium on specific three-dimensional spaciovisualization and psychomotor applications,[17,18] the same is not necessarily true for MIS-type joint replacement procedures. The simple answer to the question regarding the performance skills requirements for MIS surgery is that they are basically those that are found in standard surgical procedures but taken to a higher level. This arises from specific conditions that appear to be inherent in MIS surgery.[19]

1. In some respects, the ability to "protect" structures in the standard fashion may be altered in specific ways unique to the surgical procedure, and this may result in a directly proportional decrease in the margin of error for various intraoperative maneuvers.
2. Small errors during the course of the operation may be less easily recognized, and adjusted for, as the procedure progresses, and the implications of these small errors are potentially magnified.
3. Specific anatomic features that increase the degree of difficulty encountered in the performance of a more "open procedure" (stiffness, deformity, poor tissue quality) may

be magnified when the procedure is performed in a minimally invasive fashion.
4. Finally, and perhaps most importantly, the development of minimally invasive techniques frequently involves the removal or diminution of traditional feedback signals that surgeons normally use and have come to rely upon to make continuous adjustments to their performance. Thus, skills that are little needed, infrequently utilized, or have not been previously recognized become of greater consequence. Indeed the loss of standard cues may need to be compensated for in technique-specific ways. Ironically, in the hands of the more experienced surgeon, many of these feedback signals are no longer "conscious," having been assimilated into almost automatic motor responses; this can make the relearning process required more difficult.

Training surgeons to perform these more difficult techniques, with both less room for error and with a different set of feedback signals, would therefore seem to require the development of both traditional surgical skills as well as new ones in ways that guarantee a more demanding performance level than has traditionally been required.

The questioned need for new training methods implies two separate factors that may be driving this concern. First, are current training methods adequate to the task as currently envisioned? Second, does the conversion in the training environment from standard open to MIS procedures degrade the training experience? The answers can be found by evaluating the features of MIS procedures already noted:

1. Visibility of the surgical field is reduced, compromising visual feedback not only to the performing surgeon, but also to the learning surgeon dependent upon observation and demonstration of anatomy and surgical pathology.
2. Lowered margins for error limit the opportunities awarded to the less experienced trainee; while
3. The decreased ability of the instructor to monitor trainee performance degrades the learning environment.
4. The alteration of traditional cues and their replacement with more subtle and poorly defined feedback signals are hallmarks of MIS techniques. Thus, the replacement of standard open surgery by the MIS procedure would appear to significantly alter the training environment.

Are the traditional residency education and continuing medical education (CME) surgical training methods capable of meeting this standard? The system as currently constituted is derived (with little improvement and perhaps even development of some newer flaws) from the traditional systems of apprenticeship that began sometime between the Dark Ages and the development of city-states in the Renaissance.[20] In this pedagogical method, adapted by the German surgical schools of Kocher and Billroth, and modified in the United States by Halsted, has changed relatively little over the years. Thus, training methodologies used to teach surgical skills remain relatively primitive and have enjoyed little improvement in either theory or practice over the decades. Yet the specific technical requirements of the surgical procedures increase steadily. The combined requirements of residency education, that is, service and education, frequently seem to serve the best interest of neither. Even worse, depending on the specific setting, current training methods may be applied unevenly and randomly to the resident participants.[21] The common cliché, see one, do one, teach one, seems to summarize the cavalier approach to procedural teaching that has been the mainstay of surgical pedagogy. Moreover, when real patients are used for surgical teaching purposes, increased morbidity, prolonged intervention times, and suboptimal results may be expected.[22] It is clear that future technologies, whether they be traditionally surgical or otherwise procedurally interventional, will require more, rather than less, highly structured training and assessment methods. It has been demonstrated that laparoscopic surgery adapts poorly to the standard apprenticeship models for general surgical training. Rather, standardized skill acquisition and validation, performance goals, and a supervised, enforced, skill-based curriculum that readily can be shared between trainee and instructor are thought to be needed to replace the observation and incremental skill acquisition model used in an open surgical environment.[23]

Assuming no dramatic change in the nature of our economy and the emphasis on health care, it is not likely that the drive toward less invasive techniques will abate. As technology matures, new and improved techniques for vital structure protection, component placement and positioning, and bone and soft tissue management will come on line. As they do, the gradual development of improved skill levels in the performance of standard procedures coupled with the cautious adoption of new practices as these skills mature is warranted. An understanding of the ethical and moral responsibilities of the operating surgeon must be understood as they relate to training and surgical performance.[24] An open mind along with a critical eye will be required. The following suggestions can be offered to the surgeon who has yet to adopt these techniques.

How to Learn MIS: Practical Suggestions

It has been demonstrated that domain-specific and task-specific skills are not necessarily readily transferred to new domains or tasks in the surgical environment.[25–27] Surgeons, like other adults, learn best by doing, by practicing what they do, and by challenging themselves to take on increasingly difficult scenarios. Practice, in order to be effective, requires deconstruction of the actual procedure into key elements, each of

which is repeated until optimal results are achieved before moving onto the next element. The key ingredient to successful practice and ultimate self-improvement as a surgeon, as in other pursuits in life, is that one be self-motivated and competitive, with a strong desire to improve coupled with appropriate practice routines that can lead to improvement. This calls to mind the old joke, "Mister, How do I get to Carnegie Hall?" The answer, of course, is "practice."

Incremental Improvement Through Practice

The literature on CME provides no support for the hypothesis that didactic CME improves either practice patterns, skill levels, or patient outcomes – from this, one can infer that surgeons learn the more complex domain of surgical performance through repetition of procedures.[28] Willingness to engage in repetitive attempts at improving the quality of what one is doing is crucial. One needs to define clearly the areas requiring practice and employ a gradual, repetitive practice pattern; ultimately, one either improves or must change practice habits. This is particularly important in developing an action plan for surgeons who may not currently be performing any MIS procedures.

Practice

Correct practice begins with the break down of the procedure into its component parts, focusing performance-based exercise on those component parts, and acquiring and recognizing feedback, both during the performance in real time and after. As an example, surgeons who are the most experienced in total knee replacement arthroplasty (TKA) frequently perform the vast majority of the needed soft tissue releases to balance the knee during the initial approach and exposure of the knee. Less experienced surgeons tend to make the soft tissue releases a separate part of the technique, independent of the exposure, while the more experienced surgeon utilizes feedback throughout the procedure and employs it to guide the degree of tissue they are releasing during the exposure. In order to master the new skills that may be required in minimally invasive approaches, the surgeon must reenter the mind of the learner that was present at an earlier stage of training. The basic steps must be isolated, and renewed attention must be given to the details of procedure used to isolate those parts of the operation that require more attention, and there must be a detailed focus on accomplishing the specific tasks required at each step of the procedure, specifically, on how they present new or different challenges. Those steps that require the acquisition of new or refined skills can then receive the appropriate attention. The use of computer guidance can aggressively strengthen feedback loops for surgical technique that might otherwise take years to develop. The precision of the technology provides objective and exacting criticism.

Criticism

Another contributor to effective practice is self-grading. Over time, one increases the pressure on oneself to perform, grades the result, and seeks to improve. Self-grading requires measurement, and one needs to have some surgical goals in mind, such as tourniquet time, time to complete the procedure, or specific objective characteristics of operative performance; cement mantle quality, component position, limb alignment, etc. For more detail on this technique, see the Debriefing section below.

Varied Pressure

Surgeons can expand or contract the amount of pressure experienced, because these less invasive approaches and the procedures themselves are, for the most part, relatively extensile. Beginning a TKA as an MIS procedure does not lock the surgeon into that pathway; if, at any point, the surgeon deems the case too complex or the soft tissue considerations are becoming unexpectedly difficult, no harm is done by increasing the size of the incision to expand the exposure. Surgeons can literally "push the envelope" by working their way from the larger incision down to the smaller and, as a consequence, gradually increase the pressure on themselves. But the surgeon can also reduce that stress when desired or, more importantly, when necessary to achieve the optimal surgical outcome.

Avoid Multiple Learning Curves

It is essential to avoid combining multiple learning curves when learning a new procedure. The outcome of any surgical intervention is clearly multifactorial. Beyond the limitation of one's own surgical skill set and one's intuition, each operation encompasses a complex set of multiple factors, some of which may remain below the radar screen of the most experienced surgeon. These factors include, but are not limited to, the relative contributions of our assistants, the characteristics of the specific operating room, and the type of anesthesia being used. Multiple alterations to such a complex system are much more difficult to assimilate than the incremental addition of small changes approached one at a time. For example, it would be less than optimal to try a new technique or a new approach with new instruments, a new implant design, a new scrub technician, and a new surgical assistant all at the same time. Avoiding multiple learning curves is essential in ensuring that the pressure you exert upon yourself represents a systematic increase and not an overload; you can sequentially add more complexity and variation as you get better at what you do.

Visualization

Another important technique that has been well publicized in other areas of psychomotor skill acquisition and performance, but not as well publicized in surgery, is the use of visualization techniques. Great athletes will all admit to using visualization as an important part of their practice regimen. Similarly, most high-performing surgeons will also rehearse the operation, literally in their "mind's eye," before proceeding with the case. Most of us who perform complex surgery have the experience of repeatedly reviewing the steps and sequences in a new operation beforehand, particularly when learning something completely new.

Visualization has been used in sports, musical performance, and in other forms of physical activity, including dance and even acrobatic flying. Acrobatic pilots not only visualize the expected sequence of flight maneuvers in their minds along with the control manipulation needed to achieve them, but also assume the corresponding body postures, as if they are experiencing the forces associated with the acrobatic flight maneuver. This visualization technique combines psychomotor and cognitive skill sets. One can similarly see downhill ski racers mentally rehearsing the race course, accompanied by hand and body motion. In the same way, surgeons using similar visualization might "think through" a particular operation sequentially while imagining the potential problems, structures at risk, and specific goals of the procedure, while actually positioning their hands as if they were grasping a specific instrument for a specific task during a surgical procedure.

Debriefing

Another self-improvement method involves debriefing, a more formal model for self, group, or mentor after-activity assessment.[29,30] The classic role of debriefing is in the military, where it has been used for generations to train and improve the skills of warriors, particularly pilots. Debriefing or after-action reviews involve the meticulous creation of a specific checklist of the goals of any given performance followed by the ruthless assessment of how those goals were actually met during the performance. Debriefing techniques have applications in teaching residents and fellows as well as in improving one's own performance. Such sessions have an important role in improving performance at the step where you are at as well as in successfully ascending the ladder of surgical complexity.[31]

Team Approach—Coaching

The MIS effort generally leads to an appreciation of the importance of teamwork and its impact on surgical outcome. Perfect performance of the operation without appropriate attention given to perioperative factors, such as pain control, rehabilitation, etc., will not yield an optimal result. Similarly, increased coordination between assistants and surgeon is another requisite for the successful performance of this more demanding type of surgical procedure. Thus, a continuous focus on the need for a team approach throughout, from pre-operative considerations, to the surgical phase, and continuing through to the postoperative environment, is a key determinant of optimal outcome. Every team needs a coach, and, in most cases, the responsibility will and should rest with the surgeon. What do coaches do? Their primary role is to create a feedback loop; this is done by developing performance expectations, monitoring performance in a critical way, and, finally, providing feedback that leads to improvement and both motivates and empowers team members.

The Future

The characteristics that make up surgical performance include preoperative, intraoperative, and postoperative factors. While the focus on surgical training must be on all three arenas, it is mainly the intraoperative phase, where actual physical skills are required, that is seen by most trainees as being the area where there is the least opportunity to develop experience. Experience is ideally gained in an environment where feedback is immediate and mistakes are tolerated as part of the learning experience. One of the things that have prevented surgeons from acquiring greater levels of skill prior to entering practice or even during practice is the lack of such a practice environment.

The performance of surgery itself is dependent on performing multiple "subroutines," most of which have only been available for the surgeon to experience during the performance of actual surgical procedures and therefore presents the surgeon with no real opportunity to "practice" the psychomotor skills required during the procedure. In addition, there is little in the way of immediate information available to the surgeon during the course of the operation that would allow the surgeon to make the type of adjustments that are based on cause-effects/feedback loops. As noted earlier, even in the performance of physical skills, there are multiple

cognitive processes that must function correctly and efficiently to maximize surgical performance.

With modern technology, many of the factors that contribute to surgical performance can be simulated and repeatedly experienced with immediate feedback on the correctness of decisions and behaviors. Development and utilization of this technology would be expected to result in any given surgeon moving more rapidly along the learning curve, allowing the surgeon to perform at a higher level during the actual surgical encounter. Despite the obstacles present to the current employment of actual psychomotor skills simulation, these devices will eventually be part of the surgical training environment. In the coming era of virtual reality environments and surgical training simulators, there is good reason to believe that the coupling of these technologies to assist the surgeon in acquiring both motor and cognitive skills will result in improved surgical performance as well as improved patient outcomes as a result of the clinical encounter.

A current potential model for improving surgical responsiveness and judgment can be obtained by using the interactive video game as a model. Several features of the modern interactive video game make it both compelling and popular. One primary feature is the need for continuous involvement by the participant. Lapses of attention cause failure (or loss to an opponent). This need for continuous vigilance by the participant is structured into the gaming environment. This forcing function of involvement leads to a "flow" experience that has been described as exhilarating and involving, compelling attention and participation.

As has been demonstrated in flight simulators, the same environment, appropriately structured, can be used to improve both cognitive judgments as well as response times. The application of structured learning experiences in this type of environment might be expected to achieve remarkable improvements in information transmission, a primary goal of the educational experience.

Of additional import is the current status of computer-guided and computer-assisted procedures to the surgeon's armamentarium. As these technologies become more widely available, the surgeon will need opportunities to practice in the new environment created by the addition of a computerized guidance interface during surgical performance. Familiarity with the structure and content of guidance information, as well as integration of this information with the traditional inputs acquired during surgery, will be needed to improve the real-time intraoperative judgments and physical performance measures needed to perform surgery. This familiarity can best be accomplished in a highly integrated simulation environment.

In order to structure an environment that would provide for progressive advances in cognitive skills acquisition, several requirements must be met. The first requirement is creation of a knowledge base that will be utilized as the cognitive foundation for the simulation technology. This so-called "content knowledge" currently exists in the mind of the surgeons who currently provide education to trainees as well as in text and technique manuals. Second, the knowledge base must be structured so that it can be represented in an algorithmic format with eventual conversion of these algorithms into the type of appropriate branching chain pathways environment, which can be made accessible and modifiable at the computer interface. Third, multiple supplemental elements must be developed to provide a more challenging and robust learning environment. Fourth, an assessment module with accompanying grading mechanism must be developed to couple the quality and intensity of the learning experience to the performance level and other individual educational needs of the learner. Work on cognitive skills development, as well as visual skills acquisition, can be accomplished with little other than content knowledge coupled to appropriate software and computers. This should be the initial focus of development efforts for several reasons. First, investment need not be particularly large for the development of the cognitive skills applications of this technology. Much of the appropriate software currently exists and is utilized in the video gaming industry to structure and create complex interactive environments where multiple elements combine to provide an ever-changing and stimulating participatory environment. The addition of specific physical skills will follow.

Enhancements that will further improve surgical performance can also be introduced to this environment. Appropriately structured to approximate the real-life decisions and judgments that the surgeon will be called upon to make, the addition of creative elements, such as complication/disaster management, head-to-head or machine-based competition, continuous probing for knowledge deficits, and reinforcing functions used to transmit important supplementary and supporting content, will produce a robust learning environment that will make the educational experience engaging, stimulating, challenging, and fun.

While there have been progressive advancements in surgical technology and techniques over the past century, there is excellent evidence that exponentially increasing rates of technology growth will provide an ever more rapidly growing rate of change in the methods whereby surgery is performed. While manual skill performance is likely to remain a mainstay of the surgeons experience, increasing reliance on machine performance and even intelligence would seem to be likely. The surgeon trained today is not likely to be using technologies similar to those learned during training in the practice environment encountered in 2016. It is incumbent upon the surgeon to maintain an adaptable posture toward acquiring new skills, as well as to maintain and hone current skills in order to prepare for future developments in the field.

References

1. Peltier LF. The history of hip surgery. In: Callaghan JJ, Rosenberg AG, Rubash HE (Eds.). *The Adult Hip*. Lippincott, Phialdelphia, 1998, pp. 4–19
2. Dixon MC, Scott RD, Schai PA, Stamos V. A simple capsulorrhaphy in a posterior approach for total hip arthroplasty. J Arthroplasty 2004 19(3):373–6
3. Rogers EM. *The Diffusion of Innovation*. Free Press, New York, 5 edition, 2002
4. Fenton DS, Czervionke LF (Eds.). *Image-Guided Spine Intervention*. W B Saunders, New York, 2002
5. Castaneda-Zuniga WR, Tadavarthy SM, Qia Z. *Interventional Radiology*. Lippincott, Williams & Wilkins, Philadelphia, 3 edition, 1997
6. Tuffs A. Kurt Semm Obituary. Br Med J 2003 (327);397
7. Dincler S, Koller MT, Steurer J, Bachmann LM, Christen D, Buchmann P. Multidimensional analysis of learning curves in laparoscopic sigmoid resection: eight-year results. Dis Colon Rectum 2003;46(10):1371–8
8. Gallagher AG, Smith CD, Bowers SP, Seymour NE, Pearson A, McNatt S, Hananel D, Satava RM. Psychomotor skills assessment in practicing surgeons experienced in performing advanced laparoscopic procedures. J Am Coll Surg 2003;197(3):479–88
9. McCormick PH, Tanner WA, Keane FB, Tierney S. Minimally invasive techniques in common surgical procedures: implications for training. Ir J Med Sci 2003 172(1):27–9
10. Berger RA, Duwelius PJ. The two-incision minimally invasive total hip arthroplasty: technique and results. Orthop Clin North Am 2004 35(2):163–72
11. Hartzband, MA. Posterolateral minimal incision for total hip replacement: technique and early results. Orthop Clin North Am 2004; 35(2):119–29
12. Howell, JR, Masri, BA, Duncan, CP. Minimally invasive versus standard incision anterolateral hip replacement: a comparative study. Orthop Clin North Am 2004;35 (2): 153–62
13. Wright JM, Crockett HC, Delgado S, Lyman S, Madsen M, Sculco TP Mini-incision for total hip arthroplasty: a prospective, controlled investigation with 5-year follow-up evaluation. J Arthroplasty 2004 19(5):538–45
14. Woolson ST, Mow CS, Syquia JF, Lannin JV, Schurman DJ. Comparison of primary total hip replacements performed with a standard incision or a mini-incision. J Bone Joint Surg Am 2004 86A(7):1353–8
15. Callaghan JJ, Crowninshield RD, Greenwald AS, Lieberman JR, Rosenberg AG, Lewallen DG. Symposium: introducing technology into orthopaedic practice. How should it be done? J Bone Joint Surg Am 2005 87(5):1146–58
16. Ericsson KA Charness N Feltovich PJ, Hoffman RR. *The Cambridge Handbook of Expertise and Expert Performance*. Cambridge University Press, Cambridge, 2006
17. Wilhelm DM, Ogan K, Roehrborn CG, Cadeddu JA, Pearle MS. Assessment of basic endoscopic performance using a virtual reality simulator. J Urol 2003 170(2 Pt 1):692
18. Gallagher AG, Smith CD, Bowers SP, Seymour NE, Pearson A, McNatt S, Hananel D, Satava RM. Psychomotor skills assessment in practicing surgeons experienced in performing advanced laparoscopic procedures. J Am Coll Surg 2003 197(3):479–88
19. McCormick PH, Tanner WA, Keane FB, Tierney S. Minimally invasive techniques in common surgical procedures: implications for training. Ir J Med Sci 2003 172(1):27–9
20. Amirault RJ, Branson R. Educators and expertise: a brief history of theories and models. In: Ericsson KA, Charness N, Feltovich PJ, Hoffman RR (Eds.). *The Cambridge Handbook of Expertise and Expert Performance*. Cambridge University Press, Cambridge, 2006, pp. 72–4

21. Zhou W, Lin PH, Bush RL, Lumsden AB. Endovascular training of vascular surgeons: have we made progress? Semin Vasc Surg 2006 19(2):122–6

22. Colt HG, Crawford SW, Galbraith O. Virtual reality bronchoscopy simulation. Chest 2001 120:1333–39

23. Rosser JC, Jr, Rosser LE, Savalgi RS. Skill acquisition and assessment for laparoscopic surgery. Arch Surg 1998 133(6):657–61

24. Rogers DA. Ethical and educational considerations in minimally invasive surgery training for practicing surgeons. Semin Laparosc Surg 2002 9(4):206–11

25. Wanzel KR, HmastraSJ, AnastakisDJ, Matsumoto ED, Cusimano MD. Effect of visuo-spatial ability on learning of spatially-complex surgical skills. Lancet 2002 38:617–27

26. Naik VN, Matsumoto ED, Houston PL, Hamstra SJ, Yeung RY-M, Mallon JS, Martire TM Fibreoptic oral tracheal intubation skills: do manipulation skills learned on a simple model transfer into the operating room Anesthesiology 2001 95:343–48

27. Figert PL, Park AE, Witzke DB, Schwartz RW. Transfer of training in acquiring laparoscopic skills. J Am Coll Surg 2001 193(5):533–7

28. Norman G, Eva K, Brooks L, Hamstra S. Expertise in medicine and surgery. In: Ericsson KA, Charness N, Feltovich PJ, Hoffman RR (Eds.). *The Cambridge Handbook of Expertise and Expert Performance*. Cambridge University Press, Cambridge, 2006

29. Bond WF, Deitrick LM, Eberhardt M, Barr GC, Kane BG, Worrilow CC, Arnold DC, Croskerry P. Cognitive versus technical debriefing after simulation training. Acad Emerg Med 2006 13(3):276–83

30. Moorthy K, Munz Y, Adams S, Pandey V, Darzi A. A human factors analysis of technical and team skills among surgical trainees during procedural simulations in a simulated operating theatre. Ann Surg 2005 242(5):631–9

31. http://www.msr.org.il/R_D/Debriefing_Techniques/

Chapter 2
Overview of Shoulder Approaches: Choosing Between Mini-incision and Arthroscopic Techniques

Raymond A. Klug, Bradford O. Parsons, and Evan L. Flatow

In recent years, there has been great interest in minimally invasive orthopedic surgery. Several branches of orthopedics have embraced the principles of minimally invasive surgery, including traumatology,[1–3] spinal surgery,[4] and adult reconstruction.[5–7] By far the greatest influence has been felt in the field of sports medicine with the introduction, routine, and later obligate use of the arthroscope. Indeed, the days of the open meniscectomy or extraarticular anterior cruciate ligament (ACL) reconstruction are almost beyond us, as in these and many other cases, arthroscopic and arthroscopically assisted techniques have become the standard of care. More recently, the field of shoulder and elbow surgery has begun a similar transition; however, a single, distinct difference exists. Previously in sports medicine, the arthroscope was a new tool and standard open procedures were subsequently approached arthroscopically; however, we are currently witnessing a surge of interest in minimally invasive approaches to techniques that are not amenable to arthroscopic treatment, such as arthroplasty[5–7] or plate osteosynthesis for fractures.[1–3] This creates an interesting dilemma: when to choose arthroscopy versus minimally invasive open surgery or even more traditional open approaches.

When to Choose Arthroscopy over Other Approaches

Three key questions must be answered in order to address the above question. First, does some part of the procedure require an open incision? The most obvious example of this is arthroplasty. Because placement of the implant requires an incision at least as large as the implant itself, an open approach cannot be avoided.[8] As described in the subsequent chapters, this incision can be minimized in many cases to just that necessary for placement of the implant, but, regardless, an open approach is still required.

Second, can the necessary exposure be achieved through arthroscopic, arthroscopically assisted, percutaneous, or even mini-open approaches? If adequate exposure cannot be achieved, then conversion to an open technique is required. In many cases, this can be minimized, if not completely avoided, but it must be emphasized that the surgical result must not be compromised by an attempt at minimizing the incision. An example of this is the use of a "reduction portal" for percutaneous pinning of valgus-impacted four-part proximal humerus fractures.[9] In the hands of a skilled surgeon, the utilization of this additional "portal" can obviate the need for open surgery.

Third, can an equivalent or reasonable outcome be achieved with minimally invasive approaches when compared with the more traditional open approach? The obvious example of this, although still debated, is recurrent instability in the contact athlete.[10] While open stabilization procedures have been the gold standard, many authorities in the field disagree with this. At the 2006 annual meeting of American Association of Orthopaedic Surgeons (AAOS), an expert panel was assembled to address shoulder disorders in the contact athlete. When asked about open versus arthroscopic treatment of recurrent instability in contact athletes, 100% of the panel remarked that their preferred treatment would be arthroscopic.[11]

The Trend Toward Arthroscopy

It is clear that the trend toward arthroscopic techniques is being embraced by the orthopedic community and is not simply the hype created by a small group of arthroscopists trying to push their trade onto the remainder of the orthopedic public. In a 2003 survey of 908 members of the Arthroscopy

R.A. Klug, B.O. Parsons, and E.L. Flatow (✉)
Peter & Leni May Department of Orthopaedic Surgery,
Mount Sinai Medical Center, 5 East 98th Street, Box 1188
New York, NY 10029-6574, USA
e-mail: evan.flatow@msnyuhealth.org

G.R. Scuderi and A.J. Tria (eds.), *Minimally Invasive Surgery in Orthopedics*,
DOI 10.1007/978-0-387-76608-9_2, © Springer Science+Business Media, LLC 2010

Association of North America (AANA) and the American Orthopaedic Society for Sports Medicine (AOSSM), the 700 respondents reported that 24% routinely performed rotator cuff repair through an all-arthroscopic approach, compared with only 5% 5 years earlier. At the 2005 AAOS annual meeting, 167 attendees in a symposium on the rotator cuff were asked how they would repair a mobile, 3-cm rotator cuff tear. Sixty-two percent responded that they would repair it using all arthroscopic techniques.[12] This movement toward less invasive surgical approaches does not only apply to arthroscopy, but rather to minimally invasive open approaches as well.

The concept of pure "open" versus "mini-open" or even "arthroscopic" surgery is not well defined. Is an ACL reconstruction with a local patella tendon harvest considered "arthroscopic" if an open approach is used to harvest the graft? What if hamstring tendons are used through a separate incision? Does this make the ACL reconstruction arthroscopic, but the graft harvest open? Or mini-open? What about an arthroscopic biceps tenodesis using an interference screw that may not fit through the canula? In these and many other cases, the definitions of "open," "mini-open," and even "arthroscopic" techniques are no longer clear; in many cases, procedures that are normally considered "arthroscopic" are actually "arthroscopically assisted." More confusing is the distinction between mini-open and open approaches based on the size of the incision. As will be discussed in the subsequent chapters, varying degrees of open and arthroscopic techniques exist; there is graying of the borders between them, and several authors have begun publishing instructional monographs on making the transition from one to another, usually toward more minimally invasive techniques.[13,14]

Arthroscopy in Shoulder Surgery

Relatively uniformly in shoulder surgery, the perspective is that the gold standard is open surgery and that arthroscopic or minimally invasive techniques hope to approach these results.[15–20] Ironically, in some cases, minimally invasive surgery may actually have better results than in open cases. This may be due to a distinct advantage of arthroscopy or the lack of a distinct disadvantage inherent in traditional open surgery. Consider the example of rotator cuff repair. Although older reports have shown inferior results with arthroscopic surgery when compared with open surgery, more recent studies have begun to show equivalent results with arthroscopic techniques.[15–20] In the hands of a proficient surgeon, arthroscopy allows for several advantages over open surgery, such as the examination of concomitant intraarticular and subacromial pathology as well as better visualization and

releases of both sides of the tendon and the rotator and posterior intervals.[13,14,21,22]

Of great concern in any approach to the shoulder is damage to or detachment of the deltoid. In traditional open approaches, the deltoid is elevated off of the acromion and reattached after acromioplasty. Although uncommon, deltoid dehiscence has led to disastrous results, and meticulous repair of the deltoid origin should be done in any open approach. This complication is avoided in mini-open and arthroscopic approaches. As a result, techniques such as the open anterior acromioplasty have relatively fallen by the wayside in favor of arthroscopic subacromial decompression with mini-open rotator cuff repair or even complete arthroscopic approaches.[17,22]

In other cases, concomitant pathology may dictate the surgical approach, as in instability repair. Advantages of arthroscopic repair include preservation of the subscapularis (although splitting the subscapularis in line with its fibers may also accomplish this), ability to thoroughly evaluate and address the entire glenohumeral joint and biceps/superior labrum insertion, less immediate postoperative pain, reduced cost, and improved cosmesis.[23,24] Disadvantages include difficulty mobilizing large, medialized glenoid bone fragments and repairing capsular tears, especially humeral avulsions.[24,25] Additionally, minimally invasive approaches may be less helpful in some multidirectional cases where stretching of thin tissue rather than stiffness is more of a concern. Open repair may be necessitated by the need to perform bony procedures and has been advocated for patients with inferior glenoid bone loss who require bone grafting or coracoid transfer, and in patients with very large Hill-Sachs lesions requiring grafting or mini-surface replacement.[24,26–28] Others continue to recommend open repair for collision athletes, and in revision cases, although this may be debated.

With instability, often revision cases may be performed arthroscopically, especially when failure is due to an unaddressed or improperly (e.g., medial rather than on the glenoid rim) repaired Bankart lesion, while open approaches are used if bone grafting is needed or if subscapularis deficiency requires extensive mobilization and repair or pectoralis major transfer.[24,26–28] Often in these cases, the procedure may be performed through a concealed axillary, mini-incision approach, as described in the subsequent chapters.

As a result of the blurring of borders between open and minimally invasive approaches, the idea that open surgery is the "gold standard" in the shoulder may not be so black and white any more. Additionally, with excellent results of mini-open and arthroscopic techniques, perhaps the "gold standard" is changing.[12,18,29] Regardless of the size or number of incisions used, the surgeon must be comfortable with whichever approach is chosen and the approach must allow for all necessary pathology to be addressed. As will be seen in the subsequent chapters, excellent results can be achieved with several different techniques, and, for each procedure, there are multiple viable options. Ultimately, each surgeon must decide on an individual and case-by-case basis which approach affords the patient the highest likelihood of the best result with the least chance for complications. In many cases, this will be an all arthroscopic approach. In some cases, best results may still be achieved with traditional open approaches. However, in many cases, the best compromise may come from a minimally invasive open approach, being ever mindful that arthroscopy has not rendered open surgery obsolete. Rather, arthroscopy is yet another tool in the surgeon's armamentarium and it, like any other tool, must be used appropriately in order to ensure the patient the best possible outcome with the least chance for complications.

References

1. Janzing, H. M., Houben, B. J., Brandt, S. E., Chhoeurn, V., Lefever, S., Broos, P., Reynders, P., and Vanderschot, P. The Gotfried Percutaneous Compression Plate versus the Dynamic Hip Screw in the treatment of pertrochanteric hip fractures: minimal invasive treatment reduces operative time and postoperative pain. *J Trauma*, 2002 52(2): 293–8
2. Perren, S. M. Evolution of the internal fixation of long bone fractures. The scientific basis of biological internal fixation: choosing a new balance between stability and biology. *J Bone Joint Surg Br*, 2002 84(8): 1093–110
3. Schutz, M., Muller, M., Krettek, C., Hontzsch, D., Regazzoni, P., Ganz, R., and Haas, N. Minimally invasive fracture stabilization of distal femoral fractures with the LISS: a prospective multicenter study. Results of a clinical study with special emphasis on difficult cases. *Injury*, 2001 32(Suppl 3): SC48–54
4. Olinger, A., Hildebrandt, U., Mutschler, W., and Menger, M. D. First clinical experience with an endoscopic retroperitoneal approach for anterior fusion of lumbar spine fractures from levels T12 to L5. *Surg Endosc*, 1999 13(12): 1215–9
5. Berger, R. A., Deirmengian, C. A., Della Valle, C. J., Paprosky, W. G., Jacobs, J. J., and Rosenberg, A. G. A technique for minimally invasive, quadriceps-sparing total knee arthroplasty. *J Knee Surg*, 2006 19(1): 63–70
6. Berger, R. A., Jacobs, J. J., Meneghini, R. M., Della Valle, C., Paprosky, W., and Rosenberg, A. G. Rapid rehabilitation and recovery with minimally invasive total hip arthroplasty. *Clin Orthop Relat Res*, 2004 (429): 239–47
7. Goldstein, W. M., Branson, J. J., Berland, K. A., and Gordon, A. C. Minimal-incision total hip arthroplasty. *J Bone Joint Surg Am*, 2003 85-A(Suppl 4): 33–8
8. Blaine, T., Voloshin, I., Setter, K., and Bigliani, L. U. Minimally invasive approach to shoulder arthroplasty. In: Scuderi, G. R., Tria, A. J. Jr., and Berger, R. A., (Eds.) *MIS Techniques in Orthopaedics*. New York, NY, Springer, 2006, pp. 45–70
9. Hsu, J., and Galatz, L. M. Mini-incision fixation of proximal humeral four-part fractures. In: Scuderi, G. R., Tria, A. J. Jr., and Berger, R. A., (Eds.) *MIS Techniques in Orthopaedics*. New York, NY, Springer, 2006, pp. 32–44
10. Rhee, Y. G., Ha, J. H., and Cho, N. S. Anterior shoulder stabilization in collision athletes: arthroscopic versus open Bankart repair. *Am J Sports Med*, 2006 34(6): 979–85
11. Romeo, A. A., Arciero, R. A., and Conner, P. M. Management of the in-season collision athlete with shoulder instability. In: Burks, R. T. (Ed.) *American Shoulder and Elbow Surgeons/American Orthopaedic Society for Sports Medicine Specialty Day Joint Session*. Proceedings of the 72nd Annual Meeting of the American Academy of Orthopaedic Surgeons, Chicago, IL, 2006
12. Abrams, J. S., and Savoie, F. H. III. Arthroscopic rotator cuff repair: is it the new gold standard? In: *72nd Annual Meeting of the American Academy of Orthopaedic Surgeons*. Washington, DC, 2005, pp. 71
13. Yamaguchi, K., Ball, C. M., and Galatz, L. M. Arthroscopic rotator cuff repair: transition from mini-open to all-arthroscopic. *Clin Orthop Relat Res*, 2001 (390): 83–94
14. Yamaguchi, K., Levine, W. N., Marra, G., Galatz, L. M., Klepps, S., and Flatow, E. L. Transitioning to arthroscopic rotator cuff repair: the pros and cons. *Instr Course Lect*, 2003 52: 81–92
15. Buess, E., Steuber, K. U., and Waibl, B. Open versus arthroscopic rotator cuff repair: a comparative view of 96 cases. *Arthroscopy*, 2005 21(5): 597–604
16. Sauerbrey, A. M., Getz, C. L., Piancastelli, M., Iannotti, J. P., Ramsey, M. L., and Williams, G. R., Jr. Arthroscopic versus mini-open rotator cuff repair: a comparison of clinical outcome. *Arthroscopy*, 2005 21(12): 1415–20
17. Severud, E. L., Ruotolo, C., Abbott, D. D., and Nottage, W. M. All-arthroscopic versus mini-open rotator cuff repair: a long-term retrospective outcome comparison. *Arthroscopy*, 2003 19(3): 234–8
18. Verma, N. N., Dunn, W., Adler, R. S., Cordasco, F. A., Allen, A., MacGillivray, J., Craig, E., Warren, R. F., and Altchek, D. W. All-arthroscopic versus mini-open rotator cuff repair: a retrospective review with minimum 2-year follow-up. *Arthroscopy*, 2006 22(6): 587–94
19. Warner, J. J., Tetreault, P., Lehtinen, J., and Zurakowski, D. Arthroscopic versus mini-open rotator cuff repair: a cohort comparison study. *Arthroscopy*, 2005 21(3): 328–32
20. Youm, T., Murray, D. H., Kubiak, E. N., Rokito, A. S., and Zuckerman, J. D. Arthroscopic versus mini-open rotator cuff repair: a comparison of clinical outcomes and patient satisfaction. *J Shoulder Elbow Surg*, 2005 14(5): 455–9
21. Baker, C. L., Whaley, A. L., and Baker, M. Arthroscopic rotator cuff tear repair. *J Surg Orthop Adv*, 2003 12(4): 175–90
22. Norberg, F. B., Field, L. D., and Savoie, F. H., III. Repair of the rotator cuff. Mini-open and arthroscopic repairs. *Clin Sports Med*, 2000 19(1): 77–99
23. Caprise, P. A., Jr. and Sekiya, J. K. Open and arthroscopic treatment of multidirectional instability of the shoulder. *Arthroscopy*, 2006 22(10): 1126–31
24. Levine, W. N., Rieger, K., and McCluskey, G. M., III. Arthroscopic treatment of anterior shoulder instability. *Instr Course Lect*, 2005 54: 87–96
25. Mohtadi, N. G., Bitar, I. J., Sasyniuk, T. M., Hollinshead, R. M., and Harper, W. P. Arthroscopic versus open repair for traumatic anterior shoulder instability: a meta-analysis. *Arthroscopy*, 2005 21(6): 652–8
26. Cole, B. J., Millett, P. J., Romeo, A. A., Burkhart, S. S., Andrews, J. R., Dugas, J. R., and Warner, J. J. Arthroscopic treatment of anterior glenohumeral instability: indications and techniques. *Instr Course Lect*, 2004 53: 545–58
27. Millett, P. J., Clavert, P., and Warner, J. J. Open operative treatment for anterior shoulder instability: when and why? *J Bone Joint Surg Am*, 2005 87(2): 419–32
28. Salvi, A. E., Paladini, P., Campi, F., and Porcellini, G. The Bristow-Latarjet method in the treatment of shoulder instability that cannot be resolved by arthroscopy. A review of the literature and technical-surgical aspects. *Chir Organi Mov*, 2005 90(4): 353–64
29. Bottoni, P. C., Smith, E. L., Berkowitz, M. J., Towle, R. B., and Moore, J. H. Arthroscopic versus open shoulder stabilization for recurrent anterior instability: a prospective randomized clinical trial. *Am J Sports Med*, 2006 34(11): 1730–7

Chapter 3
Mini-incision Bankart Repair *

Edward W. Lee, Kenneth Accousti, and Evan L. Flatow

Recurrent instability has plagued physicians since ancient times, because this problem can lead to severe disability. The tenuous balance between stability and motion of the glenohumeral joint makes treatment difficult. Historically, surgical procedures to stabilize the shoulder were used mostly for recurrent, locked anterior dislocations. These included staple capsulorraphy,[1] subscapularis transposition,[2] shortening of the subscapularis and anterior capsule,[3] transfer of the coracoid,[4] and osteotomies of the proximal humerus[5] or the glenoid neck.[6] Most were successful in the sense of eliminating recurrent dislocations, but often at the cost of restricted external rotation and a resultant risk of late glenohumeral osteoarthrosis.[7–11] Furthermore, the traditional limited operative indications failed to account for the growing awareness of subluxations as a source of symptomatic instability.[12–15] Better understanding of glenohumeral joint biomechanics, the role of the capsuloligamentous structures, and their modes of failure has led to an emphasis on restoration of normal anatomic relationships.

Recent uses of minimally invasive surgery to correct a myriad of orthopedic problems through smaller incisions has included the shoulder, producing a better cosmetic appearance following surgery, and in many cases, providing decreased postoperative pain when compared with similar operations performed through standard incisions.

Anatomy and Biomechanics

The glenohumeral joint has the most range of motion of any articulation in the human body. The lack of bony restraint allows the shoulder to achieve this motion to place the hand in space but this also predisposes the shoulder to instability if the soft tissue capsuloligamentous restraints or osseous architecture is disrupted.[16,17] The rotator cuff and scapular stabilizers serve as dynamic restraints in normal shoulder biomechanics. A primary role of the rotator cuff is to resist translational forces on the joint through compression of the humeral head into the glenoid cavity.

The glenohumeral joint is composed of a relatively small glenoid that provides little inherent stability. The glenoid labrum helps to deepen the "socket" of the glenohumeral joint and increases stability to the articulation. The three major glenohumeral ligaments function as "check-reins" toward the extremes of motion while remaining relatively lax in the mid-range to allow normal joint translation. Turkel et al.[18] found that the contributions of these structures were position dependent. The superior glenohumeral ligament, coracohumeral ligament, and the rotator interval (between the leading edge of the supraspinatus and the superior edge of the subscapularis) restrain anterior humeral head translation in 0° of abduction and external rotation. With increasing abduction to 45°, the middle glenohumeral ligament provides the primary anterior restraint. Finally, the inferior glenohumeral ligament (IGHL) tightens and becomes the prime anterior stabilizer at 90° of abduction and 90° of external rotation. Biomechanical study of the IGHL has demonstrated tensile failure at the glenoid insertion or in midsubstance. Significant deformation, however, was observed in midsubstance even if the ultimate site of failure occurred at the insertion.[19]

The anterior–inferior glenoid labrum, with its attachment of the anterior band of the IGHL, provides the primary restraint to anterior humeral translation when the arm is abducted to 90° and externally rotated. The Bankart injury is a disruption of this anterior–inferior labrum and IGHL. In some cases, such as rugby players who dislocate their shoulder while in the "stiff arm" position, traumatic anterior dislocations may result in a fracture of the anterior–inferior glenoid with disruption of the labrum and IGHL. This is termed a bony Bankart injury, and X-ray examination may show a small fragment of bone along the inferior glenoid neck. This fracture can be either an avulsion injury, with the IGHL pulling the inferior glenoid off, or an impaction injury,

E.W. Lee, K. Accousti, and E.L. Flatow (✉)
Peter & Leni May Department of Orthopaedic Surgery,
Mount Sinai Medical Center, 5 East 98th Street,
New York, NY, USA
e-mail: evan.flatow@msnyuhealth.org

* Adapted from Lee EW, Flatow EL, Mini-incision Bankart Repair for Shoulder Instability, in Scuderi G, Tria A, Berger R (eds.), *MIS Techniques in Orthopedics*, New York, Springer, 2006, with kind permission of Springer Science and Business Media, Inc.

produced by the humeral head crushing the anterior glenoid lip. This marginal impaction fracture may appear as "missing bone" without a separate fragment anterior and medial to the anterior glenoid rim.

A humeral avulsion of the glenohumeral ligament (HAGL) is a disruption of the glenohumeral ligamentous complex from the humeral neck instead of the more common inferior glenoid. With anterior dislocations, the capsule (with the glenohumeral ligaments) is also stretched and this further increases the laxity of the joint. Commonly, a large pouch of loose capsule filled with synovial fluid will be seen on magnetic resonance imaging (MRI) in patients with instability of the shoulder.

Hill–Sachs lesions can occur after anterior dislocations. This is an impaction fracture on the posterior superior humeral head as the head is compressed on the anterior margin of the glenoid and is akin to a depression (Hill–Sachs) in a ping-pong ball (humeral head). If large enough, these lesions can engage the anterior glenoid rim, leading to instability secondary to loss of congruence of the glenohumeral articulation, in essence, allowing the humeral head to "fall off" the glenoid as the defect engages the anterior rim of the glenoid (engaging Hill–Sachs).

Clinical Features

Patient History

Critical to the evaluation of glenohumeral instability is a careful history and physical examination. The nature of the injury surrounding the onset of symptoms should be determined and are particularly useful in identifying the type of instability. The position of the arm at the time of injury or circumstances that provoke symptoms will often indicate the direction of instability. Reproduction of a patient's symptoms in a position of abduction, external rotation, and extension suggests anterior instability. Flexion, internal rotation, and adduction, in contrast, would more likely point to posterior instability.

In determining the degree and etiology of instability, the history should ascertain whether the initial and any subsequent episodes of instability were elicited by high-energy trauma (such as violent twisting or a fall), minimal repeated trauma (such as throwing a ball), or no trauma (such as reaching for a high shelf). An initial dislocation resulting from a single traumatic episode will frequently produce a Bankart lesion. In contrast, capsular laxity and absence of a Bankart lesion will often be found in those patients who suffer from an atraumatic dislocation, multijoint laxity, and several shoulder subluxations prior to a frank dislocation. The type of reduction required (i.e., was the shoulder self-reduced or did it require manipulation by another person?) may also provide additional information about the extent of joint laxity.

Acquired instability was described by Neer, in which cumulative enlargement of the capsule results from repetitive stress.[20] Overhead-throwing athletes may develop isolated shoulder laxity from overuse with no evidence of laxity in other joints. These patients may become symptomatic after years of microtrauma or only after a frank dislocation following a single traumatic event. This patient group demonstrates that multiple etiologies may contribute to instability and underscores the need for careful diagnosis and treatment to address coexisting pathologic entities.

Voluntary control of instability must be carefully sought out as this may change the ultimate course of treatment. Patients with psychiatric disorders may utilize a concomitant ability to dislocate the shoulder for secondary gain. While operative intervention in this situation would likely fail, treatment options exist for other forms of voluntary subluxation. Surgery may benefit patients who can subluxate the shoulder by placing the arm in provocative positions. Biofeedback techniques, however, may help those patients who sublux through selective muscular activation.[21]

A detailed record of prior treatment should also be obtained, including the type and duration of immobilization, rehabilitative efforts, and previous surgeries. Knowledge of failed interventions will help guide future treatment in the recurrent dislocator.

Pain as an isolated symptom will not typically reveal much useful information. Anterior shoulder pain may indicate anterior instability as well as other common disorders including subacromial impingement. Similarly, posterior shoulder pain is nonspecific and may represent a range of pathology from instability to cervical spine disorders. The location of the pain in combination with provoking arm positions and activities, however, may aid in making a diagnosis of instability. Altered glenohumeral kinematics in throwers, for example, may result in posterior shoulder pain during late-cocking ("internal impingement").[22]

Patients may also report other symptoms consistent with subtle shoulder instability. Rowe and Zarins[15] described a phenomenon termed the "dead-arm syndrome" in which paralyzing pain and loss of control of the extremity occurs with abduction and external rotation of the shoulder. A similar phenomenon may be seen in patients with inferior subluxation when they carry heavy loads in the affected arm.

Finally, determining the patient's functional demands and level of impairment is important prior to formulating a therapeutic plan. The different expectations of a sedentary patient with minimal functional loss versus the high-performance athlete with pain and apprehension may affect the type of prescribed treatment.

Physical Examination

A thorough physical examination is equally essential in making an accurate diagnosis and recommending the appropriate intervention. Both shoulders should be adequately exposed and examined for deformity, range of motion, strength, and laxity. Demonstration of scapular winging may accompany instability, particularly of the posterior type, and should be considered a potential cause of symptoms. Generalized ligamentous laxity may also contribute to instability and can be elicited with the ability to touch the thumb to the forearm and hyperextend the index metacarpophalangeal joint beyond 90° (Fig. 3.1). Operative reports and evidence of healed anterior or posterior scars from previous instability repairs will indicate what has been done and may provide a rationale for the patient's current symptoms.

Tenderness to palpation of the acromioclavicular joint should be sought and may represent the source of symptoms in a patient with an asymptomatic loose shoulder. Pain along the glenohumeral joint line can be associated with instability but is a nonspecific finding.

Typically, there is a full range of motion with the exception of guarding at the extremes as the shoulder approaches unstable positions. Clinical suspicion should be raised, however, in the patient older than 40 years of age who is unable to actively abduct the arm after a primary anterior dislocation. It has been shown that a high percentage of these patients will have a concurrent rupture of the rotator cuff with restoration of stability following repair.[23]

Various basic provocative tests can be used to reproduce the patient's symptoms and confirm the diagnosis. In order to minimize the effects of muscle guarding, these maneuvers should be performed first on the unaffected side and then in succession of increasing discomfort. The *sulcus test* evaluates inferior translation of the humeral head with the arm at the side and in abduction[24] (Fig. 3.2). Significant findings would include an increased palpable gap between the acromion and humeral head compared with the opposite side as well as translation below the glenoid rim. Incompetence of the rotator interval will not reduce the gap with performance of the test in external rotation.

Laxity can be further evaluated by *anterior and posterior drawer* or *load-and-shift tests*[25] (Fig. 3.3). The proximal humerus is shifted in each direction while grasped between the thumb and index fingers. Alternatively, with the patient supine, the scapula is stabilized while the humeral head is axially loaded and translated anteriorly and posteriorly. Translation greater than the opposite shoulder or translation over the glenoid rim indicates significant laxity. Only translations that reproduce the patient's symptoms are considered as demonstrating instability.

The *anterior apprehension test* is performed by externally rotating, abducting, and extending the affected shoulder while stabilizing the scapula or providing an anteriorly directed force to the humeral head with the other hand. Significant findings would include a sense of impending subluxation or dislocation, or guarding and resistance to further rotation secondary to apprehension[26] (Fig. 3.4). Pain as an isolated finding is nonspecific and may indicate other pathology such as rotator cuff disease. *Jobe's relocation test* is done in the supine position, usually accompanying the apprehension test. As symptoms are elicited with progressive external rotation, the examiner applies a posteriorly directed force to the humeral head. A positive test is signified by alleviation of symptoms[27] (Fig. 3.4).

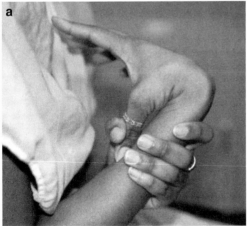
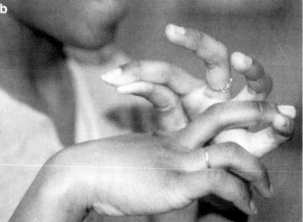

Fig. 3.1 Tests for generalized ligamentous laxity. (**a**) Thumb to forearm. (**b**) Index metacarpophalangeal joint hyperextension (From Lee EW, Flatow EL, Mini-incision Bankart Repair for Shoulder Instability. In Scuderi G, Tria A, Berger R (eds.), *MIS Techniques in Orthopedics*, New York, Springer, 2006, with kind permission of Springer Science and Business Media, Inc.)

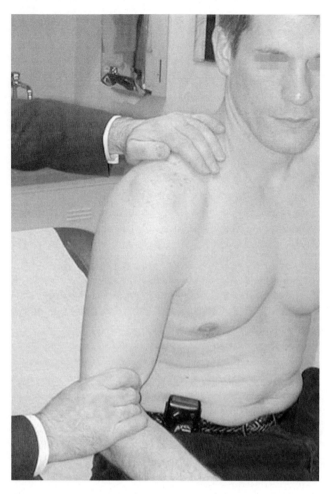

Fig. 3.2 Sulcus sign. Downward traction of the arm will create a gap between the acromion and the humeral head (From Lee EW, Flatow EL, Mini-incision Bankart Repair for Shoulder Instability. In Scuderi G, Tria A, Berger R (eds.), *MIS Techniques in Orthopedics*, New York, Springer, 2006, with kind permission of Springer Science and Business Media, Inc.)

Posterior instability can be elicited with the *posterior stress test*. As one hand stabilizes the scapula, a posteriorly directed axial force is applied to the arm with the shoulder in 90° of flexion, and adduction and internal rotation. Unlike the anterior apprehension test, the posterior stress test will usually produce pain rather than true apprehension.[28]

Radiographic Features

Although the history and physical examination are the key elements in patient evaluation, a series of radiographic studies may be helpful in confirming the diagnosis and defining associated pathology. Anteroposterior (AP) radiographs in internal and external rotation, a lateral view in the scapular plane (scapular-Y view), and a lateral of the glenohumeral joint (i.e., a standard supine axillary or Velpeau axillary view) should be obtained in the initial evaluation. A *Hill–Sachs lesion* (posterolateral impression fracture) of the humeral head is best seen on the AP radiograph in internal rotation (Fig. 3.5) or on specialized views such as the Stryker Notch view.[29] Fractures or erosions of the glenoid rim can be detected on an axillary or apical oblique view.[30]

Other more specialized imaging studies are not routinely obtained in the initial evaluation of instability but may be useful in a preoperative workup. Computed tomography (CT) results can assist in further assessment of fractures and glenoid erosions or altered glenoid version as well as detect subtle subluxation of the humeral head.[31,32] MRI and magnetic resonance (MR) arthrography can identify associated pathology of the labrum, glenohumeral ligaments, and the rotator cuff.[33–35] The addition of abduction and external rotation has been shown to increase the sensitivity

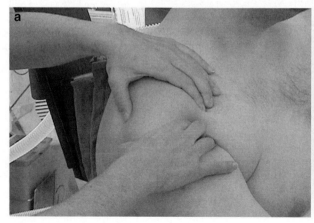
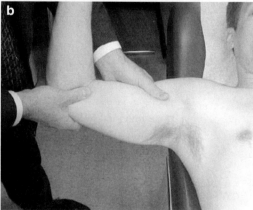
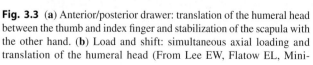

Fig. 3.3 (**a**) Anterior/posterior drawer: translation of the humeral head between the thumb and index finger and stabilization of the scapula with the other hand. (**b**) Load and shift: simultaneous axial loading and translation of the humeral head (From Lee EW, Flatow EL, Mini-incision Bankart Repair for Shoulder Instability. In Scuderi G, Tria A, Berger R (eds.), *MIS Techniques in Orthopedics*, New York, Springer, 2006, with kind permission of Springer Science and Business Media, Inc.)

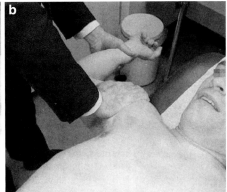

Fig. 3.4 (**a**) Apprehension test: abduction and external rotation will produce a sense of impending subluxation/dislocation with anterior glenohumeral instability. (**b**) Relocation test: posterior directed force on the humeral head will alleviate symptoms (From Lee EW, Flatow EL, Mini-incision Bankart Repair for Shoulder Instability. In Scuderi G, Tria A, Berger R (eds.), *MIS Techniques in Orthopedics*, New York, Springer, 2006, with kind permission of Springer Science and Business Media, Inc.)

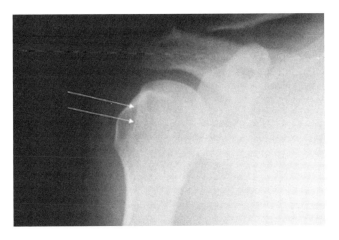

Fig . 3.5 Hill–Sachs lesion. An impaction fracture of the posterolateral humeral head associated with an anterior glenohumeral dislocation is depicted by the *small white arrows* on this internally rotated anteroposterior radiograph (From Lee EW, Flatow EL, Mini-incision Bankart Repair for Shoulder Instability. In Scuderi G, Tria A, Berger R (eds.), *MIS Techniques in Orthopedics*, New York, Springer, 2006, with kind permission of Springer Science and Business Media, Inc.)

of MR arthrography in delineating tears of the anterior labrum.[36,37] More recent radiographic modalities such as dynamic MRI currently have no defined indications but may become a useful adjunct in evaluating glenohumeral instability.[38]

Nonoperative Treatment

Although the results vary with age and associated bone and soft tissue injury, nonoperative treatment consisting of a period of immobilization followed by rehabilitation is typically successful in managing the majority of patients

with glenohumeral instability. Early studies of young (younger than 20 years old), athletic patients, however, found a recurrence rate as high as 90% after a primary dislocation.[39,40] While subsequent studies have reported lower numbers,[41,42] clearly the risk for subsequent dislocations is higher with earlier onset of instability.

The length and type of immobilization remains a matter of debate. Several published series have advocated immobilization for a few days to several weeks. However, studies by Hovelius[41] and Simonet and Cofield[42] have found no difference in outcome from either the type or length of immobilization. In general, younger patients (younger than 30 years of age) sustaining a primary dislocation are preferably immobilized for approximately 3–4 weeks. Older patients, who have a smaller risk of recurrent instability but a higher susceptibility to stiffness, may be immobilized for shorter periods.

Rehabilitation efforts are aimed at strengthening the dynamic stabilizers and regaining motion. Progressive resistive exercises of the rotator cuff, deltoid, and scapular stabilizers are recommended. Stress on the static restraints (i.e., capsuloligamentous structures) should be prevented in the immediate postinjury period by avoidance of vigorous stretching and provocative arm positions.

Operative Treatment

Failure of conservative management for glenohumeral instability is an indication for proceeding with operative intervention. Open procedures are currently the gold standard for repair of the disrupted soft tissue shoulder stabilizers.

Modern techniques emphasize anatomic restoration of the soft tissue structures. Based on the work of Perthes in 1906,[43] Bankart,[44] in 1923, popularized repair of the capsule to the anterior glenoid without shortening of the overlying subscapularis. After modifications to his original description, reconstruction of the avulsed capsule and labrum to the glenoid lip is commonly referred to today as the *Bankart repair*. Several capsulorrhaphy procedures have also been described to address capsular laxity and the increase in joint volume. These procedures allow tightening of the anterior capsule in combination with reattachment of a capsulolabral avulsion.

The inferior capsular shift was first introduced by Neer and Foster for multidirectional instability.[24] This procedure can reduce capsular volume through overlap of capsular tissue on the side of greatest instability and reducing tissue redundancy by tensioning the inferior capsule and opposite side. For anterior inferior instability, we prefer to use a modified inferior capsular shift procedure, in essence a laterally based "T" capsulorrhaphy, which allows us to adapt the repair to each individual.[45,46]

The rationale behind this universal approach to instability is predicated on several factors. First, the capsule is shaped like a funnel with a broader circumferential insertion on the humeral side. Implementing a laterally based incision allows the tissue to be shifted a greater distance and reattached to the broader lateral insertion, thus allowing more capsular overlap. Second, following intraoperative assessment of the inferior pouch and capsular redundancy, the inferior shift procedure permits variable degrees of capsular mobilization around the humeral neck to treat different grades of tissue laxity. Third, use of a "T" capsulorrhaphy permits independent tensioning of the capsule in the medial–lateral and superior–inferior directions. Medial–lateral tensioning is usually a secondary concern, and, if overdone, may result in loss of external rotation. Fourth, a lateral capsular incision affords some protection to the axillary nerve, particularly during an inferior dissection as the nerve traverses under the inferior capsule. Finally, capsular tears/avulsions from the humeral insertion, although rare, are more readily identified and repaired with a laterally based incision.

The patient is placed in a beachchair position, although slightly more recumbent than when performing a rotator cuff repair. We prefer interscalene regional block anesthesia at our institution because of its safety and ability to provide adequate muscle relaxation. Examination under anesthesia should be performed prior to breaching the soft tissues to confirm the predominant components of instability. The key to a "mini-open" Bankart procedure is the use of a concealed anterior axillary incision starting approximately 3 cm below the tip of the coracoid and extending inferiorly for 7–8 cm into the axillary recess (Fig. 3.6). Supplemental local anesthetic is injected into the inferior aspect of the wound where thoracic cross-innervation prevents a complete block in this area. Full-thickness subcutaneous flaps are mobilized until the inferior aspect of the clavicle is palpated.

The deltopectoral interval is then developed, taking the cephalic vein laterally with the deltoid. If needed, the upper 1–2 cm of the pectoralis major insertion may be released to gain further exposure. The clavipectoral fascia is then gently incised lateral to the strap muscles, which are gently retracted medially. Osteotomy of the coracoid should not be necessary and may endanger the medial neurovascular structures. A small, medially based wedge of the anterior fascicle of the coracoacromial ligament may be excised to increase visualization of the superior border of the subscapularis muscle, rotator interval, and anterior aspect of the subacromial space.

The upper and lower borders of the subscapularis are identified. The anterior humeral circumflex vessels are carefully isolated and ligated. Preservation of the inferior border of the subscapularis to provide protection to the axillary nerve has been suggested.[47] This may be a reasonable option in true unidirectional instability cases; however, inadequate exposure of the inferior capsule may compromise the ability to correct any coexisting inferior laxity component. Another approach splits the subscapularis longitudinally in line with its fibers, making visualization of the glenoid rim more difficult, but motion is less restricted postoperatively. This approach may be useful in athletes who throw, in whom any restriction in external rotation postoperatively should be avoided.[48] We prefer to detach the tendon 1–2 cm from its insertion onto the lesser tuberosity, being careful not to stray too medially into the muscle fibers and compromise the subscapularis repair. Blunt elevation of the muscle belly from the capsule medially may permit easier identification of the plane between the two structures.

Examination of the rotator interval is essential during dissection of the capsule and subscapularis. As one of the primary static stabilizers of the glenohumeral joint, the rotator interval can be an important component of recurrent anterior instability. We repair it when it is widened, aware that overly tightening the gap will limit external rotation.

The capsule is then incised laterally, leaving a 1-cm cuff of tissue for repair while placing traction sutures in the free edge. Placing the arm in adduction and external rotation maximizes the distance between the incision and axillary nerve, which should be palpated and protected throughout the procedure.

The extent of capsular dissection and mobilization will depend on the components of instability. Unidirectional anterior instability will only require dissection of the anterior capsule. Bidirectional anterior–inferior instability will require the addition of inferior capsular mobilization to eliminate the enlarged capsule. In these cases, the shoulder is gradually flexed and externally rotated to facilitate sharp dissection of the anterior and inferior capsule off of the humeral neck. A finger can be placed in the inferior recess to assess the amount of redundant capsule and the adequacy of the shift. As more capsule is mobilized and upward traction is placed

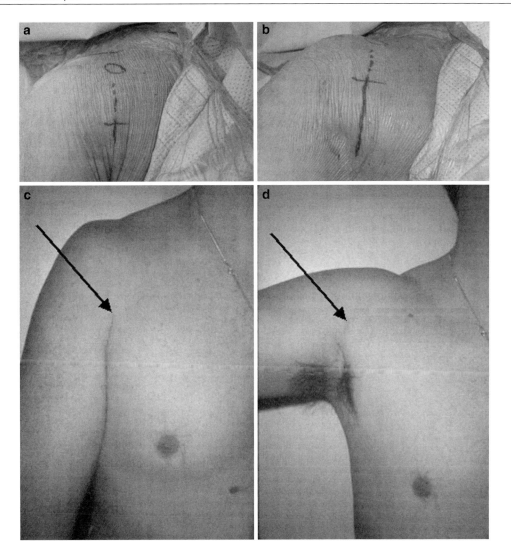

Fig. 3.6 Concealed axillary incision. (**a**) Arm at the side and (**b**) arm in abduction. The *circle* indicates coracoid process. The *solid line* indicates true concealed incision; if needed for more exposure, the *dashed line* indicates extension toward the coracoid. (**c**) and (**d**) Healed axillary incision. *Black arrows* indicate superior extent of incision (From Lee EW, Flatow EL, Mini-incision Bankart Repair for Shoulder Instability. In Scuderi G, Tria A, Berger R (eds.), *MIS Techniques in Orthopedics*, New York, Springer, 2006, with kind permission of Springer Science and Business Media, Inc.)

on the sutures, the volume of the pouch will reduce and push the finger out, indicating an adequate shift.

The inferior component in unidirectional instability is minimal, and thus, an inferior shift and the horizontal incision may be unnecessary. With a significant inferior capsular redundancy, the horizontal limb of the "T" in the capsule is made between the inferior and middle glenohumeral ligaments. A Fukuda retractor is then placed to visualize the glenoid (Fig. 3.7). If the capsule is thin and redundant medially, a "barrel" stitch can be used to tension it as well as imbricate the capsule at the glenoid rim to serve as an additional bumper to augment a deficient labrum[49] (Fig. 3.8).

Effectiveness of a shift requires anchoring of the capsule to the glenoid. When the glenohumeral ligaments and labrum are avulsed from the bone medially, they must be reattached to the glenoid rim (Fig. 3.9). The Bankart lesion must be anchored to the rim before performing the capsulorraphy because the capsule must be secured to the glenoid for the shift to be effective. This can be accomplished by inside-out anchoring the labrum with sutures through bone tunnels. After the glenoid rim is roughened with a curette or high-speed burr, two to three sets of holes are made adjacent to the articular surface and through the glenoid rim. Curved awls, angled curettes, and heavy towel clips may be used to fashion the tunnels. A small CurvTek (Arthrotek, Warsaw, IN) may also be helpful in making the holes. Number 0 nonabsorbable braided sutures (e.g., Ethibond [Ethicon/Johnson & Johnson, Somerville, NJ]) are passed through the tunnels. Both limbs are then brought inside-out through the labrum and tied on the outside of the capsule. Alternatively, suture anchors can

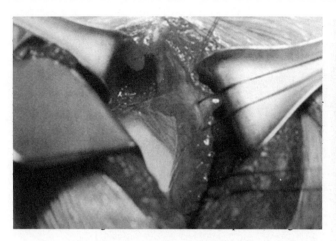

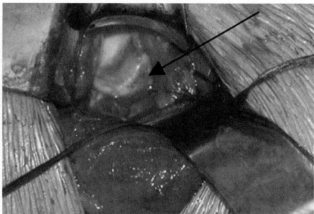

Fig. 3.7 Mobilization of the capsule and placement of traction sutures in the free edge. A Fukuda retractor is placed, allowing inspection of the glenoid (From Lee EW, Flatow EL, Mini-incision Bankart Repair for Shoulder Instability. In Scuderi G, Tria A, Berger R (eds.), *MIS Techniques in Orthopedics*, New York, Springer, 2006, with kind permission of Springer Science and Business Media, Inc.)

Fig. 3.9 Avulsion of the glenohumeral ligaments and labrum from the glenoid rim. The *solid black arrow* indicates the bare anterior glenoid rim

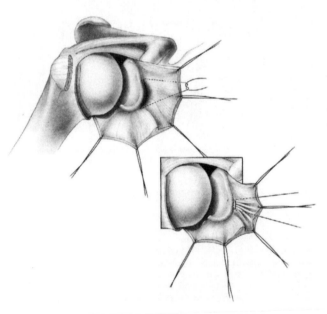

Fig. 3.8 A barrel stitch may be used medially to bunch up tissue at the glenoid rim to compensate for a deficient labrum (From Post M, Bigliani L, Flatow E, et al. The Shoulder: Operative Technique. Philadelphia: Lippincott Williams & Wilkins, 1998, p. 184.)

be utilized, placing them adjacent to the articular margin and careful not to insert them medially to avoid a step–off between the rim and the labrum.

Glenoid deficiency from a fracture of the rim or from repeated wear from chronic instability may contribute to the pathologic process. Defects representing less than 25% of the articular surface area may be repaired by reattaching the labrum and capsule back to the remaining glenoid rim. If a fragment of bone remains attached to the soft tissues, this can be mobilized and repaired back to the glenoid with sutures.

Larger fragments can be reattached with a cannulated screw, countersinking the head of the screw within the bone. Defects larger than 25% without a reparable fragment, leaving an "inverted-pear" glenoid in which the normally pear-shaped glenoid had lost enough anterior–inferior bone to assume the shape of an inverted pear,[50] should be augmented with bone. Femoral head allograft can be fashioned to reconstitute the rim. Another alternative to deepening the socket is to perform a Bristow–Laterjet procedure, transferring the coracoid tip with the attached coracobrachialis and short head of the biceps into the defect, close to the articular margin and behind the repaired capsule.[4] A cannulated screw, carefully engaging the posterior cortex of the glenoid, and a washer are used to secure the coracoid to the glenoid (Fig. 3.10).

An engaging Hill–Sachs lesion may be another source of recurrent instability requiring attention for a successful repair. Preventing the head defect from engaging the glenoid rim can be accomplished in one of three ways. First, the capsular shift can be performed to tighten the anterior structures enough to restrict external rotation. This should be done with caution as previously mentioned, given the unwanted result in overhead athletes and the risk of late glenohumeral arthrosis. Second, a size-matched humeral osteoarticular allograft or a corticocancellous iliac graft can be utilized to fill the defect. Finally, an internal rotation proximal humeral osteotomy can be performed, albeit with significant technical difficulty and potential morbidity, shifting the defect out of the arc of motion.

To perform the capsular shift, the arm is positioned in at least 20° of external rotation, 30° of abduction, and 10° of flexion while securing the tissues for the capsular shift. In overhead athletes, approximately 10° more abduction and external rotation may be used. Once any adherent soft tissues impeding excursion of the capsule are dissected from the capsule, the inferior flap should be shifted superiorly first, followed by the superior flap to a more inferior position. A suture may be placed medially to reinforce overlap of the two flaps.

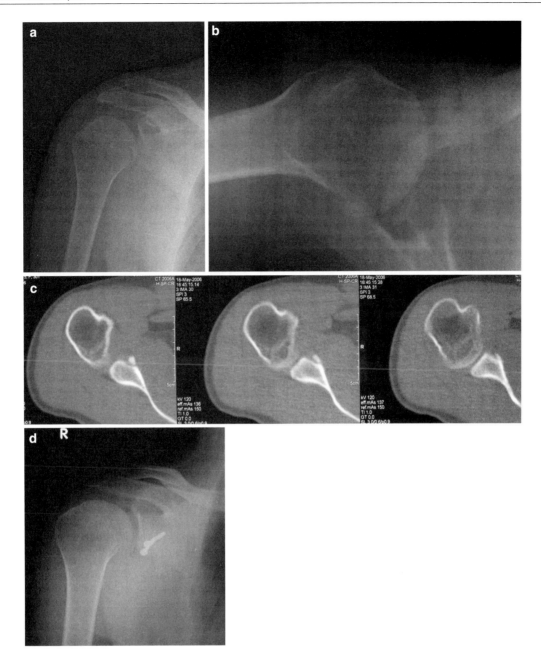

Fig. 3.10 Laterjet coracoid transfer for anterior inferior bony insufficiency. (**a**) and (**b**) Preoperative radiographs. (**c**) Preoperative axial CT images. (**d**) Postoperative scapular anteroposterior and lateral radiograph with bone block and screws in place

The subscapularis is then repaired as previously described followed by a layered closure and a subcuticular skin closure.

Postoperative Care

The challenge following an instability procedure is to find the delicate balance between early gradual motion and maintenance of stability. In general, patients are protected in a sling for 6 weeks with immediate active hand, wrist, and elbow motion and isometric shoulder exercises started at approximately 10 days. From 10 days to 2 weeks, gentle assisted motion is permitted with external rotation with a stick to 10° and elevation to 90°. From 2 to 4 weeks, motion is progressed to 30° of external rotation and 140° of elevation. From 4 to 6 weeks, external rotation to 40° and elevation to 160° are initiated in addition to light resistive exercises. Terminal elevation stretching and external rotation to 60° are permitted after 6 weeks. After 3 months, when the soft tissues have adequately healed, terminal external rotation stretches are allowed. Patients can expect a return to sport at 9–12 months postoperatively. These are broad guidelines that should be adapted to each individual case based on intraoperative findings and frequent post-operative exams. Poor tissue quality, durability of the repair, patient reliability, and future demands on the shoulder should dictate the progression of the rehabilitation program.

Results

Good results have been achieved with most open capsulorraphy techniques to treat anterior/anterior–inferior glenohumeral instability. Thomas and Matsen[51] reported 97% good or excellent results in 63 shoulders with repair of the Bankart lesion and incising both the subscapularis and capsule. Pollock et al.[46] reported 90% successful results with an anterior–inferior capsular shift in 151 shoulders with a 5% rate of recurrent instability. Bigliani et al.[45] studied 68 shoulders in athletes who underwent an anterior–inferior capsular shift with 94% of patients with good or excellent results. Fifty-eight patients (92%) returned to the major sports and 47 patients (75%) returned at the same competitive level.

Choice of Mini-incision Versus Arthroscopic Repair

With the recent advances in arthroscopic instability repair, failure rates have been comparable to open, mini-incision repair.[52,53] Many injuries can be addressed by either open or arthroscopic methods, and the limitations of arthroscopic surgery remain controversial.

Advantages of an arthroscopic repair include preservation of the subscapularis (although splitting the subscapularis in line with its fibers may also accomplish this), ability to thoroughly evaluate and visualize the entire glenohumeral joint and biceps/superior labrum insertion, less immediate postoperative pain, reduced cost, and improved cosmesis.[54–56] Disadvantages of an arthroscopic approach include difficulty mobilizing large, medialized glenoid bone fragments and repairing capsular tears, especially humeral avulsions, and the fact that a minimally invasive approach may be less helpful in some multidirectional cases where stretching out of thin tissue rather than stiffness is the most common failure mode. Furthermore, open repair has been advocated for patients with greater than 25% of inferior glenoid bone loss who require bone grafting or coracoid transfer, rare patients with extremely large Hill–Sachs requiring grafting or mini-surface replacement, collision athletes, and revision cases.[57–60]

The authors utilize arthroscopic techniques for most cases in which only labral avulsion and capsular stretch needs to be addressed. We will mobilize and repair small glenoid avulsion fragments arthroscopically, but when bone grafting of the glenoid or the Hill–Sachs lesion is required, a mini–incision

open approach is employed. Finally, revision cases may be performed arthroscopically in many cases, especially when the failure is due to an unrepaired or improperly (e.g., medial rather than on the glenoid rim) repaired Bankart lesion, but an open approach is used if bone grafting is needed or if subscapularis deficiency from a prior open approach requires extensive mobilization and repair or subcoracoid pectoralis transfer. Usually these procedures may be performed through a concealed axillary, mini-incision approach as previously described.

References

1. Du Toit GT, Roux D. Recurrent dislocation of the shoulder: a twenty-four year study of the Johannesberg stapling operation. *J Bone Joint Surg Am* 38A: 1–12, 1956
2. Magnuson PB, Stack JK. Recurrent dislocation of the shoulder. *JAMA* 123: 889–92, 1943
3. Clarke HO. Habitual dislocation of the shoulder. *J Bone Joint Surg Br* 30B: 19–25, 1948
4. Helfat AJ. Coracoid transplantation for recurring dislocation of the shoulder. *J Bone Joint Surg Br* 40B: 198–202, 1958
5. Weber BG, Simpson LA, Hardegger F. Rotational humeral osteotomy for recurrent anterior dislocation of the shoulder associated with a large Hill-Sachs lesion. *J Bone Joint Surg Am* 66(9): 1443–50, 1984
6. Saha AK. *Theory of Shoulder Mechanism: Descriptive and Applied.* Springfield, IL, Charles C. Thomas, 1961
7. Hawkins RJ, Angelo RL. Glenohumeral osteoarthrosis. A late complication of the Putti-Platt repair. *J Bone Joint Surg Am* 72(8): 1193–7, 1990
8. O'Driscoll SW, Evans DC. Long-term results of staple capsulorrhaphy for anterior instability of the shoulder. *J Bone Joint Surg Am* 75(2): 249–58, 1993
9. Samilson RL, Prieto V. Dislocation arthropathy of the shoulder. *J Bone Joint Surg Am* 65(4): 456–60, 1983
10. Steinmann SR, Flatow EL, Pollock RG, et al. Evaluation and surgical treatment of failed shoulder instability repairs. In: *38th Annual Meeting of the Orthopaedic Research Society*, p. 727, 1992
11. Young DC, Rockwood CA, Jr. Complications of a failed Bristow procedure and their management. *J Bone Joint Surg Am* 73(7): 969–81, 1991
12. Blazina ME, Satzman JS. Recurrent anterior subluxation of the shoulder in athletics: a distinct entity. *J Bone Joint Surg Am* 51A(5): 1037–38, 1969
13. Garth WP, Jr, Allman FL, Jr, Armstrong WS. Occult anterior subluxations of the shoulder in noncontact sports. *Am J Sports Med* 15(6): 579–85, 1987
14. Hastings DE, Coughlin LP. Recurrent subluxation of the glenohumeral joint. *Am J Sports Med* 9(6): 352–5, 1981
15. Rowe CR, Zarins B. Recurrent transient subluxation of the shoulder. *J Bone Joint Surg Am* 63(6): 863–72, 1981
16. Levine WN, Flatow EL. The pathophysiology of shoulder instability. *Am J Sports Med* 28(6): 910–7, 2000
17. Wang VM, Flatow EL. Pathomechanics of acquired shoulder instability: a basic science perspective. *J Shoulder Elbow Surg* 14(1 Suppl S): 2S–11S, 2005
18. Turkel SJ, Panio MW, Marshall JL, Girgis FG. Stabilizing mechanisms preventing anterior dislocation of the glenohumeral joint. *J Bone Joint Surg Am* 63(8): 1208–17, 1981
19. Bigliani LU, Pollock RG, Soslowsky LJ, Flatow EL, Pawluk RJ, Mow VC. Tensile properties of the inferior glenohumeral ligament. *J Orthop Res* 10(2): 187–97, 1992

20. Neer CS, II. Involuntary inferior and multidirectional instability of the shoulder: etiology, recognition, and treatment. *Instr Course Lect* 34: 232–38, 1985

21. Beall MS, Jr, Diefenbach G, Allen A. Electromyographic biofeedback in the treatment of voluntary posterior instability of the shoulder. *Am J Sports Med* 15(2): 175–8, 1987

22. Davidson PA, Elattrache NS, Jobe CM, Jobe FW. Rotator cuff and posterior-superior glenoid labrum injury associated with increased glenohumeral motion: a new site of impingement. *J Shoulder Elbow Surg* 4(5): 384–90, 1995

23. Neviaser RJ, Neviaser TJ. Recurrent instability of the shoulder after age 40. *J Shoulder Elbow Surg* 4(6): 416–8, 1995

24. Neer CS, II, Foster CR. Inferior capsular shift for involuntary inferior and multidirectional instability of the shoulder. A preliminary report. *J Bone Joint Surg Am* 62(6): 897–908, 1980

25. Hawkins RJ, Bokor DJ. Clinical evaluation of shoulder problems. In: *The Shoulder*, Rockwood CA, Matsen FA, (eds.), 3rd edition, pp. 149–177. Philadelphia, PA, WB Saunders, 1990

26. Speer KP, Hannafin JA, Altchek DW, Warren RF. An evaluation of the shoulder relocation test. *Am J Sports Med* 22(2): 177–83, 1994

27. Jobe FW, Tibone JE, Jobe CM. The shoulder in sports. In: *The Shoulder*, Rockwood CA, Jr, Matsen FA, (eds.), 3rd edition, pp. 961–967. Philadelphia, PA, WB Saunders, 1990

28. Hawkins RJ, Koppert G, Johnston G. Recurrent posterior instability (subluxation) of the shoulder. *J Bone Joint Surg Am* 66(2): 169–74, 1984

29. Danzig LA, Greenway G, Resnick D. The Hill-Sachs lesion. An experimental study. *Am J Sports Med* 8(5): 328–32, 1980

30. Garth WP, Jr, Slappey CE, Ochs CW. Roentgenographic demonstration of instability of the shoulder: the apical oblique projection. A technical note. *J Bone Joint Surg Am* 66(9): 1450–3, 1984

31. Itoi E, Lee SB, Amrami KK, Wenger DE, An KN. Quantitative assessment of classic anteroinferior bony Bankart lesions by radiography and computed tomography. *Am J Sports Med* 31(1): 112–8, 2003

32. Nyffeler RW, Jost B, Pfirrmann CW, Gerber C. Measurement of glenoid version: conventional radiographs versus computed tomography scans. *J Shoulder Elbow Surg* 12(5): 493–6, 2003

33. Beltran J, Rosenberg ZS, Chandnani VP, Cuomo F, Beltran S, Rokito A. Glenohumeral instability: evaluation with MR arthrography. *Radiographics* 17(3): 657–73, 1997

34. Parmar H, Jhankaria B, Maheshwari M, Singrakhia M, Shanbag S, Chawla A, Deshpande S. Magnetic resonance arthrography in recurrent anterior shoulder instability as compared to arthroscopy: a prospective comparative study. *J Postgrad Med* 48(4): 270–3; discussion 273–4, 2002

35. Shankman S, Bencardino J, Beltran J. Glenohumeral instability: evaluation using MR arthrography of the shoulder. *Skeletal Radiol* 28(7): 365–82, 1999

36. Cvitanic O, Tirman PF, Feller JF, Bost FW, Minter J, Carroll KW. Using abduction and external rotation of the shoulder to increase the sensitivity of MR arthrography in revealing tears of the anterior glenoid labrum. *AJR Am J Roentgenol* 169(3): 837–44, 1997

37. Wintzell G, Larsson H, Larsson S. Indirect MR arthrography of anterior shoulder instability in the ABER and the apprehension test positions: a prospective comparative study of two different shoulder positions during MRI using intravenous gadodiamide contrast for enhancement of the joint fluid. *Skeletal Radiol* 27(9): 488–94, 1998

38. Allmann KH, Uhl M, Gufler H, Biebow N, Hauer MP, Kotter E, Reichelt A, Langer M. Cine-MR imaging of the shoulder. *Acta Radiol* 38(6): 1043–6, 1997

39. Rowe CR. Prognosis in dislocations of the shoulder. *J Bone Joint Surg Am* 38A: 957–77, 1956

40. Wheeler JH, Ryan JB, Arciero RA, Molinari RN. Arthroscopic versus nonoperative treatment of acute shoulder dislocations in young athletes. *Arthroscopy* 5(3): 213–7, 1989

41. Hovelius L. Anterior dislocation of the shoulder in teen-agers and young adults. Five-year prognosis. *J Bone Joint Surg Am* 69(3): 393–9, 1987

42. Simonet WT, Cofield RH. Prognosis in anterior shoulder dislocation. *Am J Sports Med* 12(1): 19–24, 1984

43. Perthes G. Uber operationen bei habitueller schulterluxation. *Deutsch Ztschr Chir* 85: 199–227, 1906

44. Bankart ASB. Recurrent or habitual dislocation of the shoulder joint. *Br Med J* 2: 1132–35, 1923

45. Bigliani LU, Kurzweil PR, Schwartzbach CC, Wolfe IN, Flatow EL. Inferior capsular shift procedure for anterior-inferior shoulder instability in athletes. *Am J Sports Med* 22(5): 578–84, 1994

46. Pollock RG, Owens JM, Nicholson GP, et al. Anterior inferior capsular shift procedure for anterior glenohumeral instability: long term results. In: *39th Annual Meeting of the Orthopaedic Research Society*, p. 974, 1993

47. Matsen FA, III, Thomas SC, Rockwood CA, Jr, Wirth MA. Glenohumeral instability. In: *The Shoulder*, Rockwood CA, Jr, Matsen FA, (eds.), 3rd edition, pp. 611–754. Philadelphia, PA, WB Saunders, 1998

48. Rubenstein DL, Jobe FW, Glousman RE, et al. Anterior capsulolabral reconstruction of the shoulder in athletes. *J Shoulder Elbow Surg* 1: 229–37, 1993

49. Ahmad CS, Freehill MQ, Blaine TA, Levine WN, Bigliani LU. Anteromedial capsular redundancy and labral deficiency in shoulder instability. *Am J Sports Med* 31(2): 247–52, 2003

50. Burkhart SS, De Beer JF. Traumatic glenohumeral bone defects and their relationship to failure of arthroscopic Bankart repairs: significance of the inverted-pear glenoid and the humeral engaging Hill-Sachs lesion. *Arthroscopy* 16(7): 677–94, 2000

51. Thomas SC, Matsen FA, III. An approach to the repair of avulsion of the glenohumeral ligaments in the management of traumatic anterior glenohumeral instability. *J Bone Joint Surg Am* 71(4): 506–13, 1989

52. Carreira DS, Mazzocca AD, Oryhon J, Brown FM, Hayden JK, Romeo AA. A prospective outcome evaluation of arthroscopic Bankart repairs: minimum 2-year follow-up. *Am J Sports Med* 34(5): 771–7, 2006

53. Tjoumakaris FP, Abboud JA, Hasan SA, Ramsey ML, Williams GR. Arthroscopic and open Bankart repairs provide similar outcomes. *Clin Orthop Relat Res* 446: 227–32, 2006

54. Abrams JS, Savoie FH, III, Tauro JC, Bradley JP. Recent advances in the evaluation and treatment of shoulder instability: anterior, posterior, and multidirectional. *Arthroscopy* 18(9 Suppl 2): 1–13, 2002

55. Sachs RA, Williams B, Stone ML, Paxton L, Kuney M. Open Bankart repair: correlation of results with postoperative subscapularis function. *Am J Sports Med* 33(10): 1458–62, 2005

56. Wang C, Ghalambor N, Zarins B, Warner JJ. Arthroscopic versus open Bankart repair: analysis of patient subjective outcome and cost. *Arthroscopy* 21(10): 1219–22, 2005

57. Boileau P, Villalba M, Hery JY, Balg F, Ahrens P, Neyton L. Risk factors for recurrence of shoulder instability after arthroscopic Bankart repair. *J Bone Joint Surg Am* 88(8): 1755–63, 2006

58. Mazzocca AD, Brown FM, Jr, Carreira DS, Hayden J, Romeo AA. Arthroscopic anterior shoulder stabilization of collision and contact athletes. *Am J Sports Med* 33(1): 52–60, 2005

59. Pagnani MJ, Dome DC. Surgical treatment of traumatic anterior shoulder instability in American football players. *J Bone Joint Surg Am* 84-A(5): 711–5, 2002

60. Rhee YG, Ha JH, Cho NS. Anterior shoulder stabilization in collision athletes: arthroscopic versus open Bankart repair. *Am J Sports Med* 34(6): 979–85, 2006

Chapter 4
Mini-open Rotator Cuff Repair

W. Anthony Frisella and Frances Cuomo

Rotator cuff pathology is a common cause of shoulder pain and disability, and becomes more common with advancing patient age. Most symptomatic rotator cuff disease is seen in patients in their fifth and sixth decades. Tears of the rotator cuff are associated with pain and weakness and can result in significant disability.[1] However, it is also known that asymptomatic rotator cuff tears exist in a large percentage of patients, and the presence of asymptomatic tears increases with increasing age.[1,2] The cause of a tear of the rotator cuff is debated, but is most likely related to a combination of several factors: (1) impingement against the subacromial arch, (2) age-related degeneration or atrophy, (3) overuse, and (4) trauma.[1,3] The rationale for repairing the torn rotator cuff is derived from multiple published studies demonstrating improved function and decreased pain after rotator cuff repair and rehabilitation. Although complete healing of the tendon does not always occur, rotator cuff repair is recognized as a beneficial procedure by (1) relieving pain, (2) improving strength, and (3) improving range of motion in the affected shoulder. The earliest report of rotator cuff repair comes from Codman in 1911.[4] Since then, many studies have demonstrated good outcomes with improved pain and function following formal open repair of the rotator cuff with decompression of the subacromial space and acromioplasty.[5-12] The method by which the cuff is repaired, however, has changed over the past two decades, with a movement toward minimally invasive techniques, including both mini-open and arthroscopic repair. The mini-open or deltoid-splitting approach to the rotator cuff is a well-characterized procedure with excellent outcomes and is a useful and successful method of rotator cuff repair.

Arthroscopic visualization of joints was first described in 1931, and the advent of shoulder arthroscopy in the 1980s fundamentally changed the approach to diagnosis and treatment of pathology, including rotator cuff tears.[13-15] The rotator cuff could be visualized arthroscopically and tears could be identified and characterized. The ability to visualize the anatomy of the shoulder through the arthroscope inevitably led to strategies to treat rotator cuff tears by less invasive means. Prior to arthroscopy, rotator cuff tears were treated by formal open repair with approaches that violated the deltoid insertion on the acromion. The deltoid was removed from the acromion in order to perform an acromioplasty and decompression, and repaired to the acromion at the end of the procedure. This approach carried the risk of deltoid avulsion, a rare but catastrophic complication.[16-18] Diagnosis and characterization of tears by arthroscopy led to the description of the arthroscopically assisted, mini-open, or deltoid-splitting repair technique of rotator cuff repair.[19] The success of the mini-open technique was followed by the description of completely arthroscopic rotator cuff repair, which has also been successful. However, mini-open repair remains a viable alternative to arthroscopic repair and has advantages over both arthroscopic and formal open repair.

The mini-open rotator cuff repair represents a bridge between open and arthroscopic rotator cuff repair. It has specific advantages and disadvantages when compared with other methods of cuff repair. Advantages over open repair include the adjunctive use of arthroscopy for diagnosis and characterization of the torn cuff tendon as well as identification and treatment of associated shoulder pathology.[20,21] The arthroscopic portion of the procedure can also be used to mark the torn tendon and to assist in performing the repair. In addition, the deltoid origin is minimally disturbed, allowing for faster rehabilitation and greatly decreasing the possibility of deltoid avulsion as a complication. Mini-open repair creates less surgical trauma, facilitating early hospital discharge and decreasing postoperative pain.

Mini-open repair also has advantages over arthroscopic repair. The primary advantage is the avoidance of complex arthroscopic suture passing and tying techniques. An additional advantage of the mini-open repair is its usefulness as a bridge between the formal open and completely arthroscopic repair techniques, allowing the surgeon a means of gradual transition between the two, if desired. Like arthroscopic repair, mini-open repair with adjunctive arthroscopy allows for direct visualization of the glenohumeral joint and subacromial space for the purposes of diagnosis and allows for the

W.A. Frisella and F. Cuomo (✉)
Division of Shoulder and Elbow Surgery, Department of Orthopedics and Sports Medicine, Beth Israel Medical Center, Phillips Ambulatory Care Center, 10 Union Square East, New York, NY 10003, USA
e-mail: fcuomo98@yahoo.com

G.R. Scuderi and A.J. Tria (eds.), *Minimally Invasive Surgery in Orthopedics*,
DOI 10.1007/978-0-387-76608-9_4, © Springer Science+Business Media, LLC 2010

performance of adjunctive arthroscopic procedures, e.g., subacromial decompression, arthroscopic releases, and glenohumeral debridement. Direct arthroscopic visualization of the cuff allows the surgeon to characterize the size and orientation of the tear prior to repair. In addition, mini-open repairs have similar morbidity rates when compared with arthroscopic repairs.

Technique

There are many variations of the technique of mini-open rotator cuff repair. The basic principles are the same, however, and the steps are as follows. First, the shoulder is examined under anesthesia. The patient is then positioned and the shoulder prepped and draped as for arthroscopy. A complete diagnostic arthroscopy is performed and the presence of a cuff tear is confirmed. Associated intraarticular pathology is addressed as necessary. The subacromial space is then entered and a subacromial decompression and acromioplasty are performed. The lateral arthroscopy portal incision is then extended and the deltoid is split, exposing the cuff tear. Open repair of the tear is then performed. These steps are a general guideline. The specific approach to mini-open repair used in our center is described in detail in this section.

The patient is placed supine on the operating table. Regional anesthesia is administered, typically an interscalene block (Fig. 4.1), and may be the only anesthesia given. A light general anesthesia may be used in addition for patient comfort or per patient preference. Once adequate anesthesia is obtained, an examination under anesthesia is performed to document full range of motion. Secondary stiffness may develop in patients with rotator cuff tears, making it important to document adequate range of motion prior to the start of the procedure. If the patient has a stiff shoulder, a manipulation may be performed to release adhesions. The patient is then ready for positioning in the beachchair or sitting position. The beach chair position is characterized by (1) elevation of the torso so that the acromion is parallel to the floor, (2) elevation of the thighs above the buttocks, and (3) flexion of the knees to a comfortable position. In this position, the buttocks are in the most dependent position, ensuring that the patient is stable and will not slip down the table. The surgeon must have adequate access to the posterior shoulder to the medial border of the scapula and the anterior shoulder to the level of the mid-clavicle. The head is held gently in place with a head holder. Generally, specialized table attachments are available to facilitate adequate exposure by dropping the back of the table away from the operative shoulder.

The shoulder is prepped and draped with care taken to ensure exposure of the widest area possible, especially posteriorly. "Draping yourself out" is a common and frustrating occurrence for the inexperienced shoulder arthroscopist. A standard posterior portal is created. Finding the correct position of this portal in the medial-lateral direction may be facilitated by feeling the notch in the spine of the scapula. The slight indentation that can be palpated along the posterior spine is usually about 2 cm medial to the posterolateral corner of the acromion. The portal is then placed about 2 cm inferior to this point. A blunt trocar is used to penetrate the posterior capsule and a diagnostic arthroscopy is begun.

If necessary, an anterior portal can be created. Creation of this portal is facilitated by placing a spinal needle into the rotator interval beneath the course of the biceps tendon, above the subscapularis muscle. A thorough diagnostic arthroscopy is then performed. The glenohumeral articulation is examined for lesions and cartilage loss. The superior labrum is inspected and palpated along with the biceps tendon anchor. The anterior and inferior labrum are inspected with their associated middle and inferior glenohumeral ligaments. The axillary recess is examined, followed by the posterior labrum. Pathology is addressed as necessary, but is beyond the scope of this chapter.

Once an adequate diagnostic arthroscopy of the rest of the joint is undertaken, attention is turned to the rotator cuff. The cuff insertion is examined, starting with the anterior border of the supraspinatus tendon adjacent to the exit of the biceps tendon from the joint (Fig. 4.2). The anterior border of the supraspinatus is the starting point for most degenerative tears and must always be carefully examined. Partial-thickness tears may also be identified here, characterized by pulling away of the articular side of the cuff from its insertion. Once the cuff tear is identified, the edges of the cuff should be debrided. Gentle debridement with a shaver may facilitate an inflammatory response that enhances healing. Debridement may also be used simply to facilitate visualization of the tear.

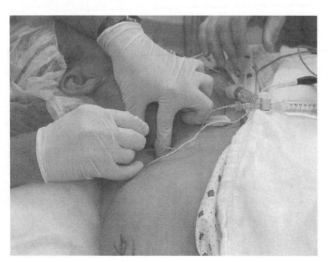

Fig. 4.1 Interscalene block is placed prior to examination under anesthesia. A general anesthesia can be used in place of, or in addition to, regional anesthesia

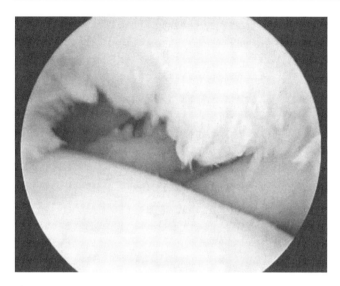

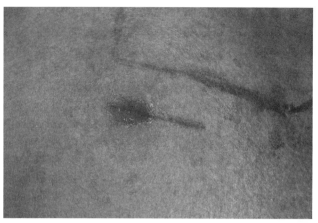

Fig. 4.3 The lateral portal is extended horizontally in line with Langer's lines. The total distance of the incision is usually between 3 and 4 cm (From Schneider JA, Cuomo F, Mini-open rotator cuff repair. In: Scuderi GR, Tria AJ, Jr., (eds.), *MIS Techniques in Orthopedics*, New York, Springer, 2006, with kind permission of Springer Science + Business Media, Inc.)

Fig. 4.2 The torn edge of the rotator cuff can be seen from the glenohumeral joint. The humeral head is inferior and the biceps tendon can be seen to the right. Most tears begin just posterior to the biceps tendon

The defect in the cuff may be marked with a percutaneously placed spinal needle, especially for a partial-thickness tear. A suture is advanced through the needle into the glenohumeral joint, allowing easier identification during the subacromial portion of the procedure and during the open repair. The arthroscope is then removed from the glenohumeral joint and the blunt trocar is used to enter the subacromial space.

Once in the subacromial space, an anterolateral portal is created 2 cm posterior and inferior to the anterolateral border of the acromion. The position of this portal may be modified to center it over the rotator cuff tear, which may be facilitated by the previously placed marking suture – the suture should be exiting the skin at the approximate location of the cuff tear. A skin incision is made in Langer's lines and a cannula is introduced and visualized in the subacromial space. There has been some controversy about the necessity of performing a subacromial decompression in the context of a rotator cuff tear. Nevertheless, we routinely perform a subacromial decompression, release the coracoacromial (CA) ligament, and perform an acromioplasty prior to cuff repair. The tear is identified using the previously placed marking suture, and further debridement is undertaken in the lateral gutter of the subacromial space. A thorough bursectomy, especially laterally, will facilitate visualization of the tear during the open portion of the procedure. The tendon edges may again be lightly debrided with a shaver.

At this point, traction sutures may be placed arthroscopically through the edge of the cuff. This may be a useful step for the surgeon who is transitioning from open to arthroscopic repairs. The arthroscopically placed sutures may then be used as traction sutures during the open portion of the repair. Alternatively, the arthroscopic portion of the procedure can be terminated and attention turned to exposure of the rotator cuff.

Arthroscopic instruments are removed and the anterolateral skin incision is extended horizontally at both ends to a total distance of 3–4 cm. The incision should be extended in such a way as to make exposure of the tear easier and thus minimize the length of skin incision (Fig. 4.3). The skin is undermined and freed from the underlying deltoid fascia. The deltoid is then split in line with its fibers, incorporating the previous arthroscopic puncture into the split. The split in the deltoid has two limits. First, the deltoid insertion should be protected and dissection should not lift the deltoid off the acromion. Second, the split in the deltoid should not extend further distal than 4 cm from the edge of the acromion to avoid injury to the axillary nerve. The nerve is located, on average, 6.3 cm from the edge of the acromion on the deep surface of the deltoid,[22] but occasionally can be found much closer.

Once the deltoid is split, the subacromial space is entered. Blunt self-retaining retractors may be helpful to hold the fibers of the deltoid apart, but care should be taken to avoid excess pressure and deltoid necrosis. Further bursectomy may be necessary to visualize the tear. Appropriate rotation of the arm is the key to positioning the cuff tear underneath the deltoid split. By varying the position of the arm, different portions of the cuff can be brought into view. If the tear is large and traction sutures had not already been placed, they can be placed to help mobilize the cuff and allow easier repair. Multiple large traction sutures can be placed through the cuff using simple stitches (Fig. 4.4). Traction sutures allow the cuff to be manipulated for releases, further suture placement, and to relieve tension while tying the definitive suture.

Extraarticular adhesions are released, allowing the cuff to be fully mobilized. The goal of release is to gain enough mobility to allow a tension-free repair with the arm at the side. Intraarticular adhesions deep to the cuff as well as the

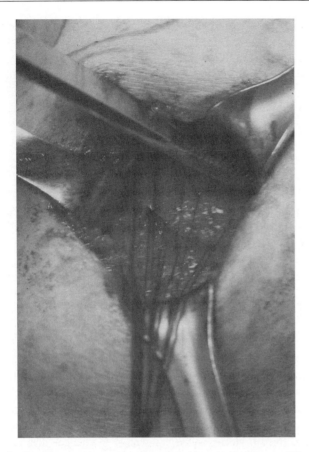

Fig. 4.4 Traction sutures have been placed into the tendon to mobilize it. Traction on the tendon allows for easier releases and better tendon excursion. The goal is to repair the tendon to bone with no tension while the arm is at the side

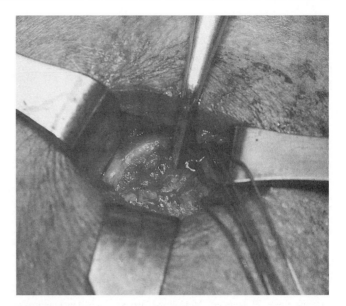

Fig. 4.5 Preparation of the greater tuberosity has been accomplished by debriding away soft tissue. Here an awl is used to create a tunnel for transosseous suture placement

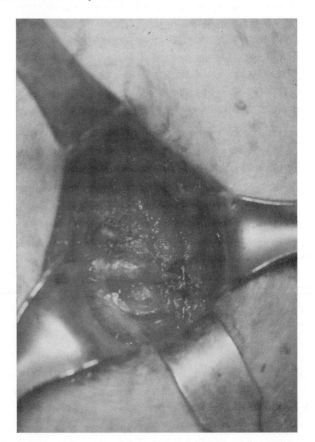

Fig. 4.6 The cuff is repaired with transosseous sutures securely down to bone

coracohumeral ligament may need to be addressed, and they can be transected as necessary. Once adequate mobilization is obtained, the size and shape of the tear is again evaluated. U-shaped tears can be repaired with a combination of side-to-side sutures and bone fixation while crescent-shaped tears are generally repaired directly to bone. Once side-to-side sutures are placed, a smaller cuff edge will be left for attachment to bone. Attention is then turned to the greater tuberosity (Fig. 4.5). The tuberosity is cleared of soft tissue, but decortication is not necessary. This is supported by the work of St. Pierre,[23] which showed in a goat model that tendon could be repaired to either cortical or cancellous bone with equal strength and equivalent histological evidence of healing.

Bony fixation can be accomplished either through transosseous tunnels or suture anchors. Bone tunnels or suture anchors are placed in the anatomic insertion or "footprint" of the cuff, and their position is chosen to allow an even repair of the tendon edge without bunching or excessive tension on one portion of the cuff. If using suture anchors, double-row fixation may be considered to better reapproximate the anatomic insertion of the cuff and to provide a stronger repair.[24,25] For cuff stitches, a grasping stitch such as a modified Mason-Allen has higher pullout strength when compared

with simple or horizontal mattress sutures.[26] Generally, braided #2 nonabsorbable sutures are used for repair. Once the anchors or drill holes have been placed and the cuff sutured, the free suture ends are sequentially tied (Fig. 4.6).

The previously placed traction sutures can be used to hold the cuff in place, without tension, and removed after tying is complete. Once the cuff has been repaired, the shoulder is taken through a range of motion to demonstrate the safe range for rehabilitation.

The wound is thoroughly irrigated and the deltoid fascia is meticulously repaired. A subcutaneous and subcuticular closure is performed and dressings are applied.

Postoperative Protocol

The patient is discharged from the hospital on the day of surgery. The patient is placed in a sling and is allowed out of the sling only for physical therapy exercises. Passive range-of-motion exercises are begun within the safe range documented at the time of surgery, including forward elevation, external rotation, and pendulum exercises. Internal rotation is not allowed until the cuff has healed. Elbow and hand exercises are also begun. The patient performs pendulum, elbow, and wrist exercises at home several times a day, while passive motion exercises are performed either at home or formally with physical therapy several times a week. The goal of early rehabilitation is to minimize stiffness without putting tension on the cuff repair. At 6 weeks postoperatively, the sling is discontinued and active-assisted range-of-motion exercises are added. Strengthening exercises are begun at 8–12 weeks postoperatively, depending on the size of the tear. A strengthening and stretching program is continued until 1 year postoperatively.

Results

Historically, good results have been reported after formal open repair of rotator cuff tears.[5–8,12] Similarly, the reported results of mini-open rotator cuff repairs have been excellent in multiple series. An early report from Levy et al. in 1990 demonstrated excellent or good results in 80% of patients and a satisfaction rate of 96%.[19] In the same year, Paulos et al. reviewed a series of 18 patients and reported 88% good or excellent outcomes and minimal complications.[27] Later reports from multiple authors revealed similar good results with this technique.[28–31] More recently, Park et al. reported on a series of 110 small or medium-sized rotator cuff repairs performed with an arthroscopically assisted mini-open technique. Excellent or satisfactory results were reported in 96% of patients at 3-year follow-up. They attributed the majority of their poor results (of which there were only four) to failure to address acromioclavicular joint pathology at the time of cuff repair.[32] Hersch et al. published a series of 22 mini-open repairs in patients with moderate- to large-sized tears. These

patients were followed an average of 40 months and demonstrated improvement in the Constant, UCLA, and ASES scores, with a high satisfaction rate of 86%.[33] The report by Shinners et al. in 2002 also demonstrated good results in a larger cohort of 41 patients at 3-year follow-up.[34]

Longer follow-up has confirmed the durability of this procedure. Posada et al. examined a cohort of patients at both 2 and 5 years after mini-open repair. Equivalent clinical outcome scores were reported at both follow-ups, demonstrating that the benefit of the procedure does not deteriorate with time.[35] A similar study examining patients at 2- and 7-year follow-up demonstrated good-to-excellent results in 74% of patients at 2 years and 84% at 7 years. Again, good results were maintained or improved with time.[36]

Several studies have compared formal open with mini-open repairs. In general, results have been comparable between the two procedures. In 1995, Baker reported on 37 shoulders, comparing 20 open repairs with 17 done through a mini-open incision. The two groups were comparable in terms of size of tear, and postoperative patient satisfaction was the same. Patients with repairs done through a mini-open approach spent less time in the hospital and they returned to work earlier.[37] Other studies have shown similar results between open and mini-open repairs.[38–40] The study by Hata et al. in 2001 showed an earlier return to activities and earlier restoration of range of motion following mini-open repair when compared with formal open repair.[39] To summarize, the published experience of mini-open rotator cuff repair demonstrates a high proportion of good to excellent results, with minimal complications in multiple small to medium series. In addition, results are comparable to open repair with earlier return of function and shorter hospital stays.

Multiple recent studies have compared the results of mini-open repair with all-arthroscopic repair of rotator cuff tears.[40–44] Ide et al. compared two groups of 50 patients who underwent either mini-open or all-arthroscopic repair. The two groups were similar in terms of the size of the cuff tear, and the outcomes as measured by the UCLA score were equivalent. Verma et al. and Youm et al. both published similar series showing the same result: equivalence of mini-open and all-arthroscopic rotator cuff repairs.[43,44] Finally, Buess et al. compared a group of patients who had mini-open and formal open repair with a second group of patients who had arthroscopic repair. The groups had similar outcomes, but the results of this study are difficult to extrapolate to mini-open repairs as both mini-open and formal open repairs were combined into one group.[41] All of these studies demonstrate methodological problems and to date no randomized controlled trial has compared outcomes for these two surgical procedures. A large multicenter randomized controlled trial is currently underway in Canada to compare mini-open with arthroscopic rotator cuff repair in small to moderate-sized tears.[45] Based on their power analysis, a total of 250 patients will be enrolled in order to detect a clinically significant difference between the two groups. This trial represents the first attempt to definitely compare the results of these two procedures.

Summary

Mini-open rotator cuff repair is a very successful procedure with multiple published studies demonstrating a high proportion of good-to-excellent results using well-validated outcomes measures. The technique is less technically demanding than all-arthroscopic repair while still retaining the advantages of arthroscopic repair. These include the ability to perform diagnostic arthroscopy, preservation of the deltoid origin, faster hospital discharge, less postoperative pain, and subsequent accelerated rehabilitation. Mini-open repair seems to be approximately equivalent to all-arthroscopic repair in multiple nonrandomized comparative studies, and a randomized trial is underway to formally address this question. Mini-open repair remains a viable option for the surgeon who wishes to use classic surgical suture passing and tying while also taking advantage of arthroscopic examination and treatment of the shoulder joint. Although there is a current trend toward using arthroscopic repair, there is no published evidence that definitively demonstrates its superiority over the mini-open procedure. The mini-open approach should remain a useful tool for rotator cuff repair for the foreseeable future.

References

1. Matsen FA, Arntz CT. Rotator cuff tendon failure. In: Rockwood CA, Matsen FA, eds. *The Shoulder*. Philadelphia: Harcourt Brace Jovanovich, Inc. 1990:647–665
2. Yamaguchi K, Middleton WD, Hildebolt CF et al. The demographic and morphological features of rotator cuff disease. A comparison of asymptomatic and symptomatic shoulders. J Bone Joint Surg 2006;88:1699–1704
3. Neer CS II. Anterior acromioplasty for the chronic impingement syndrome in the shoulder: a preliminary report. J Bone Joint Surg Am 1972;53:41–50
4. Codman EA. Complete rupture of the supraspinatous tendon: operative treatment with report of two successful cases. Boston Med Surg J 1911;164:708–710
5. Packer NP, Calvert PT, Bayley JIL et al. Operative treatment of chronic ruptures of the rotator cuff of the shoulder. J Bone Joint Surg Br 1983;65(B):171–175
6. Hawkins RJ, Misamore GW, Hobelka PE. Surgery for full thickness rotator cuff tears. J Bone Joint Surg Am 1985;67:1349–1355
7. Neer CS II, Flatow EL, Lech O. Tears of the rotator cuff. Long term results of anterior acromioplasty and repair. Orthop Trans 1988;12:735
8. Ellman H, Hanker G, Bayer M. Repair of the rotator cuff. End-result study of factors influencing reconstruction. J Bone Joint Surg Am 1986;68:1136–1144

9. Ellman H, Kay SP. Arthroscopic subacromial decompression for chronic impingement. Two to five year results. J Bone Joint Surg Br 1991;73:395–398
10. Gazielly DF, Gleyze P, Montagnon C. Functional and anatomical results of rotator cuff repair. Clin Orthop Relat Res 1994;304:43–53
11. Gupta R, Leggin BG, Iannotti JP. Results of surgical repair of full thickness tears of the rotator cuff. Orthop Clin North Am 1997;28:241–248
12. Bigliani L, Cordasco F, McIlveen S et al. Operative treatment of massive rotator cuff tears: long-term results. J Shoulder Elbow Surg 1992;1:120–130
13. Burman MS. Arthroscopy or the direct visualization of joints: an experimental cadaver study. J Bone Joint Surg Am 1931;13:669–695
14. Wantanabe M. Arthroscopy of the shoulder joint. In: Wantanabe M, ed. *Arthroscopy of Small Joints*. Tokyo: Igaku-Shoin;1985:45–46
15. Wiley AM, Older MB. Shoulder arthroscopy: investigations with a fibro-optic instrument. Am J Sports Med 1980;8:18
16. Yamaguchi K. Complications of rotator cuff repair. Tech Orthop 1997;12:33–41
17. Mansat P, Cofield RH, Kersten TE et al. Complications of rotator cuff repair. Orthop Clin North Am 1997;28:205–213
18. Karas EH, Iannotti JP. Failed repair of the rotator cuff: evaluation and treatment of complications. Instr Course Lect 1998;47:87–95
19. Levy HJ, Uribe JW, Delaney LG. Arthroscopic assisted rotator cuff repair: preliminary results. Arthroscopy 1990;6:55–60
20. Gartsman GM, Taverna E. The incidence of glenohumeral joint abnormalities associated with full thickness, repairable rotator cuff tears. Arthroscopy 1997;13:450–455
21. Miller C, Savoie FH. Glenohumeral abnormalities associated with full-thickness tears of the rotator cuff. Orthop Rev 1994;23:159–162
22. Gardner MJ, Griffith MH, Dines JS et al. The extended anterolateral acromial approach allows minimally invasive access to the proximal humerus. Clin Orthop Relat Res 2005;434:123–129
23. St. Pierre P, Olson EJ, Elliott JJ et al. Tendon healing to cortical bone compared with healing to cancellous trough. A biochemical and histological evaluation in goats. J Bone Joint Surg 1995;77:1858–1866
24. Ma CB, Comerford L, Wilson J et al. Biomechanical evaluation of arthroscopic rotator cuff repairs: double-row compared with single-row fixation. J Bone Joint Surg Am 2006;88(2):403–410
25. Fealy S, Kingham TP, Altchek DW. Mini-open RTC repair using a two-row fixation technique: outcomes analysis in patients with small, moderate, and large rotator cuff tears. Arthroscopy 2002;18:665–670
26. Bungaro P, Rotini R, Traina F et al. Comparative and experimental study on different tendinous grasping techniques in rotator cuff repair: a new reinforced stitch. Chir Organi Mov 2005;90(2):113–119
27. Paulos LE, Kody MH. Arthroscopically enhanced "miniapproach" to rotator cuff repair: preliminary results. Arthroscopy 1990;6:55–60
28. Liu SH. Arthroscopically assisted rotator cuff repair. J Bone Joint Surg Br 1994;76:592–595
29. Blevins FT, Warren RF, Cavo C, Altchek DW, Dines D, Palletta G, Wickiewicz TL. Arthroscopic assisted rotator cuff repair: results using a mini-open deltoid splitting approach. Arthroscopy 1996;12:50–59
30. Werner JJ, Goitz RJ, Irrgang JJ et al. Arthroscopic-assisted rotator cuff repair: patient selection and treatment outcome. J Shoulder Elbow Surg 1997;6:463–472
31. Pollock RG, Flatow EL. The rotator cuff: full-thickness tears: mini-open repair. Orthop Clin North Am 1997;28:169–177
32. Park JY, Levine WN, Marra G et al. Portal-extension approach for the repair of small and medium rotator cuff tears. Am J Sports Med 2000;28:312–316

33. Hersch JC, Sgaglione NA. Arthroscopically assisted mini-open rotator cuff repairs: functional outcome at two- to seven-year follow-up. Am J Sports Med 2000;28:301–311
34. Shinners TJ, Noordsij PG, Orwin JF. Arthroscopically assisted mini-open rotator cuff repair. Arthroscopy 2002;18:21–26
35. Posada A, Uribe JW, Hechtman KS et al. Mini-deltoid splitting rotator cuff repair. Do results deteriorate with time? Arthroscopy 2000;16:137–141
36. Zandi H, Coghlan JA, Bell SN. Mini-incision rotator cuff repair: a longitudinal assessment with no deterioration of result up to 9 years. J Shoulder Elbow Surg 2006;15:135–139
37. Baker CL, Liu SH. Comparison of open and arthroscopically assisted rotator cuff repairs. Am J Sports Med 1995;23:99–104
38. Weber SC, Schaefer R. "Mini-open" versus traditional open repair in the management of small and moderate size tears of the rotator cuff. Arthroscopy 1993;9:365–366
39. Hata Y, Saitoh S, Murakami N et al. A less invasive surgery for rotator cuff tear: mini-open repair. J Shoulder Elbow Surg 2001;10:11–16
40. Ide J, Maeda S, Takagi K. A comparison of arthroscopic and open rotator cuff repair. Arthroscopy 2005;21:1090–1098
41. Buess E, Steuber K, Waibl B. Open versus arthroscopic rotator cuff repair: a comparative view of 96 cases. Arthroscopy 2005;21:597–604
42. Sauerbrey AM, Getz CL, Piancastelli M et al. Arthroscopic versus mini-open rotator cuff repair: a comparison of clinical outcome. Arthroscopy 2005;21:1415–1420
43. Verma NN, Dunn W, Adler RS et al. All-arthroscopic versus mini-open rotator cuff repair: a retrospective review with minimum 2-year follow-up. Arthroscopy 2006;22:587–594
44. Youm T, Murray DH, Kubiak EN et al. Arthroscopic versus mini-open rotator cuff repair: a comparison of clinical outcomes and patient satisfaction. J Shoulder Elbow Surg 2005;14:455–459
45. Macdermid JC, Holtby R, Razmjou H et al. All-arthroscopic versus mini-open repair of small or moderate-sized rotator cuff tears: a protocol for a randomized trial. BMC Musculoskelet Disord 2006;7:11

Chapter 5
Minimally Invasive Treatment of Greater Tuberosity Fractures

Brian Magovern, Xavier Duralde, and Guido Marra

The proximal humerus tends to fracture into four distinct fragments: the humeral shaft, the greater and lesser tuberosities, and the articular surface.[1] Neer based his classification system on displacement of these fragments by greater than 1 cm or angulation of more than 45°. In a retrospective review, Neer found that 85% of fractures were considered to be minimally displaced and nonoperative management led to satisfactory results. Displaced two-part greater tuberosity fractures, according to the above criteria, were treated with open reduction and internal fixation.[1,2]

Several authors, however, have advocated treatment that is more aggressive for fractures of the greater tuberosity. Five millimeters of displacement, particularly in the superior direction, has been suggested as an indication for operative management.[3–5] The major deforming forces on the greater tuberosity are the supraspinatus, infraspinatus, and teres minor, resulting in superior and/or posterior pull of the fragment. Malunion with superior displacement may lead to painful impingement and posterior displacement may result in loss of external rotation, which can be challenging to treat.[6–8]

Minimally invasive techniques have become increasingly popular in the field of orthopedic surgery. Examples include two-incision total hip arthroplasty[9] and minimally invasive lumbar disc excision.[10] A great deal of recent research has focused on minimally invasive fracture care such as submuscular plating of long bone fractures.[11–15] When compared with conventional methods, the limited soft tissue and periosteal disruption with less invasive techniques may increase healing rates, speed recovery, and improve cosmesis. While a deltopectoral approach is most often utilized for open reduction of more complex proximal humerus fractures, several less invasive methods have been described for treatment of isolated greater tuberosity fractures. These include arthroscopic treatment,[16–21] percutaneous pinning,[22] and open reduction through a superior deltoid-splitting approach,[5,7,23,24] which will be discussed below.

B. Magovern, X. Duralde, and G. Marra (✉)
Section of Shoulder and Elbow Surgery, Loyola University
Medical Center, 2160 South First Street, Maywood, IL, USA
e-mail: gmarra@lumc.edu

Preoperative Planning/Imaging

Isolated fractures of the greater tuberosity are relatively uncommon[7] and they are frequently overlooked.[25] Up to 15% occur in association with glenohumeral dislocation[19] (Fig. 5.1) and a careful neurovascular exam is essential in the preoperative evaluation. Many patients who sustain proximal humerus fractures are elderly and have significant medical comorbidities. A proper medical evaluation should be considered as part of the standard preoperative plan.

A complete series of radiographs including anteroposterior (AP), outlet, and axillary views should be obtained (Figs. 5.2–5.4). If the patient is unable to tolerate positioning for an axillary view, a Velpeau radiograph may substitute. Rotational AP views may add additional information in determining displacement.[26] Numerous studies have documented poor interobserver and intraobserver reliability in the classification of proximal humerus fractures,[27–29] and identifying the degree of displacement of greater tuberosity fractures can be challenging. Posterior displacement of the greater tuberosity may be masked by the humeral head on the AP view and is best visualized on the axillary view.[30] Superior displacement of the greater tuberosity, on the other hand, is best appreciated on the AP view in external rotation.[26] A recent cadaveric study found significant agreement in regard to treatment recommendations of fractures of the greater tuberosity after review of a series of four standard radiographs (AP in internal and external rotation, outlet, and axillary views).[26]

The use of computed tomography (CT) may increase the reliability of fracture classification and help to determine optimal management (Fig. 5.5).[29] Other authors, however, have found CT to offer little in the evaluation and treatment of greater tuberosity fractures.[31] In all cases, high-quality radiographs must be obtained and scrutinized prior to making decisions regarding further imaging and subsequent treatment. With minimally invasive techniques of fixation, direct visualization of the reduction may be limited, and intraoperative fluoroscopy should be considered to confirm anatomic reduction.

G.R. Scuderi and A.J. Tria (eds.), *Minimally Invasive Surgery in Orthopedics*,
DOI 10.1007/978-0-387-76608-9_5, © Springer Science+Business Media, LLC 2010

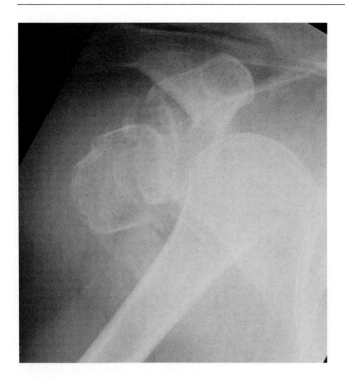

Fig. 5.1 Glenohumeral dislocation with a greater tuberosity fracture

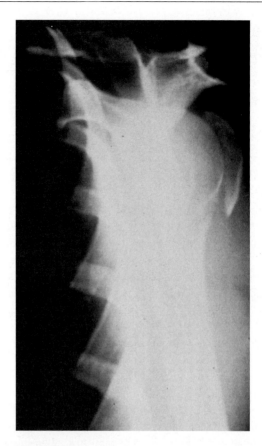

Fig. 5.3 Outlet view

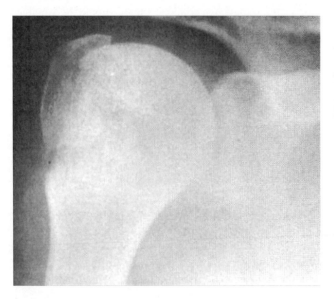

Fig. 5.2 AP view, note superior displacement

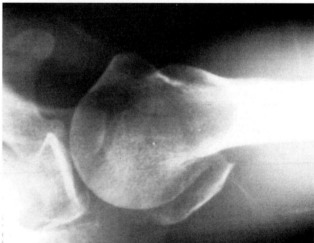

Fig. 5.4 Axillary view, note posterior displacement

Operative Treatment of Displaced Greater Tuberosity Fractures

Arthroscopic Repair of Greater Tuberosity Fractures

Shoulder arthroscopy affords excellent visualization of the glenohumeral joint and subacromial space with less morbidity than conventional open techniques. Arthroscopy has become widely accepted as a valuable and viable option in the management of a broad spectrum of shoulder pathology.[32–34] Similar to reports of arthroscopic treatment of distal radius and tibial plateau fractures,[35,36] shoulder arthroscopy may assist in the evaluation and management of fractures of the shoulder region.[16–21,37–39] Schai et al. performed diagnostic arthroscopy on 80 patients with shoulder girdle fractures. The authors identified a large percentage of secondary soft

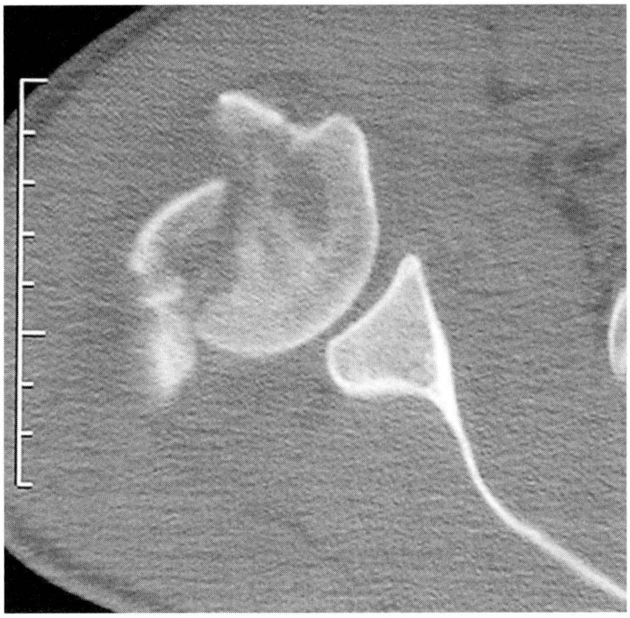

Fig. 5.5 CT scan of a greater tuberosity fracture

tissue lesions, such as labral tears, which may not have been visualized with conventional radiographic techniques.[37] Carro et al. reported an excellent outcome in a patient with a glenoid rim fracture treated with percutaneous pinning under arthroscopic visualization.[38] Kim et al. performed arthroscopy on 23 patients who had persistent pain 6 months after sustaining minimally displaced fractures of the greater tuberosity. Partial-thickness rotator cuff tears were found in all patients.[39]

Arthroscopic fixation of greater tuberosity fractures was first reported by Geissler et al. in 1994.[16] Since then, reports of arthroscopic treatment of greater tuberosity fractures have become more frequent.[18–20,21] Patients considered for this procedure must have adequate bone stock and a noncomminuted fragment that will support fixation with two or three screws.

Bonsell et al. reported four major advantages of arthroscopic treatment over traditional open reduction and internal fixation (ORIF).[19] First, arthroscopic evaluation allows the surgeon visual access to other pathology in the joint, namely Bankart lesions and articular cartilage defects. Second, evacuation of the hematoma and debridement of the fracture site is facilitated with arthroscopic instruments. Third, the magnification under arthroscopic visualization allows for a more anatomic reduction of the tuberosity fragment. Lastly, there is no dissection of the deltoid muscle, theoretically decreasing the risk of axillary nerve injury and hastening postoperative recovery of deltoid function. The procedure has been reported in both the beachchair[18,20] and lateral decubitus positions.[19,21] The technique as described by Taverna et al. is outlined below.[20]

Technique

The initial posterior viewing portal is made slightly more superior and lateral than that used classically (0.5 cm medial and 0.5 cm inferior to the posterolateral edge of the acromion). An anterior portal is created and a diagnostic evaluation of the glenohumeral joint is performed. Repair of any identified labral injuries, or other soft tissue pathology, is carried out at this time. The subacromial space is now examined and a lateral portal is created with spinal needle localization. Once the fracture has been identified and remaining hematoma has been thoroughly evacuated, the fracture bed is debrided of all fibrous tissue with a shaver and the surface is abraded with an arthroscopic burr. A blunt trocar placed through the lateral portal is used to reduce the fracture by pushing the tuberosity fragment anteriorly and inferiorly. Alternatively, a grasper placed from the anterior portal can be used to pull the cuff tendon attached to the fracture fragment in order to reduce the fracture into an anatomic position. Once reduction is obtained and confirmed fluoroscopically, two Kirschner wires are introduced percutaneously under arthroscopic guidance until they reach subchondral bone. Cannulated screws with or without a washer are then placed over the guide wires and advanced until compression across the fracture site is obtained. Again, fluoroscopy is used to evaluate the quality of the reduction. The diameter of the screws varies from 3.5 to 7.0 mm in different reports. Arthroscopic visualization confirms that the screws have not penetrated the articular surface. Wounds are closed in standard fashion.

Results

Geissler et al. performed arthroscopic fixation in 14 patients with greater tuberosity fractures.[16] Neer scores averaged 92 out of 100 at an average of 14 months postoperatively. Of note, 93% of patients had secondary soft tissue lesions identified during arthroscopy. Gartsman et al. reported on the arthroscopic treatment of an acute traumatic anterior glenohumeral dislocation with an associated greater tuberosity fracture.[18] Intraoperatively, the author performed a Bankart repair followed by fixation of the greater tuberosity fracture with one 7.0-mm cannulated screw. At the 2-year follow-up, the patient had regained full range of motion and strength, had no pain, and had radiographic evidence of fracture union. Bonsell and Buford described arthroscopic reduction and fixation of a greater tuberosity fracture in the lateral decubitus position using two 4.5-mm cannulated screws.[19] The authors noted that one advantage of the lateral decubitus position was that placement of the arm in abduction reduced the fracture to near anatomic position. The patient began pendulum exercises in the immediate postoperative period and by 2 months had complete range of motion and no limitations in his activities. The entire procedure was performed without entering the subacromial space. Taverna et al. reported that they have treated patients with this technique since 1997 and have had "remarkable clinical results."[19]

Although no controlled studies exist, these results are promising. Arthroscopic assistance and fixation of greater tuberosity fractures may decrease the morbidity associated with open techniques leading to a faster recovery, decreased pain, and improved cosmesis. Arthroscopy also allows the simultaneous management of associated pathology. The procedure, however, can be technically demanding with a steep learning curve, and not all greater tuberosity fractures are amenable to arthroscopic fixation. An anatomic reduction should not be sacrificed in order to perform a less invasive technique. The procedure must be converted to an open reduction if the fracture cannot be reduced anatomically by arthroscopic means.[18–21]

Percutaneous Fixation

Closed reduction and percutaneous pinning of proximal humerus fractures is a reliable means for stable fixation in certain patients.[22,23,40] Although it is less rigid biomechanically than plate and screw constructs,[41] percutaneous pinning may be used in patients with good bone quality and noncomminuted fracture fragments.[23] It is essential that an acceptable reduction can be obtained by closed means. Percutaneous methods of fixation posses a major advantage over open reduction and internal fixation in that there is essentially no soft tissue dissection and minimal risk of iatrogenic avascular necrosis.

Percutaneous fixation of isolated greater tuberosity fractures has rarely been reported. Chen et al. treated 19 patients with proximal humerus fractures percutaneously.[22] Two patients had isolated greater tuberosity fractures treated with a combination of percutaneous pins and screws. Both patients had excellent outcomes according to the criteria of Neer at an average of 28 months postoperatively.[22] Achieving reduction of a displaced greater tuberosity may be challenging via percutaneous methods secondary to the deforming forces contributed by the rotator cuff. If a closed reduction cannot be obtained and an open reduction is necessary, pins may be used for fixation once reduction is achieved. The pins are then placed in a manner similar to that used for more complex proximal humerus fractures.

Superior Deltoid-Splitting Approach

For the majority of displaced proximal humerus fractures, a deltopectoral approach provides the best access for open reduction. Fractures of the greater tuberosity are unique in

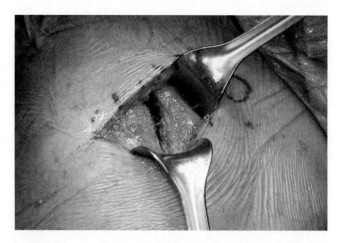

Fig. 5.6 Superior deltoid-splitting approach

that exposure may be gained by a superior deltoid-splitting approach (Fig. 5.6). In fact, this limited incision and dissection yields better visualization and allows improved manipulation and fixation of the fracture than a deltopectoral incision.[7] A lateral exposure may also decrease the risk of avascular necrosis, as there is less dissection near the bicipital groove.[42] In complex proximal humerus fractures, a two-incision technique has been proposed that uses the lateral approach for reduction of the tuberosity and a second deltopectoral approach for the remaining fragments.[43]

Surgical Approach

A 4- to 5-cm incision is made in Langer's lines off the lateral border of the acromion.[7,24] The superficial fat is bluntly dissected from the deltoid fascia. A longitudinal split is made in the deltoid fascia in line with the muscle fibers at the anterolateral border of the acromion. Alternatively, the split may be made more posteriorly depending on the size and degree of displacement of the greater tuberosity fragment. The biggest risk of this exposure is damage to branches of the axillary nerve, which have been reported to lie 3–5 cm distal to the anterolateral acromion.[44,45] A stay suture may be placed at the inferior extent of the deltoid in an effort to protect the nerve if preferred. Great care is taken not to disrupt the deltoid origin from the acromion. If necessary, this approach may be extended by axillary nerve dissection distally.[46]

Several grasping sutures are placed in the tuberosity fragment or adjacent cuff tissue to allow safe manipulation of the fragment (Fig. 5.7). Once the fragment is mobilized and reduced, several options exist for fixation, depending on bone quality, degree of comminution, and size of the fragment. These include screws,[47,48] wires, and sutures.[7] Stable anatomic fixation of displaced greater tuberosity fractures is challenged by the deforming forces of the intact rotator cuff

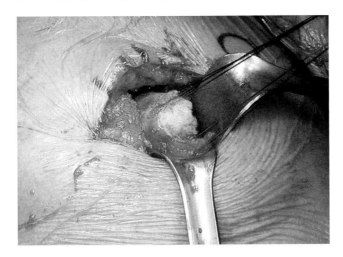

Fig. 5.7 Grasping sutures are used to manipulate the fracture fragment

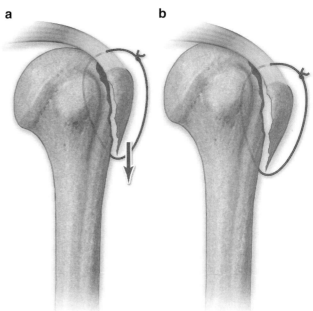

Fig. 5.8 (**a**, **b**) Overreduction of the fracture fragment

and the poor bone quality of the tuberosity.[49] In older patients, the tuberosities may consist of little more than an eggshell of cortical bone with very small amounts of cancellous bone inside and are often inadequate for screw fixation.[49,50] The strongest structure in the area may be the rotator cuff tendon itself and stable fixation requires utilization of the rotator cuff.[7,24]

Fixation with heavy nonabsorbable suture has been reported with excellent results.[7,24] The sutures are placed through multiple drill holes through bone adjacent to the fracture bed. In the section below, a two-layered suture repair utilizing suture anchors and cerclage sutures is described.

Suture Anchor Technique

Traditional techniques for repair of displaced two-part greater tuberosity fractures advocate a suture technique similar to rotator cuff repair utilizing cerclage braided nonabsorbable sutures. This technique runs the risk of over reduction of the greater tuberosity as tightening of the sutures will advance the greater tuberosity distally until the inferior edge of the greater tuberosity fragment comes into contact with the drill hole placed distally at the humeral shaft (Figs. 5.8 and 5.9). This displacement will be even greater if comminution is encountered in the tuberosity fragment allowing greater displacement of the tuberosity inferiorly and nonanatomic reduction of the rotator cuff relative to the humeral head.

This technique has been utilized in rotator cuff repair to obtain greater contact between the cuff tissue and tuberosity and this slight modification in fracture management allows anatomically precise replacement of the tendon relative to the humeral head along with excellent compression of the tuberosity fragment to obtain adequate bony healing.[24]

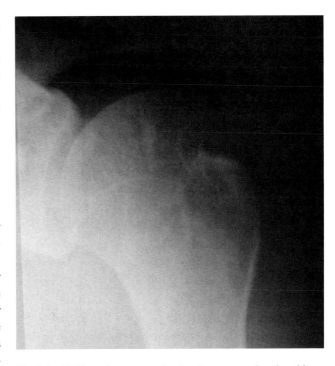

Fig. 5.9 AP X-ray demonstrates healing in an over reduced position

The superior deltoid-splitting approach is utilized to expose the displaced greater tuberosity fracture and may or may not be combined with acromioplasty depending on acromial morphology and concomitant rotator cuff disease. The greater tuberosity and rotator cuff are identified and traction sutures utilizing size 0 braided nonabsorbable sutures are placed at the margin of the rotator cuff at the junction with the greater tuberosity. The tuberosity fragment is assessed and debrided of fracture hematoma. No bone is debrided. The bed for the greater tuberosity is similarly prepared. A row of suture anchors is then placed at the junction between the bony bed of the greater tuberosity on the humerus and the articular margin (Fig. 5.10). These are placed at 45° or the "dead man's angle" into the humeral head. The sutures through the suture anchors are then passed through the rotator cuff tendons directly at the bone-tendon interface on the greater tuberosity fragment (Fig. 5.11).

A row of drill holes is then placed approximately 1 cm distal to the osseous defect on the humeral shaft. Braided nonabsorbable sutures (size 5) are then passed through these drill holes in the distal humeral shaft and through the bony bed. These sutures are then passed in a cerclage fashion through the rotator cuff tendon again at the junction of the bone-tendon interface. The suture anchor sutures are tied first, ensuring anatomic repositioning of the rotator cuff relative to the humeral head. If a significant bony defect is noted, morselized cancellous bone graft with demineralized bone matrix can be inserted into the greater tuberosity bed. The cerclage sutures are then tied over the greater tuberosity fragment to close this fragment as a book and create compression across the fragment (Figs. 5.12–5.14). Tying of the suture anchor sutures first ensures that over reduction of the greater tuberosity cannot occur. Secure closure of the deltoid is then performed using size 0 nonabsorbable braided sutures. Suction drainage is utilized if significant bleeding is noted.

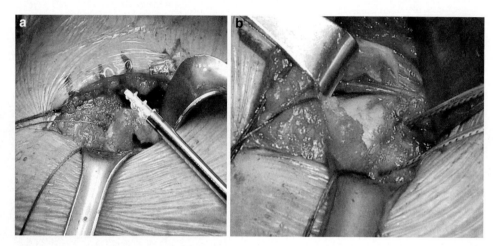

Fig. 5.10 (**a**) Suture anchor. (**b**) Placement of anchors at the articular margin

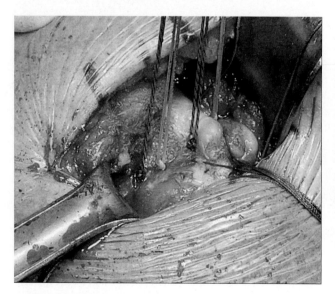

Fig. 5.11 Sutures from the anchors are placed through rotator cuff tendon and tied down

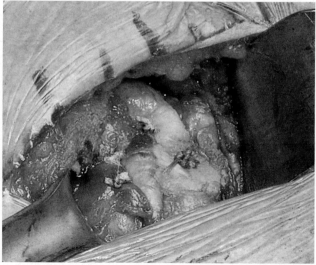

Fig. 5.12 Cerclage sutures are passed around the fragment and tied down to obtain compression across the fracture

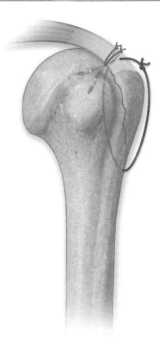

Fig. 5.13 Diagram demonstrates suture construct

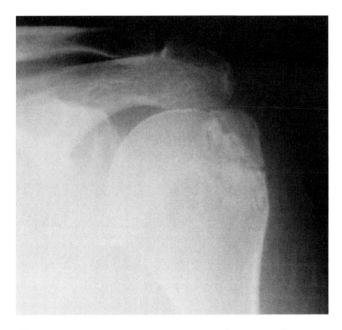

Fig. 5.14 Reduction of the tuberosity fracture in an anatomic position

Results

Few reports are dedicated solely to the management of isolated greater tuberosity fractures. Many studies group the treatment and outcomes of isolated tuberosity fractures along with more complex three- and four-part proximal humerus fractures, sometimes making outcomes difficult to discern from the literature. Flatow et al. treated 12 patients with greater tuberosity fractures using a superior deltoid-splitting approach and heavy nonabsorbable suture fixation.[7] Outcomes were excellent in all 12 of the patients at an average of 5-year follow-up. All fractures healed radiographically without loss of reduction. Active elevation and external rotation averaged 170° and 63°, respectively. Patients were able to reach behind their back, on average, to the ninth thoracic vertebra. Park et al. obtained 89% good to excellent results in a series of 27 patients with two- and three-part proximal humerus fractures treated in a manner similar to Flatow's series.[24] Although the authors did not separately list the outcomes of the two-part greater tuberosity group, they noted that there was no significant difference between different fracture types. Chun et al. reported the outcome of 137 patients with proximal humerus fractures.[48] Twenty-four patients had greater tuberosity fractures, of which, ten were treated with open reduction and internal fixation. Eight of these were treated with screw fixation. Although 8 of 11 patients had a satisfactory result, the authors did not evaluate the patients separately based on whether they received conservative or operative treatment.

Postoperative Management

Patients are placed in a sling postoperatively. Passive range of motion is instituted on postoperative day one within safe limits determined intraoperatively. These passive exercises are performed for the first 6 weeks, at which time patients are advanced to active-assisted exercises. Resistive exercises are added at approximately 10–12 weeks once bony healing has been obtained radiographically. Rehabilitation may need to be altered in the presence of other soft tissue lesions.

Complications

Complications specific to operative treatment of greater tuberosity fractures are infrequently reported in the literature. As with any surgery, infection, bleeding, and anesthetic-related complications can occur. One patient in Flatow's series sustained an axillary nerve palsy postoperatively.[7] It had completely resolved by 9 months and the patient had a good result. One patient in Park's series required arthroscopic lysis of adhesions 6 months postoperatively for adhesive capsulitis and ultimately ended up with an unsatisfactory result.[24] Obtaining an anatomic reduction and protecting the axillary nerve are two important ways to avoid complications and achieve optimal results.

Summary

Displaced fractures of the greater tuberosity may result in significant disability if not evaluated and treated appropriately. Even with modern imaging techniques, proper identification and classification of fractures can be challenging. The indication for operative repair of greater tuberosity fractures has been more aggressive than it has with other fractures of the proximal humerus. With the increased popularity of minimally invasive surgery, techniques that limit soft tissue dissection and potentially hasten recovery are becoming more attractive. Fractures of the greater tuberosity are unique in that several less invasive methods of fixation are available.

Arthroscopic and arthroscopic-assisted fixation techniques are being reported more frequently with promising clinical results. If a satisfactory reduction cannot be achieved, the procedure must be converted to an open reduction. Closed reduction and percutaneous pinning is an option, although rarely used for isolated greater tuberosity fractures. If open reduction is preferred, a superior deltoid-splitting approach offers excellent exposure and is less invasive than the deltopectoral approach used for most proximal humerus fractures. Several options for internal fixation exist, including screws and heavy sutures. Patient factors, such as poor bone stock or fracture fragmentation, may preclude the use of screw fixation. In these cases, the rotator cuff tendon is the strongest structure available for repair. Excellent clinical results have been obtained with suture fixation through bone tunnels that incorporates the rotator cuff tendon. A two-layered suture technique using suture anchors, as outlined above, allows anatomic placement and secure compressive fixation of the tendon and tuberosity fragment on the humeral head. The goal of the above techniques, identical to more traditional approaches, is stable internal fixation to allow early motion.

References

1. Neer CS II. Displaced Proximal Humeral Fractures. Part I. Classification and Evaluation. *J Bone Joint Surg* 1970;52-A:1077–1089
2. Neer CS II. Displaced Proximal Humeral Fractures. Part II. Treatment of Three-Part and Four-Part Displacement. *J Bone Joint Surg* 1970;52-A:1090–1103
3. McLaughlin HL. Dislocation of the Shoulder with Tuberosity Fracture. *Surg Clin North Am* 1963;43:1615–1620
4. Levy AS. Greater Tuberosity Fractures of the Humerus. *Orthop Trans* 1998;22:594
5. Green A, Izzi J. Isolated Fractures of the Greater Tuberosity of the Proximal Humerus. *J Shoulder Elbow Surg* 2003;12:641–649
6. Hawkins RJ, Angelo RL. Displaced Proximal Humeral Fractures. Selecting Treatment, Avoiding Pitfalls. *Orthop Clin North Am* 1987;18:421–431
7. Flatow EL, Cuomo F, Maday MG, et al. Open Reduction and Internal Fixation of Two-Part Displaced Fractures of the Greater Tuberosity of the Proximal Part of the Humerus. *J Bone Joint Surg* 1991;73-A:1213–1218
8. Berdjiklian PK, Iannotti JP, Norris TR, et al. Operative Treatment of Malunion of a Fracture of the Proximal Aspect of the Humerus. *J Bone Joint Surg* 1998;80-A:1484–1497
9. Berger RA. Total Hip Arthroplasty Using the Minimally Invasive Two-Incision Approach. *Clin Orthop Relat Res* 2003;417:232–241
10. Yeung AT, Tsou PT. Posterolateral Endoscopic Excision for Lumbar Disc Herniation: Surgical Technique, Outcome, and Complications in 307 Consecutive Cases. *Spine* 2002;27:722–731
11. Collinge CA, Sanders RW. Percutaneous Plating in the Lower Extremity. *J Am Acad Orthop Surg* 2000;8:211–216
12. Schandelmaier P, Partenheimer A, Koenemann B, et al. Distal Femoral Fractures and LISS Stabilization. *Injury* 2001;32(S3): SC55–SC63
13. Fankhauser F, Gruber G, Schippinger G, et al. Minimal-invasive Treatment of Distal Femoral Fractures with the LISS (Less Invasive Stabilization System): A Prospective Study of 30 Fractures with a Follow up of 20 Months. *Acta Orthop Scand* 2004;75:56–60
14. Anglen J, Choi L. Treatment Options in Pediatric Femoral Shaft Fractures. *J Orthop Trauma* 2005;19:724–733
15. Boldin C, Fankhauser F, Hofer HP, Szyszkowitz R. Three-Year Results of Proximal Tibia Fractures Treated with the LISS. *Clin Orthop Relat Res* 2006;445:222–229
16. Geissler WB, Petrie SG, Savoie FH. Arthroscopic Fixation of Greater Tuberosity Fractures of the Humerus (Abstract). *Arthroscopy* 1994;10:344
17. Gartsman GM, Taverna E. Arthroscopic Treatment of Rotator Cuff Tear and Greater Tuberosity Fracture Nonunion. *Arthroscopy* 1996;12:242–244
18. Gartsman GM, Taverna E, Hammerman SM. Arthroscopic Treatment of Acute Traumatic Anterior Glenohumeral Dislocation and Greater Tuberosity Fracture. *Arthroscopy* 1999;15:648–650
19. Bonsell S, Buford DA. Arthroscopic Reduction and Internal Fixation of a Greater Tuberosity Fracture of the Shoulder: A Case Report. *J Shoulder Elbow Surg* 2003;12:397–400
20. Taverna E, Sansone V, Battistella F. Arthroscopic Treatment for Greater Tuberosity Fractures: Rationale and Surgical Technique. *Arthroscopy* 2004;20:e53–e57
21. Carrera EF, Matsumoto MH, Netto NA, Faloppa F. Fixation of Greater Tuberosity Fractures. *Arthroscopy* 2004;20:e109–e111
22. Chen C, Chao E, Tu Y, et al. Closed Management and Percutaneous Fixation of Unstable Proximal Humerus Fractures. *J Trauma* 1998;45:1039–1045
23. Williams GR, Wong KL. Two-part and Three-part Fractures: Open Reduction and Internal Fixation Versus Closed Reduction and Percutaneous Pinning. *Orthop Clin North Am* 2000;31:1–21
24. Park MC, Murthi AM, Roth NS, et al. Two-part and Three-part Fractures of the Proximal Humerus Treated with Suture Fixation. *J Orthop Trauma* 2003;17:319–325
25. Ogawa K, Yoshida A, Ikegami H. Isolated Fractures of the Greater Tuberosity of the Humerus: Solutions to Recognizing a Frequently Overlooked Fracture. *J Trauma* 2003;54:713–717
26. Parsons BO, Klepps SJ, Miller S, et al. Reliability and Reproducibility of Radiographs of Greater Tuberosity Displacement. *J Bone Joint Surg* 2005;87-A:58–65
27. Sidor ML, Zuckerman JD, Lyon T, et al. The Neer Classification System for Proximal Humeral Fractures. An Assessment of Interobserver Reliability and Intraobserver Reproducibility. *J Bone Joint Surg* 1993;75-A:1745–1750
28. Siebenrock KA, Gerber C. The Reproducibility of Classification of Fractures of the Proximal End of the Humerus. *J Bone Joint Surg* 1993;75-A:1751–1755
29. Bernstein J, Adler L, Blank JE, et al. Evaluation of the Neer System of Classification of Proximal Humeral Fractures with Computerized

Tomographic Scans and Plain Radiographs. *J Bone Joint Surg* 1996;78-A:1371–1375

30. Blaine TA, Bigliani LU, Levine WN. Fractures of the Proximal Humerus. In: Rockwood CA, et al (eds.) *The Shoulder*. Philadelphia: Saunders, 2004, pp. 355–412

31. Sjoden GO, Movin T, Guntner P, et al. Poor Reproducibility of Classification of Proximal Humerus Fractures. Additional CT of Minor Value. *Acta Orthop Scand* 1997;68:239–242

32. Burkhart SS, Lo IKY. Arthroscopic Rotator Cuff Repair. *J Am Acad Orthop Surg* 2006;14:333–346

33. Kim S, Ha K, Kim S. Bankart Repair in Traumatic Anterior Shoulder Instability: Open Versus Arthroscopic Technique. *Arthroscopy* 2002;18:755–763

34. Nam EK, Snyder SJ. The Diagnosis and Treatment of Superior Labrum, Anterior and Posterior (SLAP) Lesion. *Am J Sports Med* 2003;31:798–810

35. Lubowitz JH, Elson WS, Guttmann D. Part I: Arthroscopic Management of Tibial Plateau Fractures. *Arthroscopy* 2004;20:1063–1070

36. Ruch DS, Vallee J, Poehling GG, et al. Arthroscopic Reduction Versus Fluoroscopic Reduction in the Management in the Management of Intra-articular Distal Radius Fractures. *Arthroscopy* 2004;20:225–230

37. Schai PA, Hintermann B, Koris MJ. Preoperative Arthroscopic Assessment of Fractures About the Shoulder. *Arthroscopy* 1999;15:827–835

38. Carro LP, Nunez MP, Llata JIE. Arthroscopic-Assisted Reduction and Percutaneous External Fixation of a Displaced Intra-articular Glenoid Fracture. *Arthroscopy* 1999;15:211–214

39. Kim S, Ha K. Arthroscopic Treatment of Symptomatic Shoulders with Minimally Displaced Greater Tuberosity Fracture. *Arthroscopy* 2000;16:695–700

40. Jaberg H, Warner JJP, Jakob RP. Percutaneous Stabilization of Unstable Fractures of the Humerus. *J Bone Joint Surg* 1992;74-A:508–515

41. Naidu SH, Bixler B, Capo JT, et al. Percutaneous Pinning of Proximal Humerus Fractures: A Biomechanical Study. *Orthopaedics* 1997;20:1073–1076

42. Gerber C, Schneeberger AG, Vinh T. The Arterial Vascularization of the Humeral Head: An Anatomical Study. *J Bone Joint Surg* 1990;72-A:1486–1494

43. Gallo RA, Zeiders GJ, Altman GT. Two-Incision Technique for Treatment of Complex Proximal Humerus Fractures. *J Orthop Trauma* 2005;19:734–740

44. Burkhead WZ, Scheinberg RR, Box G. Surgical Anatomy of the Axillary Nerve. *J Shoulder Elbow Surg* 1992;1:31–36

45. Hoppenfeld S, de Boer P. The Shoulder, In: Hoppenfeld S, de Boer P (eds.) *Surgical Exposures in Orthopaedics: The Anatomic Approach*. Philadelphia: Lippincott, 1994, pp. 1–50

46. Gardner MJ, Griffith MH, Dines JS, et al. The Extended Anterolateral Acromial Approach Allows Minimally Invasive Access to the Proximal Humerus. *Clin Orthop Relat Res* 2005;434:123–129

47. Paavolainen P, Bjorkenheim J, Slatis P, Paukku P. Operative Treatment of Severe Proximal Humeral Fractures. *Acta Orthop Scand* 1983;54:374–379

48. Chun J, Groh GI, Rockwood CA. Two-Part Fractures of the Proximal Humerus. *J Shoulder Elbow Surg* 1994;3:273–287

49. Hawkins RJ, Kiefer GN. Internal Fixation Techniques for Proximal Humeral Fractures. *Clin Orthop Relat Res* 1987;223:77–85

50. Earwaker J. Isolated Avulsion Fracture of the Lesser Tuberosity of the Humerus. *Skeletal Radiol* 1990;19:121–125

Chapter 6
Mini-incision Fixation of Proximal Humeral Four-Part Fractures*

Jim C. Hsu and Leesa M. Galatz

Proximal humerus fractures are notoriously difficult to treat. The surrounding rotator cuff musculature makes intraoperative assessment of the reduction of fractures, especially those involving the articular surface, difficult to assess. Even fractures fixed with open reduction and internal fixation often require intraoperative fluoroscopic guidance to ensure appropriate anatomic reduction. The anatomic relationship between the articular surface and the surrounding rotator cuff has a critical influence on the final result. Furthermore, fixation is a challenge to maintain as the rotator cuff exerts strong deforming forces on the tuberosities, which are often of poor bone quality and do not hold hardware well. In spite of this, many unstable proximal humerus fractures are treated successfully with established methods of open reduction and internal fixation.

Four-part proximal humerus fractures, as classified by Neer,[1,2] are particularly problematic. Historically, they have a very high rate of avascular necrosis following fixation. Because of this, Neer recommended hemiarthroplasty for the treatment of these fractures. However, a subgroup of four-part proximal humerus fractures, the *four-part valgus-impacted fracture*, is readily amenable to reduction and fixation. Neer did not specify this fracture in his initial classification system. In the more recent AO/ASIS classification, however, the valgus-impacted humeral head fracture is regarded as a separate type of fracture.[3] The valgus-impacted four-part fracture is an ideal fracture for minimally invasive fixation, and it is the focus of this chapter.

There has been a surge of interest in minimally invasive techniques in many different subspecialty areas of orthopedics. The recent trauma literature contains several reports of percutaneous fixation of femur, tibia, and tibial pilon fractures.[4–6] Principles of preserving blood supply and minimizing soft tissue stripping are receiving increased attention in fracture fixation. With respect to the treatment of proximal humerus fractures, there have been a few reports in the past several years of successful percutaneous reduction and fixation.[7–9] In selected fractures, percutaneous pinning allows preservation of the intact soft tissue sleeve and periosteal blood supply while obtaining and maintaining a stable reduction. Other potential advantages include smaller incisions, less dissection, and less scarring. A minimally invasive approach minimizes trauma to the rotator cuff and deltoid, and with experience can decrease operative time. While still a difficult, technically demanding procedure, percutaneous pinning of valgus-impacted four-part proximal humerus fractures shows considerable potential. This chapter discusses the unique characteristics of valgus-impacted fractures and outlines in detail the minimally invasive fixation technique.

Historical Perspective

Percutaneous pinning has been used in a variety of subtypes of proximal humerus fractures (Table 6.1). Böhler[10] originally described a method of closed reduction and pinning for the treatment of epiphyseal fractures of the proximal end of the humerus in adolescents. This technique has been modified over the years and applied to treat proximal humerus fractures more commonly seen in the older population. In 1991, Jakob[11] reported on the treatment of 19 valgus-impacted four-part proximal humerus fractures, five of which were treated closed. This is the first description of elevation of the valgus-impacted articular fragment with minimal soft tissue dissection to preserve the remaining blood supply to the proximal humerus. The valgus-impacted four-part fracture configuration became recognized as one in which there was a significantly lower rate of avascular necrosis compared

J.C. Hsu and L.M. Galatz (✉)
Department of Orthopaedic Surgery, Washington University School of Medicine, St. Louis, MO, USA
e-mail: galatzl@wustl.edu

*Adapted from Hsu J, Galatz LM, Mini-incision Fixation of Proximal Humeral Four-Part Fractures in Scuderi G, Tria A, Berger R (eds), *MIS Techniques in Orthopedics*, New York, Springer, 2006, with kind permission of Springer Science and Business Media, Inc.

with other four-part fractures. In 1995, Resch[12] reported a series of 22 patients with open reduction and internal fixation of the valgus-impacted proximal humerus fracture, further solidifying the understanding of the fracture as one that does not require hemiarthroplasty. In fact, the results of these studies showed better results after fixation than the historical results after hemiarthroplasty.

In 1992, Jaberg et al.[7] reported on percutaneous stabilization of 54 displaced proximal humerus fractures of varying types. In this series, closed reduction was performed and the fractures were stabilized with K wires placed in both antegrade and retrograde fashion. Resch et al.[8] later reported on percutaneous fixation of three- and four-part proximal humerus fractures. The authors described using a pointed hook retractor percutaneously in the subacromial space for reduction of greater tuberosity fragments and elevation of the humeral head in valgus-impacted four-part fractures.

Anatomic Considerations

Four-part valgus-impacted humerus fractures have been described as "impacted with inferior subluxation,"[13] "impacted and little displaced fractures,"[3] and minimally displaced

Table 6.1 Fractures amenable to percutaneous pinning

2-part	Surgical neck
	Greater tuberosity
	Lesser tuberosities[a]
3-part	Surgical neck/greater tuberosity
	Surgical neck/lesser tuberosity[a]
4-part	Valgus impacted

[a]Without associated posterior dislocation

fractures.[14] Fourteen percent of all humeral head fractures are valgus impacted. The articular segment is impacted into the metaphysis, causing avulsion of both the greater and the lesser tuberosities with a line of fracture through the anatomic neck (Fig. 6.1a, b). The blood supply to the articular segment via the tuberosities is therefore disrupted. The main source of vascularization for the humeral head, the ascending anterolateral branch of the anterior humeral circumflex artery,[15,16] is interrupted at its point of entry into the humeral head in the area of the intertubercular groove. The only remaining blood supply is medially via the periosteum. Numerous vessels ascend along the inferior capsule and periosteum from both the anterior and posterior humeral circumflex arteries to the calcar region of the medial portion of the anatomic neck. Any lateral displacement of the articular fragment damages the periosteal hinge and consequently interrupts this last remaining source of vascularization. Therefore, a true valgus-impacted humeral head fracture will be impacted such that the medial hinge is intact. Any lateral displacement of the head segment has been associated with a higher rate of avascular necrosis.[12]

Indications for Percutaneous Pinning

Successful outcome after operative treatment of unstable proximal humerus fractures, regardless of approach or choice of hardware, depends on a few critical factors: (1) anatomic reduction, (2) stable fixation, and (3) careful management of soft tissues. Plate fixation offers a reliably stable construct in patients with good bone quality. The surgical approach and plate application require more extensive soft tissue stripping, which may contribute to the problem of devascularization and

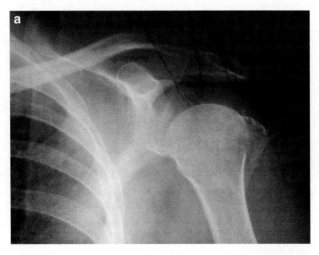
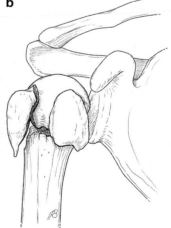

Fig. 6.1 (**a**) This anteroposterior (AP) radiograph of a valgus-impacted four-part fracture demonstrates the intact medial periosteal hinge with avulsion and lateral displacement of the greater tuberosity. (**b**) This valgus-impacted four-part fracture drawing also demonstrates the otherwise superimposed lesser tuberosity fragment fracture, making this a true four-part fracture (from Scuderi p. 34)

subsequent avascular necrosis. Intramedullary rods with cerclage wires are another alternative, and have been shown to be biomechanically stable constructs.[17] However, mechanical impingement in the subacromial space remains a potential problem.

Percutaneous pinning offers an excellent alternative to the open approach in selected fractures (Table 6.2). An anatomic reduction and stable fixation are just as important in this procedure. Patients must have good bone stock to ensure secure pin fixation. The displaced greater tuberosity fragment requiring reduction and fixation must be large and substantial enough to hold one or two screws. An intact medial calcar region is important for stability after reduction of the proximal humerus. This is the portion that must be intact in the valgus-impacted humeral head fracture to preserve the remaining vascularity.

Patient compliance is critical. Therefore, patient selection plays an important role. Postoperative rehabilitation is more conservative than after an open procedure. Patients are generally immobilized for the first couple of weeks. Patients must undergo close surveillance and consistent follow-up in order to prevent complications related to pin migration, either antegrade or retrograde, and to detect any unexpected early loss of fixation.

Percutaneous pinning is contraindicated in (1) patients with poor bone stock, (2) fracture in which there is a comminuted proximal shaft fragment, especially in the medial calcar region, (3) displaced four-part fractures (other than the valgus-impacted configuration) in elderly people requiring hemiarthroplasty, (4) noncompliant patients or patients unable or unwilling to comply with strict follow-up and rehabilitation limitations, and (5) fractures with displaced greater tuberosity fragments that are too comminuted or small for hardware fixation.

Patient Evaluation

Patient evaluation begins with a complete history and physical examination. The mechanism of injury should be noted and all associated injuries thoroughly evaluated. Most proximal humerus fractures are the result of low-energy falls in elderly patients. Another subset of fractures results from high-energy injuries in the younger population. A thorough neurovascular examination should be performed prior to any attempt at percutaneous pinning. The patient's social situation should be

Table 6.2 Conditions for successful pinning

Good bone stock
Intact medial calcar
Substantial greater tuberosity fragment
Stable reduction under fluoroscopy after pinning
Reliable, cooperative patient

assessed in order to discern whether the patient is appropriate in terms of complying with rehabilitation and close follow-up. Patients should be advised that one of the disadvantages of this procedure is that the pins may be uncomfortable in the subcutaneous position. They require subsequent removal as either an office or short operative procedure.

Radiographic evaluation consists of four standard views: an anteroposterior view of the shoulder, an anteroposterior view of the scapula, an axillary view, and a scapular Y. This combination of radiographs is helpful in evaluating posterior displacement of greater tuberosity fragments as well as anterior displacement of the shaft fragment. These X-rays are usually sufficient. A computed tomography (CT) scan can be considered if further radiographic evaluation is desirable. Three-dimensional reconstructions are rarely necessary. Studies help evaluate the suitability of the particular fracture for percutaneous reduction and fixation.

Elderly people with significant osteopenia and noncompliant patients may be better candidates for open reduction and internal fixation, a procedure that can potentially lead to more secure fixation biomechanically. Less concern exists over loss of fixation and pin migration. Preoperative consent should include possible conversion to an open procedure if the fracture cannot be adequately reduced and held with percutaneous fixation.

Surgical Procedure

Patient Positioning

The patient position must allow unencumbered access to the shoulder, both for easy visualization under fluoroscopy and for pin placement (Fig. 6.2). The patient is placed on a radiolucent operating room table with their head in a head holder such that the shoulder is proximal and lateral to the edge of the table. Adequate visualization of the shoulder under fluoroscopy should be confirmed before prepping and draping. The procedure can be performed with the patient in the supine position; however, raising the head of the bed 15–20° is often helpful for orientation and instrumentation. A mechanical arm holder is used for positioning the arm during the procedure. The holder can be useful for placing traction on the arm when necessary. The C-arm fluoroscope is positioned at the head of the bed, parallel to the patient, leaving the area lateral to the shoulder open for access and pin placement. Alternatively, the C-arm can be angled perpendicular to the patient; however, it is much more difficult to get an axillary view with the C-arm in this position. The monitor is placed on the opposite side of the patient for easy visualization by the surgeon. We recommend not using an adhesive, plastic drape directly on the skin at the operative site because

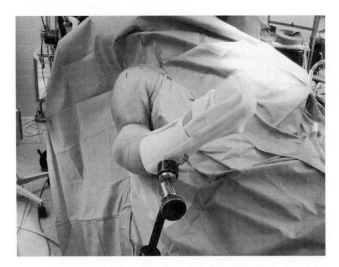

Fig. 6.2 Patient positioning allows for unencumbered access to the anterior, posterior, and lateral shoulder for easy visualization on a radiolucent table as well as pin placement. The reduction portal is drawn in its location approximately 1–2 cm distal to the anterolateral corner of the acromion

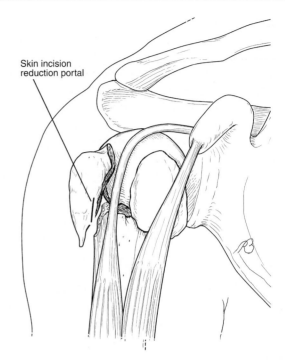

Fig. 6.3 The reduction portal is positioned distal to the anterolateral corner of the acromion at the level of the surgical neck of the humerus. This allows for easy instrumentation between the greater and the lesser tuberosity for reducing the fracture

it can become adherent to the pins inadvertently during insertion and may be introduced into the wound. The shoulder should be draped to accommodate conversion to an open procedure, should it be necessary.

Percutaneous Reduction

Bony landmarks are outlined on the skin, specifically, the acromion, clavicle, and coracoid. A small 1- to 2-cm incision is made 2–3 cm distal to the anterolateral corner of the acromion. Formation of this "reduction portal" facilitates reduction of the fracture percutaneously prior to pin fixation (Fig. 6.3). The reduction portal is positioned distal to the anterolateral corner of the acromion at the level of the surgical neck of the humerus, posterior and lateral to the biceps tendon. The fracture between the greater and the lesser tuberosities lies approximately ½–1 cm posterior to the biceps groove. Localizing the reduction portal over the split between the tuberosities enables elevation of the head fragment by placing the instrument through the natural fracture line.

The deltoid is gently and bluntly spread in order to avoid possible injury to the anterior branch of the axillary nerve in this location. A blunt-tipped elevator or a small bone tamp is placed through the *reduction portal* at the level of the surgical neck through the split in the tuberosities and under the lateral aspect of the humeral head (Fig. 6.4). The position is checked under fluoroscopy. The bone tamp or elevator is tapped with a mallet, elevating the head into the reduced position, restoring the normal angle between the humeral shaft and the articular surface of the humeral head. Characteristically, in a

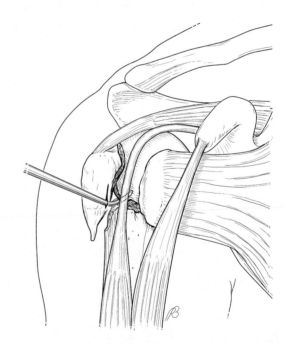

Fig. 6.4 A blunt-tipped elevator or small bone tamp is placed through the reduction portal through the split in the tuberosities and under the lateral aspect of the humeral head in order to elevate the head fragment into an anatomic position

valgus-impacted proximal humerus fracture, once the head fragment is reduced anatomically, the tuberosities naturally fall into the reduced position. Occasionally, the lesser tuberosity may still be displaced medially and can potentially require lateral traction via a small hook in the subdeltoid space to bring it into anatomic position. Final reduction is confirmed using fluoroscopic imaging.

A potential pitfall includes overly aggressive impaction with the mallet, leading to loss of cancellous bone in the head fragment and potential fracture. Valgus-impacted fractures can only be reduced using this technique before healing has taken place. Ideally, it is recommended in the first 2 weeks after the fracture. Beyond that time, more aggressive manipulation may be required in order to mobilize the head fragment.

Instrumentation

Instrumentation includes 2.5- or 2.7-mm terminally threaded pins. Terminally threaded K wires or, alternatively, guide wires from the Synthes (Synthes, Paoli, PA) 7.3-mm cannulated screw set can be used. Fully threaded pins are not used to protect the soft tissues. Terminal threads are desirable in order to prevent migration. Pins are inserted through very small incisions. Optimally, a drill guide should be used. A drill guide can be obtained from a small fragment fracture set. Alternatively, a drill guide used for arthroscopic anchor insertion can be useful.

Two to three retrograde pins are placed from the shaft into the head fragment. The pins should enter the skin distal to the site where the pins actually enter the bone in order to obtain the correct angle so that the pins do not cut out posteriorly before gaining fixation in the head fragment (Fig. 6.5). The direction of the pins is generally anterolateral to posteromedial because of the anatomic retroversion of the humeral head. Pins should not be placed directly in the coronal plane because of the normal retroversion of the humeral head. This results in pins cutting out anteriorly. The starting points of the pins should not be too close to one another to avoid a stress riser in the lateral cortex. Additionally, the pins should be multidirectional in order to stabilize the construct. Two to three pins parallel to one another will act as a single point of fixation, allowing rotation.

The tuberosities are then secured. Pins or cannulated screws can be used. We prefer fixation with cannulated screws because the ends of the pins protrude through the deltoid and can cause muscle irreparable damage. Pins, if used, must be removed before starting early range-of-motion exercises for this reason. We prefer 4.5-mm cannulated screws to secure the greater tuberosity. The 4.5-mm screws have a substantial guidewire and come in adequate lengths. The guidewire is placed under fluoroscopic guidance through the greater tuberosity approximately 1 cm below the rotator cuff insertion, engaging the medial cortex of the shaft fragment (Fig. 6.6). A screw with a washer is used, but one must be careful not to

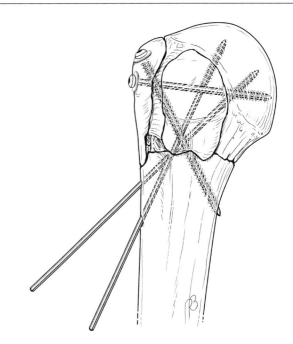

Fig. 6.5 The pins are placed in an anterolateral to posteromedial position because of the anatomic retroversion of the humeral head. Screws should be placed lateral and distal enough to avoid mechanical impingement symptoms in the subacromial space

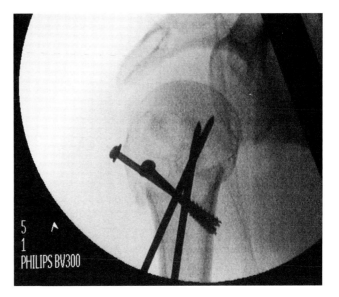

Fig. 6.6 The pins and screws are placed under fluoroscopic guidance. Reduction of the fracture as well as hardware placement can be checked using continuous fluoroscopy or spot views in multiple positions

overtighten the screw because the compression with the washer can potentially fracture the greater tuberosity. Ideally, two screws are placed. The second screw can be a cancellous screw directed into the articular fragment. Often with one antegrade screw and two retrograde pins, there is not enough room in the metaphysis for a second antegrade screw from the greater tuberosity.

Fixation of the lesser tuberosity is debatable. Once the humeral head and greater tuberosity are reduced and fixed, the lesser tuberosity is nearly always in anatomic position. If there is excessive medial displacement, a hook retractor can be used through the reduction portal in the subdeltoid space to move the fragment laterally, and a percutaneous cannulated screw can be placed from the anterior to posterior direction to secure the lesser tuberosity. We generally prefer to leave the lesser tuberosity in the reduced position without additional fixation. It has not been found to result in any functional disability postoperatively.

After percutaneous fixation, the pins are cut below the skin. This reduces the chance of superficial pin tract infection. All of these small incisions are closed using interrupted nylon suture.

Postoperative Management

After the procedure, the affected extremity is immobilized in a sling for approximately 3 weeks. Active wrist, elbow, and hand range-of-motion exercises are encouraged. Radiographs are obtained 1, 3, and 6 weeks postoperatively. If the fracture is thought to be stable, pendulum exercises can be initiated immediately; however, in many cases, pendulum exercises, passive forward flexion in the scapular plane, and external rotation are not started for 3 weeks, provided the fracture remains stable. Active assisted and active range-of-motion exercises are initiated at 6 weeks if there are signs of fracture healing. Progression to light strengthening is as tolerated at that point. The pins are removed 4–6 weeks postoperatively. In a very unstable fracture configuration, it is optimal to leave the pins in for 6 weeks; however, loosening may necessitate earlier removal. The pins are removed either as an office procedure or in the operating room under local anesthesia, depending on patient and surgeon preference.

Results

Jakob et al.[11] first presented his results of the treatment of 19 valgus-impacted four-part proximal humerus fractures. Five of these fractures were treated closed. He reported an avascular necrosis rate of 26%. Jaberg et al.[7] reported the results of 48 fractures fixed with percutaneous stabilization of unstable fractures of the proximal humerus fracture. This series had 29 fractures of the surgical neck, three of the anatomic neck, eight three-part fractures, five four-part fractures, and three fracture dislocations. They had 38 good to excellent results, ten fair, and four poor. One patient with a two-part fracture had avascular necrosis approximately 11 months postoperatively. Eight patients had localized transient avascular necrosis of the small portion of the humeral head that did not necessitate humeral head replacement.

Resch et al.[12] published his results of percutaneous pinning of 9 three-part fractures and 18 four-part fractures. None of the three-part fractures went on to avascular necrosis, and all had a good or very good result. There was an 11% incidence of avascular necrosis in the four-part fractures. Those with anatomical reconstructions did very well. Five of these patients had four-part fractures with significant lateral displacement at a humeral head. One of these required revision 1 week after surgery, and one went on to late avascular necrosis. Soete et al.[18] recommended against percutaneous pinning for the treatment of four-part proximal humerus fracture because of avascular necrosis and unsatisfactory reduction. These were not all valgus-impacted proximal humerus fractures, however.

Complications

The most worrisome complication of percutaneous pinning is nerve injury. Nerves at risk are primarily the axillary, the musculocutaneous, and, to a lesser extent, the radial nerve. The axillary nerve courses posteriorly through the quadrangular space to the undersurface of the deltoid and is located approximately 3–5 cm distal to the lateral border of the acromion. When making the anterolateral reduction portal, the deltoid should be gently and bluntly spread in order to avoid any nerve traction. This incision is generally superior to the zone where the nerve is located; however, one should still be cautious during this portion of the procedure. The axillary nerve is also at risk when placing screws through the greater tuberosity. If the screws are placed more inferiorly along the greater tuberosity, a drill guide can be inserted more superiorly and gently advanced distally in order to keep the nerve from the path of the drill.

An anatomic study of percutaneous pinning of the proximal part of the humerus[19] demonstrated that the proximal lateral retrograde pins were located a mean distance of 3 mm from the anterior branch of the axillary nerve. The screws through the tuberosity were located a mean distance of 6 and 7 mm from the axillary nerve and the posterior humeral circumflex artery. While these structures are at risk during placement, they are easily protected if the screws are placed in a careful fashion. The anterior pin is located adjacent to the long head of the biceps tendon, 11 mm from the cephalic vein, and could potentially be near the musculocutaneous nerve.[19] These findings emphasize the importance of using a drill guide. The radial nerve will not be injured as long as the retrograde pins are inserted proximal to the deltoid insertion.

The most common complication is pin migration. Most commonly, the pins back out and become prominent under the skin. Proximal migration into the joint is possible. Percutaneous pinning requires very close follow-up and strict patient compliance. Serious complications of pin migration are prevented by following patients with radiographs at regular intervals. Loss of fixation may occur as with any type of fracture fixation. In some situations, this can be treated with repeat percutaneous pinning. However, if it is believed that the fracture is in an unstable configuration and further loss of fixation may occur, open reduction and internal fixation is recommended. Malunion may result. This is usually well tolerated if the tuberosities are well reduced in relation to the humeral head. Displacement at the surgical neck is well tolerated in comparison with that of the tuberosities.

Superficial infections of the pins have been reported. Jaberg et al.[7] reported seven superficial pin tract infections, which were treated with local debridement and antibiotics. There was one deep infection in a diabetic patient. In his series, the pins were left through the skin. Because of this risk, we prefer to cut the pins deep to the skin.

Conclusion

Percutaneous pinning of proximal humerus fractures requires a thorough three-dimensional understanding of proximal humeral anatomy. Placement of the pins can be difficult and dangerous if the pins exit the bone incorrectly or penetrate nearby neurovascular structures. Assessment of reduction and stability can be challenging. The surgeon must be able to use the two-dimensional image obtained on fluoroscopy to assess a three-dimensional reduction. Success of this procedure is also dependent upon patient selection. Only fractures that can be stably reduced with pins are appropriate for this procedure. The four-part valgus-impacted proximal humerus fracture is generally very stable after reduction and is easily amenable to this type of treatment. Excessive comminution of the proximal shaft, especially the medial calcar area, indicates a fracture that may require open treatment with more secure fixation. The surgeon should always be prepared to convert to an open reduction and internal fixation if percutaneous pinning becomes difficult or impossible. In spite of the above concerns, successful percutaneous pinning in an appropriate patient offers significant advantages over open treatment in a valgus-impacted four-part proximal humerus fracture. Benefits include less dissection and the ability to take advantage of the intact soft tissue sleeve that exists in these proximal humerus fractures. The procedure is shorter in terms of operative time and results in less blood loss.

Additional advantages may include less scar formation and possibly accelerated rehabilitation. As our experience with percutaneous pinning increases and we become more familiar with this technique, we will likely see expanding indications for percutaneous pinning.

References

1. Neer CS II. Displaced proximal humeral fractures. II. Treatment of three-part and four-part displacement. J Bone Joint Surg Am, 1970. **52**(6):1090–1103.
2. Neer CS II. Displaced proximal humeral fractures. I. Classification and evaluation. J Bone Joint Surg Am, 1970. **52**(6):1077–1089.
3. Jakob RP, Kristiansen T, Mayo K, et al. Classification and aspects of treatment of fractures of the proximal humerus. In: Bateman J, Welsh R editors. Surgery of the Shoulder. Philadelphia, PA: B. C. Decker, 1984
4. Probe RA. Minimally invasive fixation of tibial pilon fractures. Oper Tech Orthop, 2001. **11**(3):205–217.
5. Kanlic EM, Pesantez RF, Pachon CM. Minimally invasive plate osteosynthesis of the femur. Oper Tech Orthop, 2001. **11**(3):156–167.
6. Morgan S, Jeray K. Minimally invasive plate osteosynthesis in fractures of the tibia. Oper Tech Orthop, 2001. **11**(3):195–204.
7. Jaberg H, Warner JJP, Jakob RP. Percutaneous stabilization of unstable fractures of the humerus. J Bone Joint Surg Am, 1992. **74-A**(4):508–515.
8. Resch H, Povacz P, Frohlich R, et al. Percutaneous fixation of three- and four-part fractures of the proximal humerus. J Bone Joint Surg Br, 1997. **79**(2):295–300.
9. Chen CY, Chao EK, Tu YK, et al. Closed management and percutaneous fixation of unstable proximal humerus fractures. J Trauma, 1998. **45**(6):1039–1045.
10. Bohler J. Perkutane oisteosynthese mit dem Rontyenbildrier-Starker. Wiener Klin Wachenschr, 1962. **74**:485–487.
11. Jakob RP, Miniaci A, Anson PS, et al. Four-part valgus impacted fractures of the proximal humerus. J Bone Joint Surg Br, 1991. **73**(2):295–298.
12. Resch H, Beck E, Bayley I. Reconstruction of the valgus-impacted humeral head fracture. J Shoulder Elbow Surg, 1995. **4**:73–80.
13. deAnquin CE, deAnquin CA. Prosthetic replacement in the treatment of serious fractures of the proximal humerus. In: Bayley I, and Lessel L, editors. Shoulder Surgery, Berlin, Springer. 1982: 207–217.
14. Stableforth PG. Four-part fractures of the neck of the humerus. J Bone Joint Surg Br. 1984. **66**(1):104–108.
15. Laing PG. The arterial supply of the adult humerus. J Bone Joint Surg Am, 1956. **38A**:1105–1116.
16. Gerber C, Schneeberger AG, Vinh TS, The arterial vascularization of the humeral head. An anatomical study. J Bone Joint Surg Am, 1990. **72**(10):1486–1494.
17. Wheeler DL, Colville MR, Biomechanical comparison of intramedullary and percutaneous pin fixation for proximal humeral fracture fixation. J Orthop Trauma, 1997. **11**(5):363–367.
18. Soete P, Clayson P, Costenoble V. Transitory percutaneous pinning in fractures of the proximal humerus. J Shoulder Elbow Surg, 1999. **8**(6):569–573.
19. Rowles DJ, McGrory JE, Percutaneous pinning of the proximal part of the humerus. An anatomic study. J Bone Joint Surg Am, 2001. **83-A**(11):1695–1699.

Chapter 7
Mini-incision Shoulder Arthroplasty

Sara L. Edwards, Theodore A. Blaine, John-Erik Bell, Chad J. Marion, and Louis U. Bigliani

Minimal disruption of soft tissue and a potential for a faster recovery are very attractive benefits of minimally invasive surgery (MIS). MIS, however, must meet the same standards and offer the same successful outcomes as traditional operations performed through larger skin incisions. While mini-incision hip and knee replacement surgery have become accepted techniques, there are no reports to date on mini-incision shoulder arthroplasty (MISA). The goals of MISA are to decrease trauma to surrounding soft tissues, accelerate postoperative rehabilitation, and decrease operative blood loss and complications. Currently, there are two techniques available to achieve the necessary exposure to perform MISA: (1) a concealed axillary incision or (2) a mini-deltopectoral incision. The use of these techniques is based upon the pathology, the severity of disease, the instrumentation, and the surgeon's experience.

Indications

Glenohumeral Arthritis

Many patients undergoing shoulder arthroplasty for arthritis require extensive releases and exposure to properly address the pathology. The decision to perform MISA vs. traditional incisions must therefore be made by the surgeon based on each individual patient's pathology, the instrumentation available, and the surgeon's experience. While MISA is becoming more common, patients who have large osteophytes, limited range of motion, or who are large and muscular may require a traditional approach. As in all cases of shoulder arthroplasty, preoperative radiographs that include a true anteroposterior (AP) and axillary view are essential for preoperative planning and in deciding whether MISA is a reasonable approach (Figs. 7.1 and 7.2). An axillary radio-

graph is especially important and a CT scan may also be required to adequately evaluate the glenoid vault. If there is excessive posterior glenoid bone erosion, then a MISA approach is not advisable, because exposure is more difficult. The ideal patient is a thin female with satisfactory range of motion (forward flexion of 100°, external rotation of 20°, and internal rotation to L3) and small osteophytes. Decreased soft tissue disruption and limited detachment of the subscapularis muscle during this approach are beneficial in terms of restoration of sub-scapularis function and accelerated rehabilitation posto-peratively.

Several reports have documented superior range of motion and better pain relief achieved in patients undergoing total shoulder arthroplasty vs. hemiarthroplasty for osteoarthritis.[1–3] Therefore, the decision to perform a hemiarthroplasty instead of total shoulder replacement (TSR) so that the operation may be done through a MISA approach is not recommended. Glenoid pathology in the setting of shoulder arthroplasty usually requires resurfacing with a glenoid component. The decision to perform humeral head replacements (HHR) vs. TSR is based on the pathology and not the approach to be used.

Four-Part Proximal Humerus Fractures

Hemiarthroplasty may be indicated for the treatment of four-part proximal humerus fractures. A minimally invasive approach in HHR for fracture needs to provide adequate exposure for secure tuberosity fixation as well as minimal soft tissue dissection to preserve the biological environment to foster bone healing. New innovative technological advances in prosthetic design aid the surgeon in achieving these goals. These include a lower profile contour of the proximal stem of the humeral prosthesis so that the tuberosity will fit anatomically. Also, the addition of tantalum, a metal that promotes ingrowth of bone, will allow bone to heal to metal as well as bone. Generally, once the hematoma has been evacuated, the rotator cuff in proximal humerus fractures is healthy and has excellent excursion, obviating the need for extensive surgical releases. We have developed

S.L. Edwards, T.A. Blaine, J. Bell and L.U. Bigliani (✉)
Columbia University, Center for Shoulder, Elbow and Sports
Medicine, 622 West 168 Street, PH 1118, New York, NY, 10032, USA
e-mail: lub1@columbia.edu

G.R. Scuderi and A.J. Tria (eds.), *Minimally Invasive Surgery in Orthopedics*,
DOI 10.1007/978-0-387-76608-9_7, © Springer Science+Business Media, LLC 2010

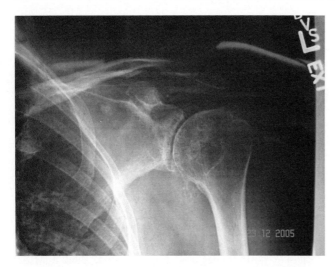

Fig. 7.1 True AP radiograph of a patient with glenohumeral osteoarthritis

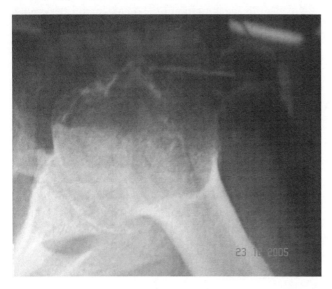

Fig. 7.2 Axillary radiograph of a patient with glenohumeral osteoarthritis

a small jig system that attaches to the prosthesis and allows the surgeon to accurately determine the retroversion and height of the humeral component. Lack of contractures combined with new technology for placement of the prosthesis and fixation of the tuberosities makes the minimally invasive approach an excellent option for these patients.

Avascular Necrosis

While total shoulder arthroplasty has had superior results to hemiarthroplasty in patients with glenohumeral arthritis in several recent series, there are some cases where hemiarthroplasty is the procedure of choice. These include avascular

necrosis (Cruess stages I-III, and sometimes IV) where the humeral head is still somewhat concentric and the glenoid is not arthritic. MISA is particularly useful in these patients, since glenoid exposure is not required.

Surgical Technique

Positioning of the arm in space to allow adequate visualization and instrumentation is critically important in all shoulder surgery, and especially in MISA. The beach chair position is used with a modified short arm board on the operative side. The arm board is placed on the distal aspect of the humerus, so the proximal humerus remains free. This allows extension of the arm for humeral shaft preparation as well as a more distal support to hold the arm in a more neutral position. Another option is the hydraulic arm positioner (SPIDER, TENET Medical Engineering, Inc., Calgary, Alberta, Canada), which eliminates the need for another assistant and also avoids inevitable assistant fatigue in holding the arm throughout the procedure (Fig. 7.3). Rotation of the humerus into both internal and external rotation is essential at different times during the procedure.

Based on cadaveric studies and clinical experience, the authors have found that the current instrumentation used for shoulder arthroplasty tends to exit the skin in a 2-in. (5-cm) arc centered and just lateral to the coracoid process (Fig. 7.4). Furthermore, we and others have also found that the average diameter of the humeral head at the surgical neck is approximately 49 mm.[4,5] Based on these findings, we think that the skin incision for shoulder arthroplasty must be at least 5 cm (2 in.) to allow placement of a humeral head component in shoulder arthroplasty, but does not necessarily need to be any larger. The authors have therefore devised a skin incision that

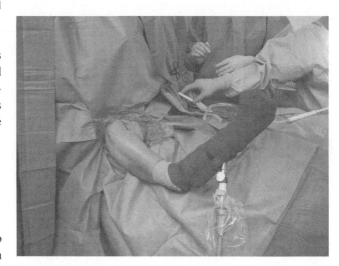

Fig. 7.3 Hydraulic arm positioner used to position the arm in space during MISA

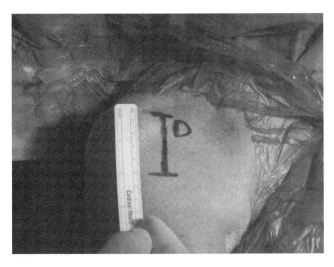

Fig. 7.4 Location of the MISA skin incision, measuring 5 cm (2 in.) just lateral to the coracoid process

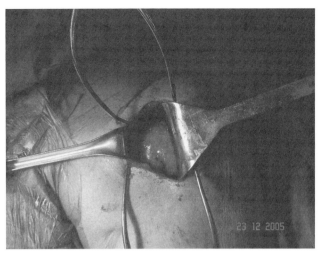

Fig. 7.5 The deltopectoral interval is entered, as per the usual deltopectoral approach

is centered just lateral to the coracoid process. This incision can be utilized in MISA for variety of diagnosis. The location of the incision allows better access to the tuberosities in fracture cases and provides adequate glenoid exposure in arthritic disorders. The incision measures approximately 2 in., just enough to deliver the humeral head from the wound. The placement of the starting incision is crucial for this approach. It has to be superior enough to provide direct access to the humeral canal for humeral preparation and placement of the prosthesis as well as allow adequate exposure of the glenoid. Alternatively, the concealed axillary incision is made within the axillary crease skin folds and begins at a point midway between the top of the coracoid and the inferior border of the pectoralis major.

The deltopectoral interval is identified and incised in a similar manner to the traditional anterior approach (Fig. 7.5). Subcutaneous dissection is necessary along the deltopectoral interval superiorly and inferiorly for adequate exposure. Care is taken to protect the attachment of the deltoid to the clavicle and acromion. The cephalic vein is generally retracted with the deltoid muscle secondary to the fact that there are more contributories superiorly from the deltoid than inferiorly from the pectoralis. The pectoralis major is retracted medially, and the deltoid with the cephalic vein is retracted laterally. The deltopectoral interval is developed and entered in a similar fashion. After exposure to the subscapularis muscle is achieved, the muscle is detached directly off the lesser tuberosity, superiorly, starting at the rotator interval (Fig. 7.6). The tendon is incised just medial to the biceps tendon, leaving a 2- to 4-mm cuff of tissue for later repair. The rotator interval is also released all the way to the base of the coracoid. In a traditional, more generous incision, the role of biceps tenotomy is debated. MISA, in most cases, requires biceps tenotomy with or without later tenodesis to provide adequate visualization (Fig. 7.7). The subscapularis

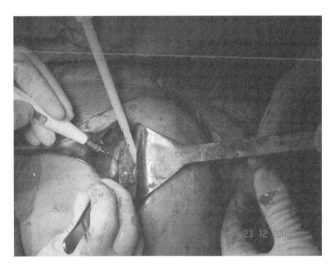

Fig. 7.6 The subscapularis is incised at its insertion to the lesser tuberosity and tagged for later repair

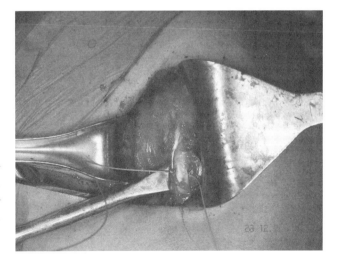

Fig. 7.7 The biceps tendon is located within its groove and tenotomized or tenodesed in the MISA approach

is detached just enough to deliver the humeral head from the wound (Fig. 7.8). Inferiorly, the subscapularis insertion may be preserved. However, if there is inferior osteophyte formation, then the inferior subscapularis insertion must be detached. The preparation of the humerus is performed with tapered reamers, which, with an incision based lateral to the coracoid, easily exit the skin (Fig. 7.9). An intramedullary cutting guide is used to make the humeral neck cut. In MISA, this cutting guide must be low profile and should have the ability to be positioned outside the skin incision if necessary (Figs. 7.10 and 7.11). Humeral trials are then performed. Correct alignment of the component is crucial and one has to have adequate visualization; the incision should be enlarged if the visualization is poor. Before placement of the final humeral prosthesis, bone tunnels are made and sutures are passed for future subscapularis repair. If TSR is performed,

attention is directed to the glenoid exposure (see following discussion).

Once the glenoid component has been replaced or if hemi-arthroplasty alone is performed, humeral trials are placed to determine appropriate sizing (Fig. 7.12); it is critical to place the humeral component in the appropriate version (usually 30° retroversion). Shoulder arthroplasty systems that allow version to be determined outside of the wound on the humeral insertors are critical for this step of the MISA procedure (Fig. 7.13). Sutures are now placed in the humeral neck for later repair of the subscapularis as per the surgeon preference.

With the advent of new humeral prostheses that promote proximal bony ingrowth, uncemented humeral components are favored, particularly with the MISA technique (Fig. 7.14). If cementation of the humeral component is performed, a cement restrictor is placed in the humeral canal 2 cm distal to

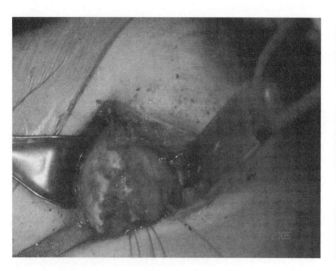

Fig. 7.8 The humeral head is delivered from the wound after releasing the subscapularis tendon insertion

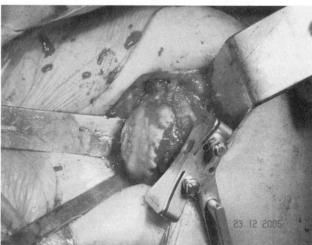

Fig. 7.10 The humeral cutting block is pinned to the humeral neck but is positioned outside the skin

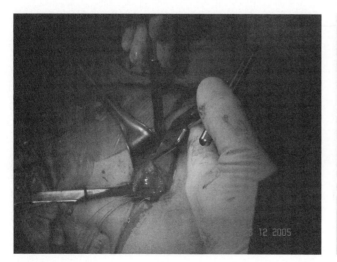

Fig. 7.9 The starter reamer is used to find the intramedullary canal of the humerus

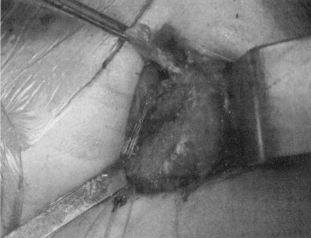

Fig. 7.11 The humeral neck cut has been made, and the humeral head removed

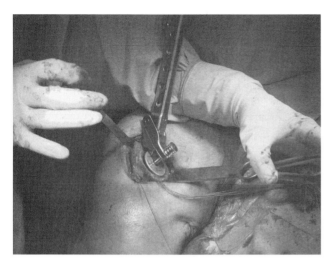

Fig. 7.12 The trial humeral prosthesis is inserted in the appropriate version, as referenced off the humeral insertor

the tip of the prosthesis. Minimal cement is typically concentrated around the metaphyseal portion of the prosthesis, since it is primarily used to control humeral component rotation.

Once the humeral component is fixed, trial head sizes are performed to reproduce the normal anatomy of the humeral head (Fig. 7.15). This typically requires an offset humeral head component with the maximal offset in the posterosuperior location. Trial reduction is then performed. An appropriate head size will allow translation of the humeral head on the glenoid of approximately 50% of the glenoid surface in any direction. It is very important to avoid overstuffing the glenohumeral joint, which can lead to persistent pain and postoperative stiffness. Once the appropriate head size is determined, the neck is dried with a clean sponge and the final humeral head is impacted on the Morse taper (Fig. 7.16).

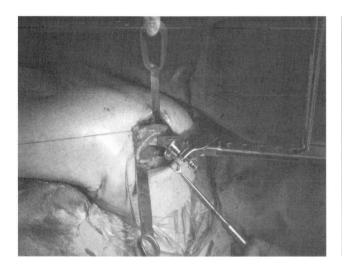

Fig. 7.13 Version rods on the humeral insertor are used to position the prosthesis in the correct version

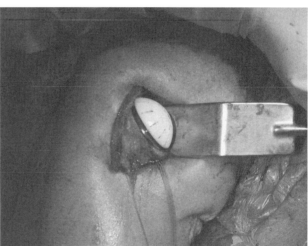

Fig. 7.15 Humeral heads are tested to determine appropriate size and offset

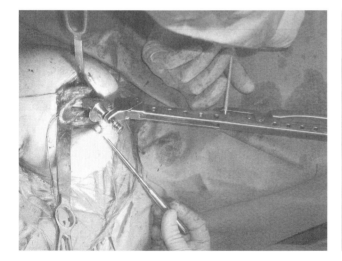

Fig. 7.14 A proximal trabecular metal prosthesis promotes bony ingrowth in the metaphysic

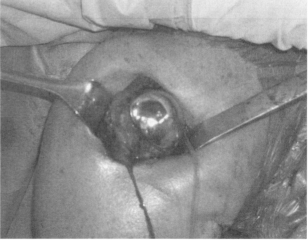

Fig. 7.16 The humeral head component of the prosthesis is impacted on the Morse taper humeral stem

Glenoid Replacement in Total Shoulder Arthroplasty

Glenoid exposure can be challenging even through the traditional incision; therefore, careful patient selection for a minimally invasive approach for total shoulder arthroplasty is required. Proper preparation of the glenoid and placement of the component is crucial. After proper humeral preparation as described previously, a Fukuda or malleable retractor is placed to assess the glenoid (Fig. 7.17). This helps retract the humerus laterally and posteriorly. An anterior spiked narrow Darrach retractor (Fig. 7.18) is then placed on the anterior rim of the glenoid. The provisional humeral stem is left in the canal during glenoid exposure and preparation. This helps to protect the integrity of the humeral stem during retraction.

To achieve adequate exposure to the glenoid, capsular release superiorly, anteriorly, and inferiorly around the glenoid is performed. Care is taken to protect the axillary nerve by staying directly on the humeral neck inferiorly and retracting the inferior capsule in an inferior direction with a Darrach retractor. For routine total shoulder arthroplasty where instability is not a problem and the rotator cuff is usually intact, an anterior capsulectomy may be performed to improve exposure. This should not proceed below the 6 o'clock position (inferior glenoid) to avoid injury to the axillary nerve. A special spiked Darrach retractor is placed anteriorly for adequate visualization. In thin patients with good range of motion and minimal glenoid deformity, this is usually enough for adequate visualization and reaming of the glenoid. Reaming is performed to achieve concentric stable fit of the glenoid component in appropriate version. Pegged or keeled glenoid components may be used. In one study, pegged glenoids were found to have superior fixation to keeled glenoids as well as decreased lucent lines, so we prefer to use pegged glenoid components. Dual-radius glenoid design can also be implemented to use smaller instruments to match a larger head size. The dual-radius implant has a small-radius base with a larger-radius articular surface, allowing easier implantation of the glenoid. Cement is pressurized in the pegged or keeled vault (Fig. 7.19).

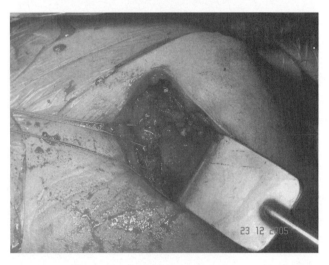

Fig. 7.17 A Fukuda retractor is placed on the posterior rim of the glenoid to allow glenoid visualization

Soft Tissue Repair and Wound Closure

Once the glenoid component is placed, attention is turned back to the humerus. The trial humeral stem is removed. A 2-mm hand-held drill is used to make three drill holes. The first hole is made on the superior aspect of the lesser tuberosity from outside to inside the humeral shaft. A #2 nonabsorbable braided suture is passed with a free needle first through the lateral cuff of tendon and then through the drill hole, from outside to in, and tagged with a free clamp. Two parallel holes are drilled across the superior half of the lesser tuberosity, in a medial to lateral direction, spaced approximately 1 cm apart.

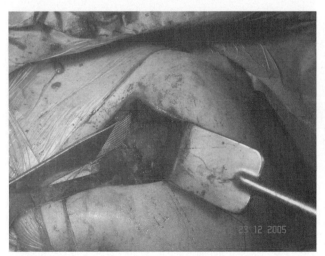

Fig. 7.18 A spiked Darrach retractor is placed on the anterior rim of the glenoid to complete glenoid visualization

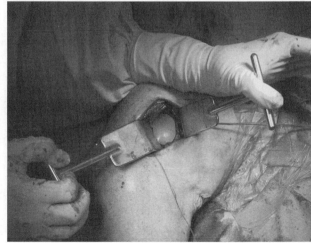

Fig. 7.19 The final glenoid component is placed through the mini-incision

Often it is necessary to drill the tunnel from both the medial and lateral side, angling slightly to allow the two sides to meet. Two #2 nonabsorbable sutures are placed in a medial to lateral direction through the tunnels. These are tagged for later use. The humeral component and the humeral head are placed as described above.

After placement of the humeral component, the arm should be placed in 20–30° of external rotation. A marking suture can be placed in the superior aspect of the tendon to set the tension for the rest of the repair. Working superiorly to inferiorly, the superior bone tunnel suture is used. This sequence is repeated with the other two bone tunnel sutures, bringing the medial edge of the suture under the corresponding tissue of subscapularis. Interrupted simple sutures are placed in the remaining superior tendon, and can be placed in between the bone tunnel sutures for added protection. More inferiorly, figure-of-eight sutures are placed. This portion of the procedure is critically important because subscapularis failure is the most common early complication of shoulder arthroplasty. Overtensioning must be avoided, because this can lead to necrosis and rupture. The rotator interval is left open to prevent stiffness in external rotation. Closure of the wound is performed in the usual fashion, with a running absorbable monofilament suture used to close the skin (Fig. 7.20). Suture tails are left out of the wound and secured with Steri-strips; these are clipped in the office at the 2-week follow-up visit. Intraoperative AP radiographs are taken in all cases to verify the size and position of the prosthesis before leaving the operating room.

Postoperative Care

Postoperative care is a critical component of managing patients after minimally invasive shoulder arthroplasty. Because of decreased soft tissue damage, patients tend to have a faster recovery time. Despite the patient's eagerness to get back to functional activities, the standard postoperative rehabilitation program must be followed at this early stage of implementation of this technique. The amount of time that is required for soft tissue healing is still the same regardless of the approach.

Results

We reviewed the results of the first 12 consecutive patients with shoulder arthroplasty performed through a mini-incision by two shoulder arthroplasty surgeons. Diagnoses included osteoarthritis (6 cases), fracture (2 cases), avascular necrosis (3 cases), and cuff tear arthropathy (1 case). There were six HHR and six TSR. One of two mini-incisions was used: (1) a 5- to 6-cm incision just lateral to the coracoid process, or (2) a 7- to 8-cm concealed axillary incision below the coracoid process. The average incision length was 6.2 cm (range 5–8 cm). A biceps tenotomy with tenodesis was performed in all patients where the biceps was present at surgery.

At the 6-month (on average) follow-up (range, 65–445 days), no patient reported significant pain postoperatively, and all but the one patient with cuff tear arthropathy had a successful result. There were two transient complications (temporary musculocutaneous nerve palsy and postoperative wound drainage), both of which resolved without incident. The musculocutaneous nerve palsy is thought to be related to excessive retraction required in the more medially based axillary incision; this incision has more recently been abandoned in favor of the incision lateral to the coracoid described in this article. Since using this incision, we have noted a high level of patient satisfaction, and the final cosmesis from this incision has been favored by our patients (Fig. 7.21).

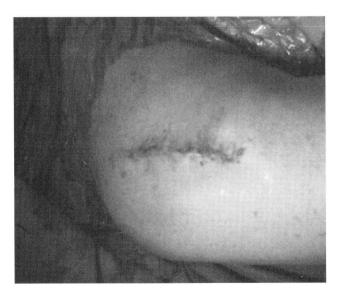

Fig. 7.20 The MISA incision is closed with an absorbable running monofilament subcuticular suture with tails left out of the wound

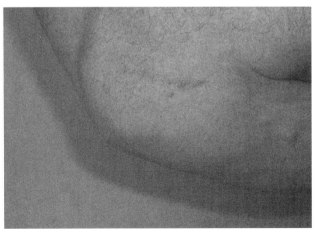

Fig. 7.21 Final appearance of the MISA incision when healed (1 year postoperatively)

Conclusions

Minimally invasive approaches for shoulder arthroplasty may offer improved patient cosmesis, faster recovery, and less soft tissue trauma. As these techniques continue to develop and patient demand increases, the development of new instrumentation (retractors, cutting guides, component insertion/removal instruments) may make MISA the preferred technique for many shoulder surgeons. Early results using currently available instruments and techniques have been encouraging and support the further advancement of minimally invasive approaches to shoulder arthroplasty.

References

1. Jain NB, Hocker S, Pietrobon R, et al. Total arthroplasty versus hemiarthroplasty for glenohumeral osteoarthritis: role of provider volume. J Shoulder Elbow Surg. 2005 Jul-Aug;14(4):361–7.
2. Rickert M, Loew M. Hemiarthroplasty or total shoulder replacement in glenohumeral osteoarthritis? Orthopade. 2007 Nov;36(11): 1013–6
3. Haines JF, Trail IA, Nuttall D, Birch A, Barrow A. The results of arthroplasty in osteoarthritis of the shoulder. J Bone Joint Surg Br. 2006 Apr;88(4):496–501
4. Blaine TA, et al. American Shoulder and Elbow Surgeons Focus Conference, November 13–16, 2003.
5. Iannotti JP, Spencer EE, Winter U, Deffenbaugh D, Williams G. Prosthetic positioning in total shoulder arthroplasty. J Shoulder Elbow Surg. 2005 Jan-Feb;14(1 Suppl S):111S–121S.

Chapter 8
Overview of Elbow Approaches: Small Incisions or Arthroscopic Portals

Bradford O. Parsons

Surgical management of patients with elbow pathology has evolved substantially in recent years. Technical improvements in fracture care, arthritis, and other pathologic conditions have led to more predictable restoration of function and relief of pain in many patients. Along with advances in elbow surgery has come the idea of "minimally invasive" surgery in orthopedics. Patients often ask for the mini-incision hip or knee surgery, and the elbow is no different. Minimally invasive techniques potentially allow for less perioperative pain, less morbidity, and faster recovery in properly selected patients. The literature is rife with reports describing less invasive surgical techniques for managing elbow conditions, especially arthroscopic techniques.[1–20] Although this "wave of enthusiasm" has led to a shift from traditional open techniques to arthroscopic surgery in many elbow conditions, the principles of surgical management must remain the same, i.e., the pathologic lesions must be appropriately addressed. This chapter serves as an overview of how we can transition from traditional open techniques to minimally invasive or arthroscopic techniques for many elbow problems.

Elbow Surgical Anatomy

The elbow is a complex joint whose main function is to enable positioning the hand in space. Morrey has described the functional range of motion of the elbow to be from 30° to 130° in flexion–extension and a 100° arc of supination and pronation (evenly divided).[21] Often patients will lose motion after trauma, and stiffness is the rule, not the exception in many situations. Stiffness can be a result of intrinsic and extrinsic contractures as well as heterotopic bone, resulting in distorted anatomy. As with any orthopedic procedure, it is critical to understand the three-dimensional anatomy and anatomical relationships of the elbow prior to performing surgery, especially

when performing minimally invasive or arthroscopic techniques, where surgical exposure is potentially limited. It is beyond the scope of this text to review all of the anatomy of the elbow, but a few principles should be discussed, specifically the location of the nerves and ligaments around the elbow.

The relationship of the neurovascular structures to the elbow is critical when attempting minimally invasive or arthroscopic elbow procedures. Portal placement around the elbow for arthroscopy is mainly based on the relationship of these structures to the osseous anatomy. The most frequently encountered nerve during elbow surgery is the ulnar nerve. The ulnar nerve lies in the cubital tunnel posterior to the medial epicondyle and therefore medial-sided procedures such as cubital tunnel release, medial column contracture release, or medial column fractures require identification of the ulnar nerve. Transposition of the nerve following trauma or other conditions may be necessary but often cannot be performed via a mini-incision.

The radial nerve is also frequently encountered, especially the posterior interosseous branch. The radial nerve usually bifurcates into superficial and posterior interosseous branches at the leading edge of the supinator. Lateral-based procedures such as two-incision biceps repair, radial head fractures, or lateral column procedures require an understanding of the location of the radial nerve. The median nerve lies medial to the bicipital aponeurosis and brachial artery. It may be encountered during medial-sided or anterior elbow approaches, such as single-incision biceps repairs, contracture release, or coronoid fractures.

The ligamentous anatomy is critical to the stability of the elbow, with the medial collateral ligament (MCL) and the lateral ulnar collateral ligament (LUCL) acting as primary stabilizers of the elbow. Violation of these ligaments iatrogenically can result in elbow instability. The MCL originates off of the anterior face of the medial epicondyle and inserts on the ulna at the sublime tubercle. It lies deep to the wrist flexor origin and is confluent with the joint capsule. The LUCL originates from an isometric point on the lateral aspect of the capitellum and courses around the posterolateral aspect of the radial head to insert on the

B.O. Parsons (✉)
Department of Orthopaedics, Mount Sinai School of Medicine, New York, NY, USA
e-mail: bradford.parsons@mountsinai.org

supinator crest of the ulna. It is also confluent with the capsule laterally and may be encountered during lateral approaches to the elbow. Regardless of the surgical approach around the elbow, the close proximity of these important structures requires a thorough understanding of their anatomy.

When to Attempt a Minimally Invasive Elbow Procedure

Although very attractive to patients and surgeons, minimally invasive approaches and procedures are often more technically challenging then their traditional open counterparts. Therefore, it is prudent to perform these minimally invasive techniques only with thorough understanding of the three-dimensional anatomy of the elbow. Additionally, a surgeon should be comfortable and competent with the principles of the traditional open techniques, as the pathology has not changed, and therefore the surgical principles must remain the same. The patient must be an appropriate candidate as well. Patients with distorted anatomy, such as end-stage rheumatoid arthritis or posttraumatic arthritis, previous surgery with scarring, or complex fractures, are often not amenable to minimally invasive techniques. Patients who are very muscular or obese also may not be candidates for minimally invasive open procedures, but arthroscopy is usually not precluded by these factors.

Pathologic entities that are amenable to minimally invasive open techniques include tennis elbow release, medial epicondylitis, collateral ligament reconstruction, biceps or triceps tendon repair, and isolated radial head, capitellar, or olecranon fractures. Advances in elbow arthroscopic technique and instrumentation have enabled many surgeons to "push the envelope" of what can safely and effectively be addressed with arthroscopy. Originally used mainly for removal of loose bodies,[7] arthroscopy has been successfully used for treatment of tennis elbow, posttraumatic contracture release, synovectomy, osteocapsular arthroplasty, osteochondral lesions, capitellar and coronoid fractures, and pediatric elbow conditions.[1–4,7,8,11–14,19,20] Although these advances have enabled experienced elbow arthroscopists and surgeons to manage increasingly complex conditions, many conditions are often not amenable to minimally invasive or arthroscopic techniques. This includes complex distal humerus or elbow fracture–dislocations, total elbow arthroplasty, complex contractures with heterotopic bone (although these can be occasionally addressed with arthroscopy in experienced hands), and revision procedures, especially when there is distorted osseous or neurovascular anatomy.

Minimally Invasive Open Approaches

As stated above, certain elbow conditions are amenable to minimally invasive open approaches. Extensile approaches to the elbow include the medial and lateral column approaches[22] and the posterior approach.[23,24] These approaches, or some variation of them, are the "workhorse" approaches to the elbow and allow excellent exposure and versatility to manage many conditions. However, they are extensile and would not be considered minimally invasive. Other approaches are less extensile and could be considered minimally invasive; these include approaches used for open tennis elbow release, one-incision or two-incision biceps tendon repairs, MCL reconstruction, and some fractures. Many of these specific entities will be discussed in later chapters and therefore we will not address them here. However, one approach is not discussed later and warrants discussion here; that is the Kocher approach to the lateral elbow.

Kocher Approach

Traditionally, the Kocher approach has been used to manage laterally based fractures or ligament injuries, such as radial head or capitellar fractures. This approach can be considered minimally invasive with small incisions in properly selected situations and patients. The Kocher approach utilizes the interval between the anconeus (posteriorly) and the extensor carpi ulnaris (ECU) (laterally). The posterior interosseous nerve (PIN) is in close proximity during the Kocher approach, and, to protect the PIN, the forearm is maintained in pronation. Although frequently used, two concerns regarding the Kocher approach should be raised. First, the classic Kocher approach is not extensile distally, as the PIN crosses the field distal to the annular ligament. Second, the interval between the ECU and anconeus traverses across the course of the LUCL, and this structure must be protected during this approach. One option is to use the interval between the extensor carpi radialis longus (ECRL) and the extensor digitorum comminus (EDC), a more anterior interval. This interval is in the anterior hemisphere of the capitellum and radial head, where most fractures occur, and will not violate the LUCL. The skin incision is made just slightly anterior then that for the Kocher along the same course.

The patient is positioned supine for the Kocher approach, with the arm on a hand table or over the chest. A tourniquet can be used if desired. The posterior and lateral osseous landmarks of the elbow are marked on the skin, including the lateral epicondyle, lateral column, radial head, and capitellum. The skin incision is marked as a curvilinear incision from just proximal to the lateral epicondyle to the radial head

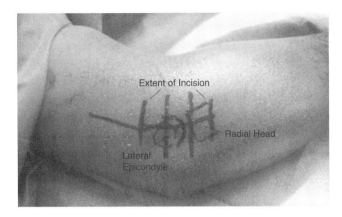

Fig. 8.1 Skin incision for the standard Kocher approach. A curvilinear incision is made over the lateral epicondyle and lateral column proximally, extending distally across the radial head

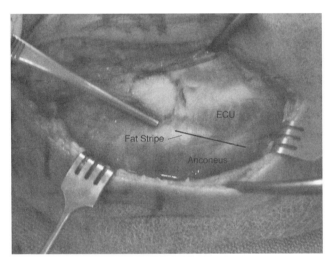

Fig. 8.2 The interval between the anconeus and ECU (Kocher's interval) can often be identified by a "fat stripe" (identified by the *forceps* and *broad solid line*)

(Fig. 8.1). The skin is incised to the level of the fascia and skin flaps are made.

The interval between the ECU and the anconeus is often identifiable by a "fat stripe" and the fascia and muscle are incised in this fat stripe (Fig. 8.2). Careful dissection can then allow for identification of the supinator muscle distally (with fibers oriented transversely vs. longitudinally for the extensors) and the capsule of the joint. Often, in trauma, the capsule is torn laterally, exposing the joint. The LUCL must be identified at this point. It is in the posterior hemisphere of the capitellum, as previously described. If an arthrotomy is necessary, it must be made at the level of the anterior half of the capitellum and radial head so as to not violate the LUCL. The joint and osseous structures of the lateral aspect of the elbow are now exposed via the arthrotomy. The capsule can be further elevated off of the distal humerus anteriorly if needed.

After completion of the procedure, it is critical to repair the capsular arthrotomy anatomically. The muscular interval must also be closed, and heavy nonabsorbable suture should be used. If injury to the LUCL has been encountered, this also must be anatomically repaired, either with anchors or (my preference) bone tunnels at the isometric point. The skin is closed in layers by surgeon preference after hemostasis has been obtained.

Elbow Arthroscopy

Elbow arthroscopy has evolved substantially over recent years. Originally performed for "simple" loose body removal or diagnostic procedures, the arthroscope now is utilized for management of complex arthritis, contractures, and some fractures of the elbow. The ability to perform these more complex procedures has been enabled by improvement in instrumentation and arthroscopic technique, and by thorough understanding of the three-dimensional anatomy of the elbow. This section details the indications and contraindications of elbow arthroscopy as well as positioning, portal placement, and technical tips on avoiding complications.

Indications

Many procedures typically performed "open" are now performed arthroscopically in experienced surgeons' hands. The pathologic entities now treated via arthroscopic techniques include tennis elbow, osteochondral lesions and loose body excision, synovectomy, capsular release, osteocapsular arthroplasty, and some intraarticular fractures.[1–4,7,8,11–14,19,20] When transitioning from open to arthroscopic techniques, the surgeon must have a thorough understanding of the surgical principles of the open procedures. It is suggested that when beginning elbow arthroscopy, one should start with less complex procedures, such as tennis elbow release or loose body removal. As surgeon experience and technical abilities increase, procedures that are more complicated can be performed.

Contraindications

Contraindications to elbow arthroscopy include patients who have significant derangement of the normal osseous and neurovascular anatomy of the elbow.[15] This would include patients who have had previous ulnar nerve transposition, as the transposed nerve lies in the path of the anteromedial portal of the elbow. In these patients, the nerve must be identified prior to medial portal placement. Additionally, patients with substantial posttraumatic or inflammatory arthritic changes with loss of the normal osseous architecture makes appropriate portal placement difficult, placing neurovascular structures at risk. Patients with substantial heterotopic ossification are often contraindicated because of the derangement of the normal neurovascular anatomy. Finally, patients with a history of previous surgery should be carefully considered for arthroscopy, as normal anatomic relationships may have been altered by the previous surgery.

Instrumentation

A standard 4.0-mm, 30°-offset arthroscope is used for elbow arthroscopy. Smaller arthroscopes are typically not necessary. It is preferable to use inflow cannulas without side vents, as the vents may lie outside the capsule and therefore can contribute to fluid extravasation and soft tissue swelling.[25] Standard arthroscopic shavers and burrs can be used, as well as standard arthroscopic graspers and biters. Cannulas help maintain portal positions and should be used routinely, and trochars should be blunt tipped to minimize iatrogenic injury of neurovascular and articular structures. Blunt-tipped switching sticks should also be available to serve as retractors for improved visualization. "Elbow arthroscopy sets" with standard instruments, including cannulated dilators, cannulas, and grasping instruments are now commercially available if desired (Arthrex, Naples, FL).

Patient Positioning

Patients can be positioned in three different manners for elbow arthroscopy, depending upon surgeon preference. We use the lateral decubitus position, with the arm placed over a post and draped free. Alternatively, the prone position can be used, and some prefer the supine position with the arm held in an extremity positioner such as the McConnel arm holder (McConnell Orthopaedics Co., Greenville, TX). Each position has its advantages and disadvantages. We will discuss the lateral position here.

Patients are positioned in lateral decubitus on a beanbag with bony prominences well padded. Care is taken to ensure that the patient is brought to the edge of the operating room table to allow for full exposure of the extremity. The contralateral arm is flexed and placed on an armrest out of the way. A tourniquet is placed on the proximal brachium, and draped out of the field. The operative arm is abducted 90° at the shoulder with the elbow flexed 90° over a post, so that the brachium is parallel to the floor and the elbow is completely free and can

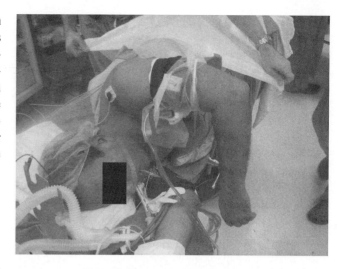

Fig. 8.3 Lateral decubitus positioning for elbow arthroscopy. The patient's operative arm is abducted 90° and the elbow is flexed over a padded post, taking care to ensure that access to the arm is not restricted. The forearm should hang free and allow for unrestricted range of motion of the elbow

be easily flexed and extended without impingement (Fig. 8.3). Care must be taken to use an arm post that will allow for easy instrumentation proximally along the brachium, and that the post is very proximal so that the elbow is completely free.

Arthroscopy Set-Up

Either pump or gravity insufflation may be used for elbow arthroscopy. If a pump is used, the pressure should be kept no higher then 30 mmHg. Unlike other joints, the elbow is subcutaneous and very susceptible to swelling of the soft tissues during arthroscopy. Once substantial soft tissue swelling has occurred, the complexity and difficulty of the elbow arthroscopy dramatically increases. Rather then increasing pump pressure to improve visualization, it is preferable to use retractors.

Outflow cannulas can be used and are set to either gravity or pump. If motorized instruments (shavers, burrs) are used, the outflow of these instruments should be set to gravity, not to suction, because exuberant suction can increase the chance that neurovascular structures may be pulled into the instrument and injured.

The osseous landmarks of the elbow are marked, including the lateral epicondyle, the radial head and capitellum, the medial epicondyle, the ulnar nerve, and the olecranon tip. The typical portals are also marked, including the proximal anteromedial, straight posterior (transtriceps), proximal posterolateral, and anterolateral. Accessory portals may be used in addition to the standard portals for retraction, etc. (Figs. 8.4 and 8.5). Each portal is discussed further below.

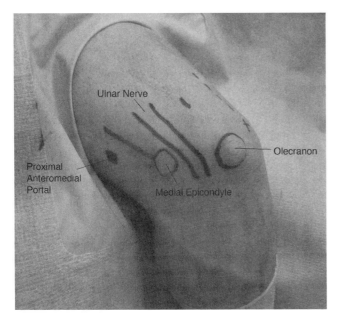

Fig. 8.4 Medial sided portals of elbow arthroscopy. The proximal anteromedial portal is approximately 2 cm proximal to the medial epicondyle and anterior to the intermuscular septum. The ulnar nerve should be marked and palpated to ensure that a subluxing nerve is not present

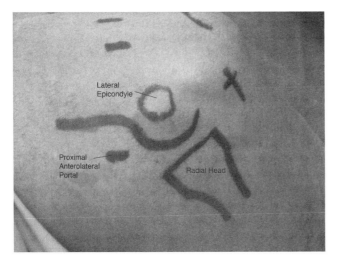

Fig. 8.5 Lateral sides portals of elbow arthroscopy. The proximal anterolateral portal is proximal to the capitellum along the column of the distal humerus. Anterolateral portals more distal (at the level of the radial head) can risk injury to the radial nerve

The joint is insufflated with ~20 mL normal saline via the lateral "soft spot" (the triangular area bounded by the lateral epicondyle, radial head, and olecranon). Realize that, in the contracted joint, insufflation may be more difficult because of the noncompliant capsule.[6,10,18,20,26] Joint insufflation is valuable in distending the capsule and increasing the distance of the neurovascular structures from the joint, but does not change the distance of these structures from the capsule,

and therefore these structures are still in close proximity when performing capsular procedures.

The elbow has two main compartments, anterior and posterior. Even in experienced hands, swelling can be an issue and therefore many surgeons will start in the compartment with greater pathology (i.e., anteriorly for a tennis elbow release, or posteriorly for an arthritic elbow with olecranon osteophytes and extension loss). Preoperative planning should assess which compartment is more pathologic and guide the surgical approach.

Similarly, some variation exists regarding which portals are used to initially visualize the joint. Anteriorly, the two standard options include visualization via the proximal anteromedial portal or via the anterolateral portal. Our standard is to use the proximal anteromedial portal to first visualize the joint, as the literature has shown that this portal is further from neurovascular structures then the lateral portals.[1,27] We then establish the lateral portal via an outside–in technique with a spinal needle. However, either option is viable and many surgeons start with the lateral portal. Posteriorly, most surgeons utilize the transtriceps (posterocentral) portal for initial visualization.

Portal Placement

Many different portals have been utilized for elbow arthroscopy, and the standard portals will be discussed. All portals are placed in an effort to avoid injury to the neurovascular structures around the elbow, but these structures are in close proximity and iatrogenic injury is possible with any of the portals.[6,10,18,26,28–34] When making portals, only the skin should be incised, and "plunging" of the scalpel should be avoided. Portals are distended with a blunt hemostat or commercially available cannulated dilators.

Proximal Anteromedial Portal

Described by Poehling et al.,[35] this portal is located anterior to the intermuscular septum and 2 cm proximal to the medial epicondyle (Fig. 8.4). The ulnar nerve is at greatest risk with this portal, and is typically located 3–4 mm posterior to this portal. After skin incision, the trochar is used to palpate the intermuscular septum and then the portal is established anteriorly. An effort should be made to enter the joint as medial as possible by bringing the trochar base close to the brachium, as this will improve visualization of the anterior compartment. Once the joint is entered, the radial head and capitellum is identified to confirm placement, and then evaluation of the anterior compartment is performed.

Proximal Anterolateral Portal

Described by Field et al.,[28] this portal is located 1–2 cm proximal to the lateral epicondyle, just anterior to the humerus (Fig. 8.5). Often this portal is made via an outside-in technique while visualizing from the medial side. The radial nerve is closest to this portal and at highest risk, although it is anterior to the sulcus between the radial head and capitellum. A "safe zone" for lateral portals includes the area bounded by the sulcus between the radial head and capitellum and the proximal anterolateral portal 2 cm proximal.[28] Proximal to the capitellum along the lateral column is safer then distally if accessory portals are needed for retractors, etc.

Transtriceps (Posterocentral) Portal

This portal is made 3 cm proximal to the olecranon process in the midline, which is proximal to the triceps muscle–tendon junction (Fig. 8.6). This is the initial portal when visualizing the posterior compartment, and the majority of the compartment can be visualized, including both medial and lateral gutters and the olecranon articulation. The posterior antebrachial cutaneous nerve and ulnar nerve are at risk with this portal but are both approximately 2 cm away.[25]

Proximal Posterolateral Portal

Often this is the initial working portal of the posterior compartment. It is made 2–3 cm proximal to the olecranon on the lateral border of the triceps (Fig. 8.6). The trochar is directed toward the olecranon fossa. The posterior and posterolateral gutter structures can be visualized via this portal. The medial and posterior antebrachial cutaneous nerves are at most risk, but are both approximately 2.5 cm away from this portal.[29]

"Soft Spot" (Direct Lateral) Portal

This portal is located in the soft spot, the triangular area bounded by the lateral epicondyle, radial head, and olecranon (Fig. 8.6). This portal is often made under direct visualization while viewing from the proximal posterolateral portal, localized with a spinal needle. The posterior antebrachial cutaneous nerve is on average 7 mm from this portal.[25] This portal allows visualization of the posterior capitellum and posterior proximal radioulnar joint. It is often utilized in the management of intraarticular plica or osteochondral lesions of the capitellum.

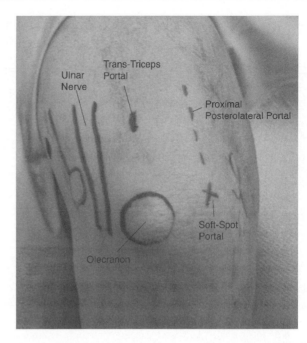

Fig. 8.6 Posterior portals of elbow arthroscopy. The transtriceps (posterocentral) portal is 2 cm proximal to the olecranon tip, in the center of the arm, whereas the accessory proximal posterolateral portal is at the same level but just lateral to the edge of the triceps tendon. Additional accessory portals are possible more distal in line with the accessory proximal posterolateral portal (*dashed lines*). The soft spot portal (marked by an "*x*") is made in the center of the triangle subtended by the radial head, olecranon, and lateral epicondyle

Tips and Tricks to Avoiding Complications

Avoiding complications centers on avoiding injury to the neurovascular structures around the elbow. The most frequent, and worrisome complication is nerve injury, and injuries to nearly all of the major nerves, or their branches, have been reported.[6,10,18,26,28–34] The risk of nerve injury has been found to be higher in patients with distorted anatomy, or soft tissue contractures, such as in advanced rheumatoid arthritis or posttraumatic arthropathies.[6] Osseous landmarks should be clearly marked before beginning, as surface landmarks will changes as the elbow swells during arthroscopy. A thorough understanding of the three-dimensional anatomy is critical to avoiding iatrogenic nerve injuries. Appropriate portal placement decreases the likelihood of nerve injury, as does the use of blunt-tipped trochars. Additionally, keeping the elbow flexed 90° helps relax the anterior capsule and soft tissues, thereby increasing the distance between the joint and neurovascular structures.

Many complications occur as soft tissue swelling distorts anatomy and visualization is compromised. Pump pressure should be kept to a minimum (<30 mmHg) or avoided all together, and intraarticular retractors should be used to increase visualization rather then increasing pump pressure.[6]

Suction on motorized shavers and burrs should not be used, as it may draw structures into harm's way. Prior to using elbow arthroscopy, a surgeon should be comfortable with similar open procedures, and, as technical skills are learned, procedures of appropriate complexity should be undertaken. It is suggested that when beginning elbow arthroscopy, one should start with less complex procedures, such as diagnostic procedures, tennis elbow release, or simple loose body excision.

Conclusions

Minimally invasive surgery is a "hot topic" in orthopedics, with many patients desiring the less invasive surgical option. This trend has been observed in nearly all fields of orthopedics, including elbow surgery. Numerous procedures traditionally performed open are now performed via "mini-incisions" or via arthroscopy about the elbow, with good results. This transition has enabled surgeons to treat patients with potentially less morbidity and faster recovery. However, minimally invasive techniques are often more technically demanding then the traditional "open" counterparts, and therefore surgeons should be very comfortable with the standard open procedures prior to attempting less invasive options. With minimally invasive elbow procedures, the key to success is found when patients are appropriately indicated, surgeons have a thorough understanding of the topographical and three-dimensional anatomy, and established techniques are utilized.

References

1. Andrews JR, Carson WG. Arthroscopy of the elbow. Arthroscopy 1985;1(2):97–107.
2. Andrews JR, St Pierre RK, Carson WG, Jr. Arthroscopy of the elbow. Clin Sports Med 1986;5(4):653–62.
3. Baker CL, Brooks AA. Arthroscopy of the elbow. Clin Sports Med 1996;15(2):261–81.
4. Brownlow HC, O'Connor-Read LM, Perko M. Arthroscopic treatment of osteochondritis dissecans of the capitellum. Knee Surg Sports Traumatol Arthrosc 2006;14(2):198–202.
5. Guhl JF. Arthroscopy and arthroscopic surgery of the elbow. Orthopedics 1985;8(10):1290–6.
6. Kelly EW, Morrey BF, O'Driscoll SW. Complications of elbow arthroscopy. J Bone Joint Surg Am 2001;83-A(1):25–34.
7. McGinty JB. Arthroscopic removal of loose bodies. Orthop Clin North Am 1982;13(2):313–28.
8. McLaughlin RE, II, Savoie FH, III, Field LD, Ramsey JR. Arthroscopic treatment of the arthritic elbow due to primary radiocapitellar arthritis. Arthroscopy 2006;22(1):63–9.
9. Morrey BF. Arthroscopy of the elbow. Instr Course Lect 1986; 35:102–7.
10. Morrey BF. Complications of elbow arthroscopy. Instr Course Lect 2000;49:255–8.
11. Moskal MJ, Savoie FH, III, Field LD. Elbow arthroscopy in trauma and reconstruction. Orthop Clin North Am 1999;30(1):163–77.
12. Mullett H, Sprague M, Brown G, Hausman M. Arthroscopic treatment of lateral epicondylitis: clinical and cadaveric studies. Clin Orthop Relat Res 2005;439:123–8.
13. Noonburg GE, Baker CL, Jr. Elbow arthroscopy. Instr Course Lect 2006;55:87–93.
14. O'Driscoll SW. Elbow arthroscopy for loose bodies. Orthopedics 1992;15(7):855–9.
15. O'Driscoll SW, Morrey BF. Arthroscopy of the elbow. Diagnostic and therapeutic benefits and hazards. J Bone Joint Surg Am 1992;74(1):84–94.
16. Ramsey ML. Elbow arthroscopy: basic setup and treatment of arthritis. Instr Course Lect 2002;51:69–72.
17. Reddy AS, Kvitne RS, Yocum LA, Elattrache NS, Glousman RE, Jobe FW. Arthroscopy of the elbow: a long-term clinical review. Arthroscopy 2000;16(6):588–94.
18. Savoie FH, III, Field LD. Arthrofibrosis and complications in arthroscopy of the elbow. Clin Sports Med 2001;20(1):123–9, ix.
19. Savoie FH, III, Nunley PD, Field LD. Arthroscopic management of the arthritic elbow: indications, technique, and results. J Shoulder Elbow Surg 1999;8(3):214–9.
20. Steinmann SP, King GJ, Savoie FH, III. Arthroscopic treatment of the arthritic elbow. J Bone Joint Surg Am 2005;87(9):2114–21.
21. Morrey BF, Askew LJ, Chao EY. A biomechanical study of normal functional elbow motion. J Bone Joint Surg Am 1981;63(6): 872–7.
22. Mansat P, Morrey BF. The column procedure: a limited lateral approach for extrinsic contracture of the elbow. J Bone Joint Surg Am 1998;80(11):1603–15.
23. Bryan RS, Morrey BF. Extensive posterior exposure of the elbow. A triceps-sparing approach. Clin Orthop Relat Res 1982(166): 88–92.
24. Wadsworth TG. A modified posterolateral approach to the elbow and proximal radioulnar joints. Clin Orthop Relat Res 1979(144):151–3.
25. Abboud JA, Ricchetti ET, Tjoumakaris F, Ramsey ML. Elbow arthroscopy: basic setup and portal placement. J Am Acad Orthop Surg 2006;14(5):312–8.
26. Adams JE, Steinmann SP. Nerve injuries about the elbow. J Hand Surg [Am] 2006;31(2):303–13.
27. Lindenfeld TN. Medial approach in elbow arthroscopy. Am J Sports Med 1990;18(4):413–7.
28. Field LD, Altchek DW, Warren RF, O'Brien SJ, Skyhar MJ, Wickiewicz TL. Arthroscopic anatomy of the lateral elbow: a comparison of three portals. Arthroscopy 1994;10(6):602–7.
29. Lynch GJ, Meyers JF, Whipple TL, Caspari RB. Neurovascular anatomy and elbow arthroscopy: inherent risks. Arthroscopy 1986;2(3):190–7.
30. Miller CD, Jobe CM, Wright MH. Neuroanatomy in elbow arthroscopy. J Shoulder Elbow Surg 1995;4(3):168–74.
31. Papilion JD, Neff RS, Shall LM. Compression neuropathy of the radial nerve as a complication of elbow arthroscopy: a case report and review of the literature. Arthroscopy 1988;4(4):284–6.
32. Ruch DS, Poehling GG. Anterior interosseus nerve injury following elbow arthroscopy. Arthroscopy 1997;13(6):756–8.
33. Stothers K, Day B, Regan WR. Arthroscopy of the elbow: anatomy, portal sites, and a description of the proximal lateral portal. Arthroscopy 1995;11(4):449–57.
34. Thomas MA, Fast A, Shapiro D. Radial nerve damage as a complication of elbow arthroscopy. Clin Orthop Relat Res 1987(215):130–1.
35. Poehling GG, Whipple TL, Sisco L, Goldman B. Elbow arthroscopy: a new technique. Arthroscopy 1989;5(3):222–4.

Chapter 9
Mini-incision Medial Collateral Ligament Reconstruction of the Elbow

Christopher C. Dodson, Steven J. Thornton, and David W. Altchek

The anterior bundle of the medial collateral ligament (MCL) of the elbow is the primary restraint to valgus load. It has been well documented that throwing athletes are prone to injury of this structure secondary to the repetitive valgus loads subjected to the elbow with overhead pitching.[1–4] Originally described in javelin throwers,[5] this injury is almost exclusively seen in overhead-throwing athletes, with baseball pitchers being the most prevalent group of patients. Injury to the MCL has also been shown in wrestlers, tennis players, professional football players, and arm wrestlers.[1,5–7] Symptomatic valgus instability can arise in these athletes after a MCL injury, thus necessitating operative intervention. Although injury to the MCL in the nonthrowing athlete can have excellent results with nonoperative intervention,[8,9] the overhead throwing athlete may find an injury to the MCL of the elbow to be a career-ending event if surgical intervention is not employed.

Biomechanics and Anatomy

The MCL complex is composed of an anterior bundle, a posterior bundle, and a transverse bundle[10] (Fig. 9.1). The anterior bundle has been shown to be the primary restraint to valgus stress at the elbow.[11–15] Injury to the anterior bundle can cause instability of the elbow with subsequent disabling pain in overhead-throwing athletes.[9,16–19] The humeral origin of both the anterior and posterior bundles is the medial epicondyle. The anterior bundle originates from the anteroinferior aspect of the medial epicondyle[10,20–22] and inserts at the sublime tubercle of the ulna.[10,22,23] On average, the anterior bundle occupies two thirds of the width of the medial epicondyle in the coronal plane.[22] It averages 4.7 mm in width and 27 mm in length.[21] The posterior bundle is triangular, smaller, and fanlike in nature; it originates from the posteroinferior aspect of the medial epicondyle and attaches to the medial olecranon margin.[14]

The anterior bundle has separate bands that function as a cam, tightening in a reciprocal fashion as the elbow is flexed and extended.[14,21,24] In a cadaveric study, Callaway et al.[10] performed sequential cutting of the MCL while a valgus torque was applied. The anterior band of the anterior bundle was the primary restraint to valgus rotation at 30, 60, and 90° of flexion. The posterior band of the anterior bundle was a coprimary restraint with the anterior band at 120°. In a separate study, Field and Altchek[25] evaluated the laxity seen with MCL injury when viewed through the arthroscope. They found that ulnohumeral joint opening was not visualized in any specimen until complete sectioning of the anterior bundle was performed. However, only 1–2 mm of joint opening was present with complete transaction of the anterior bundle, emphasizing the subtle exam findings in these athletes. It was shown that the maximum amount of valgus laxity was seen best at 60–75° of flexion.

The flexor carpi ulnaris (FCU) is the predominant muscle overlying the MCL.[26] It is the most posterior structure of the flexor–pronator mass, which places it directly overlying the anterior bundle of the MCL. Thus, the FCU is optimally positioned to provide direct support to the MCL in regards to valgus stability. Preservation of the FCU is important during reconstruction of the MCL in order to maintain one of the secondary restraints to valgus stress. This is further discussed when the surgical technique we currently use is described.

The ulnar nerve lies in close proximity to the MCL. It courses from a point posterior to the medial intermuscular septum above the medial epicondyle toward the anterior aspect of the medial elbow. Once it passes anterior to the intermuscular septum, the ulnar nerve then courses posterior to the medial epicondyle within the cubital tunnel. It then progresses distally to a point just posterior to the sublime tubercle. At this point, the ulnar nerve dives into the FCU, which it innervates. It is important to be familiar with the anatomy of this vulnerable structure during MCL reconstruction in order to avoid an iatrogenic injury.

History and Physical Examination

In the evaluation of overhead athletes with medial-sided elbow complaints, it is important to first obtain a detailed history. Questions should be posed as to the chronicity of the

C.C. Dodson, S.J. Thornton, and D.W. Altchek (✉)
Sports Medicine and Shoulder Service, Hospital for Special Surgery, New York, NY, 10021, USA
e-mail: altchekd@hss.edu

G.R. Scuderi and A.J. Tria (eds.), *Minimally Invasive Surgery in Orthopedics*,
DOI 10.1007/978-0-387-76608-9_9, © Springer Science+Business Media, LLC 2010

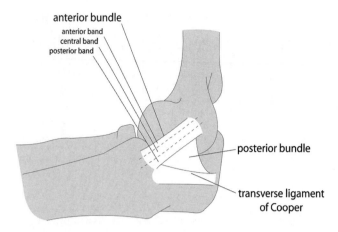

anterior bundle
anterior band
central band
posterior band

posterior bundle

transverse ligament
of Cooper

Fig. 9.1 Schematic drawing of the MCL complex. Note that the anterior bundle is composed of three bands. The anterior band of the anterior bundle is the primary restraint to valgus stress. (From Dodson CC, Altchek DW. The Management of Medial Collateral Ligament Tears in the Athlete. Oper Tech Sports Med:14(2): 75–80, 2006, with permission)

symptoms as well as its effect on overhead activity. Issues regarding velocity, accuracy, and stamina are important to the throwing athlete and should, therefore, be addressed. It is important to note that many of these athletes will modify their pitching techniques to compensate for the pain; however, these athletes will not be able to reach their maximal throwing velocity secondary to the altered mechanics being implemented. The phase of throwing in which the pain occurs is another important aspect. Conway et al. have shown that nearly 85% of athletes with medial elbow instability will complain of discomfort during the acceleration phase of throwing, in contrast to less than 25% of athletes that will experience pain during the deceleration phase.[1] This same study also showed that up to 40% of patients with MCL injuries may also suffer from ulnar neuritis;[1] therefore, a history of ulnar nerve symptoms should be ascertained as well as information pertaining to the position in which these symptoms are most prevalent.

Patients will present either with an acute event or with an acute on chronic episode. In an acute event, the patient reports having heard a "pop," and subsequently experienced acute medial pain with the inability to continue pitching. In an acute on chronic event, the patient will have experienced an innocuous onset of medial-sided elbow pain over an extended period of time with overhead throwing. This would preclude the acute event as described previously with an inability to continue with full-velocity pitching.

Both passive and active range of motion of the elbow should be documented. During the range of motion testing, attention should be turned to the detection of any crepitus, pain, or mechanical blocks. Patients with valgus overload will frequently develop posteromedial osteophytes that will present as a bony block to full extension. A possible loose body may also present with a similar exam.

Direct palpation of the origin of the MCL is unreliable secondary to the overlying flexor–pronator mass. However, an attempt should be made to elicit discomfort in this region with palpation. The ulnar nerve should be palpated (e.g., Tinel's) to assess for ulnar neuritis or subluxation of the nerve resulting in paresthesias. The medial epicondylar insertion of the flexor pronator mass should also be palpated for tenderness. If the flexor pronator tendon is involved, pain will be reproduced with resisted forearm pronation. This resisted maneuver can help distinguish a MCL injury from a flexor pronator tendonitis.

Several tests to test the MCL have been described. Generally speaking, we typically find the valgus stress test and the moving valgus stress test to be the most specific. To perform the valgus stress test, the examiner places the player's distal forearm under their axilla and applies a valgus load to the elbow in 30° of flexion while palpating the MCL (Fig. 9.2). If the patient complains of increased medial-sided elbow pain or if valgus instability is present, then the test is considered positive. However, it must be noted that the amount of instability present in these cases is sometimes too small to be picked up by this maneuver. Therefore, pain may be the only indication of a MCL injury with this test. The moving valgus stress test was originally described by O'Driscoll.[27] This test is performed by applying a valgus stress to the elbow in the flexed position and then quickly extending the elbow. (Fig. 9.3) A positive test produces

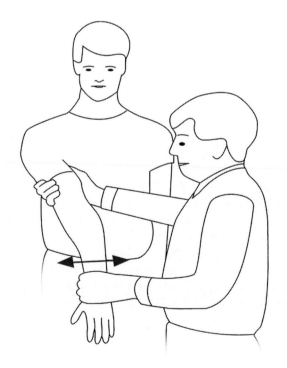

Fig. 9.2 Valgus stress test. While one hand of the examiner supports the elbow, valgus stress is applied with the elbow in approximately 30° of flexion. Tenderness to palpation over the MCL as well as valgus laxity are assessed

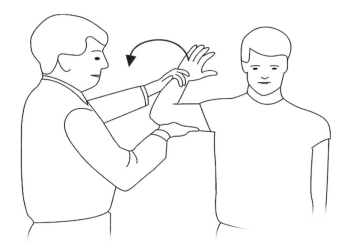

Fig. 9.3 The moving valgus stress test is performed by applying a valgus stress to the maximally flexed elbow and then quickly extending the elbow. A positive test usually produces pain between 120° and 70° of flexion

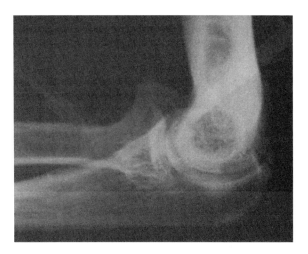

Fig. 9.4 Lateral radiograph of the elbow showing a prominent osteophyte at the tip of the olecranon. Patients who have X-ray results consistent with valgus extension overload need an MRI scan to assess the MCL. (From Dodson CC, Altchek DW. The Management of Medial Collateral Ligament Tears in the Athlete. Oper Tech Sports Med:14(2):75–80, 2006, with permission)

medial pain typically between 120° and 70° of flexion as a result of shear stress on the MCL. Finally, we also sometimes use the "milking maneuver," which is performed by pulling on the patients thumb with the forearm supinated, the shoulder extended, and the elbow flexed to 90°. A feeling of instability and apprehension along with pain is a positive finding and indicates insufficiency of the posterior band of the anterior bundle.

Posterior impingement secondary to posteromedial olecranon osteophytes should also be assessed. This is accomplished through the valgus extension overload test. The examiner uses one hand to apply a valgus force across the elbow while stabilizing the elbow joint with the opposite hand. The forearm is placed in a pronated position and the elbow is then quickly brought to full extension while the valgus load is applied. A positive test is indicated by pain in the posteromedial aspect of the elbow.

Imaging

Plain radiographs remain the gold standard for initial evaluation of the elbow. Routine anteroposterior (AP), lateral, and oblique views should be obtained. These standard radiographic views may reveal calcifications in the MCL, medial spurs on the humerus and ulna at the joint line, spurs on the posterior olecranon tip, or loose bodies present in the olecranon fossa (Fig. 9.4). Stress radiographs have been advocated to aid in the diagnosis of MCL tears,[28, 29] but we do not routinely use them.

We recommend getting a magnetic resonance imaging (MRI) scan on every patient with a suspected MCL tear. Some studies have shown that the sensitivity of MRI in detecting partial MCL tears is increased by injecting the elbow joint with saline prior to imaging.[30] At the Hospital for Special Surgery, however, we currently use three-dimensional volumetric gradient-echo and fast spin-echo techniques, which enables thin section (<3 mm) imaging of the elbow, thus improving visualization of partial tears of the MCL and obviating the need for contrast injection.[31, 32] Partial tears can be seen on MRI scans as areas of focal interruption that do not extend through the full thickness of the ligament. Complete tears can be seen on coronal MRI scans as increased signal intensity and focal disruption of the normally hypointense, vertically oriented ligament (Fig. 9.5). In chronic ligament injuries without tears, the MCL will appear thickened without focal discontinuity, but with global increased signal intensity. Because arthroscopic evaluation of the MCL is limited in its ability to visualize the anterior bundle and humeral or ulnar insertions,[25] MRI is an effective technique for distinguishing ligament tears from flexor or pronator tendinopathy. In addition, ulnar neuritis may be observed with enlargement and increased signal intensity in the nerve. Osteochondral impaction injuries to the radiocapitellar joint may also be seen, which emphasizes the importance of obtaining appropriate cartilage pulse sequencing.

Development of the Docking Procedure

Early experience of MCL reconstruction at the Hospital for Special Surgery led to some concerns about the original procedure as described by Jobe.[3] These concerns included (1) the ability to adequately tension the graft at the time of final fixation, (2) potential complications from detachment of the

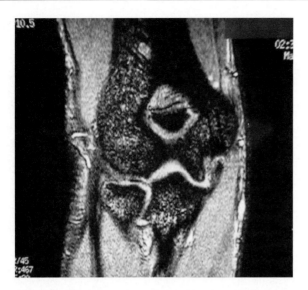

Fig. 9.5 Coronal MRI scan shows abnormal signal intensity and structure of the humeral insertion of the MCL, indicating a complete tear. (From Dodson CC, Altchek DW. The Management of Medial Collateral Ligament Tears in the Athlete. Oper Tech Sports Med:14(2):75–80, 2006, with permission)

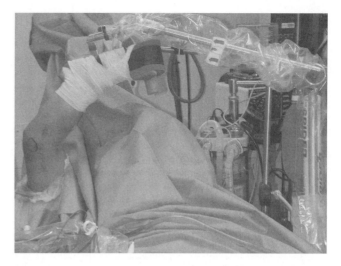

Fig. 9.6 The humerus and forearm are positioned across the chest and held in an arm holder to facilitate arthroscopic examination of the elbow

flexor origin, (3) potential complications from the placement of three large drill holes in a limited area on the epicondyle, (4) complications from routine ulnar nerve transposition, and (5) the strength of suture fixation of the free tendon graft. Therefore, in 1996, the senior author (DWA) began to look for alternative methods to reconstruct the MCL in order to address these concerns. The resulting procedure is referred to as the docking technique and highlights the following: (1) routine arthroscopic evaluation of the anterior and posterior compartments of the elbow to observe the degree of joint laxity and to evaluate and treat posterior medial lesions secondary to valgus extension overload, (2) using a muscle-splitting "safe zone" approach, (3) avoiding routine transposition of the ulnar nerve, (4) reducing the number of large drill holes from three to one in the medial epicondyle, and (5) addressing tendon length to ensure proper tensioning and fixation in bony tunnels.[33]

Surgical Technique

At our institution, the procedure is generally performed under regional anesthesia. After the block is administered, the patient remains in the supine position, a tourniquet is placed, and the involved upper extremity is prepped and draped in the usual sterile fashion. Using an arm holder (Spider, TENET Medical Engineering, Calgary, Canada), the humerus and forearm are positioned across the patient's chest for the arthroscopic evaluation of the elbow (Fig. 9.6).

The joint is insufflated with approximately 40–50 mL of saline and an anterolateral portal is established, which facilitates arthroscopic examination of the articular surfaces and the remaining anterior compartment. An arthroscopic stress test is typically done at this point. With the elbow at 90° of flexion, the forearm is pronated and a valgus stress is applied. A positive test results in medial opening between the ulna and the humerus greater than 2 mm and is indicative of MCL insufficiency[25] (Fig. 9.7).

After evaluating the anterior compartment, attention is then turned to the posterior compartment of the elbow. A posterolateral portal is established and the olecranon and the humeral fossae are examined for loose bodies or bone spurs. The trochlea is also examined for articular injury. Lastly,

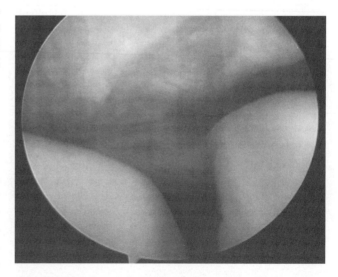

Fig. 9.7 Arthroscopic picture of a positive valgus stress test. Note the increased opening between the ulna (left) and the humerus (right), which is indicative of MCL insufficiency

the posterior radiocapitellar joint is evaluated by advancing the arthroscope down the lateral gutter. A transtriceps portal can be created through the center of the triceps tendon at the level of the olecranon tip, which allows for removal of loose bodies, osteophyte debridement, and microfracture of chondral lesions.

Once the arthroscopy has been completed, the arm is released from the arm holder and placed on the hand table. In cases where the palmaris longus tendon is absent, the gracilis tendon is harvested at this time. Otherwise, the ipsilateral palmaris longus tendon is harvested through a 1-cm incision in the volar wrist flexion crease over the tendon. At the time of harvest, the visible portion of the tendon is tagged with a No. 1 Ethibond suture (Ethicon, Inc., Johnson & Johnson) in a Krackow fashion and the remaining tendon is then harvested using a tendon stripper (Fig. 9.8a, b). The incision is then closed with interrupted nylon sutures and the tendon is placed in a moist sponge on the back table.

After the arm is exsanguinated to the level of the tourniquet, an 8- to 10-cm incision is created from the distal third of the intermuscular septum across the medial epicondyle to a point 2 cm beyond the sublime tubercle of the ulna. While exposing the fascia of the flexor–pronator mass, care is taken to identify and preserve the antebrachial cutaneous branch of the medial nerve, which frequently crosses the operative field. A muscle-splitting approach is then utilized through the posterior one third of the common flexor pronator mass within the most anterior fibers of the FCU muscle. This approach is beneficial because it utilizes a true internervous plane, allows for adequate exposure of the native MCL, and is less traumatic than detaching the entire flexor-pronator mass from its origin.[34] The anterior bundle of the MCL is now incised longitudinally to expose the joint.

The tunnel positions for the ulna are exposed first. The posterior tunnel requires that the surgeon subperiosteally expose the ulna 4–5 mm posterior to the sublime tubercle while meticulously protecting the ulnar nerve. Using a 3-mm burr, tunnels are made anterior and posterior to the sublime tubercle such that a 2-cm bridge exists between them. The tunnels are connected using a small, curved curette, taking care not to violate the bony bridge. A suture passer is used to pass a looped suture through the tunnel. To expose the humeral tunnel position, the incision within the native MCL is extended proximally to the level of the epicondyle. A longitudinal tunnel is then created along the axis of the medial epicondyle using a 4-mm burr; care is taken not to violate the posterior cortex of the proximal epicondyle. The upper border of the epicondyle, just anterior to the intramuscular septum, is then exposed, and two small exit punctures are made with a 1.5-mm burr. They should be approximately 5 mm to 1 cm apart from each other. Again a suture passer is used from each of the two exit punctures to pass a looped suture, which will be used later for graft passage. With the elbow reduced, the incision in the native MCL is repaired using a 2–0 absorbable suture.

With the forearm supinated and applying a mild varus stress to the elbow, the graft is then passed through the ulnar tunnel from anterior to posterior (Fig. 9.9). The limb of the graft on which sutures have already been placed is then passed into the humeral tunnel with the sutures exiting one of the small humeral exit punctures. This first limb of the graft is now securely "docked" in the humerus. With the elbow reduced, the graft is tensioned in flexion and extension to determine what length would be optimal by placing the second limb of the graft adjacent to the humeral tunnel. Final length is determined by referencing the graft to the exit hole

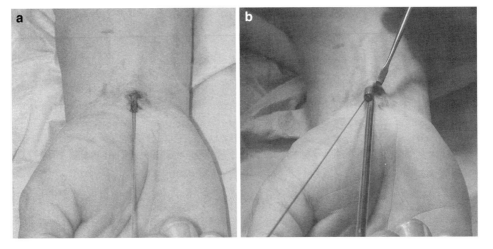

Fig. 9.8 (a) When present, the palmaris longus is harvested for graft reconstruction. The visible portion of the tendon is tagged with a suture. (b) A tendon stripper is used to harvest the remaining tendon once it has been identified and tagged

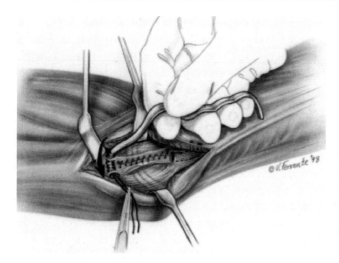

Fig. 9.9 The graft is passed through the ulnar tunnel from anterior to posterior. The limb of the graft with sutures is then docked into the humeral tunnel with the sutures exiting one of the exit holes

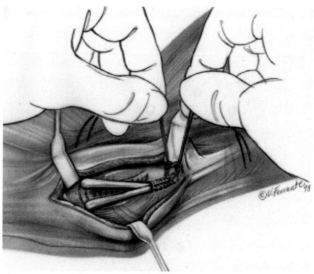

Fig. 9.11 Once both limbs of the graft have been successfully docked into the humeral tunnel, the graft sutures are tied down. (From Rohrbough et al.[33])

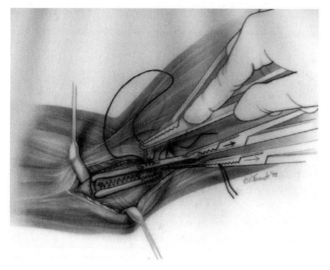

Fig. 9.10 The final length of the tendon is marked on the graft and another tagging stitch is placed. (From Rohrbough et al.[33])

in the humeral tunnel. This point is marked on the graft and a No. 1 Ethibond suture is placed in a Krackow fashion (Fig. 9.10). The excess graft is then excised immediately above the Krackow stitch and this end of the graft is then docked securely in the humeral tunnel, with the sutures exiting the free exit puncture.

Final graft tensioning is now performed by taking the elbow through a full range of motion. Once the surgeon is satisfied, the two sets of graft sutures are tied over the bony bridge on the humeral epicondyle (Fig. 9.11). After the tourniquet is deflated and hemostasis achieved, an ulnar nerve transposition is performed if indicated. We only do this when the preoperative exam is consistent with ulnar neuritis. Otherwise, the fascia over the flexor pronator mass is reapproximated and the remaining wound is closed in layers. The elbow is then placed in a plaster splint at 45° of flexion and neutral rotation with the hand and wrist free.

Postoperative Management

Immediately after surgery, the patients' arm is placed in a plaster splint for approximately 1 week. At the first postoperative visit, the sutures are removed and the elbow is placed in a hinged brace. Initially, motion is only allowed from 30° of extension to 90° of flexion. In the third to fifth week, motion is advanced to 15° of extension and 105° of flexion. Wrist flexion of the contralateral limb is also encouraged if the palmaris longus was harvested from that forearm. At 6 weeks, the brace is discontinued and formal physical therapy is begun, which focuses on shoulder and forearm strengthening as well as elbow range of motion. By 12 weeks, the patient is advanced to an aggressive physical therapy program that includes trunk strengthening as well as shoulder and scapula strengthening. A formal tossing program is begun at 16 weeks. Initially, throwing starts at a distance of 45 ft and is advanced at regular stages. If pain occurs during any stage, the patient is instructed to back up to the previous stage of therapy. If at 9 months the patient can throw pain free from 180 ft, they are allowed to begin pitching from a mound. We generally discourage competitive pitching until 1 year postoperatively.

Results

Conway et al.[1] conducted the first outcome study on the original procedure, as described by Jobe,[3] which included detachment of the flexor–pronator mass and routine transposition of the ulnar nerve. Only 68% of the athletes in that series were able to return to either their previous or a higher level of competition. In addition, 21% of the patients were observed to develop postoperative ulnar nerve neuropathies.

Thompson and Jobe were the first to report on 83 athletes who underwent MCL reconstruction using a muscle-splitting approach without transposition of the ulnar nerve. Of these 83 patients, 33 were followed for at least 2 years. The surgical result was excellent in 27 (82%) of 33 patients, good in 4 patients (12%), and fair in 2 patients (6%). These results improved to 93% excellent when those patients who had had a prior procedure were excluded.[7] Several authors have since reported on MCL reconstruction, using a muscle-splitting approach or transposing the ulnar nerve subcutaneously, and noted lower ulnar nerve-related complication rates, ranging from 8 to 9%.[35, 36]

We have recently reported on 100 consecutive MCL reconstructions using the docking technique with an average follow–up of 3 years.[37] No patients were lost to follow-up. Ninety (90%) of 100 patients returned to or exceeded their previous level of competition for at least 1 year, meeting the Conway-Jobe classification criteria of "excellent." Additionally, seven patients had a good result, which means that they were able to compete at a lower level for at least 12 months. Two patients (2%) had poor results and were not able to return to throwing.

In our series, 22% of patients underwent a subcutaneous transposition with fascial sling at the time of surgery. None of these patients suffered postoperative complications. Two athletes (2%) required transposition postoperatively after they had returned to throwing for at least 1 year. Neither patient had preoperative symptoms, and both had excellent results at the time of follow-up.[37]

As previously stated, we routinely perform an arthroscopic evaluation both anteriorly and posteriorly of all patients prior to reconstruction. It is not unusual for this patient group to develop intraarticular pathology secondary to the mechanics of valgus extension overload. In our recent series, 45 (45%) of 100 patients had associated intraarticular pathology that were all managed arthroscopically just before reconstruction.[37] Detection of the lesions on preoperative imaging studies occurred in only 25 of these 45 cases. Without arthroscopy, a posterior arthrotomy is necessary to treat such pathology, which necessitates transposition of the ulnar nerve. Arthroscopy is a more minimally invasive approach and has the added benefit of avoiding obligatory transposition of the nerve. Before our use of routine arthroscopy, we had patients who required repeat surgery for conditions that were unrecognized and could have been treated arthroscopically at the time of the initial procedure.

Summary

We think that the modifications described in the "docking technique" have resulted in excellent outcomes for athletes at all levels of play and that this technique has proven to be a minimally invasive and reliable method of reconstruction of the MCL.

References

1. Conway JE, Jobe FW, Glousman RE, Pink M. Medial instability of the elbow in throwing athletes. Treatment by repair or reconstruction of the ulnar collateral ligament. J Bone Joint Surg Am 1992; 74(1): 67–83.
2. Hamilton CD, Glousman RE, Jobe FW, Brault J, Pink M, Perry J. Dynamic stability of the elbow: electromyographic analysis of the flexor pronator group and the extensor group in pitchers with valgus instability. J Shoulder Elbow Surg 1996; 5(5): 347–354.
3. Jobe FW, Stark H, Lombardo SJ. Reconstruction of the ulnar collateral ligament in athletes. J Bone Joint Surg Am 1986; 68(8): 1158–1163.
4. Tullos HS, Erwin WD, Woods GW, Wukasch DC, Cooley DA, King JW. Unusual lesions of the pitching arm. Clin Orthop 1972; 88: 169–182.
5. Waris W. Elbow injuries of javelin-throwers. Acta Chir Scand 1946; 93: 563–575.
6. Kenter K, Behr CT, Warren RF, O'Brien SJ, Barnes R. Acute elbow injuries in the National Football League. J Shoulder Elbow Surg 2000; (9): 1–5.
7. Thompson WH, Jobe FW, Yocum LA, Pink MM. Ulnar collateral ligament reconstruction in athletes: muscle-splitting approach without transposition of the ulnar nerve. J Shoulder Elbow Surg 2001; 10(2): 152–157.
8. Josefsson O, Gentz CF, Johnell O, et al. Surgical versus non-surgical treatment of ligamentous injuries following dislocation of the elbow joint. J Bone Joint Surg Am 1987; 69: 605–608.
9. Miller CD, Savoie FH, III. Valgus Extension Injuries of the Elbow in the Throwing Athlete. J Am Acad Orthop Surg 1994; 2(5): 261–269.
10. Callaway GH, Field LD, Deng XH, Torzilli PA, O'Brien SJ, Altchek DW, et al. Biomechanical evaluation of the medial collateral ligament of the elbow. J Bone Joint Surg Am 1997; 79(8): 1223–1231.
11. Hotchkiss RN, Weiland AJ. Valgus stability of the elbow. J Orthop Res 1987; 5(3): 372–377.
12. Morrey BF, An KN. Articular and ligamentous contributions to the stability of the elbow joint. Am J Sports Med 1983; 11(5): 315–319.
13. Morrey BF, Tanaka S, An KN. Valgus stability of the elbow. A definition of primary and secondary restraints. Clin Orthop 1991; 265: 187–195.
14. Regan WD, Korinek SL, Morrey BF, An KN. Biomechanical study of ligaments around the elbow joint. Clin Orthop 1991; 271: 170–179.

15. Sojbjerg JO, Ovesen J, Nielsen S. Experimental elbow instability after transaction of the medial collateral ligament. Clin Orthop 1987; 218: 186–190.

16. Andrews JR, Whiteside JA. Common elbow problems in the athlete. J Orthop Sports Phys Ther 1993; 17(6): 289–295.

17. Glousman RE, Barron J, Jobe FW, Perry J, Pink M. An electromyographic analysis of the elbow in normal and injured pitchers with medial collateral ligament insufficiency. Am J Sports Med 1992; 20(3): 311–317.

18. Timmerman LA, Schwartz ML, Andrews JR. Preoperative evaluation of the ulnar collateral ligament by magnetic resonance imaging and computed tomography arthrography. Evaluation in 25 baseball players with surgical confirmation. Am Sports Med 1983; 11(2): 83–88.

19. Wilson FD, Andrews JR, Blackburn TA, McCluskey G. Valgus extension overload in the pitching elbow. Am J Sports Med 1983; 11(2): 83–88.

20. Fuss FK. The ulnar collateral ligament of the human elbow joint. Anatomy, function, and biomechanics. J Anat 1991; 175: 203–212.

21. Morrey BF, An KN. Functional anatomy of the ligaments of the elbow. Clin Orthop 1985; 201: 84–90.

22. O'Driscoll SW, Jaloszynski R, Morrey BF, An KN. Origin of the medial ulnar collateral ligament. J Hand Surg Am 1992; 17(1): 164–168.

23. Timmerman LA, Andrews JR. Undersurface tear of the ulnar collateral ligament in baseball players. A newly recognized lesion. Am J Sports Med 1994; 22(1): 33–36.

24. Schwab GH, Bennett JB, Woods GW, Tullos HS. Biomechanics of elbow instability: the role of the medial collateral ligament. Clin Orthop 1980; 146: 42–52.

25. Field LD, Callaway GH, O'Brien SJ, Altchek DW. Arthroscopic assessment of the medial collateral ligament complex of the elbow. Am J Sports Med 1995; 23(4): 396–400.

26. Davidson PA, Pink M, Perry J, Jobe FW. Functional anatomy of the flexor pronator muscle group in relation to the medial collateral ligament of the elbow. Am J Sports Med 1995; 23(2): 245–250.

27. O'Driscoll SW, Lawton RL, Smith AM. The "Moving Valgus Stress Test" for medial collateral ligament tears of the elbow. Am J Sports Med 2005; 33(2): 231–239.

28. Ellenbecker TS, Mattalino AJ, Elam EA, Caplinger RA. Medial elbow joint laxity in professional baseball pitchers. A bilateral comparison using stress radiography. Am J Sports Med 1998; 26(3): 420–424.

29. Rijke AM, Goitz HT, McCue FC, Andrews JR, Berr SS. Stress radiography of the medial elbow ligaments. Radiology 1994; 191(1): 213–216.

30. Schwartz ML, Al Zahrani S, Morwessel RM, Andrews JR. Ulnar collateral ligament injury in the throwing athlete: evaluation with saline-enhanced MR arthrography. Radiology 1995; 197(1): 297–299.

31. Gaary EA, Potter HG, Altchek DW. Medial elbow pain in the throwing athlete: MR imaging evaluation. Am J Roentgenol 1997; 168(3): 795–800.

32. Potter HG. Imaging of posttraumatic and soft tissue dysfunction of the elbow. Clin Orthop 2000; 370: 9–18.

33. Rohrbough JT, Altchek DW, Hyman J, et al. Medial collateral ligament reconstruction of the elbow using the docking technique. Am J Sports Med 2002; 30(4): 541–548.

34. Smith GR, Altchek DW, Pagnani MJ, Keeley JR. A muscle-splitting approach to the ulnar collateral ligament of the elbow. Neuroanatomy and operative technique. Am J Sports Med 1996; 24(5): 575–580.

35. Azar FM, Andrews JR, Wilk KE, et al. Operative treatment of ulnar collateral ligament injuries of the elbow in athletes. Am J Sports Med 2000; 28: 16–23.

36. Elattrache NS, Bast SC, Tal D. Medial collateral ligament reconstruction. Tech Shoulder Elbow Surg 2001; 2(1): 38–49.

37. Dodson CC, Thomas A, Dines JS et al. Medial collateral ligament reconstruction of the elbow in throwing athletes. Am J Sports Med 2006; 34: 1926–1932.

Chapter 10
Mini-incision Distal Biceps Tendon Repair

Bradford O. Parsons and Matthew L. Ramsey

Rupture of the biceps tendon from its distal insertion has historically been considered a rare injury, and early management was mainly nonoperative, with early reports citing satisfactory results.[1] However, more recent literature has recognized the persistent deficits of supination strength and endurance, and to a lesser degree flexion, in active high-demand patients, and has implicated these outcomes as an indication for acute repair.[2-6] Distal biceps ruptures currently seem to be encountered more frequently then historically reported, possibly due to increased awareness, and most surgeons now recommend early repair to maintain supination and flexion strength and endurance.

Complete distal biceps ruptures have been classified chronologically, with acute tears being recognized within 4 weeks from rupture, while chronic repairs are diagnosed after 4 weeks. With chronic tears, the integrity of the lacertus fibrosis may play a role in the degree of retraction and therefore the reparability of the tendon rupture. More recently, partial tears of the distal biceps have been recognized, and are classified by location, either insertional or intrasubstance.[7-10] Traditionally managed nonoperatively, some series have begun to elucidate the role of operative management of high-grade, symptomatic partial tears in certain patients.[8]

When indicated for repair, two operative approaches are most commonly used, either a one-incision repair utilizing suture anchors or other devices to secure the biceps to the radial tuberosity, or, more commonly, a two-incision technique that utilizes a bone trough and tunnels in the tuberosity, as a modification of the original Boyd-Anderson technique.[11] Much debate has occurred in the orthopedic literature regarding one-incision versus two-incision techniques for repair of distal biceps ruptures, and numerous studies have been performed attempting to identify which approach is "better."[12-16] Proponents of the two-incision technique think that it is a stronger repair then the one-incision technique, because it reattaches the tendon directly into a bony trough. Additionally, the two-incision technique has historically been thought to have a lower likelihood of neurovascular complications.[16-18] Those who favor one-incision approaches think that the repair is as strong as the two-incision technique, but minimizes the risk of heterotopic bone and radioulnar synostosis because the tendon is not passed between the radius and ulna during repair.[14,19,20] Suffice it to say that the controversy still rages to some degree, and therefore we will present both the one-incision and two-incision techniques, both of which allow the use of mini-incisions to repair acute distal biceps ruptures.

Pathoanatomy

Most distal biceps ruptures occur at the insertion of the tendon onto the radial tuberosity, often in the presence of preexisting tendon degeneration or partial tearing. The biceps muscle is the most anterior muscle in the anterior compartment of the arm and contributes to the formation of the lacertus fibrosis (the bicipital aponeurosis) at the level of the muscle–tendon junction. The lacertus arises off of the medial aspect of the biceps muscle and fans out across the antecubital fossa, connecting with the fascia of the proximal flexor muscles of the forearm, finally attaching to the subcutaneous border of the ulna. Deep to the lacertus, the biceps tendon travels distally to its insertion onto the radial tuberosity.

An understanding of the neurovascular structures around the elbow, especially the lateral antebrachial cutaneous nerve, median nerve, radial nerve, and posterior interosseous nerve (PIN), is critical to avoiding injury to these structures during surgical repair. The lateral antebrachial cutaneous nerve, which is the terminal sensory branch of the musculocutaneous nerve, sits lateral to the biceps tendon in the antecubital fossa. The median nerve lies medial to the biceps tendon in the antecubital fossa. The radial nerve lies between the brachialis and brachioradialis proximal to the elbow, then divides, giving off a superficial (sensory) and deep branch (PIN). The PIN dives into the supinator on the lateral side of the proximal radius, while the superficial branch sits under the brachioradialis as it travels distally into the forearm.

B.O. Parsons (✉) and M.L. Ramsey
Department of Orthopaedics, Mount Sinai School of Medicine,
One Gustave Levy Place, Box 1188 New York NY, 10029, USA
e-mail: Bradford.parsons@mountsinai.org

G.R. Scuderi and A.J. Tria (eds.), *Minimally Invasive Surgery in Orthopedics*,
DOI 10.1007/978-0-387-76608-9_10, © Springer Science+Business Media, LLC 2010

With complete ruptures, the biceps tendon will retract, often either to the level of the lacertus fibrosis, which if intact may tether the tendon distally, or more proximally in situations where the lacertus has been compromised. With retraction, the biceps tendon often "rolls-up" on itself, forming a ball of tendon, which, if not identified early, can degenerate, making late (>4 weeks) primary repair difficult or impossible. The biceps' tunnel (between the proximal radius and ulna) to the tuberosity is narrow, and varies in size depending upon the rotation of the forearm. In pronation, the biceps takes up 85% of the space in the tunnel, while, in supination, more space is available between the radius and ulna.[21]

Diagnosing Distal Biceps Ruptures

Acute ruptures of the biceps are often made by history and physical examination. As stated, the distal biceps most frequently ruptures off of the radial tuberosity, usually during a rapid or sudden eccentric contraction of the biceps, most frequently in men around the age of 50 years. Patients often report a "pop" and immediate pain in the antecubital fossa following injury, and may develop ecchymosis after injury. Rupture often results in a deformity of the contour of the biceps muscle belly, which may be accentuated when a biceps contraction is attempted. However, in a patient with large arms, it may be difficult to clinically appreciate a muscular deformity, and therefore clinical examination is critical to the appropriate diagnosis.

Palpation of the antecubital fossa often elicits tenderness along the course of the normal biceps tendon. A defect in the fossa is indicative of a full rupture. Integrity of the lacertus fibrosis should also be assessed. As stated previously, if the lacertus is ruptured, the biceps tendon can retract further proximally. In the acute phase, pain often prohibits normal flexion of the elbow or rotation of the forearm, but as the pain and swelling subside, motion improves. Often flexion strength will be nearly equal to the contralateral side, but may elicit discomfort, or accentuate deformity of the biceps contour. Provocative testing of supination is more diagnostic. Patients with full ruptures will have weakness when asked to hold a supinated position against forceful pronation, and will also fatigue quickly as the supinator fatigues. It is important to assess cyclic strength in someone who has good strength on initial testing, as this can be helpful in identifying partial tears as well.

Radiographs are not very helpful in the diagnosis of a distal biceps rupture, as the results are most often normal. Magnetic resonance imaging (MRI) may be helpful, although not necessary in patients where history and clinical examination confirm a rupture. MRI may be used to identify partial tears, although differentiating partial tearing versus bicipital aponeurosis or tendonosis can be difficult.[10] In chronic cases, or when the history and exam do not yield an obvious diagnosis, an MRI scan can help confirm the diagnosis.

Indications for Repair

Most surgeons currently recommend surgical repair of distal biceps ruptures in the active patient.[2–4,6,17,22] Once a full rupture is identified, patients should be counseled on the likely outcome of nonoperative and operative treatment. It is well established in the literature that early repair offers the best opportunity for preserving flexion and supination strength and endurance.[2–4,6,17,22] Although some patients with low demands of their injured extremity may have a satisfactory outcome with nonoperative treatment, most distal biceps ruptures occur in active, middle-aged men, who often poorly tolerate the functional loss and symptoms associated with the results of nonoperative treatment. Patients who are identified acutely following rupture, especially in the first 10 days, are often amenable to a minimally invasive approach to repair.[18] However, with further delay in diagnosis, especially after 1–2 months, a more extensive dissection and exposure is required, and tendon grafts may be needed to reconstruct the tendon defect.[6]

Patients with high-grade partial tears who are symptomatic and have failed nonoperative modalities including therapy are also amenable to repair of their partial tear. As awareness of this clinical entity has increased, these patients are more frequently being identified, and early reports have found successful outcomes with completion and repair of their high-grade partial biceps tears.

Contraindications

Patients who are low demand may refuse surgical repair. Additionally, patients who cannot safely undergo surgery because of medical comorbidities should be managed nonoperatively. As opposed to acute tears, patients who have chronic tears, especially those who are months removed from their injury date, may not be amenable to primary repair. With chronic tears, the biceps tendon scars and may degenerate, thereby shortening and making anatomic repair difficult or impossible. Additionally, the bicipital tunnel often fills with scar tissue, making identification difficult, which may require a more extensive exposure to identify and protect the neurovascular structures of the antecubital fossa. Rarely are these patients amenable to a "mini-incision" type of approach. Often they require an extensive exposure and tendon grafts for reconstruction.

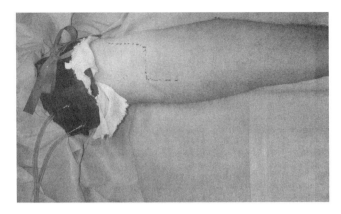

Fig. 10.1 Traditional skin incision employed in the original Boyd-Anderson technique. The proximal extent of the incision is often not necessary in acute tears. The distal extent is may be necessary for single-incision techniques

When to Attempt Mini-incision Repairs of The Distal Biceps

Ruptures addressed within 4 weeks from injury, especially if they are within the first 2 weeks, can often be surgically repaired using mini-incisions with either a one-incision or a two-incision technique. The original Boyd–Anderson anterior incision involved a large L-shaped incision along the lateral border of the biceps proximally and a transverse distal component in the flexion crease (Fig. 10.1).[11] This type of anterior incision is usually not necessary in the acute setting, especially when the lacertus fibrosis is intact. Often, a single transverse incision located in the flexion crease is sufficient for the anterior exposure (Fig. 10.2). If performing a two-incision technique, the anterior incision can be as small as

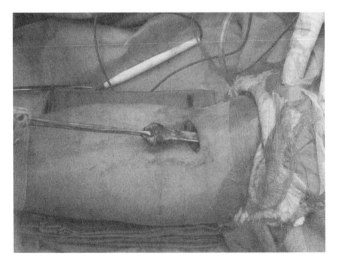

Fig 10.2 A straight horizontal incision measuring approximately 2 cm in the anterior flexion crease is usually sufficient for identification and mobilization of acute tears

2 cm, but may need to be slightly wider if performing a one-incision technique (to allow additional exposure to the radial tuberosity).

Familiarity with the typical course of the biceps tendon between the radius and ulna, and its usual point of retraction when torn, helps in keeping incisions small. Typically, the biceps retracts just proximal to the flexion crease and is often more superficial than most think. The distal stump of tendon can usually be palpated proximally just beneath the skin. If there is substantial proximal retraction, as in the case of chronic tears, or where the lacertus fibrosis has been ruptured, then an L-type incision, as originally described by Boyd and Anderson, may be necessary.

Surgical Procedure: The Two-Incision Technique

Patient Positioning

Patients are positioned supine with the affected arm on a hand table. Either regional or general anesthesia can be used. Tourniquet control may be helpful, and should be placed on the proximal arm. The tourniquet is not inflated initially, as it may inhibit excursion of the biceps tendon, and an attempt should be made to perform the repair without tourniquet inflation initially. The extremity is draped free, and the hand covered with stockinet. The anterior incision is marked in the flexion crease of the antecubital fossa of the elbow. As stated above, a 2- to 3-cm incision is often sufficient, depending upon the size of the arm.

Instrumentation

Certain instruments and equipment are necessary to perform the two-incision technique. A bipolar cautery and standard cautery should both be available. We routinely use two #2 Fiberwire sutures (Arthrex, Naples, FL) to reattach the tendon, but any heavy, nonabsorbable suture may be used. A 2.0-mm drill bit and drill is used to make bone tunnels in the radial tuberosity, and a 3.1-mm round tip burr is used to make a trough in the tuberosity. A Hewson suture-passing device can be used to pass sutures through bone tunnels.

Procedure

Once the patient is anesthetized, positioned, and prepped and draped, a 2- to 3-cm skin incision is made in the flexion crease. Dissection is carried into the subcutaneous tissue, to the level of the deep fascia. The lateral antebrachial cutaneous nerve is identified on the lateral aspect of the incision and it should be retracted laterally. Often, a rent in the deep fascia is observed, and digital palpation will identify the bicipital tunnel to the radial tuberosity. If the fascia is intact, it should be incised and then the biceps stump should be identified. The biceps tendon will often retract to the level of the lacertus fibrosis, but may retract more proximally if the aponeurosis is torn. In most acute tears, the biceps stump can often be palpated just proximal to the incision, on the undersurface of the fascia. Once identified, the stump is passed into the wound distally, freshened, and secured with two running Krakow-type sutures utilizing #2 Fiberwire (or other stout, nonabsorbable sutures). The sutures should be cut to slightly different lengths to identify matched pairs easily once they have been passed posteriorly. The sutures are then clamped for later passage to the posterior incision.

As stated, the tunnel for the biceps is often easily identifiable in the acute setting. Keeping the forearm in maximal supination, the biceps tuberosity can be palpated deep in the antecubital fossa. A blunt hemostat is then passed between the radius and ulna, hugging the radial tuberosity, into the subcutaneous tissue of the posterolateral forearm (Fig. 10.3). Care must be taken to stay on the medial surface of the radius, and to not violate the ulnar periosteum, in an effort to minimize the risk of radioulnar synostosis. Once the hemostat has been passed around the radial tuberosity, the arm can be pronated, and attention turned to the posterolateral second incision.

The posterior incision utilized in a two-incision technique is also a "mini-incision." Morrey's modification of the Boyd–Anderson approach utilizes a muscle-splitting approach to minimize the chance of radioulnar synostosis (Fig. 10.3).[4] The location of the posterior incision is identified by a hemostat passed through the radioulnar joint at the level of the radial tuberosity. The skin incision is centered over the hemostat, and usually a 3-cm skin incision is sufficient in most patients. The incision is carried down to the fascia sharply, and then an electrocautery is used to perform a muscle-splitting approach down to the tuberosity. This is done in maximal pronation, to protect the PIN.

The superficial fascia and common extensor muscle is incised in line with the skin incision. The supinator can be identified as the fibers travel obliquely across the wound. Keeping the forearm in maximal pronation, the supinator fibers are incised over the radial tuberosity, which is often palpable at this point. The tuberosity is then exposed and cleaned of soft tissue. Self-retaining retractors are placed to keep the incision open, and small Homan retractors are placed anterior and posterior to the tuberosity. Utilizing a 3.1-mm round-tipped, high-speed burr, a 1.5-cm by 5-mm trough is made in the radial tuberosity, large enough to place the biceps tendon stump into. Using a 2.0-mm drill bit, three drill holes are made in the posterior cortex of the radial tuberosity, exiting in the bone trough, with care taken to ensure at least a 5-mm bone bridge between holes (Fig. 10.4). Copious irrigation is used to remove all bony debris, in an effort to minimize heterotopic bone formation.

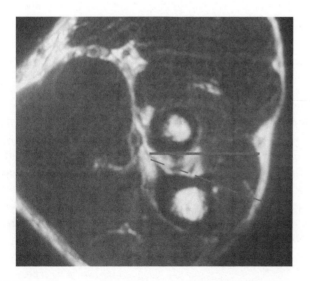

Fig. 10.3 Care is taken to develop the posterior interval (with a hemostat or other blunt instrument) around the proximal radius to the posterior aspect of the forearm (*red solid line*) so that it does not contact the ulna or disrupt the ulnar periosteum (*red dashed line*). This ensures that the posterior approach to the tuberosity is performed through a muscle-splitting approach to minimize the chance of radioulnar synostosis

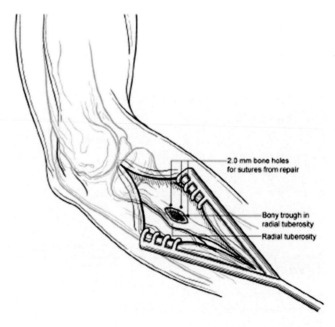

Fig. 10.4 Once the radial tuberosity is exposed, a bony trough is made to receive the freshened tendon end. Three 2.0-mm drill holes are made along the posterior cortex of the tuberosity, with care taken to ensure an adequate bone bridge between drill holes

The arm is then supinated, and, using a curved hemostat, the Fiberwire sutures are passed through the biceps tract, hugging the radial tuberosity, and into the posterior skin incision. Care is taken to ensure that the lateral antebrachial cutaneous nerve remains lateral to the biceps tendon at all times and does not become tethered around the tendon. The arm in pronated, and the elbow flexed to deliver the sutures posteriorly. Using a suture-passing device, the proximal limb of the proximal Krakow suture is passed through the proximal drill hole of the radial tuberosity, followed by the two middle sutures (one from each Krakow) into the middle hole, and finally the distal limb into the distal hole. Once passed, the slack is taken out of the sutures and the biceps is delivered into the bone trough. The appropriate paired sutures (identified by their slightly different lengths) are then tied over the posterior bone bridge.

At completion of the repair, the elbow is gently ranged while in supination, assessing the excursion of the repair, in an effort to guide rehabilitation. The wounds are irrigated and closed sequentially. The anterior skin incision is closed in layers, utilizing a subcuticular stitch for the skin. If the biceps rupture is more chronic and shortening of the tendon has occurred, it may be advantageous to close the anterior skin incision after the biceps sutures have been passed posteriorly, but before they have been tied, as elbow extension and exposure to the anterior incision may be compromised. Similarly, the posterior skin incision is also closed in layers, utilizing a running subcuticular skin closure. Drains are usually not necessary. The elbow is immobilized in 90° flexion with the forearm in supination.

Surgical Procedure: The One-Incision Technique

Patient Positioning

As with the two-incision technique, patients are positioned supine, with the extremity on a hand table. A tourniquet is placed on the upper arm but often is not inflated. The arm is prepped and draped free.

Instrumentation

Many variations of the one-incision technique have been described, utilizing suture anchors, EndoButtons, pullout sutures over an external button, interference screws, etc. As such, it is beyond the scope of this text to describe all of these various techniques utilizing all of the possible fixation

methods. We will describe the technique utilizing suture anchors in the radial tuberosity as an illustrative example of the one-incision technique. Any anchor single-loaded with a heavy, nonabsorbable suture is adequate, and most techniques describe using metal anchors versus bioabsorbable anchors. A high-speed burr can be used to decorticate the tuberosity in an effort to improve tendon healing to bone.

Procedure

Once the patient is anesthetized, positioned, and prepped and draped, an upside-down L incision is made, with the horizontal limb in the elbow flexion crease, and the vertical limb extending from the medial aspect of the horizontal limb along the medial volar forearm (see Fig. 10.1). As described in the two-incision technique, a proximal extension along the volar–lateral arm is often not necessary as the biceps can often be identified and pulled distally in the acute setting by palpation in the subcutaneous tissue. However, the greater the chronicity of the injury (especially after 4 weeks), the greater the likelihood that the incision will need to be extended proximal to the elbow crease (making the inverted L into an S).

After the skin incision, dissection is carried into the subcutaneous tissue, to the level of the deep fascia. The lateral antebrachial cutaneous nerve is identified on the lateral aspect of the incision and it should be retracted laterally. Often, a rent in the deep fascia is observed, and digital palpation will identify the bicipital tunnel to the radial tuberosity. If the fascia is intact, it should be incised and then the biceps stump should be identified. The biceps tendon will often retract to the level of the lacertus fibrosis, but may retract more proximally if the aponeurosis is torn. In most acute tears, the biceps stump can often be palpated just proximal to the incision, on the undersurface of the fascia. Once identified, the stump is passed into the wound distally, freshened, and secured with a traction suture. Any adhesions around the tendon are removed so as to gain maximal excursion of the tendon.

As stated, the tunnel for the biceps is often easily identifiable in the acute setting. Keeping the forearm in maximal supination, the biceps tuberosity can be palpated deep in the antecubital fossa. In the acute setting, it is often not necessary to expose the radial nerve or PIN, but often these can be gently retracted laterally. The radial recurrent vessels often overlie the tuberosity and obscure visualization, therefore necessitating ligation. The radial artery is retracted medially after ligation of the recurrent vessels. It is important to maintain excellent hemostasis for visualization. The tuberosity is then cleaned of soft tissue and a high-speed burr is used to decorticate the surface of the tuberosity to yield a bed for tendon healing. The wound is copiously irrigated to remove all bone debris in an effort to minimize the chance of heterotopic bone formation.

Two suture anchors loaded with nonabsorbable sutures are then placed into the tuberosity under direct visualization in the center of the burred bed. Once placed, the anchor integrity in bone is tested and tensioned. If the anchors do not have good fixation, an alternative method of fixation may be required, such as an EndoButton, pullout sutures, tenodesis screw, etc. The inner limb of suture from each anchor is then passed into the biceps tendon in a running Krakow configuration on the respective medial and lateral aspect of the tendon. These sutures are then tied together at the proximal extent of the biceps tendon (Fig. 10.5).

Keeping the elbow flexed and the forearm in supination, the biceps tendon is delivered to the tuberosity by pulling tension on both of the remaining suture limbs (Fig. 10.6). This applies equal medial and lateral tension and brings the tendon cut surface down flush to the tuberosity bed and the anchors. Once the tendon is flush with the tuberosity bed, these two remaining suture limbs are then tied together after being appropriately tensioned. The wound is again irrigated and the integrity of the repair is evaluated to guide rehabilitation. Keeping the forearm in supination, the elbow is gently extended to test the limits of range of motion. The wound is then closed in layers. Drains are usually not necessary. The elbow is immobilized in a posterior splint in maximal supination after the wound is dressed.

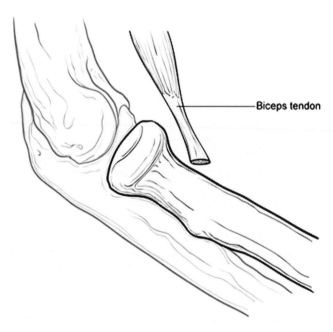

Fig. 10.5 After placement of the anchors in the radial tuberosity, the inner limb from each anchor is passed through the end of the tendon proximally in a Krakow fashion. After sufficient passage of suture, these proximal limbs are then tied together

Postoperative Protocol

Acute repairs (within 4 weeks) are immobilized in flexion and supination in a posterior splint for 7–10 days and then the arm is placed in a hinged orthosis that maintains supination and can gradually be brought out to extension over the next few weeks. In settings where there is no tension on the repair in extension intraoperatively, the patient may be allowed to be without splint immobilization after the first postoperative visit at 7–10 days, although if any concern exists, the repair should be protected and elbow extension gradually regained. Extension is gradually regained after 8 weeks in the orthosis, following which, the patient is allowed unrestricted motion and gradual strengthening. Heavy lifting and sports are restricted until 5 months after repair.

We routinely place patients on oral indomethacin (75 mg daily) for 6 weeks following distal biceps repair to minimize the chance of heterotopic bone formation. Although the likelihood of heterotopic ossification may be less with the one-incision technique, we would use indomethacin in these patients as well.

Results

Historical management of distal biceps ruptures was often nonoperative or nonanatomic, with mixed results. Morrey and colleagues identified some of the functional deficiencies associated with biceps ruptures, including loss of flexion and supination strength, and reported near full restoration of flexion (97%) and supination (95%) strength compared with the uninvolved extremity.[4] More recent analyses have corroborated these findings.[3,6,17,23] A recent comparison of the outcome following acute repairs (<8 days) against delayed repairs (>3 weeks) found excellent results of nine patients undergoing acute repair (all of whom returned to preinjury activity levels) and nine of ten excellent results in the late repair group.[6] Outcomes were classified as excellent if flexion and supination strength was 95% of the contralateral limb, and range of motion was normal. A meta-analysis performed by the same investigators of 147 repairs found 90% excellent results following anatomic repair compared with 14% in nonoperative repairs.

Although the indication and results of acute repair have been well established, the controversy over one-incision versus two-incision techniques still rages. Numerous biomechanical studies have been performed in an attempt to identify which repair is "strongest."[13–16] Pereira and colleagues compared repairs using suture anchor repairs to bone tunnels in cadaveric specimens and found that the repair through bone tunnels was significantly stiffer and stronger, but

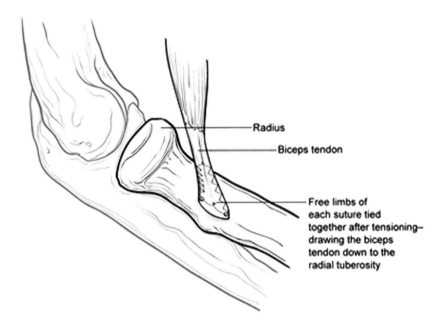

Fig. 10.6 The distal limbs of the suture anchor can then be tightened, drawing the tendon edge into the bony bed where the anchors have been placed, and, once reduced into the bony bed, they are tied, reattaching the biceps tendon

weaker then the native tendon–bone interface.[16] Conversely, Lemos et al. found suture anchor repair using two suture anchors to be significantly stronger then bone tunnels in their biomechanical analysis (263 N vs. 203 N).[15] Other fixation techniques have also been examined. Idler and colleagues found the failure strength and stiffness of an interference screw technique to be significantly greater then a repair through bone tunnels in cadaveric specimens.[14] Greenberg et al. reported that a repair using the EndoButton was significantly stronger then either suture anchor or bone tunnels (584 N vs. 254 N and 178 N, respectively).[13]

Although these studies shed some light on repair strength and options available for fixation, the use of cadaveric specimens for biomechanical testing has some inherent flaws, such as bone quality. Therefore, it is important to take the data in proper context. Until a randomized, prospective trial comparing one-incision to two-incision technique has shown conclusive data, either approach is a viable option when repairing a distal biceps rupture.

Complications

Early reports of the original Boyd–Anderson two-incision repairs found an unacceptable incidence of heterotopic ossification and radioulnar synostosis.[4,24] Other early reports highlighted some of the neurovascular complications that occurred following anterior single-incision repairs, including median and radial nerve palsy.[18,25–27] A recent study by

Kelly and colleagues at the Mayo Clinic reviewed the complication rate of 74 consecutive biceps repairs (acute, subacute, and delayed) using a modified two-incision technique.[18] The overall complication rate was 31% and included five sensory nerve paresthesias (three lateral antebrachial cutaneous, two superficial radial nerve), one PIN palsy (resolved), six patients with anterior-based elbow pain, and four cases of anterior heterotopic ossification. No patients developed radioulnar synostosis. Interestingly, the rate of neurologic complication in this series was similar to the rate following one-incision repairs.

The authors found when they subdivided acute (<10 days) from subacute (10 days to 3 weeks) and delayed (>3 weeks), the likelihood of complications was significantly greater in patients with subacute and delayed repairs. In fact, all patients with postoperative paresthesias were subacute or delayed repairs requiring a formal extended anterior Henry approach. As a result, they concluded that delayed repairs often require more extensive exposure, potentially placing neurovascular and other structures at greater risk.

Conclusion

Rupture of the distal biceps from its insertion on the radial tuberosity often leads to disability and weakness of supination and flexion of the involved extremity. Surgical repair, especially in the acute setting, has been found to reliably reestablish strength and function in the extremity. As such, most authors currently advocate acute surgical repair, although the choice of approach remains controversial. As with most other aspects of orthopedic surgery, a push has been made to perform more minimally invasive techniques for a multitude of conditions, and distal biceps ruptures are no different. The patient with an acute tear, especially those within 10 days from injury, often can be treated with a minimally invasive repair utilizing either a one-incision or a two-incision technique, depending upon surgeon preference.

References

1. Kron SD, Satinsky VP. Avulsion of the distal biceps brachii tendon. Am J Surg 1954;88(4):657–9
2. Baker BE, Bierwagen D. Rupture of the distal tendon of the biceps brachii. Operative versus non-operative treatment. J Bone Joint Surg Am 1985;67(3):414–7
3. D'Alessandro DF, Shields CL, Jr, Tibone JE, Chandler RW. Repair of distal biceps tendon ruptures in athletes. Am J Sports Med 1993;21(1):114–9
4. Morrey BF, Askew LJ, An KN, Dobyns JH. Rupture of the distal tendon of the biceps brachii. A biomechanical study. J Bone Joint Surg Am 1985;67(3):418–21
5. Ramsey ML. Distal biceps tendon injuries: diagnosis and management. J Am Acad Orthop Surg 1999;7(3):199–207
6. Rantanen J, Orava S. Rupture of the distal biceps tendon. A report of 19 patients treated with anatomic reinsertion, and a meta-analysis of 147 cases found in the literature. Am J Sports Med 1999;27(2):128–32
7. Bourne MH, Morrey BF. Partial rupture of the distal biceps tendon. Clin Orthop Relat Res 1991;(271):143–8
8. Kelly EW, Steinmann S, O'Driscoll SW. Surgical treatment of partial distal biceps tendon ruptures through a single posterior incision. J Shoulder Elbow Surg 2003;12(5):456–61
9. Norman WH. Repair of avulsion of insertion of biceps brachii tendon. Clin Orthop Relat Res 1985;(193):189–94
10. Rokito AS, McLaughlin JA, Gallagher MA, Zuckerman JD. Partial rupture of the distal biceps tendon. J Shoulder Elbow Surg 1996;5(1):73–5
11. Boyd HaA, LD. A method for reinsertion of the distal biceps brachii tendon. J Bone Joint Surg Am 1961;43:1041–3
12. Berlet GC, Johnson JA, Milne AD, Patterson SD, King GJ. Distal biceps brachii tendon repair. An in vitro biomechanical study of tendon reattachment. Am J Sports Med 1998;26(3):428–32
13. Greenberg JA, Fernandez JJ, Wang T, Turner C. EndoButton-assisted repair of distal biceps tendon ruptures. J Shoulder Elbow Surg 2003;12(5):484–90
14. Idler CS, Montgomery WH, III, Lindsey DP, Badua PA, Wynne GF, Yerby SA. Distal biceps tendon repair: a biomechanical comparison of intact tendon and 2 repair techniques. Am J Sports Med 2006;34(6):968–74
15. Lemos SE, Ebramzedeh E, Kvitne RS. A new technique: in vitro suture anchor fixation has superior yield strength to bone tunnel fixation for distal biceps tendon repair. Am J Sports Med 2004;32(2):406–10
16. Pereira DS, Kvitne RS, Liang M, Giacobetti FB, Ebramzadeh E. Surgical repair of distal biceps tendon ruptures: a biomechanical comparison of two techniques. Am J Sports Med 2002;30(3):432–6
17. El-Hawary R, Macdermid JC, Faber KJ, Patterson SD, King GJ. Distal biceps tendon repair: comparison of surgical techniques. J Hand Surg (Am) 2003;28(3):496–502
18. Kelly EW, Morrey BF, O'Driscoll SW. Complications of repair of the distal biceps tendon with the modified two-incision technique. J Bone Joint Surg Am 2000;82-A(11):1575–81
19. Lintner S, Fischer T. Repair of the distal biceps tendon using suture anchors and an anterior approach. Clin Orthop Relat Res 1996;(322):116–9
20. Sotereanos DG, Pierce TD, Varitimidis SE. A simplified method for repair of distal biceps tendon ruptures. J Shoulder Elbow Surg 2000;9(3):227–33
21. Seiler JG, III, Parker LM, Chamberland PD, Sherbourne GM, Carpenter WA. The distal biceps tendon. Two potential mechanisms involved in its rupture: arterial supply and mechanical impingement. J Shoulder Elbow Surg 1995;4(3):149–56
22. Louis DS, Hankin FM, Eckenrode JF, Smith PA, Wojtys EM. Distal biceps brachii tendon avulsion. A simplified method of operative repair. Am J Sports Med 1986;14(3):234–6
23. McKee MD, Hirji R, Schemitsch EH, Wild LM, Waddell JP. Patient-oriented functional outcome after repair of distal biceps tendon ruptures using a single-incision technique. J Shoulder Elbow Surg 2005;14(3):302–6
24. Failla JM, Amadio PC, Morrey BF, Beckenbaugh RD. Proximal radioulnar synostosis after repair of distal biceps brachii rupture by the two-incision technique. Report of four cases. Clin Orthop Relat Res 1990;(253):133–6
25. Dobbie R. Avulsion of the lower biceps brachii tendon. Analysis of fifty-one previously unreported cases. Am J Surg 1941;51:662–83
26. Friedmann E. Rupture of the distal biceps brachii tendon. Report on 13 cases. JAMA 1963;184:60–3
27. Meherin JH, Kilgore BS, Jr The treatment of ruptures of the distal biceps brachii tendon. Am J Surg 1960;99:636–40

Chapter 11
Minimally Invasive Approaches for Complex Elbow Trauma

Raymond A. Klug, Jonathon Herald, and Michael R. Hausman

The use of arthroscopic approaches in complex elbow trauma has several advantages over more traditional open approaches. Arthroscopy results in less soft tissue dissection and may reduce postoperative pain and ease rehabilitation. Additionally, arthroscopy allows for improved visualization of intraarticular fractures and may improve anatomic reduction of the articular surface. Aside from standard diagnostic or therapeutic arthroscopy, there are several indications for arthroscopy in addressing fractures about the elbow.

Indications

The indications are pediatric lateral condyle fractures, coronoid fractures without associated radial head fractures, capitellum fractures, and radial head fractures. In our institution, we routinely use arthroscopy in the treatment of all of these indications with the exception of radial head fractures because we think this a technically more demanding procedure with increased risk for neurovascular injury. The following chapter focuses on arthroscopic treatment of coronoid fractures, pediatric lateral condyle fractures, and fractures of the capitellum.

Arthroscopically Assisted Treatment of Coronoid Fractures

The coronoid process of the ulna is of critical importance to elbow stability.[1-7] Although occasionally isolated injuries, fractures of the coronoid most commonly occur in association with ligamentous injury and result in varying degrees of elbow instability. The Regan and Morrey classification described three types of coronoid fractures based on the level

of coronoid detachment in the coronal plane.[8] Type III fractures involve more than 50% of the coronoid process and require open reduction and internal fixation to avoid recurrent elbow instability from loss of bony constraint.[8] More recently, it has been recognized that late elbow instability resulting from soft tissue damage may occur with smaller fracture fragments and that these injuries may be more complex than previously thought (Fig. 11.1).[1, 6, 7]

In patients with apparently isolated type I or II coronoid fractures who have had computed tomography (CT) scans, we have noted the presence of a "sag sign" in the ulnohumeral joint that may be indicative of ligamentous injury due to an associated lateral ulnar collateral ligament (LUCL) or medial collateral ligament (MCL) injury resulting in posterolateral or posteromedial "sagging" of the elbow joint (Fig. 11.2).[7] Additionally, other authors have appreciated the complexity of injury patterns associated with smaller coronoid fractures; open reduction and internal fixation techniques are being performed more frequently for type I and II fractures as associated elbow instability is being recognized more often.[2, 3]

Persistent elbow instability is a challenging problem. Treatment of gross instability, such as that associated with a "terrible triad" type of injury, may require fixation of the coronoid and repair of the anterior capsule, as repair or reconstruction of the radial head and collateral ligaments alone may not adequately stabilize the elbow.[1, 7] Although recurrent frank dislocation is uncommon following surgical treatment of these injuries, lesser degrees of instability may result in premature degenerative changes. Fixation of the coronoid, capsular repair, and stabilization of the joint could potentially decrease this complication, although compelling evidence for this is currently lacking.

The combination of small fracture fragments, comminution, and soft tissue stripping may result in marginal fixation and residual instability despite open reduction. Additionally, there may be loss of the capsule as a stabilizing structure. A less invasive approach achieving accurate reduction and stable fixation may be advantageous when operative fracture treatment is indicated. Repair of the anterior capsule may also be important, particularly when the coronoid fragment is small or comminuted.

R.A. Klug, J. Herald, and M.R. Hausman (✉)
Department of Orthopaedics, Mount Sinai School of Medicine,
One Gustave Levy Place, Box 1188, New York, NY, 10029, USA
Michael.hausman@mountsinai.org

G.R. Scuderi and A.J. Tria (eds.), *Minimally Invasive Surgery in Orthopedics*,
DOI 10.1007/978-0-387-76608-9_11, © Springer Science+Business Media, LLC 2010

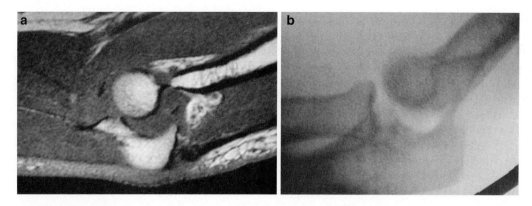

Fig. 11.1 Nonconcentric reduction of ulnohumeral joint with type I coronoid fracture suggesting additional capsuloligamentous injury. (**a**) MRI scan. (**b**) Fluoroscopic examination

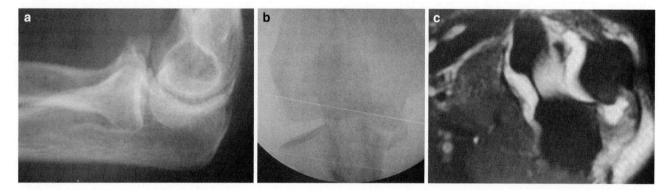

Fig. 11.2 Static varus instability in a patient with type II coronoid fracture. (**a**) Lateral view. (**b**) Anteroposterior (AP) view. (**c**) Axial MRI scan showing posteromedial subluxation

Indications

Doornberg and Ring suggest that Regan-Morrey type I or II coronoid fractures may be associated with a more guarded prognosis than type III fractures because the former are usually, if not always, associated with capsular disruption and/or ligamentous injury. This is not typically the case with type III fractures, which are more commonly purely bony injuries without associated ligamentous disruption.[1, 9]

Various methods of coronoid and capsular repair are available. Medial coronoid compression fractures may be fixed by a medial approach and use of small screws and plates (Fig. 11.3).[7] Larger fragments, such as the type III injury associated with a Monteggia-type fracture-dislocation, may be reduced and fixed from the posterior approach.[10] "Terrible triad" injuries frequently necessitate radial head arthroplasty. In these cases, the coronoid and anterior capsule are accessible from the lateral approach once the radial head is removed (Fig. 11.4).

Conventional open reduction and internal fixation requires extensive exposure and frequently, detachment of residual anterior capsular attachments.[3, 4] With open approaches, a portion of the anterior capsule is detached from the proximal ulna to facilitate exposure of the fracture site. This is technically

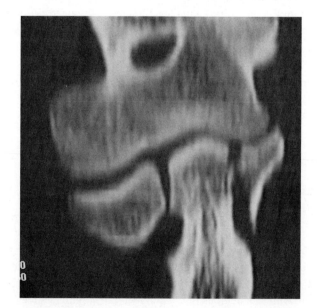

Fig. 11.3 Medial coronoid fracture

difficult and may jeopardize the vascularity of the fracture fragment. More difficult to treat are coronoid fractures with demonstrable, but lesser degrees of instability without radial head fractures or with fracture patterns less amenable to open reduction and internal fixation. In such cases, coronoid repair may be desirable, but repair by open means would require a more extensive surgical approach than would otherwise be needed (Fig. 11.4). The most relevant example of this is the "terrible triad" injury in which fracture of the radial head essentially necessitates open exposure of the lateral side of the elbow. Once the radial head is exposed, it can be retracted or removed to facilitate approach to the coronoid. Without fracture of the radial head, open exposure may no longer be necessary. In such situations, arthroscopically assisted reduction may be of greatest benefit, as it permits fixation of the coronoid and capsular repair without an otherwise unnecessary extensive surgical approach. In addition, repair of small or multiple fragments may only be feasible by capsular repair and this may be technically more feasible by arthroscopic means in those patients not requiring radial head resection for arthroplasty.

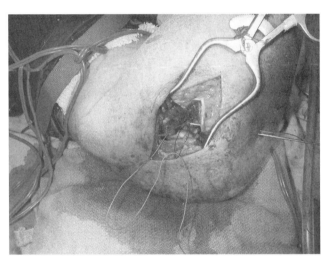

Fig. 11.4 Lateral approach after radial head removal showing capsular repair sutures being passed with a Hewson suture passer

Operative Technique

Patient Positioning

The procedure is performed under nondepolarizing general or regional anesthesia. Patients are placed in the supine position with the affected arm in an arm support (McConnell arm holder, McConnell Orthopaedic Manufacturing Company, Greenville, TX) (Fig. 11.5). The involved extremity is draped free. The shoulder of the involved extremity is positioned at the edge of the bed so that the remainder of the arm can hang free over the edge. The main tube of the C-arm is sterilely draped so that the upper arm and elbow can lie on the base of C-arm, which serves as the operating table.

Arthroscopic Reduction

After marking the major landmarks and confirming the location of the ulnar nerve, a standard proximal anteromedial viewing portal is created using a blunt technique. Low infusion pressures of 25–30 mmHg are used to avoid excessive fluid extravasation. Under arthroscopic visualization, an anterolateral working portal is created and a cannula is introduced into the elbow joint. The anterior compartment of the elbow is inspected first, and a 4.5-mm shaver is used to remove any clot or fracture debris. The coronoid fragment is then visualized and the fracture site is prepared using the soft tissue shaver (Fig. 11.6g). Intraarticular retractors can be used to help with exposure. A trial reduction of the fracture fragment is attempted using an arthroscopic grasper through the anterolateral portal (Fig. 11.6h).

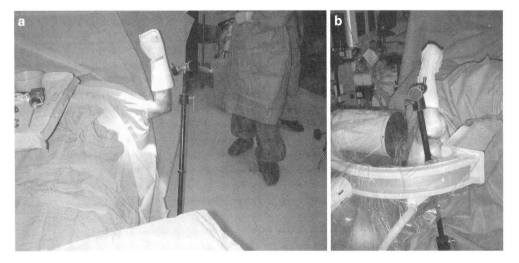

Fig. 11.5 Operating suite setup with McConnell arm holder (**a**) and Mini C-arm (**b**)

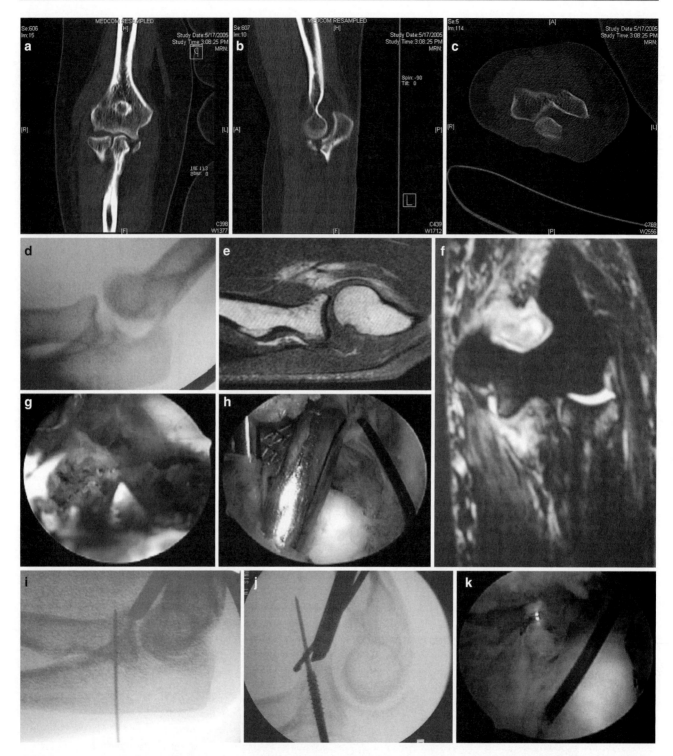

Fig. 11.6 Case example: 53-year-old woman with type II coronoid fracture, posteromedial subluxation, and varus instability. (**a**) Preoperative coronal CT scan showing type II fracture. (**b**) Sagittal cut showing fracture fragments and ulnohumeral subluxation. (**c**) Axial cut showing ulnohumeral subluxation. (**d**) Preoperative fluoroscopic examination. (**e**) Sagittal MRI scan. (**f**) Coronal MRI scan showing intact lateral ulnar collateral ligament. (**g**) Arthroscopic view of fracture site with hema-toma. (**h**) Fracture reduction held with arthroscopic grasper. (**i**) Fluoroscopic view of guide wire placement. (**j**) Reduction held with arthroscopic clamp during drilling and screw placement. (**k**) Arthroscopic monitoring of guide wire placement. (**l**) Placement of capsular repair suture. (**m**) Intraoperative AP view showing fracture reduction and screw placement. (**n**) Intraoperative lateral view showing reduction and screw placement. (**o**) Patient range of motion 6 weeks after surgery

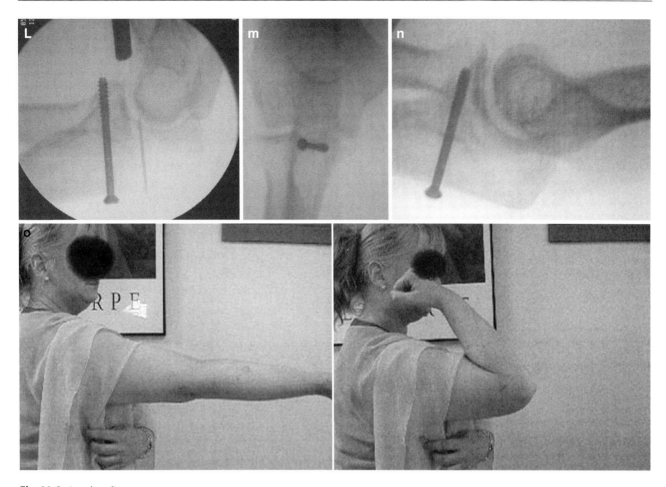

Fig. 11.6   (continued)

Percutaneous Fixation

Next, a 1- to 2-cm incision is made over the posterior aspect of the proximal ulna. Under fluoroscopic control, two guide pins are advanced from the posterior ulnar shaft into the base of the coronoid. Arthroscopic visualization is used to ensure that one guide wire exits centrally in the coronoid fragment. The guide wires are then backed out, and the fracture anatomically reduced and held with an arthroscopic grasper. The wires are then advanced into the coronoid fragment (Fig. 11.6i). The central wire is used for cannulated screw placement while the other wire is for derotational purposes. If the fragment is sufficiently large, two screws may be used, although most type I or II fractures are too small to accept two screws. After fluoroscopic confirmation of the position of the guide wires and the reduction, the screw length is measured with an additional identical guide wire. The original wires are then advanced slightly to avoid inadvertent withdrawal after drilling. If necessary, the wires can be grasped with an alligator clamp for stabilization. A cannulated 2.5-mm drill and tap are used and a 3.5- or 4.0-mm, short threaded cannulated screw is placed while anatomic reduction is monitored under arthroscopic visualization (Fig. 11.6k). An arthroscopic grasper or small gynecological ring curette is used to help reduce and hold the coronoid fragment or fragments in position during drilling and screw placement (Fig. 11.6j).

Capsular Repair

In type I or comminuted fractures, the coronoid fragment may be too small for screw placement. In these cases, the fixation is done with pull-out mattress sutures tied posterolaterally. To do this, an arthroscopic suture passing instrument is used to pass one or two 2–0 Proline (Ethicon, Somerville, NJ) or Fiberwire (Arthrex, Naples, FL) sutures through the anterior capsule and around the coronoid fragments. We have used the Opus suture system (ArthroCare Corp., Austin, TX) and the Spectrum soft tissue repair system (Linvatech Corp., Largo, FL) to place the sutures. Once placed, a Hewson suture retriever or a looped suture is inserted to retrieve the sutures. The sutures are then tied over the posterior, subcutaneous border of the ulna and reduction is confirmed radiographically (Fig. 11.7). This technique can also be used to augment the screw fixation techniques described above. In this case, suture retrieval is done through the cannulated screws (Fig. 11.6l). Postoperatively, all patients are immobilized in a splint for 2–3 weeks and then gradually started with physical therapy for range of motion.

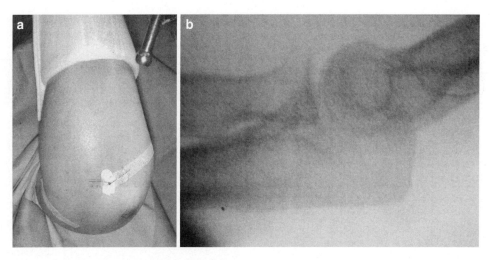

Fig. 11.7 (**a**) Pull-out suture placed for capsular repair. (**b**) Reduction is confirmed fluoroscopically

Results

Preliminary results in our institution have been encouraging. In a study of four consecutive patients with Regan–Morrey type I or 2 coronoid fractures evaluated at a mean of 23.7 weeks, anatomic reduction was achieved in all patients, and all patients went on to osseous union by 6 weeks postoperatively. At final follow-up, all patients had full flexion; three patients had full extension and one patient lacked 10°. The average range of motion was 2.5–140°, with full pronation/supination. There was no residual or recurrent instability, neurovascular injury, infection, or other complications. Stress testing showed no residual varus, valgus, posteromedial, or posterolateral instability. Fluoroscopic examination revealed no instability throughout the range of motion. One patient who did not undergo screw fixation had subsequent removal of a prominent Fiberwire suture over the subcutaneous border of the ulna. One other patient complained of a prominent screw head on the subcutaneous border of the ulna, but opted against hardware removal.

Arthroscopically Assisted Treatment of Pediatric Lateral Humeral Condyle Fractures

Fractures and dislocations about the elbow are second in frequency only to distal forearm injuries in children.[11] Specifically, lateral humeral condyle fractures account for up to 17% of elbow fractures in children.[12, 13]

Pediatric lateral humeral condyle fractures were classified by Milch[13] as type I or II based on the position of the fracture line in relation to the trochlear groove. Salter and Harris[14] further classified those fractures that exit medial to the trochlear groove as type IV according to their classification scheme. Nondisplaced Milch type I fractures can be treated nonoperatively; however, in our experience, truly nondisplaced

fractures are rare. Type I fractures with intraarticular displacement, and all type II fractures require anatomic reduction of the articular surface.

Currently, anatomic reconstitution of the joint surface is done percutaneously following arthrography. If anatomic reduction of the joint surface cannot be achieved with this method, an open Kocher approach to the lateral side of the distal humerus is required. Open approaches not only require dissection of the fine capsulosynovial attachments, but also elevation of the periosteum of the distal fragment, both of which can compromise the vascularity of the distal fragment and lead to avascular necrosis. Arthroscopic reduction of the lateral condyle fracture may avoid this catastrophic complication while still obtaining an anatomic articular reduction. The fracture is then percutaneously pinned and immobilized for 4–6 weeks, per the standard treatment protocol.

Elbow arthroscopy can be performed safely and effectively in the pediatric population by experienced small joint arthroscopists. Micheli et al. have reported the diagnostic and therapeutic benefits of elbow arthroscopy in athletically active pediatric patients.[15] Of their 49 patients, none experienced nerve injury, infection, or postoperative loss of motion. Additionally, Dunn et al. reported good results using arthroscopic synovectomy to reduce hemarthroses in various joints including the elbow for hemophilic joint disease in the pediatric population.[16]

Complications of lateral condyle fractures include avascular necrosis and cubitus valgus deformity. Avascular necrosis, often seen in cases treated with late open reduction is likely due to the extensive soft tissue dissection necessary in healed or partially healed malunited fractures.[17, 18] The primary blood supply to the lateral condyle is a branch of the radial recurrent artery entering along the posterior aspect of the distal humerus. This branch is commonly disrupted by fracture of the lateral condyle. A secondary blood supply arises from the anterolateral capsule and the synovial fold along the lateral border of the capitellum and may be injured during surgical approach. As a result, avascular necrosis may occur with fragmentation of the

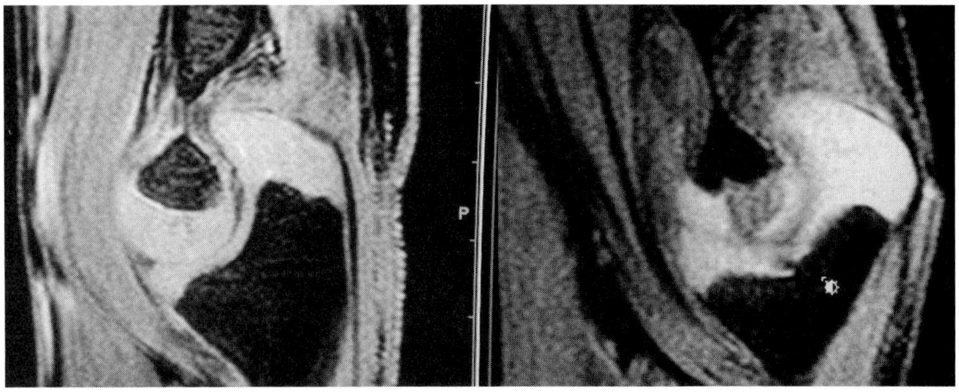

Fig. 11.8 MRI scan showing cartilaginous contribution to the elbow joint and intimate relationship of soft tissue attachments to the distal humerus

capitellum and lateral condyle, resulting in permanent deformity. Regardless of the presence of avascular necrosis, cubitus valgus deformity may occur as a result of fracture malunion or less commonly secondary to lateral condylar epiphysiodesis.

Indications

Although nonoperative treatment can be considered for nondisplaced Milch I fractures, articular surface incongruity must be ruled out. This can be confirmed by arthrogram or possibly via computer tomography. If displaced or unstable fractures are treated nonoperatively, nonunion or malunion may ensue. Operative fixation is indicated in Milch II fractures, as well as displaced Milch I fractures. Great care must be taken to ensure that anatomic reduction is obtained to prevent development of irregularity at the articular surface. Because these fractures involve the physis, nonanatomic reduction may also result in complete or partial growth arrest and/or late deformity.[19]

In order to ensure anatomic articular reduction, most surgeons have resorted to open approaches for displaced lateral humeral condyle fractures. Although great care is taken to preserve the posteriorly based blood supply to the capitulum, the dissection involves detachment of capsulosynovial structures and periosteum that are critical to the vascularity of the distal fracture fragment. These technical difficulties may contribute to the etiology of nonunion, malunion, valgus angulation, and avascular necrosis (Fig. 11.8).[20]

Operative Technique

Patient Positioning

The procedure is performed under nondepolarizing general anesthesia in all patients. The patients are positioned supine with the involved extremity draped free. The shoulder of the

involved extremity is positioned at the edge of the bed so that the remainder of the arm can hang free over the edge. The main tube of the C-arm is sterilely draped so that the upper arm and elbow can lie on the base of the C-arm, which serves as the operating table.

Arthroscopic Reduction

After sterile preparation and draping of the involved upper extremity, standard landmarks for elbow arthroscopy are carefully marked, including the ulnar nerve and the medial epicondyle. A number 15 blade is used to incise the skin and establish a standard anteromedial portal. An atraumatic technique that involves only incision to the dermis with subcutaneous spreading to protect the cutaneous sensory nerves and a special, blunt trocar to enter the joint is used. The joint is usually distended by fracture hematoma and easily entered. A 2.5-mm wrist arthroscope is used for smaller patients (usually below age 3 years), while a standard 4.5-mm arthroscope is used beyond this age. After irrigation of the fracture hematoma, an anterolateral portal is established and used to insert a 3.5-mm shaver to further debride and facilitate visualization of the fracture site. Identification of landmarks on the lateral side is difficult and the lateral portal, if necessary, is made under arthroscopic visualization from the inside–out to avoid erroneous placement.

Percutaneous Pinning

Once the fracture line is visualized, the distal fragment is anatomically reduced under arthroscopic visualization. Manual pressure over the lateral condyle is used to reduce the fracture and 0.062 K-wires are used as joysticks. Any interposed soft tissue blocking the reduction may be debrided or extracted from the fracture site using a probe, an arthroscopic grasper, or a shaver. Then, 0.062 K-wires are inserted into the lateral condyle fragment in a retrograde manner.

Two K-wires are placed in the distal–lateral portion of the fragment and advanced proximally and medially, engaging the medial cortex proximal to the fracture in a standard fashion. A third K-wire is placed at the level of the center of rotation of the capitellum in a lateral to medial direction. This wire is inserted into the trochlea transversely, in a trajectory similar to that employed in fixation of an adult intercondylar fracture, and serves three purposes regarding rotation. First, it allows visualization of the degree of rotational correction needed. Second, it is used to help derotate the fragment, and third, it allows improved fixation stability by preventing rotation around the retrograde wires (Fig. 11.9). The position and trajectory of the K-wires is confirmed fluoroscopically while maintenance of anatomic articular reduction is confirmed arthroscopically.

Postoperative Management

All patients are placed in a long arm cast postoperatively for 4–6 weeks. Patients are followed weekly with radiographs to ensure maintenance of reduction for the first 6 weeks postoperatively. The pins and cast are removed at 4 weeks postoperatively, at which time motion is begun.

Results

Preliminary results in six consecutive patients at our institution have been encouraging. All patients had full active and passive range of motion of the involved elbow from at least 5–130°. There was no statistically significant difference in flexion, extension, or arc range of motion compared with the uninvolved side ($p < 0.05$). There was no difference in carrying angle between the involved and uninvolved sides ($p < 0.05$). One patient had a slight lateral prominence. All patients were pain free at final evaluation. All fractures healed radiographically by 4 weeks. There were no cases of nonunion or malunion. One patient developed radiolucency of the capitulum, which may represent avascular necrosis.

Arthroscopically Assisted Treatment of Capitellum Fractures

Capitellar fractures may be deceptively severe; injuries and complications such as avascular necrosis, malunion, and nonunion may be more common than previously appreciated.

Operative Technique

Patient Positioning

The procedure is performed under nondepolarizing general anesthesia in all patients. The patients are positioned supine with the involved extremity draped free. The shoulder of the involved extremity is positioned at the edge of the bed so that the remainder of the arm can hang free over the edge. The main tube of the C-arm is sterilely draped so that the upper arm and elbow can lie on the base of C-arm, which serves as the operating table. The upper extremity is draped over the chest of the patient for screw placement and lateral fluoroscopic views (Fig. 11.10).

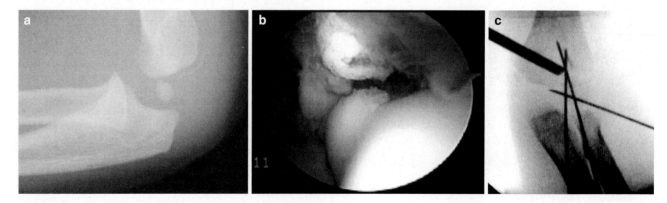

Fig. 11.9 Case example. (**a**) Preoperative lateral view showing subtle displacement of lateral condyle fracture. (**b**) Arthroscopic view showing intraarticular extension of lateral condyle fracture. (**c**) Intraoperative view showing pin placement. Note lateral to medially placed transverse pin

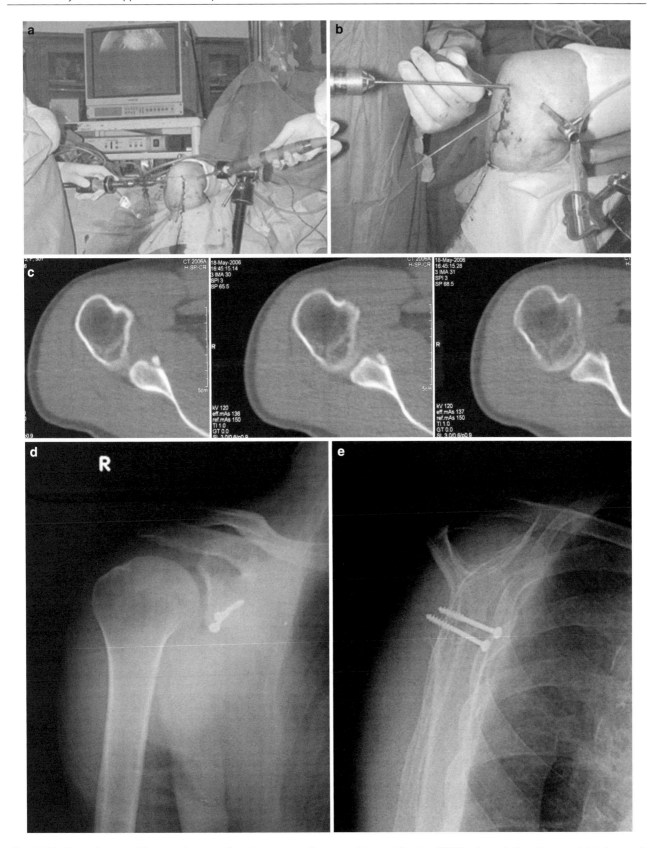

Fig. 11.10 Typical setup of the operating room for arthroscopic reduction and internal fixation (ARIF) of a capitellum fracture. (**a**) Arthroscopic reduction and pin placement. (**b**) Drilling over cannulated wires. (**c**) Fluoroscopic evaluation of guide wire position

Fracture Reduction

Fracture reduction can usually be performed by closed means (Fig. 11.11). The elbow is placed in extension and pronated with a varus stress. If the fragment is reduced, the elbow is then flexed and the forearm supinated to "lock" the capitellar fr agment in place with the radial head.

If the capitellum does not reduce in extension or the radial head remains too prominent to ride over the edge of the capitellar fragment, the capitellum may be manipulated using a 0.062 K-wire joystick. Arthroscopic visualization is rarely necessary at this point. If reduction cannot be achieved, a proximal anteromedial portal can be made for debridement of the hematoma with a curette. Once this is done, a posterior portal can be established proximal to the displaced capitel-

lum. This should be done with great care as distortion of the anatomy may place the radial nerve at increased risk.

One common source of trouble is "plastic deformation" of the distal part of the lateral condyle that prevents anatomic reduction of the displaced coronoid fragment, resulting in an ovoid-shaped capitellum, rather than the desired sphere. Sagittal cuts on a limited CT scan may help anticipate this problem. If present, preliminary curettage of the posterior capitellum from a "soft spot" portal and compaction molding with a Frier or small Cobb elevator may be necessary (Fig. 11.12).

Once preliminary reduction is achieved, standard anteromedial and anterolateral portals are established and debridement is completed. The fracture line through the articular surface is the best indicator of the accuracy of reduction, and intraoperative fluoroscopy cannot always discriminate residual superior and anterior displacement of the distal edge of the capitellum.

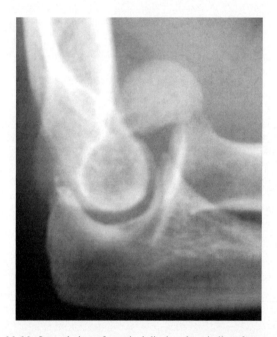

Fig. 11.11 Lateral view of a typical displaced capitellum fracture

Fracture Fixation

Once accuracy of the reduction is confirmed, guide wires are inserted in a posterior to anterior direction into the capitellum for cannulated screw placement. A minimum of two screws should be used. An elevator or trochar should be inserted in the radiocapitellar joint to maintain compression across the fracture site as the wires are advanced (Fig. 11.13).

After measuring the required screw length, the wires are advanced into the radial head to prevent inadvertent extraction. The 2.5-mm cannulated drill is used, taking care not to penetrate the subchondral bone, and short threaded 3.5- or 4-mm cannulated screws are inserted. The reduction is checked once again with the arthroscope and the elbow is extended to ensure the articular surface has not been violated (Fig. 11.14).

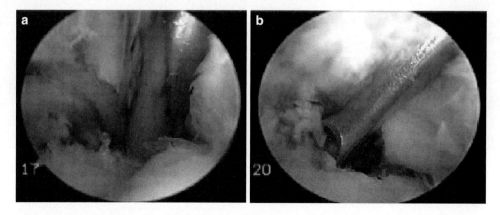

Fig. 11.12 (**a**) Malreduction of the distal edge of the capitellum is seen in this view from the posterolateral portal, passing the arthroscope down the lateral gutter. (**b**) A curette is used to remove debris blocking anatomic reduction

Fig. 11.13 Placement of guide wires. The screws may cross or be placed parallel to one another. The first screw should be placed distal to proximal to compress the fracture site and help reduce any residual displacement of the fragment

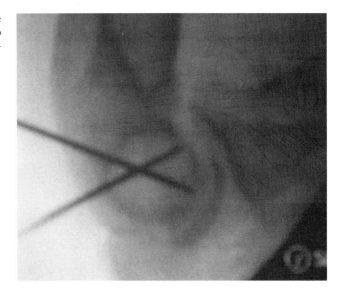

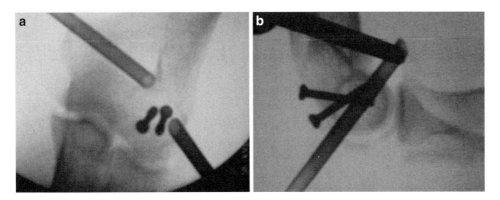

Fig. 11.14 Placement of cannulated screws for fixation of the fragment. (**a**) AP view. (**b**) Lateral view

Headed screws are utilized to take advantage of the additional support and purchase afforded by cortical bone posteriorly. This is particularly important when there is only a thin shell of posterior bone. Thin anterior osteochondral fragments remain challenging even with anterior to posterior screws and may be best treated by immobilization to allow some healing and subsequent arthroscopic release of any residual contracture, rather than risking loss of a substantial portion of the articular surface. Postoperatively, all patients are immobilized in a splint for 2–3 weeks and then gradually started with physical therapy for range of motion.

addressing these injuries. We have begun using arthroscopic techniques in specific fracture patterns in an attempt to decrease some of these complications. In the hands of a skilled arthroscopist, these techniques can provide excellent visualization and enable anatomic repair of some intraarticular elbow fractures with minimal surgical dissection. Arthroscopy also allows for the preservation of soft tissue attachments. Improved instrumentation and surgical technique has expanded the indications for arthroscopy in soft tissue and bony repair in elbow trauma. Our preliminary data is encouraging, however, long-term studies and larger series are necessary.

Summary

Intraarticular fractures about the elbow are often difficult injuries to treat. Several complications have been described, including malunion, nonunion, infection, avascular necrosis, heterotopic ossification, stiffness, and partial or complete growth arrest in children. Many of these complications may be related to the extensile surgical approaches sometimes necessary in

References

1. Doornberg JN, Ring D. Coronoid fracture patterns. J Hand Surg Am 2006; 31:45–52
2. Sanchez-Sotelo J, O'Driscoll SW, Morrey BF. Medial oblique compression fracture of the coronoid process of the ulna. J Shoulder Elbow Surg 2005; 14:60–64
3. Pugh DM, Wild LM, Schemitsch EH, King GJ, McKee MD. Standard surgical protocol to treat elbow dislocations with radial

head and coronoid fractures. J Bone Joint Surg Am 2004; 86: 1122–1130

4. Cage DJ, Abrams RA, Callahan JJ, Botte MJ. Soft tissue attachments of the ulnar coronoid process. An anatomic study with radiographic correlation. Clin Orthop Relat Res 1995 Nov; (320):154–158

5. Closky RF, Goode JR, Kirschenbaum D, Cody RP. The role of the coronoid process in elbow instability. A biomechanical analysis of axial loading. J Bone Joint Surg Am 2000; 82:1749–1755

6. O'Driscoll SW, Bell DF, Morrey BF. Posterolateral rotatory instability of the elbow. J Bone Joint Surg Am 1991; 73:440–446

7. O'Driscoll SW, Jupiter JB, Cohen MS, Ring D, McKee MD. Difficult elbow fractures: pearls and pitfalls. Instr Course Lect 2003; 52:113–134

8. Regan W, Morrey BF. Fractures of the coronoid process of the ulna. J Bone Joint Surg Am 1989; 71:1348–1354

9. Broberg MA, Morrey BF. Results of treatment of fracture-dislocations of the elbow. Clin Orthop Relat Res 1987 Mar;(216):109–19.

10. Ring D, Jupiter JB, Simpson NS. Monteggia fractures in adults. J Bone Joint Surg Am 1998 Dec;80(12):1733–44

11. Lichtenburg R. A study of 2532 fractures in children. Am J Surg 1954; 87:330–338

12. Flynn JC, Richards JF, Saltzman RI. Prevention and treatment of nonunion of slightly displaced fractures of the lateral humeral

13. condyle in children. An end-result study. J Bone Joint Surg Am 1975; 57:1087–1092

13. Milch H. Fractures and fracture-dislocations of humeral condyles. J Trauma 1964; 4:592–607

14. Salter R, Harris W. Injuries involving the epiphyseal plate. J Bone Joint Surg Am 1963; 45:587–592

15. Micheli LJ, Luke AC, Mintzer CM, et al. Elbow arthroscopy in the pediatric and adolescent population. Arthroscopy 2001; 17(7): 694–699

16. Dunn AL, Busch MT, Wyly JB, et al. Arthroscopic synovectomy for hemophilic joint disease in a pediatric population. J Pediatr Orthop 2004; 24(4):414–426

17. Haraldsson S. On osteochondrosis deformas juvenilis capituli humeri including investigation of intraosseous vasculature in distal humerus. Acta Orthop Scand Suppl. 1959; 38:1–23

18. Jakob R, Fowles JV, Rang M, et al. Observations concerning fractures of the lateral humeral condyle in children. J Bone Joint Surg Br 1975; 57:430–436

19. Bernstein SM, King JD, Sanderson RA. Fractures of the medial epicondyle of the humerus. Contemp Orthop 1981; 12:637–641

20. Skak SV, Olsen SD, Smaabrekke A. Deformity after fracture of the lateral humeral condyle in children. J Pediatr Orthop B 2001; 10(2):142–152

Chapter 12
Minimally Invasive Approaches for Lateral Epicondylitis

Bradford O. Parsons and Michael R. Hausman

Lateral epicondylitis is a painful condition that affects the lateral aspect of the elbow, usually centered around the epicondyle of the humerus. Historically called tennis elbow, this condition occurs in both men and women, usually in the 35- to 50-year age range, and rarely in tennis players. Patients present with laterally based elbow pain, exacerbated with repetitive stresses to the wrist and finger extensors, specifically the extensor carpi radialis brevis (ECRB) and extensor digitorum communis (EDC). A distinct pathoetiology has not been elucidated, and as such most patients have an idiopathic source, although some patients report "work-related" causes. Direct trauma is rarely a source of tennis elbow pain, neither is tennis, as only 5–10% of patients with lateral epicondylitis are tennis players.[1] Most patients report an insidious onset with pain associated with gripping, carrying, and holding objects with the forearm in pronation and the elbow in extension.

The natural history of tennis elbow is that it will usually resolve over time, but often with a protracted course. Numerous nonoperative and operative modalities to treat lateral epicondylitis have been described in the literature, although determining the "best" treatment is difficult if not impossible based on the literature.[1–15] Currently, most patients who are indicated for operative treatment of their painful tennis elbow are managed with one of two procedures, a formal open release, as described originally by Hohmann, and modified by Nirschl, or an arthroscopic release.[6,9] A review of the literature will reveal support for both open and arthroscopic techniques, and until a well-designed prospective, randomized trial comparing these techniques is available, many surgeons are guided by "their subjective viewpoint and clinical experience."[16] As such, we will describe the open and the arthroscopic procedures to treat patients with tennis elbow, both of which adhere to the principles of minimally invasive procedures.

Pathoanatomy

Lateral epicondylitis pain is located near the origin of the extensor muscles at the lateral epicondyle, most frequently at the origin of the ECRB and EDC. The ECRB originates on the anterior aspect of the lateral epicondyle, deep to the EDC and inferior to the extensor carpi radialis longus (ECRL), which originates proximally on the flare of the lateral column just above the lateral epicondyle. The ECRL muscle is the most superficial and proximal muscle observed during tennis elbow open surgery, and serves as a guide to the ECRB, which is deep and distal to the muscle.

Although the ECRB has historically been implicated in lateral epicondylitis, anatomically there is no distinct division between the ECRB and EDC origins. Often, the pathologic lesion is observed in this confluent area. Additionally, the tendinous origins of the EDC and ECRB are confluent with the lateral ulnar collateral ligament (LUCL), which may be palpable as a stout band deep to the muscle.[17] Iatrogenic LUCL injuries following tennis elbow procedures have been reported and an understanding of the normal ligamentous anatomy of the lateral elbow is critical to preventing ligament injury and elbow instability.[18,19] The LUCL originates off of the lateral epicondyle and inserts on the proximal ulna. The lesion associated with lateral epicondylitis is usually anterior to the LUCL and can be treated without damaging this critical structure.

Although often misrepresented as an inflammatory process, lateral epicondylitis does not involved acute inflammation. Biopsy specimen analyses of the pathologic tissue found at the ECRB and EDC origin have not shown acute or chronic inflammation, but have shown vascular proliferation, hyaline degeneration, and granulation tissue.[2,8,15,20–23] Some have hypothesized that the changes seen on specimen analysis may be a result of some of the nonoperative treatments of lateral epicondylitis, such as cortisone injections.[16]

Degeneration of the ECRB/EDC origin may not be the sole etiology of symptoms in patients who are diagnosed with lateral epicondylitis. Recently, one of us[8] described a meniscal-like fold of tissue that extends off of the radiocapitellar capsule and impinges on the radial head or interposes

B.O. Parsons (✉) and M.R. Hausman
Department of Orthopaedics, Mount Sinai School of Medicine, One Gustave Levy Place, Box 1188, New York, NY, 10029, USA
e-mail: Bradford.parsons@mountsinai.org

G.R. Scuderi and A.J. Tria (eds.), *Minimally Invasive Surgery in Orthopedics*,
DOI 10.1007/978-0-387-76608-9_12, © Springer Science+Business Media, LLC 2010

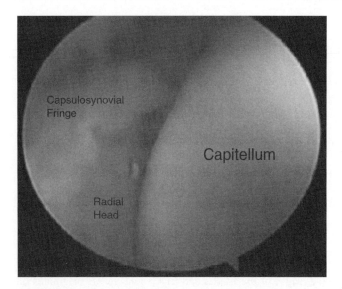

Fig. 12.1 Capsulosynovial fringe of tissue seen arthroscopically in many patients with lateral epicondylitis. Often this tissue can be found to be impinging on the radial head articular cartilage, causing synovitis and pain

in the radiocapitellar joint in patients with symptoms of lateral epicondylitis, similar to a "snapping plica" lesion described by others (Fig. 12.1).[2,24,25] This capsulosynovial fringe of tissue was found in a large subset of patients, and a cadaveric study also identified this same tissue in many specimens. In their series, the authors resected the pathologic fringe of tissue back to the native annular ligament. Subsequent to surgery, 28 of 30 patients subjectively graded their outcome as either better (4 patients) or much better (24 patients). The exact role this tissue has in patients with lateral epicondylitis remains to be seen, but an open technique often does not allow the identification of such pathologic lesions.

Diagnosing Lateral Epicondylitis

Lateral epicondylitis is diagnosed by a careful history and physical examination. Patients often report a specific *event* that heralds the onset of their symptoms, but often, upon further investigation, an insidious onset is appreciated. As mentioned previously, rarely are patients tennis players. History should identify exacerbating activities, such as carrying objects with the wrist extended and the forearm pronated. Painful symptoms with gripping activities, such as turning a doorknob or holding objects (even as small as a toothbrush), should be elicited.

Mechanical symptoms, such as locking or clicking, may describe an intraarticular source, such as loose bodies, or a capsulosynovial fold. Additionally, any symptoms of instability,

especially in the face of failed open tennis elbow surgery, should be elicited. Often, these patients will describe vague pain with activities that mimic the lateral pivot shift maneuver, such as rising out of an armchair by pushing off with the triceps. Patients who report numbness or tingling or shooting pains often have a neurologic source of their pain, such as radial tunnel. Often the subtle differences in radial tunnel and tennis elbow can be identified by physical examination.

Patients with tennis elbow have tenderness at the ECRB/EDC origin, often one fingerbreadth distal and anterior to the tip of the lateral epicondyle. Pain is exacerbated with provocative maneuvers. These include pain with resisted wrist extension, more so with the elbow in extension versus flexion. Pain can also be elicited with resisted long finger extension. Gripping with the elbow in extension can also evoke painful symptoms. Often, symptoms are less dramatic with these provocative maneuvers performed in elbow flexion versus elbow extension, especially gripping tests.

Clicking over the radiocapitellar joint while moving the elbow through an arc of motion, or tenderness over the joint line, may indicate an intraarticular source, such as loose bodies or a plica. A provocative test for a symptomatic plica can be performed by moving the elbow through an arc of motion while the patient holds their forearm in pronation and wrist in resisted extension.[24] This maneuver causes a large plica to "snap" back and forth into the radiocapitellar joint.

Patients with lateral epicondylitis need to be differentiated from those with radial tunnel syndrome. Radial tunnel syndrome is caused by compression of the posterior interosseous nerve in the radial tunnel. These patients often have more poorly localized pain, often distal to the epicondyle, and may also have wrist aching or complaints of "heaviness" in the forearm or wrist. Tenderness is elicited in the area of the radial tunnel, not over the ECRB/EDC origin. Pain may be exacerbated by resisted supination or resisted long finger extension. It is possible for patients to have findings of both lateral epicondylitis and radial tunnel, and differentiating the primary problem may be difficult. An injection of local anesthetic, with or without cortisone, can be helpful in determining the exact source of symptoms.

Plain radiograph results of the elbow are often normal in patients with lateral epicondylitis, but may reveal a degenerative changes or loose bodies. Magnetic resonance imaging (MRI) is used in patients whose diagnosis is not obvious, or in those patients where suspicion that an intraarticular lesion, such as a plica, may be present. However, the utility of MRI in evaluation of these patients has not been validated, and is often not necessary. Electromyogram (EMG) analysis is not usually helpful in diagnosing radial tunnel syndrome, which remains a diagnosis based on the history and physical examination.

Nonoperative Management

Most patients with symptoms of lateral epicondylitis will improve with nonoperative measures and time, although a long course is often observed. Numerous nonoperative modalities have been attempted, with little validation of their success, including bracing, acupuncture, ultrasound, extracorporeal shock wave therapy, and laser treatment, among many others.[4,5,7,12,14] We find that a mainstay of nonoperative management is patient education and activity modification in an effort to diminish inciting or exacerbating activities. Patients should learn to carry objects with the forearm supinated and wrist straight. Avoiding grip or wrist extension often is helpful in alleviating symptoms. Laborers who perform repetitive activities, especially those requiring substantial force across the extensor origin, should have duties restricted and modified. Additionally, the use of tools that generate vibratory forces should be restricted.

Patients may benefit from a home-based physical therapy regimen aimed at stretching and strengthening the extensors, while using modalities such as ice and heat to reduce pain and improve mobility. Additionally, counterforce braces are often used to relieve pressure on the ECRB origin, thereby (in theory) allowing the body to heal the degenerative tissue. Finally, patients with acute painful processes may get symptomatic relief from a steroid injection, although most series report temporary relief in patients, often those previously untreated for their symptoms.[11,26]

Surgical Indications

While some[21] have outlined specific indications for surgical management of patients with tennis elbow, many patients "fail" nonoperative measures because of the impact symptoms have on their ability to work or their quality of life. Such patients, especially if temporary relief was obtained with a steroid injection, are candidates for operative treatment. All patients are initially managed nonoperatively with a rehabilitation program and steroid injection, and those patients whose symptoms do not improve enough or within an acceptable modicum of time are offered surgery.

Determining which surgery to perform for patients with lateral epicondylitis can be more difficult then choosing which patients should be indicated. No consensus of procedure, whether percutaneous, open, or arthroscopic can be clearly gleaned from the current literature. Nearly all procedures currently utilize mini-incisions and avoid extensive exposures. Therefore, we describe both the traditional open approach as well as the arthroscopic procedure we use.

Patients who have classic signs and symptoms of lateral epicondylitis are amenable to an open release, as are those with recurrent symptoms. Additionally, any patients with symptoms of posterolateral rotatory instability will require open surgery, as ligament reconstruction is likely to be required. Conversely, those with signs and symptoms of intraarticular lesions, such as mechanical symptoms, are indicated for arthroscopic management. In our practice, we have transitioned to performing nearly all tennis elbow procedures arthroscopically because of the ability to evaluate the joint and look for synovial folds and plicas, as well as debride the ECRB origin (if pathologic).

Contraindications

There are no specific contraindications for surgical management of patients with lateral epicondylitis. Most errors of management come following inaccurate diagnosis or failure to appreciate subtle instability or joint derangement. Obviously, patients who are unable to undergo anesthesia are not candidates, and are managed nonoperatively.

Surgical Procedure: Open Lateral Epicondylitis Debridement

Patient Positioning

Patients are positioned supine with the arm on a hand table. Either regional or general anesthesia can be used. A tourniquet is placed on the upper arm, and the extremity is draped free distal to the tourniquet. The hand is covered with a stockinet.

Procedure

Once the patient is anesthetized and draped, the incision is marked out. The lateral epicondyle and radiocapitellar joint is identified and marked, and the incision is marked along a line from the epicondyle toward Lister's tubercle distally, measuring 2–3 cm (Fig. 12.2). The arm is exsanguinated and the tourniquet is inflated to 100 mmHg above systolic blood pressure. The incision is carried down to the fascia of the extensor muscles. Identification of the ECRL fascia is the landmark to finding the ECRB. The thin fascia with muscle tissue present is the ECRL, while the thicker fascia posteriorly represents the EDC. The ECRB fascia will be deep and anterior to the ECRL fascia.

At this point, the fascial septae are palpated to discern the orientation of the LUCL, which divides the radiocapitellar

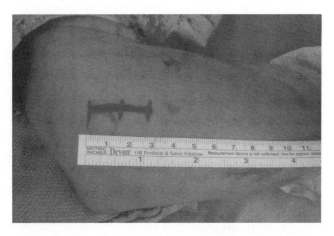

Fig. 12.2 Skin incision for open tennis elbow release. The incision is along a line from the anterior aspect of the lateral epicondyle to Lister's tubercle in the wrist. Usually, a few centimeters are sufficient

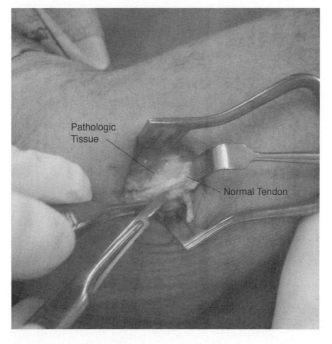

Fig. 12.3 Pathologic tissue often observed during open tennis elbow release

joint into two hemispheres. The LUCL will feel as a thickened band of the fascia. The fascia of the ECRL is then incised just anterior to the LUCL, along the length of the skin incision. The ECRB/EDC origins are now exposed. Often at this point, the degenerated, pathologic tissue of lateral epicondylitis can be identified in the origin (Fig. 12.3). The pathologic tissue is excised sharply starting distally at the boundary of pathologic and normal tissue, extending proximally to the origin off of the lateral epicondyle. Often the entire thickness of the portion of

the ECRB/EDC involved is removed, although care should be taken to not violate the joint capsule at this point.

The anterior limit of dissection is the muscle of the ECRL, while posteriorly it is the normal portion of the EDC tendinous origin. Some authors have advocated burring or drilling the bone of the lateral epicondyle after all pathologic tissue has been removed.[3,9,21] In theory this helps bring fresh blood into the area and help healing, but we have found, as have others,[27,28] that this increases perioperative pain and may delay recovery. Therefore, we do not decorticate the lateral epicondyle at the origin of the ECRB.

Patients with suspected intraarticular pathology should have the joint inspected through a small capsulotomy, although exposure is limited through this mini-incision approach, and therefore an arthroscopic evaluation may be more appropriate. To expose the joint, the anterolateral capsule of the radiocapitellar joint is incised from the anterior column distally. Utmost care should be taken to not violate the LUCL, which originates on the epicondyle. By incising the anterolateral capsule of the radiocapitellar joint, the capsulotomy will remain in the anterior hemisphere of the joint and should not violate the LUCL. The supinator muscle fibers are often encountered distally over the radiocapitellar joint and can be bluntly dissected off of the capsule and retracted to give a little more distal exposure. This will allow limited exposure of the radiocapitellar joint.

The wound is then irrigated with normal saline and the joint capsule (if opened) is closed with 3–0 Vicryl suture. The anterior and posterior fascial edges are then approximated together with a 2–0 Vicryl suture. We do not repair the fascia back to the epicondyle through bone tunnels or using suture anchors, but rather repair the fascia together in a side-to-side method. The skin is repaired using a 3-0 Monocryl suture in the dermis and a 4-0 running subcuticular stitch. The wound is dressed with Steri-Strips and a bandage. The elbow is initially immobilized in a long arm splint in 90° flexion and the wrist in slight dorsiflexion.

Rehabilitation

The splint is removed at the first postoperative visit at 7–10 days, and active range of motion exercises of the elbow, wrist, and hand are started. Additionally, the patient is allowed to use the extremity for activities of daily living. A removable wrist splint with dorsiflexion cock-up is given for comfort if needed. Strengthening exercises are begun at 6 weeks with unrestricted use of the extremity beginning at 3 months.

Surgical Technique: Arthroscopic Lateral Epicondylitis Release

Patient Positioning

Either regional or general anesthesia may be used. Arthroscopic release may be performed in either the lateral decubitus or supine position, as preferred by the surgeon. The lateral decubitus positioning will be described here. The patient is positioned lateral decubitus on a beanbag with care to pad the all bony prominences and ensure no pressure is placed on the peroneal nerve of the contralateral leg. A tourniquet is placed around the upper arm and the extremity is draped free with a stockinet placed over the hand. The extremity is placed over a lateral elbow positioner so that the arm is parallel to the floor, and the elbow flexed 90°. The arm is positioned so that the holder is at the midpoint of the humerus, just distal to the tourniquet. Care should be taken to ensure further flexion is possible without impingement of the hand against the operating table, and that instruments can be utilized without impingement against the holder prior to draping.

Instrumentation

Standard arthroscopic instruments are used, including a 4.0-mm, 30° arthroscope and 5.5-mm unfenestrated cannulas. A full radius 3.5-mm shaver is used, as is an electrocautery ablation device. Extra switching sticks (preferably pointed, not blunt tip) are used to retract during arthroscopy. A spinal needle is used to localize portal placement from an inside-out technique. Occasionally a banana blade is also used to remove a capsulosynovial fringe when present.

Procedure

After the patient is positioned, standard arthroscopic portals are marked, including a proximal anteromedial, an anterolateral, a trans-triceps posterior, and a posterolateral portal (a detailed discussion of portal placement in elbow arthroscopy is discussed in Chapter 8). Additionally, the palpable landmarks are also marked, including the medial epicondyle, medial intermuscular septum, capitellum, radial head, and the course of the ulnar nerve (Fig. 12.4). The arm is then exsanguinated and the tourniquet raised to 100 mmHg over systolic pressure.

The joint is then insufflated with 25 cc of normal saline via the direct lateral "soft spot" (the center of a triangle formed by the lateral epicondyle, radial head, and olecranon). The proximal anteromedial portal is incised and bluntly developed with a clamp, taking care to remain anterior to the intermuscular septum. The 4.0-mm trochar and camera sleeve are then placed into the joint just above the trochlea, with joint penetration confirmed by backflow of fluid through the cannula outflow.

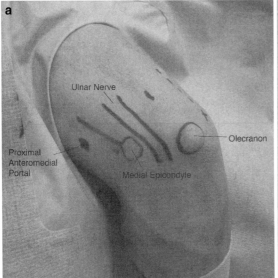 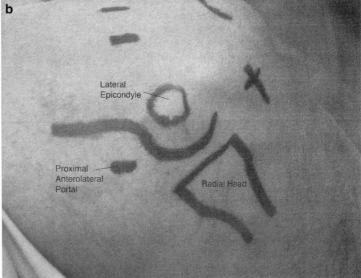

Fig. 12.4 Position and surface landmarks for arthroscopic tennis elbow release. (**a**) The medial landmarks include the medial epicondyle (*circle*), ulnar nerve, and medial intramuscular septum (*line*). (**b**) Laterally, the epicondyle (*circle*), radial head, and capitellum are landmarks. Standard portals are marked

The 4.0-mm, 30° arthroscopic camera is then introduced and a diagnostic arthroscopy is performed of the anterior joint. Under direct visualization, the working anterolateral portal is made by introducing a spinal needle into the joint so that it enters just anterior to the junction of the capitellum and lateral column, at the ECRB-capsular attachment to the lateral column. The portal should be made proximal enough to allow an angle of approach to the anterior capsular tissue of the radiocapitellar joint. Once established, a smooth cannula is introduced over a pointed switching stick into the lateral portal. The 3.5-mm shaver is then used through the lateral working portal to debride any synovitis and clean the anterolateral capsule.

Often a capsulosynovial fold will be observed adherent to the annular ligament and radial head, occasionally interposing into the radiocapitellar joint (Fig. 12.1). When observed, this tissue is removed to expose the native annular ligament and uncover the radial head. It has been one of our experiences that this often seems to be the source of pain in these patients. The aberrant capsular tissue is removed using a combination of shaver, electrocautery ablation, and occasionally a banana blade for tough, resistant tissue. Care is taken to protect the radial head articular cartilage, which, once exposed, often reveals areas of contact degeneration as a result of direct pressure from the pathologic capsular folds (Fig. 12.5).

After removal of this tissue, attention is then turned to the anterolateral capsule and overlying ECRB/EDC origin. Often this area is synovitic in patients with tennis elbow. The capsule is removed with electrocautery, starting proximally at the junction of the anterior capitellum and lateral column. The capsule is removed from deep to superficial, at which

point the tendon of the ECRB and EDC is visible. The capsule is removed distally to the level of the radiocapitellar joint, taking care to remain in the anterior hemisphere of the capitellum to protect the LUCL. Once the capsule is removed, the ECRB/EDC tendon origins are removed with the shaver until healthy muscle fibers (ECRL) are exposed.

Often, patients with intraarticular-based symptoms or synovitis anteriorly will have posterior or posterolateral compartment involvement as well. The posterior trans-triceps portal is developed, along with a proximal posterolateral (working) portal to evaluate the posterior compartment of the elbow. The olecranon and olecranon fossa are evaluated, and if normal attention is taken, to the posterolateral gutter, especially in patients who had the aforementioned pathologic capsulosynovial fold compressing the radiocapitellar joint. This tissue frequently extends posterolaterally to encroach on the radial head and radiocapitellar joint, and if the posterolateral gutter is not visualized, this tissue will be missed.

The posterolateral gutter is entered by placing the arthroscope in the proximal posterolateral (working) portal, and passing it posterior to the capitellum, just lateral to the olecranon. Once confirmation of location is obtained by visualizing the radial head and sigmoid notch of the ulna, a distal posterolateral (accessory or radiocapitellar) portal is made under direct visualization. Any synovitis or pathologic capsular tissue is removed by shaving and electrocautery. Care is taken to not violate the LUCL, which travels along the lateral aspect of the joint, from the epicondyle around the radial head onto the ulna. By working more medially along the lateral surface of the ulna and around the radial head, the LUCL can be avoided.

After all debridement is completed, the joint is copiously irrigated with fluid and the portals are closed with interrupted nylon stitches, with care taken to obtain a watertight closure in an effort to prevent sinus formation. The wounds are dressed and the elbow is placed in a posterior splint for immobilization.

Rehabilitation

One of the advantages of an arthroscopic debridement is that the only "healing" that needs to occur is the skin of the portals. As there is no fascial repair, the elbow does not need to be protected. As such, the splint and bandages are removed after 3 days by the patient, and the patient is allowed to use the elbow for activities of daily living within their limits of discomfort. Stitches are removed at the first postoperative visit in 7–10 days. As perioperative pain resolves, the patient is allowed to resume all activities, including athletics. Formal rehabilitation is reserved for the rare patient who develops perioperative stiffness of the elbow.

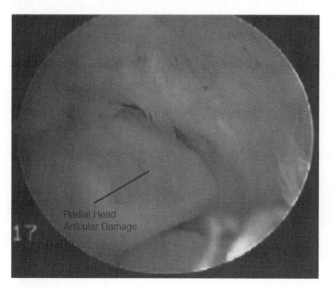

Fig. 12.5 Damaged radial head articular cartilage observed after resection of impinging capsulosynovial fringe of pathologic tissue during elbow arthroscopy

Results

Many patients with tennis elbow improve with time and nonoperative measures, however, patients with recalcitrant symptoms often undergo surgical treatment. The surgical management of lateral epicondylitis has been the source of much debate, with multiple procedures described, most with similar results. Most series report 80–85% of patients obtaining "good to excellent" results, with few prospective series available for analysis.[3,6,8–10,15,16,21,27–30] Hohmann reported 86–88% satisfactory results following the original description of open release of patients with tennis elbow in 1933.[6] Nirschl and Pettrone cited 85% good to excellent results in their review of 88 elbows treated with their modified open release, which included isolated debridement of the pathologic tendon tissue, decortication of the epicondyle, and repair of the ECRL.[9] Additionally, 85% of their patients returned to full activity, including sports. Subsequently, the Nirschl technique became the "gold standard" in the surgical management of patients with tennis elbow.

Similar reports are found with more recent analyses of open procedures. Zingg and Schneeberger reported 81% of 21 patients had a satisfactory outcome with no or mild pain.[28] However, they voiced concern over the prolonged perioperative recovery following open release using the modified Nirschl method. They found similar results to Khashaba, who reported increased pain and greater stiffness in patients who had decortication and drilling of the epicondyle compared with those who had just release in a prospective, randomized series of 23 elbows.[27] Based on these recent investigations, we currently debride the pathologic tissue during open release, but do not decorticate or drill the epicondyle.

Concerns over perioperative pain and delayed recovery following open repair, as well as allowing for an intraarticular evaluation, led many surgeons to perform arthroscopic releases of the ECRB/EDC origin to manage tennis elbow.[8,10,29,30] Peart et. al. found that 72% of arthroscopic releases had good to excellent outcomes, similar to the 69% following open release, but the patients treated arthroscopically recovered and returned to work faster.[10] Stapleton and Baker reported faster recovery and quicker return to sports in a review of open versus arthroscopically treated elbows (35 vs. 66 days for return to sport).[30] They also found that 60% of patients treated arthroscopically had associated intraarticular disorders. A later study by Kaminsky and Baker reported that 95% of 39 patients were "better" or "much better" following arthroscopic release.[29] Similarly, in a series performed at our institution, Mullet et al. reported 93% of patients were "better" or "much better" following arthroscopic debridement. The patients in this series returned to work at an average of 7 days.[8]

We have found arthroscopic release allows for the potential of quicker recovery, often resulting in less need for rehabilitation. Additionally, associated intraarticular lesions, especially any capsulosynovial folds impinging on the radiocapitellar joint, can be removed, whereas they may be missed following an open release. Although having many potential advantages, elbow arthroscopy is technically challenging and has a substantial learning curve, and is not without complication, such as nerve injury. As such, until a prospective, randomized trial examining arthroscopic versus open release is performed, a clear answer as to the "gold standard" approach will be lacking.

Conclusion

Most patients with lateral epicondylitis will obtain symptomatic improvement with nonoperative modalities. Occasionally, however, patients cannot tolerate their symptoms, or are not improving expeditiously enough and can benefit from surgical intervention. As with many other areas of orthopedic surgery, a trend toward minimally invasive surgical techniques has occurred, and the treatment of tennis elbow is no different. Traditional open techniques involve minimally dissection and exposure, and with more surgeons becoming comfortable with arthroscopic elbow surgery, the surgical management of tennis elbow has become truly minimally invasive. Arthroscopy offers many advantages, including visualization of the entire joint, faster recovery (including return to work), and results compare favorably to many of the reports of traditional open techniques.

References

1. Assendelft WJ, Hay EM, Adshead R, Bouter LM. Corticosteroid injections for lateral epicondylitis: a systematic overview. Br J Gen Pract 1996;46(405):209–216
2. Bosworth DM. The role of the orbicular ligament in tennis elbow. J Bone Joint Surg Am 1955;37-A(3):527–533
3. Dunkow PD, Jatti M, Muddu BN. A comparison of open and percutaneous techniques in the surgical treatment of tennis elbow. J Bone Joint Surg Br 2004;86(5):701–704
4. Haker E, Lundeberg T. Pulsed ultrasound treatment in lateral epicondylalgia. Scand J Rehabil Med 1991;23(3):115–118
5. Harding W. Use and misuse of the tennis elbow strap. Phys Sportsmed 1992;20:65–74
6. Hohmann G. Das Wesen und die Behandlung des sogenannten Tennisellbogens. Munch Med Wochesnschr 1933;80:250–252
7. Molsberger A, Hille E. The analgesic effect of acupuncture in chronic tennis elbow pain. Br J Rheumatol 1994;33(12):1162–1165
8. Mullett H, Sprague M, Brown G, Hausman M. Arthroscopic treatment of lateral epicondylitis: clinical and cadaveric studies. Clin Orthop Relat Res 2005;439:123–128

9. Nirschl RP, Pettrone FA. Tennis elbow. The surgical treatment of lateral epicondylitis. J Bone Joint Surg Am 1979;61(6A):832–839

10. Peart RE, Strickler SS, Schweitzer KM, Jr. Lateral epicondylitis: a comparative study of open and arthroscopic lateral release. Am J Orthop 2004;33(11):565–567

11. Price R, Sinclair H, Heinrich I, Gibson T. Local injection treatment of tennis elbow - hydrocortisone, triamcinolone and lignocaine compared. Br J Rheumatol 1991;30(1):39–44

12. Rompe JD, Hopf C, Kullmer K, Heine J, Burger R, Nafe B. Low-energy extracorporal shock wave therapy for persistent tennis elbow. Int Orthop 1996;20(1):23–27

13. Smidt N, van der Windt DA, Assendelft WJ, Deville WL, Korthals-de Bos IB, Bouter LM. Corticosteroid injections, physiotherapy, or a wait-and-see policy for lateral epicondylitis: a randomised controlled trial. Lancet 2002;359(9307):657–662

14. Vasseljen O, Jr, Hoeg N, Kjeldstad B, Johnsson A, Larsen S. Low level laser versus placebo in the treatment of tennis elbow. Scand J Rehabil Med 1992;24(1):37–42

15. Verhaar J, Walenkamp G, Kester A, van Mameren H, van der Linden T. Lateral extensor release for tennis elbow. A prospective long-term follow-up study. J Bone Joint Surg Am 1993;75(7):1034–1043

16. Boyer MI, Hastings H, II. Lateral tennis elbow: "Is there any science out there?" J Shoulder Elbow Surg 1999;8(5):481–491

17. Cohen MS, Hastings H, II. Rotatory instability of the elbow. The anatomy and role of the lateral stabilizers. J Bone Joint Surg Am 1997;79(2):225–233

18. Kalainov DM, Cohen MS. Posterolateral rotatory instability of the elbow in association with lateral epicondylitis. A report of three cases. J Bone Joint Surg Am 2005;87(5):1120–1125

19. Morrey BF. Reoperation for failed treatment of refractory lateral epicondylitis. J Shoulder Elbow Surg 1992;1:47–55

20. Bosworth DM. Surgical treatment of tennis elbow; a follow-up study. J Bone Joint Surg Am 1965;47(8):1533–1536

21. Nirschl RP. Elbow tendinosis/tennis elbow. Clin Sports Med 1992;11(4):851–870

22. Potter HG, Hannafin JA, Morwessel RM, DiCarlo EF, O'Brien SJ, Altchek DW. Lateral epicondylitis: correlation of MR imaging, surgical, and histopathologic findings. Radiology 1995;196(1):43–46

23. Regan W, Wold LE, Coonrad R, Morrey BF. Microscopic histopathology of chronic refractory lateral epicondylitis. Am J Sports Med 1992;20(6):746–749

24. Antuna SA, O'Driscoll SW. Snapping plicae associated with radiocapitellar chondromalacia. Arthroscopy 2001;17(5):491–495

25. Duparc F, Putz R, Michot C, Muller JM, Freger P. The synovial fold of the humeroradial joint: anatomical and histological features, and clinical relevance in lateral epicondylalgia of the elbow. Surg Radiol Anat 2002;24(5):302–307

26. Solveborn SA, Buch F, Mallmin H, Adalberth G. Cortisone injection with anesthetic additives for radial epicondylalgia (tennis elbow). Clin Orthop Relat Res 1995;(316):99–105

27. Khashaba A. Nirschl tennis elbow release with or without drilling. Br J Sports Med 2001;35(3):200–201

28. Zingg PO, Schneeberger AG. Debridement of extensors and drilling of the lateral epicondyle for tennis elbow: a retrospective follow-up study. J Shoulder Elbow Surg 2006;15(3):347–350

29. Kaminsky SB, Baker CL, Jr. Lateral epicondylitis of the elbow. Tech Hand Up Extrem Surg 2003;7(4):179–189

30. Stapleton TR, Baker, CL. Arthroscopic treatment of lateral epicondylitis: a clinical study [abstract]. Arthroscopy 1996;12:365–366

Chapter 13
Overview of Wrist and Hand Approaches: Indications for Minimally Invasive Techniques

Steve K. Lee

Orthopedic surgery has seen a recent explosion of minimally invasive techniques[1–7] and the wrist and hand are no exception. These techniques range from percutaneous, endoscopic, arthroscopic, to mini-open procedures. The main topics covered in the following chapters include minimally invasive fixation for wrist fractures, endoscopic carpal tunnel release, minimally invasive trigger finger release, and minimally invasive treatment of finger fractures. Indications and advantages of minimally invasive wrist and hand surgery will be discussed as well as detailed descriptions of these new surgical techniques.

Similar to advantages proposed in other regions of orthopedic surgery, the advantages of minimally invasive techniques for surgery of the wrist and hand include shorter recovery times, earlier return to work, and less scar tissue formation with potentially improved outcomes.[8,9] Advances in visualization via endoscopic and arthroscopic cameras and improved anatomic knowledge for increased safety during minimally invasive approaches have helped expand the use and experience in these techniques.

Regarding wrist fractures, the surgeon has a wide range of options for distal radius fracture operative treatment, such as external fixation, open reduction and internal fixation with fixed-angle plates and other devices, and minimally invasive techniques of percutaneous intrafocal Kapandji pinning, mini-open reduction and bone grafting, and arthroscopic reduction and fixation, among others.[10–16] Distal to the radial platform, the main paradigm for minimally invasive carpal bone fracture treatment is arthroscopic reduction and internal fixation of scaphoid fractures championed by Slade and others.[17–21]

Endoscopic carpal tunnel release has been shown to decrease recovery times with earlier return to work.[8,9] Generally, outcomes are similar to open carpal tunnel release after 3 months.[22] Potential complications range from failure of surgery from incomplete release to reversible and irreversible nerve injury.[23–27] There are two major types of endoscopic carpal tunnel release: the one-incision technique of Agee,[28] and the two-incision technique of Chow.[29,30]

Trigger finger release has classically been performed with an open technique of a 1- to 2-cm incision, either transversely, obliquely, or longitudinally placed. Minimally invasive techniques include percutaneous with a hypodermic needle, endoscopic, and mini-open with special trigger digit devices.[31–40]

Regarding hand fractures, it is generally accepted that the less dissection and open exposure is performed, the better the results. Open approaches run the risk of increased scarring between bone and the soft tissues of tendon, ligament, and skin. When possible, closed reduction and internal fixation (usually by percutaneous pinning) is preferable.[41–44] Percutaneous pinning minimizes scarring, the hardware is inexpensive and readily available, and the hardware is easy to remove in the office. Recent new reduction clamps with built-in pin guides help simplify the pinning.

External fixation and other minimally invasive techniques have been described.[45–49] Arthroscopic reduction and internal fixation has been described for intraarticular fractures of the metacarpophalangeal joints of the thumb and fingers,[50] the carpometacarpal joint of the thumb (basal joint), and the proximal interphalangeal joints of the fingers. Small joint arthroscopy is a relatively new technique and does not enjoy as widespread use as its larger cousins. Continued advances in miniature optics and surgical techniques will spawn new advances in minimally invasive treatment techniques of hand fractures.

The following chapters discuss in depth specific techniques of minimally invasive wrist and hand surgery. Special emphasis will be on indications, advantages of minimally invasive techniques, anatomy, surgical technique, and pearls and pitfalls.

S.K. Lee (✉)
Division of Hand Surgery, Department of Orthopaedic Surgery,
The New York University Hospital for Joint Diseases,
New York, NY, USA; Department of Orthopaedic Surgery,
The New York University School of Medicine, New York, NY, USA;
Hand Surgery Service Bellevue Hospital Center, New York, NY, USA
e-mail: steve.lee@nyumc.org

G.R. Scuderi and A.J. Tria (eds.), *Minimally Invasive Surgery in Orthopedics*,
DOI 10.1007/ 978-0-387-76608-9_13, © Springer Science+Business Media, LLC 2010

References

1. Bottner F, Delgado S, Sculco TP. Minimally invasive total hip replacement: the posterolateral approach. American Journal of Orthopedics (Belle Mead, N.J.) 2006;35(5):218–24

2. Egol KA. Minimally invasive orthopaedic trauma surgery: a review of the latest techniques. Bulletin (Hospital for Joint Diseases (New York, N.Y.)) 2004;62(1–2):6–12

3. Klein GR, Parvizi J, Sharkey PF, Rothman RH, Hozack WJ. Minimally invasive total hip arthroplasty: internet claims made by members of the Hip Society. Clinical Orthopaedics and Related Research 2005 Dec;(441):68–70

4. Langlotz K. Minimally invasive approaches in orthopaedic surgery. Minimally Invasive Therapy and Allied Technologies 2003;12(1):19–24

5. Lehman RA, Jr., Vaccaro AR, Bertagnoli R, Kuklo TR. Standard and minimally invasive approaches to the spine. The Orthopedic Clinics of North America 2005;36(3):281–92

6. Nogler M. Navigated minimal invasive total hip arthroplasty. Surgical Technology International 2004;12:259–62

7. Wall EJ, Bylski-Austrow DI, Kolata RJ, Crawford AH. Endoscopic mechanical spinal hemiepiphysiodesis modifies spine growth. Spine 2005;30(10):1148–53

8. Saw NL, Jones S, Shepstone L, Meyer M, Chapman PG, Logan AM. Early outcome and cost-effectiveness of endoscopic versus open carpal tunnel release: a randomized prospective trial. The Journal of Hand Surgery (Edinburgh, Lothian) 2003;28(5):444–9

9. Trumble TE, Diao E, Abrams RA, Gilbert-Anderson MM. Single-portal endoscopic carpal tunnel release compared with open release: a prospective, randomized trial. The Journal of Bone and Joint Surgery American 2002;84-A(7):1107–15

10. Weil WM, Trumble TE. Treatment of distal radius fractures with intrafocal (kapandji) pinning and supplemental skeletal stabilization. Hand Clinics 2005;21(3):317–28

11. Duncan SF, Weiland AJ. Minimally invasive reduction and osteosynthesis of articular fractures of the distal radius. Injury 2001;32(Suppl 1):SA14–24

12. Ring D, Jupiter JB. Percutaneous and limited open fixation of fractures of the distal radius. Clinical Orthopaedics and Related Research 2000 Jun;(375):105–15

13. Geissler WB, Fernandes D. Percutaneous and limited open reduction of intra-articular distal radial fractures. Hand Surgery 2000;5(2):85–92

14. Auge WK, II, Velazquez PA. The application of indirect reduction techniques in the distal radius: the role of adjuvant arthroscopy. Arthroscopy 2000;16(8):830–5

15. Trumble TE, Wagner W, Hanel DP, Vedder NB, Gilbert M. Intrafocal (Kapandji) pinning of distal radius fractures with and without external fixation. The Journal of Hand Surgery 1998;23(3):381–94

16. Naidu SH, Capo JT, Moulton M, Ciccone W, II, Radin A. Percutaneous pinning of distal radius fractures: a biomechanical study. The Journal of Hand Surgery 1997;22(2):252–7

17. Slade JF, III, Grauer JN, Mahoney JD. Arthroscopic reduction and percutaneous fixation of scaphoid fractures with a novel dorsal technique. The Orthopedic Clinics of North America 2001; 32(2):247–61

18. Slade JF, III, Jaskwhich D. Percutaneous fixation of scaphoid fractures. Hand Clinics 2001;17(4):553–74

19. Slade JF, III, Gutow AP, Geissler WB. Percutaneous internal fixation of scaphoid fractures via an arthroscopically assisted dorsal approach. The Journal of Bone and Joint Surgery American 2002;84-A(Suppl 2):21–36

20. Slade JF, III, Geissler WB, Gutow AP, Merrell GA. Percutaneous internal fixation of selected scaphoid nonunions with an arthroscopically assisted dorsal approach. The Journal of Bone and Joint Surgery American 2003;85-A (Suppl 4):20–32

21. Slade JF, III, Dodds SD. Minimally invasive management of scaphoid nonunions. Clinical Orthopaedics and Related Research 2006 Apr;(445):108–19

22. Macdermid JC, Richards RS, Roth JH, Ross DC, King GJ. Endoscopic versus open carpal tunnel release: a randomized trial. The Journal of Hand Surgery 2003;28(3):475–80

23. Thoma A, Veltri K, Haines T, Duku E. A meta-analysis of randomized controlled trials comparing endoscopic and open carpal tunnel decompression. Plastic and Reconstructive Surgery 2004; 114(5):1137–46

24. Kretschmer T, Antoniadis G, Borm W, Richter HP. [Pitfalls of endoscopic carpal tunnel release]. Der Chirurg; Zeitschrift fur alle Gebiete der operativen Medizen 2004;75(12):1207–9

25. Thoma A, Veltri K, Haines T, Duku E. A systematic review of reviews comparing the effectiveness of endoscopic and open carpal tunnel decompression. Plastic and Reconstructive Surgery 2004;113(4):1184–91

26. Uchiyama S, Yasutomi T, Fukuzawa T, Nakagawa H, Kamimura M, Miyasaka T. Median nerve damage during two-portal endoscopic carpal tunnel release. Clinical Neurophysiology 2004; 115(1):59–63

27. Varitimidis SE, Herndon JH, Sotereanos DG. Failed endoscopic carpal tunnel release. Operative findings and results of open revision surgery. The Journal of Hand Surgery (Edinburgh, Lothian) 1999;24(4):465–7

28. Agee JM, Peimer CA, Pyrek JD, Walsh WE. Endoscopic carpal tunnel release: a prospective study of complications and surgical experience. The Journal of Hand Surgery 1995;20(2):165–71; discussion 172

29. Chow JC, Hantes ME. Endoscopic carpal tunnel release: thirteen years' experience with the Chow technique. The Journal of Hand Surgery 2002;27(6):1011–8

30. Chow JC. Endoscopic release of the carpal ligament for carpal tunnel syndrome: long-term results using the Chow technique. Arthroscopy 1999;15(4):417–21

31. Slesarenko YA, Mallo G, Hurst LC, Sampson SP, Serra-Hsu F. Percutaneous release of A1 pulley. Techniques in Hand & Upper Extremity Surgery 2006;10(1):54–6

32. Ragoowansi R, Acornley A, Khoo CT. Percutaneous trigger finger release: the "lift-cut" technique. British Journal of Plastic Surgery 2005;58(6):817–21

33. Wilhelmi BJ, Mowlavi A, Neumeister MW, Bueno R, Lee WP. Safe treatment of trigger finger with longitudinal and transverse landmarks: an anatomic study of the border fingers for percutaneous release. Plastic and Reconstructive Surgery 2003;112(4):993–9

34. Wilhelmi BJ, Snyder NT, Verbesey JE, Ganchi PA, Lee WP. Trigger finger release with hand surface landmark ratios: an anatomic and clinical study. Plastic and Reconstructive Surgery 2001;108(4):908–15

35. Blumberg N, Arbel R, Dekel S. Percutaneous release of trigger digits. The Journal of Hand Surgery (Edinburgh, Lothian) 2001; 26(3):256–7

36. Ha KI, Park MJ, Ha CW. Percutaneous release of trigger digits. The Journal of Bone and Joint Surgery 2001;83(1):75–7

37. Dunn MJ, Pess GM. Percutaneous trigger finger release: a comparison of a new push knife and a 19-gauge needle in a cadaveric model. The Journal of Hand Surgery 1999;24(4):860–5

38. Cihantimur B, Akin S, Ozcan M. Percutaneous treatment of trigger finger. 34 fingers followed 0.5–2 years. Acta Orthopaedica Scandinavica 1998;69(2):167–8

39. Bain GI, Turnbull J, Charles MN, Roth JH, Richards RS. Percutaneous A1 pulley release: a cadaveric study. The Journal of Hand Surgery 1995;20(5):781–4; discussion 785–6

40. Pope DF, Wolfe SW. Safety and efficacy of percutaneous trigger finger release. The Journal of Hand Surgery 1995;20(2):280–3

41. Geissler WB. Cannulated percutaneous fixation of intra-articular hand fractures. Hand Clinics 2006;22(3):297–305, vi

42. Sawaizumi T, Nanno M, Nanbu A, Ito H. Percutaneous leverage pinning in the treatment of Bennett's fracture. Journal of Orthopaedic Science 2005;10(1):27–31

43. Galanakis I, Aligizakis A, Katonis P, Papadokostakis G, Stergiopoulos K, Hadjipavlou A. Treatment of closed unstable metacarpal fractures using percutaneous transverse fixation with Kirschner wires. The Journal of Trauma 2003;55(3):509–13

44. Klein DM, Belsole RJ. Percutaneous treatment of carpal, metacarpal, and phalangeal injuries. Clinical Orthopaedics and Related Research 2000 Jun;(375):116–25

45. Freeland AE, Orbay JL. Extraarticular hand fractures in adults: a review of new developments. Clinical Orthopaedics and Related Research 2006 Apr;(445):133–45

46. Mader K, Gausepohl T, Pennig D. [Minimally invasive management of metacarpal I fractures with a mini-fixateur]. Handchir Mikrochir Plast Chir 2000;32(2):107–11

47. McCulley SJ, Hasting C. External fixator for the hand: a quick, cheap and effective method. Journal of the Royal College of Surgeons of Edinburgh 1999;44(2):99–102

48. Drenth DJ, Klasen HJ. External fixation for phalangeal and metacarpal fractures. The Journal of Bone and Joint Surgery 1998;80(2):227–30

49. Seitz WH, Jr., Gomez W, Putnam MD, Rosenwasser MP. Management of severe hand trauma with a mini external fixateur. Orthopedics 1987; 10(4):601–10

50. Slade JF, III, Gutow AP. Arthroscopy of the metacarpophalangeal joint. Hand Clinics 1999;15(3):501–27

Chapter 14
Minimally Invasive Surgical Fixation of Distal Radius Fractures

Phani K. Dantuluri

The advent of improved surgical instrumentation and advances in healthcare have driven the rapidly evolving field of orthopedics. There has been a trend toward minimally invasive surgery in order to improve cosmesis, minimize soft tissue trauma, and allow superior fracture healing by minimally disturbing the biological environment around the fracture. Minimally invasive joint replacement surgery, arthroscopic surgery, and locking screw technology have been some of the newer developments in orthopedics that have significantly altered patient care and potentially the outcomes that can be achieved. In this regard, fractures of the distal radius have also been reexamined to see if minimally invasive surgery would be possible in treating this increasingly common fracture of the upper extremity and one of the leading reasons for visits to the emergency room.

Standard treatment for distal radius fractures not too long ago was cast immobilization. Closed reduction and percutaneous pinning and external fixation were some of the earlier methods used to treat fractures of the distal radius.[1,2] However, there were limits to the types of fractures that could be treated closed, leading to increasing recognition of the importance of restoring articular congruity and fracture alignment.[3,4] This needed to be done in an open fashion, and open reduction and internal fixation became much more common. Various types of plate and screw constructs were used to treat fractures of the distal radius. Plates were applied internally to the distal radius, as the idea of rigid fracture fixation with an internal implant was appealing to surgeon and patient alike.[5]

This trend has accelerated rapidly over the last decade and, at this point, the most commonly used implant to treat fractures of the distal radius has become the volar plate.[6] Other pioneers in the field of upper extremity surgery have championed the cause of column-specific fixation with smaller implants addressing specific load-bearing areas of the distal radius in an attempt to provide more rigid fixation

with smaller implants.[7] These methods have all been tremendously successful in treating fractures of the distal radius, however, problems still remain.[8]

There is a thin soft tissue envelope surrounding the distal radius and the neurovascular structures are in very close proximity. Tendon and nerve complications are quite common with surgery of the distal radius despite advances in implant technology and lower profile implants.[9,10] Locking screw technology has definitely improved fracture fixation and allowed for less complications as implants are lower profile, however, significant problems remain with tendon irritation and rupture as well as nerve problems, scar formation, stiffness, and the occasional need to remove implants.

The only type of implant that could potentially avoid these types of complications is an intramedullary one, as the implant could be seated completely underneath the cortical surface and not cause impingement on neighboring soft tissue and neurovascular structures. In addition, these implants can be inserted in the most minimally invasive fashion.

As modern medicine has rapidly surged forward, a greater understanding of the basic science of fracture healing has resulted. It has become clear that preservation of the blood supply to fracture fragments can greatly aid in fracture healing and lead to better clinical results. If one could successfully reduce a fracture and maintain its alignment with a minimal amount of soft tissue trauma while preserving the vascularity of fracture fragments, this would be optimal.

It has been known for quite some time that intramedullary implants have become the standard of care for diaphyseal fractures of the tibia and the femur in patients who need operative fixation.[11] These have been shown to have excellent results. The benefits of intramedullary fixation include less soft tissue trauma, preservation of the vascularity of fracture fragments, and an implant that acts as a load-sharing device rather than a load-bearing one. Some prior investigators have examined the concept of intramedullary fixation for fractures of the distal radius, but no specific completely intramedullary implant for the distal radius had been developed.[12–19]

In an attempt to avoid many of the mentioned complications associated with the current surgical treatment of distal

P.K. Dantuluri (✉)
Department of Orthopaedics, Thomas Jefferson University Hospital, Jefferson Medical College, The Philadelphia Hand Center, 834 Chestnut Street, Suite G114, Philadelphia, PA, 19106, USA
e-mail: pkdantuluri@handcenters

G.R. Scuderi and A.J. Tria (eds.), *Minimally Invasive Surgery in Orthopedics*,
DOI 10.1007/ 978-0-387-76608-9_14, © Springer Science+Business Media, LLC 2010

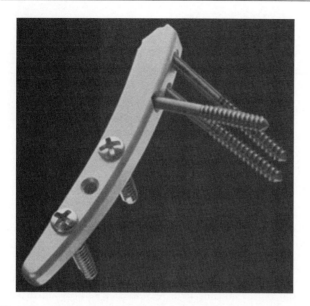

Fig. 14.1 MICRONAIL distributed by Wright Medical Technologies, Inc., demonstrating purple distal fixed-angle locking screws and gold proximal bicortical screws (From Dantuluri P. Distal Radius Fractures, An Issue of Atlas of the Hand Clinics, November 2006, with permission of Elsevier, Inc.)

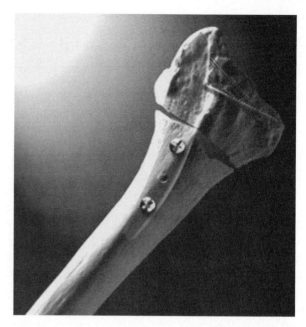

Fig. 14.2 Virtual image demonstrating ideal intramedullary nail position (From Dantuluri P. Distal Radius Fractures, An Issue of Atlas of the Hand Clinics, November 2006, with permission of Elsevier, Inc.)

radius fractures, several investigators in conjunction with Wright Medical Technologies, Inc. have developed a novel intramedullary device (MICRONAIL) for fixation of distal radius fractures (Fig. 14.1). This implant utilizes fixed-angle locking screw technology in conjunction with an intramedullary construct in order to rigidly stabilize fractures of the distal radius while preserving fracture fragment vascularity and minimizing soft tissue trauma.

Indications

Intramedullary nail fixation is best indicated for extraarticular distal radius fractures that are unstable and cannot be maintained with closed reduction (Fig. 14.2). Simple intraarticular fractures of the distal radius can also be treated with this device, but the fracture should have a minimum number of stable articular fragments and should not have extensive articular comminution. Fractures should also not have excessive metaphyseal-diaphyseal comminution with proximal extension, as the proximal fixation point for the device could be compromised, resulting in a loss of reduction. The device is an excellent choice for malunion surgery and is best indicated for extraarticular malunions of the distal radius. The device can provide an immediate rigid construct in malunion surgery and better disperse loading forces through the distal radius as it is a load-sharing device rather than a load-bearing one. This is of great benefit in malunion surgery as the resulting cortical defect that exists after surgical

correction can take several months to reintegrate and, during this time, plate and screw constructs are subjected to tremendous loads that can lead to implant failure. It is necessary to carefully evaluate the initial injury and postreduction films to determine the appropriate patients amenable to intramedullary fixation.

Preoperative Planning

The preoperative radiographic evaluation follows a detailed history and physical examination and includes standard anteroposterior (AP), lateral, and oblique radiographs of the injured wrist (Fig. 14.3). Careful assessment of the ipsilateral upper extremity, particularly the elbow and forearm, are necessary to rule out more complex injury patterns, e.g., Essex-Lopresti injuries. Further radiographs of the forearm and elbow can be acquired if deemed necessary from the physical examination and history. A thorough neurovascular examination is of necessity and a careful assessment of the associated soft tissue injury is of paramount importance.

Contralateral radiographs of the opposite wrist are recommended in order to carefully evaluate each patient's individualized anatomy of the distal radius and are useful in preoperative templating for implant selection. Postreduction radiographs, if available, should also be evaluated to further assess fracture stability (Fig. 14.4). Prior history of injury or malunion of the injured distal radius needs to be addressed

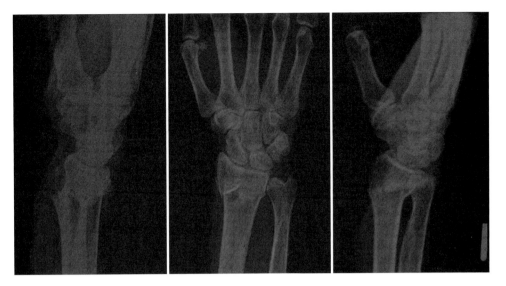

Fig. 14.3 Initial injury films demonstrating dorsal angulation, radial shortening, and loss of radial inclination (From Dantuluri P. Distal Radius Fractures, An Issue of Atlas of the Hand Clinics, November 2006, with permission of Elsevier, Inc.)

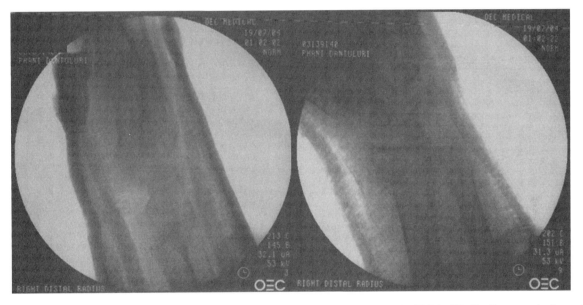

Fig. 14.4 Postreduction films demonstrate fracture instability and lack of alignment (From Dantuluri P. Distal Radius Fractures, An Issue of Atlas of the Hand Clinics, November 2006, with permission of Elsevier, Inc.)

preoperatively as significant alteration in the normal parameters of the distal radius may prevent implant insertion.

Necessary Equipment

The minimally invasive surgical technique for intramedullary nail fixation of distal radius fractures described below requires the following specific equipment: (1) Wright Medical Intramedullary Implant System, (2) one 0.62 Kirshner wire and two 0.45 Kirshner wires, (3) K-wire driver, (4) drill, (5) small rongeur, and (6) intraoperative fluoroscopy.

Surgical Technique

Operative Setup

The versatility of the intramedullary system is that nail fixation can be performed if necessary in the multiply injured patient, in the supine, lateral decubitus, or prone positions. If there is no contraindication, surgery is most easily performed with the patient in the supine position. A standard arm board is attached to the side of the operating room table and is used to support the operative extremity (Fig. 14.5). However, a hand table can also alternatively be used, but the single arm

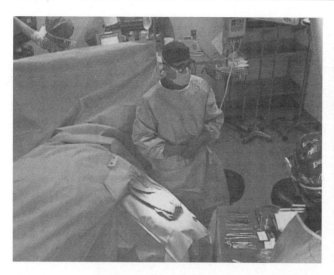

Fig. 14.5 Patient positioning with a single arm board for an injured extremity demonstrated (From Dantuluri P. Distal Radius Fractures, An Issue of Atlas of the Hand Clinics, November 2006, with permission of Elsevier, Inc.)

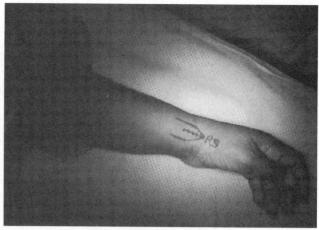

Fig. 14.6 Lateral view of injured extremity demonstrating contours of radial styloid (*RS*) and proposed surgical incision (From Dantuluri P. Distal Radius Fractures, An Issue of Atlas of the Hand Clinics, November 2006, with permission of Elsevier, Inc.)

board is the more versatile as it can be moved out of the way during the procedure when the fluoroscopic unit is in use. A mini-C arm fluoroscopy unit is preferred due to its decreased radiation exposure, but a standard fluoroscopy unit can be used as well.

Surgical Landmarks

Once the patient has been properly positioned and the arm prepped and draped in the usual sterile fashion, several key surgical landmarks should be identified. The radiocarpal and radioulnar joints should be palpated and identified. The tip and dorsal and volar contours of the radial styloid should also be identified. If excessive soft tissue swelling makes this difficult, fluoroscopy can be used to determine these critical landmarks and these areas can be marked on the skin to aid in the proper placement of surgical incisions.

Surgical Approach

Prior to the sterilely draped injured extremity being properly positioned on the arm board, the arm board should be adequately covered with a sterile drape, allowing the surgeon to grasp the arm board and move it without the risk of contamination. The fluoroscopic unit is then used to assess the fracture to confirm that it can easily be reduced or is able to be reduced with minimal percutaneous incisions. After it has been confirmed that the fracture can be reduced anatomically, the tip of the radial styloid is palpated and identified. A 2- to 3-cm longitudinal incision is then made centered over

the tip of the radial styloid and midline between the dorsal and volar contours of the styloid (Fig. 14.6). Surgical dissection proceeds carefully at this point, and any branches of the radial sensory nerve that are in the field are identified and carefully retracted. No skeletonization of these nerve branches should be done, and they should be retracted with their neighboring fat and vessels to avoid any radial sensory nerve problems postoperatively.

After the edges of the first and second dorsal extensor tendon compartments are identified, the periosteum between them is then incised in line with the skin incision, and the cortical surface of the radial styloid is exposed just enough for the entrance hole for the intramedullary nail. The periosteum should be preserved if possible so that it can be closed over the entrance hole later to prevent any adherence of the tendons or nerve branches to the nail underneath, which should be recessed below the cortical surface of the styloid.

Preliminary Reduction

It is of benefit to the surgeon to have an anatomic reduction of the fracture, which is held with K-wire fixation prior to nail insertion for a number of reasons. First, once the external jig is in place, it can be difficult to visualize the joint line and alignment of the fracture as both the jig and the nail are radio-opaque. Second, the nail may have a degree of intramedullary fill, which, while helping the stability of the fracture reduction, can prevent any fine tuning of the reduction once the implant is in place, particularly in terms of dorsal or volar translation or restoration of volar tilt. Thus, it is recommended that the fracture be anatomically reduced and held prior to nail insertion.

This can generally be easily done and fluoroscopy should be used to verify the anatomic reduction. Once the fracture is reduced, the distal fragment is then preliminarily pinned with a 0.62 K-wire inserted through the radial styloid with fixation in the shaft proximally. This K-wire should inserted, if possible, in the volar portion of the styloid so that it will not interfere with insertion of the nail, but provides very stable fixation of the distal fragment and also helps to protect and retract the tendons of the first dorsal extensor compartment and sensory branches of the radial sensory nerve (Fig. 14.7). This can be a difficult K-wire to insert, but is well worth the effort as it makes the rest of the procedure much easier.

A second percutaneous 0.45 K-wire is then inserted dorsally, typically between the fourth and fifth dorsal extensor compartments. A small 1-mm stab incision can be made here to ensure that the correct interval has been entered and that the K-wire does not entangle tendons or sensory nerve branches. Typically, a guide can be slid down over the K-wire once it is in the proper 4–5 interval prior to insertion to prevent any soft tissues from wrapping around the wire. This K-wire should capture the dorsal ulnar corner of the distal fragment and, in conjunction with the 0.62 K-wire through the radial styloid, provide rigid 90/90 fixation of the distal fragment (Fig. 14.8).

It is recommended to achieve this anatomic rigid 90/90 fixation prior to nail insertion, as while insertion of the nail should be a gentle process, it can disrupt the preliminary reduction if inadequate K-wire fixation is achieved. The rigid 90/90 fixation provided by the two K-wires best resists any displacement forces created through the nail insertion process (Fig. 14.9).

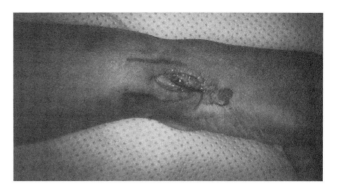

Fig. 14.7 Demonstration of surgical exposure and placement of 0.62 K-wire volarly in the styloid (From Dantuluri P. Distal Radius Fractures, An Issue of Atlas of the Hand Clinics, November 2006, with permission of Elsevier, Inc.)

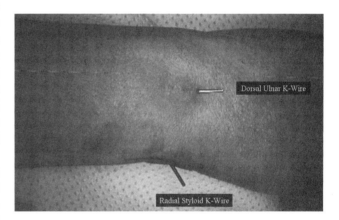

Fig. 14.8 Preliminary reduction maintained with dorsal ulnar and radial styloid K-wires providing rigid 90/90 fixation (From Dantuluri P. Distal Radius Fractures, An Issue of Atlas of the Hand Clinics, November 2006, with permission of Elsevier, Inc.)

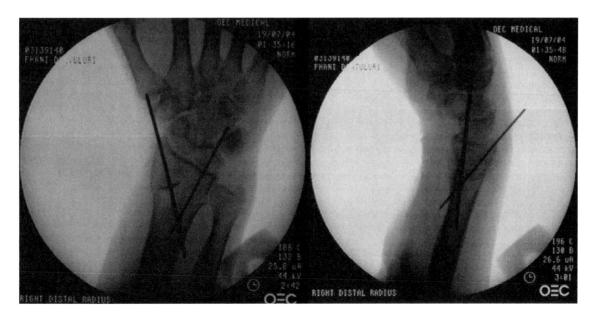

Fig. 14.9 Fluoroscopic images demonstrating typical K-wire positions to maintain preliminary reduction. Note volar position of 0.62 K-wire in the lateral view and note the dorsal ulnar position of the 0.45 K-wire in the posteroanterior (PA) (From Dantuluri P. Distal Radius Fractures, An Issue of Atlas of the Hand Clinics, November 2006, with permission of Elsevier, Inc.)

If the reduction of the fracture cannot be achieved by closed means, one can utilize the anticipated small dorsal incision for the proximal locking screws as a window to help with the reduction without making any additional incisions. The nail can be placed on the dorsal surface of the skin in its expected intramedullary position with the wrist in a posteroanterior position on the fluoroscopic unit. Fluoroscopy will reveal the anticipated incision site for the proximal locking screws. A Freer elevator can then be inserted through this incision to help reduce difficult fractures, particularly in the region of the sigmoid notch as well as simple articular fractures. Once reduction has been achieved, the K-wires should be inserted as previously described.

Nail Insertion

At this point, the tip of the radial styloid is identified and a cortical window is made in the styloid approximately 5 mm proximal to the tip of the styloid. This cortical window must be made proximal enough in the styloid to prevent violation of the articular surface of the scaphoid facet with successive broaching, but not be too proximal to prevent adequate subchondral support with the distal locking screws. An awl or the 6.1 cannulated drill bit can be used to make this entrance hole in the styloid (Fig. 14.10). Fluoroscopy should be used at this critical step to ensure the proper entrance hole for insertion of the intramedullary implant.

After the cortical window has been made, a small rongeur can be used to expand the window typically in the proximal direction longitudinally in line with the radius for about 5 mm in order to allow atraumatic broach insertion. A small canal finder is then inserted gently into the intramedullary canal (Fig. 14.11). It is critical that the canal finder should stay along the radial cortex during insertion in order to prevent penetration of the ulnar cortex of the radial shaft. Using fluoroscopy to ensure proper entry, a small broach is then inserted across the fracture site and advanced proximally across the metaphyseal-diaphyseal junction (Fig. 14.12). Increasingly larger broaches are then inserted sequentially until the broach is large enough within the canal to resist spinning when rotational torque is applied as well provide reasonable intramedullary fill. Preoperative templating using the contralateral wrist radiographs should also provide the surgeon with valuable information as to which size implant is the likely size that will be used.

After the last broach has been removed, the implant is then mounted on the external jig and then gently inserted following the path of the prior broach (Fig. 14.13). The nail should be carefully inserted toward the sigmoid notch far enough medially into the radius so that no part of the nail is protruding above the radial cortex (Fig. 14.14). This will prevent any contact between the nail and the undersurface of

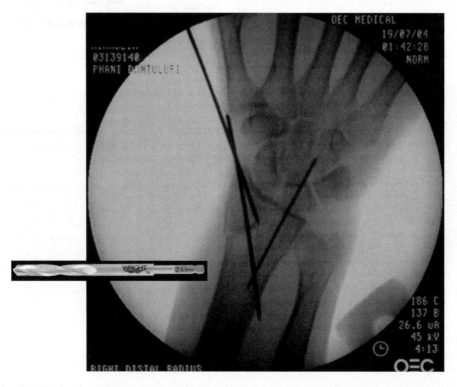

Fig. 14.10 Guide wire placed in tip of styloid for cannulated drill insertion to create entrance hole for implant (From Dantuluri P. Distal Radius Fractures, An Issue of Atlas of the Hand Clinics, November 2006, with permission of Elsevier, Inc.)

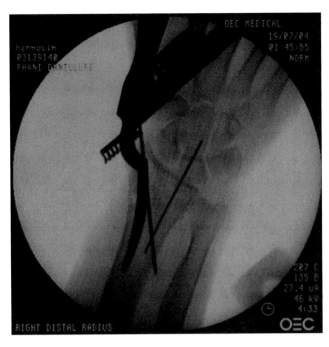

Fig. 14.11 Canal finder insertion. Note that the canal finder hugs the radial cortex to prevent ulnar cortical perforation (From Dantuluri P. Distal Radius Fractures, An Issue of Atlas of the Hand Clinics, November 2006, with permission of Elsevier, Inc.)

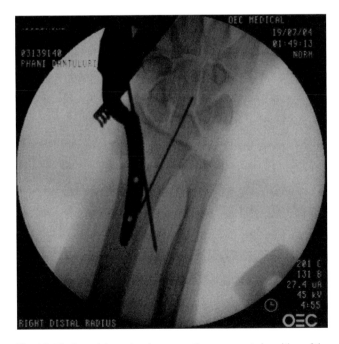

Fig. 14.12 Broach insertion demonstrating an expected position of the intramedullary nail (From Dantuluri P. Distal Radius Fractures, An Issue of Atlas of the Hand Clinics, November 2006, with permission of Elsevier, Inc.)

the tendons of either the first or second compartment. In addition, the nail is inserted gently proximally enough so that the distal-most locking screw will be just underneath the subchondral bone supporting the radiocarpal articular surface. A K-wire or a drill bit can be inserted through the distal-most

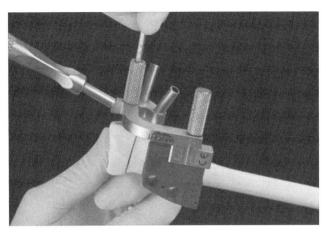

Fig. 14.13 Close up view of external jig demonstrating screw alignment guides for proximal and distal screw insertion in sawbones model (From Dantuluri P. Distal Radius Fractures, An Issue of Atlas of the Hand Clinics, November 2006, with permission of Elsevier, Inc.)

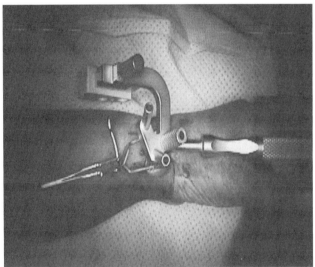

Fig. 14.14 External jig in place with intramedullary nail insertion (From Dantuluri P. Distal Radius Fractures, An Issue of Atlas of the Hand Clinics, November 2006, with permission of Elsevier, Inc.)

drill guide and then checked under fluoroscopy to ensure that the distal-most locking screw will be in the desired subchondral position (Fig. 14.15).

At this point, the distal locking screw holes are drilled and measured and three distal locking screws are inserted into the nail with the distal-most screw inserted first (Fig. 14.16). Fluoroscopy should also be used when measuring the length of the screws to ensure that they do not penetrate the sigmoid notch and enter the distal radioulnar joint (Fig. 14.17). It is important to remember that the sigmoid notch has a concavity for the distal ulna so that a screw may appear to be safely out of the distal radial ulnar joint on the fluoroscopic view, but may still actually be penetrating this joint. Therefore, it is best to have these screws err on the side of being 2 mm short

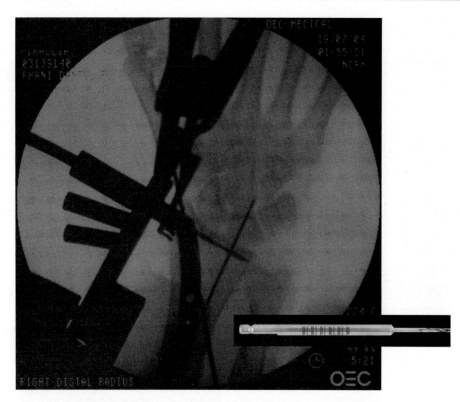

Fig. 14.15 Drilling of distal locking screws with care to avoid penetration of radiocarpal and radioulnar joints (From Dantuluri P. Distal Radius Fractures, An Issue of Atlas of the Hand Clinics, November 2006, with permission of Elsevier, Inc.)

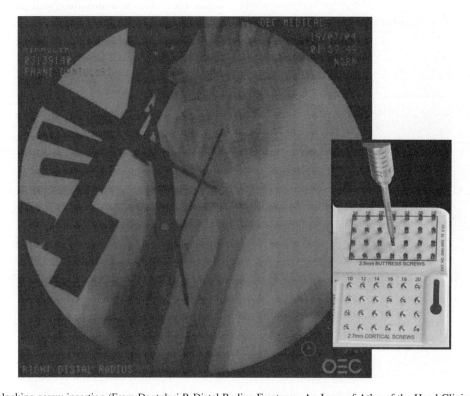

Fig. 14.16 Distal locking screw insertion (From Dantuluri P. Distal Radius Fractures, An Issue of Atlas of the Hand Clinics, November 2006, with permission of Elsevier, Inc.)

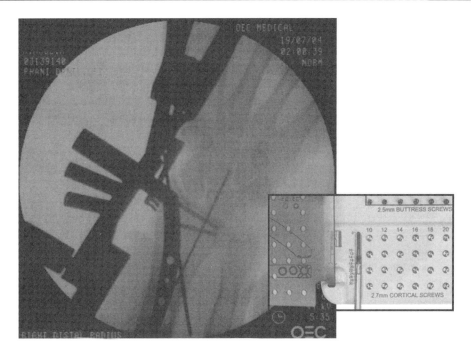

Fig. 14.17 Insertion of remaining distal locking screws keeping them short of the sigmoid notch to avoid penetration (From Dantuluri P. Distal Radius Fractures, An Issue of Atlas of the Hand Clinics, November 2006, with permission of Elsevier, Inc.)

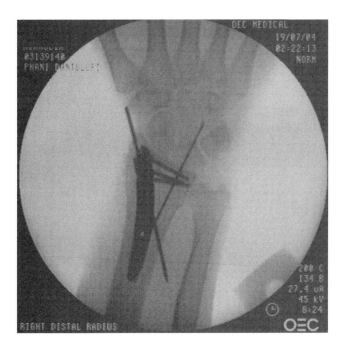

Fig. 14.18 Fluoroscopic image after completed distal locking screw insertion demonstrating ideal distal locking screw positions (From Dantuluri P. Distal Radius Fractures, An Issue of Atlas of the Hand Clinics, November 2006, with permission of Elsevier, Inc.)

and be sure to check for crepitus. Once all of the distal locking screws have firmly locked into the nail, the fracture reduction should be carefully assessed (Fig. 14.18). If there has been a slight loss of reduction of the fracture due to nail insertion, an attempt can now be made to gently reduce the fracture anatomically prior to proximal screw insertion.

At this stage, a 0.45 K-wire is then inserted through the dorsal cortex and the nail to rigidly hold the implant in place and prevent subtle displacement of the implant within the canal or loss of reduction. The proximal screws can then be inserted through two small 1-cm incisions or one single 2-cm dorsal incision. The appropriate drill guide and sleeves are used to drill and insert the proximal screws (Fig. 14.19). These screws achieve bicortical purchase and lock the implant in place. It is important to prevent any soft tissue such as extensor tendons from being trapped under the screw heads. Also, it is *critical* not to compromise purchase of the proximal locking screws by overtightening as there are only two proximal locking screws and they are crucial in maintaining implant position and proximal fixation, especially if there is not good intramedullary fill of the implant. A good technique to avoid stripping these screws is retracting the drill guides for the last few turns so that this can done under direct visualization so that it is clear when the screw heads are down tight on the dorsal cortex of the radius.

Final fluoroscopic images are used to verify that the reduction of the fracture has been accomplished and that the implant and all screws are in appropriate positions (Fig. 14.20). The periosteum is then closed over the cortical window in the radial styloid if possible to prevent any contact of the nail with the surrounding soft tissues. The deeper subcutaneous tissues are closed with a minimum of 2.0 Vicryl suture and the skin is closed with 3.0 Monocryl subcuticular suture (Fig. 14.21). Benzoin and Steri-strips are then applied and patient's arm is placed into a temporary short arm splint for comfort.

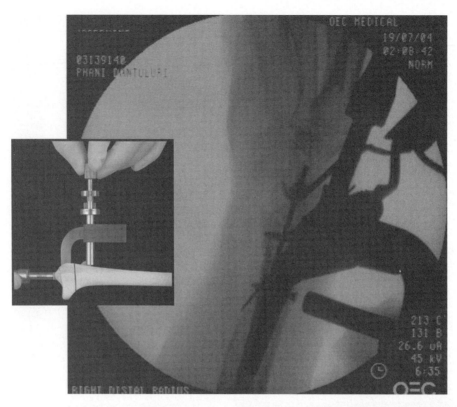

Fig. 14.19 Proximal locking insertion demonstrating how the drill guide can be withdrawn for the final few turns to allow direct visualization and avoid stripping of the screws (From Dantuluri P. Distal Radius Fractures, An Issue of Atlas of the Hand Clinics, November 2006, with permission of Elsevier, Inc.)

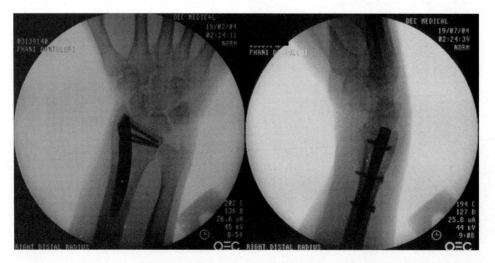

Fig. 14.20 Completed intramedullary fixation of distal radius fracture demonstrating anatomic reduction and ideal implant placement (From Dantuluri P. Distal Radius Fractures, An Issue of Atlas of the Hand Clinics, November 2006, with permission of Elsevier, Inc.)

Postoperative Care

Patients are instructed to begin immediate postoperative finger, elbow, and shoulder range of motion to avoid stiffness and reduce swelling. Patients are typically seen for their first postoperative visit at a week to 10 days. At that visit, they are given a removable orthoplast short arm splint only for comfort. At this point, unrestricted active range of motion is allowed for the wrist as well and patients are also instituted in occupational therapy to monitor and aid in their rehabilitation. Patients are followed with serial radiographs to evaluate bony union, which typically occurs at approximately 6 weeks postoperatively (Fig. 14.22). New

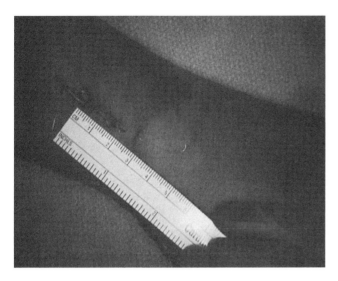

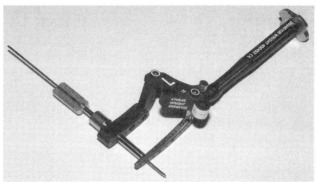

Fig. 14.24 Improved proximal fixation is allowed by having three proximal screws that engage the distal radius and also go through the intramedullary nail (From Dantuluri P. Distal Radius Fractures, An Issue of Atlas of the Hand Clinics, November 2006, with permission of Elsevier, Inc.)

Fig.14.21 Postoperative closure demonstrating 2-cm incision for nail insertion (From Dantuluri P. Distal Radius Fractures, An Issue of Atlas of the Hand Clinics, November 2006, with permission of Elsevier, Inc.)

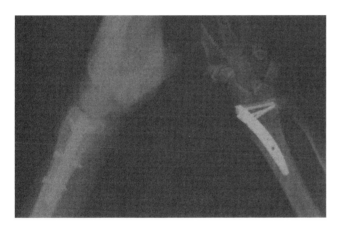

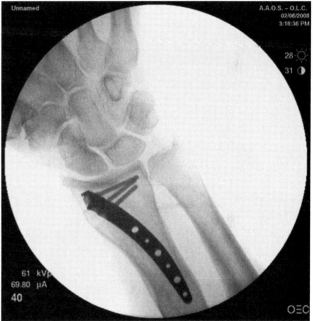

Fig. 14.22 Early postoperative radiographs demonstrating maintenance of reduction (From Dantuluri P. Distal Radius Fractures, An Issue of Atlas of the Hand Clinics, November 2006, with permission of Elsevier, Inc.)

Fig. 14.25 Example of newer intramedullary design with implant in place demonstrating the three proximal screw fixation points (From Dantuluri P. Distal Radius Fractures, An Issue of Atlas of the Hand Clinics, November 2006, with permission of Elsevier, Inc.)

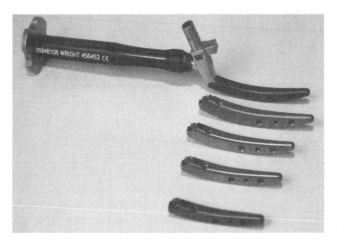

Fig. 14.23 New developments in intramedullary nail fixation include longer intramedullary nails allowing better proximal fixation (From Dantuluri P. Distal Radius Fractures, An Issue of Atlas of the Hand Clinics, November 2006, with permission of Elsevier, Inc.)

developments in the instrumentation system include the development of longer intramedullary nails (Fig. 14.23) to provide better proximal fixation. Having three proximal screws allows superior fixation of the implant and prevents proximal migration of the nail (Figs. 14.24 and 14.25). The most significant new development is the introduction of a radiolucent guide, which allows better visualization of the fracture lines, allowing superior fracture reductions (Fig. 14.26). In this example case, one can see the superior visualization afforded by the radiolucent guide of the distal radius, particularly on the lateral view, allowing anatomic reductions of both the radiocarpal and distal radioulnar joints (Fig. 14.27).

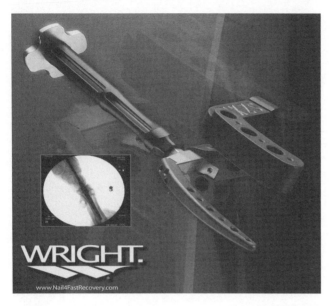

Fig. 14.26 Development of a new radiolucent guide allows superior visualization of the fracture and allows more precise placement of the distal and proximal screws (From Dantuluri P. Distal Radius Fractures, An Issue of Atlas of the Hand Clinics, November 2006, with permission of Elsevier, Inc.)

Follow-Up Results and Complications

It has been shown, at least in short-term follow-up, that distal radius fractures can be successfully treated with intramedullary fixation. Tan et al. presented a prospective study of 23 consecutive fractures treated with intramedullary fixation using the MICRONAIL.[20] This study showed that outcomes were excellent at 6-month follow-up in terms of maintenance of alignment of the distal radius, range of motion, and improvement of grip strength. Outcome measurements using standardized outcome tools (DASH) also demonstrated excellent results. There were relatively few complications and these consisted of three transient radial sensory nerve injuries, and three patients who had loss of fracture reduction, but these patients all had more complex intraarticular fracture types. As with any surgical implant, improperly measured screws can lead to soft tissue complications or loss of reduction. Screws not placed just underneath the articular surface of the distal radius can result in possible fracture subsidence and loss of alignment. Penetration of either the radiocarpal or radioulnar joints with screws can lead to irreversible articular damage. It is clear in early follow-up that intramedullary fixation of distal radius fractures is not only possible, but can lead to excellent results in properly selected patients.[21]

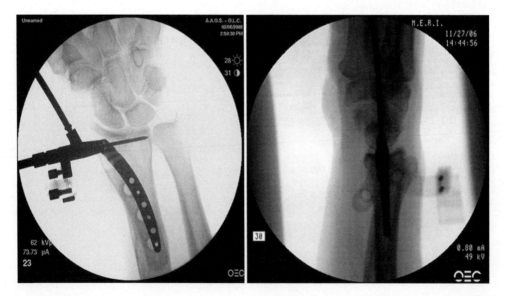

Fig.14.27 Example of the radiolucent guide in place demonstrating the views afforded of the distal radius. Much more of the bony landmarks of the distal radius can be visualized with the radiolucent guide, which will allow for superior fracture reductions and exact screw placement (From Dantuluri P. Distal Radius Fractures, An Issue of Atlas of the Hand Clinics, November 2006, with permission of Elsevier, Inc.)

Conclusions

Despite the success of open reduction and internal fixation of distal radius fractures, problems persist, including loss of reduction, hardware failure, tendon and nerve injuries, and infection. Significant scarring of tendons and neurovascular structures can occur with extensive surgical dissection, leading to limitation of function. The thin soft tissue envelope surrounding the distal radius and the close proximity of tendons, nerves, and vascular structures to the distal radius may contribute to the development of some of these complications. Minimally invasive surgical fixation of the distal radius has been developed using an intramedullary nail as a new treatment option for fractures of the distal radius in an attempt to minimize these potential complications. It is clear that careful surgical technique and proper patient selection can lead to successful outcomes in patients with distal radius fractures treated with intramedullary nail fixation.[21]

References

1. Simic P, Weiland A. Fractures of the distal aspect of the radius; changes in treatment over the past two decades. *J Bone Joint Surg (Am)* 2003;85:552–564
2. McQuuen MM. Redisplaced unstable fractures of the distal radius. A randomized prospective study of bridging versus non-bridging external fixation. *J Bone Joint Surg* 1998;80B:665–669.
3. Knirk JL, Jupiter JB. Intraarticular fractures of the distal end of the radius in young adults. *J Bone Joint Surg* 1986;68:647–659
4. Lafontaine M, Hardy D, Delince P. Stability assessment in distal radius fractures. *Injury* 1989;20:208–210
5. Ruch DS, Papadonikolakis A. Volar versus dorsal plating in the management of intraarticular distal radius fractures. *J Hand Surg (Am)* 2006;31(1):9–16
6. Orbay JL, Fernandez DL. Volar fixed-angle plate fixation for unstable distal radius fractures in the elderly patient. *J Hand Surg* 2004;29:96–102
7. Ring D, Prommersberger K, Jupiter JB. Combined dorsal and volar plate fixation of complex fractures of the distal part of the radius. *J Bone Joint Surg Am* 2004;86:1646–1652
8. Jakob M, Rikli DA, Regazzoni P. Fracture of the distal radius treated by internal fixation and early function. A prospective study of 73 consecutive patients. *J Bone Joint Surg* 2000;82: 340–344
9. Rozental TD, Beredjiklian PK, Bozentka DJ. Functional outcome and complications following two types of dorsal plating for unstable fractures of the distal part of the radius. *J Bone Joint Surg Am* 2003;85:1956–1960
10. Rozental TD, Blazar PE. Functional outcome and complications after volar plating for dorsally displaced, unstable fractures of the distal radius. *J Hand Surg (Am)* 2006;31(3):359–365.
11. Tarr RR, Wiss DA. The mechanics and biology of intramedullary fracture fixation. *Clin Orthop Relat Res* 1986;212:10–17
12. Pritchett JW. External fixation or closed medullary pinning for unstable Colles' fractures? *J Bone Joint Surg* 1995;77:267–269
13. Saeki Y, Hashizume H, Nagoshi M, Tanaka H, Inoue H. Mechanical strength of intramedullary pinning and transfragmental Kirschner wire fixation for Colles' fractures. *J Hand Surg (Br)* 2001;26: 550–555
14. Sato O, Aoki M, Kawaguchi S, Ishii S, Kondo M. Antegrade intramedullary K-wire fixation for distal radius fractures. *J Hand Surg* 2002,27:707–713
15. Street DM. Intramedullary forearm nailing. *Clin Orthop Relat Res* 1986;212:219–230
16. Van der Reis WL, Otsuka NY, Moroz P, et al. Intramedullary nailing versus plate fixation for unstable forearm fractures in children. *J Pediatr Orthop* 1998;18:9–13
17. Gao H, Luo CF, Zhang CO, Shi HP, Fan CY, Zen BF. Internal fixation of diaphyseal fractures of the forearm by interlocking intramedullary nail: short term result in eighteen patients. *J Orthop Trauma* 2005;19(6):384–391
18. Sasaki S. Modified Desmanet's intramedullary pinning for fractures of the distal radius. *J Orthop Sci* 2002;7(2):172–181
19. Bennett GL, Leeson MC, Smith BS. Intramedullary fixation of unstable distal radius fractures: a method of fixation allowing early motion. *Orthop Rev* 1989;18(2):210–216
20. Tan V, Capo JT, Warburton M. Distal radius fracture fixation with an intramedullary nail. *Tech Hand Up Extrem Surg* 2005;9(4): 195–201
21. Brooks KR, Capo JT, Warburton M, Tan V. Internal fixation of distal radius fractures with novel intramedullary implants. *Clin Orthop Relat Res* 2006 Apr;(445):42–50

Chapter 15
Minimally Invasive Fixation for Wrist Fractures

Louis W. Catalano, Milan M. Patel, and Steven Z. Glickel

There are multiple techniques for treating distal radius fractures. Closed reduction and percutaneous pinning remains a valid and well-accepted method of surgical treatment for displaced and unstable fractures. Pinning has been described for both intraarticular and extraarticular fractures and it represents a relatively simple, minimally invasive, and cost-effective method of treatment. This technique may become more appealing as complications from volar plating are being reported in the literature.

Indications and Contraindications

The goal of surgical treatment of distal radius fractures is to obtain and maintain anatomic reduction in order to maximize the patient's functional outcome. Percutaneous pinning can be used for both extraarticular (AO/ASIF type A2 and A3) and intraarticular fractures, including three- and four-part fractures (AO/ASIF type C1 and C2). Pinning is most effective for fractures that can be closed reduced by traction, manipulation, and ligamentotaxis. Contraindications for percutaneous pinning alone (without augmentation, using external fixation or open reduction and internal fixation) include severe metaphyseal or intraarticular comminution (AO/ASIF type C3), poor bone stock, and shear fractures (AO/ASIF type B). Fixation of these fractures with percutaneous pinning can lead to loss of reduction and subsequent malunions.

Techniques for Radial Pinning

Several techniques of percutaneous pinning of distal radius fractures have been described in the literature. Techniques of radial pinning have included one or multiple pins placed

obliquely through the radial styloid (Fig. 15.1a), crossed pinning from the radial styloid and dorsoulnar cortex (Fig. 15.1b), intrafocal pinning within the distal radius fracture site (Fig. 15.1c), and oblique and horizontal pins placed through the radial styloid (Fig. 15.2). In 1907, Lambotte[1] described using a single radial styloid pin as a method of stabilization, and in 1959, Willenegger and Guggenbuhl[2] further reported on their experience with this method in 25 patients. In 1975, Stein and Katz,[3] and in 1984, Clancey[4] described crossed pinning of the radius, using one or more pins through the radial styloid and another pin through the dorsal and ulnar corner of the distal radius. This technique stabilized the dorsoulnar radial fragment and provided orthogonal pin configuration, inherently more stable than pins in one plane. Fernandez and Geissler[5] described another method for stabilizing the dorsoulnar fragment. In addition to two oblique radial styloid pins, they placed transverse pins in the subchondral bone from the radial styloid to the ulnar fragment, avoiding entering the distal radioulnar joint (DRUJ). The transverse pin supported the intraarticular fracture fragments, preventing displacement. In 1976, Kapandji[6] reported a technique of intrafocal pinning using two pins in the fracture site for reduction and buttress fixation of the fracture and modified this in 1987, using three-pin intrafocal pinning.[7]

Practically, these techniques of closed reduction and percutaneous pinning are used alone or in combination depending on the particular fracture pattern. The number of pins, size of the pins, and configuration within the distal radius are adapted to the fracture pattern. In a biomechanical study, Naidu et al.[8] demonstrated that crossed pinning with at least 0.062-in.-diameter K-wires was more rigid than two parallel radial styloid pins alone. Rogge et al.[9] corroborated this finding in their study using mathematical and computer-generated finite element modeling. Our approach and technique is described below.

A pneumatic tourniquet is placed on the arm and the hand and arm are prepped and draped with a stockinette and a prefabricated extremity drape. The procedure is performed using a radiolucent hand table to which an outrigger for longitudinal traction can be incorporated. We currently use the Carter hand surgery table (Innovation Sport, Foothill Ranch, CA)

L.W. Catalano(✉), M.M. Patel, and S.Z. Glickel
Department of Orthopaedic Surgery, Attending Hand Surgeon,
C.V. Starr Hand Surgery Center, New York, NY, USA
e-mail: catalano@msn.com

L.W. Catalano(✉)
Columbia College of Physicians and Surgeons, St. Luke's - Roosevelt Hospital Center, New York, NY, USA
e-mail: louiscatalano@aol.com

G.R. Scuderi and A.J. Tria (eds.), *Minimally Invasive Surgery in Orthopedics*,
DOI 10.1007/978-0-387-76608-9_15, © Springer Science+Business Media, LLC 2010

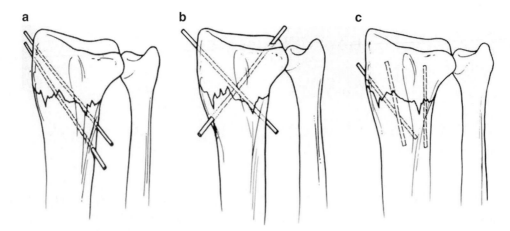

Fig. 15.1 (**a**) Multiple pins placed obliquely through the radial styloid. (**b**) Crossing pins from the radial styloid and dorsoulnar corner. (**c**) Intrafocal pinning into the distal radius fracture (From Fernandez DL, Jupiter JB. Fractures of the Distal Radius. A Practical Approach to Management, 2nd ed., New York: Springer, 2002, p. 153, with kind permission of Springer Science and Business Media.)

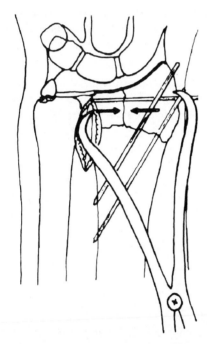

Fig. 15.2 Multiple pins placed obliquely through the radial styloid are combined with transverse pins to capture the dorsoulnar radial fragment. Subchondral pins can also help buttress the depressed lunate facet. The dorsoulnar radial fragment can be reduced through a small incision utilizing a bone tenaculum (From Fernandez DL, Jupiter JB. Fractures of the Distal Radius. A Practical Approach to Management, 2nd ed., New York: Springer, 2002, p. 153, with kind permission of Springer Science and Business Media.)

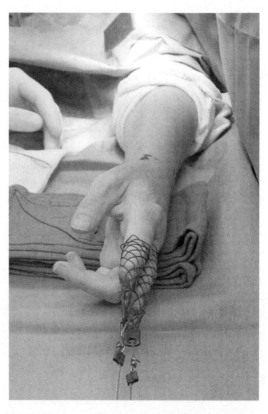

Fig. 15.3 Fingertraps are placed on the index and middle fingers. Ten pounds of traction is placed through the fingertraps to aid with the reduction and to keep the fracture out to length

for the traction set-up. Finger traps on the index and long fingers are attached to a wire, which runs over the pulley of the traction outrigger. Depending on the size of the patient, five or ten pounds of weight are applied for longitudinal traction with the limb horizontal on the hand table (Fig. 15.3).

The head and arm of the image intensifier are sterilely draped. The image intensifier is brought into the operative field and posteroanterior (PA) and lateral images of the distal radius are obtained. The fracture is manipulated with volarly directed pressure on the dorsum of the distal fracture fragment in an effort to restore length and volar tilt. Volar tilt can also be regained by translating the carpus volarly. In instances where the distal fracture fragment is radially translated, ulnarly directed pressure on the radial styloid and/or ulnar translation of the wrist by ulnar deviation and manual translation of the hand can facilitate reduction. The reduction is monitored fluoroscopically. If it is thought that reduction is achievable, the surgeon proceeds with the planned percutaneous pin fixation. If the fracture is not reducible closed, open reduction and internal fixation may be required.

Fractures treated 2–3 weeks after injury may be difficult to reduce simply with manipulation and manual pressure (Fig. 15.4). In that case, an intrafocal pin may be used to assist in the reduction. If the fracture is shortened and the distal articular surface dorsally tilted, an intrafocal pin is placed into the fracture dorsally at an angle from proximal to distal. The position of the pin is confirmed fluoroscopically and the pin is used to manually advance the distal fracture fragment distally and volarly by levering the pin distally, changing the obliquity of the pin from distal to proximal. Usually, this can be done percutaneously. The exception is a fracture close to 3-weeks old that is healed enough that a 0.062-in. K-wire is not sufficiently rigid to accomplish the goal of mobilization of the distal fracture fragment. In that case, a small Freer elevator can be used percutaneously in the same manner (Fig. 15.5a, b). An intrafocal wire can than be placed from dorsal to volar in order to maintain the reduction that was created by breaking up the healing callus.

A similar intrafocal technique can be used to restore loss of radial inclination. This should be done under direct vision to avoid injury to the superficial radial nerve and the tendons of the first compartment. A 0.062-in. K-wire is placed into the fracture at an angle from proximal to distal. The pin is levered distally, forcing the fracture fragment distally as well as translating it ulnarly. Once the reduction is felt to be satisfactory, percutaneous pin fixation is achieved using the technique described previously. The surgeon may opt to leave the intrafocal pin in place and drive it proximally into the ulnar cortex of the radius, proximal to the fracture site. This intrafocal K-wire helps prevent loss of radial inclination, which can produce irritating cosmetic concerns for the patient.

Our preference is to place two to three pins from the radial styloid. The pins are 0.062-in. in diameter. We place the pins under direct vision in order to avoid injury to the superficial radial nerve or the tendons of the first dorsal compartment. A 1.5-cm-long longitudinal incision is made extending from the tip of the radial styloid distally (Fig. 15.6). The superficial radial nerve is identified and retracted. The pins are usually placed just dorsal to the first extensor compartment but may be placed volar to the compartment depending upon the pattern of the fracture and the location of the nerve. There is frequently some loss of reduction of the fracture once manual pressure on the distal fracture fragment is released in order to begin pin placement. Therefore, the first pin is placed in the distal fracture fragment, not crossing the fracture line. The pin is always placed through a soft tissue protector in

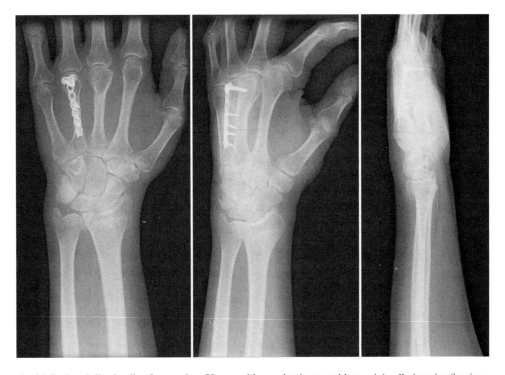

Fig. 15.4 A 3-week-old displaced distal radius fracture in a 50-year-old man that is amenable to minimally invasive fixation

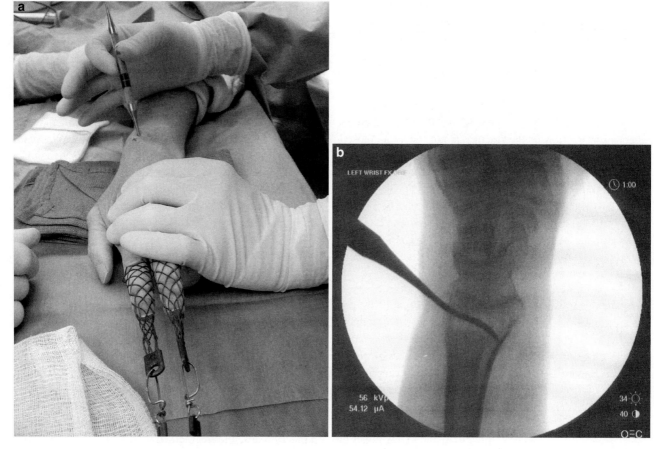

Fig. 15.5 (**a**, **b**) A small elevator is placed through a stab incision into the fracture site to aid with restoration of the normal volar tilt of the distal radius

order to avoid wrapping up adjacent soft tissues structures. The first pin is started at the tip of the radial styloid and directed at a fairly shallow angle obliquely, with the goal of crossing the fracture line and engaging the ulnar cortex of the radius proximal to the fracture. Once the pin is driven into the distal fracture fragment with a K-wire driver, the fracture is re-reduced and the reduction confirmed with PA and lateral radiographs. When the fracture is anatomically reduced, the K-wire is driven across the fracture and the distal radial metaphysis engaging the ulnar cortex proximal to the fracture line. Postfixation fluoroscopic images are obtained (Fig. 15.7a, b). Usually, a second 0.062-in. K-wire is placed at a slightly more proximal starting point and at a slightly different angle than the initial pin, directing it more dorsally or volarly within the medullary canal and aiming more proximally (Fig. 15.8a, b). Reduction and fixation are confirmed with the image intensifier.

For two-part fractures, another set of pins is placed perpendicular to the radial styloid pins. Generally, we place those pins beginning from the dorsal rim of the distal radius just distal to Lister's tubercle. The pins should be started just distal to the tubercle or slightly radial to it. Beginning the pin

ulnar to that point runs the risk of tethering or otherwise injuring the extensor pollicis longus (EPL) tendon. The wrist is placed in position to obtain a lateral image and the starting point of the pin at the dorsal rim of the radius is confirmed (Fig. 15.9). The authors find it easier to manually insert the K-wire and feel the dense, solid dorsal rim of the distal radius. It is important to start the pin in the solid bone of the dorsal rim of the radius as opposed to the more proximal metaphyseal region where the cortex is thinner and may be comminuted from the fracture. The pin is driven obliquely from dorsal to volar across the fracture line, engaging the volar cortex of the radius proximal to the fracture. In some patients, a second pin may be placed in a similar manner beginning just proximal to the first pin and directed at a slightly different angle to enhance the fixation.

Some modifications of this basic pinning technique are used in specific fractures to assist with the reduction or provide fixation for the ulnar fracture fragment in three-part fractures. If the fracture has three parts and there is any proximal subsidence of the lunate fossa creating a step off, this may be addressed percutaneously as well. If there is proximal displacement of the lunate fossa fragment, it can be advanced

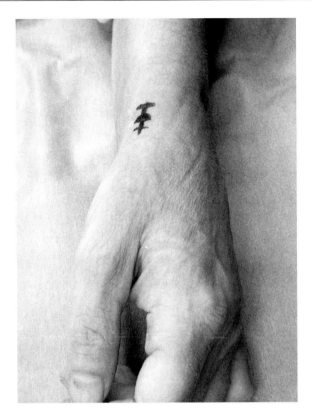

Fig. 15.6 The incision to identify the superficial radial nerve and first dorsal compartment is marked out at the radial styloid

distally using an intrafocal pin placed percutaneously into the dorsum of the fracture as described previously. The pin is angled from proximal to distal and the fracture fragment advanced distally as the pin is pushed in an arc from proximal to distal. Fixation of the lunate fossa fragment can be achieved in one of two ways. Proximal subsidence of the fracture can be prevented by placing two transverse pins from the radial styloid across the distal radial metaphysis just proximal to the subchondral bone (see Fig. 15.2). One pin is placed volarly and the other pin is placed dorsally across the distal radius. The tips of the pins are driven to engage the ulnar cortex of the radius in the area of the sigmoid notch but the pins should not extend beyond the cortex into the DRUJ. An alternative is to fix the lunate fossa fragment with a pin placed percutaneously from the dorsoulnar corner of the distal radius, driving it obliquely in a dorsovolar direction to engage the volar cortex proximal to the fracture line. In general, that pin is started in the interval between the fourth and fifth extensor compartments and the starting point of the pin is confirmed fluoroscopically prior to advancing the pin.

Once the distal radius fracture is stabilized, the DRUJ is examined to assess stability (Fig. 15.10). If the joint is unstable, and there is no ulnar styloid fracture, the DRUJ is stabilized by pinning the ulna to the radius with two 0.062-in. Kirscher wires placed transversely proximal to the joint. If the ulnar styloid is fractured at its base, consideration is given to fixing the fracture using a tension band construct.

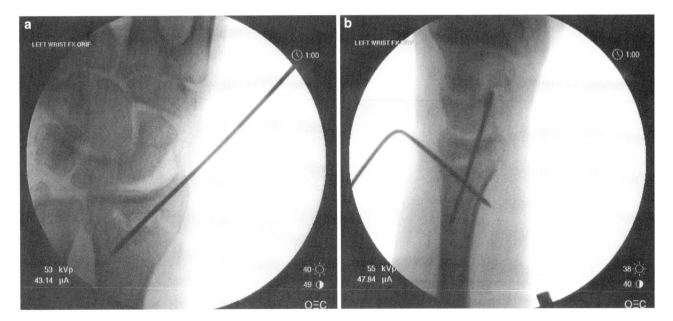

Fig. 15.7 (**a**) A 0.062-in. K-wire is placed obliquely through the radial styloid and across the fracture site. (**b**) The second K-wire is driven as an intrafocal wire to maintain the volar tilt

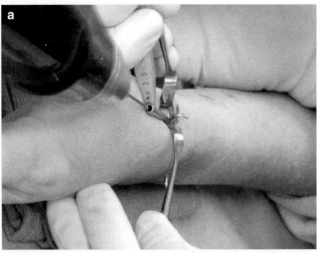

Fig. 15.8 (**a**) A second oblique wire is placed through the radial styloid at a slightly different angle and a soft tissue protector is used to avoid wrapping up the adjacent structures. (**b**) The radial styloid incision with the obliquely directed K-wires and an adjacent superficial vein and the superficial radial nerve

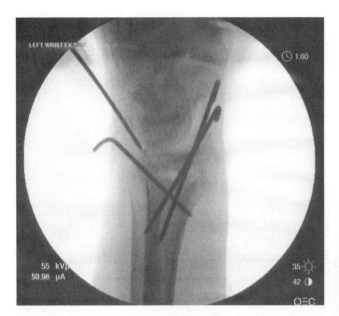

Fig. 15.9 Another perpendicular 0.062-in. K-wire is placed from just distal to Lister's tubercle starting on the solid bone of the dorsal rim

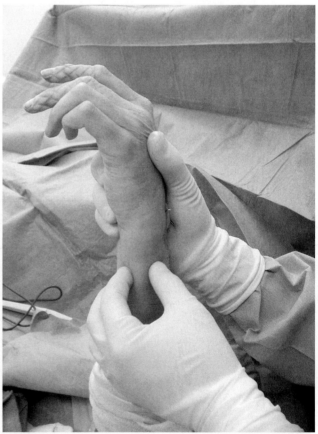

Fig. 15.10 The DRUJ is tested for instability after the fixation of the radius is finalized

The reduction and fixation is assessed with final fluoroscopic images in at least two planes (Fig. 15.11a, b). The pins are left superficial to the skin and are bent using pliers to prevent migration. The radial styloid pins may be left through the incision. If the K-wires tent the skin, the skin either needs to be released with a secondary incision or the pin can be cut and, before bending it, placed through the skin adjacent to the incision obviating the need for relaxing incisions.

The radial styloid incision is closed with interrupted absorbable sutures thereby precluding suture removal.

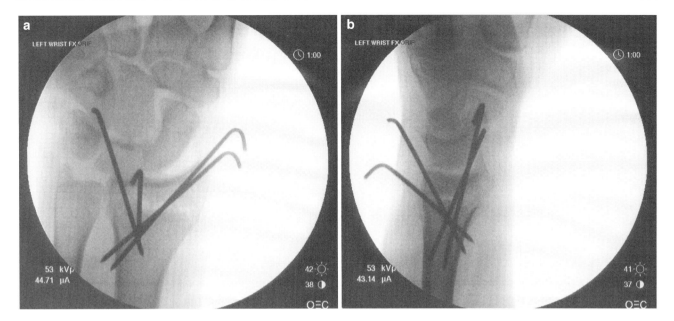

Fig. 15.11 (**a**, **b**) Final postoperative fluoroscopic scans after the K-wires are cut, bent, and left outside of the skin

Postoperative Care and Rehabilitation

The fracture is usually immobilized for the first 2 weeks postoperatively in a sugar tong splint. It is our impression that immobilizing the forearm for 2 weeks is useful to allow the skin around the pins to begin healing. This may help to prevent irritation of the pin sites. Alternatively, the wrist can be immobilized in dorsovolar splints. The splints are secured with Coban (3M, St. Paul, MN) or another self-adhering wrap with no tension (Fig. 15.12). After the initial 2 weeks of immobilization, the patient is seen back in the office for follow-up radiographs. The wrist is then immobilized in a short arm cast if the DRUJ was stable at surgery or a long arm cast if the DRUJ was unstable and needed to be pinned during the surgery. Patients are then seen biweekly in order to obtain new radiographs. The cast is removed and the pin sites are examined only if the patient has complaints or if there is a concern about pin site infection or pin migration. Immobilization is usually continued for a total of 5–6 weeks postoperatively. We never immobilize a fracture of the distal radius for longer than 6 weeks. At that point, the cast is removed. If the fracture is nontender and if radiographs confirm maintenance of reduction and healing of the fracture, the K-wires are removed. The patient is referred to the hand therapist for a prefabricated wrist-resting splint, which is used for support and protection of the wrist for the 2 weeks after immobilization is discontinued. The patient removes the splint to work on range of motion exercise and scar massage. Range of motion can usually be regained within 4–6 weeks after the cast removal. Two weeks after immobilization is discontinued, gentle strengthening exercise with putty

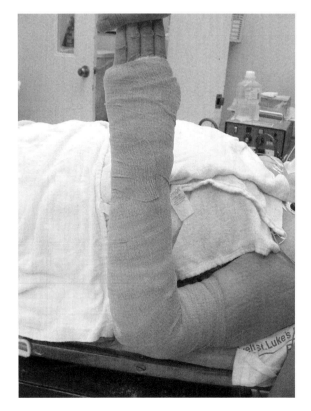

Fig. 15.12 The final dressing is placed consisting of a plaster sugar tong splint and overwrapped with Coban (3M, St. Paul, MN)

and a hand gripper is started. At 1-month after immobilization, light resistive exercises can be started using a 1- to 3-lb. dumbbell and progressing as the patient tolerates. At 3

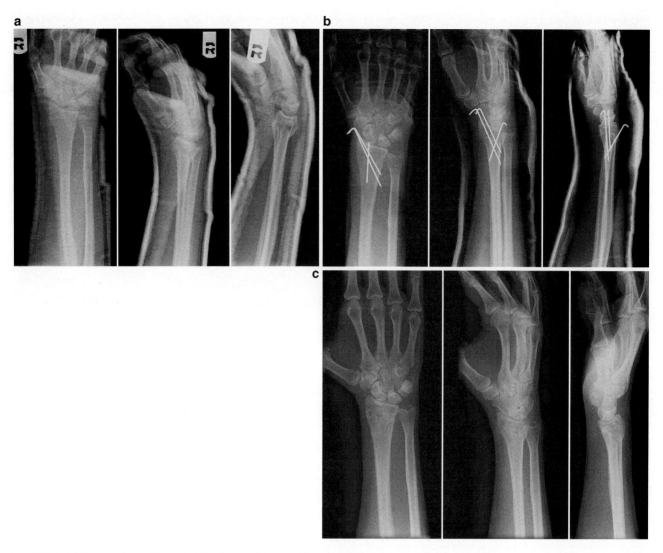

Fig.15.13 (**a**) Preoperative radiographs of a 46-year-old man with an unstable distal radius fracture. (**b**) Radiographs after minimally invasive fixation of the distal radius. (**c**) Final radiographs of the healed fracture 8 weeks after the initial injury

months after fracture, they can resume all activities (Fig. 15.13a–c).

Results and Complications

Several recent prospective studies demonstrated the effectiveness of closed reduction and percutaneous pinning when the pins were placed in an orthogonal configuration.[10,11] Follow-up studies in the past have shown variable results and have reported several instances of loss of reduction when fractures were solely pinned through the radial styloid.[12–14]

In a prospective randomized study with 100 patients, Strohm et al.[15] compared two different procedures for pinning of distal radius fractures. One method of pinning was with two K-wires inserted at the styloid process as described by Willenegger and Guggenbuhl2. The technique to which it was compared was a modified Kapandji method as described by Fritz et al.,[16] using two dorsal intrafocal pins and one radial styloid pin. They found the functional and radiographic outcomes to be significantly better in the patients who had intrafocal pinning and attributed the results, in part, to a shorter immobilization period in those patients. Complications were not significantly different between the groups. In total, 12 patients had nerve irritations that resolved after pin removal. Eight patients between the groups had wire migration, but none of the patients had tendon injury or rupture. One patient in each group developed carpal tunnel syndrome and one patient in each group developed reflex sympathetic dystrophy (RSD).

Minimally invasive fixation for distal radius fractures may also become a more desirable option than volar plating in amenable fractures as the long-term results are being reported. Rozental and Blazar[17] reported on 41 patients who underwent volar plating and who were followed for a minimum of 12 months. While all of the patients had good to excellent results, there was a 22% complication rate, of which 7% was hardware-related tendon irritation. Two patients had symptomatic subluxation of the flexor pollicis longus tendon over the plate and one patient experienced dorsal swelling and irritation caused by a prominent screw. Each patient had some improvement after hardware removal.

In our experience, we have been very satisfied with closed reduction and percutaneous pinning for unstable distal radius fractures. Complications are rare and include pin tract irritation and superficial infection, loss of reduction, and superficial radial nerve irritation. Fortunately, superficial radial nerve complaints have been minimal and resolve after pin removal, and we think this is directly related to visualization of the nerve during pin placement. It is also the authors' opinion that more complications from volar plating such as palmar cutaneous nerve injuries and flexor pollicis longus and EPL tendon ruptures will be reported in the future as the long-term results are reviewed.

Conclusion

Closed reduction and percutaneous pinning is a valuable technique for treating displaced and unstable distal radius fractures. The method is relatively simple, minimally invasive, and reliable. Good to excellent results can usually be achieved when the procedure is performed for the proper indications and biomechanically sound pin configuration is used. Complication rates have been low and manageable and have included pin tract infections and skin irritation. These problems can usually be treated effectively with oral antibiotics or pin removal. Injury to the superficial radial nerve is also a commonly reported complication that can be avoided with direct visualization of the nerve.

Acknowledgment Special thanks to Benjamin Chia, BA, for his assistance with preparation of the manuscript.

References

1. Lambotte A. *L'Intervention opératoire dans les fractures récentes et anciennes.* Paris: A. Maloine; 1907
2. Willenegger H, Guggenbuhl A. [Operative treatment of certain cases of distal radius fracture.]. *Helv Chir Acta.* 1959;26(2):81–94
3. Stein AH, Jr., Katz SF. Stabilization of comminuted fractures of the distal inch of the radius: percutaneous pinning. *Clin Orthop Relat Res.* May 1975(108):174–181
4. Clancey GJ. Percutaneous Kirschner-wire fixation of Colles fractures. A prospective study of thirty cases. *J Bone Joint Surg Am.* 1984;66(7):1008–1014
5. Fernandez DL, Geissler WB. Treatment of displaced articular fractures of the radius. *J Hand Surg (Am).* 1991;16(3):375–384
6. Kapandji A. [Internal fixation by double intrafocal plate. Functional treatment of non articular fractures of the lower end of the radius (author's transl)]. *Ann Chir.* 1976;30(11–12):903–908
7. Kapandji A. [Intra-focal pinning of fractures of the distal end of the radius 10 years later]. *Ann Chir Main.* 1987;6(1):57–63
8. Naidu SH, Capo JT, Moulton M, Ciccone W, II, Radin A. Percutaneous pinning of distal radius fractures: a biomechanical study. *J Hand Surg (Am).* 1997;22(2):252–257
9. Rogge RD, Adams BD, Goel VK. An analysis of bone stresses and fixation stability using a finite element model of simulated distal radius fractures. *J Hand Surg (Am).* 2002;27(1):86–92
10. Harley BJ, Scharfenberger A, Beaupre LA, Jomha N, Weber DW. Augmented external fixation versus percutaneous pinning and casting for unstable fractures of the distal radius - a prospective randomized trial. *J Hand Surg (Am).* 2004;29(5):815–824
11. Ludvigsen TC, Johansen S, Svenningsen S, Saetermo R. External fixation versus percutaneous pinning for unstable Colles' fracture. Equal outcome in a randomized study of 60 patients. *Acta Orthop Scand.* 1997;68(3):255–258
12. Habernek H, Weinstabl R, Fialka C, Schmid L. Unstable distal radius fractures treated by modified Kirschner wire pinning: anatomic considerations, technique, and results. *J Trauma.* 1994; 36(1):83–88
13. Mah ET, Atkinson RN. Percutaneous Kirschner wire stabilisation following closed reduction of Colles' fractures. *J Hand Surg (Br).* 1992;17(1):55–62
14. Munson GO, Gainor BJ. Percutaneous pinning of distal radius fractures. *J Trauma.* 1981;21(12):1032–1035
15. Strohm PC, Muller CA, Boll T, Pfister U. Two procedures for Kirschner wire osteosynthesis of distal radial fractures. A randomized trial. *J Bone Joint Surg Am.* 2004;86-A(12):2621–2628
16. Fritz T, Wersching D, Klavora R, Krieglstein C, Friedl W. Combined Kirschner wire fixation in the treatment of Colles fracture. A prospective, controlled trial. *Arch Orthop Trauma Surg.* 1999; 119(3–4):171–178
17. Rozental TD, Blazar PE. Functional outcome and complications after volar plating for dorsally displaced, unstable fractures of the distal radius. *J Hand Surg (Am).* 2006;31(3):359–365

Chapter 16
Endoscopic and Minimally Invasive Carpal Tunnel and Trigger Finger Release

Mordechai Vigler and Steve K. Lee

Minimally Invasive Carpal Tunnel Release

Carpal tunnel syndrome (CTS) is the most common peripheral entrapment neuropathy,[1,2] with a lifetime incidence estimated at up to 10%.[3] The pathophysiology of CTS is thought to be due to compression of the median nerve in the region of the carpal tunnel.[4,5] When symptoms are recalcitrant to conservative management, surgical intervention is indicated. The goal of surgery is to decompress the median nerve in the carpal tunnel by transecting the deep transverse carpal ligament (TCL).

Surgical options include open or endoscopic division of the TCL. The gold standard of operative intervention has been the open carpal tunnel release (CTR), which was first popularized by Phalen et al.[6,7] In the open technique, this division is typically carried out through a longitudinal palmar incision. Direct vision allows a safe division of the palmar fascia, following which, the TCL is identified and divided longitudinally, with care taken to protect the underlying median nerve.

The most common complications after open procedure are hypertrophic or painful scars and pillar pain (pain in the nar or hypothenar eminences).[8,9] In an effort to decrease these complications, limited or short palmar incisions as well as endoscopic techniques have evolved, because these methods are thought to result in reduced morbidity versus more extensive approaches that violate all tissue levels over a greater distance.[10,11] Proposed advantages of using a limited incision are decreased pillar tenderness and earlier return to work or avocational activities.[12,13] According to several studies, endoscopic carpal tunnel release (ECTR) results in a notably more rapid return to work and daily activities, more rapid return of postoperative grip and pinch strengths, and less scar tenderness than open CTR.[14–18]

The objective of this chapter is to describe the technical details of performance of the limited incision as well as two basic types of ECTR, namely the single-portal and two-portal techniques.

Limited Incision Carpal Tunnel Release

Security Clip Enclosed Carpal Tunnel Release System (Biomet Orthopedics, Inc.)

Indications. Patients whose CTS symptoms are unresponsive to conservative treatment after 2–3 months may be considered for operative release using the Security Clip or standard open incision. Contraindications for the Security Clip include patients with a known palmar carpal canal mass, previous displaced wrist fracture, or any other condition that may have altered wrist morphology. A relative contraindication is a patient requiring concomitant open palmar flexor tenosynovectomy.

Surgical Technique. Local anesthesia is administered followed by pneumatic tourniquet inflation. The landmarks for the surgical incision are the distal border of the thenar muscles and the radial border of the ring finger. A line is drawn over the distal extent of the TCL in line with the longitudinal axis of the radial border of the ring finger. A second line is drawn diagonally from the thenar musculature. The point of intersection of the two lines approximates the most distal edge of the TCL (Fig. 16.1). The skin incision is approximately 1.5 cm in length. It is designed to be approximately two thirds proximal and one third distal to the extended thenar muscle line.

A self-retaining retractor is introduced (Holtzheimer or Biomet CTR retractor). A blunt, right angle proximal retractor is utilized to retract the soft tissue proximally exposing the distal edge of the TCL. The superficial palmar arterial arch is usually visualized and easily protected throughout the procedure. The distal aspect of the TCL is longitudinally incised for a distance of 1.5 cm using a scalpel under direct visualization (Fig. 16.2). The carpal tunnel contents can now

M. Vigler and S.K. Lee (✉)
Division of Hand Surgery, Department of Orthopaedic Surgery,
The New York University Hospital for Joint Diseases, The New York
University School of Medicine, Hand Surgery Service, Bellevue
Hospital Center, New York, NY, USA
e-mail: steve.lee@nyumc.org

G.R. Scuderi and A.J. Tria (eds.), *Minimally Invasive Surgery in Orthopedics*,
DOI 10.1007/978-0-387-76608-9_16, © Springer Science+Business Media, LLC 2010

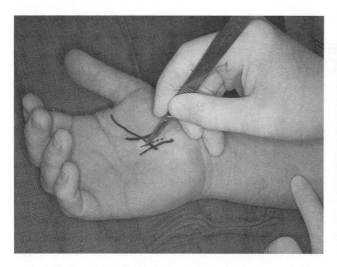

Fig. 16.1 Landmarks for the surgical incision. The incision is two thirds proximal and one third distal to the extended thenar muscle line and in line with the radial border of the ring finger (Courtesy of James W. Strickland, MD, Carmel, IN, with permission)

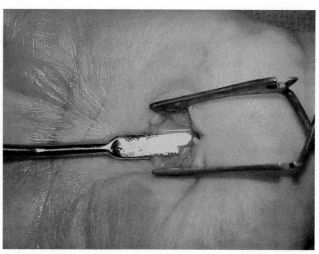

Fig. 16.3 The Blunt Single Pilot is passed beneath the transverse carpal ligament (Courtesy of James W. Strickland, MD, Carmel, IN, with permission)

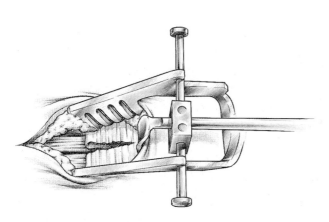

Fig.16.2 Incision of the distal 1.5 cm of the transverse carpal ligament under direct vision. The specially designed, three-sided Biomet retractor facilitates exposure (Courtesy of Biomet Orthopedics Inc., Warsaw, IN, with permission)

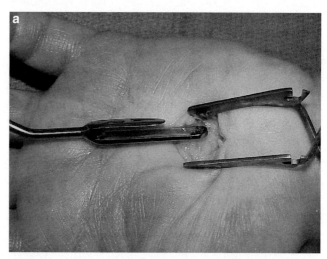

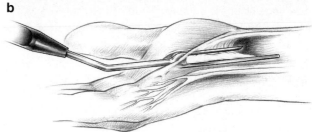

Fig. 16.4 (**a**) The Palmar Stripper with its long blunt lower skid and a short sharp upper skid. (Courtesy of James W. Strickland, MD, Carmel, IN, with permission.) (**b**) Completed passage of the Palmar Stripper after it has prepared a channel through the dense palmar connective tissue (Courtesy of Biomet Orthopedics Inc., Warsaw, IN, with permission)

be seen and protected throughout the remainder of the procedure.

Three instruments are used to clear any tissues adherent to the TCL. The first instrument, the Blunt Single Pilot, has a smooth edge and flat plane (Fig. 16.3). The purpose of the tool is to create a clear plane between the ligament and the underlying contents of the carpal tunnel. The pilot is placed just deep to the V-shaped notch created by incising the distal 1.5 cm of the TCL. The instrument is passed from distally to proximally, just deep to the TCL. The Pilot and all subsequent instruments must be directed slightly ulnarward to avoid injury to the radially vectored median nerve.

After removal of the pilot, the Palmar Stripper is placed into the wound. It is a double-sided instrument with a long blunt lower skid and a short sharp upper skid (Fig. 16.4a). The tool is

designed to prepare a channel through the dense superficial fascia immediately palmar to the TCL. The distance between the two skids is 3 mm, approximating the thickness of the ligament at its distal third. This allows the instrument to straddle the ligament as it is passed from distally to proximally. Under direct visualization, the tool is inserted into the notch created by distal division of the ligament. The lower skid is placed deep to the TCL and passed proximally. The sharper shorter upper skid will pass palmar to the TCL. The stripper is passed until the blunt center post meets the edge of the V-shaped defect of the ligament (Fig. 16.4b).

After withdrawing the Palmar Stripper, the Double Pilot is introduced. The tool has long blunt upper and lower skids (Fig. 16.5a). There are no sharp edges on the skids that could injure surrounding anatomical structures (the Palmar Stripper is shorter and has a sharp upper skid). The Double Pilot enters the V-shaped notch created by the incision in the distal ligament. It straddles the ligament and is passed proximally to establish a pathway for the Security Clip. The Double Pilot is passed until the blunt center post is fully engaged against the distal edge of the ligament (Fig. 16.5b). It is critical that the instruments are passed sequentially using the same ulnar vector. All instruments should be moistened prior to passage to provide better sliding characteristics. If some difficulty is encountered when passing the Double Pilot, it may be passed several times in a slightly different direction to be sure that there is an adequate channel for Security Clip passage.

The Security Clip is designed to protect the soft tissues on both the palmar and dorsal sides of the ligament. The lower skid has the same length as that of the Double Pilot. An upper skid is present, which converges on the lower skid terminally (Fig. 16.6a). The distance between the proximal end of the clip and the terminal closure of the upper skid is 3.5 cm. With this

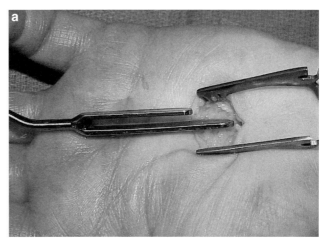

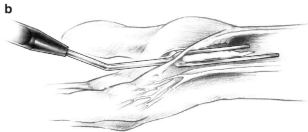

Fig. 16.5 (**a**) The Double Pilot with its blunt upper and lower skids. (Courtesy of James W. Strickland, MD, Carmel, IN, with permission.) (**b**) Completed passage of the Double Pilot with the skids straddling the transverse carpal ligament (Courtesy of Biomet Orthopedics Inc., Warsaw, IN, with permission)

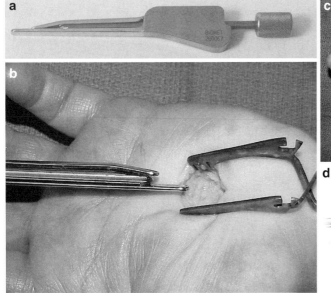

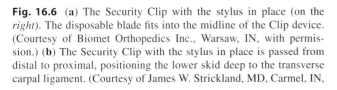

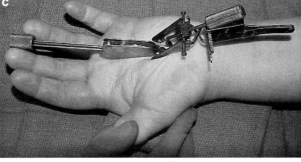

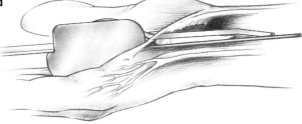

Fig. 16.6 (**a**) The Security Clip with the stylus in place (on the *right*). The disposable blade fits into the midline of the Clip device. (Courtesy of Biomet Orthopedics Inc., Warsaw, IN, with permission.) (**b**) The Security Clip with the stylus in place is passed from distal to proximal, positioning the lower skid deep to the transverse carpal ligament. (Courtesy of James W. Strickland, MD, Carmel, IN, with permission.) (**c**) As the Security Clip is fully seated, the stylus is automatically backed out of the device. (Courtesy of James W. Strickland, MD, Carmel, IN, with permission.) (**d**) The Security Clip fully engaged with the TCL contained between the upper and lower skids (Courtesy of Biomet Orthopedics Inc., Warsaw, IN, with permission)

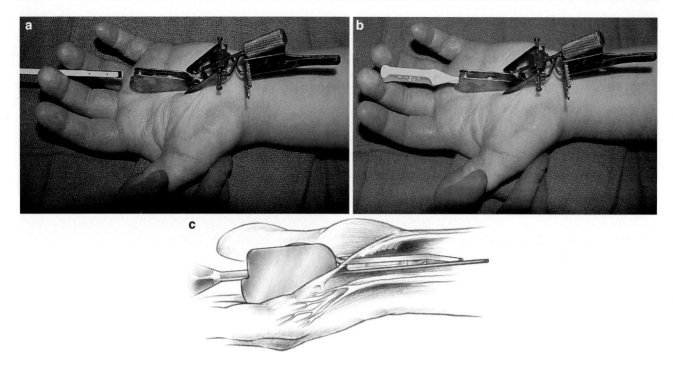

Fig. 16.7 (**a**) The disposable blade is positioned into the clip and passed distal to proximal between the upper and lower skids. (Courtesy of James W. Strickland, MD, Carmel, IN, with permission.) (**b**) Advancement of the blade continues until it is fully seated within the Security Clip. (Courtesy of James W. Strickland, MD, Carmel, IN, with permission.) (**c**) The Security Clip with the disposable blade fully seated within the device. The blade is positioned between the upper and lower skids protecting the surrounding tissue. The transverse carpal ligament has been transected at this point. (Courtesy of Biomet Orthopedics Inc., Warsaw, IN, with permission)

configuration, the Security Clip straddles the ligament, creating a closed system that is consistent with the usual morphology of the TCL. Prior to passing the Security Clip, a stylus is introduced into its central track, creating a 3-mm separation between the lower and upper skids (Fig. 16.6b). This facilitates positioning of the Security Clip into the prepared channel across the ligament. As the assembly is advanced from distal to proximal across the TCL, the stylus will automatically be backed out by the edge of the ligament, and the distal tips of the instrument will close together on the ligament (Fig. 16.6c). When fully seated, the Security Clip will contain the entire TCL between its skids, and all other adjacent tissues will be safely out of harm's way (Fig. 16.6d).

With the Security Clip straddling the ligament, a disposable blade is inserted into the track of the device and passed from distally to proximally between the upper and lower skids (Fig. 16.7a). The blade is passed down the Security Clip, completely dividing the TCL. The upper and lower skids serve to protect the tissues dorsal and palmar to the ligament. Advancement of the blade continues until the disposable device fits flush with the Security Clip (Fig. 16.7b, c). Once the blade is fully seated, it is withdrawn. The Security Clip is then removed from the wound.

The soft tissues are carefully retracted proximally to confirm complete decompression of the TCL. A Freer elevator may also be used to confirm the interval between the transected edges of the TCL.

Endoscopic Carpal Tunnel Release

ECTR, introduced by Oksuto, et al. in 1989,[19,20] has been promoted as an alternative to the open technique, largely to minimize the theoretical disadvantages of an incision through glabrous palmar skin and palmar fascia. There are two basic types of ECTR: single-portal and two-portal techniques.[11,14,21–26] Both techniques approach the carpal tunnel either proximally or proximally and distally from the limits of the thick region of the TCL. The endoscope permits constant visualization of the deep surface of the TCL, which is sharply divided through the same incision. The overlying palmar skin, subcutaneous fat, palmar fascia, and palmaris brevis muscle are preserved.

The overriding principle of ECTR is that it is of value in viewing and dividing the TCL but nothing else. It is not designed to explore the contents of the carpal tunnel. Patient selection, therefore, requires careful preoperative evaluation to exclude those individuals with pathology requiring direct inspection or surgical treatment of their carpal tunnel contents.

Excluded are patients with rheumatoid synovitis, fracture, nonunion, congenital malformation of the hook of the hamate, calcific tendonitis, or deposits of gout or amyloid.[27]

The techniques of ECTR are initially technically challenging and the surgeon should attend a formal instructional course prior to introduction of these techniques into clinical practice.[28] Additionally, one should be prepared to abort to the standard open technique if technical difficulties arise, such as inadequate views or difficulty in clearing tendinous structures from the field of view.

Endoscopic Carpal Tunnel Release (Two-Portal Technique)

Chow published his two-portal technique in 1989 and followed this with a report of his clinical results in 1990.[10,14] The original Chow technique was a transbursal technique in which the cannula system enters and exits the flexor tendon bursa. Since then, the modified Chow or extrabursal technique in which the bursa is not entered has been used. Nagle et al.[29] reviewed both techniques and concluded that the transbursal technique was associated with a higher complication rate and a higher rate of conversion to open CTR. Others have also concluded that the extrabursal technique is preferable.[30]

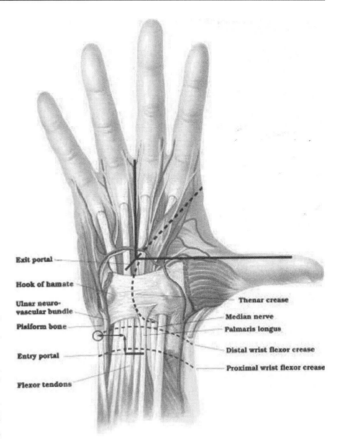

Exit portal
Hook of hamate
Ulnar neurovascular bundle
Pisiform bone
Entry portal
Flexor tendons

Thenar crease
Median nerve
Palmaris longus
Distal wrist flexor crease
Proximal wrist flexor crease

Fig. 16.8 Entry and exit portals of the two-portal endoscopic carpal tunnel release technique (Courtesy of Smith & Nephew, Andover, MA, with permission)

Surgical Technique: Extrabursal Two-Portal Technique of ECTR (ECTRA System: Smith & Nephew)

As a prerequisite to surgery, it is necessary that the patient be able to hyperextend the wrist and fingers in order to perform this technique safely.[31] After adequate general anesthesia, regional block, or local anesthesia has been administered, the hand is prepared for surgery in the usual manner. A pneumatic tourniquet is inflated over the arm. A sterile skin marker is used to map landmarks and locate entry and exit portals (Fig. 16.8).

Entry Portal. The pisiform is palpated on the volar surface of the wrist within the flexor carpi ulnaris tendon at the distal wrist crease. A line from the proximal tip of the pisiform is drawn radially, approximately 1.0–1.5 cm in length. From this point, a second line is drawn proximally 0.5 cm. A third line is then drawn from the proximal end of the second line radially 1.0 cm. This last line, which represents the entry portal incision, should be just ulnar to the palmaris longus tendon, if present (approximately at the level of the proximal wrist flexor crease) (Fig. 16.8). Average dimensions of these lines vary slightly, depending on the overall size of the hand.

Exit Portal. The patients thumb is placed in full abduction. A line is drawn across the palm from the distal border of the thumb to the approximate center of the palm. A second line is drawn from the web space between the middle and ring fingers to meet the first line, forming a right angle. A line bisecting this right angle is extended proximally 1.0 cm proximal from the vertex. This represents the exit portal (Fig. 16.8). Again, dimensions of these lines may vary slightly, depending on the overall size of the hand.

Creation of portals and placement of the cannula: A 1.0-cm transverse incision is made at the marked entry portal site, extending just through the skin. Subcutaneous tissue is bluntly dissected off the volar forearm fascia and retracted with Ragnell retractors (Fig. 16.9a). Care must be taken to avoid damage to the subcutaneous blood vessels. A transverse incision is then made through the fascia. The long blade of a Ragnell retractor is passed just beneath the fascia in a distal direction (Fig. 16.9b). The retractor should pass easily into the proximal aspect of the carpal tunnel. A Curved Dissector is passed into the carpal tunnel just under the TCL and above the carpal tunnel tenosynovium (Fig. 16.10a). It is important to keep the Curved Dissector pointed toward the planned exit portal to avoid inadvertent entry into Guyon's canal.

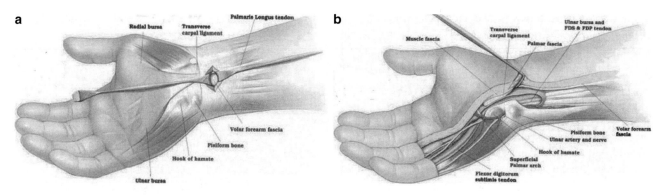

Fig. 16.9 (**a**) Incision for the proximal entry portal. Retraction of subcutaneous tissue. (**b**) Long blade of the Ragnell retractor passed beneath palmar fascia in a distal direction (Courtesy of Smith & Nephew, Andover, MA, with permission)

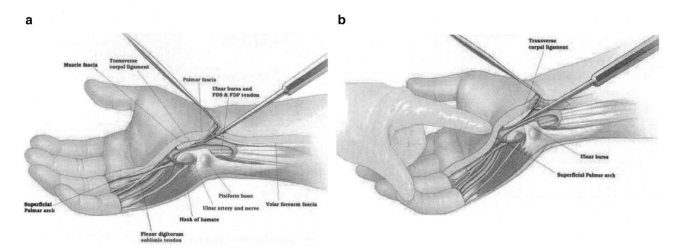

Fig. 16.10 (**a**) The Curved Dissector is passed into the carpal tunnel just under the TCL and above the carpal tunnel tenosynovium. (Courtesy of Smith & Nephew, Andover, MA, with permission.) (**b**) Tip of the Curved Dissector palpated just distal to the TCL (Courtesy of Smith & Nephew, Andover, MA, with permission)

The tenosynovium is often adherent to the TCL within the carpal tunnel. The tenosynovium should be bluntly dissected with the Curved Dissector off the carpal ligament and distal forearm fascia, from the proximal incision to the distal extent of the TCL. When the TCL is adequately prepared, drawing the Curved Dissector over the TCL should result in a type of "washboard" feeling.

The tip of the Curved Dissector should be palpated just distal to the TCL (Fig. 16.10b) and the location noted in relation to the planned distal incision. The Curved Dissector is then removed. A Slotted Cannula Assembly can now be guided into the space vacated by the Curved Dissector, following the route of entry created by its removal. The Slotted Cannula Assembly is advanced into the carpal tunnel on the underside of the TCL just radial to the hook of the hamate, staying to the ulnar side of the carpal tunnel (Fig. 16.11).

The hand and Cannula Assembly are now moved as a unit and placed on the Hand Holder with the wrist and fingers

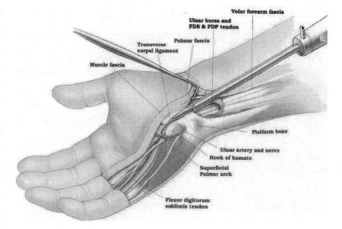

Fig. 16.11 The Slotted Cannula Assembly is passed into the carpal tunnel just under the TCL, superficial to flexor tenosynovium in the space made by Curved Dissector. Stay just radial to the hook of the hamate in line with the radial aspect of the ring finger (Courtesy of Smith & Nephew, Andover, MA, with permission)

in full hyperextension. The hyperextended hand is now strapped into the Hand Holder, following which, the Cannula Assembly is advanced along the underside of the TCL in line with the radial aspect of the ring finger until the tip of the Cannula Assembly can be easily palpated in the area of the mark for the distal incision (Fig. 16.12). The tension created by hyperextension, as well as the shape of the Cannula Assembly, causes the flexor tendons and other tissues to deflect from the pathway.

Care should be taken to avoid plunging the cannula assembly too deeply into the hand in a distal orientation. When the tip glides past the distal border of the TCL, it has entered the subcutaneous tissue. An incision is made just over the palpable Cannula Assembly tip. The incision is made only through the dermis and not into the subcutaneous tissue. The tip should exit proximally and superficially to the superficial palmar arch. The palmar skin and soft tissue is depressed using the Palmar Arch Suppressor, and the Cannula

Assembly tip is then pushed into the receptacle of the Palmar Arch Suppressor (Fig. 16.13a).

The obturator is now removed from the cannula. If positioned correctly, the Slotted Cannula should lie just below the TCL, superficial to the palmar arch and the branches of the median nerve (Fig. 16.13b). The slotted window of the cannula permits a safe cutting zone, isolating the TCL. The walls of the cannula guard vital tissues and delicate structures such as the median nerve and flexor tendons (Fig. 16.14).

Visualizing the TCL. The VideoEndoscope is inserted into the Slotted Cannula at the proximal portal. A thin bursal membrane may be seen above the Cannula's slotted opening. To gain access to the ligament, this portion of the bursa is dissected with a probe inserted through the Slotted Cannula's distal opening.

The TCL should now be identified by its fibers that run in a transverse direction. A white tissue with a swollen appearance, running longitudinally on the radial side of the opening,

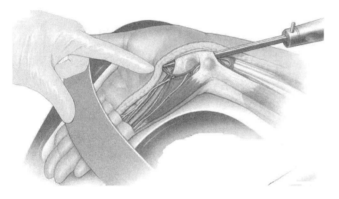

Fig. 16.12 The hand and wrist are positioned in hyperextension on the hand holder. The Slotted Cannula Assembly is advanced along the underside of the TCL in line with the radial aspect of the ring finger until the tip of the Cannula Assembly can be easily palpated in the area of the mark for the distal incision (Courtesy of Smith & Nephew, Andover, MA, with permission)

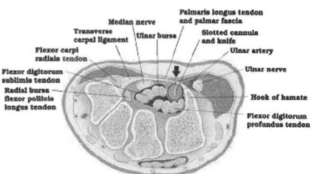

Fig. 16.14 Cross-section of the wrist. Slotted cannula and knife are shown in position within the carpal tunnel. The *arrow* indicates the site of TCL release. The cannula protects the contents of the carpal tunnel (Courtesy of Smith & Nephew, Andover, MA, with permission)

a

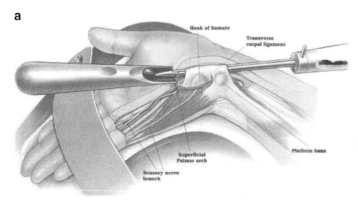

b

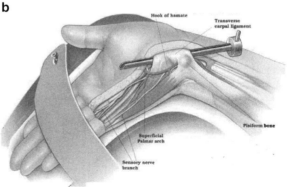

Fig. 16.13 (**a**) Palmar skin and soft tissue is depressed with the Palmar Arch Suppressor. The Slotted Cannula Assembly is pushed into the receptacle of Palmar Arch Suppressor. (**b**) Positioned correctly, the

Slotted Cannula Assembly lies just below the TCL, but superficial to the palmar arch and branches of the median nerve (Courtesy of Smith & Nephew, Andover, MA, with permission)

a
b

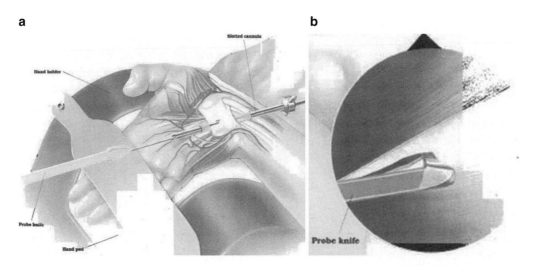

Fig. 16.15 (a) The Probe Knife, inserted in the distal portal, for forward cutting of the distal edge of the TCL. (Courtesy of Smith & Nephew, Andover, MA, with permission.) (b) The Probe Knife cutting the distal edge of the TCL, distally to proximally (Courtesy of Smith & Nephew, Andover, MA, with permission)

may also be seen. This is either the ulnar edge of the median nerve or the tendon sheath of the flexor tendons. It should be protected from injury.

The area is then probed in a distal to proximal direction until the entire TCL has been visualized. The TCL must be clearly seen with no other tissue visible between the ligament and the cannula. If difficulty in accessing the ligament is experienced, the VideoEndoscope should be removed. The TCL should be further prepared by the Curved Dissector. The Cannula Assembly should then be reinserted, the Obturator removed, and the VideoEndoscope reinserted.

Release of the TCL. The Probe Knife, which permits forward cutting only, is inserted into the distal portal (Fig. 16.15a). The blunt surface of the knife can be used to probe proximally to distally along the ligament. The cutting edge is then used to release the distal edge of the ligament (Fig. 16.15b). The Triangle Knife is then inserted through the distal opening of the slotted cannula to the midsection of the TCL, and an upward cut is made (Fig. 16.16). The Retrograde Knife is now positioned into the distal opening and its blunt tip is gently inserted through the incision made by the Triangle Knife. The cutting edge of the Retrograde Knife is drawn distally, making an incision that joins the previous two cuts, thereby completing the release of the distal aspect of the TCL (Fig. 16.17).

The VideoEndoscope is then moved from the proximal to the distal opening of the Slotted Cannula. The probe is inserted in the proximal opening. The Triangle Knife is used to initiate a longitudinal cut in the proximal fascia. The Probe Knife is then used to further extend the proximal cut. The Retrograde Knife is inserted into the midsection of the TCL from the proximal portal, then drawn proximally to join the previous cuts (Fig. 16.18). This completes the release of the TCL (Fig. 16.19).

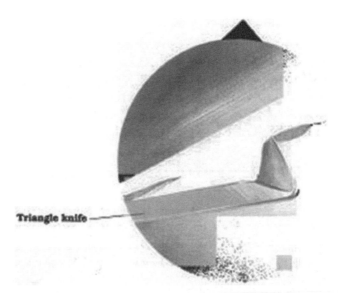

Fig. 16.16 The Triangle Knife allowing a controlled upward cut for incising the midsection of the TCL (Courtesy of Smith & Nephew, Andover, MA, with permission)

Single-Portal Surgical Technique (MicroAire Surgical Instruments, LLC)

The first commercial version of the Hand Biomechanics Lab, Inc., device designed by Agee had a blade design that did not allow viewing of the point of penetration of the blade into the ligament. This limitation, combined with a problem related to blade elevation, led to a voluntary recall of the device. The blade assembly was redesigned to permit viewing of the point of entry of the blade into the ligament, and the device was reintroduced to the market in 1992. General or regional anesthesia is recommended, although the procedure can be done under local anesthesia.[27] A pneumatic tourniquet is inflated over the arm.

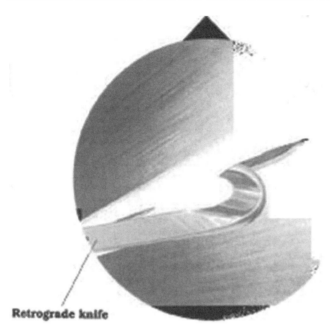

Fig. 16.17 The Retrograde Knife is drawn distally to join the previous two cuts, completing the distal release of the TCL (Courtesy of Smith & Nephew, Andover, MA, with permission)

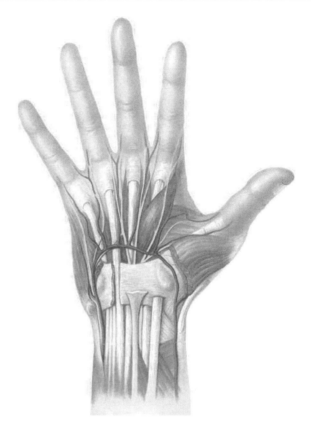

Fig. 16.19 Complete release of the TCL (Courtesy of Smith & Nephew, Andover, MA, with permission)

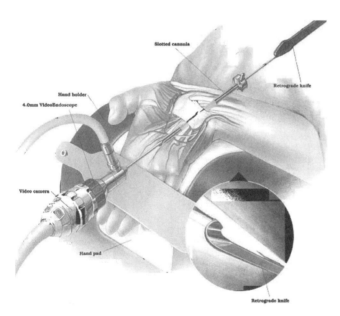

Fig. 16.18 The VideoEndoscope in the distal portal. The Retrograde Knife is used to join the previously made distal and proximal cuts (Courtesy of Smith & Nephew, Andover, MA, with permission)

Skin Incision

In a typical patient with two or more wrist creases, an incision in a more distinct distal crease produces a better cosmetic result, whereas an incision in a more proximal crease is technically easier to use because of thinner subcutaneous fat. Of note, an incision in the more distal crease increases the possibility of inadvertently inserting the device into

Guyon's canal. In addition, some patients have distal flexor creases that extend into the glabrous palmar skin on their ulnar extent. Wound in this glabrous skin should be avoided to prevent the possibility of a tender postoperative scar. The skin incision itself is made transversely between the adjacent borders of the flexor carpi radialis and flexor carpi ulnaris tendons (Fig. 16.20). It is centered over the palmaris longus, if it is present. The incision stops short of the subcutaneous tissues and their cutaneous nerves. A longitudinal spreading dissection is used to protect the subcutaneous nerves and expose the volar forearm fascia. The palmaris longus, if present, is retracted radially to protect the palmar cutaneous branch of the median nerve.

Critical surgical plane and release of TCL. A U-shaped, distally based flap of volar forearm fascia is incised and elevated (Fig. 16.21). The flexor tendon tenosynovium is then separated from the underside of the TCL by first the Synovium Elevator (Fig. 16.22) and then the Rounded Probe (Fig. 16.23). These tools should remain aligned with the ring finger, just radial to the hook of the hamate, and remain snugly apposed to the deep surface of the TCL. This positioning defines a path for the Blade Assembly.

With the wrist in slight extension, the Blade Assembly is inserted into the carpal tunnel and its viewing window is pressed snugly against the deep surface of the TCL (Fig. 16.24).

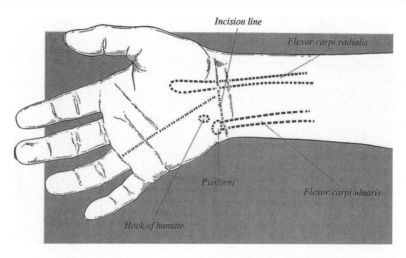

Fig. 16.20 Skin markings for the incision (Courtesy of MicroAire Surgical Instruments LLC, Charlottesville, VA, with permission)

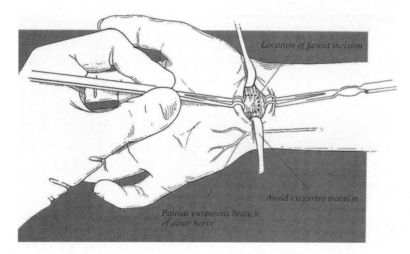

Fig. 16.21 U-shaped [**Comp: sans serif U**], distally based flap of forearm fascia is incised and elevated (Courtesy of MicroAire Surgical Instruments LLC, Charlottesville, VA, with permission)

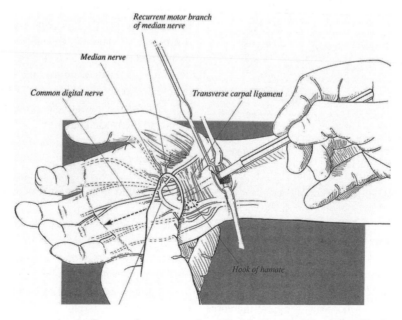

Fig. 16.22 Synovium Elevator separating the flexor tendon tenosynovium off of the deep surface of the TCL (Courtesy of MicroAire Surgical Instruments LLC, Charlottesville, VA, with permission)

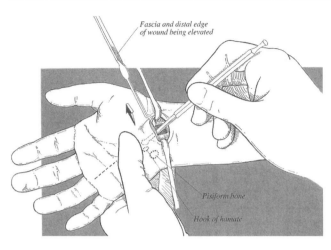

Fig. 16.23 The Rounded Probe is passed down the ulnar side of carpal tunnel to define a path for insertion of the Blade Assembly (Courtesy of MicroAire Surgical Instruments LLC, Charlottesville, VA, with permission)

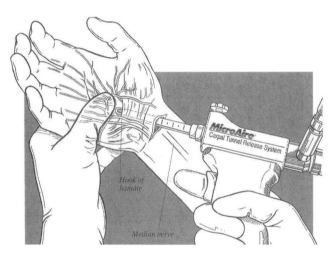

Fig. 16.24 Insertion of the Blade Assembly into the carpal tunnel (Courtesy of MicroAire Surgical Instruments LLC, Charlottesville, VA, with permission)

Maintaining alignment with the ring finger, the blade assembly is advanced distally while hugging the hook of the hamate to ensure an ulnar position. The distal advancement is to a depth of <3.0 cm to avoid injury to the superficial palmar arch or the common digital nerve to the fourth web space. Proximal-to-distal passes are used to define the distal edge of the TCL.[32] Multiple techniques are used to define the distal end of the TCL: the video picture, ballottement, and light through the skin. With the Blade Assembly correctly positioned, the trigger is depressed to elevate the cutting blade and the Blade Assembly is withdrawn proximally, incising the ligament (Fig. 16.25). Several passes may be required when the TCL is very thick. A Ragnell retractor is used to protect the distal skin edge from laceration by the blade.

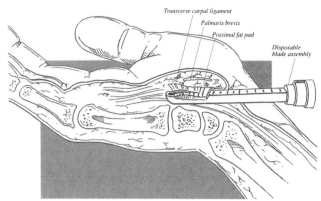

Fig. 16.25 Incision of the TCL (Courtesy of MicroAire Surgical Instruments LLC, Charlottesville, VA, with permission)

With the blade retracted, the Assembly is reinserted to inspect for completeness of ligament division. Completeness of ligament division is assessed by multiple techniques in addition to the video image. These techniques include palpation of the divided ligament with the Blade Assembly and the Rounded Probe, sensing the reduced pressure on the Blade Assembly when it is reinserted into the decompressed carpal tunnel, noting a more subcutaneous course of the Blade Assembly after ligament division, and direct inspection obtained by inserting one or two suitable right-angle retractors into the proximal end of the tunnel.

Endoscopic Assessment of the Completeness of Division of the Transverse Carpal Ligament

When viewed endoscopically, the partially divided ligament separates on its deep surface creating a V-shaped defect (Fig. 16.26). This is due to the superficial fibers of the TCL remaining intact. Subsequent cuts create a trapezoidal defect that is evident with complete ligament division when the two "halves" spring apart in radial and ulnar directions (Fig. 16.27). The retracted fully cut ligament exposes transverse fibers of palmar fascia intermingled with globules of fat and muscle that can be forced to protrude by pressing on the overlying skin.

Release of Volar Forearm Fascia

TCL release is followed by palmar displacement of the carpal tunnel contents.[33] If the volar forearm fascia proximal to the carpal tunnel is left intact, this palmar displacement occurs distal to the fascia, thereby possibly kinking the median nerve on the undivided edge of the fascia. This fascia should be released under direct vision with tenotomy

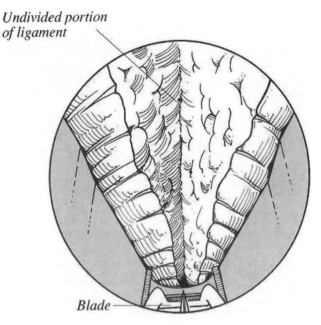

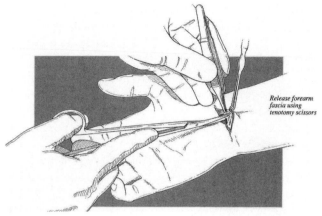

Fig. 16.28 Release of volar forearm fascia with tenotomy scissors (Courtesy of MicroAire Surgical Instruments LLC, Charlottesville, VA, with permission)

Fig. 16.26 Partially divided transverse carpal ligament, separated on its deep surface creating a V-shaped defect [**Comp: sans serif V**] (Courtesy of MicroAire Surgical Instruments LLC, Charlottesville, VA, with permission)

Minimally Invasive Trigger Finger Release

Trigger finger, or stenosing tenosynovitis of the thumb or finger flexor tendon, frequently occurs in adults. Triggering is produced by thickening (fibrocartilaginous metaplasia) of the fibrous sheath through which the tendon glides or by thickening of the tendon's normally thin synovial covering. Symptoms of triggering may also be produced by a tendon nodule[34] or by an enlarged tendon that locks the flexor tendon at the level of the first annular pulley (A1 pulley). Patients typically complain of pain, swelling, and in some cases of having to grasp the digit with the other hand to extend the digit from its locked flexed position.

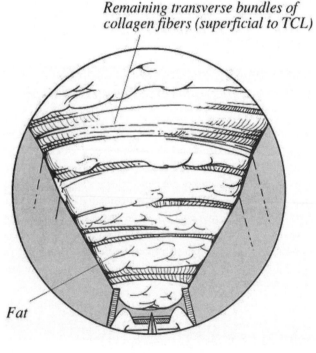

Fig. 16.27 Complete TCL division (Courtesy of MicroAire Surgical Instruments LLC, Charlottesville, VA, with permission)

scissors to ensure complete median nerve decompression (Fig. 16.28). The volar forearm fascia is divided for 2–3 cm in line with the ulnar aspect of the palmaris longus to avoid injury to the palmar cutaneous branch of the median nerve.

Numerous methods for treating trigger fingers have been developed. Nonsurgical treatments include extension splinting, administration of nonsteroidal anti-inflammatory drugs, and steroid injections. When nonoperative treatment fails, surgical release of the A1 pulley is indicated. Open release is typically performed via a small palmar incision under local anesthesia; the A1 pulley is completely visualized and incised. Although the success rate of open release is 97–100% with a recurrence rate of only 3%,[35–38] complication rates of 7–28% have been described.[35,39] These include digital nerve injury,[39] infection,[39] stiffness,[40] weakness,[39] scar tenderness,[39] and bowstringing of the flexor tendons.[41] The open procedure requires an operative facility, and the surgical site requires wound care and can remain painful for up to 2 weeks.[42]

Percutaneous release, using a fine tenotome, was first described by Lorthioir,[43] who obtained good outcomes with no complications. A few decades later, Eastwood, et al.,[44] reported the use of a needle tip instead of a tenotome and reported 94% excellent results. Several recent studies of the percutaneous release have also demonstrated favorable results.[44–47] Although percutaneous release for trigger digits is a quicker procedure[36] than the open approach, incomplete release or the need to convert to open release with this technique ranges from 0 to 11%.[44,48,49] Gilberts et al.[36,38] concluded that percutaneous release was a quick procedure, was less painful, and obtained considerable better outcomes in rehabilitation than open surgery in the short term. One potential disadvantage is that it is a blind method; therefore, the approach can cause nerve or tendon damage. Nerve damage has not been reported with the percutaneous procedure, although it has been reported at the radial side of the thumb following open release.[39,42,44,48–50] Cadaveric studies of percutaneous needle release have found superficial longitudinal lacerations along the flexor tendons in 88% of fingers and in all thumbs.[45,50] This does not appear to have any significant consequences in most patients.[46]

In this chapter we describe the technical details of the performance of the percutaneous needle and knife methods as well as the endoscopic method for trigger finger release.

Percutaneous Needle Release

Surgical Technique

Percutaneous release can be performed in the office setting. Local anesthetic is administered and the palmar base of the affected finger is prepared sterilely. The patient is asked to flex the affected digit actively. The surgeon then hyperextends the finger. This brings the flexor tendon sheath directly under the skin and allows the neurovascular bundles to displace to either side.

An 18-gauge needle is inserted at the proximal aspect of the A1 pulley. Care should be taken to stay centered over the flexor tendon sheath to avoid neurovascular structures and to enter the skin perpendicularly with the bevel of the needle parallel to the tendon. Alternatively, some investigators (and the authors' preferred method) have advocated inserting the needle slightly more distally in the middle of the pulley and then proceeding with release proximally and distally.

The proximal edge of the A1 pulley is located near the distal horizontal palmar crease for the small, ring, and middle fingers. For the index finger, it is located at the proximal horizontal palmar crease. Release of the ring and middle fingers is believed to be relatively safe. The oblique course of the flexor tendons and neurovascular structures to the index and small finger, however, pose a greater challenge. Wilhelmi et al.[51] (Fig. 16.29) described reliable landmarks for the small finger flexor tendon sheath in the area of the A1 pulley as lying underneath a line connecting the ulnar border of the scaphoid tubercle proximally to the center of the proximal digital crease distally. For the index finger, the landmarks were the radial border of the pisiform proximally

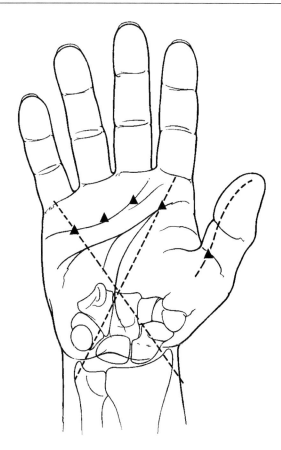

Fig. 16.29 Surface landmarks for percutaneous A1 pulley release. Index finger: at the proximal palmar crease at a line connecting the radial border of the pisiform and the center of the proximal digital crease of the index finger. Middle finger: at the distal palmar crease in the midaxis of the finger. Ring finger: at the distal palmar crease in the midaxis of the digit. Small finger: at the distal palmar crease at a line connecting the ulnar border of the scaphoid tubercle with the center of the proximal digital crease of the small finger. Thumb: at the proximal digital crease in the midaxis of the thumb (Courtesy of Biomet Orthopedics Inc., Warsaw, IN, with permission)

and the midline of the proximal digital crease distally. By using these landmarks in a cadaver study, the A1 pulley was reliably transected. None of the digital nerves or arteries was transected. In the thumb, the intersection of the proximal thumb digital crease and a perpendicular line up the central axis of the palmar aspect of the thumb is the preferred insertion site.

The needle may be inserted into the tendon. This is confirmed by needle movement when the patient flexes and extends the distal phalanx. The needle is withdrawn slowly until this motion ceases. The needle tip is now in the A1 pulley. The A1 pulley is cut by moving the needle forward and back while advancing it in line with the longitudinal axis of the flexor tendon sheath. A grating sensation indicates the A1 pulley is being cut. Once the surgeon thinks the pulley has been released adequately, the needle is withdrawn and the patient is asked to flex and extend the digit to show relief from triggering.

Percutaneous Trigger Finger Knife (Biomet Orthopedics, Inc.)

Unlike percutaneous needle release, the Trigger Finger Knife is designed to avoid damage to the flexor tendons, avoiding possible complications of scarring and recurrent triggering.

Surgical Technique

Local anesthesia is used. Use a ruler to mark 1-cm-wide transverse lines, 1 cm and 2 cm proximal to the proximal finger crease. The approximate location of the A1 pulley is between these lines. The skin incision is made as a transverse line 3-mm wide and 3-cm proximal to the proximal finger crease (Figs. 16.30 and 16.31). A small pair of scissors may be used to gently spread the incision and palmar fascia if entrance is difficult.

The Trigger Finger Knife is inserted longitudinally, parallel to the flexor tendons (Fig. 16.32). The knife is guided distally until the proximal end of the A1 pulley is palpated. The surgeon's thumb is placed firmly on the distal skin marking to prevent passage of the knife into the A2 pulley (Fig. 16.32). The Trigger Finger Knife is gently advanced through

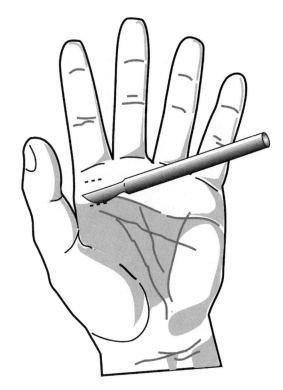

Fig. 16.31 The skin incision is at the most proximal of these marks (Courtesy of Biomet Orthopedics Inc., Warsaw, IN, with permission)

the A1 pulley. A grating sensation may be felt and will stop when the pulley is completely released. The knife is removed. Confirm complete release by asking the patient to flex and extend the finger. Movement should be free and smooth without any triggering.

Endoscopic Tendon Sheath Release for Trigger Finger (Smith & Nephew)

Proponents of endoscopic trigger finger release argue that it maximizes patient outcome by being a minimally invasive approach and yet releasing the A1 pulley under direct endoscopic visualization.

Surgical Technique

The procedure is performed under local anesthesia and the use of a pneumatic tourniquet. Two transverse incisions, each 2.5 mm in length, are made. The proximal incision is made 1 cm proximal to the proximal edge of the A1 pulley and the distal incision is located on the

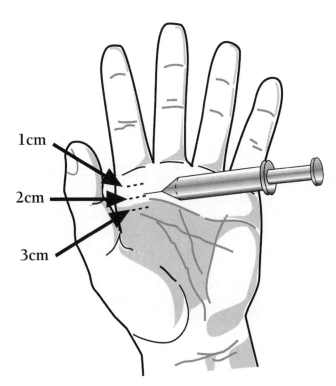

Fig. 16.30 Skin markings 1 cm, 2 cm, and 3 cm proximal to proximal finger crease. Local anesthesia is injected (Courtesy of Biomet Orthopedics Inc., Warsaw, IN, with permission)

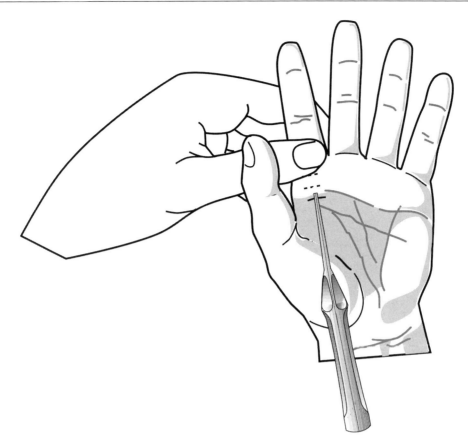

Fig. 16.32 The Trigger Finger Knife is inserted longitudinally, parallel to the flexor tendons. The surgeon's thumb is placed firmly on the distal skin marking to prevent passage of the knife into the A2 pulley (Courtesy of Biomet Orthopedics Inc., Warsaw, IN, with permission)

proximal palmar digital crease. The metacarpophalangeal joints are positioned in hyperextension. Separation of the flexor tendon and subcutaneous tissue is performed using a Curved, Blunt Dissector (Fig. 16.33). This is inserted proximally at the proximal incision site, and swept distally to create a channel.

The Window Cannula Assembly is inserted subcutaneously along the flexor tendon sheath from the proximal portal and advanced until it passes through the distal portal (Fig. 16.34). The obturator is then removed. A 2.7-mm, 30° Light Post Opposite Endoscope is passed into the proximal portal to confirm the extent of the stenosed A1 pulley, and to examine the anatomy through the cannula window (Fig. 16.35). A probe can be used to palpate tissue, confirm anatomical structures, and pinpoint the proximal edge of the A1 pulley. A retrograde knife is inserted from the distal portal. The proximal edge of the A1 pulley is hooked and the entire length is sectioned under direct endoscopic vision, revealing the underlying flexor tendon.

After completion of the A1 pulley release, the synovial sheath may be released if the flexor tendon is longitudinally covered with synovium. This is achieved by use of

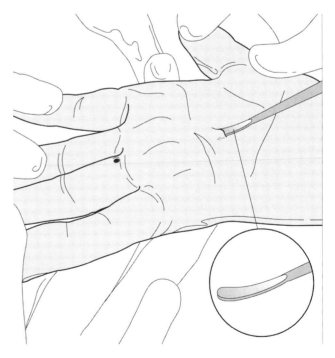

Fig. 16.33 A Curved Blunt Dissector is inserted distally to create a channel (Courtesy of Smith & Nephew, Andover, MA, with permission)

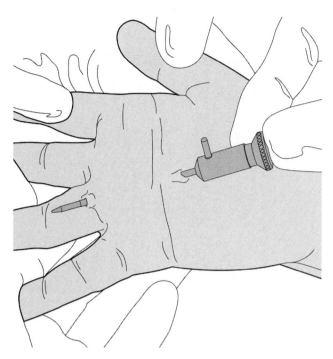

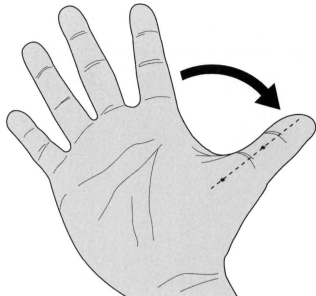

Fig. 16.36 Skin markings on the thumb for incision location (Courtesy of Smith & Nephew, Andover, MA, with permission)

Fig. 16.34 The Window Cannula Assembly is inserted subcutaneously along the flexor tendon sheath from the proximal to distal portal (Courtesy of Smith & Nephew, Andover, MA, with permission)

Endoscopic Trigger Thumb Release

Thumb portal locations are more distal than those in the fingers (Fig. 16.36). The distal incision is located at the midpoint between the interphalangeal and metacarpophalangeal joints. The thumb should be in full abduction when making the proximal incision over the flexor pollicis longus tendon, 1 cm proximal to the proximal palmar thumb crease. The thumb procedure proceeds as above. It is performed in full abduction to avoid digital nerve injury.

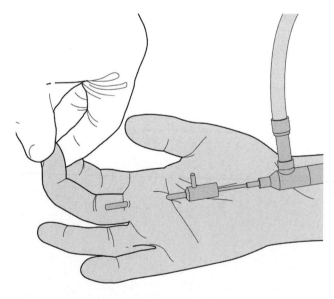

References

1. Duncan K.H., et al., Treatment of carpal tunnel syndrome by members of the American Society for Surgery of the Hand: results of a questionnaire. J Hand Surg (Am), 1987 **12**(3): p. 384–91
2. Pfeffer, G.B., et al., The history of carpal tunnel syndrome. J Hand Surg (Br), 1988 **13**(1): p. 28–34
3. Stevens, J.C., et al., Carpal tunnel syndrome in Rochester, Minnesota, 1961 to 1980. Neurology, 1988 **38**(1): p. 134–8
4. Gelberman, R.H., et al., The carpal tunnel syndrome. A study of carpal canal pressures. J Bone Joint Surg Am, 1981 **63**(3): p. 380–3
5. Cobb, T.K., et al., The carpal tunnel as a compartment. An anatomic perspective. Orthop Rev, 1992 **21**(4): p. 451–3
6. Phalen, G.S., W.J. Gardner, and A.A. La Londe, Neuropathy of the median nerve due to compression beneath the transverse carpal ligament. J Bone Joint Surg Am, 1950 **32A**(1): p. 109–12
7. Phalen, G.S., The carpal-tunnel syndrome. Clinical evaluation of 598 hands. Clin Orthop Relat Res, 1972 **83**: p. 29–40
8. Semple, J.C. and A.O. Cargill, Carpal-tunnel syndrome. Results of surgical decompression. Lancet, 1969 **1**(7601): p. 918–9

Fig. 16.35 The Light Post Opposite Endoscope is inserted into the cannula after the obturator has been removed (Courtesy of Smith & Nephew, Andover, MA, with permission)

the triangle knife. Complete A1 pulley release is confirmed by smooth gliding of the flexor tendon during passive motion of the finger and absence of triggering during active motion.

9. Seradge, H. and E. Seradge, Piso-triquetral pain syndrome after carpal tunnel release. J Hand Surg (Am), 1989 **14**(5): p. 858–62

10. Chow, J.C., Endoscopic release of the carpal ligament: a new technique for carpal tunnel syndrome. Arthroscopy, 1989 **5**(1): p. 19–24

11. Agee, J.M., et al., Endoscopic release of the carpal tunnel: a randomized prospective multicenter study. J Hand Surg (Am), 1992 **17**(6): p. 987–95

12. Nathan, P.A., K.D. Meadows, and R.C. Keniston, Rehabilitation of carpal tunnel surgery patients using a short surgical incision and an early program of physical therapy. J Hand Surg (Am), 1993 **18**(6): p. 1044–50

13. Lee, W.P. and J.W. Strickland, Safe carpal tunnel release via a limited palmar incision. Plast Reconstr Surg, 1998 **101**(2): p. 418–24; discussion 425–6

14. Chow, J.C., Endoscopic release of the carpal ligament for carpal tunnel syndrome: 22-month clinical result. Arthroscopy, 1990 **6**(4): p. 288–96

15. Trumble, T.E., et al., Single-portal endoscopic carpal tunnel release compared with open release: a prospective, randomized trial. J Bone Joint Surg Am, 2002 **84-A**(7): p. 1107–15

16. Palmer, D.H., et al., Endoscopic carpal tunnel release: a comparison of two techniques with open release. Arthroscopy, 1993 **9**(5): p. 498–508

17. Brown, R.A., et al., Carpal tunnel release. A prospective, randomized assessment of open and endoscopic methods. J Bone Joint Surg Am, 1993 **75**(9): p. 1265–75

18. Kerr, C.D., M.E. Gittins, and D.R. Sybert, Endoscopic versus open carpal tunnel release: clinical results. Arthroscopy, 1994 **10**(3): p. 266–9

19. Okutsu, I., et al., Endoscopic management of carpal tunnel syndrome. Arthroscopy, 1989 **5**(1): p. 11–8

20. Okutsu, I., et al., Measurement of pressure in the carpal canal before and after endoscopic management of carpal tunnel syndrome. J Bone Joint Surg Am, 1989 **71**(5): p. 679–83

21. Adams, B.D., Endoscopic carpal tunnel release. J Am Acad Orthop Surg, 1994 **2**(3): p. 179–84

22. Bande, S., L. De Smet, and G. Fabry, The results of carpal tunnel release: open versus endoscopic technique. J Hand Surg (Br), 1994 **19**(1): p. 14–7

23. Brown, M.G., B. Keyser, and E.S. Rothenberg, Endoscopic carpal tunnel release. J Hand Surg (Am), 1992 **17**(6): p. 1009–11

24. Erdmann, M.W., Endoscopic carpal tunnel decompression. J Hand Surg (Br), 1994 **19**(1): p. 5–13

25. Feinstein, P.A., Endoscopic carpal tunnel release in a community-based series. J Hand Surg (Am), 1993 **18**(3): p. 451–4

26. Resnick, C.T. and B.W. Miller, Endoscopic carpal tunnel release using the subligamentous two-portal technique. Contemp Orthop, 1991 **22**(3): p. 269–77

27. Agee, J.M., H.R. McCarroll, and E.R. North, Endoscopic carpal tunnel release using the single proximal incision technique. Hand Clin, 1994 **10**(4): p. 647–59

28. Berger, R.A., Endoscopic carpal tunnel release. A current perspective. Hand Clin, 1994 **10**(4): p. 625–36

29. Nagle, D.J., et al., A multicenter prospective review of 640 endoscopic carpal tunnel releases using the transbursal and extrabursal chow techniques. Arthroscopy, 1996 **12**(2): p. 139–43

30. Seiler, J.G., III, et al., Endoscopic carpal tunnel release: an anatomic study of the two-incision method in human cadavers. J Hand Surg (Am), 1992 **17**(6): p. 996–1002

31. Chow, J.C., Endoscopic carpal tunnel release. Two-portal technique. Hand Clin, 1994 **10**(4): p. 637–46

32. Viegas, S.F., A. Pollard, and K. Kaminksi, Carpal arch alteration and related clinical status after endoscopic carpal tunnel release. J Hand Surg (Am), 1992 **17**(6): p. 1012–6

33. Richman, J.A., et al., Carpal tunnel syndrome: morphologic changes after release of the transverse carpal ligament. J Hand Surg (Am), 1989 **14**(5): p. 852–7

34. Hueston, J.T. and W.F. Wilson, The aetiology of trigger finger explained on the basis of intratendinous architecture. Hand, 1972 **4**(3): p. 257–60

35. Bonnici, A.V. and J.D. Spencer, A survey of 'trigger finger' in adults. J Hand Surg (Br), 1988 **13**(2): p. 202–3

36. Gilberts, E.C., et al., Prospective randomized trial of open versus percutaneous surgery for trigger digits. J Hand Surg (Am), 2001 **26**(3): p. 497–500

37. Benson, L.S. and A.J. Ptaszek, Injection versus surgery in the treatment of trigger finger. J Hand Surg (Am), 1997 **22**(1): p. 138–44

38. Gilberts, E.C. and J.C. Wereldsma, Long-term results of percutaneous and open surgery for trigger fingers and thumbs. Int Surg, 2002 **87**(1): p. 48–52

39. Thorpe AP, Results of surgery for trigger finger. J Hand Surg (Br), 1988 **13**(2): p. 199–201

40. Hodgkinson JP, et al. Retrospective study of 120 trigger digits treated surgically. J R Coll Surg Edinb, 1988 **33**(2): p. 88–90

41. Heithoff, S.J., L.H. Millender, and J. Helman, Bowstringing as a complication of trigger finger release. J Hand Surg (Am), 1988 **13**(4): p. 567–70

42. Fu, Y.C., et al., Revision of incompletely released trigger fingers by percutaneous release: results and complications. J Hand Surg (Am), 2006 **31**(8): p. 1288–91

43. Lorthioir, J., Jr., Surgical treatment of trigger-finger by a subcutaneous method. J Bone Joint Surg Am, 1958 **40-A**(4): p. 793–5

44. Eastwood, D.M., K.J. Gupta, and D.P. Johnson, Percutaneous release of the trigger finger: an office procedure. J Hand Surg (Am), 1992 **17**(1): p. 114–7

45. Bain, G.I. and N.A. Wallwork, Percutaneous A1 pulley release a clinical study. Hand Surg, 1999 **4**(1): p. 45–50

46. Blumberg, N., R. Arbel, and S. Dekel, Percutaneous release of trigger digits. J Hand Surg (Br), 2001 **26**(3): p. 256–7

47. Bara T, and T. Dorman, [Percutaneous trigger finger release]. Chir Narzadow Ruchu Ortop Pol, 2002 **67**(6): p. 613–7

48. Cihantimur, B., S. Akin, and M. Ozcan, Percutaneous treatment of trigger finger. 34 fingers followed 0.5–2 years. Acta Orthop Scand, 1998 **69**(2): p. 167–8

49. Patel, M.R. and V.J. Moradia, Percutaneous release of trigger digit with and without cortisone injection. J Hand Surg (Am), 1997 **22**(1): p. 150–5

50. Pope, D.F. and S.W. Wolfe, Safety and efficacy of percutaneous trigger finger release. J Hand Surg (Am), 1995 **20**(2): p. 280–3

51. Wilhelmi, B.J., et al., Safe treatment of trigger finger with longitudinal and transverse landmarks: an anatomic study of the border fingers for percutaneous release. Plast Reconstr Surg, 2003 **112**(4): p. 993–9

Chapter 17
Round Table Discussion of Minimally Invasive Surgery Upper Extremity Cases

Evan L. Flatow, Bradford O. Parsons, and Leesa M. Galatz

Case 1

Dr. Flatow: This first case is a 55-year-old, right hand-dominant ex-police detective who was injured in a motor vehicle accident in 1978. We don't have the initial films of the shoulder fracture, but he was evidently treated with olecranon-pin traction for 5 weeks. We first saw him in 1988, when he was virtually ankylosed and had moderate pain. The pain became gradually worse over the ensuing 18 years, and is now unbearable (requiring narcotic pain medications). He is also frustrated with the stiffness: he has elevation of 90°, external rotation to negative 10°, and internal rotation with the hand reaching the buttocks posteriorly. Dr. Parsons, are there any joint-sparing options for this patient?

Dr. Parsons: Joint-sparing procedures such as arthroscopic capsular release and osteoplasty, or open debridement procedures, are options in cases of glenohumeral arthritis in patients with mild arthrosis without substantial articular deformity. These types of procedures can be very helpful in decreasing pain and improving motion in properly selected patients, especially patients who are too young or too physically active to undergo shoulder replacement. Gerry Williams has had success with open debridement and a biological resurfacing of the glenoid with capsular tissue in carefully selected patients; younger, more active patients with primary glenohumeral osteoarthritis. However, once there are extensive arthritic changes, especially in posttraumatic arthritis where significant deformity exists, the success of these options is less predictable. In a patient such as this, I would offer two main options: continuing to live with the shoulder the way it is or considering replacement arthroplasty.

Dr. Flatow: I came to the same conclusion. With this degree of posttraumatic arthritis, I felt at least the humeral side required replacement. In some younger, more active patients, we have tried to avoid a polyethylene glenoid. Initially we tried just reaming the glenoid, but these have not

done well, so we have moved to biological resurfacing, either with capsule or fascia as described by Burkhead, or with a meniscal allograft as described by Levine and Yamaguchi. However, the results are not always predictable, and this 55-year-old, though still active, was willing to modify his activities, and I felt a total replacement made sense.

Dr. Galatz: I agree – placing a glenoid offers the most reliable pain relief and does have proven longevity. However, there are technical challenges: the shaft malunion will make use of a traditional stemmed implant difficult.

Dr. Flatow: This was a problem. In mild malunions, variable anatomy prostheses have been advocated to allow adjusting the implant to the distorted anatomy. However, I have not seen the logic in turning a bone malunion into a metal one. I have preferred, when possible, to use a cutting guide to reset the prosthetic head to the tuberosity and shaft axis, ignoring the malunited head, and aiming to restore more normal mechanics. When the distortions are severe, as in this case, I have resorted to resurfacing replacements.

Dr. Galatz: The use of a resurfacing arthroplasty is an excellent choice in this situation. The use of this particular prosthesis is bone preserving. In this young patient, this offers the advantages of future reconstructive options.

Dr. Flatow: One big disadvantage of resurfacing is it is harder to expose the glenoid. In some cases, we have used the superior approach advocated by Copeland, **XX** but in this case we were able to perform releases, which allowed exposure through a deltopectoral approach. A minimally invasive axillary skin incision can often be used, although we used a standard deltopectoral in this case. This patient went on to excellent pain relief and substantial but not complete improvement in motion. His latest range of motion is as follows: he has elevation of 140°, external rotation to 40°, and internal rotation behind the back to L1 posteriorly.

Case 2

Dr. Flatow: This 57-year-old, right hand-dominant man fell more than 5 ft. off of a ladder, landing on his left shoulder. He is a retired police captain and an active golfer. There is no

E.L. Flatow (✉), B.O. Parsons, and L.M. Galatz
Peter & Leni May Department of Orthopaedic Surgery, Mount Sinai Medical Center, 5 East 98th Street, Box 1188, New York, NY, 10029-6574, USA
e-mail: evan.flatow@msnyuhealth.org

G.R. Scuderi and A.J. Tria (eds.), *Minimally Invasive Surgery in Orthopedics*,
DOI 10.1007/978-0-387-76608-9_17, © Springer Science+Business Media, LLC 2010

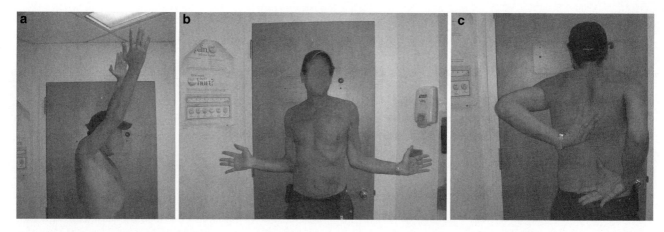

Fig.17.1 (**a–c**) A locking plate was used to repair a proximal humerus fracture in a 57-year-old man who fell off a ladder. This patient went on to have to excellent function and reasonable motion

neurovascular deficit. He has ecchymoses in his arm and axilla. Dr. Galatz, you are one of the pioneers of percutaneous fixation of proximal humerus fractures – would these techniques be helpful here?

Dr. Galatz: This particular fracture is not a good one for percutaneous pinning. The reason is because of the comminution along the medial shaft and calcar area. Comminution in this area is a contraindication to percutaneous pin fixation, as it will lead to an unstable reduction.

Dr. Flatow: Dr. Parsons, would intramedullary devices such as locked rods be an option?

Dr. Parsons: Intramedullary rods are an option in some proximal humeral fractures. These implants, when used, are most successful when good bone and stout proximal fixation in the humeral head enables a stable construct. In a comminuted fracture such as this, especially when the greater tuberosity is involved, I would be concerned about blowing out the tuberosities during insertion of the rod, and about my proximal fixation once the rod was implanted. As a result, I don't think a rod is a great option for this patient.

Dr. Flatow: We elected a locking plate. It allowed us to secure the greater tuberosity with sutures to the plate holes, and to rigidly fix the head to the shaft.

Dr. Galatz: The use of a locking plate is an excellent choice as this affords stability needed for this difficult fracture.

Dr. Flatow: Some surgeons have advocated an extended superior deltoid-split approach, exposing and protecting the circumflex branch of the axillary nerve as needed. However, I have generally preferred the deltopectoral approach. He went on to excellent function and reasonable motion (Fig. 17.1a–c).

Case 3

Dr. Flatow: This 62-year-old, right hand-dominant woman presented 10 days after being struck by a car. She had rib fractures and this left proximal humerus fracture.

Dr. Galatz: This fracture is a valgus-impacted fracture configuration and is very amenable to percutaneous pin fixation. This is an excellent choice in this case. On the fluoroscopic views, the valgus deformity is not yet reduced, however, it is reduced in the final X-rays. Reduction of the valgus deformity by upward impaction using the described technique is critical for allowing the greater tuberosity to fall into anatomic position. The pins are best placed low along the surgical neck to engage the head.

Case 4

Dr. Flatow: This is a 31-year-old, right hand-dominant woman who suffered a traumatic anterior right dislocation 6 years ago when she fell down a mountain. It took 6 h to get help and have the shoulder reduced. She has had four subsequent dislocations, all requiring manual reductions. The second also happened after a fall, but the last three were positional (e.g., reaching for a nightstand). On examination, she has classic anterior apprehension with abduction and external rotation, normal strength and motion, and mild generalized laxity (her elbows hyperextend to 12° of recurvatum and she can just approximate her thumbs to her forearms). Dr. Parsons – is she a candidate for a minimally invasive capsular procedure?

Dr. Parsons: The traditional surgical management of anterior glenohumeral instability has been an open labral repair with capsular shift if capsular laxity is apparent. Currently, many surgeons are performing arthroscopic repairs for instability with success, but there is still a role for open stabilization, especially in patients with glenoid bone loss or in patients with previous failed stabilization procedures. When indicated, these open procedures can be performed through a small, "minimally invasive" incision in the axillary skin crease that is very cosmetic and allows excellent exposure.

Dr. Flatow: Dr. Galatz, would you consider arthroscopic management?

Dr. Galatz: The use of arthroscopic stabilization for instability remains a controversial topic. However, there are several advantages of an arthroscopic approach. One is preserving subscapularis integrity and function. Even though subscapularis healing is reliable after instability surgery, there still is likely some compromise and this is somewhat substantiated in the literature. Another advantage of arthroscopy is the preservation of proprioceptive ability, which is easily disrupted, especially in people with some underlying intrinsic laxity.

Dr. Flatow: We did go in arthroscopically, and found not only a huge Bankart avulsion but a large SLAP tear, both of which we fixed along with some capsular tensioning.

Dr. Galatz: This highlights another advantage of arthroscopy: it allows treatment of concurrent pathology – in this case, the SLAP lesion, which can be very difficult to fix through an open approach.

Case 5

Dr. Flatow: This is an active 37-year-old, right hand-dominant man with right shoulder pain since an overuse incident working out with weights. Radiographs show an enchondroma (which had been biopsied) and no other abnormalities. He has marked external rotation weakness on examination, and an electromyogram (EMG) documenting suprascapular nerve dysfunction.

Dr. Parsons: External rotation weakness is usually due to one of two pathologic entities, a massive rotator cuff tear or suprascapular nerve palsy. In a young patient without history of trauma, the likelihood of a large rotator cuff tear is very low. Isolated suprascapular nerve palsy is often the result of a ganglion cyst in either the suprascapular or spinoglenoid notch. When I see patients with isolated external rotation weakness, I check both an magnetic resonance imaging scan (MRI) and an EMG. Prior to MRI, we probably missed many cysts that were impinging on the nerve and causing weakness. When ordering the MRI, I make sure to tell the radiologist to go medial enough to include the suprascapular notch in the MRI field, or you may miss a cyst there. The EMG is also helpful in localizing the lesion. A suprascapular notch lesion will affect both supra and infra, while a spinoglenoid notch lesion would only effect the infraspinatus. The EMG also helps rule out a more global nerve dysfunction such as Parsonage–Turner syndrome, which, although rare, I have seen.

Dr. Flatow: Many approaches for suprascapular nerve release have been described. A small incision and a split of the trapezius directly over the suprascapular notch can allow release of the nerve at that location, while a small incision over the scapular spine allows exposure of the nerve from the suprascapular notch (by elevating a bit of trapezius and lifting up the supraspinatus) to below the spinoglenoid notch (by elevating a bit of deltoid and rolling the infraspinatus back). However, when compression is due to a cyst, also called a ganglion, most of us would use an arthroscopic approach.

Dr. Galatz: I agree. Spinoglenoid notch cysts are very easily treated arthroscopically. The cyst is the result of a SLAP lesion, which allows some synovial fluid to be compressed into the spinal glenoid notch area, putting pressure on the suprascapular nerve. If left alone, this can result in atrophy of infraspinatus primarily, but also of the supraspinatus if the cyst is higher, near the suprascapular notch. The cyst can be decompressed through an arthroscopic approach and the most important component of the repair is repair of the SLAP lesion. If this is not addressed then the source of the problem will not be eliminated.

Dr. Flatow: This is what we did, and the patient regained full external rotation strength at 6-month follow-up. He continues to have mild pain and weakness with overhead activities, but reports that he is much better than prior to surgery. He has returned to work on restricted duty.

Chapter 18
Anterolateral Mini-incision Total Hip Arthroplasty

Sanaz Hariri and Andrew A. Freiberg

Anterolateral Approach

Historical Perspective and Evolution

At the advent of the total hip arthroplasty (THA), Charnley advocated the transtrochanteric approach ("the lateral exposure with elevation of the greater trochanter") for THAs.[1] However, surgeons such as Müller and Harris argued that there were many advantages to performing primary THAs without a trochanteric osteotomy, including a shortened operative time, less blood loss, elimination of the need to perform a trochanteric repair, avoidance of common trochanteric complications (e.g., nonunion and painful bursitis due to the irritation caused by the metal fixation wires), and earlier return to unsupported weight bearing.[2,3] The most popular alternatives to the transtrochanteric approach are the posterior or posterolateral, the direct lateral, and the anterolateral approaches.

In his 1935 description of femoral neck fracture treatment, Watson-Jones described the anterolateral approach entailing an exposure of the femoral neck through the interval between the gluteus medius and the tensor fasciae femoris. To provide better exposure, he describes dissecting the anterior fibers of the gluteus medius insertion off of the trochanter. In cases where still further exposure is needed, he advocated driving an osteotome into the front of the trochanter and levering out on its intact posterior margin. He warns surgeons not to fully separate the trochanter to avoid bleeding.[4]

In 1966, McKee and Watson-Farrar further described the anterolateral approach. Their skin incision started at the anterior superior iliac spine, extended down to the greater trochanter tip, and then continued down the femoral shaft approximately 2–3 in., curving the incision slightly anteriorly. The interval between the tensor fasciae latae (TFL) anteriorly and the gluteus minimus and medius posteriorly was developed. They suggested first developing this plane distally where it is most easily found by the finger after incision of the deep fascia. Proximally, the muscles are more intimately blended and sharp dissection between them is necessary. The reflected head of the rectus femoris and anterior half of the hip joint are then visible and excised, revealing the head of the femur.[5]

While a classic anterolateral approach involves an intermuscular dissection between the TFL and gluteus medius, most versions of the anterolateral approach involve some degree of intraoperative detachment and subsequent repair of at least a portion of the anterior abductor mechanism. Surgeons either divide the anterior 25–50% of the gluteus medius and minimus, or they anteriorly reflect that portion of the abductors in continuity with a sleeve of vastus lateralis, bridging the two muscles with fascia or a small wafer of greater trochanter bone.[6]

Several surgeons have modified the anterolateral approach, differing mainly in the degree of abductor disruption. The difference between an anterolateral approach and a direct lateral approach is often blurred both in conversation and in the literature. Although most anterolateral approaches dissect through the abductors, these approaches are generally more anterior to the direct lateral approach described by Hardinge.[7]

In 1974, Mallory compared the transtrochanteric and anterolateral approaches. He found that pain relief was consistent in both groups. However, at 1-year postoperatively, the transtrochanteric group did better in terms of loss of limp, improved walking endurance, and active abduction against gravity.[8] In 1975, when comparing these two approaches, Thompson and Culver concluded that the anterolateral approach was indicated for most uncomplicated primary THAs in light of the trochanteric complications they encountered (e.g., nonunion and irritation caused by fixation wires). They did note that the trochanteric osteotomies were still "invaluable" for "the difficult, previously operated on hip" and in particular with patients with fixed flexion deformities greater than 30°, fixed external rotation deformities greater than 10°, or "gross distortion of normal pelvi-femoral relations."[9]

Advantages of the anterolateral approach include a historically lower dislocation rate than the posterior approaches, ease of surgery with one or no assistants, and avoidance of the sciatic nerve. An early study comparing the anterolateral, transtrochanteric, and posterior surgical approaches in primary THAs revealed that the dislocation rate was four times more common in the pos-

S. Hariri and A.A. Freiberg (✉)
Department of Orthopedics, Massachusetts General Hospital, Yawkey Center for Outpatient Care, 55 Fruit Street, Suite 3700, Boston, MA, 02114-2696, USA
e-mail: afreiburg@partners.org

G.R. Scuderi and A.J. Tria (eds.), *Minimally Invasive Surgery in Orthopedics*,
DOI 10.1007/978-0-387-76608-9_18, © Springer Science+Business Media, LLC 2010

terior approach than in the other two groups and the incidence of trochanteric bursitis was twice as high in the transtrochanteric approach compared with the other two approaches.[10]

Another study comparing just the posterolateral and anterolateral approaches confirmed a significantly higher rate of dislocation in the posterolateral group (4.21% versus 0%). The authors used Mulliken's "modified direct lateral approach" as their anterolateral exposure, with a split of the gluteus medius/minimus tendons in continuity with the vastus lateralis at the junction between the anterior one third and posterior two thirds of the gluteus medius. With this approach, the anterolateral group had a higher incidence of limp of any severity (29% versus 17%) and a higher incidence of a moderate or severe limp (7% versus 4%).[11] Thus, the classic concept of a trade-off between instability (posterior approach) and limp (anterior approach) was established. This concept has recently been challenged.

With the popularization of a posterior soft tissue repair (i.e., the posterior capsule and short external rotators) in the posterior approaches, the difference in dislocation rates between the anterolateral and posterior approaches has been reported to be reduced. A metaanalysis of studies comparing posterior approaches with and without posterior soft tissue repairs revealed a dislocation rate of 0.49% and 4.46%, respectively. A systemic review of the literature showed a dislocation rate of 0.70% for the anterolateral approach and 1.01% for the posterior approach with a capsular repair.[12] However, a posterior capsular repair is not always possible in the posterolateral approach.

Recent modifications to the anterolateral approach have similarly decreased the likelihood of a postoperative limp. Postoperative abductor weakness, resulting in a Trendelenburg gait, is caused by either inadequate repair of the abductors and/or damage to the superior gluteal nerve innervating the gluteus medius and minimus. Jacobs and Buxton identified a "safe area" for the superior gluteal nerve encompassing a band of the gluteus medius approximately 5-cm wide immediately proximal to the greater trochanter.[13] Limiting proximal longitudinal dissection of the gluteus medius minimizes risk to the superior gluteal nerve. Recent modifications that limit the portion of anterior gluteus medius detached from the greater trochanter tip minimize postoperative abductor dysfunction.

Mini Anterolateral Approach

The mini anterolateral approach by definition entails a skin incision of 10 cm or less. In 2004, Bertin and Röttinger described a mini anterolateral approach ("a modified Watson-Jones approach") that dissects between the gluteus medius and the TFL to expose the anterior capsule, preserving the integrity of the abductors. They noted that, using this interval, there is a danger of excessive acetabular anteversion and difficulty with femoral exposure. They proposed releasing sufficient capsule (posteriorly to the area of the piriformis insertion and inferiorly to the

medial border of the femoral neck) to facilitate exposure. Overall, after having performed more than 300 of these approaches, they noted that it is "an excellent anterior approach without muscle damage through a small incision," although they have yet to formally present their results.

Most surgeons performing the mini anterolateral approach dissect the anterior portion of the abductors off the greater trochanter to some degree. In general, however, the mini anterolateral approach involves less abductor disruption than the conventional anterolateral approaches. This less invasive abductor approach theoretically should decrease postoperative abductor weakness and, thus, limp.

Indications and Contraindications

The most important consideration in performing a THA is adequate exposure. Retractors and instruments specifically designed for minimally invasive surgery are strongly preferred as they protect soft tissues and allow reaming and broaching without compromise in position. Surgeons may routinely start with a small incision, but they should not hesitate to extend the incision if the exposure is deemed inadequate or if there is extensive skin traction. Ideal patients for mini anterolateral THAs are female, less muscular, low body mass index (BMI) patients. However, as surgeons gain more experience, their indications for a mini anterolateral approach can vastly expand. Patients with large retained hardware that must be removed (e.g., blade plates or dynamic hip screws), dysplasias requiring femoral osteotomies, severe dysplasia or congenital dislocations requiring a trochanteric osteotomy, and revision THAs involving more than a simple liner exchange are not candidates for this approach.

In developing one's practice, we agree with Berger's conservative, progressive approach. Surgeons should begin with the incision with which they are most comfortable and gradually shorten it as they gain more experience. When starting to use mini approaches, the surgeon should choose smaller, less muscular patients with minimal deformity and few osteophytes. Specialized retractors and instrumentation (e.g., fiberoptic lighted retractors and low-profile acetabular reamers with shells that are more than hemispheric) should be sought to facilitate the approach.[14] Modification to the deep exposure can accompany smaller skin incisions as well.

Technique and Potential Pitfalls

A beanbag, peg board, or clamp-type positioner holds the patient in a lateral position on a standard operating room table. Stable positioning of the patient is critical for proper component position. The operative table must be flat and the patient must be in a true lateral position to maintain accurate bony landmarks. The anesthesiologist must be warned not to adjust the table without the surgeon's knowledge. Patient positioning devices cannot impede full flexion or adduction of the hip or else they will compromise exposure during femoral preparation.

One third of the approximately 10-cm incision is posterior and proximal to the palpable tip of the greater trochanter; two thirds of the incision is anterior and distal to this point. The incision progresses distally from posterior to anterior at a 30° angle from horizontal, resulting in the anterior limb of the incision being distal (Figs. 18.1, 18.2, and 18.3). To make this incision even smaller, the incision can be more acutely angled closer to 45° from the horizontal.

The TFL is then exposed and cleared using a Cobb elevator, defining it for later closure. The fascia is then incised in line with the skin exposure. Acetabular exposure can be compromised by a fascial incision that is either too posterior or not long enough. An anterior curve of the incision's distal extent relaxes the tension on this layer.

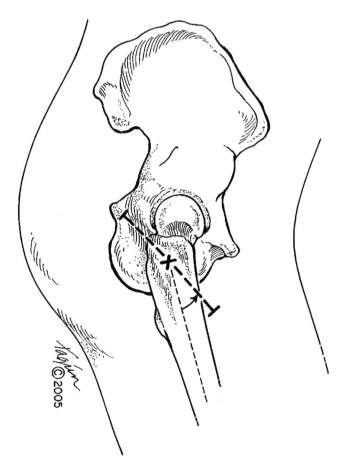

Fig. 18.1 Schematic view from above of the patient in the lateral position. There is a *dotted line* marking the femoral shaft axis. The "*X*" marks the palpable tip of the greater trochanter. The incision (*dotted line* with *bars* at endpoints) is made at a 30° angle to the axis of the femoral shaft. One third of the incision is proximal and posterior to the "*X*," two thirds of the incision is distal and anterior to the "*X*" (From Freiberg AA. Anterolateral mini-incision total hip arthroplasty. *Oper Tech Orthop.* 2006;16:87–92, with permission of Elsevier)

The gluteus maximus is now visible proximally and split in line with the fascial incision approximately 3–4 cm using electrocautery. The bursa deep to the gluteus maximus must carefully be excised without compromising the surrounding tissue.

Based on patient factors (i.e., BMI and degree of muscle mass) and surgeon experience, the surgeon must decide what percentage of the anterior gluteus medius to reflect. In the case of a surgeon with relatively less experience or a patient who is obese or very muscular, a larger portion of the gluteus medius may be reflected off the greater trochanter for enhanced exposure. We routinely dissect approximately 10–30% of the anterior abductor muscle mass off of the greater trochanter, translating into approximately a 1-cm transverse distance. The thickest portion of the gluteus medius and minimus tendon, and therefore the most effective area for later repair, is anterior, with the thickest portion in fact slightly anterior to the greater trochanter's bony border (Figs. 18.4 and 18.5).

Electrocautery is used to split the gluteus medius longitudinally approximately 3 cm from the trochanteric tip, creating an L-shaped gluteus medius incision when viewed in combination with the transverse release of the tendon off the greater trochanter. A dull retractor is then placed to posteriorly retract the gluteus medius, exposing a layer of adipose tissue between the gluteus medius and minimus. A vascular bundle often lies in this interval and should be coagulated before incising the gluteus minimus tendon. The gluteus minimus tendon and anterior hip joint capsule are then incised in line with the femoral neck and head all the way up proximally to the acetabular edge without stopping at the anterior osteophytes. An anterior capsulotomy is then performed using a Cushing forceps and electrocautery. To ease hip dislocation, the anterior–inferior capsule must be thoroughly incised or excised. The hip is then flexed, adducted, and externally rotated to deliver the femoral head anteriorly into the wound.

In order to establish another useful bony landmark, the lesser trochanter can be better exposed by releasing the capsule above it or by more aggressive external rotation of the hip. It is worthwhile to expose the lesser trochanter to ensure that the femoral cut is sufficiently distal to facilitate later acetabular exposure. The femoral neck osteotomy is then performed, the femoral head is freed up with sharp transection of the ligamentum teres, and the femoral head is removed.

A Hibbs retractor placed superiorly and a short cerebellar retractor placed deep and proximal offers excellent acetabular exposure. With the leg in a neutral position on the operating room table, the acetabular labrum and any impinging capsule is excised. Standard or, preferably, low-profile reamers are used to prepare the acetabulum. Osteophytes are removed. The cup is then placed in 40–45° of abduction and 10–20° of anteversion.

A cerebellar retractor is placed anteriorly and a curved femoral elevator is placed posteriorly to offer exposure for the femoral preparation. The leg is placed into the anterior leg bag and hyper-externally rotated to both protect the abductors and prevent soft tissue impingement that could cause excessive anteversion (Fig.

Fig. 18.2 Illustration of the hip musculature as it relates to the mini anterolateral incision (From Freiberg AA. Anterolateral mini-incision total hip arthroplasty. *Oper Tech Orthop.* 2006;16:87–92, with permission of Elsevier)

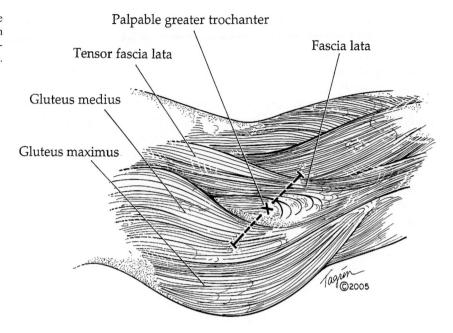

Fig. 18.3 Cross-sectional anatomy of the femoral head and neck as it relates to the mini anterolateral incision (From Freiberg AA. Anterolateral mini-incision total hip arthroplasty. *Oper Tech Orthop.* 2006;16:87–92, with permission of Elsevier)

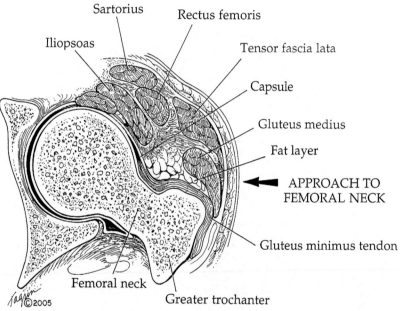

18.6). The canal is broached using offset broach handles, the trial femoral stem placed, the trial femoral head is placed, and the hip is carefully relocated, making sure not to impinge on skin, fascia, or musculature as this can result in a femoral fracture. Actual components are then placed if the hip is deemed stable and has acceptable range of motion.

The capsule has been incised, and therefore the gluteus minimus is first repaired. The anterior portion of the gluteus medius is meticulously repaired with Mersilene sutures in the abductors threaded through two 2.4-mm drill holes in the greater trochanter (Fig. 18.7). The Mersilene sutures are covered and augmented with multiple Vicryl or Ethibond sutures. Covering the heavy Mersilene sutures minimizes the risk of them rubbing against the fascial repair and subsequently causing trochanteric bursitis (Fig.

18.8). The abductor repair sutures are each tightened down with the leg slightly abducted and internally rotated to approximately 10–20°. A drain is only used for patients with a BMI greater than 30. The patient is made weight bearing as tolerated. Daily subcutaneous injections of low-molecular weight heparin are used for thromboembolic prophylaxis.

The anesthetic protocol is critical to ease and expedite functional recovery. We utilize preoperative narcotics and intraoperative regional anesthesia supplemented by intraoperative injections of local anesthetic into the musculature, fascia, and subcutaneous tissue at the end of the case. Perioperative oral or intravenous anti-inflammatory drugs in doses high enough to control pain are administered to avoid the potential debilitating side effects of narcotics (e.g., nausea, constipation, and altered mental status).

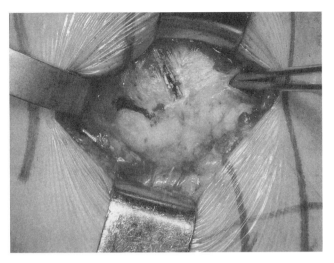

Fig. 18.4 The inferior border of the gluteus medius (marked with the *hemostat tip*) is identified via palpation (From Freiberg AA. Anterolateral mini-incision total hip arthroplasty. *Oper Tech Orthop*. 2006;16:87–92, with permission of Elsevier)

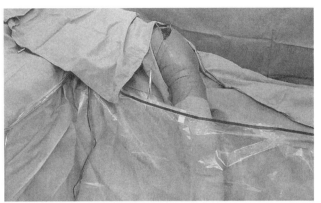

Fig. 18.6 The leg is placed into an anterior sterile leg bag for femoral preparation (From Freiberg AA. Anterolateral mini-incision total hip arthroplasty. *Oper Tech Orthop*. 2006;16:87–92, with permission of Elsevier)

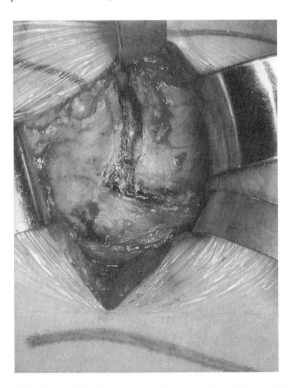

Fig. 18.5 Up to 30% of the anterior gluteus medius will be split from the posterior 70% of the tendon essentially in line with the femoral neck (planned split marked by *electrocautery* in the Fig.) (From Freiberg AA. Anterolateral mini-incision total hip arthroplasty. *Oper Tech Orthop*. 2006;16:87–92, with permission of Elsevier)

Results

In presenting results of the mini anterolateral approach, it is important to specify to what degree the abductors are dissected away from the greater trochanter. In a 2003 review of 212 uncemented THAs performed using the anterolateral approach,

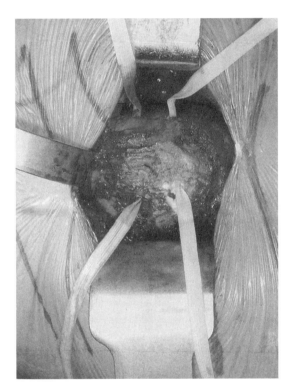

Fig. 18.7 2.4-mm drill holes are made in the proximal greater trochanter to secure the gluteus medius repair with Mersilene tape (From Freiberg AA. Anterolateral mini-incision total hip arthroplasty. *Oper Tech Orthop*. 2006;16:87–92, with permission of Elsevier)

Higuchi et al. split the gluteus medius just proximally to the tip of the greater trochanter using finger dissection then sharply divided the vastus lateralis longitudinally just distal from the greater trochanter.[14] Both muscles were divided for the anterior border of the greater trochanter in continuity. They found that, with a shorter incision length, there was a statistically significant decrease in operative duration and intraoperative blood loss. There were no significant differences in postoperative bleeding and complications between the mini and conventional anterolat-

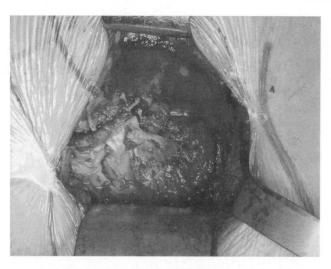

Fig. 18.8 Additional Vicryl or Ethibond sutures augment the repair (From Freiberg AA. Anterolateral mini-incision total hip arthroplasty. *Oper Tech Orthop.* 2006;16:87–92, with permission of Elsevier)

eral groups. They always initially started with a short skin incision and extended the incision as necessary during the surgery. They found that a longer incision was more commonly needed for those with a high BMI and for male patients.

In 2004, Berger compared two groups of 100 consecutive patients: (1) a standard anterolateral approach (removing 50% of the abductor off the trochanter) and (2) a mini-incision anterolateral (removing only 20–25% of the abductor off the trochanter).[15] The blood loss, length of hospital stay, and rate of transfer home (as opposed to a rehabilitation facility) were significantly lower in the mini anterolateral group. There was no difference in operative time or complications between the groups. Neither group had a dislocation.[15]

In 2006, Jerosch et al. reported on 75 consecutive THAs performed through a mini anterolateral approach. They incised the iliotibial band longitudinally over the greater trochanter and dissected anterior to the gluteus medius, preserving its attachment to the greater trochanter. The average Harris hip score improved from 44 preoperatively to 90 at 1-year follow-up. There were no wound complications, no dislocations, and two patients with a slight Trendelenburg sign.[16]

Summary

The anterolateral approach entails a spectrum of dissections. At one extreme is an intermuscular dissection between the TFL anteriorly and the anterior border of the gluteus medius posteriorly. However, most surgeons either release between 25 and 50% of the abductors from the greater trochanter or anteriorly retract this portion of the abductors in continuity with a portion of the vastus lateralis inferiorly, bridging the two muscles with either fascia or a wafer of greater trochanter bone. The advantages of the anterolateral approach are classically a lower dislocation rate

than the posterolateral approach, although this difference has probably been narrowed by the advent of posterior capsular repairs. Potential disadvantages of the anterolateral approach include abductor dysfunction (either through damaging the superior gluteal nerve or a failed stable repair of the abductors back to the greater trochanter), resulting in a Trendelenburg gait.

The mini anterolateral approach involves a skin incision of 10 cm or less and less dissection of the abductors off the greater trochanter, theoretically decreasing intraoperative blood loss and minimizing abductor dysfunction, thus expediting rehabilitation. We describe a mini anterolateral approach typically involving 10–20% of anterior gluteus medius dissection off of the greater trochanter. There is a paucity of literature reporting on the outcomes of this approach, but the literature available shows that the mini anterolateral approach is a safe approach offering significant advantages over the conventional anterolateral approach in terms of operative time, blood loss, and speed of functional recovery.

References

1. Charnley J. Total hip replacement by low-friction arthroplasty. *Clin Orthop Relat Res.* 1970;72:7–21
2. Harris WH. A new approach to total hip replacement without osteotomy of the greater trochanter. *Clin Orthop Relat Res.* 1975(106): 19–26
3. Muller ME. Total hip prostheses. *Clin Orthop Relat Res.* 1970;72: 46–68
4. Watson-Jones R. Fractures of the neck of the femur. *Br J Surg.* 1935–36;23:787–808
5. McKee GK, Watson-Farrar J. Replacement of arthritic hips by the McKee-farrar prosthesis. *J Bone Joint Surg Br.* 1966;48:245–259
6. Dall D. Exposure of the hip by anterior osteotomy of the greater trochanter. A modified anterolateral approach. *J Bone Joint Surg Br.* 1986;68:382–386
7. Hardinge K. The direct lateral approach to the hip. *J Bone Joint Surg Br.* 1982;64:17–19
8. Mallory TH. Total hip replacement with and without trochanteric osteotomy. *Clin Orthop Relat Res.* 1974:133–135
9. Thompson RC, Jr, Culver JE. The role of trochanteric osteotomy in total hip replacement. *Clin Orthop Relat Res.* 1975(106):102–106
10. Vicar AJ, Coleman CR. A comparison of the anterolateral, transtrochanteric, and posterior surgical approaches in primary total hip arthroplasty. *Clin Orthop Relat Res.* 1984(188):152–159
11. Ritter MA, Harty LD, Keating ME, Faris PM, Meding JB. A clinical comparison of the anterolateral and posterolateral approaches to the hip. *Clin Orthop Relat Res.* 2001(385):95–99
12. Kwon MS, Kuskowski M, Mulhall KJ, Macaulay W, Brown TE, Saleh KJ. Does surgical approach affect total hip arthroplasty dislocation rates? *Clin Orthop Relat Res.* 2006;447:34–38
13. Jacobs LG, Buxton RA. The course of the superior gluteal nerve in the lateral approach to the hip [see comment]. *J Bone Joint Surg Am.* 1989;71(8):1239–1243
14. Higuchi F, Gotoh M, Yamaguchi N, et al. Minimally invasive uncemented total hip arthroplasty through an anterolateral approach with a shorter skin incision. *J Orthop Sci.* 2003;8(6):812–817
15. Berger RA. Mini-incision total hip replacement using an anterolateral approach: technique and results. *Orthop Clin North Am.* 2004;35: z143–151
16. Jerosch J, Theising C, Fadel ME. Antero-lateral minimal invasive (ALMI) approach for total hip arthroplasty technique and early results. *Arch Orthop Trauma Surg.* 2006;126:164–173

Chapter 19
Minimally Invasive Total Hip Arthroplasty with the Anterior Surgical Approach

B. Sonny Bal and Joel Matta

Total hip arthroplasty (THA) with less surgical trauma is of interest to surgeons and patients because early recovery parameters are improved over standard techniques, and the procedure can be done with less surgical trauma and with shorter insicions.[1,2] So-called minimally invasive THA (MIS-THA) procedures have been described with two small incisions, and in the hands of selected surgeons, the two-incision MIS-THA offers accelerated hospital discharge, and an earlier return to function when compared with traditional methods of performing THA.[3,4] In the two-incision technique, the anterior incision and dissection are performed in the Smith-Petersen surgical interval. THA done with this method is a true muscle-sparing approach that is less invasive than any other method that divides or detaches tendons. Excellent outcomes of THA done with other variations of the anterior approach have been reported previously.[5–7]

Unlike the more commonly utilized posterior and direct lateral approaches to THA in the United States, the Smith-Petersen surgical approach allows access to the hip joint without dividing tendons or splitting muscle fibers. The two-incision MIS-THA is performed by implanting the acetabular component placement through the Smith-Petersen interval; femoral component placement is similar to an intramedullary rod placement during blind nailing of the femur.[8] The advantage of the single-incision anterior approach is that implantation of both acetabular and femoral components can be achieved with a single incision alone. This chapter will describe the key steps in the single-incision anterior THA technique, identify potential dangers, and discuss the early clinical outcomes. The authors' reasons for adopting this particular technique for routine primary THA were: (1) preservation of the hip musculature, (2) ability to accurately position prosthetic components and judge leg lengths, (3) to decrease complications, such as posterior hip dislocation, and (4) to increase patient satisfaction with THA.

Learning the Technique

Hip surgeons in the United States, while generally unfamiliar with the anterior approach to THA, can quickly recognize its advantages. The single-incision anterior THA is performed through a portion of the Smith-Petersen surgical interval.[9] For surgeons inexperienced with performing THA in the supine position and through the anterior surgical approach, a thorough review of the relevant anatomy is essential. Following review of anatomic details, cadaver training and live surgery with an experienced mentor will facilitate learning and minimize the risk of complications. If intraoperative fluoroscopy is desired, training in the interpretation of fluoroscopic images showing implant positioning relative to reference points in the pelvis is mandatory. Finally, unless the surgeon is familiar with the THA in the supine position, it is safest to use instrumented guides, direct visualization, and intraoperative fluoroscopy to assure proper implant positioning early in the learning curve. With experience, component implantation can be done with or without intraoperative fluoroscopy.

Equipment

An orthopedic table (PRO*fx* or HANA model, OSI, Union City, CA) can be used to perform anterior THA. Some authors have described anterior THA without the use of the table, by extending and externally rotating the ipsilateral hip and using special instruments to implant the prosthesis.[10] Both methods are variations on the same theme; the principal advantage of an orthopedic table is that it serves as a passive retraction device, allowing easy positioning of the leg in the optimal position for the surgeon. By facilitating surgical exposure, the orthopedic table makes it possible to perform anterior primary THA through the Smith-Petersen interval on nearly all patients with degenerative arthritis of the hip. Without the table, it is difficult to perform anterior THA on short and obese patients, and the surgeon must be more selective.

In addition to the table, lighted Hohmann retractors, and specially angled instruments to facilitate acetabular cup

B.S. Bal (✉) and J. Matta
Department of Orthopaedic Surgery, University of Missouri-Columbia, 204 N. Keene Street, Columbia, MO, 65212, USA
e-mail: balb@health.missouri.edu

G.R. Scuderi and A.J. Tria (eds.), *Minimally Invasive Surgery in Orthopedics*,
DOI 10.1007/978-0-387-76608-9_19, © Springer Science+Business Media, LLC 2010

insertion and femoral preparation will facilitate the operation. Fluoroscopic imaging during surgery can be useful to ensure accurate component positioning in both MIS two-incision THA,[11] and anterior THA performed on the orthopedic table.[7,12] The surgeon should recognize that intraoperative radiographs can easily mislead the unwary surgeon, unless careful attention is paid to subtle variations in patient positioning, spinal curvature, and skeletal anatomy of the pelvis.[13] As an alternative to intraoperative fluoroscopic imaging, direct visualization of the skeletal anatomy during surgery, careful preoperative templating of radiographs, and the use of custom alignment guides for cup alignment and orientation can be used, such that anterior THA can be done safely and reliably without intraoperative fluoroscopy.

Surgical Technique

Patient Positioning and Extremity Draping

The patient is positioned supine on the orthopedic (HANA) table. The operative foot must be firmly secured in the table to avoid it slipping out from the foot holder during surgery. The ipsilateral arm can be folded over the chest and taped in position. The HANA table is optimized for anterior THA, and has a special motorized lift to allow femoral elevation during the procedure. This motorized lift can be positioned for a left or a right THA, and the mechanism should be tested to ensure proper functioning before the procedure is started. Almost all patients who are candidates for primary anterior THA can undergo surgery through the anterior approach on the orthopedic table.

Leg lengths should be estimated by palpating the patellae on either leg, with the feet in neutral rotation. This check is readily performed before and after draping. An alternative method of accurate leg length determination is to insert a Steinmann pin in the readily palpable ridge of the iliac wing, and use this fixed landmark to measure the distance to another fixed point on the femur, such as a pin inserted in the calcar. Comparison of the linear distance between bony landmarks before and after total hip replacement will allow determination of leg length changes.

The circulating nurse can be trained to operate the table; this equipment is simple to learn and can be operated by a normal-sized person. Draping of the surgical field is simpler with the anterior surgical approach when compared with any other THA procedure. The skin should be prepped from the ipsilateral knee to approximately one hand-breadth above the iliac crest (Fig. 19.1). Skin preparation should extend from the groin to the buttock; the supine position ensures that buttock fat is suspended freely, and situated well away

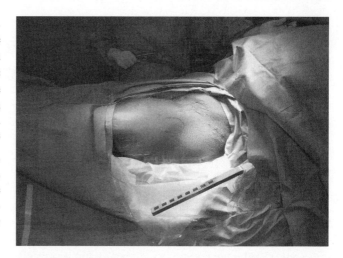

Fig. 19.1 Positioning on the HANA orthopedic table with a fracture drape covering the operative left leg. The motorized femoral left is shown attached to the table

from the surgical field. The palpable greater trochanter and anterior superior iliac spine (ASIS) are marked with a surgical pen. Then, a self-adhesive hip fracture plastic drape is used first, with the Betadine-impregnated adhesive section covering the prepped area.

In some patients with truncal obesity, the abdominal pannus will fall over the iliac crest. In such cases, the abdominal fat should be taped out of the way using adhesive tape before the skin preparation. The groin crease must be visualized clearly in this procedure, without overhanging abdominal fat covering this area. After the plastic hip fracture drape, an abdominal drape is applied over the surgical site, with the open rectangular area positioned over the operative area. The plastic pouch built into the fracture drape is brought out through the rectangular opening in the second drape; this will capture blood and irrigation during the operation (Fig. 19.1). This simple two-step draping (credited to Tom Calvin, CST) is sufficient for anterior THA; other drapes can be used to cover the periphery if necessary.

After draping, a hole is cut in the drapes, and a sterile bracket for the femoral hook arm is attached to the motorized arm below the drapes. The hole is sealed over with sterile vinyl drape to restore the sterile field, and the instrument used to cut the hole is handed off the sterile field (Fig. 19.1).

Surgical Dissection

The ASIS and greater trochanter are palpable in nearly every patient; these structures will have been outlined by the surgical marker previously. In very rare cases, if these anatomic landmarks cannot be palpated in the very obese individual, they can be identified and localized using an intraoperative X-ray.

The incision is made in a straight line, extending in an oblique direction from approximately 3 cm distal and lateral to the ASIS to a point 2 cm anterior and distal to the greater trochanter (Fig. 19.2). In obese patients, and those with a varus femoral neck, it may be necessary for the incision to cross the groin crease. A longer incision is preferable to forcibly stretching the proximal incision during stem insertion, which can lead to skin maceration and delayed healing. Especially early in the surgeon's experience, it is safer to err on the side of a longer incision for adequate surgical visualization, particularly since the length of the skin incision does not contribute to early recovery. With experience, it is possible to perform anterior THA using an 8- to 12-cm incision in nearly all patients, without resorting to skin stretching.

A self-retaining retractor is positioned to expose the subcutaneous fat, which is sharply divided until the thin, translucent fascia overlying the tensor fascia lata muscle is visible (Fig. 19.3). This fascia should be incised sharply to reveal the fibers of the tensor. Deep to the anterior fascial flap, a sharp elevator is used to gently separate the tensor muscle fibers adherent to the underside of the fascia, such that a palpating finger can be slipped over the medial border of the tensor, and into the interval between the superior femoral capsule and the abductors. A variation on this approach is to split the fibers of the tensor muscle and access the hip joint by splitting the muscle in the direction of its fibers.[14] A cobra retractor is next placed between the superior femoral capsule and the tensor, such that the tensor muscle is retracted laterally (Fig. 19.4).

The anterior hip capsule is visualized by sharply elevating the rectus femoris and psoas muscles off the hip capsule, and retracting these muscles behind a second cobra or lighted Hohmann retractor that is placed around the medial hip capsule (Fig. 19.4). Another Hohmann retractor is next placed on the anterior acetabular wall to improve exposure; this instrument must be placed directly on bone to protect the femoral nerve from inadvertent injury. The anterior Hohmann retractor can be placed deep to the insertion of the rectus femoris tendon on the anterior acetabular wall. In some cases, it may be helpful to release this insertion instead to gain visualization. Distal exposure of the hip capsule requires identification of the lateral femoral circumflex vessels; these must be coagulated and divided to avoid inadvertent avulsion and bleeding during surgery. Dividing these vessels allows the exposure to proceed safely in a distal direction, until the entire anterior hip capsule and the intertrochanteric ridge are identified.

The interval between the tensor and the rectus femoris must be developed distally using blunt finger dissection. This step will mobilize the tensor muscle distally. In very muscular individuals with a well-developed tensor, it may also be necessary to sharply release the tense adhesions between the tensor and rectus femoris insertion near the ASIS. The goal is to allow safe retraction of the tensor muscle laterally with

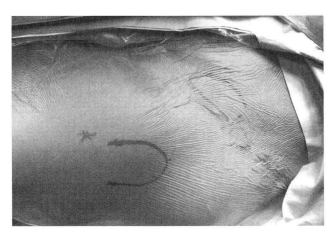

Fig. 19.2 The ASIS and greater trochanter are marked on the left hip. The incision uses these two landmarks

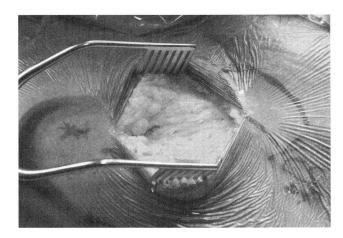

Fig. 19.3 Incision taken through the superficial fat with the fascia over the tensor muscle exposed

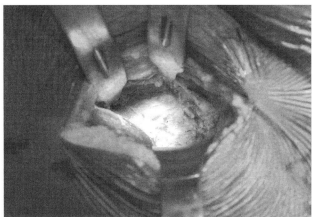

Fig. 19.4 Anterior hip capsule exposed in left hip with retractors holding the tensor laterally and the rectus femoris/psoas muscles medially and anteriorly

a cobra retractor. Aggressive retraction can lacerate the muscle belly of the tensor, especially in muscular individuals. The surgeon should proceed further with the operation only when the tensor can be retracted with minimal tension, without risk of amputating or otherwise injuring the muscle with the retractor.

The anterior hip capsule is opened with two flaps that are retracted superiorly and inferiorly with the cobra retractors that are repositioned inside the capsular flaps (Fig. 19.5). In very arthritic hips with a flexion contracture, it may be necessary to excise the anterior hip capsule. With the hip capsule removed or retracted, the leg is rotated externally by the unscrubbed assistant. Using a curved osteotome, a few millimeters of the anterior acetabular wall and calcified labrum should be removed. This is especially useful in the retroverted acetabulum; this step will facilitate the placement of a hip skid between the femoral head and the acetabulum, and allow anterior dislocation of the femoral head.

Femoral Head Extraction

A skid is placed in the hip joint by applying light traction to the leg, opening the joint cavity, and slipping the skid inside the hip joint, using light impaction with a mallet if necessary. With the hip externally rotated, and with no traction on the leg, a drill hole is placed in the femoral head and a T-handled corkscrew is threaded securely into this hole. With assistance from the hip skid and anterior traction on the corkscrew, the femoral head is dislocated anteriorly (Fig. 19.6).

Only gentle external femoral rotation is needed for this step; the risk in dislocating the hip joint anteriorly is inadvertent fracture of the ankle or femur. This is particularly important in the severely arthritic hip joint, or a degenerative hip

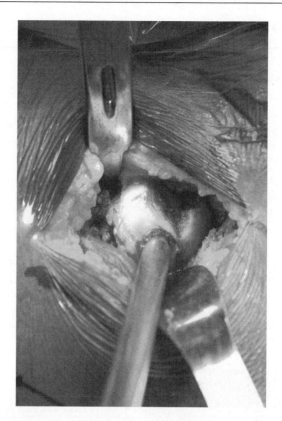

Fig. 19.6 Head dislocated anteriorly with corkscrew; note that a part of the head is osteotomized to ease insertion of the hip skid and anterior dislocation

with a protrusion deformity. If the assistant forcibly rotates the leg to dislocate the head, an iatrogenic fracture can occur. To avoid this complication, the surgeon should ensure proper placement of the corkscrew, ensure traction on the leg, insert a skid or similar device in the hip joint, and pull the femoral head out anteriorly with the T-handle. These steps should be preceded by removal of a part of the arthritic anterior acetabular wall. By methodically following this sequence, it is possible to anteriorly dislocate even the severely arthritic hip joint, without forcibly rotating the leg.

An alternative to femoral head dislocation is osteotomy of the femoral neck in situ, followed by removal of the osteotomized neck fragment, and subsequent extraction of the femoral head.[11] This is an acceptable variation, although dislocating the femoral head anteriorly will facilitate subsequent steps, including calcar osteotomy, femoral exposure, and identification of the lesser trochanter. Nonetheless, hip dislocation is not essential to performing THA with the anterior approach.

With the hip dislocated anteriorly, the vastus lateralis muscle origin near the distal femoral neck is retracted with a narrow Hohmann retractor, and the calcar region of the proximal femur is exposed subperiosteally, until the lesser trochanter is clearly identified (Fig. 19.7). This is an essential step if no intraoperative fluoroscopy is used, since preoperative

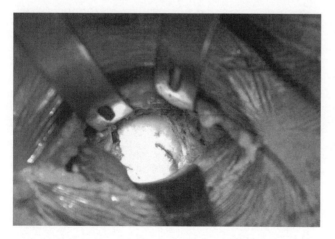

Fig. 19.5 Anterior hip capsule opened with capsular flaps retracted, to show the femoral head in the acetabulum

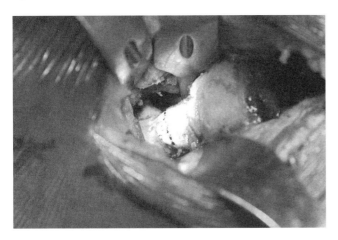

Fig. 19.7 Femoral neck and lesser trochanter exposed, with a pen mark showing the anticipated calcar cut

templating can identify the distance from the calcar cut to the lesser trochanter, thereby allowing reproduction of leg lengths.[13] An alternative is to use intraoperative fluoroscopy to guide the level of the calcar cut, so that it matches the preoperative plan based on templating.

Once the lesser trochanter is visible, the level of calcar cut anticipated from preoperative templating is marked on the bone, and the calcar cut is made with the head dislocated anteriorly. The cut is stopped approximately two thirds of the way through the bone, and the hip is relocated in the acetabulum. The second, lateral cut is placed just medial to the greater trochanter, oriented obliquely from proximal to distal. An osteotome is used to complete the cut, rather than risk an aggressive cut through the calcar that could extend into the greater trochanter. The corkscrew is reinserted into the drill hole previously placed in the femoral head, and the head–neck fragment is extracted from the hip joint.

Acetabular Exposure and Reconstruction

The lateral cobra retractor is repositioned in an opening cut into the posterior–superior hip capsule. The goal is to keep the tensor muscle retracted, without tension on the muscle, and also to retract the proximal femur downward toward the floor, to ease acetabular exposure. Preferably, a sponge should protect the muscle, rather than direct pressure on the tensor muscle belly with a metal retractor. A spiked Hohmann retractor is next placed on the anterior–inferior acetabular wall, and a second Hohmann retractor is placed on the anterior acetabulum, with the spike of this retractor directly positioned on bone, rather than on soft tissue. The femur is externally rotated with slight traction on the leg to facilitate acetabular exposure. Visualization of the bony socket is excellent with this technique, and complete circumferential

exposure of the acetabulum allows osteophyte excision, safe reaming, and accurate cup placement (Fig. 19.8).

Reaming can be performed with standard hemispherical reamers, although special cutout reamers optimized for minimally invasive surgery are easier to use (Fig. 19.9). Care must be taken not to lever the reamer handle on the thigh, thereby reaming out the anterior acetabular wall. The safe direction of reaming in the supine position is in the posterior direction, after the bony socket has been medialized by initial reaming. The fovea of the acetabulum should be identified and exposed; this is a landmark that can reliably orient the surgeon to the location of the medial wall. An alternative is to use intraoperative fluoroscopy to guide acetabular reaming and reamer position. Proper fluoroscopic interpretation requires close attention to the bony landmarks, pelvic tilt and rotation, and overall pelvic symmetry (Fig. 19.10).

If no intraoperative fluoroscopy is used, then cup insertion and positioning are achieved with instrument guides that can facilitate accurate alignment, and by visualizing the bony

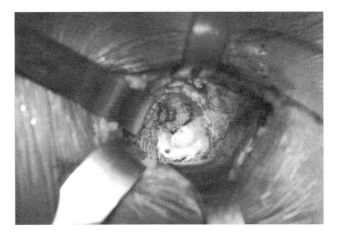

Fig. 19.8 Left hip acetabular exposure, with retractors placed around the socket, and the medial acetabular wall seen clearly

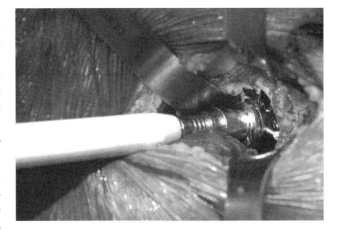

Fig. 19.9 Reaming of the acetabular cavity under direct vision

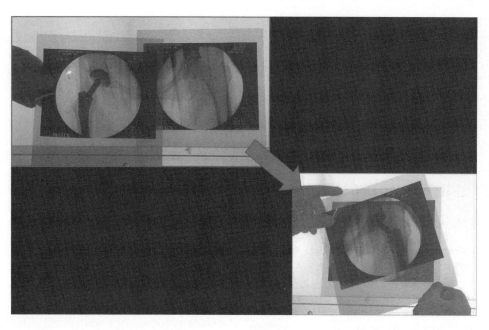

Fig. 19.10 Intraoperative fluoroscopy and X-ray overlay technique to measure trial offset, leg lengths, and implant orientation

anatomy of the socket during cup placement. In the supine patient, the typical pitfalls in cup positioning for the surgeon unaccustomed to supine THA are vertical placement of the cup, and too much anteversion. Screw fixation of the cup is optional if adequate press-fit is not achieved. After insertion of the acetabular bearing, and removal of acetabular osteophytes, attention is directed to femoral stem implantation.

Femoral Exposure

The HANA orthopedic table is equipped with a bone hook that is designed to fit the motorized elevator built into the table, and safely elevate the proximal femur. This sterile hook is placed around the proximal femur, just distal to the greater trochanter. Slight internal rotation of the hip will facilitate this step. The hook allows the surgeon to lift up the femur and estimate tissue tension, which varies by individual. By pulling laterally on the hook, the surgeon can also maneuver the femur to ensure that the greater trochanter is not caught behind the posterior acetabular wall. With the femur pulled laterally, and lifted up, the leg is externally rotated and gently lowered to the floor by the unscrubbed assistant, thereby placing the limb in extension at the hip joint.

The surgeon should conceptualize both the bone hook and the externally rotated position of the leg as passive retraction devices that are designed to facilitate the operation. This is an important concept to understand, and will help avoid the pitfalls of inadvertent trochanter or proximal femur fracture. Safe retraction during THA requires mobilization of the soft tissues, followed by placement of retractors to hold the mobilized soft

tissues safely out of the way. Forcing a retractor to compel surgical exposure is dangerous, and this principle should be kept in mind while exposing the proximal femur during anterior THA. External rotation of the femur is achieved incrementally, and should be done only after the surgeon can rotate the ipsilateral knee with the hand. Likewise, manual elevation of the femur hook should always precede operation of the motorized hook elevator. By dissecting the superior and medial hip capsule, incremental external rotation of the leg can be gained steadily. The femoral hook and HANA table are designed to maintain the safe exposure thus gained.

External femoral rotation and proximal femoral elevation are critical to exposing the femur during anterior THA. Femoral preparation should not be attempted before this exposure is achieved. Release of the thick hip capsule off the greater trochanter from anterior to posterior while protecting the abductors with a Hohmann retractor is the first step in mobilizing the proximal femur. Next, a subperiosteal release of soft tissues off the medial surface of the greater trochanter tip, and off the medial femoral neck, should be done sequentially. If necessary, the piriformis, followed by the obturator internus tendons, can be released, and this will bring the externally rotated proximal femur into satisfactory view in all cases. The obturator externus tendon should be preserved since it applies a medial pull on the femur, and contributes to hip joint stability (Fig. 19.11). Previous exposure of the lesser trochanter and release of the medial capsule off the calcar will facilitate external femoral rotation and elevation. The exact amount of soft tissue release will vary by patient and anatomy, but by proceeding sequentially and patiently, excellent proximal femoral exposure is possible in all cases. Femoral exposure is more difficult in the short, obese,

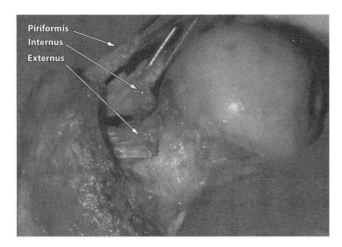

Fig. 19.11 Anatomic specimen showing location of piriformis, obturator externus, and obturator internus tendons on the posterior aspect of the proximal femur

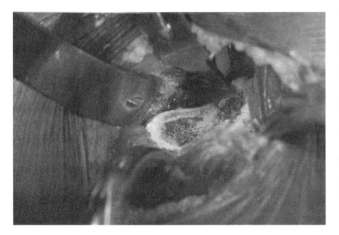

Fig. 19.12 Proximal femoral exposure with the orthopedic table

and muscular patient; in such cases, the table can be placed in a Trendelenburg position that can allow the leg to be lowered further on the floor, thereby allowing greater femoral elevation for added exposure.

The surgeon should avoid the pitfalls of using the femoral hook to forcibly elevate the femur, and using the orthopedic table to forcibly rotate the leg. Proper exposure should be instead achieved by a methodical, step-by-step process, and the surgeon should not use the femoral hook or the orthopedic table as tools to gain exposure; they are passive retraction devices that are used only to maintain exposure otherwise obtained by the surgeon.

Femoral Preparation and Prosthesis Insertion

Once sufficient exposure of the proximal femur is achieved (Fig. 19.12), a Hohmann retractor is placed behind the greater

trochanter, protecting the proximal part of the skin incision and the underlying abductors from femoral broaches. The canal is opened with a curved awl; the position of the knee can assist in properly estimating the direction of the femoral canal and avoiding the pitfall of canal perforation. The author has used uncemented press-fit femoral stems that require rasping of the femur, without canal reaming. Both the Corail system (DePuy, Warsaw, IN), and the ML taper stem (Zimmer, Warsaw, IN) have been used with excellent results. Rasps and stem inserters are mounted on special instruments that are angled to clear the soft tissues proximally.[10]

Unrecognized calcar fracture is avoided with this method since the calcar is visualized during stem insertion (Fig. 19.13). If a calcar crack develops, a cerclage wire can be placed around the proximal femur. Femoral head trials and neck trial segments (on stems with modular necks) can be inserted easily on the seated femoral broaches for trial reductions.

Leg lengths are determined by examining the positions of the patellae, and ensuring that the calcar cut is made at the level consistent with preoperative templating. If desired, a pin can be driven into the iliac crest, with a second pin driven into a drill hole placed into the anterior proximal femur. The two fixed reference points will allow measurement of preoperative and postoperative leg lengths with certainty. With the use of intraoperative fluoroscopy, leg lengths and hip joint offset can be determined very accurately, particularly by overlaying an X-ray image over an image of the contralateral hip on the X-ray screen (Fig. 19.11). This technique is powerful, as long as the surgeon is knowledgeable about the pelvis bony landmarks, pelvic tilt, lumbar spine curvature, and overall pelvic symmetry.

Hip stability is assessed by maximally externally rotating the femur following trial reduction, and checking for impingement or subluxation of the femoral head (Fig. 19.14). This is relevant since anterior dissection destabilizes the hip anteriorly. Posterior stability can also be tested by removing the

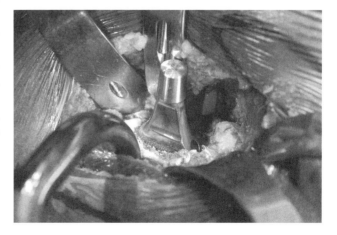

Fig. 19.13 Femoral stem is seated with direct visualization of the calcar

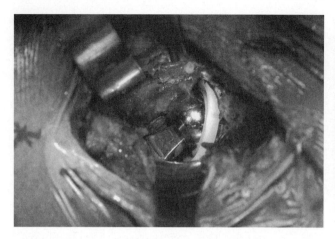

Fig. 19.14 Prosthesis is reduced; external rotation will test anterior stability

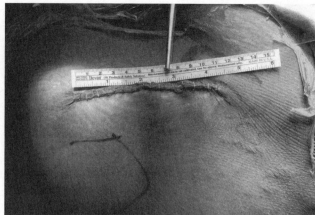

Fig. 19.15 Final closure of the skin incision following a left anterior THA

boot from the orthopedic table, but this has been unnecessary in the author's experience and contributes no useful information, as long as leg length and offset of the reconstruction have been restored. With large diameter femoral heads, the procedure described here is inherently stable, and the risk of dislocation is very low. In a multicenter retrospective trial of 1,277 anterior THAs conducted by one of the authors (JMM), the rate of hip dislocations was 0.6%.

Wound Closure

The anterior hip capsule can be closed anatomically to reduce dead space, or the capsular flaps can be left to fall in place. A drain can be left deep in the joint space and brought out distally and laterally; a potential pitfall is exiting the drain trocar too medially and placing the femoral neurovascular structures at risk of injury. The surgical approach described is anatomically correct in that the overlying tensor and rectus muscles fall in place as the retractors are removed. The thin fascia over the tensor is closed, followed by skin closure (Fig. 19.15). Local anesthetic is injected into the skin edges and subcutaneous tissues.

Rehabilitation

With spinal anesthesia, local wound infiltration with anesthetic agents, and preemptive treatment of nausea and pain by appropriate medications, the anterior THA method described here is associated with very little postoperative pain. For prophylaxis against venous thrombosis, the method described here allows the application of foot and calf intermittent pumps to both lower extremities even before the operation is begun. Patients with anterior THA do not require pain pumps or

intramuscular narcotics; oral anti-inflammatory and narcotic medications are sufficient to control postoperative pain.

Physical therapy and patient mobilization are started on the first postoperative day, or on the day of surgery for procedures done early in the day. No hip precautions are prescribed, and patients can fully weight-bear with an assistive device for balance and safety. Patients are discharged home on the second postoperative day, with follow-up at 4 weeks postoperatively. In the month following surgery, home health visits ensure wound checks, compliance with anticoagulation therapy, suture removal, and hip exercises. No outpatient physical therapy is prescribed after home health visits are complete. We use dose-adjusted warfarin for antithrombotic prophylaxis, along with compression stockings, early patient mobilization, and intermittent foot and calf pumps that are applied intraoperatively.

Outcomes

In a consecutive series of 100 patients who had 100 anterior THAs without intraoperative fluoroscopy by one of the authors (BSB), minimum 6-month follow-up data showed only two complications. One patient developed a pulmonary embolism while in the hospital; this complication required prolonged anticoagulation. This patient also developed increased wound drainage after the anticoagulation dose was increased to address the pulmonary embolism, but the drainage resolved spontaneously. Another patient developed an undisplaced calcar fracture during femoral stem insertion; this was stabilized with a single cerclage wire without any change in the rehabilitation protocol.

No patient who was a candidate for a primary THA was excluded from the above consecutive series. The mean patient age was 62.3 years (range 32–91 years); the mean patient body mass index (BMI) was 29.1 (range 18.0–54.9); intraoperative blood loss was 189 cc (range 75–556 cc); the mean hospital stay was 2.2 days (range 1–5 days), and all patients were discharged home. Early hospital discharge was not particularly encouraged, and no patients underwent preoperative teaching to promote early discharge. The mean operative time was 52 min (34–88 min). The mean incision length was 10.5 cm (range 7.7–13.7 cm), and no skin maceration or excessive drainage occurred, with the exception of the one patient described above. No patient required a change in intraoperative plans because of the anterior supine position.

Thigh numbness was present on objective testing in only seven patients, and was clinically insignificant in that it could not be detected at the most recent clinic visit. No patient complained of thigh numbness. All patients had resumed reasonable activities of daily living by a month after the procedure, and reported satisfaction with the outcome. Participation in light sports and recreational activities was permitted at 8 weeks after the procedure.

Component migration was defined as a >3-mm subsidence of the femoral implant, a >3° change in stem alignment relative to the femoral canal, or a >3° change in orientation of the acetabular component. By these criteria, no component migration occurred in this series. The mean acetabular component abduction was 42.6° (range 36.3–51.9°), the mean cup anteversion on the true lateral radiograph was 15.1° (range 5.8–28.2°), and all but three femoral components were within ±3° of varus/valgus alignment relative to the diaphyseal femoral shaft.

Three femoral stems were in >3° of varus relative to the diaphyseal femur on the anteroposterior (AP) hip radiograph. Varus stem positioning in these three cases was probably the result of inadequate lateralization of the entry point during femoral preparation. The significance, if any, of this radiographic finding in the stem design used in this series is uncertain. All implants were radiographically stable and none of the three patients with varus stem positioning reported hip pain.

Intraoperative fractures, repeat surgery, nerve injury, excessive blood loss, prolonged operative times, skin maceration, and component instability are serious complications associated with MIS-THA.[15–18] These complications are not unique to minimally invasive surgery, in that they have been described with THA performed with standard techniques as well. None of these adverse outcomes were encountered in series described above. These data show that THA with the anterior approach is safe and predictable, with excellent short-term clinical outcomes.

Advantages Over Minimally Invasive Two-Incision THA

Despite the excellent outcomes with the two-incision technique documented by developer surgeons,[4,19] the single-incision anterior THA has distinct advantages over the two-incision method. One advantage is that the second, posterior incision is avoided entirely. Some authors have suggested that blind canal preparation and component placement during two-incision THA may lead to unrecognized muscle injury.[20,21] A related complication encountered twice by one of the authors in a consecutive series of two-incision THAs was a postoperative intramuscular buttock hematoma. By avoiding blind instrumentation of the femur through a small buttock incision, these complications can be avoided during anterior THA.

The risk of thigh numbness may be decreased by placing the anterior incision more laterally during the procedure described here. Lateral placement of the incision, when compared with the two-incision THA technique, can lead to a reduced risk of inadvertent injury to the branches of the lateral femoral cutaneous nerve.[5] Since the incision is further from the femoral neurovascular bundle as well, it is possible that the risk of femoral nerve injury is also decreased with anterior THA.

Intraoperative blood loss may be less with anterior THA when compared with two-incision THA. Since the femur is placed over the other leg in two-incision THA, intramedullary blood runs down and into the hip joint as the femur is prepared. In contrast, during anterior THA, the proximal femur is positioned above the knee joint. In our experience, intraoperative blood loss during canal preparation is less during anterior THA, even with identical stem design, possibly because of this difference in femur position.

Because the two incisions are combined into one single anterior incision, the surgical exposures of the acetabulum and the femur are superior during the single-incision anterior approach, when compared with the MIS two-incision THA. Since proximal femur is directly visualized, the risk of unrecognized fracture is avoided, and timely cerclage wiring is possible if a fracture is detected. Finally, during anterior THA, the broach can be left in the femur, while trial neck/head combinations can be used to optimize the neck length and hip offset. With two-incision THA, the femoral stem usually must be implanted first, and trial reductions with the femoral broach are not possible. The single-incision anterior THA may be particularly advantageous if a femoral stem with a modular neck piece is used. The surgeon can test various combinations of offsets and neck lengths to achieve a precise hip reconstruction.

The improved surgical exposure and avoidance of blind femoral preparation also make the anterior THA more amenable to teaching in a residency training environment. Surgical exposure is relatively simple, and circumferential visualization of the acetabulum is readily obtained. Femoral instrumentation and preparation are done under direct visualization, and selected portions of the operation can be performed by supervised assistants while the surgeon maintains control of the procedure. This method also addresses the popular patient demand for muscle-sparing surgery with small skin incisions. Since only minimal thigh fat is present over the anterior thigh, the skin incision can be relatively short with anterior THA.

A disadvantage of any anterior THA is diminished access to the posterior column. Accordingly, if the patient has a deficient posterior acetabular wall from previous hardware or trauma, or if posterior acetabular augmentation is necessary, THA with an anterior approach is contraindicated. Another disadvantage of anterior THA is the necessity of an orthopedic table and the added expense and training with this device. In our experience, however, the investment is worth the superior clinical outcomes, expeditious surgery, and easier surgical exposure. Also, the table is useful for commonly performed orthopedic trauma procedures, such as the operative fixation of proximal femur fractures.

Conclusions and Future Directions

The minimally invasive single-incision anterior approach based on the Smith-Petersen interval provides the optimal combination of sufficient exposure, simplicity, safety, consistency, and preservation of muscle and tendons when compared with any other surgical approach for primary THA.[5,13,19] Dissection is entirely within intermuscular planes, without disruption of tendinous insertions.[7,22] The preservation of tendon and muscles is unique to the anterior approach to THA, and makes this method less invasive than any other technique for total hip replacement, independent of incision length. Trial reduction and consistent component positioning are possible. Intraoperative fluoroscopy is an option at the discretion of the surgeon. The supine patient position is more physiologic for the patient and anesthesiologist.

Regardless of these advantages, most US surgeons are unfamiliar with the anterior approach for hip arthroplasty. Accordingly, the investment, risk, and difficulty that are inherent in new learning may discourage widespread dissemination of anterior THA. Nonetheless, the outcomes of this procedure in terms of patient acceptance, less pain and disability, and rapid return to function make it ideal for THA. Proper learning of this procedure should include a thorough familiarity with the anatomy of the anterior and lateral thigh,t practice with cadaver dissection, and training with an experienced surgeon to learn, recognize, and avoid the pitfalls that are associated with any new surgical procedure. In our practice, the anterior THA method illustrated and described here is the standard procedure for primary THA in all patients.

Since the supine patient position is readily amenable to total hip computer navigation systems, navigated positioning of the components and assessment of intraoperative variables such as leg lengths, offset, and arc of motion is a likely future enhancement of anterior THA.[23] For experienced surgeons, this will allow further shortening of the incision length, thereby improving on the cosmetic appeal of this procedure, while optimizing the safety and tissue-sparing benefits of this technique.

The anterior surgical approach is also amenable to performing hip resurfacing; a particular advantage of this method is that the posterior blood supply to the femoral head is preserved and surgical trauma is decreased.[24] The challenges are in developing new teaching and training methods that allow dissemination of anterior THA to residency training programs, and to seminars for practicing surgeons.

References

1. Sculco TP. Minimally invasive total hip arthroplasty: in the affirmative. J Arthroplasty 2004;19(4 Suppl 1):78–80
2. Dorr LD, Maheshwari AV, Long WT, et al. Early pain and functional results comparing minimally invasive to conventional total hip arthroplasty: a prospective, randomized blinded study. J Bone Joint Surg Am 2007;89(6):1153–60
3. Berger RA. Total hip arthroplasty using the minimally invasive two-incision approach. Clin Orthop Relat Res 2003;(417):232–41
4. Duwelius PJ. Two-incision minimally invasive total hip arthroplasty: techniques and results to date. Instr Course Lect 2006;55:215–22
5. Light TR, Keggi KJ. Anterior approach to hip arthroplasty. Clin Orthop Relat Res 1980;441:255–60
6. Sahm DF, Critchley IA, Kelly LJ, et al. Evaluation of current activities of fluoroquinolones against gram-negative bacilli using centralized in vitro testing and electronic surveillance. Antimicrob Agents Chemother 2001;45(1):267–74
7. Matta JM, Shahrdar C, Ferguson T. Single-incision anterior approach for total hip arthroplasty on an orthopaedic table. Clin Orthop Relat Res 2005;441:115–24
8. Hoppenfield S, deBoer P. Surgical Exposures in Orthopaedics: The Anatomic Approach, 3rd edition. Philadelphia: Lippincott Williams & Wilkins; 2003
9. Smith-Petersen MN. Approach to and exposure of the hip joint for mold arthroplasty. J Bone Joint Surg 1949;31A:40
10. Nogler M, Krismer M, Hozack WJ, Merritt P, Rachbauer F, Mayr E. A double offset broach handle for preparation of the femoral cavity in minimally invasive direct anterior total hip arthroplasty. J Arthroplasty 2006;21(8):1206–8
11. Berger RA. The technique of minimally invasive total hip arthroplasty using the two-incision approach. Instr Course Lect 2004;53:149–55
12. Matta J. A one incision anterior MIS approach. In: Advances in Arthroplasty: Battle of the Bearing Surfaces and Surgical Techniques; Boston; Harvard Advances in Arthroplasty Course 2004
13. Ballesta S, Conejo MC, Garcia I, Rodriguez-Martinez JM, Velasco C, Pascual A. Survival and resistance to imipenem of Pseudomonas aeruginosa on latex gloves. J Antimicrob Chemother 2006;57(5):1010–2
14. Kennon RE, Keggi JM, Wetmore RS, et al. Total hip arthroplasty through a minimally invasive anterior surgical approach. J Bone Joint Surg Am 2003;85-A(Suppl 4):39–48
15. Chambers LW, Rhee P, Baker BC, et al. Initial experience of US Marine Corps forward resuscitative surgical system during Operation Iraqi Freedom. Arch Surg 2005;140(1):26–32
16. Woolson ST, Mow CS, Syquia JF, et al. Comparison of primary total hip replacements performed with a standard incision or a mini-incision. J Bone Joint Surg Am 2004;86-A(7):1353–8
17. Ogonda L, Wilson R, Archbold P, et al. A minimal-incision technique in total hip arthroplasty does not improve early postoperative outcomes. A prospective, randomized, controlled trial. J Bone Joint Surg Am 2005;87(4):701–10

18. Pagnano MW, Leone J, Lewailen DG, Hanssen AD. Two-incision THA had modest outcomes and some substantial complications. Clin Orthop Relat Res 2005;441:86–90
19. Berger RA, Duwelius PJ. The two-incision minimally invasive total hip arthroplasty: technique and results. Orthop Clin North Am 2004;35(2):163–72
20. Mardones R, Pagnano MW, Nemanich JP, Trousdale RT. The Frank Stinchfield Award: muscle damage after total hip arthroplasty done with the two-incision and mini-posterior techniques. Clin Orthop Relat Res 2005;441:63–7
21. McConnell T, Tornetta P, III, Benson E, Manuel J. Gluteus medius tendon injury during reaming for gamma nail insertion. Clin Orthop 2003;(407):199–202
22. Matta JM, Ferguson TA. The anterior approach for hip replacement. Orthopedics 2005;28(9):927–8
23. Weil Y, Mattan Y, Kandel L, Eisenberg O, Liebergall M. Navigation-assisted minimally invasive two-incision total hip arthoplasty. Orthopedics 2006;29(3):200–6
24. Beaule PE, Campbell P, Lu Z, et al. Vascularity of the arthritic femoral head and hip resurfacing. J Bone Joint Surg Am 2006;88(Suppl 4):85–96

Chapter 20
The Watson-Jones Approach to Minimally Invasive Total Hip Arthroplasty

Stephen M. Walsh and Richard A. Berger

The current interest in minimally invasive total hip arthroplasty stems from the potential to improve postoperative recovery. This is accomplished by utilizing mobile windows to reduce soft tissue trauma and preserve intact musculotendinous units. Minimally invasive techniques have been developed for the anterolateral (Hardinge) and posterior approaches with each retaining respective advantages and disadvantages. Many surgeons prefer the Hardinge approach due to the historically lower dislocation rate when compared with posterior surgery. However, the necessary violation of the anterior abductor insertion on the greater trochanter can result in weakness and gait alteration in some patients. The desire to minimize postoperative dislocation risk while maximizing functional recovery and maintenance of abductor strength has led to the development of the minimally invasive Watson-Jones approach. The objective of this chapter is to describe the surgical technique in detail. This challenging approach uses a combination of new instrumentation and positioning which, while more difficult than the classic Watson-Jones approach, aims to provide patients with a low risk of dislocation, improved maintenance of abductor strength, and more rapid rehabilitation without compromising long-term outcomes.

The classic Watson-Jones approach for total hip arthroplasty avoids dissection of posterior soft tissues with concomitant low dislocation rate. However, the technique mobilizes the anterior abductors from both the greater trochanter and the ilium en route to the hip. This disruption of the abductor musculotendinous unit often results in weakness and limp.

The minimally invasive Watson-Jones approach for total hip arthroplasty retains advantages of the classic technique while avoiding detachment of the abductors. The approach, originally described by Bertin and Röttinger,[1] uses the same interval but allows preservation of the abductors. This exploits the low dislocation rate of an anterolateral interval with less risk of postoperative weakness and limp.

This chapter describes, in detail, the minimally invasive Watson-Jones approach for total hip arthroplasty. This will be accomplished by a thorough discussion of indications and preoperative planning, patient positioning, dissection, femoral and acetabular preparation, implantation, and wound closure. Finally, potential complications and pitfalls will be addressed.

Indications and Preoperative Planning

The learning curve associated with any new procedure places great importance on careful patient selection. As the surgeon gains experience, more and more challenging cases may be tackled. The easiest patients for the minimally invasive Watson-Jones approach are, not surprisingly, the easiest patients for any total hip arthroplasty. Specifically, women who are thin, non-muscular, with a small bone structure and atrophic degeneration are most amenable to perfecting the technique. Heavy, muscular men with a large bone structure, varus neck, and hypertrophic degeneration are some of the most challenging. The in situ neck osteotomy utilized with this technique is made difficult by a varus neck deformity. Femoral preparation requires adequate mobilization, which can be encumbered by large, low anteriorly inserting abductors.

Most patients who are candidates for total hip arthroplasty are appropriate for the minimally invasive Watson-Jones approach. However, certain patient scenarios may be better served by more traditional approaches. Patients suffering from morbid obesity create a particular challenge with this procedure. Significant anatomic abnormalities, complete dislocation, and prior surgical procedures provide additional challenges that require careful consideration of more extensile approaches.

Preoperative planning is of paramount importance and involves patient assessment and X-ray templating. The minimally invasive nature of the modified Watson-Jones approach limits visualization of extraarticular landmarks and places particular importance on preparation. Patient evaluation implies not only surgical indications but appropriateness of surgical approach as described previously. Careful radiographic evaluation allows the surgeon to plan for optimal acetabular and femoral implants based on assessment of the

S.M. Walsh and R.A. Berger (✉)
Department of Orthopedic Surgery, Rush–Presbyterian–St. Luke's Medical Center, 1725 West Harrison Street, Suite 1063, Chicago, IL 60612, USA
e-mail: r.a.berger@sbcglobal.net

G.R. Scuderi and A.J. Tria (eds.), *Minimally Invasive Surgery in Orthopedics*,
DOI 10.1007/978-0-387-76608-9_20, © Springer Science+Business Media, LLC 2010

patient's unique anatomy. Additionally, femoral neck osteotomy level, prosthetic neck length, and femoral offset are determined and care is taken to ensure that the implants are available.

As with any total hip arthroplasty, appropriate postoperative leg length is best assured by preoperative assessment. The anterior-posterior (AP) pelvis X-ray provides the most common method of evaluation. Further imaging such as scanogram or computed tomography (CT) scan may be helpful in cases of distorted anatomy. Significant varus of the proximal femur or other cases of unusually high offset may preclude anatomic restoration. In these rare cases, limb lengthening may be necessary to obtain stability via soft tissue tension. Limb length discrepancy can be a source of postoperative patient dissatisfaction, emphasizing the importance of preoperative planning to identify this potential issue and counsel patients regarding the true goals of the procedure.

Surgical Technique

Patient Positioning

The procedure is performed with the patient in the lateral decubitus position. A standard pelvic positioning system is employed that supports the symphysis and contralateral anterior-superior iliac spine anteriorly and the sacrum posteriorly (Fig. 20.1). Care is taken to ensure that the anterior-superior iliac spines are perpendicular to the floor. Femoral preparation requires extension, adduction, and external rotation of the operative leg. A table that allows removal of the posterior leg section makes proper positioning possible. Finally, an attachment supporting the operative leg in approximately 15° of abduction sufficiently de-tensions the hip abductors during the initial exposure.

At our institution, we employ the Universal Jupiter Table (TRUMPF Inc., Farmington, CT), which allows independent removal of the right and left leg sections distal to the patients waist. The nonoperative leg rests on the remaining section in slight flexion. This configuration facilitates femoral preparation with leg preparation as previously described (Fig. 20.1). A workable alternative involves positioning the patient distally on a standard operative table and attaching a hand table or other extension to support the nonoperative leg.

Approach

Incision placement is crucial in order to optimize the effect of a mobile window. The lateral borders of the greater trochanter must be accurately identified, a task made easier by using a 22-gauge spinal needle in heavy patients. When possible, the anterior border of the gluteus medius is palpated and marked on the skin. The incision is typically 3.5-in. long with one third distal to the tip of the greater trochanter and the remainder proximal (Fig. 20.2). The distal incision is parallel to the femur and slightly posterior to the anterior border of the greater trochanter. At the tip of the trochanter, the incision is curved anteriorly approximately 30° to follow slightly posterior to the anterior edge of the gluteus medius.

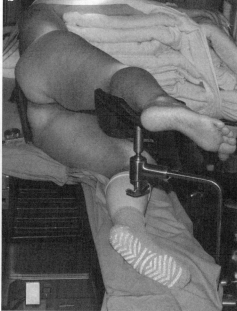

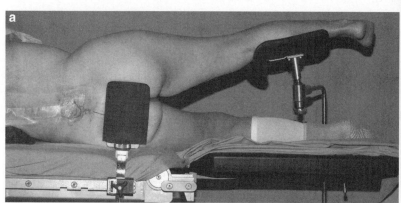

Fig. 20.1 Lateral decubitus position with 15° abduction leg support (**a**). Leg extension removed to allow extension, adduction, and external rotation of operative leg (**b**)

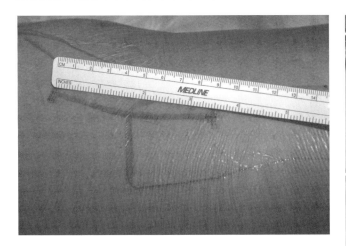

Fig. 20.2 Curvilinear incision, 3.5 in. in length, over the anterior border of the gluteus medius

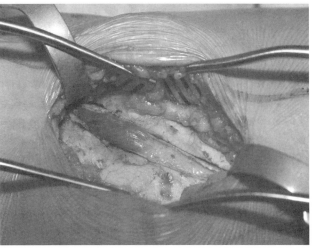

Fig. 20.4 Fascial incision: gluteus medius muscle fibers seen proximally and fatty tissue between medius and tensor fasciae lata seen distally

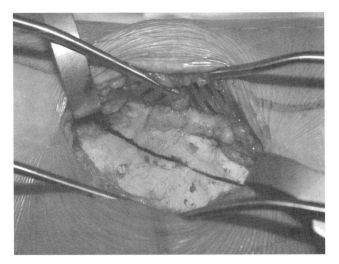

Fig. 20.3 *Solid line* marking fascial incision over the anterior border of the gluteus medius

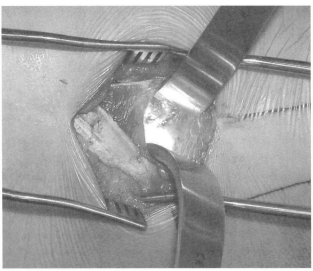

Fig. 20.5 Adductor tensor interval being developed by slowly spreading retractors

After sharp incision of the skin, we utilize electrocautery to dissect the subcutaneous tissues. The subcutaneous dissection must proceed following the curve of the skin incision to allow adequate exposure. When the fascia overlying the gluteus medius and tensor fascia lata muscles is reached, the intermuscular interval is identified (Fig. 20.3). The fascia is then divided longitudinally just anterior to the edge of the greater trochanter. Deep to the fascia, adipose tissue between the abductor and tensor is found distal to the tip of the greater trochanter and muscle fibers of the gluteus medius are found proximally as they course from the trochanter to the ilium (Fig. 20.4).

Deeper dissection proceeds with identification of the gluteus medius and minimus. The surgeon directs his or her finger anteroinferiorly along the anterior border of the medius until it falls on the femoral neck. Lit retractors (#1, Zimmer, Dover, OH, MIS Watson-Jones retractor set) are then placed

through this interval, first posterior and then anterior to the femoral neck, taking care not to violate the abductors. The interval between the abductors and the tensor is developed by gently spreading the retractors (Fig. 20.5). The occasional robust fascial attachment is divided with electrocautery.

The fatty layer superficial to the capsule, if not opened by retractor placement, is excised for improved visualization. The capsule is then incised or excised from the acetabular rim, along the superior neck, anteroinferiorly along the intertrochanteric line, and finally back to the rim along the inferior neck. In muscular patients, improved exposure is obtained with a Hohmann-type retractor placed along the superior acetabular rim, which also serves to protect the abductors.

A right-angle retractor may aid in protecting the vastus musculature inferiorly. Once the rim, head, and neck are exposed, the #1 retractors are replaced intracapsularly over the acetabular rim prior to removing the femoral head (Fig. 20.6).

Femoral Neck Osteotomy

Removal of the femoral head represents a diversion from traditional techniques that rely on dislocation, a step that is extraordinarily difficult in this case. The femoral head is therefore removed in sequential steps with the oscillating saw, starting with a very thin (2–3 mm) wafer at the dome (Fig. 20.7). The remainder of the head is removed in slices (Fig. 20.8), and, with each cut, the tension decreases, allowing removal of larger slices of bone. The final provisional cut is at the head-neck junction. Care is taken to remove all of the posterior femoral head, which will allow adequate mobilization and identification of the lesser trochanter (Fig. 20.9). When resecting the head, care is taken to avoid plunging with the saw into the acetabulum. With experience, femoral head removal in this fashion allows the surgeon to quickly and safely overcome inability to dislocate the native head.

Once the head is completely removed, the leg is removed from the support and reoriented in the figure of four position (flexed and externally rotated) (Fig. 20.10). A right-angle retractor is utilized to mobilize the vastus off of the calcar, and the lesser trochanter is identified. The final neck cut is then made based on preoperative templating. A #3 double-pronged retractor (Zimmer, MIS Watson-Jones retractor set) placed around the lesser trochanter improves visualization.

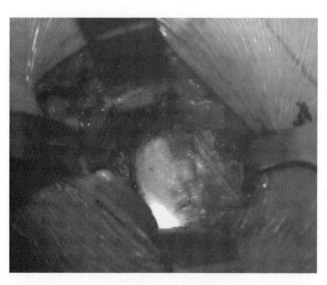

Fig. 20.6 Exposure of femoral head and acetabulum

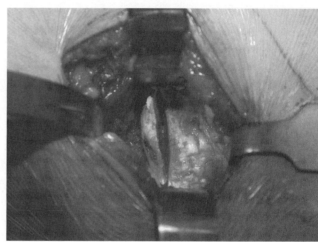

Fig. 20.7 Small wafer of femoral head from initial osteotomy

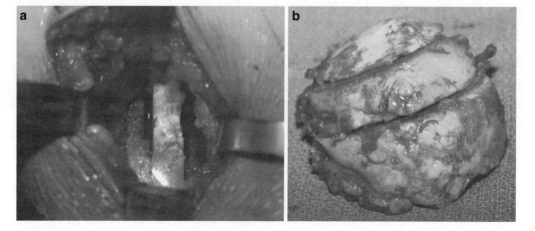

Fig. 20.8 Second slice of femoral head, slightly larger (approximately 1 cm) (**a**). The femoral head is approached in successive cuts, which greatly facilitates head removal (**b**)

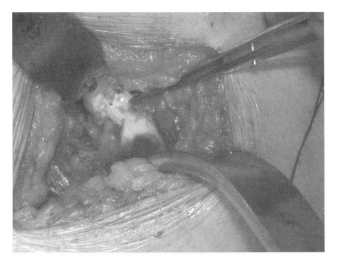

Fig. 20.9 Lesser trochanter easily visible to align final neck cut

Acetabulum

Accurate retractor placement is of paramount importance in acetabular exposure. The #3 double-pronged retractor, placed posteriorly, holds the proximal femur out of view. The tip of the retractor lies over the acetabular rim, resting on the ischium. The anteroinferior capsule is retraced with a standard cobra retractor. Finally, the abductors are retracted postero-superiorly with a lit #2 retractor. The acetabular rim is fully exposed by resecting the labrum and periacetabular tissues. The acetabular floor is exposed by removing any remaining pulvinar and ligamentum (Fig. 20.11). Cutout reamers and an offset reamer handle (Zimmer, MIS hip set) are used, with care taken to ensure proper abduction and anteversion. It is possible to ream with a straight handle by placing the leg in abduction and flexion. We choose a 2-mm press-fit with a porous cup on an offset inserter (Fig. 20.12) augmented with

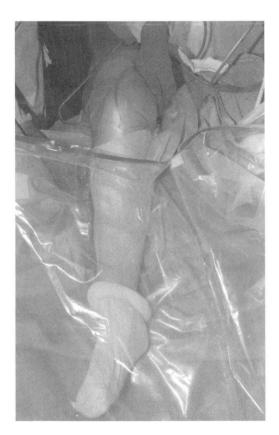

Fig. 20.10 Operative leg flexed, externally rotated, and placed in the sterile drape bag for final neck cut

A standard Hohmann retractor is then placed at the junction of the femoral neck and greater trochanter (saddle point). We direct our neck cut from the appropriate medial position to the saddle point, negating the need to recut remaining lateral neck. After a satisfactory neck cut is complete, the leg is repositioned on the support to allow acetabular exposure.

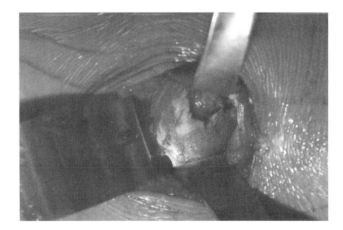

Fig. 20.11 Acetabular exposure noting clear view of cotyloid fossa

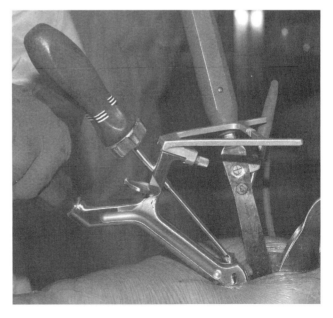

Fig. 20.12 View of the offset acetabular insertion handle

screws. After placing the liner, the locking mechanism is easily visualized and verified (Fig. 20.13).

Femur

Femoral preparation requires reposition of the leg into extension, adduction, and external rotation. Femoral exposure is the most challenging part of this technique and careful attention to positioning of the extremity is necessary. The assistant must adduct the leg as much as possible, placing the patient's foot close to the floor. We employ a plastic "kangaroo" pouch clipped to the assistant's waist (Fig. 20.14). This allows unrestricted mobility and maintains sterility.

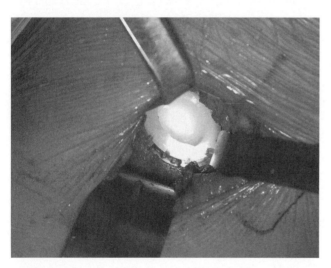

Fig. 20.13 Visualization of the acetabular shell, liner, and locking mechanism

As stated previously, exposure is most challenging in muscular men. The well-developed abductors restrict access to the femoral canal. Femoral mobilization typically requires release of the posterior–superior capsule from the posterior femoral neck. Occasionally the piriformis must be released as well.

Similar to acetabular exposure, accurate retractor placement is a key to femoral preparation. The calcar is elevated with a #3 lit double-pronged retractor placed anteriorly. The abductors are retracted with a #4 single-pronged Hohmann retractor with the tip placed over the posterior acetabular rim. Finally, a right-angle retractor may by used to protect the vastus lateralis (Fig. 20.15). The femoral canal is accessible with the combination of careful retractor placement and leg positioning as previously described. We utilize a curved awl to localize the femoral canal. The curve helps to avoid the tendency to direct instruments posterolaterally with risk of metaphyseal perforation.

The need to mobilize the abductor bulk, especially in muscular male patients, is eased by using a curved, tapered femoral stem. Such a stem is introduced in a relative varus position and aligned to neutral as it is fully seated. We routinely employ the Zimmer ML taper stem (Zimmer). Regardless of the implant, care is taken to avoid damage to the abductor musculature during broaching. This is facilitated with careful retraction and by using offset broach handles (Fig. 20.16). Careful positioning and retraction allows adequate visualization of the femoral neck and calcar to ensure appropriate femoral component version (Fig. 20.17).

Implantation of the final implant is accomplished by inserting the stem by hand until it is completely within the incision prior to tamping the component further. This helps to avoid trauma to the proximal skin and soft tissue. The final position is visualized directly (Fig. 20.18). Trial reductions are undertaken, as usual, with varied neck lengths to obtain appropriate stability prior to impacting the final head onto the trunnion.

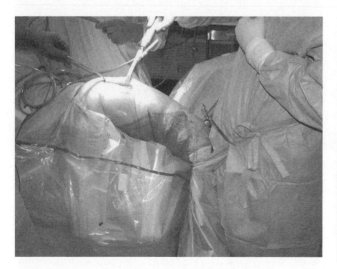

Fig. 20.14 Operative leg placement in the "kangaroo" pouch allowing extension, adduction, and external rotation

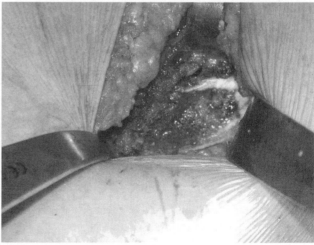

Fig. 20.15 Retraction of the vastus lateralis and visualization of the femoral neck

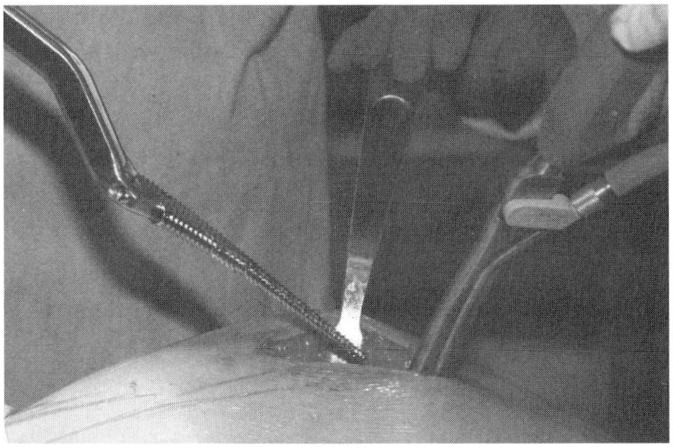

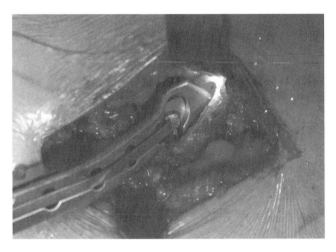

Fig. 20.16 Offset broach handle prior to insertion

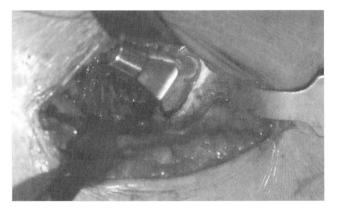

Fig. 20.17 Assessment of femoral broach version and insertion depth

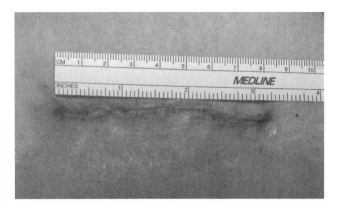

Fig. 20.19 Final incision length of 3.25 in.

Closure

Deep closure is not necessary. We begin by closing the fascia overlying the tensor with a #1 absorbable suture. Closure follows in layers including the adipose tissue, deep dermis, and skin. We prefer to close the skin with a #3–0 absorbable running suture followed by polymer adhesive (Fig. 20.19). Once the polymer has cured, a small sterile bandage is applied.

Complications and Pitfalls

As with any other operation, there are potential complications at every stage of this procedure. With attention to detail they can all be minimized if not eliminated.

Anesthesia

Regional anesthesia is typically utilized to minimize postoperative nausea and vomiting and to facilitate pain management. However, the relative increase in muscle tone compared with general anesthesia makes the procedure technically more difficult. For this reason, we recommend general anesthesia while gaining experience with the technique to take advantage of the superior muscle relaxation before transitioning to regional anesthesia.

Dissection

Appropriate location and orientation of the skin incision are essential. If the incision is placed too posteriorly relative to the anterior border of the abductor, the skin itself will limit exposure and the incision will have to be lengthened. Division of the fascia overlying the tensor should be performed just posterior to the anterior border of the medius. Again, if this

![Fig. 20.18]

Fig. 20.18 Final femoral component position

Once the hip is reduced with final components and the stability is again tested, the wound is closed. Violation of a small portion (5–10%) of the anterior borders of the gluteus medius and minimus is not uncommon. Careful attention to leg position and retractor placement limits this soft tissue damage and we have not noted a clinical consequence when a small violation occurs.

is too posterior, mobilization of the abductor unit will be compromised. Frequent identification of the abductor and trochanteric borders during the dissection will help to optimize skin and fascial incisions.

Retraction

One of the goals of the procedure is to maintain abductor integrity. For this reason, it is imperative to retract the entire abductor unit posteriorly and to avoid splitting the muscle. Initial retraction of the abductor unit should allow unobstructed visualization of the joint capsule. Any muscle fibers visible in the interval typically represent an abductor split and require retractor reassessment and repositioning.

Joint Capsule

Varus femoral neck orientation increases the difficulty of capsular incision or excision. In many cases, this leads to capsular division in a superior position on the ilium. This can be avoided by incising the capsule along the superior femoral neck from the saddle point toward the acetabulum until the acetabular rim is encountered.

Femoral Resection

It is necessary to adequately identify and expose the acetabular rim prior to making the initial femoral head cut. Failure to do this often results in an initial cut that is too large and the wafer of bone becomes incarcerated. Should this happen, the wafer can be split and removed in sections prior to proceeding with sequential head and neck cuts.

Reaming the Acetabulum

Care must be taken when reaming the acetabulum to avoid levering the reamer handle on the femur, a position that can force the reamer anteriorly. This is especially true when a long femoral neck is retained. The combination of an offset reamer handle and careful manual direction of the reamer helps to avoid eccentric reaming.

Cup Positioning

There is a tendency to place the acetabular cup in exaggerated anteversion and adduction. Using an offset cup inserter can assist in reproducing native acetabular version.

Femoral Preparation

Lateral soft tissues may inhibit delivery of the proximal femur into the incision. Release of the posteromedial capsule from the femur allows elevation of the proximal femur and improved access to the canal. Care must taken to aim the starting awl toward the knee to avoid posterolateral perforation. Finally, use of a curved femoral component helps to avoid placement of the prosthesis in varus, particularly in muscular patients.

Conclusion

The minimally invasive Watson-Jones approach for total hip arthroplasty was designed to facilitate postoperative recovery, maintain a low dislocation rate, and to improve abductor strength while not compromising long-term outcomes. In order for this technique to enjoy success and reproducibility, the surgeon must employ proper instrumentation and an altered operating table. Training, preparation, and the use of general anesthesia will all aid the surgeon when adapting to this technique. Acetabular exposure is straightforward in almost all patients, but femoral preparation can be a challenge in muscular males, emphasizing the importance of patient selection when embarking on the learning curve. The minimally invasive Watson-Jones approach, while more difficult than the classic Watson-Jones or Hardinge approaches, retains the benefit of the anterolateral interval while maintaining abductor integrity and providing patients with the potential for more rapid rehabilitation.

Reference

1. Bertin KC, Röttinger H. Anterolateral mini-incision hip replacement surgery: a modified Watson-Jones approach. Clin Orthop Relat Res. 2004 Dec;(429):248–55

Suggested Readings

Bertin KC, Röttinger H. Anterolateral mini-incision hip replacement surgery: a modified Watson-Jones approach. Clin Orthop Relat Res. 2004 Dec;(429):248–55

Cech O, Dzupa V. The European school of total hip arthroplasty and 35 years of total hip arthroplasty in the Czech Republic. Acta Chir Orthop Traumatol Cech. 2005;72(1):57–76

de Beer J, McKenzie S, Hubmann M, Petruccelli D, Winemaker M. Influence of cementless femoral stems inserted in varus on functional outcome in primary total hip arthroplasty. Can J Surg. 2006;49(6):407–11

Graf R, Mohajer MA. The Stolzalpe technique: a modified Watson-Jones approach. Int Orthop. 2007 31(Suppl 1):S21–4

Laffosse JM, Chiron P, Accadbled F, Molinier F, Tricoire JL, Puget J. Learning curve for a modified Watson-Jones minimally invasive approach in primary total hip replacement: analysis of complications and early results versus the standard-incision posterior approach. Acta Orthop Belg. 2006;72(6):693–701

Lazovic D, Zigan R. Navigation of short-stem implants. Orthopedics. 2006 29(10 Suppl):S125–9

Pflüger G, Junk-Jantsch S, Schöll V. Minimally invasive total hip replacement via the anterolateral approach in the supine position. Int Orthop. 2007 31(Suppl 1):S7–11

Stähelin T. [Abductor repair failure and nerve damage during hip replacement via the transgluteal approach. Why less invasive methods of joint replacement are needed, and some approaches to solving the problems]. Orthopade. 2006;35(12):1215–24 (German)

Chapter 21
Posterolateral Mini-incision Total Hip Arthroplasty

Gregg R. Klein and Mark A. Hartzband

The posterior approach to the hip was first popularized by Von Langenbeck in the 1870s and later modified by Moore,[1] Gibson,[2] and Marcy.[3] All of these modifications included release of the posterior soft tissue sleeve posterior to the gluteus medius and minimus muscles. They varied with respect to the precise location of skin incision and the exact description of the soft tissue exposure. All resulted in a posterior dislocation of the femoral head in relationship to the acetabulum.

In the United States today, the posterior approach is one of the most commonly used exposures for total hip arthroplasty. The posterior approach is familiar to most arthroplasty surgeons and is quickly and easily performed. This approach minimizes damage to the abductor musculature and has a low rate of heterotopic ossification. In addition, the posterolateral approach may be readily extended during total hip arthroplasty into a more expansile exposure if necessary. However, dislocation after the posterior approach remains a concern.[4–6] More recently, the posterolateral approach for total hip arthroplasty has been modified to include a posterior capsular repair to decrease the incidence of dislocation. With the incorporation of a capsular repair, the incidence of dislocation approaches that of the anterior approaches.[7–10]

The posterior mini-incision is more than just a small skin incision. It incorporates minimal soft tissue dissection and modified limb positioning, and it eliminates portions of the surgical exposure that are unnecessary for accurate and reproducible implant placement. The senior author's (MAH) experience with posterolateral mini-incision total hip arthroplasty has been evolving since 1996.[11] As more experience was gained, the incision length was progressively shortened. As the incisions became shorter, it became clear that modification of traditional instrumentation was necessary. Although similar to traditional instruments, these newer instruments aid in exposure while protecting the soft tissues. Incision and exposure size should be progressively diminished over time as more experience with these techniques is obtained. It is important to

understand that all parts of the hip should be readily visualized throughout this approach. In many cases, all portions of the hip are not, however, visualized as the same instant. Manipulation of a mobile window or the limb may be necessary at any given time to properly expose the hip.

Indications

Mini-incision posterolateral total hip arthroplasty can be performed on a large percentage of patients indicated for hip replacement. However, appropriate patient selection, especially in the early part of the learning curve, is imperative. As experience is gained, more and more patients are candidates for this technique. Thin women with a general lack of muscular development are the easiest candidates for mini-incisions. A varus femoral neck tends to facilitate this approach, while long valgus femoral necks are more difficult, especially in muscular men. Hypertrophic arthritis patterns and protrusio deformity make mini-incision surgery more difficult and should not be attempted until more experience has been gained. Mild degrees of hip dysplasia, i.e., Crowe I and II hips, can be readily approached through a posterolateral mini-incision. Flexion and external rotation contractures make exposure more difficult. As in all posterior approaches, large muscular males are the most difficult patients.

Preoperative Planning

Any type of total hip arthroplasty should begin with precise preoperative planning. Predicted component placement and leg length assessment should be made preoperatively. An anteroposterior (AP) X-ray of the pelvis and lateral of the hip are essential. Meticulous preoperative templating is the most accurate method for obtaining appropriate postoperative leg lengths. Standard intraoperative neck cutting guides may be easily used through a small incision, and leg length confirmation systems of choice may be used with this exposure.

G.R. Klein and M.A. Hartzband (✉)
Hartzband Center for HIP and Knee Replacement, 10 Forest Avenue, Paramus, NJ, 07652, USA
e-mail: info@HartzbandCenter.com

G.R. Scuderi and A.J. Tria (eds.), *Minimally Invasive Surgery in Orthopedics*,
DOI 10.1007/ 978-0-387-76608-9_21, © Springer Science+Business Media, LLC 2010

Surgical Technique

Patient Positioning

The patient is positioned in the lateral decubitus position with any one of the commercially available hip-holding devices. It is critical that the operative limb is able to move freely. Bony prominences should be appropriately padded. It is imperative not to restrict movement of the contralateral extremity, as it will need to be repositioned during femoral preparation. The pelvis must be secured rigidly in the hip-holding device. Any unappreciated change in the position of the pelvis during the surgery may compromise acetabular component positioning. A carpenter's level is applied to the table to make sure that the table is horizontal to the floor and not tilted anteriorly or posteriorly. The level is then placed on the hip positioner to ensure that the pelvis is perpendicular to the floor. It is important to realize that most standard pelvic-holding devices apply up to 20° of flexion to the pelvis and therefore require a corresponding modification in acetabular component position in order to obtain appropriate acetabular anteversion. The patient is then prepped and draped in the routine fashion.

Landmarks

Correct incision placement is essential when performing mini-incision arthroplasty (Fig. 21.1). Incorrect positioning may significantly compromise exposure of the acetabulum, femur, or both. In addition, if an inappropriate incision location is chosen, the incision most likely will need to be extended in order to appropriately position the components. The true high point of the pelvis (i.e., the point at which the lumbar paraspinal muscles meet the lateral border of the posterior ilium) is identified and marked. Next, a second point approximately two fingerbreadths posterior to the high point of the pelvis and directed toward the center of the greater trochanter is marked. This line generally represents a good approximation of the acetabular anteversion angle. The proximal, anterior, and posterior borders of the greater trochanter are marked. In larger patients, it may be difficult to identify the trochanter. A 22-gauge, 3.5-in. spinal needle may be used to identify the borders of the greater trochanter. A 6- to 8-cm incision 10–20° oblique to the long axis of the femur is marked. This is usually parallel to the line approximating the anteversion angle. The incision is positioned so that approximately 80% of the incision is distal to the most proximal border of the greater trochanter. The incision is also placed slightly posterior (5 mm) to the midline of the greater trochanter. It is often necessary to translate the incision somewhat posteriorly and perhaps 1 cm proximally in patients with large amounts of adipose tissue. However, excessive posterior positioning of the incision will greatly compromise visualization of the anterior aspect of the acetabulum. Proximal positioning of the incision makes femoral preparation technically easier in these patients. The incisions should be translated distally (so the entire incision is distal to the most proximal border of the greater trochanter) in patients with hip dysplasia (Crowe I and II) and lateral subluxation of the hip.

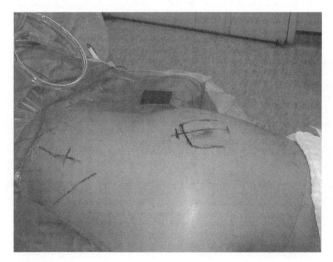

Fig. 21.1 Landmarks and location of incision for mini-posterolateral total hip arthroplasty (From Hartzband MA, Posterolateral minimal incision for total hip replacement: technique and early results, in Scuderi GR, Tria AJ, Jr., Berger RA (eds.), MIS Techniques in Orthopedics, New York, Springer, 2006, with kind permission of Springer Science + Business Media, Inc.)

Surgical Exposure

Using the previously defined landmarks, the skin incision is made and dissection is carried through the subcutaneous tissue in line with the skin incision. Only the fascia in line with the skin incision is exposed, care is taken not to expose an excess amount of fascia; this will create a potential dead-space for hematoma collection postoperatively. The gluteus maximus fascia and fascia latae are incised in the direction of their fibers. Proximally the gluteus maximus muscle is bluntly divided. The sciatic nerve is identified but not formally exposed. Extension of the fascial incision beyond the limits of the skin incision is rarely necessary. Extending the fascial incision may make closure more difficult. A modified Charnley retractor is then placed below the fascia. The Charnley blades must be radiused so as to maximize exposure of the deeper structures through the mobile skin window. In addition, the blades of the Charnley have been lengthened to allow engagement in very short incisions.

The short external rotators are identified. The limb is placed in extension, gravity adduction, and forced internal rotation. In contrast to the traditional posterior approach using a flexion, adduction, and internal rotation, this approach uses extension to keep the proximal femur central in the mobile window. In addition, extension minimizes potential pressure on the sciatic nerve under the tendon of the gluteus maximus (which is not released in this approach).[12] The short external rotators and posterior capsule are divided with electrocautery from their insertion at the piriformis fossa (Fig. 21.2). Bending the tip of the electrocautery will facilitate division of the rotators and the capsule from their bony insertions. The limb is progressively internally rotated to release the rotators. The short external rotators are deliberately not mobilized from the pericapsular fat or capsule. This facilitates closure of this layer at the conclusion of the procedure.

The superior border of the piriformis is identified, and a Cobb elevator is placed along its superior border and then slid anteriorly to separate the gluteus minimus from the hip capsule. The piriformis tendon is then released from the piriformis fossa and a radial capsulotomy is performed along the superior border of the piriformis to the acetabular rim. Next, the superior capsule may be incised with a long scalpel blade under the protection of the previously placed Cobb elevator to the zenith of the acetabulum (for a right hip this is from the 10 o'clock to the 12 o'clock position). With division of this posterior–superior portion of the capsule, a dramatic increase in posterior laxity will be noted. The hip is gently dislocated in 15° of flexion, adduction, and internal rotation. A bone hook may be used if dislocation is difficult (Fig. 21.3).

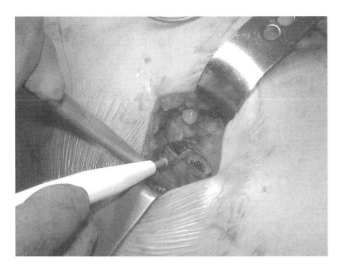

Fig. 21.2 Elevation of the posterior capsular flap including the short external rotators and piriformis (From Hartzband MA, Posterolateral minimal incision for total hip replacement: technique and early results, in Scuderi GR, Tria AJ, Jr., Berger RA (eds.), MIS Techniques in Orthopedics, New York, Springer, 2006, with kind permission of Springer Science + Business Media, Inc.)

Femoral Osteotomy

Once the hip is dislocated, the proximal femur is positioned to perform the femoral osteotomy. This femoral neck cut is marked based on the previously templated measurements from the proximal aspect of the lesser trochanter (Fig. 21.3b). Extension of the limb aides in visualization of the lesser trochanter. Occasionally, 5–10 mm of quadratus femoris may be released to improve exposure. Any of the traditional neck cutting guides may be used in this approach. Alternatively, a broach of the templated femoral component size may be used. The vertical distance form the tip of the greater trochanter or the shoulder of the femoral neck is also a valuable guide to

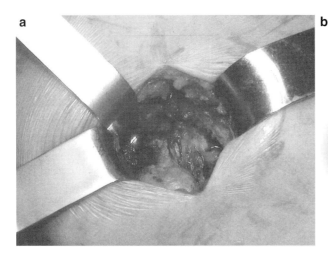 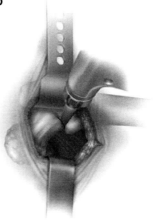

Fig. 21.3 (a) Posterior dislocation of the femoral head. (b) Femoral neck osteotomy with a reciprocating saw (a, from Hartzband MA, Posterolateral minimal incision for total hip replacement: technique and early results, in Scuderi GR, Tria AJ, Jr., Berger RA (eds.), MIS Techniques in Orthopedics, New York, Springer, 2006, with kind permission of Springer Science + Business Media, Inc.; b, courtesy of Zimmer, Warsaw, IN)

assist in proper location of the neck osteotomy. Starting at the medial calcar, a reciprocating saw with teeth on only one side is used to make the neck osteotomy. This blade is critical in the exposure to avoid inadvertent injury to the posterior structures such as the sciatic nerve and other soft tissues in this region. As the neck cut progresses from the medial calcar, the first assistant gradually flexes the hip to 45° to bring the greater trochanter into view. At this point it is important to avoid notching the greater trochanter thus preventing a potential greater trochanteric fracture or abductor injury. With more flexion, the vertical limb of the neck cut is made from the piriformis fossa distally along the medial aspect of the greater trochanter to the previous osteotomy.

Once the osteotomy is completed, the limb is brought back into extension. This exposes the cut cancellous surface of the osteotomized head and neck, which can be easily grasped with a bone-holding clamp and removed. Release of capsule or soft tissue attachments such as the ligamentum teres may be necessary. In very small incisions with large femoral heads, it may be necessary to remove the Charnley retractor in order to facilitate the removal of the femoral head.

Acetabular Exposure

Once the femoral head has been removed, the acetabulum can be exposed (Fig. 21.4). A Kocher clamp is placed on the internal aspect of the posterior capsular flap at the posterior superior corner of the posterior capsular incision (at the level of the piriformis tendon). This clamp serves to retract the

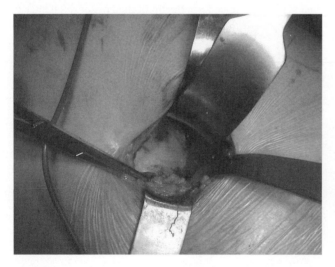

Fig. 21.4 Acetabular exposure with retractors in place. Note the Kocher clamp posteriorly retracting the posterior capsule (From Hartzband MA, Posterolateral minimal incision for total hip replacement: technique and early results, in Scuderi GR, Tria AJ, Jr., Berger RA (eds.), MIS Techniques in Orthopedics, New York, Springer, 2006, with kind permission of Springer Science + Business Media, Inc.)

posterior soft tissues during the acetabular exposure and is maintained throughout acetabular preparation.

One of a number of radiused anterior retractors is placed into the acetabulum and then walked up the anterior acetabular wall. If desired, a lighted retractor may be used to improve visualization. The retractor is then pushed through the anterior capsule to retract the proximal femur anteriorly. In large muscular men, retraction of the femur anteriorly may be difficult. An anterior capsulotomy may be performed to improve exposure. Under direct visualization, a scalpel blade is advanced, beginning at the superior pole of the previous capsular incision and continued anteriorly and distally until adequate capsular relaxation has been obtained. Generally, by the time an additional 70–90° of capsule has been released, the anterior femoral capsule should relax and adequate acetabular exposure should be obtained. The acetabular bed is exposed in a traditional manner. A long-handled knife and Kocher clamp may be used to remove any remaining labrum. The pulvinar can be excised using a large curette or rongeuer. If a large medial osteophyte is present, a curette or osteotome may be used to identify the true medial wall. The medial wall osteophyte, when it exists, is keyholed with a rongeuer to the level of the transverse acetabular ligament. The inferior aspect of the acetabulum and transverse acetabular ligament is then defined. A large, self-illuminated, blunt Hohmann retractor bent to 45° is directed from within the acetabulum deep to the transverse acetabular ligament. This is brought inferiorly and distally to provide inferior acetabular exposure.

The operative limb is allowed to lay dependent on the opposite leg in a position that allows optimal acetabular exposure. The limb may be slightly internally rotated to improve exposure. If necessary, the foot may be placed on a padded Mayo stand to maintain the limb in internal rotation. A single assistant on the contralateral side of the table holds the anterior and inferior retractors. No additional assistants are necessary.

Acetabular Preparation

Reaming (Fig. 21.5a) should begin with a reamer a few millimeters smaller than the templated acetabular size. Side cut, hemisphere plus reamers have been created to facilitate insertion through a limited exposure. These reamers are very aggressive and, as such, minimize the number of "passes" required to machine the acetabulum adequately. If significant medial wall or shelf osteophytes exist, it is important to ream medially to bring the center of rotation back to the anatomic position. Reaming progresses sequentially in 2-mm increments until a concentric reaming is obtained. It is important to avoid inadvertent levering of the reamer on the posterior border of the proximal femur as this may create eccentric

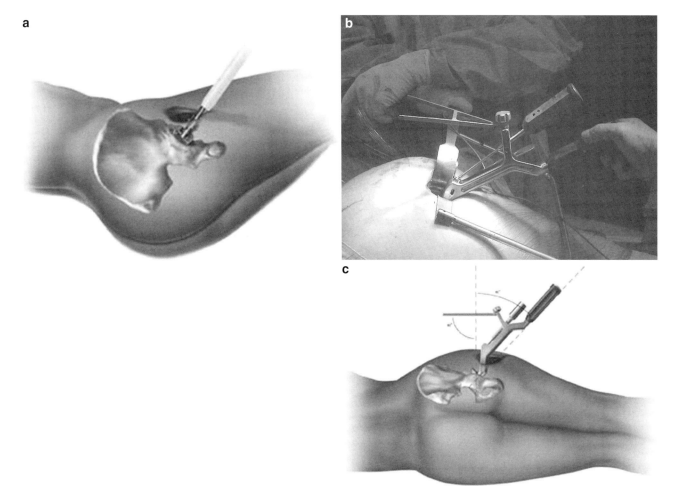

Fig. 21.5 (a) Acetabular inserter in position. (b) Acetabular reamer in position. Note impingement of the reamer on the distal aspect of the incision. This may result in excessive vertical reaming and positioning of the implant. (c) Offset acetabular inserter in position. Note the inserter does not impinge on the soft tissue thus decreasing the chance of improper component position. (a and c, courtesy of Zimmer, Inc., Warsaw, IN; b, from Hartzband MA, Posterolateral minimal incision for total hip replacement: technique and early results, in Scuderi GR, Tria AJ, Jr., Berger RA (eds.), MIS Techniques in Orthopedics, New York, Springer, 2006, with kind permission of Springer Science + Business Media, Inc.)

posterior reaming of the acetabulum and possibly compromise the posterior wall or column. It is also important to ensure that the reamer does not damage the soft tissue and skin at the distal pole of the mini-incision. If necessary, the limb may be internally rotated to improve visualization while reaming. A number of offset reamers are available; however, these are typically unnecessary if the incision has been made in the appropriate location. Acetabular cup size is based on the last reamer used and the specifics of the individual acetabular shell chosen.

The acetabular shell is now inserted (Fig. 21.5b, c). In small-incision surgery, it is important to try to minimize contact between the implant and the skin edges so as to avoid contamination. The shell should be oriented with its internal surface directed posteriorly and its external convex surface directed anteriorly. The radiused surface of the anterior acetabular retractor is used to guide the implant into the wound. This is particularly important with larger implants

and small incisions. Once at the level of the acetabulum, the shell is oriented to the desired position (Fig. 21.6). The ideal implant position has been debated, but is roughly 40–45° of lateral opening and 20° of true acetabular anteversion. It is important to ensure there is no soft tissue entrapment between the acetabulum and the shell prior to final impaction. There is a tendency early in one's experience with small incisions for the acetabular impactor to impinge on the distal skin incision, resulting in a more vertical acetabular component. Most implant manufacturers now make an offset acetabular inserter to avoid soft tissue impingement and prevent vertical cup positioning.

Anterior and anterior–inferior peripheral osteophytes are generally removed prior to insertion of the acetabular liner. This is best accomplished with a 1.5-cm curved osteotome. Posterior and posterior-inferior osteophytes are most easily removed after the trial femoral component is in place and the hip is reduced. The acetabular liner may be inserted at this

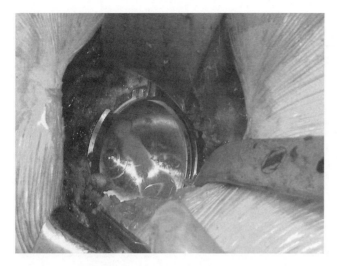

Fig. 21.6 Acetabular shell impacted in place. Note the position of the locking mechanism (From Hartzband MA, Posterolateral minimal incision for total hip replacement: technique and early results, in Scuderi GR, Tria AJ, Jr., Berger RA (eds.), MIS Techniques in Orthopedics, New York, Springer, 2006, with kind permission of Springer Science + Business Media, Inc.)

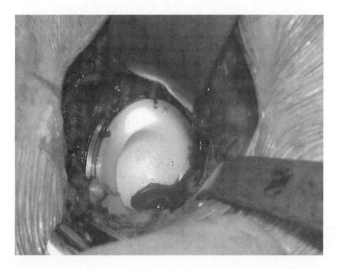

Fig. 21.7 Acetabular liner inserted (From Hartzband MA, Posterolateral minimal incision for total hip replacement: technique and early results, in Scuderi GR, Tria AJ, Jr., Berger RA (eds.), MIS Techniques in Orthopedics, New York, Springer, 2006, with kind permission of Springer Science + Business Media, Inc.)

point. The surgeon's bearing surface of preference can be used with this technique. The liner is inserted free hand and dialed to the appropriate rotation. It is important to ensure that there is not capsule or soft tissue caught between the liner and shell prior to seating. The liner is then impacted into place with firm impaction with the appropriately sized liner impactor (Fig. 21.7). The security of the liner locking mechanism should be checked prior to removing the acetabular retractors and the Kocher clamp.

Femoral Preparation

After the acetabular retractors are removed, the limb is placed in extension, adduction, and internal rotation. Previously described posterior approaches require flexion for femoral preparation. Extension is utilized in a mini-posterior approach. Because of the location and angle of the skin incision, flexion would direct the femur under the skin incision. By keeping the limb in near full extension, the long axis of the femur is maintained along the long axis of the skin incision, thus maximizing femoral exposure and, at the same time, minimizing tension on the soft tissues. Additionally, the extra benefit of minimizing pressure on the sciatic nerve below the gluteus maximus tendon insertion onto the femur is realized. The contralateral extremity should be flexed to allow the operative leg to be extended and adducted. During patient positioning, it is important not to restrain the contralateral extremity, as intraoperative modified positioning may be necessary. A combination proximal skin protector and proximal femoral elevator have been designed to elevate the proximal femur into the wound and simultaneously protect the proximal corner of the skin incision. This retractor is placed beneath the anterior aspect of the femur and is used to elevate the proximal femur out of the wound. With the proximal femoral elevator held in place by the surgeon, the initial hand starter reamer is positioned centrally and laterally into the cancellous surface of the neck and femoral canal and directed down the femoral shaft (Fig. 21.8). Care must be taken to avoid an excessively posterior starting point for this initial canal reamer, as this may tend to direct the tip of the prosthesis anteriorly and theoretically increase the risk of impingement of the distal

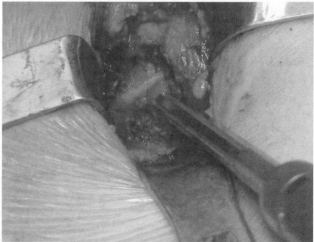

Fig. 21.8 Initial hand starter reamer inserted centrally and laterally. The limb is extended, adducted, and internally rotated (From Hartzband MA, Posterolateral minimal incision for total hip replacement: technique and early results, in Scuderi GR, Tria AJ, Jr., Berger RA (eds.), MIS Techniques in Orthopedics, New York, Springer, 2006, with kind permission of Springer Science + Business Media, Inc.)

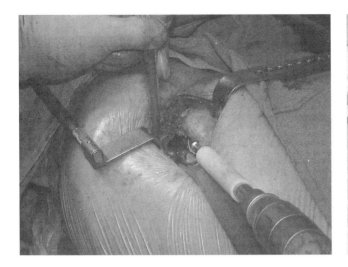

Fig. 21.9 A side-cutting reamer is used to lateralize the femoral starting point (From Hartzband MA, Posterolateral minimal incision for total hip replacement: technique and early results, in Scuderi GR, Tria AJ, Jr., Berger RA (eds.), MIS Techniques in Orthopedics, New York, Springer, 2006, with kind permission of Springer Science + Business Media, Inc.)

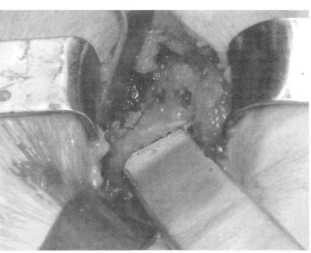

Fig. 21.10 The femoral broach is seated in position. Note the femoral elevator is displaced medially during broaching (From Hartzband MA, Posterolateral minimal incision for total hip replacement: technique and early results, in Scuderi GR, Tria AJ, Jr., Berger RA (eds.), MIS Techniques in Orthopedics, New York, Springer, 2006, with kind permission of Springer Science + Business Media, Inc.)

tip of the stem on the endosteal femur, with the subsequent potential risk of femoral fracture or thigh pain. If the body habitus is such that the initial hand reamer cannot be readily passed in a coaxial position down the femoral canal, then the proximal corner of the skin incision should be extended without hesitation.

A box chisel or lateralizing reamer (Fig. 21.9) is then placed into the femoral shaft and directed laterally into the piriformis fossa in appropriate rotation. Lateralization will decrease the likelihood of varus positioning of the femoral component. At this point, the femur, which is now held in extension, adduction, and internal rotation, is slightly flexed to bring the greater trochanter and piriformis fossa into a central position in the wound. A deliberate search is then made for any remaining fibrous tissue, capsule, or piriformis tendon stump in the area of the piriformis fossa and, if identified, it is excised with a scalpel blade or cautery.

Broaching of the femoral canal (Fig. 21.10) is now performed according to the technique of the implant desired. Modified broach handles have been developed to minimize impingement on the posterior superior edge of the skin incision. There remains a slight tendency for the proximal pole of the incision to apply a retroverting force onto the broach handle. As such, it is important to use a Tommy bar (or other means of broach handle rotational control) and to exert constant vigilance during the broaching and femoral canal preparation process so as to avoid component malposition.

Proximal wound problems remain a concern when a mini-incision technique is used. There are a number of ways in which the proximal pole of the skin incision is protected from broach abrasion during this portion of the procedure.

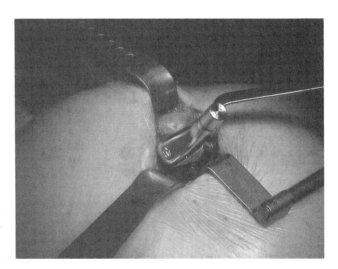

Fig. 21.11 The femoral component is initially introduced in relative retroversion (From Hartzband MA, Posterolateral minimal incision for total hip replacement: technique and early results, in Scuderi GR, Tria AJ, Jr., Berger RA (eds.), MIS Techniques in Orthopedics, New York, Springer, 2006, with kind permission of Springer Science + Business Media, Inc.)

Maintaining the hip in extension is extremely helpful. Another useful technique is to initially introduce the broach in retroversion (Fig. 21.11). A major advantage of using a proximally coated, robustly tapered femoral component is that rotation of the rasp handle during the first 5 or 6 cm of its introduction has no effect on final component interfaces. The broach is inserted in 60–90° of retroversion and as soon as its proximal teeth have progressed beyond the proximal pole of the skin incision, the broach can be rotated into its definitive, appropriate anteversion. Additionally, the use of the proximal femoral elevator is critical to protection of the superior pole of the wound during this phase of femoral preparation. The elevator is applied in its normal fashion, parallel to the long axis of the shaft of the femur until the broach has seated below the proximal margin of the skin wound. The retractor is then allowed to slide directly posteriorly and thereby protects the proximal posterior corner of the wound and soft tissue from any incidental broach-induced abrasion. The concave geometry of this retractor allows it to remain in this posterior position.

The broaches are successively increased in 1- to 2-mm increments until an appropriate sense of fit and fill has been achieved and the broach has been demonstrated to be rotationally stable. Once the definitive broach has been selected and the actual prostheses determined, a provisional reduction is performed with the trial femoral stem in place so as to fine tune leg length and offset. The actual prosthesis is opened, the broach is removed, and a dilation and curettage (D&C) curette is lightly applied to the internal surface of the lateral femoral endosteal cortex corresponding to Gruen zone 1. In this way, any fibrous tissue that may have been inadvertently introduced down the femoral canal is removed (as a rule, irrigation is not performed at this point as noncemented implants are typically utilized). The stem is guided down the canal by hand and introduced initially, similar to the broach, in substantial retroversion. The stem is then dialed into appropriate anteversion as it moves down the femoral canal. Care must be used to place the stem in the same version at which the broaches were placed to prepare the femur. This lessens the chances of intraoperative femoral fracture. On occasion, particularly in cases with a small incision and a large femoral component, the hip must be hyperextended to facilitate reduction of the neck of the femoral component below the level of skin and fascia.

Femoral head trials are then sequentially applied until appropriate leg length and hip joint tension and stability have been achieved (Fig. 21.12). Side-mounting femoral head trials have been designed to simplify this portion of the procedure. The taper is then cleaned and dried. The femoral head is then placed onto the taper, twisted, and struck with a modified, offset head impactor. Traditional straight head impactors cannot be used safely in a mini-posterior approach. The hip is reduced and then evaluated to ensure that there is not soft tissue interposition in the joint.

Wound Closure

An enhanced posterior capsular closure is then performed (Fig. 21.13). A figure-of-eight suture is placed through the posterior superior corner of capsule and the piriformis tendon

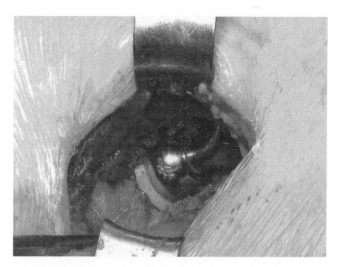

Fig. 21.12 Acetabular and femoral components in position (From Hartzband MA, Posterolateral minimal incision for total hip replacement: technique and early results, in Scuderi GR, Tria AJ, Jr., Berger RA (eds.), MIS Techniques in Orthopedics, New York, Springer, 2006, with kind permission of Springer Science + Business Media, Inc.)

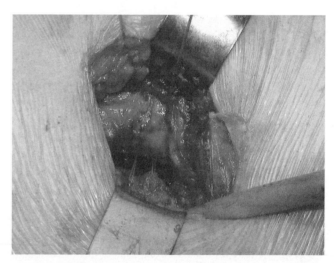

Fig. 21.13 Enhanced posterior capsular repair (From Hartzband MA, Posterolateral minimal incision for total hip replacement: technique and early results, in Scuderi GR, Tria AJ, Jr., Berger RA (eds.), MIS Techniques in Orthopedics, New York, Springer, 2006, with kind permission of Springer Science + Business Media, Inc.)

at the point at which the radial and longitudinal portions of the capsulotomy meet. A second suture is placed approximately 1 cm distal to this through the posterior limb of capsule and the conjoined tendon. It is important to avoid large bites of posterior soft tissue during this portion of the procedure to prevent injury to the sciatic nerve. Drill holes are then placed through the trochanter into the piriformis fossa taking care that the starting point is at least 1 cm below the tip of the trochanter and 1 cm lateral to the medial border of the trochanter.

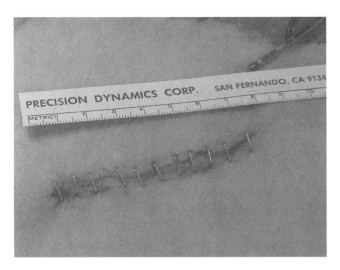

Fig. 21.14 Final wound closure (From Hartzband MA, Posterolateral minimal incision for total hip replacement: technique and early results, in Scuderi GR, Tria AJ, Jr., Berger RA (eds.), MIS Techniques in Orthopedics, New York, Springer, 2006, with kind permission of Springer Science + Business Media, Inc.)

Number 4 (22-gauge) wires are then placed through the drill holes, and are used as suture passers. The sutures are tied to each other with the limb in neutral rotation and 15–20° of abduction. All wounds are closed over a reinfusion drainage system (Fig. 21.14).

Postoperative Protocol

Patients are generally out of bed and ambulating on the evening of surgery. Hospital length of stay ranges from 18 to 48 h. Patients are allowed full weight as tolerated but are encouraged to use a walker or crutches for support during the first 2 postoperative weeks. They are then advanced to a single-prong cane for an additional 4 weeks. Antigravity abductor strengthening is begun within a few days of the procedure. Standard hip precautions are maintained for 3 months. The patient is advised to use an extended toilet seat and to avoid sleeping in other than a supine position with a pillow between the legs for the first 6 weeks.

All patients are bolused with 1,000–2,000 U of intravenous heparin at the time of skin incision, with the actual dose relating to body weight. Surgery is performed with a spinal anesthetic. All patients are administered 10 mg of Coumadin on the night of surgery and rapidly brought up to an INR of 2–2.5. Coumadin therapy is maintained for 2 weeks and is followed by 325 mg of aspirin daily for a total of 3 months. Patients undergo bilateral lower extremity venous imaging at the first postoperative visit (approximately 10–14 days). Vascular surgical consultation is obtained in all cases with a positive Doppler.

Summary

Minimally invasive techniques for total hip arthroplasty have gained increasing popularity over the past few years. A number of authors have published their personal experience with differing techniques concluding that there are multiple advantages to this concept for total hip arthroplasty. Our perception is that the advantages of minimally invasive posterolateral approach total hip arthroplasty are multiple. They include more rapid mobilization and more prompt return to activities of daily living. A concomitant decrease in hospital stay has been noted. Patients undergoing the procedure today have an average length of hospital stay of 1.2 days. Decreased operative time and improved cosmesis have also been positive results of this technique. It has been shown that a decrease in operative time results in a lower infection rate.[13] Although wound cosmesis has traditionally been ignored in arthroplasty surgery, it may now be appropriate to include improved cosmesis as at least a minor factor to be considered in selection of technique.

Surgeons performing this procedure require familiarity with the local anatomy, as the technique is certainly more demanding than traditional arthroplasty. It is perhaps a technique best applied by surgeons performing hip arthroplasty on a regular basis. The two keys to successful application of the technique are adequate surgical training and use of specialized instrumentation. With respect to component positioning, there may be a tendency to vertical cup placement early in one's experience. This is avoided by proper location of the skin incision and by use of an offset acetabular component inserter, which facilitates proper positioning of the component in spite of the prominence of the distal angle of the skin incision. A tendency to eccentric reaming of the acetabulum may be noted if the proximal femur is not adequately retracted anteriorly. One must beware of inadvertent levering of the acetabular reamers on the posterior aspect of the retracted femur resulting in eccentric reaming of the acetabulum.

Finally, there remains a risk of proximal skin abrasion, particularly when one is beginning to decrease the incision length in posterolateral approach to total hip arthroplasty. The evolution of proximal femoral elevators and skin protectors has dramatically reduced this complication in the hands of experienced surgeons. There has been no instance of skin abrasion in our last 1,000 cases.

Conclusion

A new surgical technique for posterolateral minimal incision total hip arthroplasty is described. The technique of minimally invasive posterolateral total hip arthroplasty represents more than a shortened skin incision. It represents a decrease in soft tissue dissection and trauma during the arthroplasty. This minimal dissection has been greatly aided by well-modified retractors that allow illumination of the deep layers and maximize visualization through the mobile window while being considerate to the surrounding soft tissues. Despite the potential benefits, one must always remember that the goal of total hip arthroplasty is to achieve accurate and reproducible implant placement with long-term survival of the hip arthroplasty. In addition, if the perceived implant position is compromised by the limited exposure or visualization, the mini-posterior incision is easily extended if necessary.

References

1. Moore AT. The self-locking metal hip prosthesis. J Bone Joint Surg Am 1957; 39-A:811–27
2. Gibson A. Posterior exposure of the hip joint. J Bone Joint Surg Br 1950; 32-B:183–6
3. Marcy GH, Fletcher RS. Modification of the posterolateral approach to the hip for insertion of femoral-head prosthesis. J Bone Joint Surg Am 1954; 36-A:142–3
4. Jolles BM, Bogoch ER. Posterior versus lateral surgical approach for total hip arthroplasty in adults with osteoarthritis. Cochrane Database Syst Rev 2006; 3:CD003828
5. Masonis JL, Bourne RB. Surgical approach, abductor function, and total hip arthroplasty dislocation. Clin Orthop Relat Res 2002; 405:46–53
6. Woo RY, Morrey BF. Dislocations after total hip arthroplasty. J Bone Joint Surg Am 1982; 64:1295–306
7. Pellicci PM, Bostrom M, Poss R. Posterior approach to total hip replacement using enhanced posterior soft tissue repair. Clin Orthop Relat Res 1998; 355:224–8
8. Suh KT, Park BG, Choi YJ. A posterior approach to primary total hip arthroplasty with soft tissue repair. Clin Orthop Relat Res 2004; 418:162–7
9. Ko CK, Law SW, Chiu KH. Enhanced soft tissue repair using locking loop stitch after posterior approach for hip hemiarthroplasty. J Arthroplasty 2001; 16:207–11
10. Hedley AK, Hendren DH, Mead LP. A posterior approach to the hip joint with complete posterior capsular and muscular repair. J Arthroplasty 1990; 5 Suppl:S57–66
11. Hartzband MA. Posterolateral minimal incision for total hip replacement: technique and early results. Orthop Clin North Am 2004; 35:119–29
12. Hurd JL, Potter HG, Dua V, Ranawat CS. Sciatic nerve palsy after primary total hip arthroplasty: a new perspective. J Arthroplasty 2006; 21:796–802
13. Leong G, Wilson J, Charlett A. Duration of operation as a risk factor for surgical site infection: comparison of English and US data. J Hosp Infect 2006; 63:255–62

Chapter 22
Minimally Invasive Approach to Metal-on-Metal Total Hip Resurfacing Arthroplasty

Slif D. Ulrich, Michael A. Mont, David R. Marker, and Thorsten M. Seyler

Resurfacing is a type of total hip arthroplasty in which the femoral head is mostly preserved and the resurfacing component caps the top of the head in a manner similar to which a dentist caps a tooth. Modern day resurfacing involves metal-on-metal articulations with the resurfacing femoral component presently mated with a metal acetabular component. The acetabular components used in resurfacing are typically one piece, but are generally similar to acetabular components that are used for standard total hip replacements. The use of these metal on-metal resurfacings have become more popular recently with the advent of new metallurgy, which promises that these devices may have low wear rates and hence excellent longevity. Present day resurfacing results are at a maximum of close to 10 years. The early results are excellent, with complication rates that approach the results for standard total hip arthroplasty.[1,2]

Many authors have reported on the early complications of these procedures, which primarily are femoral head or acetabular loosening, as well as femoral neck fractures.[3–5] Although it is important to know the indications for this technique with substandard indicated patients leading to higher complication rates, most complications have been noted to be technique related.[6] This addresses the importance of knowledge of surgical approaches and the nuances of the procedure. Most authors have described increased difficulty in performing resurfacing when compared with standard total hip replacements.[7] It is the present authors' contention that, with knowledge of the techniques and experience, resurfacing can be similar in technical difficulty to standard total hip replacement. Often the procedure is described as utilizing a large incision and not soft tissue preserving. This chapter describes a minimally invasive, soft tissue-preserving technique that can be used with small incisions for metal-on-metal resurfacing.

Indications for Resurfacing

The indications for total hip resurfacing arthroplasty are similar to the indications for any standard total hip replacement for arthritis. Previously, a number of conditions have been semi-contraindicated or fully contraindicated for resurfacing. Recently, some of these conditions that were contraindicated for resurfacing have been reported on as having successful results. These include patients with rheumatoid arthritis, osteonecrosis of the hip, Perthes disease, and patients older than 50 years of age.[8–11] It is still too early to know the long-term results of this procedure in any of these conditions or for arthritis in general, but the indications have expanded.

Various authors have reported the worst results in patients with osteopenia, which remains a relative contraindication.[12] Lack of femoral head bone stock, which includes massive cysts of the femoral head or neck, would be a contraindication for the procedure. Some authors have advocated assessment of bone stock adequacy made through preoperative DEXA scans. Previously, patients with deficient acetabulae would have been considered not candidates, as resurfacing acetabular components were not typically made with screws. More recently, various companies have introduced various screws or other ancillary fixation spikes for more rigid fixation and there should be fewer patients with bone deficiency on the acetabular side who would not be candidates.

Preoperative Templating

The authors encourage surgeons to preoperatively template patients concerning the size of components. Not all companies make a large range of sizes and there may be individuals who are too small or too large and thus are not appropriate candidates for resurfacing. Another factor to consider when templating is that leg length inequalities are much harder, if not impossible, to make up for in resurfacing in comparison to standard total hip replacements. One must appreciate that there is no modularity at the present for modern day resurfacing.

S.D. Ulrich, M.A. Mont (✉), D.R. Marker, and T.M. Seyler
Rubin Institute for Advanced Orthopaedics, Center for Joint
Preservation and Reconstruction, Sinai Hospital of Baltimore, 2401
West Belvedere Avenue, Baltimore MD, 21215, USA
e-mail: mmont@lifebridgehealth.org, rhondamont@aol.com

G.R. Scuderi and A.J. Tria (eds.), *Minimally Invasive Surgery in Orthopedics*,
DOI 10.1007/ 978-0-387-76608-9_22, © Springer Science+Business Media, LLC 2010

Equipment

Minimally invasive metal-on-metal resurfacing can be performed with current instrumentation. Certainly the use of specialized retractors for minimally invasive approaches to standard hip replacement may make the procedure easier. The authors presently use the following instruments, in addition to standard resurfacing instrumentation to perform this minimally invasive approach: sharp Hohmann retractors, Bennett and Richardson retractors, Weitlander retractors, Cobb elevators, two Meyerding retractors, and a Taylor retractor for acetabular exposure.

Placement of Incision and Initial Exposure

The incision is very important, especially when contemplating minimally invasive approaches. The authors advocate an incision that starts 15–20 cm long when initially performing resurfacing and then building down toward the minimally invasive 6- to 10-cm incision when one has mastered the techniques. To mark the appropriate incision, the greater trochanter should be marked and a line co-equal with the anterior superior iliac spine should be made (Fig. 22.1). In the traditional anterolateral approach, from the anterior superior iliac spine to the top of the greater trochanter will be approximately 8 cm and will represent half of the incision (Fig. 22.2). Then, from the top of the greater trochanter down along the shaft will be the other wing of the distal part of the incision, for a total of approximately 16 cm in normal-sized individuals. To make a small incision, this approach can then be reduced by two thirds by making the small incision and undermining

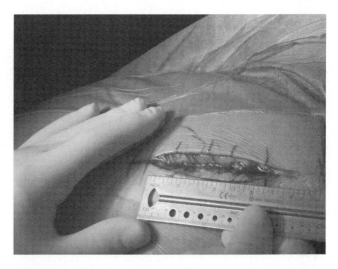

Fig. 22.2 Opening of the wound should aim for a 6- to 8-cm (3- to 4-in.) incision

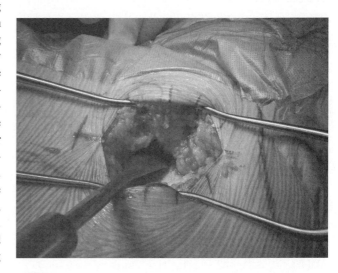

Fig. 22.3 Cobb elevator is used to perform subcutaneous tissue dissection of the fascia latae

the subcutaneous tissue so that the procedure can be performed through a mobile window, pulling this window proximally when one needs to see distally (for the femoral component) and pulling the incision distally when one needs to see proximally (for the acetabular component) (Figs. 22.3 and 22.4). The incision is made through the subcutaneous tissue down to the fascia over the tensor fascia latae muscle, as well as the fascia over the gluteus maximus (Fig. 22.5). For this approach, one should lift the leg before incising the fascia lata so that incision is made more anteriorly then if the leg is left adducted. By incising the fascia anteriorly, one can avoid any of the muscle fibers of the gluteus maximus. For some patients, after incising the fascia, more exposure may be needed and the authors would advocate T-ing the fascia lata posteriorly and superiorly. Superiorly is used above the greater trochanter so that patients do not end up at a later date having

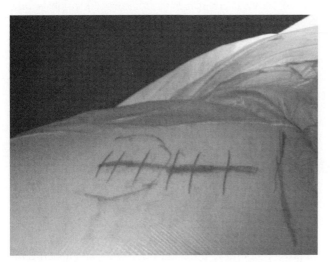

Fig. 22.1 Fig. showing the landmarks used for placement of the initial skin incision. The superior extent is co-equal to the anterior superior iliac spine. Halfway down leads to the top of the greater trochanter

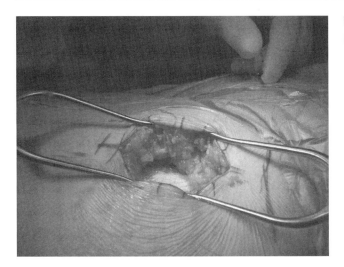

Fig. 22.4 The development of a plane over the tensor fascia lata undermining the subcutaneous tissue allows mobilization of the incision proximally and distally

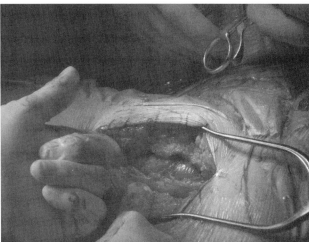

Fig. 22.6 A finger is placed under the edge of the gluteus medius and minimus muscle palpating the capsule

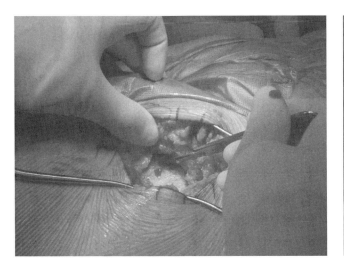

Fig. 22.5 The hip is abducted and the incision is made in the anterior edge of the tensor fascia lata

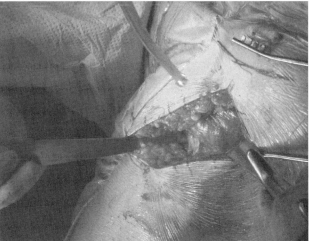

Fig. 22.7 A retractor is placed anterior to the femoral neck

trochanteric bursitis if the split is made too close to the trochanter. As in all parts of the case, one should obtain excellent hemostasis. Small Weitlander retractors are usually used to visualize the next steps.

Deep Exposure

The anterior 20% of the gluteus medius muscle is identified. One finger can be put on the anterior edge to lift this up and a few millimeters-long incision in this leading anterior edge of the gluteus medius muscle is made (Fig. 22.6). This allows for palpating the anterior capsule of the hip underneath the gluteus minimus muscle. When this is palpated, a sharp

Hohmann retractor can be placed around the femoral neck to define the anterior limits of the exposure (Fig. 22.7). The incision is then continued in the anterior 20% of the gluteus medius muscle in a beefy area of the muscle insertion to allow for later reattachment of the muscle insertion rather than leaving a bare area on the greater trochanter, which makes later reattachment more difficult (Fig. 22.8). The posterior 70–80% of the gluteus medius is left as a sharp incision is made in the gluteus medius insertion and then the trapdoor in the gluteus medius muscle is lifted up, exposing the gluteus minimus muscle. The gluteus minimus muscle can then easily be lifted off, exposing the hip capsule (Fig. 22.9). Once this is done, a posterior retractor around the posterior part of the femoral neck is then placed and further dissection exposing the whole acetabular rim is made (Fig. 22.10). Occasionally, it is necessary to lift off the fibers of the reflected head of the rectus femoris muscle anteriorly to gain

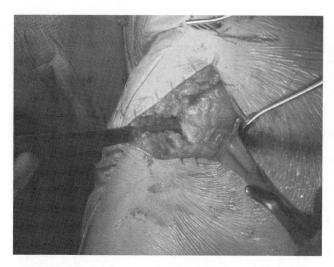

Fig. 22.8 Anterior 20% of the gluteus medius muscle is elevated

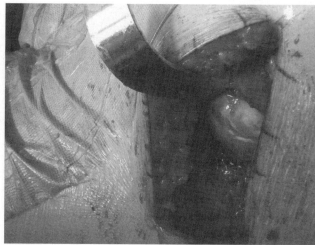

Fig. 22.11 The head is easily dislocated with external rotation once the capsule is excited

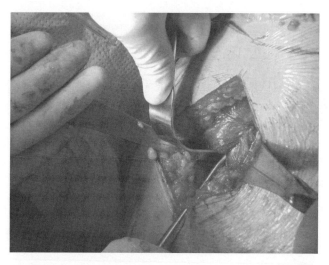

Fig. 22.9 The trapdoor of the gluteus medius and minimus lifted to reveal the capsule underneath

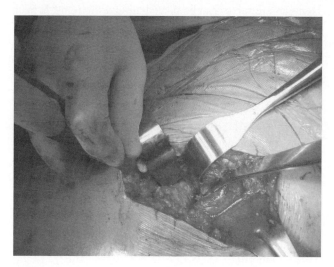

Fig. 22.10 The capsule of the head and neck is exposed

further exposure of the femoral head (Fig. 22.11). Once the anterior capsule is dissected free of any minimus fibers, the capsulectomy is then performed. The capsule is excised from anterior to posterior. This is usually sufficient to be able to get great exposure and to facilitate easy dislocation of the femoral head. In certain cases the surgeon can use a Smillie meniscal knife both anterior and posteriorly if the surgeon needs to release more capsule. This is usually unnecessary and the surgeon should be careful not to penetrate the femoral neck, even with a Smillie knife, as this could lead to a stress riser in the neck that could lead to a fracture as a complication. When the hip is ready to be dislocated, all of the retractors are pulled out except that one Meyerding retractor is left to see the femoral head. A Bennett retractor is then placed behind the greater trochanter to keep the fascia lata posteriorly and then the assistant across from the surgeon externally rotates the hip to dislocate the femoral head. Because of the exposure that was previously performed, this should not be extremely difficult. The authors do not advocate using a bone hook because the point of the hook can penetrate the femoral neck, again leading to a possible unnecessary stress riser (Fig. 22.12). Please note also that the posterior limb of the tensor fascia lata will prevent dislocation unless a retractor is placed on the bone to keep this posteriorly and not anterior to the greater trochanter.

Initial Femoral Preparation

Initially, the femoral head and neck is debrided of any remaining exposed capsule. The capsule that is posterior to the incision is left in place because this may be providing blood supply to the femoral head and neck. The authors think that it is important to make a neck measurement at this point

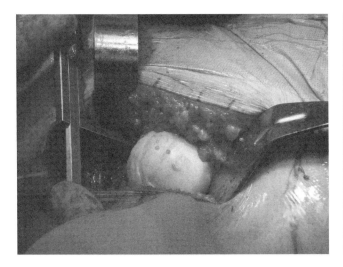

Fig. 22.12 Dislocated head with variety of retractors used to protect overlying skin

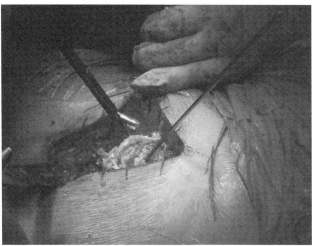

Fig. 22.14 After a circumferential guide ensures centralization of the guide pin and cylindrical reaming of the femoral head, excessive bone is taken away by a Rongeur to prevent impingement

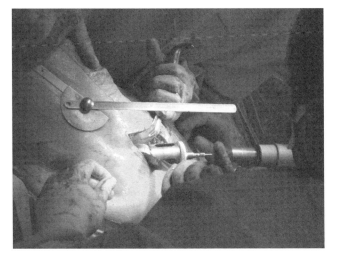

Fig. 22.13 Use of goniometer to confirm neck shaft angle at 140° (±5°)

in the case to determine what should be the minimum acetabular shell side that can be used. By knowing the femoral neck width and knowing what reamer would be necessary to avoid notching the femoral neck, one can then extrapolate what size acetabulum will be needed. The neck diameter should be measured in two planes to get the best measurement of the neck diameter to avoid notching (Fig. 22.13). This is a key step in resurfacing and cannot be overemphasized because femoral neck notching can lead to the surgeon converting a resurfacing case to a standard total hip replacement. The surgeon can further debride any neck osteophytes when one is sizing the neck (Fig. 22.14). Care should be made to avoid debriding osteophytes unnecessarily or bone that may be exposing cancellous bone in the neck, which could lead to a stress riser or femoral neck fracture at a later date. The authors also do not advocate preparation of the femoral head at this time because even though this may facilitate exposure

of the acetabulum, retraction on the weakened femoral head and neck could lead to a fracture. The authors do advocate taking a sliver of bone that is anterior to the femoral neck off the femoral head, which will facilitate later acetabular exposure. This is more important in cases where there is a moderate slip of the femoral head as in slipped capital femoral epiphysis, where this anterior part of the bone could impede visualization of the acetabulum.

Exposing the Acetabulum

In the authors' opinion, exposure of the acetabulum is the most difficult part of resurfacing. Actually, reaming and preparation of the acetabulum is the same as for standard total hip replacement, but one is doing this preparation while retaining the femoral head. Typically, the hip is flexed 30° and externally rotated to allow for the head to be retracted posteriorly. An anterior retractor is placed anteroinferiorly at approximately the five o'clock position (Fig. 22.15). A Meyerding is next placed superiorly and then a posterior Hohmann retractor is placed in the posterior inferior position at approximately seven o'clock. These retractors provide the entrance for reaming the acetabulum (Fig. 22.16). It is often necessary to make an incision in the medial and inferior capsule, which allows for separation of the retractors to visualize the acetabulum. In addition, a spike or Taylor retractor typically replaces the superior Meyerding retractor. When incising the inferior capsule, one should note the presence of the psoas tendon, to avoid cutting it. The remaining capsule pulvinar tissue and labrum can then be incised to provide adequate exposure for acetabular reaming.

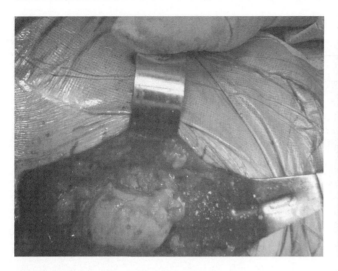

Fig. 22.15 The anterior edge of the femoral head can be initially excised to facilitate acetabular exposure

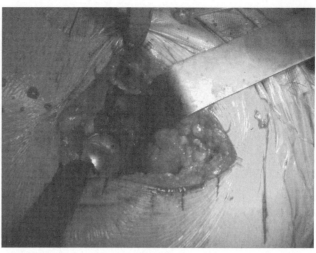

Fig. 22.17 Acetabular cup has been placed. Ready for osteophytes to be removed

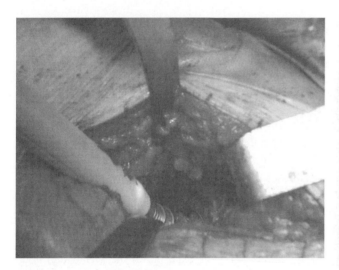

Fig. 22.16 An angled anterior retractor, angled posterior Hohmann retractor, and a spiked Taylor retractor permit appropriate visualization and reaming of the acetabulum

Reaming then proceeds as for any hip replacement. There are now cups on the market that allow for screw or spike placement for additional stability (Fig. 22.17). Certainly, many of the resurfacing components have no holes and it is not easy to know for sure when the cup is exactly bottomed out. The authors do advocate using fluoroscopy to make sure that the cup is fully seated (Fig. 22.18). After the insertion of the cup, another important step is to remove all peripheral osteophytes, especially inferior ones that would lead to later impingement. This can be done with simple straight or curved osteotomes, but sometimes a burr can facilitate removal of excess bone. One should always perform this removal of osteophytes at this point in the case because it is much more difficult to do this later after the femoral head resurfacing component has been placed.

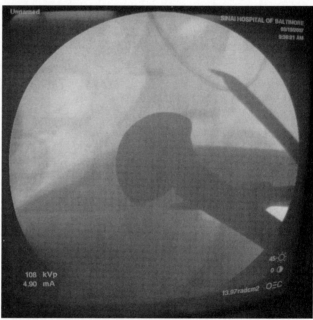

Fig. 22.18 Fluoroscopy allows visualization of the seated acetabular component

Femoral Head Resurfacing

The hip is placed in a figure-of-four position with the leg externally rotated to visualize the femur. The skin may be protected by various Hohmann retractors (Bennett and Richardson retractors). The critical step for the femoral head resurfacing is correct pin placement. We typically use a smooth 32-mm pin that is aligned with a goal of 140° using an intraoperative goniometer (see Fig. 22.13). Initially, the leg is rotated externally to facilitate exposure of the head and the surgeon must visualize straight down to ensure that the pin is being placed at 140°.

The surgical assistant on the other side is in the most appropriate position to make sure that the pin is siting down the femoral neck co-equal with the axis of the neck (see Fig. 22.14). Once the pin is initially placed, the leg can then be made horizontal to the floor by making sure that the epicondylar axis of the knee is placed straight up. The pin angle is then rechecked, trying to aim for 140°, accepting an angle between 135° and 145°. Note that higher angles may lead to greater increases in neck length or limb length, but may have a predisposition for notching the lateral neck, which can be ominous. Smaller angles less than 135° lead to varus placement of the resurfacing component and have been noted in most studies to lead to premature failure (neck collapse). Various instrumentation systems have "spin around" devices that can confirm that the pin is centrally located around the neck, including around osteophytes to avoid notching. If the potential for notching exists, the pin should be translated in the appropriate direction without changing the 140° angle. If one is changing pins, one can always recheck this angle with a goniometer. Once the angle is appropriate and the location around the femoral neck is also confirmed to be appropriate, reaming can then commence. Typically, surgeons will ream with a reamer that is 4–8 mm larger than the actual diameter that will be used as a further check. After this initial skin cut around the femoral head and neck, one can then readjust, if necessary, the position of the final reaming of the component. The final cylindrical reaming of the component should be taken down appropriately, but not too far to hit into the top of the greater trochanter or into the femoral neck medially. Most systems allow for cutting off the very top of the femoral head with a "donut" guide or various types of "cheese grater" type reamers. After this step, there are typically devices that allow for drilling for the short stem and then final Chamfer reamers are used (Fig. 22.19). Certainly, trial heads can be used to make sure that the resurfacing is performed correctly, but these trials should not be reduced into the actual acetabulum as this

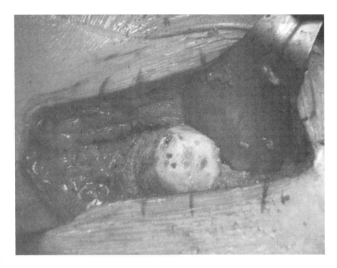

Fig. 22.19 Final head preparation with extra drill holes for cement penetration

may lead to unnecessary scratching of the acetabular component. The next step involves cementing the femoral head component, which may differ depending on the device that is used. Once the cement is cured, hip motion should be completely checked to make sure that there is no neck impingement (Fig. 22.20). In resurfacing, more femoral pistoning can be accepted than for total hip replacement because of the large femoral head size.

Closure involves two 5-0 Ethibond sutures for the gluteus minimus muscle that are put through the greater trochanteric bone (Fig. 22.21). The gluteus medius muscle is then reattached with size 0 Vicryl sutures directly to the soft tissue sleeve that was taken off. A drain can be used in this layer below the tensor fascia lata. The tensor fascia lata is closed with interrupted size 0 Vicryl sutures. The subcutaneous tissue is closed with 2-0 Vicryl sutures and the skin is typically closed with staples (Fig. 22.22).

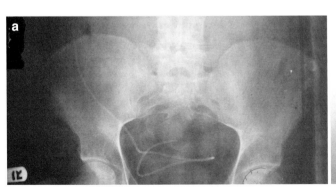
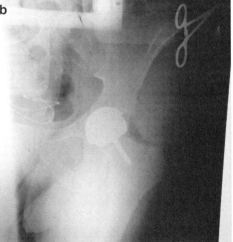

Fig. 22.20 (**a**, **b**) Preoperative and postoperative radiographs of the left hip with osteonecrosis

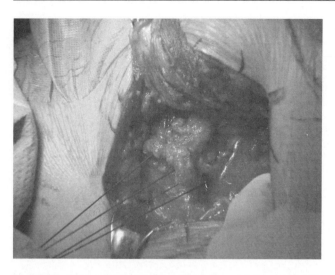

Fig. 22.21 Ethibond sutures to close the gluteus minimus muscle with Krackow-type interlocking suture

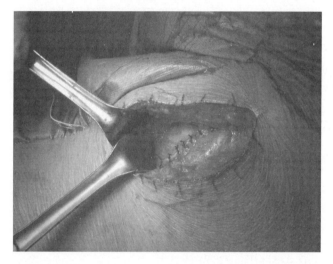

Fig. 22.22 Gluteus medius muscle sleeve closed with interrupted 2-0 Vicryl suture

Postoperative Rehabilitation

Typically, patients with resurfacings are rehabilitated in a similar manner as for standard hip replacements. Our protocol is for 50% weight bearing for the first 5 weeks using a cane or a crutch in the opposite hand. Patients are then progressed to full weight bearing as tolerated after 5 weeks. Hip precautions (not bending past 90° and not crossing the leg) are utilized for the first 10 weeks. After the 10-week period, no precautions are used for any resurfacing patient. Patients are encouraged to do strengthening exercises of their hip abductors, flexors, and extensors for approximately 20 min every other day for their lifetime.

Discussion

The minimally invasive anterolateral approach used for resurfacing has been recently studied. A comparison of 25 patients (25 hips) with resurfacing done with this approach was made to a cohort of 25 hips who had a standard procedure.[13] The minimally invasive approach included all patients with shorter than 15-cm incisions with the approach described in this technique. These patients were compared with patients with incisions that were longer than 15 cm and were not tissue sparing. The average length of the incision in the minimally invasive approach was 10 cm (range, 8–15 cm) and, in the standard group, the average was 20 cm (range, 18–25 cm). The results showed that the mean intraoperative time was not significantly longer for the minimally invasive group, which had a mean of 148 min versus a mean of 124 min for the standard incision group. The minimally invasive group had less blood loss. Neither group had differences in transfusion rates. The minimally invasive group also had better 3-month Harris Hip scores, but at the final follow-up, which was a mean of 19 months (range, 17–22 months), there were no differences in mean Harris Hip scores or radiographic outcomes. In summary, the authors found that this approach could be used safely as a possible alternative to standard approaches. However, they could not conclude that there would necessarily be anything more than a cosmetic advantage to using these minimally invasive approaches.

The authors presently use this minimally invasive approach for all metal-on-metal resurfacing surgeries, with the incision size usually ranging from 8 to 12 cm. Typically, using these techniques, the procedure can be done between 45 and 90 min. This has certainly been part of the learning curve, as these procedures initially averaged more than 120 min. However, the learning curve has led to reductions in time.

In the future, this anterolateral approach as well as posterior minimally invasive approaches will be facilitated by various technological advances. Presently, there are a number of studies using various targeting devices for the femoral head resurfacing to make this part of the case easier and computer-assisted techniques may become important in the future. Various companies have introduced new retractors and lighting systems to facilitate minimally invasive approaches for resurfacing. In addition, for the very difficult part of the case, special curved acetabular reamers, as well as new inserting devices, have been developed by various companies to facilitate component positioning and placement.

In summary, metal-on-metal resurfacing total hip arthroplasty has traditionally utilized large incisions and has been described as not soft tissue sparing, even though it is bone sparing on the femoral side. With many of the techniques mentioned in this article, this technique can be considered minimally invasive and should offer no more difficulty to the surgeon than a standard hip replacement. In addition, the techniques described can be performed in a soft tissue-sparing manner.

References

1. Mont MA, Seyler TM, Ragland PS, Starr R, Erhart J, Bhave A. Gait analysis of patients with resurfacing hip arthroplasty compared with hip osteoarthritis and standard total hip arthroplasty. *J Arthroplasty* 2007;22(1):100–108
2. Vail TP, Mina CA, Yergler JD, Pietrobon R. Metal-on-metal hip resurfacing compares favorably with THA at 2 years followup. *Clin Orthop Relat Res* 2006;453:123–131
3. Amstutz HC, Campbell PA, Le Duff MJ. Fracture of the neck of the femur after surface arthroplasty of the hip. *J Bone Joint Surg Am* 2004;86-A(9):1874–1877
4. Beaule PE, Harvey N, Zaragoza E, Le Duff MJ, Dorey FJ. The femoral head/neck offset and hip resurfacing. *J Bone Joint Surg Br* 2007;89(1):9–15
5. Shimmin AJ, Bare J, Back DL. Complications associated with hip resurfacing arthroplasty. *Orthop Clin North Am* 2005;36(2):187–193
6. Mont MA, Ragland PS, Etienne G, Seyler TM, Schmalzried TP. Hip resurfacing arthroplasty. *J Am Acad Orthop Surg* 2006;14(8):454–463
7. Eastaugh-Waring SJ, Seenath S, Learmonth DS, Learmonth ID. The practical limitations of resurfacing hip arthroplasty. *J Arthroplasty* 2006;21(1):18–22
8. Amstutz HC, Ball ST, Le Duff MJ, Dorey FJ. Resurfacing THA for patients younger than 50 years: results of 2- to 9-year followup. *Clin Orthop Relat Res* 2007;460:159–164
9. Mont MA, Seyler TM, Marker DR, Marulanda GA, Delanois RE. Use of metal-on-metal total hip resurfacing for the treatment of osteonecrosis of the femoral head. *J Bone Joint Surg Am* 2006;88(Suppl 3):90–97
10. Revell MP, McBryde CW, Bhatnagar S, Pynsent PB, Treacy RB. Metal-on-metal hip resurfacing in osteonecrosis of the femoral head. *J Bone Joint Surg Am* 2006;88(Suppl 3):98–103
11. Schmalzried TP. Total resurfacing for osteonecrosis of the hip. *Clin Orthop Relat Res* 2004 Dec;(429):151–156
12. Shimmin AJ, Back D. Femoral neck fractures following Birmingham hip resurfacing: a national review of 50 cases. *J Bone Joint Surg* 2005;87(4):463–464
13. Mont MA, Ragland PS, Marker D. Resurfacing hip arthroplasty: comparison of a minimally invasive versus standard approach. *Clin Orthop Relat Res* 2005 Dec;(441):125–131

Chapter 23
MIS Approach for Hip Resurfacing

Francesco Falez and Filippo Casella

Minimally Invasive Surgery and Hip Resurfacing

The minimally invasive surgical (MIS) technique represents one of the most exciting trends in hip arthroplasty. However, the question remains, is it more conservative and clinically favorable to have a minimally invasive soft tissue procedure, or is it better to conserve the bone stock and femoral architecture? This question was important, because these two philosophies, until recently, have been impossible to combine, since a minimally invasive soft tissue approach provides limited exposure, whereas a bony conservative philosophy requires a larger incision with significant soft tissue disruption. These limits became dramatically evident as resurfacing hip arthroplasty and minimally invasive soft tissue procedures became popular. Because of its focus on bone preservation, resurfacing hip arthroplasty requires a wide soft tissue exposure, that is, the ability to permit epiphyseal preparation and acetabular visualization. Additionally, even if the skin incision is reduced, the most common approach for resurfacing hip arthroplasty (posterolateral or posterior) requires detachment of short external rotators from the greater trochanter and a partial release of the gluteus maximus insertion, which obviously is contrary to truly minimally invasive soft tissue exposures (mini-Watson-Jones,[1] mini-anterior,[2] minimally invasive two-incision approach[3]). Furthermore, limited visualization in a mini-incision may pose increased risks of vascular complications (surgical damage of the femoral head blood supply is not uncommon with posterior exposure). As a result, different strategies have been developed; reduction of skin incisions with more limited muscular dissection (adapting instrumentation and developing specific surgical techniques) and development of techniques to accomplish resurfacing hip arthroplasty through intermuscular surgical approaches.

Anatomic Considerations

Resurfacing hip arthroplasty is dependent on maintaining the vascular supply to the proximal femur and neurovascular preservation of hip muscles. The medial circumflex artery and inferior gluteal bundle are key elements for maintenance of these principles in posterior-based approaches. Relatively recent anatomic studies[4] provided a more accurate description of the topographic location of these structures, relating it with hip surgical exposures. In minimally invasive resurfacing hip arthroplasty, the surgery should minimally impact these neurovascular structures. Only then can the biological survivorship of femoral epiphysis and proper function of reconstructed hip be optimized.

Mini-incision Resurfacing Hip Arthroplasty Through the Posterior Approach

Technique

The exposure for hip arthroplasty through the posterior approach has been described by McMinn et al.[5] This is a minimally invasive variation of his original operative technique. The patient is positioned on lateral position on the unaffected side. The skin is marked at the tip and posterior margin of the greater trochanter.

The skin incision is directed obliquely, from a backward direction, from a point approximately 5 cm distal to the tip of the grater trochanter and tangent to its posterior margin, through a line extended proximally for 10 cm (angled at approximately 20–30° to the posterior margin of greater trochanter) (Fig. 23.1). Cutaneous and subcutaneous layers are developed until the gluteal fascia beneath the gluteus maximus is identified. After fascia incision (that can be extended 1 cm more than the skin incision if necessary), gluteus maximus fibers are divided bluntly in line with the skin incision and in line with the fibers. A Charnley retractor is then placed (Fig. 23.2). Palpation of the sciatic nerve is recommended before positioning the Charnley posterior blade.

F. Falez (✉) and F. Casella
Department of Orthopaedic and Traumatology, S. Spirito in Sassia Hospital, L.go tevere in Sassia 3, Rome, Italy
e-mail: F.falez@flashnet.it

G.R. Scuderi and A.J. Tria (eds.), *Minimally Invasive Surgery in Orthopedics*,
DOI 10.1007/978-0-387-76608-9_23, © Springer Science+Business Media, LLC 2010

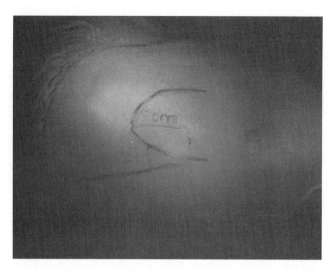

Fig. 23.1 Landmarks and skin incision for minimally invasive resurfacing hip replacement

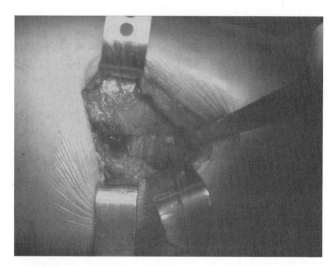

Fig. 23.2 Gluteus maximus division with a Charnley retractor to expose the trochanteric plane. A temporary suture identifies the piriformis tendon

With the retractor in place, the femoral insertion of gluteus maximus should be incised to reduce tension during rotation of the femur. This also makes femoral exposure easier and reduces compression on the sciatic nerve.

The deep muscular plane is then developed, usually as with conventional exposure: anterior retraction of the gluteus medius and separation of the piriformis from the gluteus minimus with release of the latter from the iliac bone. Care is taken not to interrupt the fibers of the gluteus medius. Finally, a pin is inserted in the ilium to retract the gluteus medius and minimus forward from the external rotators. With the separation of the piriformis and short external rotators from the abductors, they are incised close to their insertion and retracted backward to protect the sciatic nerve. Taking special

care of the soft tissues envelope on the posterior femoral neck is important during this dissection to preserve the femoral bloody supply.

After the capsule has been exposed, the posteroinferior section is retracted and held with a second pin, while the anterosuperior section is divided; the femoral head can now be dislocated. A complete acetabular exposure is then obtained with a retractor positioned at the 5 o'clock and 7 o'clock positions. The femur is dislocated anteriorly (Fig. 23.3).

Acetabular preparation and component placement are performed using modified instruments specifically designed for mini-incision: offset acetabular reamers and an offset cup introducer. This preparation and insertion is the same as with any mini-incision technique (Fig. 23.4a, b).

With the acetabulum finished, attention is returned to the femur. To prepare the femoral epiphysis, the femur is internally rotated until the posterior neck and intertrochanteric crest are directly visualized. With the Charnley retractor loosened, the lesser trochanter is exposed with a retractor. On the intertrochanteric crest, the pin insertion point for the femoral jig with proper varus-valgus alignment is marked. The distance between this point and lesser trochanter should be preoperatively measured with templates on the preoperative radiographs (Fig. 23.5). This distance is then reproduced intraoperatively with a hooked guidewire or specifically designed instrument (Fig. 23.6). This pin placement is different from a conventional approach, usually inserted on the lateral aspect of the proximal femur, which reduces the required length of the skin incision and deep dissection.

The dislocated hip is then internally rotated again, which hides the pin in the soft tissues. Then the femoral epiphysis is exposed, and the long arm of the jig is adjusted for lateral alignment (Fig. 23.7). The next steps of femoral preparation

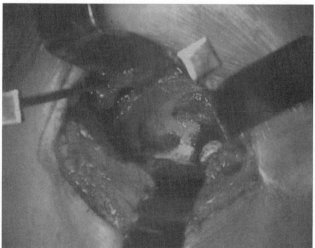

Fig. 23.3 Acetabular exposure: Anterior retraction of abductors (gluteus medius and minimus) with a pin inserted in the iliac bone. The capsule is retracted by a second pin with Hohmann retractors at 5 o'clock and 7 o'clock positions. The femur is dislocated anteriorly

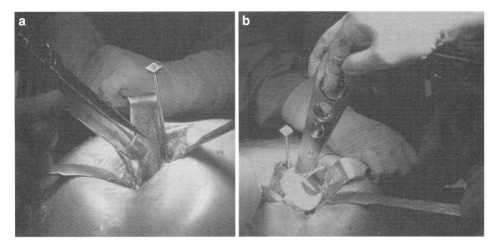

Fig. 23.4 (**a**) Offset acetabular reamer. (**b**) Offset cup introducer

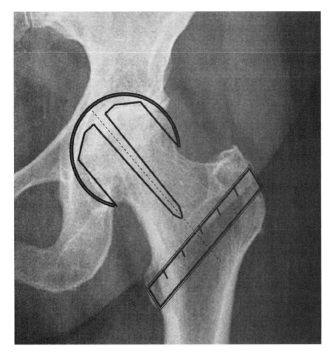

Fig. 23.5 Templating of component size and site of pin placement on the intertrochanteric crest. This is done by measuring the distance of the axis of the femoral component on the template from the lesser trochanter

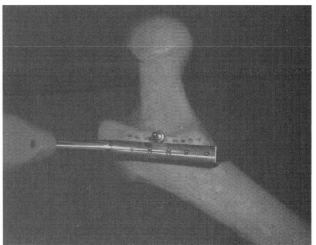

Fig. 23.6 Placement of a hooked guide wire to reproduce distance templated on the intertrochanteric crest

Clinical Application and Comments

McMinn has presented the largest clinical experience available in a paper published in 2005.[5] He reported 232 consecutive procedures, performed between January and December 2004. This was a retrospective comparative study. The MIS posterolateral procedure showed a surprising reliability with wide applicability in patients with different body mass indexes, ranging from 17.6 to 46.7. There was no significant difference in mean operative time compared with the traditional approach (67 vs. 71 min). Furthermore, there was good reproducibility of skin incision length (mean 11.8 cm), with 77% of incisions between 9 and 12 cm.

Acetabular component placement was within the target range (35–45°) in most cases. In the traditional exposure group, acetabular component placement was 44 ± 6°, with a range of 28° to 58°. This compared favorably with the minimally

follow the traditional technique of implantation (Fig. 23.8). These steps include circumferential removal of cartilage with maintenance of the head-neck junction, confirmation of the top of femoral head, and multiple hole drilling. Before seating the prosthetic component, application of a suction vent through the lesser trochanter is recommended to reduce systemic embolization and intraosseous vessel embolization.

With the final components in place and the hip reduced, closure is begun. The short rotators are reattached as with conventional exposures. Finally, the deep fascia is closed, and the skin is then closed (Fig. 23.9).

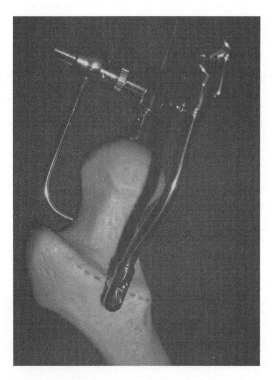

Fig. 23.7 Compass position for the jig lateral alignment

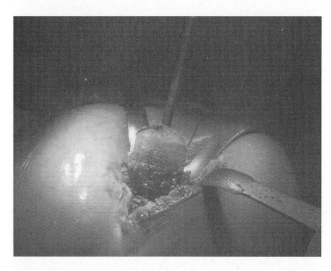

Fig. 23.8 Femoral exposure and preparation is done with special care for the soft tissues enveloping the posterior femoral neck

invasive group, which had an average of 40° ± 4.4, with a range of 29–52°. In the minimally invasive group, the femoral component placement was in neutral position in 194 hips, mild valgus occurred in 29 hips, marked valgus in 8 hips, and mild varus in 1 hip. Most importantly, there was no component in a marked varus position.

Clinical advantages of the MIS technique were shortening of hospital stay (7.2 days compared with 5.8 days, respectively

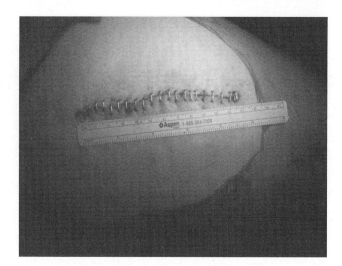

Fig. 23.9 Wound closed

for traditional and MIS), less postoperative pain, faster recovery, and better cosmesis. Furthermore, patient perception of minimally invasive resurfacing arthroplasty of hip compared with traditional resurfacing hip replacement in subjects undergoing bilateral hip reconstruction before and during 2004 was compared. When asked about pain, recovery rate, wound complications, cosmesis, and recommendation of minimally invasive resurfacing arthroplasty of hip to a friend; minimally invasive resurfacing arthroplasty of hip was significantly preferred in every category.

McMinn emphasized that the steep learning curve could lead to suboptimal component placement, which could adversely affect future outcomes. In his developing series with minimally invasive resurfacing arthroplasty of hip (2002–2003, 114 implants), McMinn reported two early failures caused by femoral neck fracture as a result of either varus positioning or femoral neck notching. However, with further practice and refinements of these techniques, this is no longer a clinical problem.

In femoral and acetabular positioning, important variations exist in surgical MIS technique compared with traditional surgery. A different pin insertion is needed for the femoral jig, and an offset reamer and cup introducer for acetabular preparation and seating are also needed.

In MIS resurfacing hip replacement, fluoroscopy is usually not necessary because of a direct visualization; however, computer navigation does represent a fascinating perspective with the ability to improve reliability of the procedure.[6] This has the potential of providing real-time numeric and image control of instruments and prosthetic component positioning, which may improve results.

Finally, and most importantly, surgeons should have no hesitation in extending the incision if difficulty is encountered. Extending the incision is performed rather than compromising component position.

Trochanteric Slide Osteotomy-Digastric Trochanteric Osteotomy

Technique

An alternative exposure has been proposed by Ganz[7] and other authors that was originally used for intracapsular hip procedure and can be applied to resurfacing hip arthroplasty. It is based on the medial femoral circumflex artery and its vital role for epiphysis survivorship.

The most important landmark in the technique is the piriformis tendon (Fig. 23.10). The final anastomosis between the medial femoral circumflex artery and the inferior gluteal

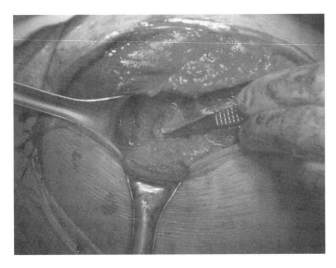

Fig. 23.10 The piriformis tendon is shown, which is the landmark for deep dissection. All dissection is proximal to this structure

artery is located at the inferior margin of this structure, while the superior acetabular branch of the superior gluteal artery runs at the superior edge of the piriformis. These anatomic considerations explain why surgical dissection of the hip capsule should be proximal to this defining structure. Moreover, during dislocation of the hip, the femoral head blood flow is not damaged if the obturator externus tendon remains intact. During a conventional, or even a MIS approach, release of all of the short external rotators is mandatory to achieve a sufficient mobilization of proximal femur, which may interrupt the blood supply of the head. However, with a trochanteric slide osteotomy, the dissection can stay proximal to the piriformis and maintain the blood supply more reproducibly.

A trochanteric slide osteotomy is thought to minimize soft tissue release around the femoral neck to achieve joint access. This technique involves a posterolateral skin incision, and osteotomy of the greater trochanter, with subsequent cephalad abductor turndown with the bony insertion (Fig. 23.11). The deep muscular plane is developed over the piriformis tendon taken posteriorly to the gluteus minimus tendon, which is dissected and retracted forward without disruption of its fibers or detachment of its insertion. This then exposes the capsule, which is incised (Fig. 23.12). Finally, anterior dislocation of femoral head can be performed (Fig. 23.13).

Clinical Application and Comments

This surgical exposure provides an excellent visualization of the proximal femur and acetabulum. It is also used for open reduction and internal fixation of Pipkin fractures.[8] This technique has been successfully used for hip resurfacing.[4]

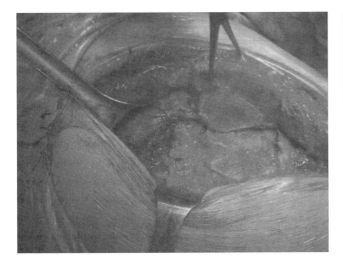

Fig. 23.11 Greater trochanter osteotomy and cephalad abductor turndown

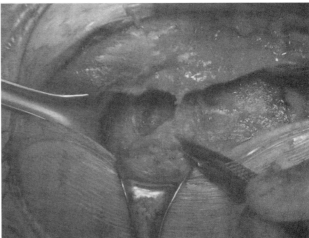

Fig. 23.12 Development of muscular plane over the piriformis and posteriorly to the gluteus minimus tendon to expose the capsule

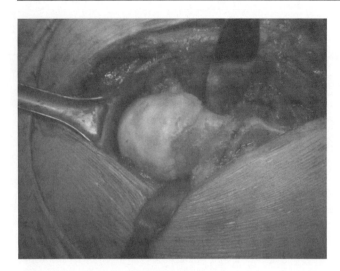

Fig. 23.13 Anterior dislocation of femoral head

The trochanteric osteotomy has generated a debate between surgeons performing minimally invasive procedures. Some think that a larger bone osteotomy may have more favorable outcomes due to maintenance of the femoral head blood supply and maintenance of the external rotators. Other think that soft tissue-sparing surgery is best because it yields a shorter skin incision, less deep structure separation, and is less aggressive for bone.

Unfortunately, there is no definitive answer to this question. Personal experience of the authors using the trochanteric slide osteotomy approach of surgical exposure for other intracapsular procedures confirms the biological suppositions that it does reliably give good exposure with maintenance of the blood supply to the femoral head. However, to date, we do not have the experience to comment on which technique will be better in the long term for resurfacing arthroplasty. We need published studies that detail specific clinical experiences with MIS resurfacing hip replacement matched with the trochanteric slide osteotomy approach.

References

1. Bertin KC, Rottinger H. Antero-lateral mini-incision hip replacement surgery: a modified Watson-Jones approach. Clin Orthop Relat Res. 2004 Dec;(429):248–55.
2. Kennon RE, Keggi JM, Wetmore RS, Zatorski LE, Huo MH, Keggi KJ.Total hip arthroplasty through a minimally invasive anterior surgical approach. J Bone Joint Surg Am. 2003;85-A(Suppl 4):39–48.
3. Berger RA.Total hip arthroplasty using the minimally invasive two-incision approach. Clin Orthop Relat Res. 2003 Dec;(417):232–41.
4. Nork SE, Schar M, Pfander G, Beck M, Djonov V, Ganz R, Leunig M. Anatomic considerations for the choice of surgical approach for hip resurfacing arthroplasty. Orthop Clin North Am. 2005;36(2): 163–70.
5. McMinn DJ, Daniel J, Pynsent PB, Pradhan C. Mini-incision resurfacing arthroplasty of hip through the posterior approach. Clin Orthop Relat Res. 2005 Dec;(441):91–8.
6. Ganz R, Gill TJ, Gautier E. Surgical dislocation of the adult hip: a technique with full access to the femoral head and acetabulum without the risk of avascular necrosis. J Bone Joint Surg Br 2001;83 (8):1119–24.
7. Allison C. Minimally invasive hip resurfacing. Issues Emerg Health Technol. 2005;(65):1–4.
8. Kloen P, Siebenrock K, Raaymakers E, Marti RK, Ganz R. Femoral head fractures rivisited. Eur J Trauma 2002;28:221–233.

Chapter 24
Minimally Invasive Total Hip Arthroplasty Using the Two-Incision Approach*

Richard A. Berger

Minimally invasive hip replacement has the potential for minimizing surgical trauma, pain, and recovery in total hip replacement. These minimally invasive approaches for total hip surgery include single-incision and two-incision techniques. These approaches minimize sacrificing muscle and tendon yet still allow direct or indirect visualization for preparation and component placement.

Specifically, searching for an approach to avoid transecting any muscle or tendon, thereby minimizing morbidity and recovery, a new approach was developed; the minimally invasive two-incision total hip procedure. This technique uses an anterior incision for preparation and insertion of the acetabular component and a posterior incision for preparation and insertion of the femoral component. This novel, minimally invasive, fluoroscopy-assisted, two-incision total hip arthroplasty uses a number of new instruments that have been developed to facilitate exposure and component placement. Standard implants with well-established designs are used to maintain the present expectation for implant durability. The following text describes the technique of the minimally invasive two-incision technique; combining an anterior, Smith-Peterson approach and a posterior incision that is like an intra medually (IM) femoral nail.

Surgical Technique

The anesthesia of choice for this minimally invasive total hip arthroplasty procedure is a regional anesthesia with supplemental sedation. An epidural anesthesia with intravenous Propofol is the combination of choice. Propofol is a very short-acting agent that is rapidly eliminated from the body and the epidural allows the medication to be titrated. This combination allows rapid recovery from the anesthesia, facilitating recovery.

The patient is placed in the supine position on a radiolucent operating room table. A special operating room table is not required; however, a pure radiolucent table is preferable. A small bolster, approximately 2 in., is placed under the ischium on the effected side; this elevates the acetabulum to aid in acetabular preparation and allows the posterior buttock to be prepped and draped (Fig. 24.1a). The entire leg and hip is prepped up to the chest wall including the posterior hip. After prepping, the leg is placed in impervious sterile stockinet and is wrapped with an Ace bandage from the foot to above the knee. The hip area is then draped superiorly from above the iliac crest, posteriorly to the posterior hip, and anteriorly to almost the midline of the patient (Fig. 24.1b).

After the prepping is completed, the fluoroscope is used to define the femoral neck. The femoral neck lays approximately two fingerbreadths distally from the anterior superior iliac spine. A metal marker is used to mark the midline of the femoral neck from the junction of the head distally 1.5–2.0 in. (Fig. 24.2). This incision is then made through the skin and the subcutaneous fat, directly over the femoral neck from the base of the femoral head distally. Care must be taken, as the subcutaneous fat in this area is very thin. The fascia is exposed. The sartorius muscle is present in the proximal medial incision, while the tensor fascia lata lies at the distal lateral tip of the incision. The sartorius muscle and tensor fascia lata can be seen beneath the fascia. The fascia at the medial boarder of tensor fascia lata is incised longitudinally parallel to the tensor fascia lata. The lateral femoral cutaneous nerve is located over the sartorius muscle; therefore, an incision made lateral to sartorius, at the medial boarder of the tensor fascia lata avoids the lateral femoral cutaneous nerve. The nerve should not be dissected out, as postoperative scaring may cause a lateral thigh hypoesthesia. After the fascia is incised, a retractor is used to retract the sartorius medially. A second retractor is used to retract the tensor fascia lata laterally. This exposes the lateral boarder of the rectus femoris (Fig. 24.3a). The medial retractor is repositioned to retract the rectus muscle medially (Fig. 24.3b). This exposes the

R.A. Berger (✉)
Department of Orthopedic Surgery, Rush–Presbyterian–St. Luke's Medical Center, 1725 West Harrison Street, Suite 1063, Chicago, IL 60612, USA
e-mail: r.a.berger@sbcglobal.net

*Adapted from Berger RA, Minimally invasive total hip arthroplasty using the two-incision approach, in Scuderi GR, Tria AJ, Berger RA (eds.), MIS Techniques in Orthopedics, 2006, New York, Springer, with kind permission of Springer Science + Business Media, Inc.

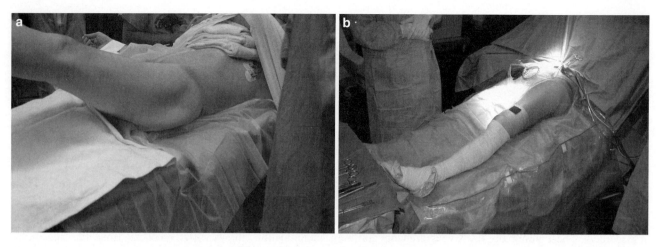

Fig. 24.1 Prep and drape for two-incision minimally invasive total hip. (**a**) Small bolster under the ischium on the effected side elevating the pelvis. (**b**) The entire leg prepped and draped to allow access to the anterior and posterior incision

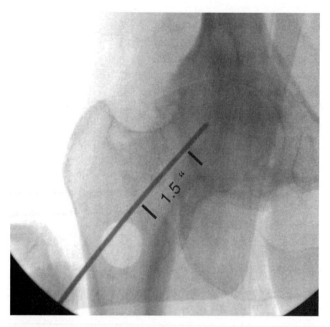

Fig. 24.2 Fluoroscope picture of the incision site over the femoral neck. The incision is made from the head/neck junction distally to the intertrochanteric line; approximately 1.5 in

fascia overlying the lateral circumflex vessels and the femoral capsule. This thin fascia lying over the lateral circumflex vessels is incised carefully as the lateral circumflex vessels are adherent to the undersurface. The lateral circumflex vessels are then carefully found within the small fat pad over the capsule of the femoral neck. The lateral femoral vessels are carefully coagulated with an electrocautery. The fat pad is then incised in the line of the femoral neck and gently moved medially and laterally off the femoral neck, exposing the capsule over the femoral neck.

Two curved lit Hohmann retractors, part of the minimally invasive instrument set (Zimmer), are then placed extracapsularly around the femoral neck perpendicular to the femoral neck. These lit retractors afford an excellent view of the capsule (Fig. 24.4a). After being identified, the capsule is incised in line with the femoral neck just lateral to the middle of the femoral neck. This incision is made from the edge of the acetabulum distally to the intertrochanteric line (Fig. 24.4b). If necessary for enhanced exposure, the capsule can be elevated approximately 1 cm medially and laterally along the intertrochanteric line. The femoral neck and femoral head are now visible.

The two curved lit Hohmann retractors, which were extracapsular, are now placed intracapsularly along the femoral neck, one medially and one laterally. The lit retractors in place afford excellent visualization of the femoral neck (Fig. 24.5). The femoral neck should now be visualized from the acetabulum distally to the intertrochanteric line. With the two curved lit Hohmann retractors still in place, a high neck cut is made at the equator of the femoral head with an oscillating saw. This is made perpendicular to the axis of the femoral neck. A second cut is then made 1 cm distal to the first cut in the femoral head (Fig. 24.6). First, the small 1-cm wafer of bone is removed using a threaded Steinmann pin; gentle traction placed on the leg will facilitate removing this piece of bone (Fig. 24.7). Next, a threaded Steinmann pin or corkscrew is placed into the femoral head and is used to slightly dislocate the femoral head. A curved Cobb elevator osteotome is used to transect the ligamentum Teres. Again, gentle traction placed on the leg usually allows the femoral head to be removed completely (Fig. 24.7). If the femoral head cannot be completely removed due to osteophytes or soft tissue attachments, the head may be morselized in situ, but this is unusual.

The fluoroscope is used to assess the angle and length of the femoral neck resection based upon the lesser trochanter. Based upon preoperative templating, the final neck resection is then made. The resection length is checked with fluoroscopy. Alternatively, flexing and externally rotating the hip in

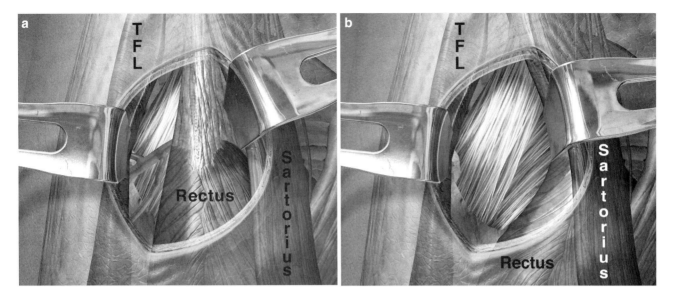

Fig. 24.3 Illustration of the anterior dissection. (**a**) Illustration of the sartorius and tensor fascia latae after being retracted. Note the rectus femoris. (**b**) Illustration of the rectus femoris retracted, exposing the capsule

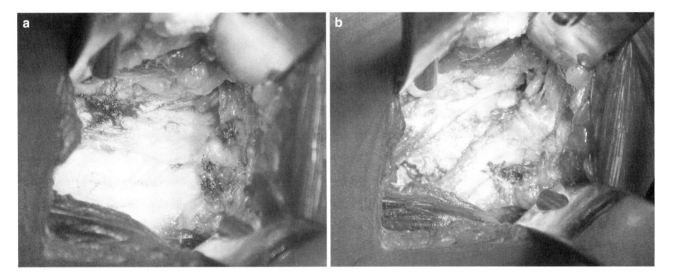

Fig. 24.4 (**a**) Picture of the lit Hohmann retractors positioned around the capsule and exposing the hip capsule. (**b**) The hip capsule is incised in line with the femoral neck, exposing the femoral head and neck

a figure-of-four can directly visualize the lesser trochanter. In this position, the lesser trochanter is easily seen and is used as a landmark to measure the neck resection. Alternatively, the fluoroscope can be used to check the angle of resection as well as the length of resection based upon the lesser trochanter (Fig. 24.8). If an additional neck cut is needed, the oscillating saw is used to make the final neck resection and a sagittal saw is then used to make a longitudinal neck cut as to not disrupt the trochanteric bed. This final thin wafer of bone is then removed. Again, the resection length is checked with fluoroscopy or by rotating the hip in a figure-of-four position, exposing the lesser trochanter.

With the final neck resection made, attention is turned to acetabular preparation. Having the pelvis elevated (with the bolster) allows the femur to fall posteriorly, facilitating access to the acetabulum. Three curved lit Hohmann retractors are placed around the acetabulum, one directly superiorly in the line of the incision is placed over the brim of the acetabulum, a second is placed anteriorly at the anterior margin of the transverse acetabular ligament, and a third is placed posteriorly around the acetabulum. This allows excellent retraction of the entire capsule. The lit retractors in these positions allow excellent visualization of the acetabulum. However, unlike conventional exposure, where the entire

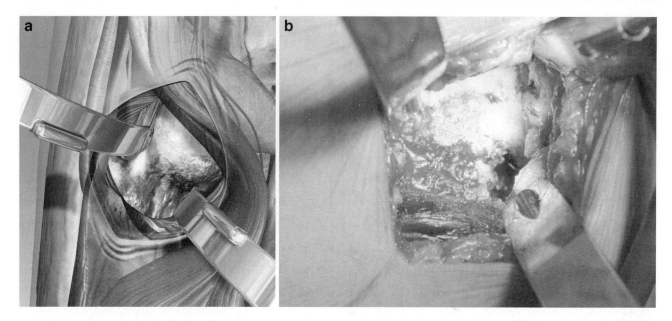

Fig. 24.5 (**a**) Illustration of the of Hohmann retractors intracapsular around the femoral neck, exposing the femoral head and neck. (**b**) Picture of the femoral head and neck. The hip capsule is incised in line with the femoral neck and the Hohmann retractors are placed intracapsularly around the femoral neck, exposing the femoral head and neck

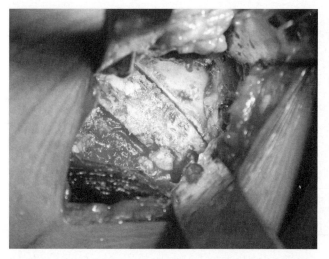

Fig. 24.6 Picture of the of Hohmann retractors intracapsular around the femoral neck, exposing the femoral head and neck. Two lines show the placement of the initial two cuts in the femoral head and neck

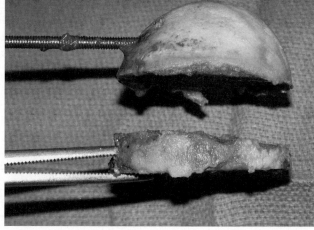

Fig. 24.7 Picture of the removed femoralhead and upper neck in two pieces to facilitate removal

acetabulum can be seen in one view, with this exposure, only about three quarters of the acetabulum can be seen at one time. To visualize the entire acetabulum, the retractors can be shifted slightly anteriorly or posteriorly to see anteriorly or posteriorly as needed. With this technique, the acetabulum is assessed (Fig. 24.9). Of note, pulling hard on opposing retractors paradoxically limits visualization by shortening the incision. Gentile retraction of one retractor should be associated with a release of the opposite retractor.

The labrum and redundant synovium is then excised around the entire periphery of the acetabulum. After the

superior acetabulum is excised, the superior retractor can be removed and repositioned more inferiorly, allowing better visualization of the inferior acetabulum. The remaining labrum and redundant synovium is then removed, exposing the entire peripheral of the acetabulum (Fig. 24.9). The acetabulum, now clear of invaginating soft tissue, is prepared for reaming.

At this point, acetabular reaming is begun. The anterior and posterior retractors are left in place and the superior retractor is removed. Specially designed, low-profile reamers, which are cut out on the sides, are used to ream the acetabulum (Fig. 24.10a). These reamers are especially aggressive, with

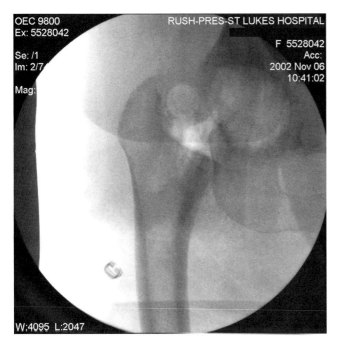

Fig. 24.8 Fluoroscopy picture of final femoral neck cut

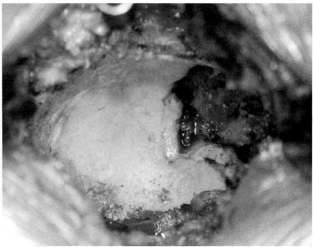

Fig. 24.9 Picture showing lit Hohmann retractor placement and superior view of acetabulum

square cutting teeth; therefore, it is useful to start with a reamer that is very close in size to the intended final reamer. It is useful to ream with as few reamers as necessary to avoid inserting and extracting reamers. In addition, the open design of these reamers allows good visualization of the acetabulum during reaming. The reamer is inserted in line with the femoral neck, with the cutouts of the reamer aligned with the two retractors. This position allows the reamer to be easily inserted. Gentle traction on the leg facilitates the reamer into the acetabulum (Fig. 24.10b).

With the reamer at 45° of abduction and 20° of anteversion, the acetabulum is reamed. The fluoroscope is used for visualization as the acetabular as bone is gradually removed (Fig. 24.10c). The acetabulum is appropriately reamed and the reamer is then removed. The lit retractors, which remain in replace around the acetabulum, afford good visualization. Any redundant tissue that had been invaginated due to reaming can be removed at this time. The acetabulum is sequentially reamed until good bleeding bone is present throughout the entire acetabulum. Any remaining pulvinar is cut away from the fossa with an electric cautery. Again, the entire acetabulum rim is fully evaluated and care is taken to remove any excess labrum.

A specialized dogleg acetabular inserter with the supine positioner is used to place an acetabulum shell that is 2 mm larger than the last reamer used. This will give a 2-mm press-fit. The two the acetabular retractors, one anterior and one posterior, are left in place as gentle traction is placed on the leg. The acetabular component is then inserted into the acetabulum (Fig. 24.11a). The bolster beneath the pelvis is

then removed and the patient is now directly supine on the operating room table. Fluoroscopy is again used to check to make sure that the pelvis is flat and does not have any obliquity. The fluoroscope should also be rotated so that the pelvis is directly horizontal. This allows proper assessment of the abduction angle of the acetabular component.

The acetabular shell is then manipulated in place; the retractors keep the capsule from invaginating. The retractors are then removed. The acetabulum is viewed with the fluoroscope as the cup is positioned in 45° of abduction and 20° of anteversion. The cup is impacted in place, keeping the cup in 45° of abduction and 20° of anteversion (Fig. 24.11b). When the cup is fully seated, the dogleg acetabulum inserter is removed (Fig. 24.11c).

The curved lit acetabular retractors are replaced around the acetabulum. The lit retractor allows excellent visualization of the acetabular shell. Stability of the shell can hen be assessed. Two screws may be placed in the posterior superior quadrant of the shell, up the wing of the ileum and slightly posteriorly over the sciatic notch. These screws usually measure 30 mm and 35 mm. Finally, a small curved osteotome is used to remove any osteophytes around the rim of the acetabulum, and the liner is then impacted in place. With the acetabulum complete, all retractors are removed from the acetabulum and attention is turned to the femur.

The femur is placed back in a figure-of-four and a burr is used to mark the medial apex of the calcar. This mark is then used for palpation and visualization for femoral component rotation. The leg is then fully adducted and placed in neutral rotation. A finger is placed into the piriformis fossa to allow assessment of where to make the starting point on the skin on the posterior lateral buttocks. This point is colinear with the piriformis fossa to allow access to the femoral canal. A small stab wound is made in the posterior lateral buttock

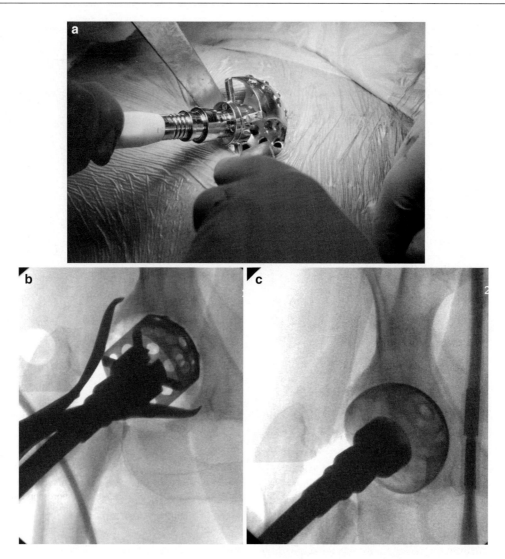

Fig. 24.10 Reaming the acetabulum. (**a**) Picture of the cutout reamer being inserted through the soft tissue. (**b**) Fluoroscope view of reamer seated in acetabulum ready to begin reaming. (**c**) Fluoroscope view of reamer seated in acetabulum while reaming. Note that, during reaming, the cutout reaming appears hemispherical

corresponding to the location of the piriformis fossa to allow access to the femoral canal. A Charnley awl is then used as a finger in the piriformis fossa. The Charnley awl is guided posteriorly, posterior to the abductors and anterior to the piriformis under direct palpation. The Charnley awl is then manipulated down the femur with the aid of fluoroscopy.

The initial insertion point into the femur is usually slightly medial to the desired starting point. Specially designed side-cutting reamers are used to enlarge this starting hole and position the starting point lateral against the trochanteric bed. The reamers are used sequentially starting with the smallest, 9-mm reamer. This reamer is placed in the canal from the posterior, within the same track the Charnley awl made. The reamers are used with visualization from the fluoroscope to allow lateralization of the starting hole to the lateral edge of the femoral canal (Fig. 24.12). The initial stab wound is

opened in line with the femur neck extending approximately 1.25 in. A self-retaining retractor is used to spread the fat, and the fat is cauterized. The lateralization reamers are then used sequentially from 9 mm to up to the intended size of the stem. Fluoroscopy is used to assure that the starting point is lined up with the lateral cortex of the femur. This point corresponds to the tip of the trochanter in most patients, but it should be based on the preoperative templating. Care is taken with periodic fluoroscopy views of the leg in a frog position lateral to make sure the starting point is well centralized anteriorly and posteriorly. In addition, palpation from posterior straight down the canal can be used to palpate the anterior and the posterior wall of the trochanter to make sure that the starting point is well centralized anteriorly and posteriorly.

With the starting point being fully lateralized, flexible reamers are used to gently ream the canal starting until cortical

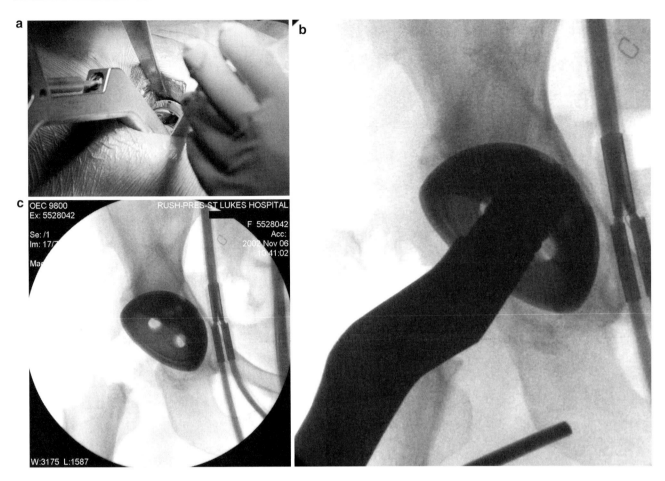

Fig. 24.11 Inserting the acetabulum. (**a**) Picture of the acetabulum being inserted through the soft tissue. (**b**) Fluoroscope view of acetabular component with the inserter seated in the acetabulum. (**c**) Fluoroscope view of final acetabular component placement

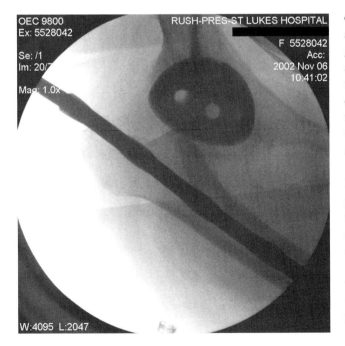

Fig. 24.12 Fluoroscope view of the lateralization reamer clearing the trochanteric bed, getting to a neutral alignment

chatter is obtained. Straight reamers with a tissue-protecting sleeve are then used to ream down the femoral shaft until good cortical chatter is obtained. Fluoroscopy is used to assure the reamers are well centralized both on the anterior fluoroscopy view as well as the lateral radiograph fluoroscopy view (Fig. 24.13). A full-coated stem is used; therefore, the cortex is reamed 0.5 mm less than the stem that is chosen. Good cortical chatter is must be obtained before reaming is discontinued.

After reaming is completed, broaching is performed. The leg remains adducted and in neutral rotation while rasps are placed down the canal. The rasps have a medial groove cut in them that can be palpated as the rasp is introduced. The rasp is aligned, by palpation or visualization though the anterior incision, to the mark that was made in the calcar. The rasp is fully seated and checked with fluoroscopy. Rasps are then sequentially introduced and seated, ending with the size stem that was reamed (Fig. 24.14). When the final rasp is seated, the rotation of the rasp should be viewed through the anterior incision to ensure that it is aligned with the apex of the calcar.

At this point, the rasp handle is removed and a trial reduction can be performed. Traction is placed on the leg to pull

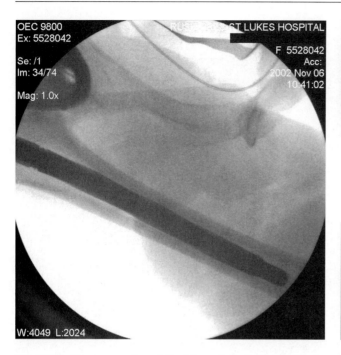

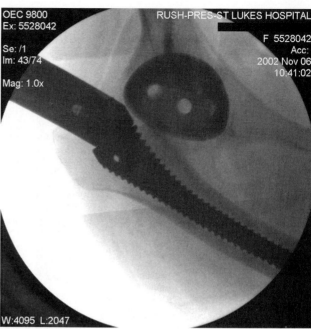

Fig. 24.13 Fluoroscope view of distal femoral diaphysis showing the fill and alignment of stem

Fig. 24.14 Fluoroscope view of final femoral rasp being seated

the rasp completely within the capsule of the hip. The trial neck and head is placed on the neck from the anterior wound. Externally rotate the hip, and a bone hook around the neck gently pulls the neck anteriorly through the wound. Traction on the leg at this point can make placing the head more difficult. The head is placed on the neck and then the leg is pulled with gentle traction as internal rotation is placed on the leg; this locates the hip. If the calcar requires trimming, this is done from the anterior incision with a sagittal saw. The calcar is easily accessed from the anterior incision with the leg in external rotation. The hip is then put through a range of motion to assess stability. The hip should be stable in full extension with 90° of external rotation as well as 90° of flexion and 20° of adduction with at least 50° of internal rotation. The fluoroscope can be used to assess leg lengths by comparing the level of the lesser trochanters to the obturator foramen. In addition, with the patient in the supine position, the medial malleoli may be checked to assess leg length. When the trial reduction is complete, the head and neck is removed though the anterior incision and the rasp is removed through the posterior incision.

Hohmann retractors are placed into the posterior wound, placed anterior around the femoral neck. This will keep the anterior soft tissue clear from the stem as it is placed into the femoral canal. Gravity keeps the posterior soft tissue clear from the stem as it is placed into the femoral canal. The stem is then introduced into the femoral canal from the posterior incision (Fig. 24.15). The stem is rotationally aligned

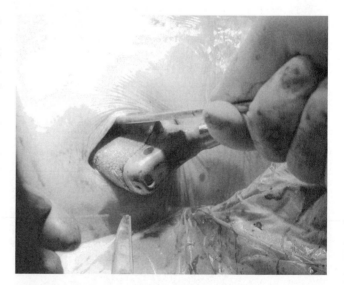

Fig. 24.15 Inserting the femoral component through the skin in the posterior incision

as the rasp is placed, this should be in line with the mark that was made on the tip of the calcar. The stem is impacted in place until approximately 1 cm from being seated. Gentle traction is then placed on the leg, with the leg in neutral abduction. This allows the soft tissue to come around the neck of the prosthesis. In addition, this pulls the entire femoral component though the capsule to lie within the hip. In this position, the version of the femoral component can be

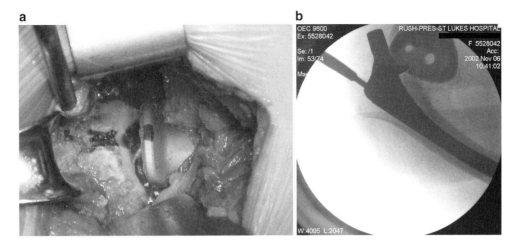

Fig. 24.16 Inserting the femoral component. (**a**) The femoral rotation as seen through the anterior incision, aligning the stem with the apex of the calcar. (**b**) Fluoroscope view of the femoral component during insertion. The component is seated to the final position

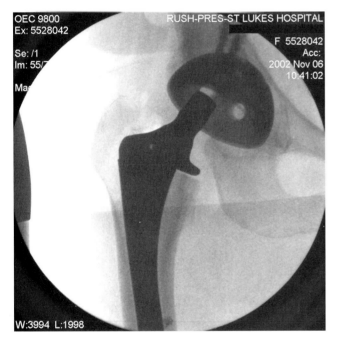

Fig. 24.17 Fluoroscope view of the femoral component with the neck reduced into the acetabulum

easily assessed through the anterior incision (Fig. 24.16a). The leg is then put back into abduction and care is taken to make sure all soft tissue is cleared from around the collar and around the neck. The stem is then impacted into place and seated (Fig. 24.16b).

If the neck is not fully through the capsule, traction is again placed on the leg, which brings the neck through the capsule lying into the acetabulum (Fig. 24.17). Care is taken again to look in the anterior incision to assure that no soft tissue is caught between the calcar and the collar as well as making sure the rotation of the stem is correct, being aligned with the apex of the calcar and that mark that was placed.

A trial reduction is performed, placing the heads from the anterior incision. The hip should be stable in full extension with 90° of external rotation as well as 90° of flexion and 20° of adduction with at least 50° of internal rotation. The fluoroscope can be used to assess leg lengths by comparing the level of the lesser trochanters to the obturator foramen. In addition, with the patient in the supine position, the medial malleoli may be checked to assess leg length. When the trial reduction is complete, the head is removed though the anterior incision.

Prior to placing the final head, two stitches are put in the capsule, one on the medial and one on the lateral sides. This is done prior to reducing the head, as the capsule can become invaginated posteriorly once the hip is located. With the hip in external rotation and the bone hook around the neck, the neck is gently pulled anteriorly through the anterior incision and the final head is then placed on the neck and gently impacted in place. Then the leg is pulled with gentle traction as internal rotation is placed on the leg and the hip is located. During the location process, the two stitches that were put on the medial and lateral capsule are kept taut so the capsule does not invaginate posteriorly. With the hip located, it is again put through a full range of motion and stability and leg length is assessed.

Both anteriorly and posteriorly, a total of 40–60 ml of 0.25% Marcaine with epinephrine is infiltrated in the capsule, the surrounding tissue, and the skin. Care is taken not to infiltrate the femoral nerve. The two sutures in the capsule are tied and one or two additional stitches are used to fully close the capsule anatomically. The fascia is closed between the sartorius and tensor fascia lata. Care is taken not to entrap the lateral femoral cutaneous nerve. A few 2–0 Vicryl stitches are placed into the fat layer and then the skin is closed anteriorly with 2–0 Vicryl and staples. Posteriorly, the small rent in the maximus fascia is closed with 2–0 Vicryl and a few deep sutures are put in with 2–0 Vicryl in the subcutaneous fat. The skin is then closed with 2–0 Vicryl and staples. Two 2 × 2-in. bandages with Tegaderm are used to cover the incisions (Fig. 24.18). Figure 24.19 shows the preoperative and postoperative radiographs of a patient who received a total hip with this minimally invasive two-incision approach.

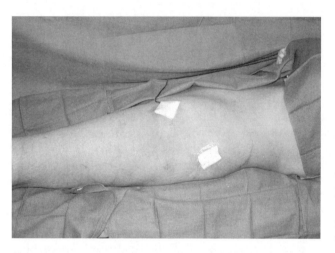

Fig. 24.18 Final dressing on minimally invasive two-incision total hip with two 2 × 2-in. bandages with Tegaderm covering the incisions

Summary

Minimally invasive surgery has the potential for minimizing surgical trauma, pain, and recovery in total hip arthroplasty. This two-incision minimally invasive total hip procedure was found to be safe and facilitated a rapid patient recovery. In the first 100 minimally invasive two-incision total hip arthroplasties performed at Rush Presbyterian St Luke's hospital, the 1% complication rate was acceptable, a single femoral fracture. There have been no dislocations, no failure of ingrowth, and no re-operations. Since initiating an accelerated hospital pathway to allow a shorter length of stay, 85% of patients have chosen to go home the same day with no patient staying for longer than a 23-h admission. Furthermore, there have been no readmissions for any reason and no postdischarge complications. Lastly, radiographically, since fluoroscopy is used during insertion, the overall alignment and ingrowth of the components have been excellent.

In conclusion, this two-incision minimally invasive total hip technique has demonstrated great results; however, this technique is technically extremely challenging and is very different from a standard total hip technique. When performed in the hands of a trained surgeon, the minimally invasive two-incision procedure achieves excellent success; nevertheless, the minimally invasive two-incision procedure employs novel procedures that must be learned. Optimizing patient outcomes using the minimally invasive two-incision approach requires meticulous surgical technique, specialized instrumentation, and special instruction. As such, active participation in the pretraining exercises, anatomy labs, cadaver training, and proctoring program are essential to minimize complications and ensure success of this procedure.

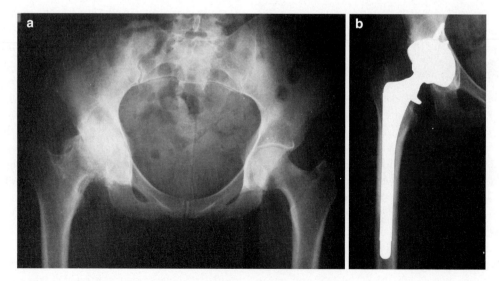

Fig. 24.19 Radiographs of a patient who received a total hip with this minimally invasive two-incision approach. (**a**) Preoperative radiograph shows a patient with an arthritic right hip. (**b**) Postoperative radiographs show with the minimally invasive two-incision total hip arthroplasty (THA) reconstruction

Chapter 25
Round Table Discussion of Mini-incision Total Hip Arthroplasty

Richard Berger: Many different minimally invasive total hip arthroplasty (THA) techniques have become popular in the last few years. Let's start by defining what is a minimally invasive total hip arthroplasty? Is it a skin incision length, a soft tissue procedure, or a systematic approach to THA?

Andrew Freiberg: As you know, most of us believe that there really is no single approach for a minimally invasive total hip replacement. Moreover, what started as only a surgical approach now has matured to encompass an entire philosophy for patient care that concentrates on rapid recovery. To me, minimally invasive surgery (MIS) can be summarized as a combination of preoperative teaching, anesthesia, pain management and prevention, discharge education and planning, and finally the actual surgical procedure. To answer your question, I think the skin incision length is the least important part of the actual surgical procedure; however, it's the most visibly definable aspect. Patients' and their family all key in on incision length, and it really affects how many people feel about the job we performed. I believe that how the hip joint is exposed, minimizing the trauma to the deep tissues by gentle handling, has the greatest impact on early pain and return to function.

Richard Berger: There is minimally soft tissue dissection (MIS) and then there is minimally bone invasion (surface replacement). How do you compare these conflicting parameters? Which is more important to you?

Michael Mont: Minimally invasive can encompass any or all of the following three broad categories: (1) skin incision length, (2) soft tissue invasion – usually talking about the least trauma to muscles, but this may also encompass how much soft tissue trauma there is, such as dislocating or not dislocating the joint, and (3) bone conservation – whether we are talking about resurfacing or even small stems. I think one has to look at each individually, although most would agree that incision length is least important – just do the least incision necessary for the individual patient or procedure. Unfortunately, with the current generation of surface replacements, stems, and techniques, you do have to choose; do you want to conserve bone or soft tissue. Perhaps in the future we will be able to minimize both soft tissue disruption and bone invasion with a single procedure; however, not today.

Francesco Falez: Why should we make a choice and not try to combine the two options? I am not convinced that one excludes the other; both aspects are important and, if carried out at the same time in the same procedure, they both contribute to achieve a tissue-sparing surgery procedure. Probably this term is more appropriate to indicate the real goal of a modern procedure as a combination of a minimally invasive approach (i.e., mini Watson-Jones (WJ), anterior, or simply mini standard approaches) associated with a bone-retaining implant (i.e., short metaphyseal stems or neck-retaining stems). This is probably the most actual attitude in Europe and I do believe it will, within a few years, represent the standard procedure for total hip replacement.

Richard Berger: Is there a minimally invasive THA technique for every patient? Tell me who is the optimal patient and who is the most difficult patient for minimally invasive THA.

Mark Hartzband: I think that there is a minimally invasive THA technique available for the vast majority of primary arthroplasty patients. The optimal patient is obviously someone who is thinner, more mobile, with an atrophic pattern of arthritis and the relative absence of significant contractures. Large muscular men, especially those with contractures, are generally the most difficult patients for a minimally invasive or, for that matter, conventional THA. Severe osteoporosis and extremely poor-quality soft tissues, for example, in steroid-dependent patients, require special care when performing MIS procedures, or, for that matter, any procedure.

Richard Berger: With these variables in mind, Sonny, which patients may be better served with a more traditional/extensile approach?

Sonny Bal: The minimally invasive philosophy can and should be used in all patients; this includes making incisions no longer than they need to be, optimizing anesthesia and pain control regimens, and minimizing the takedown of muscles and tendons. Early in the surgeon's experience, and in patients in whom obesity or excessive muscle development is combined with a short stature, and a varus femoral neck, a more extensile approach may be safer. Also, patients with prior hip surgery, existing hardware, or congenital abnormalities are better served with traditional surgical approaches.

G.R. Scuderi and A.J. Tria (eds.), *Minimally Invasive Surgery in Orthopedics*, DOI 10.1007/ 978-0-387-76608-9_25, © Springer Science+Business Media, LLC 2010

Rich Berger: I believe that almost any surgeon, with proper training, can become proficient at minimally invasive THA. Getting started with minimally invasive THA should be done with a stepwise approach. I recommend first becoming accustomed to your minimally invasive instruments using whichever approach you are most familiar with. Then as you become facile with the instruments, begin making a smaller incision and dissecting less muscles. If you experience difficulty during a case, simply extend the incision and dissection. With more experience, further reduce the incision and really concentrate on a minimal dissection under the skin. All of these steps will be facilitated either by a formal course at the AAOS or by one of the implant companies, or by visiting one of the experts in your approach. If a surgeon wants to learn a new approach, what are your recommendations for beginning to learn a completely new technique and learn all the perioperative protocols that go along with this?

Andrew Freiberg: Taking the time to learn a new technique is well worth the effort as it is personally renewing to sit down and study hip anatomy and reexamine what you as an experienced surgeon actually do. There is no doubt that surgeon mentoring is a key aspect of learning a new procedure and for making it safe for all involved. When I've learned a new technique, my approach has been to restudy the anatomy, visit experienced surgeons, and attend at least one formal course where there is a chance to use cadavers under the direction of people experienced in that particular procedure. Sometimes it takes more than one visit or one course for a surgeon to feel safe with a new technique. With advanced procedures like two-incision total hip procedure, it can be very valuable to have other experienced surgeon available for your first one.

Richard Berger: I believe, the more exposure you have, the more trauma you are causing for the patient; therefore, some struggle is necessary to help your patient recover more rapidly postoperatively. Mark, now that you know how to do different MIS THA approaches, can you tell us which you choose, which give better exposure, and the difference to your patients.

Mark Hartzband: My principle MIS approaches are the mini posterior and the two-incision THA. Acetabular exposure is excellent with both techniques once some experience has been obtained, especially in terms of incision location and proper retractor placement. Direct femoral exposure is obviously superior with the mini posterior approach and, for that reason, I tend to use a mini posterior approach in dysplastic patients who have significant version anomalies of the proximal femur and obviously for those with proximal femoral hardware. The difference to my patients primarily relates to the speed of recovery and the length of hospital stay. Although a small percentage of my mini posterior patients are discharged on the day of surgery, the vast majority stay in hospital for one night. In contrast, the two-incision patients are almost invariably discharged on the day of surgery. The two-incision patients are more rapidly independent, first to drive, see more rapid results in rehabilitation, and return to work earlier.

Richard Berger: Mark, I agree with you. In a prospective randomized study, I have had a quicker recovery with less use of narcotic using the two-incision approach compared with a single-incision approach. Ideally, there should be little difference in the approaches if all approaches used very small instruments, did not stress the surrounding tissues, and did not forcibly dislocate the hip. Any approach under these conditions should similarly benefit our patients. Unfortunately, many approaches can potentially damage the underlying soft tissues. Perhaps there is less muscle damage with the two-incision approach. Sonny, you have done many of the two-incision approaches and have done some research on muscle damage with the two-incision approach. Can you tell us how this approach compares with the anterolateral and posterolateral approach for muscle damage?

Sonny Bal: The elegance and attractiveness of the two-incision approach is that it is based on the Smith-Peterson surgical interval, which allows access to the hip joint without disrupting muscles or tendon insertions. Our clinical outcomes and MRI data obtained after surgery validate the advantages of the two-incision method as a muscle-sparing technique. In this sense, the two-incision method is based on a true muscle-sparing approach. Posterior insertion of the femoral stem, if done appropriately, can also navigate an intermuscular path, much like blind insertion of a femoral nail. In contrast, the anterolateral technique based on the Hardinge approach directly disrupts the abductor mechanism. The posterolateral approach requires takedown of the short external rotators; repair of these structures has been recommended to restore hip stability.

Richard Berger: You have more recently moved away from the two-incision approach to a single anterior approach. Why the change and how is this working for you now?

Sonny Bal: The single-incision anterior MIS–THA promoted by Joel Matta is, in my opinion, a variation on the MIS two-incision method. Both operations are based on the muscle-sparing Smith-Peterson approach. The single-incision anterior approach allows me to use a fracture table as a retractor and positioning device, thereby facilitating exposure. The proximal femoral exposure allows broaches to be left in place, and trial femoral necks and heads can be used when testing the components. Hip resurfacing is theoretically possible with the single-incision anterior THA. In terms of outcomes, the single-incision is similar to the two-incision method, in that patients recover quickly, without hip precautions, and actively recommend this method to other prospective patients. So, the switch to the single-incision method was driven by my curiosity, the availability of a fracture table, and my desire to attempt a variation of the two-incision method.

Richard Berger: Andy, you have done the anterolateral, mini WJ, and two-incision approaches. How do you see these three approaches in your hands? Which was easiest to learn, which is best for your patients? How do you choose?

Andrew Freiberg: The anterolateral is the easiest to learn and for me to teach residents and fellows. I moved away from the posterior approach because of a persistent low rate of dislocation. The mini WJ is easier to learn than the two incision, but I think it's much harder to do surgically. My patients' early recovery with the mini WJ is slightly better than with the anterolateral, but I use the anterolateral because I don't need an additional assistant or specialized bed, it uses minimal retractors, and visualization for acetabular and femoral preparation is outstanding. In my hands, the anterolateral is safer than the mini WJ with a lower risk of femoral fracture. Either way, acetabular preparation and component placement are straightforward. The two incision has outstanding early recovery and allows for fantastic early function and pain relief. Surgeons who have never done a two incision are really missing an opportunity to learn how powerful MIS techniques can be.

Richard Berger: When you are not doing a surface replacement, what approach do you prefer for THA and why? How import is navigation with surface replacements?

Francesco Falez: Confirming my previous statement, a mini WJ is the first-choice approach because preserving all the muscular insertion, if in combination with a conservative stems, offers to the patient a real tissue trauma surgery THA. Resurfacing definitively benefits in terms of navigation by achieving a more precise positioning of the femoral component, but I do not believe that this improvement will solve the problems related to hip resurfacing; it's my opinion that this procedure deserves a better understanding of the unacceptable high failure rate.

Michael Mont: When I'm not doing a surface replacement, I still use the anterolateral approach with very small incisions – 2–3 in. – primarily because it's easy, I've rarely had a dislocation, and I can get a great repair of what I've detached.

Richard Berger: Michael, how often are you doing surface replacements and how are these patients doing in the short term and long term?

Michael Mont: In my practice, I'm about 60% resurfacing, but this is because of several factors: I've always many young patients referred to me with dysplastic hips as well as osteonecrosis and I'm well known for resurfacing. Therefore, I'm not sure the 60% means anything - I think that the true practice considering typical ages of patients getting hip replacements in this country of 70 years average would lead to a resurfacing advocate surgeon to do no more than 30–40% maximum if they were using appropriate indications.

Short-term results past the initial learning curve are excellent – comparable to standard total hip replacement in my hands as well as for most high-volume resurfacing surgeons.

We really don't have follow-up past 7–8 years right now. They were first implanted in the United States in 1999–2000 and, even in Europe, the devices were changed shortly before this. So far, they are holding up, but we really won't know long-term follow-up past 10 years for a few years.

Richard Berger: Francesco and Michael, what would you do for the patient who wanted the quickest recovery so they could return to their desk job? How long would you expect this person to be in the hospital and to return to work?

Francesco Falez: First, please understand that, in Europe, the length of stay and return to work is much longer that in the United States. However, with a tissue-sparing approach, definitely the right choice to reduce the length of hospitalization, our length of stay has been reduced to 2 or 4 days. In addition, the recovery is shortened; return to active work is accomplished in 3 or 4 weeks.

Michael Mont: Like Francesco, either resurfacing or standard THA would be similar with a hospital stay for 2–3 days and return to work in 7–14 days. Incidentally, my hospital doesn't want me to do outpatient surgery; it adverse effects how they get reimbursed.

Richard Berger: Reimbursement aside, I do outpatient total hip replacement every day. This is accomplished with a comprehensive approach to the patient. This includes the surgery, perioperative anesthesia and pain management, preoperative patient education, and rapid rehabilitation protocols. The combination of less soft tissue injury with less medication allows patients to ambulate with only a cane or no assistive device within a few hours after the procedure in most cases. With little pain and little functional deficients, most of my patients choose to go home the day of surgery. Mark, Michael, and Andy, what are you doing for your perioperative pathway and what is your length of stay?

Andrew Freiberg: All of our patients attend a surgeon-specific preoperative educational program so people really understand what will happen. Our experience has been that patient and family expectations and anxiety are the most powerful impediments to early discharge. More specifically, we use intraoperative IV ketorolac (Toradol), several measures to prevent nausea, generous use of bupivacaine (Marcaine) with epinephrine in the periarticular tissues (minimal in the skin), and oral long-acting narcotics supplemented with shorter-acting ones for breakthrough pain. In the past 2 years, we have not used oral cox-2 inhibitors because of concern about the cardiovascular risks. Our average length of stay for two incisions has been 1 day (our target). For anterolateral procedures, all patients, the average length of stay is 2.5 days.

Mark Hartzband: As Andy mentioned, the most important in my comprehensive approach to short-stay total hip replacement is preoperative education. The patients are instructed that they can expect to be discharged on the day of or the morning following the surgical procedure depending on which MIS approach is planned. The patients typically receive celecoxib (Celebrex), oxycodone and acetaminophen (Percocet), metoclopramide (Reglan), and ondansetron (Zofran) preoperatively. A scopolamine patch is applied on admission to the hospital and 8 mg of prednisone is given intravenously prior to the surgical procedure. Also very important to a shortened hospital stay is rapid ambulation and, in my practice, patients are typically ambulating within 4 h of their surgical procedure.

Michael Mont: For surface replacements, we have a 2-day pathway to home or rehab, which leads to my average length of stay of 2.3 days.

Richard Berger: Sonny, how has your patient's recovery changed from the two-incision approach to the single-incision anterior approach?

Sonny Bal: Patient recovery may be marginally better with the single-incision method, but it is hard to tell since I do not have randomized data. My impression is that the posterior incision does not add to the surgical trauma, therefore, the recovery is about the same as a single incision. Specifically, in nearly 400 two-incision THAs in my practice, two patients had a buttock hematoma that resolved without surgery, and one patient had prolonged drainage from the posterior incision; this person resumed professional diving in a lake to retrieve objects dropped in the water only 1 week after surgery with the staples in place. The posterior incision became macerated and took longer to heal; the anterior incision was unaffected by exposure to lake water. Other than these three patients, the posterior incision has never been an issue; in fact, many patients have to be reminded that they have a second incision on the buttock. So, whether it is done with two incisions or one, the Smith-Peterson THA offers excellent outcomes.

Richard Berger: I have completely moved away from cemented stems. In part due to poorer results and in part due to difficulty with the technique in MIS approaches. Is there still a role for cemented stems with an MIS THA approach?

Andrew Freiberg: Rich, I'm with you on this one. The most common reason I have had to do a revision in my own practice has been for intermediate-term failure of a cemented stem. My strong preference is to use mediolateral taper wedge stems in the great majority of patients. Cemented stems can be easily performed through the MIS anterolateral or posterolateral approach. I have never tried it through the Mini WJ, but suspect it would be difficult to avoid cement mantle defects because of the angle of insertion. I strongly advise against an attempted use of cemented stems for a two incision.

Richard Berger: What is your stem of choice for these MIS approaches? Does your stem of choice change with your approach or with your patient?

Mark Hartzband: I prefer a fully coated straight cylindrical stem for my two-incision THAs. As the femoral preparation is performed with very little direct visualization of the canal, I think that it is most reasonable to employ a stem that takes advantage of the ability to consistently obtain predictable cylindrical contact with this approach. At this time, I am using the Epoch composite femoral stem, which has all the advantages of a fully coated stem and has a 10-year track record for minimizing stress shielding. I am presently using a mix of different tapered designs for my mini posterior cases, including a new modular stem system with a neck module that greatly facilitates very small posterior approaches and avoids sacrifice of the piriformis tendon.

Richard Berger: I agree, I use different stems partly based on approach and partly based on the patient bone type and morphology. The last question I have for you is what is the one major change you can see in the next few years that will improve total hip replacement and recovery.

Mark Hartzband: Over the last 10 years, we have seen improvements in total hip replacement and recovery based primarily on modifications in surgical technique and perioperative clinical pathways. I think in the next few years we will see significant changes in component design that will further facilitate minimized approaches and their associated accelerated postoperative recovery. The concepts of modularity in the neck segment and composite stem structure both will have significant effects on MIS techniques.

Andrew Freiberg: As Mark said, I think we will have smaller stems that are stable and easier to place through small surgical approaches, which will change the techniques we use and how our patients recover. In addition, as we better understand pain pathways and the biochemistry of muscle trauma, we will likely have drugs that revolutionize our ability to do outpatient surgery. Within a decade or two, we will have polymeric materials that can be combined with biologics and used to resurface joints.

Michael Mont: Yes, and much more rigorous rehabilitation pathways will be developed that enhance the strides made in anesthesia and pain management. This will be important for the patient's ultimate outcome as tightness/contractures not addressed early (first 6–12 weeks) are harder if not impossible to rehabilitate later.

Francesco Falez: As Mark and Andy have said, we have a lot to improve in stem design and bearing surfaces; probably these two will make the difference for total hip replacement in the next few years, on the other hand, recovery will always be influenced by the quality of surgery and even if we are mowing in the right direction by reducing surgical damages, surgery will always affect some how and at some level functional anatomy.

Sonny Bal: I would go one step further; I envision a marriage of hip arthroscopy and the MIS techniques that we are using today. The future will bring several "disruptive" technologies together that make incisions smaller, relying on indirect visualization of the hip joint, and improve recovery following THA. The goal is to develop a true outpatient procedure with virtually immediate return to function after a hip replacement. I believe that our methods, techniques, and technology will keep driving us toward this goal. I also see MIS techniques applied to hip resurfacing, to minimize the surgical trauma associated with that procedure.

Richard Berger: It sounds like we are in agreement that the future will introduce new stem designs that are more readily implanted through small incisions and that conserve more bone than the current generation of total hip components. This advancement will then make further refinements in our pathways possible, resulting in a very rapid recovery and return to function. Lastly, new bearing will allow this component to continue to function or decades. This agreement, I thank you all for participating.

Section III
The Knee

Chapter 26
MIS Unicondylar Arthroplasty: The Bone-Sparing Technique

John A. Repicci and Jodi F. Hartman

Minimally invasive (MIS) unicondylar knee arthroplasty (UKA) and total knee arthroplasty (TKA) each have specific indications and distinctive roles in the senior author's algorithm for the treatment of knee osteoarthritis (OA). MIS UKA is not a substitute for TKA, which is the procedure of choice for treatment of advanced stages of OA. This philosophy is supported by Thornhill and Scott, who assert that UKA should be considered in the "continuum of surgical options for the treatment of the osteoarthritic patient."[1] In cases of earlier, nonadvanced OA, the two procedures may act in conjunction with one another, with MIS UKA serving as a supplement to future TKA. Together, these devices may be considered as a "knee prosthetic system."[2]

With the limited survivorship of TKA and the aging of the active baby boomer population, there is a need for a procedure in addition to TKA to address the treatment of earlier, nonadvanced stages of OA and to extend the survivability of knee prosthetics. Because knee prosthetics have a finite life span, a single device cannot encompass the entire spectrum of survivability necessary for many patients. Under the senior author's serial replacement concept, a procedure such as MIS UKA performed at an earlier age, before TKA use and as a supplement to TKA, will absorb approximately 10 years of functional capacity so that when and if future arthroplasty is required, the survivability of the entire knee prosthetic system is lengthened.[2,3] By following this philosophy, the use of MIS UKA in conjunction with a future TKA may increase the functional capacity of the entire knee prosthetic system to 20–30 years. The fundamental goal of this serial prosthetic replacement is to decrease the likelihood of a complex revision procedure in the patient's lifetime.

Minimally Invasive UKA Program

A unique feature of this serial replacement philosophy is the MIS UKA program that was introduced by the senior author in 1992.[4] This program is significantly different from simply the use of a small incision or implementation of a MIS surgical approach. Instead, it combines the following MIS concepts into a single program.

Adjunct Use of Arthroscopy

This multipronged MIS approach begins with arthroscopic evaluation prior to arthroplasty, which allows assessment of the articular cartilage in the contralateral compartment and permits the evaluation of the contralateral meniscus. The contralateral meniscus cannot be visualized through traditional surgical exposure alone. If the contralateral compartment has advanced OA or if the contralateral meniscus is not intact, the preplanned MIS UKA procedure may be abandoned in favor of TKA.

Verification of a fully functioning, intact, contralateral meniscus is critical for successful UKA, as the load-bearing surface area and the stability of the knee joint are enhanced by intact menisci.[5–11] Due to the lower tibiofemoral contact area compared with TKA designs, a certain degree of cold flow is permissible in UKA designs, but an absent contralateral meniscus will result in an inadequate amount of tibiofemoral contact. If UKA is performed in spite of an absent contralateral meniscus, the continued osteoarthritic progression may hasten the rate of degeneration of the untreated contralateral side, possibly leading to early failure of the UKA device.[12] Thus, although eliminating overcorrection has reduced the incidence of UKA failures in recent years,[1,6,12–25] contralateral compartment degeneration and early UKA failure remain a concern if the contralateral meniscus is not intact and the cruciate ligaments are not properly balanced.

Minimally Invasive Surgical Approach Avoiding Patellar Dislocation

A distinction must be made between a MIS surgical approach and a "mini incision," which merely is a small hole and may result in significant distortion of soft tissue. A MIS surgical approach requires preservation of all possible tissues required

J.A. Repicci (✉) and J.F. Hartman
Joint Reconstruction Orthopedic Center, 4510 Main Street, Buffalo, NY 14226, USA
e-mail: repicci@adelphia.net

G.R. Scuderi and A.J. Tria (eds.), *Minimally Invasive Surgery in Orthopedics*, DOI 10.1007/978-0-387-76608-9_26, © Springer Science+Business Media, LLC 2010

for any future restoration, including the suprapatellar pouch, the quadriceps tendon, the patella, and the medial tibial buttress. The only UKA system meeting these criteria is the MIS bone-sparing UKA technique. By combining UKA with a MIS surgical approach, a reduction in postoperative morbidity and pain, a decrease in rehabilitation time without the need for formal physical therapy, and the ability to perform the procedure on a same-day or short-stay basis are possible.[4,26–31] Compared with traditional open UKA, MIS UKA is associated with faster rates of recovery and earlier discharge.[29,30,32] In addition, equal reliability, without compromising proper component placement or long-term survivorship, has been demonstrated between a MIS surgical approach and a wide incision.[26,29,32] The diminished postoperative pain and decreased rehabilitation time associated with MIS UKA most likely is a result of preservation of the quadriceps tendon and not the short skin incision itself.[32]

Resurfacing UKA Design with Inlay Tibial Component

Another key feature of the senior author's MIS UKA program is the use of a resurfacing UKA design with an inlay tibial component. A significant problem in the conversion of UKA to TKA is medial tibial bone loss.[33,34] The use of an all-polyethylene inlay tibial component requires minimal bone resection and preserves the medial buttress and, therefore, is advantageous compared with use of their modular, saw-cut tibial counterparts, which are thicker and require significantly more bone resection. Due to the minimally invasive nature of the bone-sparing UKA technique, conversion to a TKA may be considered as a delayed primary TKA. An additional source of bone resection with other UKA systems is the full exposure often required for jig instrumentation. Finally, because many saw-cut tibial designs employ peg or fin fixation, tibial bone is further compromised upon implant removal and may necessitate the use bone grafts, special custom devices, or metal wedge tibial trays to stabilize the tibia during conversion to TKA.[33–37]

Pain Management with Local Anesthetic and Without Use of Narcotics

Outpatient status is possible with the advocated MIS UKA program due to a structured pain management protocol. Spinal or general anesthesia is used in all cases. During surgery, 30 mg ketorolac tromethamine (15 mg for patients older than 65 years of age) is administered either intramuscularly or intravenously and is repeated after 5 h in patients with normal renal function.

All incised tissues are infiltrated with long-acting local anesthetics to further pain relief. Additional components of the pain management protocol include patient education, avoidance of cerebral-depressing injectable narcotics, and the preemptive use of scheduled oral 400 mg ibuprofen every 4 h and oral 500 mg acetaminophen/5 mg hydrocodone bitartrate every 4 h for the first 3 days postoperatively.

As a result of this multimodal pain management program, patients are fully alert in the recovery room and have no local knee pain. Because pain is absent, the patients are able to perform straight leg raises and to actively participate in the postoperative rehabilitation process. The use of local anesthetic and avoidance of narcotics are credited for shortening the recovery and rehabilitation time, permitting the procedure to be performed on an outpatient basis.

Patient Selection

Proper patient selection is a significant factor contributing to the success of UKA for both MIS and traditional techniques. According to the senior author's selection criteria, all patients between 50 and 90 years of age who are diagnosed with OA, have failed nonoperative treatment, present with weight-bearing pain that significantly impairs quality of life, and have weight-bearing radiographs with complete loss of medial joint space are considered candidates for MIS UKA. During the preoperative evaluation, radiographic assessment identifies pathological changes and establishes the extent of OA; physical examination determines the degree of pain, function, and deformity; and patient discussion divulges activities of daily living limitations, as well as occupational and functional demands, which are of particular importance in electing UKA.[17,38] Although this preoperative evaluation assists in selecting potential UKA candidates, the decision to perform UKA may only be finalized at the time of surgery, at which point the status of the contralateral compartment and meniscus are evaluated.

A thorough radiographic analysis is critical to the patient selection process. In addition to obtaining weight-bearing anteroposterior, lateral, and patellofemoral radiographs, the Ahlback classification routinely is used to grade the progression of medial compartment OA.[39] The anatomic tibiofemoral alignment averages 6° varus for medial disease.[40] To qualify for UKA, OA must be confined to a single tibiofemoral compartment on weight-bearing radiograph. According to Sisto et al., the key to UKA success is being absolutely certain that OA is confined only to the involved compartment that is to be replaced.[41] Slight degenerative changes in the contralateral compartment, however, may be permissible and do not seem to adversely affect the results of UKA provided that the articular cartilage on the weight-bearing surface of the contralateral compartment appears adequate.[15,20,21,42,43] The presence of large osteophytes on the femoral condyle of the uninvolved compartment, however, may be indicative of bi- or tri-compartmental disease and, hence, is a contraindication to UKA.[1,20,44]

Because the joint line becomes elevated by several millimeters in the weight-bearing position, most patients with medial OA exhibit an altered patellofemoral compartment, which is not considered a contraindication for UKA.[20,21,42] UKA should not be an option, however, if the Merchant's view demonstrates sclerosis with marked loss of lateral patellofemoral joint space.[40]

Although the majority of patients selected for UKA demonstrate Ahlback stage 2 (absence of joint line) or stage 3 (minor bone attrition), the procedure may be considered in select cases with Ahlback stage 4 (moderate bone attrition).[40] Patients with Ahlback stage 1 should be excluded from consideration, as the disease progression is in its early stages. Ahlback stage 5 patients have advanced OA with gross bone attrition, and, therefore, are more appropriately treated with TKA.[40]

For Ahlback stage 2, 3, and 4 patients to be considered as UKA candidates, range of motion must be at least 10–90°.[2,3] Instability, such as a compromised anterior cruciate ligament (ACL), is a relative contraindication to medial UKA,[1–3,23,43,45–47] but an absolute contraindication to lateral UKA.[2,3] Rheumatoid arthritis, extensive avascular necrosis, and active or recent infection are absolute contraindications.[2,3] As long as absolute indications are met, certain relative contraindications, including obesity and high activity, do not appear to significantly affect UKA survivorship.[22,25,47]

Whereas other surgeons adhere to strict selection criteria,[18,48–50] concentrating on absolute indications and contraindications, the senior author follows a broad approach,[3,31] considering patient choice rather than definitive criteria. In accordance to the serial replacement concept, MIS UKA is used to treat patients with unicompartmental OA who wish to avoid or postpone TKA. If TKA is required in the future, the UKA may be converted to a primary TKA, which may survive the duration of the patient's life.

In the senior author's 25 years of offering MIS UKA, patients with unilateral OA readily accept the concept of a temporizing arthritis bypass to delay or prevent TKA. When presented with a choice between UKA and TKA, patients tend to opt for the less invasive procedure.[3,31] In a study by Hawker et al. assessing the need for and willingness to undergo arthroplasty, less than 15% of patients with severe arthritis were definitely willing to undergo arthroplasty, which led to the conclusion that patients' preferences and surgical indications must be considered mutually when evaluating the need and appropriateness of arthroplasty.[51] Because most patients with unicompartmental OA are inconvenienced by pain, but remain involved in recreational or professional interests, UKA is an appealing alternative to TKA as a means of not only reducing symptoms, but also of allowing continued participation in their desired activities.

Preoperative Discussion and Informed Patient Consent

A comprehensive preoperative discussion is an integral component of this treatment approach. The serial replacement concept must be explained to the patient so that he or she understands that most knee prosthetics, including UKA and primary TKA devices, have a finite survivorship. If MIS UKA is selected, the patient must be aware that it may be the first component of a serial knee prosthetic system that will be used to treat knee OA. This is of particular importance to the young, heavier, or more active patient, who must be advised that the effectiveness of his or her UKA may be shorter than the 10-year duration experienced by the average UKA patient.[31,52,53] Conversely, UKA in an older or less active patient may function well beyond 10 years.[31,52] Finally, the surgeon should explain that the most appropriate treatment option, UKA or TKA, will be determined at the time of surgery. Because of the possibility of performing TKA if OA is too advanced, all patients scheduled to undergo surgery should be encouraged to sign informed consents for both UKA and TKA.[1,54]

MIS Bone-Sparing UKA Surgical Technique

The MIS bone-sparing UKA surgical technique has been previously described.[2,4,40,55] The technique for medial implantation is summarized below, as medial compartment OA is the most common indication for UKA. The goal of the procedure is to replace the medial tibiofemoral compartment and balance the forces so that body weight is equally dispersed between the replaced compartment and the opposite compartment.

Patient Preparation

General, spinal, or regional anesthesia may be employed; however, the anesthesia team must be cognizant of the goal for outpatient or short-stay rehabilitation, which requires walking within 2–4 h postsurgery. Patient preparation is performed per standard protocols, with patient placement in a supine position. A thigh holder with an arterial tourniquet set at 300 mmHg is used to secure the leg. A standard operating table is used, with the foot end of the table placed in a flexed position. The MIS surgical approach requires continuous repositioning of the knee to optimize visualization, as certain structures are better visualized at low or high degrees of flexion. Because knee positioning from 0 to 120° of flexion is necessary, the lower leg and knee are drape-free.

Diagnostic Arthroscopy

Prior to commencing MIS UKA, the preoperative diagnosis of unicompartmental OA is confirmed through arthroscopy using a medial portal. In addition to verifying that the contralateral compartment is unaffected, the status of the contralateral meniscus must be inspected, as it cannot be visualized through the flexion gap during the open procedure. The extent of medial compartment damage and the status of the ACL also should be noted.

The UKA procedure should proceed only if the OA is limited to one tibiofemoral compartment and the contralateral meniscus is functional. If the disease process is more progressive, the surgeon must be prepared to perform a TKA, the potential of which should be preoperatively discussed and consented to by the patient.

Exposure with Posterior Femoral Condyle Resection

To proceed with the MIS UKA, a limited 7- to 10-cm skin incision is developed from the superomedial edge of the patella to the proximal tibial region, incorporating the arthroscopic portal. A subcutaneous dissection, producing a 2- to 5-cm skin flap surrounding the entire incision, improves skin mobility and visualization.

A medial parapatellar capsular arthrotomy is created from the superior pole of the patella to the tibia. A 2-cm transverse release of the vastus medialis tendon further enhances visualization. If additional exposure to the femoral condyle is required, a 2- to 3-cm segment of the medial parapatellar osteophyte may be resected with a sagittal saw. This medial parapatellar capsular arthrotomy is fundamental to the MIS surgical technique, as it does not violate the extensor mechanism nor does it dislocate the patella. By avoiding patellar dislocation, the suprapatellar pouch remains intact and able to unfold the required four times in length during knee flexion to 90°.[40,55,56] On the contrary, during traditional open TKA or UKA procedures, the suprapatellar pouch is damaged when the patella is everted, necessitating extensive physical therapy to reverse the iatrogenic damage.

Because medial compartment OA is an extension gap disease (Fig. 26.1), with no defect in flexion gap, approximately 10 mm of space must be created in the flexion gap to accommodate the prosthesis. The first step in generating this space is a 5- to 8-mm resection of the posterior femoral condyle. The articular defect is located at the distal femur and the anterior tibia. An area of preserved articular cartilage, located by flexing the knee 90°, causing the femur to roll back onto the tibia, serves as an excellent reference point for reconstruction (Fig. 26.2).

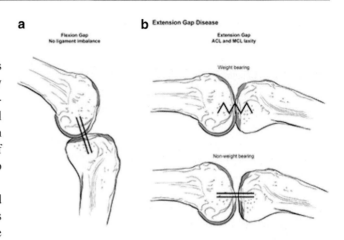

Fig. 26.1 Medial unicompartmental osteoarthritis is an extension gap disease. (**a**) No articular surface loss is present in the flexion gap. (**b**) In contrast, approximately 5 mm of articular surface is lost in the extension gap. This narrowing of the medial compartment joint space is evident on radiographic evaluation and is responsible for many of the clinical observations characteristic of medial unicompartmental osteoarthritis, including ACL and medial collateral ligament (MCL) laxity, lateral tibial thrust, or varus deformity, present in the extension gap; and absence of deformity in the flexion gap

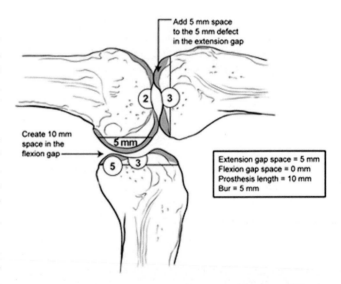

Fig. 26.2 Illustration depicting the creation of several internal landmarks, which assist in the necessary femoral and tibial resections

Distraction with Tibial Inlay Preparation and Resection

Curved distractor pins are inserted at the femoral and tibial levels to allow placement of a joint distractor, which improves visualization of the tibial plateau. At the posterior tibia, adjacent to the posterior tibial rim, a high-speed bur is buried 5 mm into normal cartilage to create the additional 4–5 mm of space in the flexion gap necessary for prosthetic insertion. In the anterior tibial region, corresponding to the area of articular cartilage loss and sclerotic bone formation, the medial tibial buttress is preserved by burying the bur at half-depth (3 mm). The bur holes are connected, creating a guide slot (Fig. 26.3).

During tibial resection, it also is critical to preserve a 2- to 3-mm circumferential rim, which aids in component stabilization. This entire resection process creates a bed for the all-polyethylene tibial inlay component. The natural location of femoral weight transfer at the anterior tibial level is indicated by the use of a crosshatch. The tibia inlay component then is fitted and adjusted as necessary.

Preservation of the layer of sclerotic bone creates a stable platform for the tibial component and minimizes medial tibial bone loss, which is a major cause of UKA revision.[33,34] The importance of preserving this medial tibial buttress is analogous to the preservation of the posterior acetabular rim in total hip arthroplasty in that, if absent, future reconstruction is severely compromised. The use of resurfacing UKA designs with tibial inlay components is advantageous compared with the use of other UKA designs that require saw-cut resections and, hence, sacrifice the valuable layer of sclerotic bone, i.e., the medial tibial buttress (Fig. 26.4).

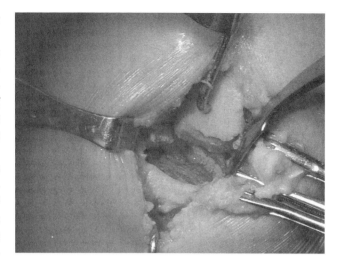

Fig. 26.4 Final preparation of the tibia. Unlike polyethylene saw-cut tibial components that require more aggressive bone resection, the use of an all-polyethylene inlay tibial component allows limited bone resection with preservation of the medial tibial buttress

Femoral Preparation and Resection

Femoral preparation begins by creating a depth gauge using a 5.5-mm round bur drilled to a half-depth of 3 mm into the femoral extension gap surface (Figs. 26.2 and 26.5). An additional full-depth of 5 mm is created at the junction with the previous saw cut and the distal femoral surface, which will allow the curved portion of the femoral component to set midway between the flexion and extension gaps (45° flexion position). Four 3-mm drill-hole guides are created and bulk bone is resected to the guide depth (Fig. 26.6). This method of femoral resection allows adequate space for component insertion, while preventing settling.

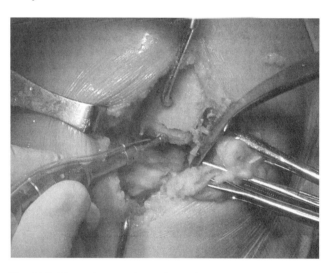

Fig. 26.5 Femoral preparation and resection

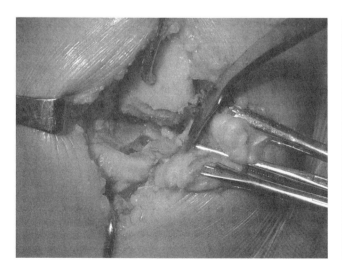

Fig. 26.3 Creation of a guide slot for tibial component insertion

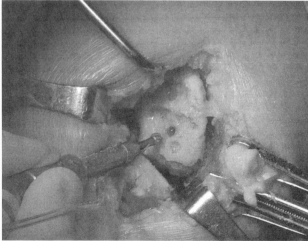

Fig. 26.6 Creation of drill hole guides to aid in femoral resection

Femoral-Tibial Alignment

With the knee in full extension and flexion, methylene blue marks are created on the sclerotic tibial bone and on the corresponding area of the femoral condyle to indicate both the desired center of rotation, or contact point, of the femoral component in relation to the tibial component and the desired center point of the femoral component (Fig. 26.7). A femoral drill guide with a large central slot to visualize component alignment is inserted to assist in the creation of a center femoral drill hole. Referencing the methylene blue markings, a keel-slot for the fin of the femoral component is created using a sagittal saw or side-cutting bur. The trial femoral component is placed using the femoral inserter.

Trial Reduction and Local Anesthetic Injection

Trial reduction is performed to evaluate range of motion through 115° of flexion and to assess soft tissue balancing. Lack of complete extension or flexion indicates inadequate tibial or femoral preparations. Insertion and proper alignment of appropriately sized implants should result in ligament balancing. If, however, the ligaments are tight only in the extension gap, tension may be adjusted by further bone removal at the distal femoral level. If tension is present in both the flexion and extension gaps, additional tibial bone may be resected, as previously described, in 1-mm increments until proper tension is achieved.

After satisfactory range of motion and proper soft tissue balancing are achieved, the trial components are removed, the joint is irrigated thoroughly, and a dry field is established. At this stage, both the femoral and tibial preparations are visible. Prior to component insertion, all incised tissues are infiltrated with

anesthesia (0.25% bupivacaine and 0.5% epinephrine solution) for postoperative pain relief and hemostasis (Fig. 26.8).

Component Insertion and Final Preparation

After irrigation with pulse lavage and antibiotic solution, methylmethacrylate cement is used to insert all components into gauze-dried bone (Fig. 26.9). To dry the field and to aid in cement removal, sponge packs are placed in the suprapatellar pouch, posterior to the femoral condyle, and on the femoral and tibial surfaces. Excess cement is removed from the posterior recess and perimeter of the tibial component after insertion, but before femoral component placement, using a narrow nerve hook. After femoral component placement, excess cement is removed from the perimeter using a dental pick.

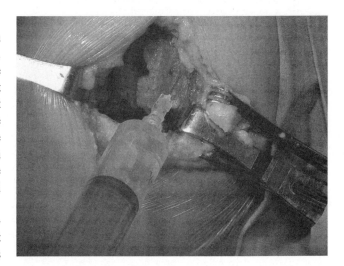

Fig. 26.8 Local anesthetic injection

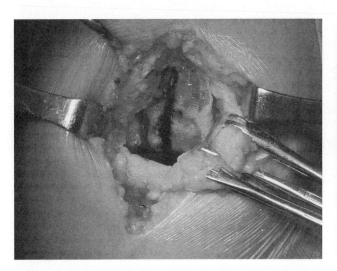

Fig. 26.7 Femoral-tibial alignment

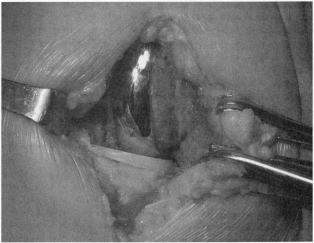

Fig. 26.9 Implantation of the UKA resurfacing prosthesis

Range of motion is performed following final prosthetic implantation to evaluate the flexion-extension gaps. Cement is cured with the knee in full extension. After the cement mantle has hardened, any remaining osteophytes should be removed. Patella contouring or notchplasty also may be performed, if necessary. As a final step, the joint is thoroughly irrigated with sterile saline.

The tourniquet is deflated and hemostasis is achieved with electrocautery. A tube drain is inserted into the contralateral component via a stab wound. Capsular closure is performed with size 0 Vicryl suture (Ethicon Company; Somerville, NJ). Subcuticular size 0 Prolene suture and sterile dressing is used for skin closure. Before exiting the operating room, a circumferential ice cuff, a pneumatic compression device, and an immobilizer are applied.

Surgical Technique for Conversion of MIS Bone-Sparing UKA to TKA

UKA Prosthesis Removal

The Repicci II unicondylar knee system (Biomet Inc., Warsaw, IN) is designed to extend the life of a natural knee, while preserving bone. As OA advances into the lateral femoral condyle, which may occur 10 years after the UKA procedure, conversion to TKA may be necessary. The MIS nature of this particular UKA design, along with the surgical technique described below for the removal of the UKA prosthetic system, results in minimal bone loss. Because resections equivalent to those performed in a primary TKA are produced, this conversion to a TKA may be considered as a delayed primary TKA.

Patient Preparation and Exposure

Anesthesia and patient preparation are performed per routine TKA protocols. A standard medial parapatellar approach is used, incorporating the previous UKA incision. The quadriceps tendon is split to the apex of the suprapatellar pouch. Four loops of size 0 Vicryl suture are placed at the apex to prevent tearing into the quadriceps muscle. A standard medial parapatellar approach is used to complete the exposure. The undersurface of the patella is resected to allow visualization with minimal soft tissue exposure.

Femoral Preparation

Overgrown bone is removed from the medial aspect of the femoral component. A drill hole is created in the distal femur

for insertion of a standard intermedullary guide rod. A standard TKA distal femoral resection guide then is fixated into position. The femoral prosthesis should not be removed at this time. A standard, thick saw blade is used to resect the distal femur at the 9-mm level. It is important to resect all bone visible around the prosthetic system, taking caring to undermine the bone adjacent to the fin of the prosthesis (Fig. 26.10). A small saw blade is used to strip all remaining bone visible around the prosthetic system. A small osteotome then is used to remove the excess bone that has been previously undermined from the initial saw cut.

The femoral prosthesis is 3 mm in thickness and the femoral cutting guide is set at 9 mm; therefore, 5–6 mm of fin and post are exposed by this technique, with the surface of the femoral prosthesis sitting 5–6 mm proud of the distal femoral surface cut (Fig. 26.11). The remaining exposed bone is removed from the fin and the posterior aspect of the femoral

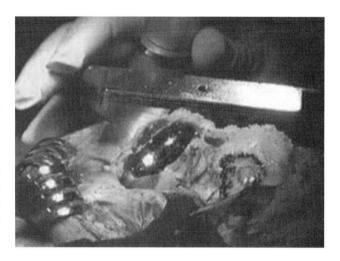

Fig. 26.10 Femoral preparation during conversion of a UKA to a delayed primary TKA. The distal femoral is resected at 9 mm, taking care to resect all bone visible around the femoral component and undermining the bone adjacent to the fin

Femoral Resection Necessary for Conversion to TKA

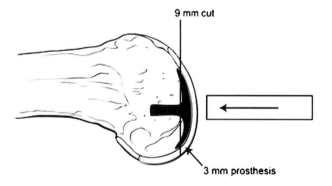

Fig. 26.11 Illustration depicting the femoral resection necessary for conversion to TKA in relation to the thickness of the UKA femoral prosthetic component

prosthesis with a small saw blade. The saw is placed posteriorly along the posterior aspect of the femoral condyle to ensure that the bony interface has been properly exposed.

At this time, any attempt to drive the femoral prosthesis off the femur risks the development of a serious fracture or loss of a significant portion of the femoral condyle. The surface of the prosthesis, therefore, is tapped into the distal femur with a hammer. The post of the prosthesis acts as a punch and is driven somewhat into the bone. The fin serves as an osteotome, allowing disruption of the bone–cement interface without damage to the condyles or bone loss (Fig. 26.12). The femoral prosthesis then is grasped and removed from the femoral condyle without bone loss.

Tibial Preparation

The all-polyethylene inlay tibial component is 6.5 mm in thickness. The standard TKA tibial cutting guide is set at 10 mm for 10 mm of resection. It is not necessary to remove the prosthesis. By simply cutting below it, the medial tibial buttress is preserved, which allows adequate bone support for TKA (Fig. 26.13). This step is performed prior to the final femoral resection to allow adequate space for insertion of the distal femoral resection guide.

Final Femoral Preparation

The distal femoral resection guide is applied using Whiteside's anteroposterior (AP) axis line as a mid-guide due to the

defect in the posterior aspect of the femoral condyle. Standard saw cuts are used to create the necessary distal surfaces. As when performing a standard TKA, it is important to remove the posterior femoral osteophytes.

At this point, the UKA prosthetic system as been removed with minimal bone loss and the appropriate femoral and tibial preparations are complete (Fig. 26.14). The TKA may proceed with insertion of the desired TKA prosthetic design per standard procedures.

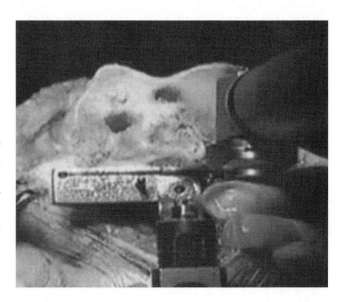

Fig. 26.13 Tibial resection with removal of the UKA tibial prosthetic component

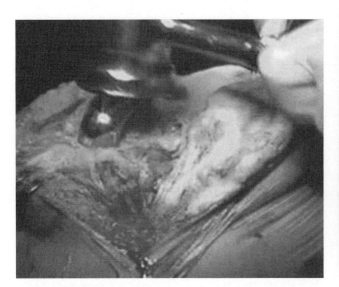

Fig. 26.12 Removal of the UKA femoral prosthetic component, using the post of the prosthesis as a punch and the fin as an osteotome. This technique disrupts the bone–cement interface without damage to the femoral condyles or bone loss

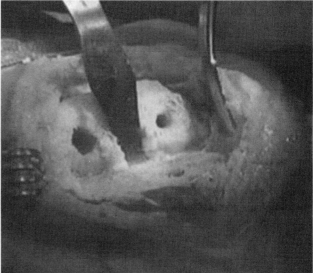

Fig. 26.14 Completion of femoral and tibial preparations in preparation of insertion of the TKA prosthetic system. Because the UKA prosthetic system has been removed with minimal bone loss, this conversion procedure may be considered as a delayed primary TKA

Results

This MIS UKA approach with medial inlay preparation was utilized in a retrospective study comprised of 136 patients classified with Ahlback stages 2, 3, or 4 OA.[31] A resurfacing UKA design, the Repicci II unicondylar knee system, was used in all cases. All patients ambulated with a walker within 4 h after surgery and most (98%) were discharged from the hospital within 23 h. The overall revision rate to TKA was 7% at 8 years. Primary TKA designs were used in the eight cases requiring revision, with good (25%) or excellent (75%) Knee Society clinical ratings at follow-up. These results support the safety and efficacy of this MIS UKA technique, illustrate its decreased recovery and rehabilitation time, and substantiate the relative ease of conversion to TKA, if required.

Conclusion

The senior author's multipronged MIS UKA program results in minimal interference in physiology, lifestyle, and future treatment options. The thorough preoperative clinical and radiographic evaluation, which is corroborated by diagnostic arthroscopy, assists in excluding patients with more advanced stages of OA, for whom TKA is the more appropriate treatment choice, thereby reducing morbidity and increasing survivorship of MIS UKA. Because the MIS surgical approach avoids patellar dislocation and nonessential tissue dissection, interference in physiology is averted, which results in lower morbidity and rapid rehabilitation. The resurfacing UKA design diminishes bone resection compared with other UKA designs and, consequently, does not limit future treatment options. Therefore, this MIS UKA may be used in a broader range of patients, including younger, heavier, or more active patients. Combined with the structured pain management program, MIS UKA may be performed on an outpatient basis, with full independence achieved within 4 h postoperatively. The resulting rapid rehabilitation and return to activities of daily living address patient desire to minimize lifestyle interference, thereby enhancing patient satisfaction.

The long-term survivorship of MIS UKA is variable and dependent on many factors, including the stage of OA at insertion, the amount of tibial bone support, and material limitations, such as polyethylene deformity and wear. However, because the single most important factor affecting UKA survivorship, regardless of design or use of a MIS approach, is precise surgical technique, proper instructional training is critical in ensuring the surgical expertise required for a successful UKA. Although combining a MIS approach with UKA is appealing, due to lower morbidity and decreased rehabilitation, it adds a significant variable to an already demanding surgical procedure. Proper component positioning and accurate cement removal in the face of decreased visualization is essential. However, once the technique is mastered, this UKA bone-sparing technique combined with the multipronged MIS program is a highly desirable treatment option for patients suffering from unicompartmental OA and has a distinctive role in the orthopedic surgeon's knee prosthetic armamentarium.

References

1. Thornhill TS, Scott RD. Unicompartmental total knee arthroplasty. Orthop Clin North Am 1989;20(2):245–256
2. Repicci JA, Hartman JF. Minimally invasive unicondylar knee arthroplasty for the treatment of unicompartmental osteoarthritis: an outpatient arthritic bypass procedure. Orthop Clin N Am 2004;35:201–216
3. Repicci JA, Hartman JF. Unicondylar knee replacement: the American experience. In: Fu FH, Browner BD, editors. *Management of osteoarthritis of the knee: an international consensus*, 1st edition. Rosemont, IL: American Academy of Orthopaedic Surgeons, 2003. pp. 67–79
4. Repicci JA, Eberle RW. Minimally invasive surgical technique for unicondylar knee arthroplasty. J South Orthop Assoc 1999;8(1): 20–27
5. Fithian DC, Kelly MA, Mow VC. Material properties and structure-function relationships in the menisci. Clin Orthop Relat Res 1990 Mar;(252):19–31
6. Grelsamer RP. Current concepts review. Unicompartmental osteoarthrosis of the knee. J Bone Joint Surg Am 1995;77(2):278–292
7. Ihn JC, Kim SJ, Park IH. In vitro study of contact area and pressure distribution in the human knee after partial and total meniscectomy. Int Orthop 1993;17(4):214–218
8. Johnson RJ, Kettelkamp DB, Clark W, et al. Factors affecting late results after meniscectomy. J Bone Joint Surg Am 1974;56(4):719–729
9. Kurosawa H, Fukubayashi T, Nakajima H. Load-bearing mode of the knee joint: physical behavior of the knee joint with or without menisci. Clin Orthop Relat Res 1980 Jun;(149):283–290
10. Shrive NG, O'Connor JJ, Goodfellow JW. Load-bearing in the knee joint. Clin Orthop Relat Res 1978 Mar-Apr;(131):279–287
11. Walker PS, Erkman MJ. The role of the menisci in force transmission across the knee. Clin Orthop Relat Res 1975;(109):184–192
12. Marmor L. Results of single compartment arthroplasty with acrylic cement fixation. A minimum follow–up of two years. Clin Orthop Relat Res 1977 Jan–Feb;(122):181–188
13. Bohm I, Landsiedl F. Revision surgery after failed unicompartmental knee arthroplasty. A study of 35 cases. J Arthroplasty 2000;15(8): 982–989
14. Goodfellow JW, Kershaw CJ, Benson MK, et al. The Oxford knee for unicompartmental osteoarthritis. The first 103 cases. J Bone Joint Surg Br 1988;70(5):692–701
15. Goodfellow JW, Tibrewal SB, Sherman KP, et al. Unicompartmental Oxford meniscal knee arthroplasty. J Arthroplasty 1987;2(1):1–9
16. Kennedy WR, White RP. Unicompartmental arthroplasty of the knee. Postoperative alignment and its influence on overall results. Clin Orthop Relat Res 1987 Aug;(221):278–285
17. Kozinn SC, Scott R. Unicondylar knee arthroplasty. J Bone Joint Surg Am 1989;71(1):145–150
18. Laskin RS. Unicompartmental tibiofemoral resurfacing arthroplasty. J Bone Joint Surg Am 1978;60(2):182–185
19. Marmor L. Marmor modular knee in unicompartmental disease. Minimum four year follow-up. J Bone Joint Surg Am 1979;61(3): 347–353

20. Marmor L. Unicompartmental knee arthroplasty. Ten- to 13-year follow-up study. Clin Orthop Relat Res 1988 Jan;(226):14–20

21. Murray DW, Goodfellow JW, O'Connor JJ. The Oxford medial unicompartmental arthroplasty: a ten-year survival study. J Bone Joint Surg Br 1998;80(6):983–989

22. Squire MW, Callaghan JJ, Goetz DD, et al. Unicompartmental knee replacement. A minimum 15 year follow-up study. Clin Orthop Relat Res 1999 Oct;(367):61–72

23. Stockelman RE, Pohl KP. The long-term efficacy of unicompartmental arthroplasty of the knee. Clin Orthop Relat Res 1991 Oct;(271):88–95

24. Swank M, Stulberg SD, Jiganti J, et al. The natural history of unicompartmental arthroplasty. An eight-year follow-up study with survival analysis. Clin Orthop Relat Res 1993 Jan;(286):130–142

25. Tabor OB, Jr, Tabor OB. Unicompartmental arthroplasty: a long-term follow-up study. J Arthroplasty 1998;13(4):373–379

26. Brown A. The Oxford unicompartmental knee replacement for osteoarthritis. Issues Emerg Health Technol 2001;23:1–4

27. Deshmukh RV, Scott RD. Unicompartmental knee arthroplasty: long-term results. Clin Orthop Relat Res 2001 Nov;(392):272–278

28. Keys GW. Reduced invasive approach for Oxford II medial unicompartmental knee replacement-a preliminary study. Knee 1999; 6(3):193–196

29. Murray DW. Unicompartmental knee replacement: now or never? Orthopedics 2000;23(9):979–980

30. Price A, Webb J, Topf H, et al. Oxford unicompartmental knee replacement with a minimally invasive technique. J Bone Joint Surg Br 2000;82(Suppl 1):24

31. Romanowski MR, Repicci JA. Minimally invasive unicondylar arthroplasty. Eight-year follow-up. Am J Knee Surg 2002;15(1): 17–22

32. Price AJ, Webb J, Topf H, Dodd CA, Goodfellow JW, Murray DW. Rapid recovery after Oxford unicompartmental arthroplasty through a short incision. J Arthroplasty 2001;16(8):970–976

33. Barrett WP, Scott RD. Revision of failed unicondylar unicompartmental knee arthroplasty. J Bone Joint Surg Am 1987;69(9): 1328–1335

34. Padgett DE, Stern SH, Insall JN. Revision total knee arthroplasty for failed unicompartmental replacement. J Bone Joint Surg Am 1991;73(2):186–190

35. Insall J, Dethmers DA. Revision of total knee arthroplasty. Clin Orthop Relat Res 1982 Oct;(170):123–130

36. Lai CH, Rand JA. Revision of failed unicompartmental total knee arthroplasty. Clin Orthop Relat Res 1993 Feb;(287):193–201

37. Rand JA, Bryan RS. Results of revision total knee arthroplasties using condylar prostheses. A review of fifty knees. J Bone Joint Surg Am 1988;70(5):738–745

38. Kozinn SC, Scott RD. Surgical treatment of unicompartmental degenerative arthritis of the knee. Rheum Dis Clin North Am 1988;14(3):545–564

39. Ahlback S. Osteoarthrosis of the knee. A radiographic investigation. Acta Radiol Diagn 1968;277(Suppl):7–72

40. Romanowski MR, Repicci JA. Unicondylar knee surgery: development of the minimally invasive surgical approach. In: Scuderi GR, Tria AJ, Jr, editors. MIS of the hip and the knee: a clinical prospective. New York: Springer, 2004. pp. 123–151

41. Sisto DJ, Blazina ME, Heskiaoff D, et al. Unicompartmental arthroplasty for osteoarthrosis of the knee. Clin Orthop Relat Res 1993 May;(286):149–153

42. Carr A, Keyes G, Miller R, et al. Medial unicompartmental arthroplasty. A survival study of the Oxford meniscal knee. Clin Orthop Relat Res 1993 Oct;(295):205–213

43. Jackson RW. Surgical treatment. Osteotomy and unicompartmental arthroplasty. Am J Knee Surg 1998;11(1):55–57

44. Marmor L. Unicompartmental knee arthroplasty of the knee with a minimum ten-year follow-up period. Clin Orthop Relat Res 1988 Mar;(228):171–177

45. Cartier P, Sanouiller JL, Grelsamer RP. Unicompartmental knee arthroplasty surgery. 10-year minimum follow-up period. J Arthroplasty 1996;11(7):782–788

46. Christensen NO. Unicompartmental prosthesis for gonarthrosis. A nine-year series of 575 knees from a Swedish hospital. Clin Orthop Relat Res 1991 Dec;(273):165–169

47. Voss F, Sheinkop MB, Galante JO, et al. Miller-Galante unicompartmental knee arthroplasty at 2- to 5-year follow-up evaluations. J Arthroplasty 1995;10(6):764–771

48. Berger RA, Nedeff DD, Barden RM, et al. Unicompartmental knee arthroplasty. Clinical experience at 6- to 10-year follow-up. Clin Orthop Relat Res 1999 Oct;(367):50–60

49. Bert JM. 10-year survivorship of metal-backed, unicompartmental arthroplasty. J Arthroplasty 1998;13(8):901–905

50. Capra SW, Jr., Fehring TK. Unicondylar arthroplasty. A survivorship analysis. J Arthroplasty 1992;7(3):247–251

51. Hawker GA, Wright JG, Coyte PC, et al. Determining the need for hip and knee arthroplasty: the role of clinical severity and patients' preferences. Med Care 2001;39:206–216

52. Knutson K, Lewold S, Robertsson O, et al. The Swedish knee arthroplasty register. A nation-wide study of 30,003 knees 1976–1992. Acta Orthop Scand 1994;65:375–386

53. Scott RD, Cobb AG, McQueary FG, et al. Unicompartmental knee arthroplasty. Eight- to 12-year follow-up evaluation with survivorship analysis. Clin Orthop Relat Res 1991 Oct;(271):96–100

54. Keblish PA. The case for unicompartmental knee arthroplasty. Orthopedics 1994;17:853–855

55. Repicci JA, Hartman JF. Minimally invasive surgery for unicondylar knee arthroplasty: the bone-sparing technique. In: Scuderi GR, Tria AJ, Jr, Berger RA, editors. MIS techniques in orthopedics. New York: Springer Science + Business Media, Inc., 2006. pp. 193–213

56. Kapandji IA. The physiology of the joints, 5th edition, volume 2. New York: Churchill Livingstone, 1987

Chapter 27
Minimally Invasive Surgery for Unicondylar Knee Arthroplasty: The Intramedullary Technique*

Richard A. Berger and Alfred J. Tria

Minimally invasive surgery (MIS) for unicondylar knee arthroplasty (UKA) was instituted in the early 1990s by John Repicci.[1,2] While there had been a long history of UKA dating back to the early 1970s,[3–6] the techniques and surgical approaches were modeled after total knee arthroplasty (TKA). The results were not equal to TKA and many surgeons abandoned the procedure. The MIS approach introduced a new method to perform the surgery and helped to improve the results by emphasizing the differences between TKA and UKA. MIS forced the surgeon to consider UKA as a separate operation with its own techniques and its own principles.

Preoperative Planning

The preoperative evaluation of the patient should include the history, physical examination, and X-ray. It is critical to choose the correct patient for the operation and to observe the limitations that it imposes. The patient should identify a single compartment of the knee as the primary source of the pain. The physical examination should correlate with the history. Tenderness should be isolated to one tibiofemoral compartment and the patellofemoral exam should be negative. The posterior cruciate and collateral ligaments should be intact with distinct endpoints. The literature suggests that the anterior cruciate ligament (ACL) should be intact;[7] however, the authors will accept some ACL laxity when implanting a fixed bearing UKA. If a mobile bearing device is planned, the ACL should be intact or the knee should have enough

R.A. Berger (✉) and A.J. Tria
Department of Orthopedic Surgery, Rush–Presbyterian–St. Luke's Medical Center, 1725 West Harrison Street, Suite 1063, Chicago, IL 60612, USA
e-mail: r.a.berger@sbcglobal.net

*Adapted from Berger RA, Tria AJ, Jr., Minimally invasive surgery for unicondylar knee arthroplasty: the intramedullary technique, in Scuderi GR, Tria, AJ, Jr., Berger RA (eds.), MIS Techniques in Orthopedics, 2006, with kind permission of Springer Science + Business Media.

anterior to posterior stability to eliminate the need for the ACL. Any existing varus or valgus deformity does not have to be completely correctable to neutral; but the procedure is more difficult to perform with fixed deformity. The range of motion in flexion should be greater than 105°.

The standing X-ray is the primary imaging study (Fig. 27.1). While it is ideal to have a full view of the hip, knee, and ankle, it is not absolutely necessary. The 14 × 17-in. standard cassette allows measurement of the anatomic axes of the femur and the tibia, which will permit adequate preoperative planning for the surgical procedure. An anteroposterior flexed knee view (notch view) is helpful to rule out any involvement of the opposite condyle. The patellar view, such as a Merchant, will allow evaluation of that area of the knee and will confirm that there is no significant malalignment. The lateral X-ray is used to further judge the patellofemoral joint and to measure the slope of the tibial plateau (Fig. 27.2). The tibial slope can vary from 0 to 15° and can be changed during the surgery to adjust the flexion-extension gap balancing.

The X-rays are important guidelines for the surgery. The varus deformity should not exceed 10°; the valgus should not exceed 15°; and the flexion contracture should not exceed 10°. It is ideal if the varus or valgus deformity corrects to neutral with passive stress. Deformities outside these limits will require soft tissue releases and corrections that are not compatible with UKA. There should be minimal translocation of the tibia beneath the femur (Fig. 27.3) and the opposite tibiofemoral compartment, and the patellofemoral compartment should show minimal involvement. Translocation indicates that the opposite femoral condyle has degenerative changes and this will certainly compromise the clinical result. While Stern and Insall indicated only 6% of all patients satisfy the requirements for the UKA,[8] the authors have found the incidence to be approximately 10–15%. This incidence is, however, decreasing as the minimally invasive TKAs are beginning to flourish. It is best to observe the strict limitations for the procedure because it will insure a higher rate of success in the cases that are performed.

Magnetic resonance imaging (MRI) is sometimes helpful for evaluation of an avascular necrosis of the femoral condyle or to confirm the integrity of the meniscus in the opposite

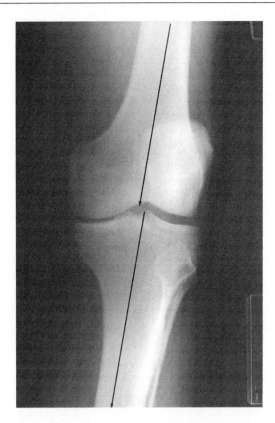

Fig. 27.1 Anteroposterior standing X-ray of a left knee (From Choi YJ, Tanavalee A, Chan A, et al. Unicondylar knee arthroplasty: Surgical approach and early results of the minimally invasive surgical approach, in Scuderi GR, Tria AJ Jr, (eds.), MIS of the Hip and the Knee: A Clinical Perspective. New York, Springer, 2004, with kind permission of Springer Science + Business Media.)

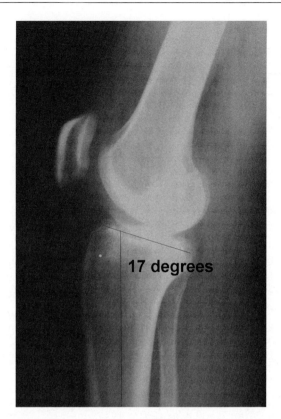

Fig. 27.2 Lateral X-ray of the knee showing a 17° tibial slope (From Choi YJ, Tanavalee A, Chan A, et al. Unicondylar knee arthroplasty: Surgical approach and early results of the minimally invasive surgical approach, in Scuderi GR, Tria AJ Jr, (eds.), MIS of the Hip and the Knee: A Clinical Perspective. New York, Springer, 2004, with kind permission of Springer Science + Business Media.)

compartment when the patient complains of an element of instability. However, MRI is not necessary on a routine basis.

Scintigraphic studies are sometimes helpful to identify the extent of involvement of one compartment versus the other. However, once again, this is not a routine diagnostic test.

Surgical Technique (Intramedullary Approach)

The operation can be performed with epidural, spinal, or general anesthesia. Femoral nerve blocks have become very popular but the authors do have some hesitation concerning the technique because of the occasional associated motor block that inhibits the patient's ability to move the knee through active range of motion immediately after the surgical procedure. It is important that the anesthesia team understands that the patients will be required to walk and begin physical therapy within 2–4 h of the completion of the operation and the anesthesia must be in harmony with this approach

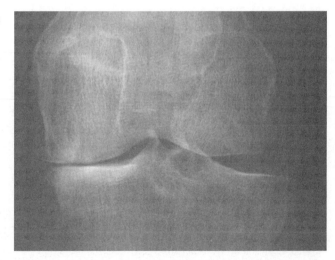

Fig. 27.3 Translocation of the lateral tibial spine contacting the lateral femoral condyle on a standing anteroposterior X-ray of the knee. This is a relative contraindication to UKA (From Choi YJ, Tanavalee A, Chan A, et al. Unicondylar knee arthroplasty: Surgical approach and early results of the minimally invasive surgical approach, in Scuderi GR, Tria AJ Jr, (eds.), MIS of the Hip and the Knee: A Clinical Perspective. New York, Springer, 2004, with kind permission of Springer Science + Business Media.)

and with possible discharge to home on the day of the surgical procedure.

The surgery is usually performed with an arterial tourniquet; however, this is not mandatory. The limited MIS incision necessitates continuous repositioning of the knee. The surgeon should be prepared for this and the authors have found that a leg-holding device facilitates the exposure (Fig. 27.4).

The incision is made on either the medial or the lateral side of the patella (depending on the compartment to be replaced) at the superior aspect and is carried distally to the tibial joint line. It is typically 7- to 10-cm long. The incision should not be centered on the joint line because this will

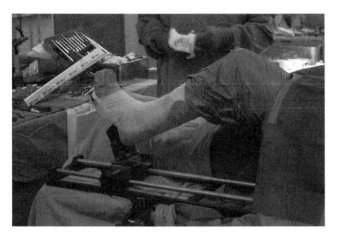

Fig. 27.4 The leg holder (Innovative Medical Products, Inc., Plainville, Connecticut) allows flexion and extension of the knee along with internal and external rotation (From Choi YJ, Tanavalee A, Chan A, et al. Unicondylar knee arthroplasty: Surgical approach and early results of the minimally invasive surgical approach, in Scuderi GR, Tria AJ Jr, (eds.), MIS of the Hip and the Knee: A Clinical Perspective. New York, Springer, 2004, with kind permission of Springer Science + Business Media.)

limit the exposure to the femoral condyle. In the varus knee, the arthrotomy is performed in a vertical fashion and the authors initially included a short, transverse cut in the capsule approximately 1–2 cm beneath the vastus medialis (Fig. 27.5). The capsular extension is helpful when the surgeon's experience is limited and when exposure is difficult in the "tight" knee. With greater experience, the extension is not necessary. The transverse cut is not a subvastus approach and is an incision in the capsule of the knee midway between the vastus medialis and the tibial joint line. The deep MCL is released on the tibial side to improve the exposure of the joint. The release is not performed for the purposes of alignment correction. This is the beginning of the divergence of the UKA from the TKA surgery. It is important to remember that the surgery is only performed on one side of the joint. The goal of the surgery is to replace one side and to balance the forces so that the arthroplasty and the opposite compartment share the weight bearing equally. If the medial ligamentous complex is released, there is the potential for overloading the opposite side, with resultant pain and failure.

In the lateral UKA, the "T" extension is not necessary. The vertical incision is taken down to the tibial plateau and the iliotibial band (ITB) is sharply released from Gerdy's tubercle and elevated posteriorly (Fig. 27.6). The arthrotomy is closed in a vertical fashion and the ITB is left to scar down to the tibial metaphysis.

The patella is not everted in the procedure and the vastus medialis is not violated either by a dividing incision or a subvastus approach. The sparing of the surrounding soft tissue structures and the preservation of the extensor mechanism in its entirety makes the procedure minimally invasive.

With the completion of the arthrotomy, the peripheral osteophytes should be removed from the femoral condyle and the tibial plateau. All compartments of the joint should

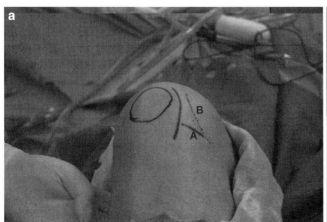
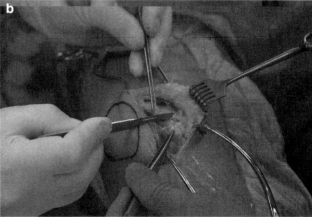

Fig. 27.5 (**a**) The medial incision extends from the top of the patella to just below the tibial joint line (*A*). *B* is the outline of the margin of the medial femoral condyle. (**b**) The medial arthrotomy can include a "T" in the capsule (made with the tip of the knife blade) (From Scuderi GR, Tria AJ Jr, MIS of the Hip and the Knee: A Clinical Perspective. New York, Springer, 2004, with kind permission of Springer Science + Business Media.)

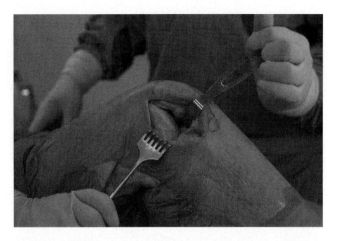

Fig. 27.6 The lateral view of a right knee shows the anterior tibial joint line after the iliotibial band has been released and retracted posteriorly (From Choi YJ, Tanavalee A, Chan A, et al. Unicondylar knee arthroplasty: Surgical approach and early results of the minimally invasive surgical approach, in Scuderi GR, Tria AJ Jr, (eds.), MIS of the Hip and the Knee: A Clinical Perspective. New York, Springer, 2004, with kind permission of Springer Science + Business Media.)

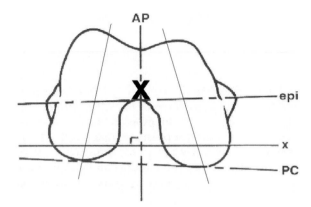

Fig. 27.7 The intramedullary hole is located just above the roof of the intercondylar notch (marked with the letter "*X*") (Adapted from Choi YJ, Tanavalee A, Chan A, et al. Unicondylar knee arthroplasty: Surgical approach and early results of the minimally invasive surgical approach, in Scuderi GR, Tria AJ Jr, (eds.), MIS of the Hip and the Knee: A Clinical Perspective. New York, Springer, 2004, with kind permission of Springer Science + Business Media.)

be inspected. It is not unusual to see some limited arthritic involvement in the other compartments of the knee. The preoperative evaluation should be thorough enough to preclude a conversion to a TKA. Diagnostic arthroscopy is not necessary but can sometimes be included to confirm the anatomy of the opposite side in an unusual case. The addition of this procedure should be undertaken with care to avoid the possibility of increasing the associated infection rate.

The intramedullary technique requires an entrance hole centered just above the roof of the intercondylar notch (Fig. 27.7). The intramedullary canal is suctioned free of its contents to decrease fat embolization and the instrument is set into the canal. The depth of the distal femoral cut affects the extension gap and also the anatomic valgus of the distal femur (Fig. 27.8). The angle (or tilt) of the cut determines the perpendicularity of the component to the tibial plateau surface in full extension (Fig. 27.9). This angle can be precisely determined by measuring the difference between the anatomic and mechanical axis of the knee on long standing X-ray films. In the clinical setting, the authors arbitrarily choose a 4° angle for the varus knee and a 6° angle for the valgus knee.

Flexion contractures of the knee can be corrected with the medial UKA but not with the lateral replacement. If there is a flexion contracture and the distal anatomic femoral valgus is 5° or less in the varus knee, the standard amount of bone is removed to be replaced millimeter for millimeter with the prosthesis. If the distal femoral valgus is 6° or more in the varus knee, 2 mm of additional bone is removed from the distal femur to decrease the excess valgus and to increase the space in full extension. Increasing the space in full extension helps to correct the flexion contracture and enables the surgeon to decrease the associated depth of the tibial cut.

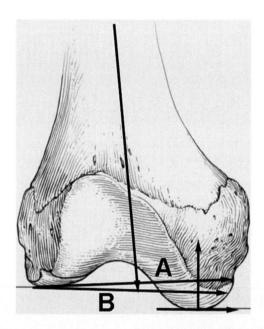

Fig. 27.8 The two cuts on the medial femoral condyle show that the deeper resection (line "*A*") results in less valgus than line "*B*" (3° versus 5°). This also allows for more space in full extension (From Tria AJ, Klein KS. An Illustrated Guide to the Knee. New York, Churchill Livingstone, 1992, with permission of Elsevier, Inc.)

The deeper femoral cut saves 2 mm of bone on the tibial side and results in a total distal femoral resection of 8 mm. The resection does not elevate the femoral joint line as it would in a TKA. Most TKA femoral components remove a minimum of 9 mm for the prosthesis so that this change does not adversely affect revision to a TKA.

In the valgus knee, the maximum acceptable deformity is 15° and the distal femur is cut millimeter for millimeter for replacement. The deformity will be slightly decreased with a

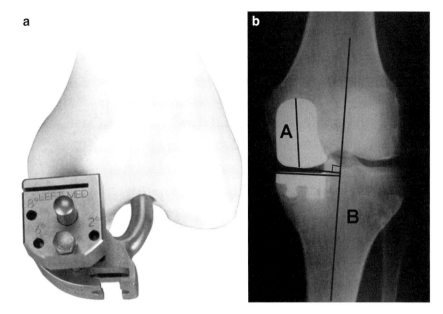

Fig. 27.9 (**a**) The intramedullary guide allows for a distal cut of 2, 4, 6, or 8°. This setting adjusts the angle of the femoral component with relation to the tibial plateau cut surface. It does not adjust the overall varus or valgus of the knee because it is only cutting one condyle. (**b**) The femoral component "tilt" is defined as the angle between the long axis of the component (line "*A*") referenced to the axis of the tibial shaft (line "*B*"). (**a**, From Berger RA, Tria AJ Jr, Minimally invasive surgery for unicondylar knee arthroplasty: the intramedullary technique, in Scuderi GR, Tria AJ Jr, Berger RA (eds.), MIS Techniques in Orthopedics, 2006, with kind permission of Springer Science + Business Media.)

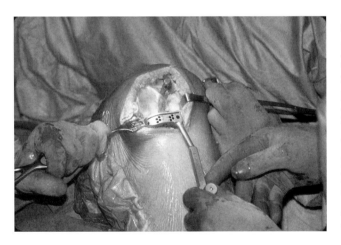

Fig. 27.10 The tibial cut is complete with an extramedullary guide (From Berger RA, Tria AJ Jr, Minimally invasive surgery for unicondylar knee arthroplasty: the intramedullary technique, in Scuderi GR, Tria AJ Jr, Berger RA (eds.), MIS Techniques in Orthopedics, 2006, with kind permission of Springer Science + Business Media.)

standard resurfacing because the prosthesis and the cement mantle are slightly thicker than the bone that is removed. Because the lateral femoral condyle is less prominent than the medial condyle in full extension, flexion contractures cannot be corrected as easily on the lateral side. A deeper cut on the lateral femoral condyle will only increase the distal femoral valgus without changing the extension gap significantly.

After completing the distal femoral cut, it is easier to proceed to the tibial preparation because this in turn opens up the space in 90° of flexion and makes the femoral finishing cuts much easier. The tibial cut is made with an extramedullary instrument (Fig. 27.10). In the MIS setting, intramedullary instrumentation is difficult on the tibial side without everting the patella. The tibial cut can be angled from anterior to posterior. Most systems favor a 5–7° posterior slope for roll back. The slope of the cut also affects the flexion–extension balancing. The balancing is not the same as the techniques for TKA. In the UKA surgery, the flexion gap is usually larger than the extension gap because of the flexion contracture that is present in almost all arthritic knees. As the flexion contracture increases to 10°, the extension gap becomes tighter. If the slope of the tibial cut is decreased from the anatomic slope of the preoperative tibial X-ray, the cut can be made deeper anteriorly to give greater space in extension while maintaining the same flexion gap posteriorly (Fig. 27.11). This is the alternate technique for flexion contracture correction if the distal femoral valgus is normal at 5° or less.

With the completion of the tibial cut, the remainder of the femoral cuts can be completed with the appropriate blocks for guidance of the saws. An intramedullary retractor can be used to retract the patella (Fig. 27.12). The femoral runner should be a slight bit smaller than the original femoral condyle surface and it should be perpendicular to the tibial plateau at 90° of flexion and centered medial to lateral on the condyle. If the femoral condyle divergence is extreme in 90° of flexion, the femoral component should be positioned perpendicular to the tibial cut surface (parallel to the long axis

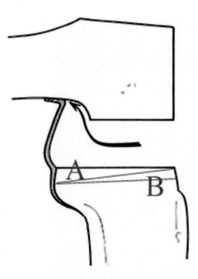

Fig. 27.11 The slope of the tibial cut can be changed to correct flexion-extension imbalance. The flexion gap is often larger than the extension gap. The cut "*A*" can be lowered anteriorly and the slope decreased to line "*B*," which will equalize the gaps. (From Berger RA, Tria AJ Jr, Minimally invasive surgery for unicondylar knee arthroplasty: the intramedullary technique, in Scuderi GR, Tria AJ Jr, Berger RA (eds.), MIS Techniques in Orthopedics, 2006, with kind permission of Springer Science + Business Media.)

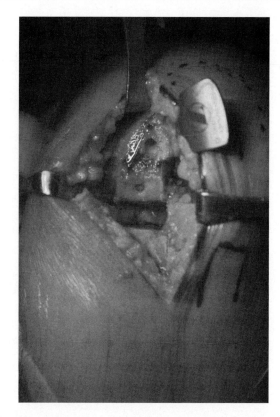

Fig. 27.12 The intramedullary retractor is useful to visualize the joint (labeled with "*Z*")

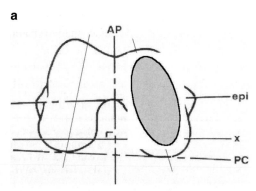

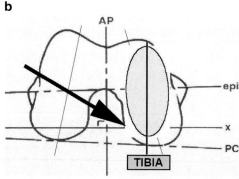

Fig. 27.13 (**a**) If the femoral component is aligned with the cut articular surface of the femur, the divergence of the condyles may be too great and the subsequent position may lead to edge loading on the polyethylene tibial insert. (**b**) The femoral component should be perpendicular to the tibial insert even if this leads to a non-anatomic position on the femoral surface and slight overhang of the component into the intercondylar notch

of the tibia). This positioning may result in some overhang of the femoral runner into the intercondylar notch (Fig. 27.13).

The tibial tray should cover the entire cut surface out to the cortical rim without overhang on the medial or lateral side of the tibia. The component is not inlayed and any degree of varus positioning should be avoided. The inlay technique depends upon the subchondral bone surface for support and if this is violated during the tibial preparation, sinkage of the component will certainly follow. Varus inclination can lead to early component loosening and should be avoided.

Once the cuts are completed, the flexion–extension gap should be tested with the trial components in position. In the ideal case, there should be 2 mm of laxity in both positions (Fig. 27.14). It is best not to over tighten the joint and to accept greater rather than less laxity. Excess tightness may lead to early polyethylene failure and also contributes to increase pressure transmission to the opposite side. Three separate items determine the overall varus or valgus of the knee: the depth of the tibial cut, the tibial polyethylene thickness, and the depth of the femoral cut. The tibia can be cut

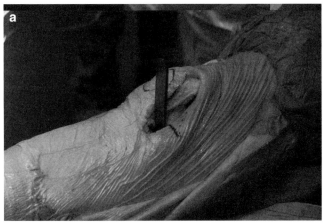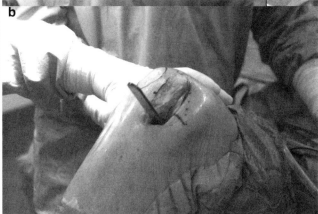

Fig. 27.14 (**a**) The tongue depressor is 2-mm thick and demonstrates the proper laxity in full extension of the knee. (**b**) The tongue depressor demonstrates the matching proper laxity in 90° of flexion (From Choi YJ, Tanavalee A, Chan A, et al. Unicondylar knee arthroplasty: Surgical approach and early results of the minimally invasive surgical approach, in Scuderi GR, Tria AJ Jr, (eds.), MIS of the Hip and the Knee: A Clinical Perspective. New York, Springer, 2004, with kind permission of Springer Science + Business Media.)

exactly perpendicular and the distal femoral cut can be set in 4° of valgus; but with the insertion of an excessively thick polyethylene, the knee can be shifted into 6 or more degrees of valgus and overcorrected despite properly aligned bone cuts. In the setting of the TKA, changing the thickness of the tibial insert affects spacing in full extension and 90° of flexion but it does not affect the varus or valgus of the knee, which remain the same.

If the UKA spacing is not symmetric, the tibial cut should be altered. Typically, the extension space will be smaller than the flexion space. This can be corrected by starting the tibial cut slightly deeper on the anterior surface and decreasing the slope angle. Once again, in TKA, the extension space is easily increased by removing more bone from the distal femur. In UKA, deepening the femoral cut will change the distal femoral valgus and will also increase the size of the component because the anteroposterior surface will be increased. This may lead to poor bone contact with the new femoral component and possible early loosening. Thus, it is best to modify the spacing with changes on the tibial side. If the space in extension is larger than the flexion space, this usually means that the slope of the tibial cut was made too shallow and the slope should just be increased.

After testing the components for stability, range of motion, and flexion–extension balance, the final components are cemented in place. Cementless fixation for UKA has not been very successful and the authors do not recommend that approach. When the tibial component is a modular design, the metal tray can be cemented in place first and this allows excellent visualization of the posterior aspect of the joint and also allows more space for the femoral component cementing. The all-polyethylene insert does give more thickness to the prosthesis. However, the thicker polyethylene blocks visualization for the cementing; and, if full thickness

polyethylene failure occurs, the exchange will require invasion of the underlying tibial bone. The modular tibial tray allows polyethylene exchange without bone invasion and backside wear is not a problem in UKA surgery. The femoral runner is cemented after the tibial tray, and the polyethylene is inserted last.

The tourniquet is released before the closure and adequate hemostasis is established. The closure is completed in the standard technique with special attention to be sure that the vastus medialis is well reattached to the patella to allow early and rapid range of motion of the knee.

At the time of the closure, the posterior capsule and the surrounding structures can be infiltrated with anesthetic agents to help with the early postoperative physical therapy.

Results

At present there are few reports using the MIS surgical approach. Berger's report[9] included a 10-year follow-up with 98% longevity using standard open arthrotomy techniques. The average age of the patients was 68 years old and the indications for the procedure were quite strict. His second report extended the follow up to 13 years with a survival rate of 95.7%.[10] Price reported early follow-up of an abbreviated incision for UKA with good results.[11] He compared 40 Oxford UKAs using an MIS-type incision with 20 Oxford UKAs performed with a standard incision. The average rate of recovery of the MIS UKAs was twice as fast. The accuracy of the implantation was evaluated using 11 variables on fluoroscopically centered postoperative X-rays and was found to be the same as the open UKAs. Price concluded that more rapid recovery was possible with less morbidity. The technique did not compromise the final result of the UKA. Repicci reported on 136 knees with 8 years of follow-up using the MIS technique.[2] There were ten revisions (7%): three for technical errors, one for poor pain relief, five for advancing disease, and one for fracture. The revisions for technical errors occurred from 6 to 25 months after surgery. The revisions for advancing disease occurred from 37 to 90 months after surgery. Repicci concluded that MIS UKA is "... an initial arthroplasty procedure (that) relieves pain, restores limb alignment, and improves function with minimal morbidity without interfering with future TKA."

The senior author has performed 385 UKAs using the Miller-Galante Unicondylar Knee Arthroplasty (Zimmer, Warsaw, IN). Fifty-seven patients underwent UKA in the first year (2000). Forty-one (72%) patients have 2 or more years of follow up.[12] There were 24 women and 17 men, including six bilateral surgeries, four simultaneous, and two staged 6–8 weeks apart. There were 47 knees, 45 varus and 2 valgus. The average age was 68 years old, with a range from 42 to 93 years. Ten patients (30%) were younger than age 60 years and eight patients (20%) were older than age 75 years. The average weight was 189 pounds. The range of motion went from 120° before the operation to 132° after the surgery. One knee was converted to a TKA because of patellar subluxation occurring 9 months after the surgery. The revision was performed at 14 months after the original TKA. One knee was revised to a TKA 5 years after the original surgery because of increasing patellofemoral arthritis. One patient sustained an undisplaced tibial plateau fracture 2 weeks after surgery and this healed without intervention. All patients obtained their full range of motion within 3 weeks. The overall revision rate is 2 (4%) of 47 knees at 6 years after surgery.

In the entire group of 385 UKAs that have been performed since 2000, there have been seven revisions. Five of these revisions were for advancing patellofemoral arthritis, one was for the patellar subluxation mentioned previously, and one was for a femoral component loosening. The femoral component failed because it was too large and impinged upon the patellofemoral joint. While these are very early results, most of the series with poor results started to see the failures within the first 2–5 years following the procedure.

Conclusions

The results of UKA have improved steadily since the late 1990s. The MIS technique has fostered better results and has helped to set UKA apart from TKA in the minds of the operating surgeons. The intramedullary instrumentation has been well adapted to the MIS technique. As the prosthetic designs and surgical techniques continue to improve, MIS UKA should have results similar to those of TKA in the first 10–15 years and give patients a choice before TKA that will permit greater activity and improved quality of life without compromising the result of a later TKA.

References

1. Repicci JA, Eberle RW. Minimally invasive surgical technique for unicondylar knee arthroplasty. J South Orthop Assoc 8(1): 20–27, 1999
2. Romanowski MR, Repicci JA. Minimally invasive unicondylar arthroplasty, eight year follow-up. J Knee Surg 15(1): 17–22, 2002
3. Marmor L. Marmor modular knee in unicompartmental disease. Minimum four-year follow-up. J Bone Joint Surg Am 61A(3): 347–353, 1979
4. Insall J, Walker P. Unicondylar knee replacement. Clin Orthop Relat Res ; (120): 83–85, 1976 Oct
5. Laskin RS Unicompartment tibiofemoral resurfacing arthroplasty. J Bone Joint Surg Am 60A: 182–185, 1978
6. Goodfellow J, O'connor J. The mechanics of the knee and prosthesis design. J Bone Joint Surg Br 60B: 358–369, 1978
7. Goodfellow JW, Kershaw CJ, Benson MK, O'Connor JJ. The Oxford knee for unicompartmental osteoarthritis. The first 103 cases. J Bone Joint Surg Br 70: 692–701, 1988
8. Stern SH, Becker MW, Insall J. Unicompartmental knee arthroplasty. An evaluation of selection criteria. Clin Orthop Relat Res 286: 143–148, 1993
9. Berger RA, Nedeff DD, Barden RN, Sheinkop MN, Jacobs JJ, Rosenberg AG, Galante JO. Unicompartmental knee arthroplasty. Clin Orthop Relat Res 367: 50–60, 1999
10. Berger RA, Meneghini RM, Jacobs JJ, Sheinkop MB, Della Valle CJ, Rosenberg AG, Galante JO. Results of unicompartmental knee arthroplasty at a minimum of ten years of follow-up. J Bone Joint Surg Am 87: 999–1006, 2005
11. Price AJ, Webb J, Topf H, Dodd CAF, Goodfellow JW, Murray DW, Oxford Hip and Knee Group. Rapid recovery after Oxford unicompartmental arthroplasty through a short incision. J Arthroplasty 16: 970–976, 2001
12. Gesell MW, Tria AJ, Jr. MIS unicondylar knee arthroplasty: surgical approach and early results. Clin Orthop Relat Res 428: 53–60, 2004

Chapter 28
The Extramedullary Tensor Technique for Unicondylar Knee Arthroplasty*

Paul L. Saenger

The extramedullary (EM) tensor tools and surgical technique were developed to orient cutting guides for the implantation of the M/G unicompartmental prosthesis with greater ease and accuracy and to reduce the surgical morbidity of this limited reconstruction. Unicompartmental knee replacement attempts to reduce pain and improve function by restoring the extremity's alignment and the joint's soft tissue balance with the positioning of an implant limited to that compartment. All unicompartmental implants, be they monoblock wafers, mobile bearing devices, or fixed articular prostheses, must effect this restoration to enjoy whatever success they may provide.

Various surgical techniques for their implantation are available. Instrument systems without direct linkage of the femoral and tibial cuts require intuitive estimates. With such a technique, the implant must, in effect, be retrofitted. The cuts are made and then a device of a given volume and width is chosen that best fits the flexion and extension gaps created. Those cuts were not predetermined for a given implant and thus are approximations. Approximations can work well should there be unlimited prosthetic sizes from which to choose.

The relationship between the bone cuts and the subsequent insertion of an implant with its particular geometry filling the created extension and flexion gaps, it should be remembered, is the key to the angular and soft tissue balance one is attempting to achieve. Instruments now exist that allow the anticipated cuts to be positioned relative to a knee's corrected posture. There is a direct relationship such that the cuts made are specific for a given implant's dimensions. The EM tensor technique herein described uses patented instrumentation with direct linkage, referencing off the femur and tibia simultaneously. Knowing the dimensions of the intended implant in both extension and flexion allows then the use of cutting guides that create spatial dimensions, that is, extension and flexion gaps, to accommodate a particular composite implant.

The Tensor

The tensor device is an adjustable interposed spacer with incorporated tibial and femoral cutting surfaces that is positioned in extension between the femur and tibia while their articular surfaces are held in a corrected position. The space to be created for a given implant can then be made with a specific width and slope oriented at will prior to setting the surface cutting guides. The relationship of the two cut surfaces is set with respect to a preachieved correction of the soft tissue tension and overall limb alignment (Fig. 28.1).

Predetermined flexion and extension gaps lesson the need to modify or compensate for an imbalance potentially created by guesswork. The need for subsequent *eyeball* revisions is reduced. Alignment instruments that measure first and cut second attempt to eliminate the inaccuracies and secondary complexities of the bone preparation.

Minimally Invasive Surgery

Central to developing the EM tensor system was the desire to lessen the morbidity associated with this limited reconstruction. The invasiveness of any surgical procedure is certainly more than the length or the incision. In the case of knee reconstruction, the extent of the quadriceps division, the intrusion of the intramedullary canal,[1,2] or the use of a tourniquet add to the morbidity of the effort. To avoid or limit such compromising elements is the goal of MIS. The tensor technique requires a small skin incision, usually 4–7 cm,

P.L. Saenger (✉)
Private Practice, Blue Ridge Bone & Joint Clinic,
PA, 129 McDowell Street, Asheville, NC, 28801, USA
e-mail: kcherry@brbj.com

*Adapted from Saenger PL, Minimally invasive surgery for unicondylar knee arthroplasy: The extramedullary approach, in Scuderi GR, Tria AJ, Berger RA (eds.), MIS Techniques in Orthopedics, 2006, with kind permission of Springer Science+Business Media.

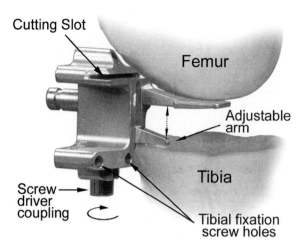

Fig. 28.1 The tensor device

a modest division of the vastus medialis oblique (VMO), no intrusion of the intramedullary canal, and there is no need for a tourniquet.

The instruments and implants detailed in this chapter will likely be soon replaced with new versions. However, the concept and use of artificial implants that adhere to the host bone so as to anatomically reconstruct articular surfaces will likely endure. Their surgical implantation will require an ever more accurate and less morbid technique. Understanding the nature of this implant, the Zimmer M/G unicompartmental, and its attendant EM tensioning instrumentation and technique is apropos to the consideration of future developments.

The Implant

Unicompartmental knee reconstruction using femoral and tibial implants that mimic the original geometry of the host articular surfaces and that are secured to cut bone with cement has been shown to offer reliably good to excellent results.[3–8] Several series have demonstrated the M/G unicompartmental (Zimmer, Inc., Warsaw, IN) prosthesis to offer success for at least 10 years equal to or better than total knee arthroplasty (TKA) in middle aged or older populations.[9–11] The prosthesis consists of a biconvex chrome cobalt femoral component with three precoated backside facets. It is cemented to three matching cut femoral bone surfaces; planed cuts that determined the implant's position and orientation. The tibial implant, either monoblock or modular, is available in incremental widths of 8, 10, 12, and 14 mm. It, too, is cemented to a cut, planed surface (Fig. 28.2).

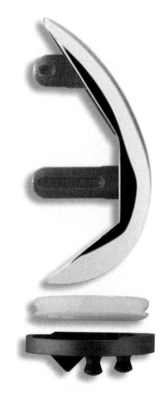

Fig. 28.2 The M/G unicompartmental prosthesis

Measure First, Cut Second

Regardless of future navigational aids for yet-to-be-designed implants, the procedure will likely require orienting the bone preparation for a given implant relative to a specifically corrected and thereafter maintained joint and limb posture.

The tensor technique uses a space-filling tensioner that serves as an adjustable expansive unit between the femur and tibia that maintains the corrected alignment and tissue balance in extension. With that done, the femoral and tibial cutting blocks, using shared fixation screws, are set so as to create a space equal to the intended implant's composite width. The orientation of the surfaces to be cut can be accurately established. As presently configured, those surfaces are parallel to one another in the coronal plane. In the sagittal plane, the slope on the tibia is adjustable to 3, 5, or 7°. These cut surface relationships could be readily altered if it is determined to be otherwise optimal (Fig. 28.3a, b).

How Much Correction?

Occasionally, unicompartmental pathology does not involve significant deformity of the joint space and thus the alignment and tissue balance is intact. In that case, maintaining the existing

a   **b**

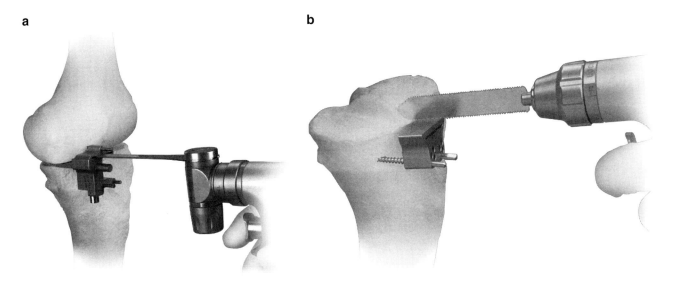

Fig. 28.3 (**a**) The tensor serves as the distal femoral cutting block held with tibial fixation screws that then (**b**) support and orient the tibial cutting block

dynamic geometric relationships is a fundamental goal of the procedure. More often, with the eccentric loss of articular and meniscal cartilage seen in unicompartmental disease, the knee falls into varus or valgus. This intraarticular loss secondarily affects the ligamentous stability. By restoring the intraarticular spacing, the ligaments are again tensioned. Assuming there is no soft tissue contracture, replacing the lost cartilage and bone with an implant of equal dimensions should restore both the joint's soft tissue tension and overall alignment relative to the mechanical and anatomical axes.

Alignment and soft tissue balance are critical to the success of TKAs, too. However, it must be understood that the alignment of the extremity as a whole in TKA is a function of the angle of the cuts. That is not true for unicondylar knee arthroplasty (UKA). For instance, in TKA, a 6° femoral cut combined with a standard 0° cut on the tibia can be expected to result in a femoral-tibial angle of 6°. Varying the thickness of the plastic insert will affect the soft tissue tension but not the angle of the extremity's alignment.

Varying the thickness of the insert in a UKA directly affects the soft tissue tension as well. But, unlike the TKA, in a UKA it is an eccentric variation and changes the alignment, too. In that sense, it is similar to the angular alteration seen with wedge resection or insertion used in high tibial osteotomies (HTO). However, unlike HTO, a unicompartmental insert is intraarticular and thus the addition of a thicker implant will, once the soft tissues are already snug, *overstuff* the joint. Too wide a prosthesis creates intraarticular compressive forces detrimental to not only the implant, but to the uninvolved compartment as well and can be expected to be deleterious to both.[12] It is very important to avoid *overstuffing*

the joint throughout its arc of movement from extension to flexion.

The mechanical axis of the lower extremity is that line that passes through the center of the hip, knee, and ankle. This system assumes that a mechanical axis of 0° is a reference point, not a target. It is thought that knees that fall into varus for want of medial cartilage were likely in some varus relative to a 0° mechanical axis even before the pathology notably altered the alignment. Thus, to force that knee to 0° would presumably go beyond what was once normal and in so doing would tighten the medial ligaments beyond their norm. Therefore, when using the mechanical axis as a guide, the correction will typically fall slightly short of full correction to 0°.[13]

While the two, alignment and soft tissue tension, are directly related and can each be used to help assess the correction, it is the latter, the soft tissue tension, that is thought to be most critical. Until such time as a more sophisticated method of measuring intracompartmental pressure is used, the present system relies on the manual and visual perceptions of the surgeon such that a valgus stress (or varus in the case of lateral reconstruction) should allow approximately 2 mm of opening. Regardless of the alignment, if the ligaments are too tight and the knee *overstuffed*, the long-term success of the procedure is likely to be compromised.

In the author's experience, most knees thought to be appropriate for this procedure can be adequately corrected without soft tissue release. Indeed, for many knees, there may be little or no angular or ligamentous deformity. However, in selected cases, a correction toward an improved alignment and appropriate soft tissue tension requires the release of the soft tissue contracture (Fig. 28.4a, b).

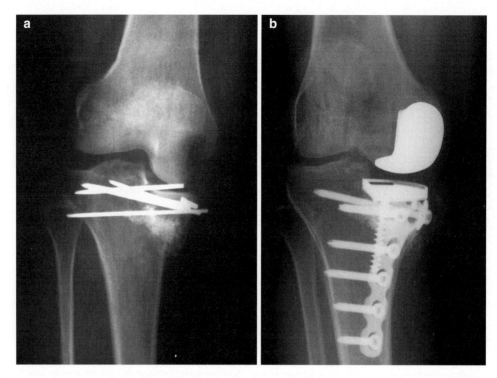

Fig. 28.4 (a) Nonunion with varus 9 months after inadequate fixation of a medial tibial plateau fracture in a 51-year-old woman. (b) Four-year postoperative X-ray of a unicompartmental reconstruction with soft tissue release for a contracture using a Sulzer Natural Knee Uni. Preoperative range of motion (ROM), 5–65°; postoperative ROM, 3–122°

Surgical Technique

Medial unicompartmental degenerative joint disease can be seen as a disease of extension.[14] Cartilage loss on the femur, for instance, is often minimal on the posterior condyle where it articulates with the tibia in flexion. Rather, the more profound compromise occurs on the distal end of the condyle in the area that articulates with the tibia as the knee extends. Genu varum is an extension deformity. The correction to be made is in extension (Fig. 28.5).

Keying off the distal femur with a cutting guide that allows the reestablishment of the appropriate joint line, the EM tensor, a variable spacing block inserted into the involved compartment, is adjusted to maintain a corrected extension alignment. Secured to both femur and tibia by shared fixation posts, coordinated cutting blocks serve to allow the distal femoral and then the tibial cuts to be made in a directly linked fashion that will prepare this predetermined space to be filled by an anticipated implant (Fig. 28.6a–e).

With the extension pathology restructured, it is time to balance the flexion gap. It is important that the knee not be compromised in flexion by overtensioning or undertensioning the flexion gap with inappropriate bone preparation or inaccurate femoral sizing. To avoid that complication, a gauge is used to predict the ensuing flexion gap. This ensures that the

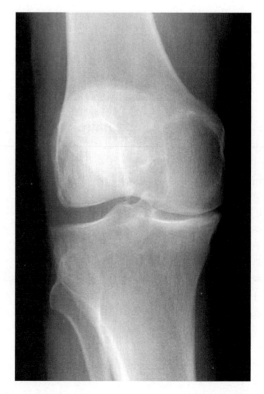

Fig. 28.5 X-ray of medial degenerative joint disease (DJD) with varus deformity

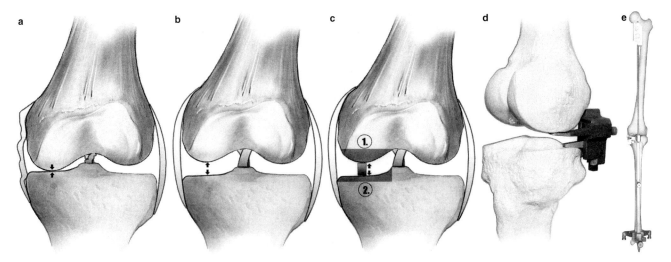

Fig. 28.6 (**a**) The narrowed medial compartment is opened until (**b**) the medial ligaments are tensioned. (**c**) The space is filled with the tensor. (**d**) Setting parallel cuts (1 and 2) for the intended implant. (**e**) Attached alignment rods confirm orientation

subsequent cut on the posterior femur combined with the cut already made on the tibia creates a flexion space whose soft tissue tension is consistent with that established for extension.

The EM tensor technique is intended to follow sequential steps. Altering the sequence may compromise the end result. With experience, the procedure can be regularly accomplished with a 4- 7-cm skin incision, the extent of which has the potential to shrink further with future innovation.

Given the restricted space, the intact ligaments, and the modest incision, adequate exposure requires that the limb be postured and manipulated in specific ways to facilitate the various steps. For instance, knee extension relaxes the quad mechanism and allows displacement of the patella not possible with even slight flexion with the VMO intact. Thus, certain steps are best done in full extension whereas other steps require flexion to as much as 120°. In that case, maintaining a valgus stress while holding the leg externally rotated for a medial reconstruction will, along with the wise use of retractors, enhance greatly the exposure.

The following description of the surgical technique reflects one surgeon's way of doing things. It represents a considered effort to minimize the morbidity and ensure proper implant positioning. It involves obtaining a preoperative anteroposterior (AP) hip X-ray with markers over the hip joint in an effort to determine accurately the mechanical axis as a reference point for limb alignment. Also, the use of a tourniquet is thought to be unnecessary. That unicompartmental procedures are routinely done successfully without X-rays and with tourniquets is recognized. It is also known that large numbers of prosthetic devices of this and similar design have been implanted with reported good results using indirectly linked cutting or measuring guides. That is a credit

to the skill and understanding of those surgeons implanting the prosthesis. It also suggests the potential and adaptability of these secured implants. The EM tensor technique was developed to lessen the guesswork by providing accurate, reproducible cuts with minimally invasive instruments that can diminish many of the complexities inherent to this procedure.

The great majority of unicompartmental reconstructions are done medially and, of those, most are in middle-aged to older men and women with a narrowed medial compartment secondary to osteoarthritis as seen on physical examination and standing X-rays. The procedure is thus described for that compartment with that pathology in mind and assumes some varus misalignment with associated medial ligament laxity that allows correction without soft tissue release. The steps of the procedure are the same whether this deformity is a little or a lot. Lateral reconstruction is essentially the same other than the incision is made lateral to the patella.

Surgical Steps

Incision

The length and position of the incision is dependent on the exposure required for certain surgical steps done in flexion (Table 28.1). In extension, the arthrotomy is a window that can be moved about for better viewing. In flexion, however, the quad is tight and the patella locked into the trochlea. Knowing what must be seen in flexion, that is, the anterior aspect of the distal femur down to the tibial joint line just medial to the patellar tendon, can then serve to guide the

Table 28.1 Surgical steps for extramedullary tensor technique for unicondylar knee arthroplasty

1. Incision
2. Removal of the anterior boss of the tibia
3. Alignment correction
4. Distal femoral cut
5. Tibial cuts
6. Flexion and extension gaps
7. Anterior femoral marking
8. Femoral finishing guide sizing and positioning
9. Tibial sizing and finishing
10. Testing and cementing

proximal and distal extent of the skin and retinaculum incision.

Therefore, with the knee flexed, an incision is made slightly medial to the midline from near the superior pole of the patella to just a few millimeters below the joint line. Likewise, divide the medial retinaculum and fat pad. Excise a portion of the fat pad in the area along with the anterior third of the meniscus. Use electrocautery for hemostasis. Excise osteophytes found on the femur, tibia, and patella. For exposure now and whenever the knee is flexed, use a 90° bent sharp Hohmann retractor positioned in the notch and a similar retractor or two along the medial tibia. Importantly, this also protects the cruciates and medial collateral ligament (MCL) while using saw blades (Figs. 28.7 and 28.8).

Removal of the Anterior Boss of the Tibia

Positioning and manipulating the tensor is made easier by removing the anterior tibial boss normally encountered. With the reciprocating saw, make a 2- or 3-mm-deep cut along the medial edge of the tibial spine parallel to the tibial axis. Then, with the oscillating saw, remove the tibial boss perpendicular to the tibial axis to a depth of approximately 3 mm. This additional space makes easier the insertion of the spacer arms and also improves the interface between the active (it moves) tibial arm and the surface of the anterior tibial plateau (Fig. 28.9).

Alignment Correction

The tensor and alignment rods are positioned with the knee in extension. To ease their assembly, put the tensor into the joint with the connecting tower attached. Clamp the tibial alignment rod to the distal leg with the locking screws loose so as to allow multidirectional adjustments. Now, insert the tibia's square alignment rod into the square hole in the tower by manipulating the tensor and tower with the round femoral rod held proximally (Fig. 28.10).

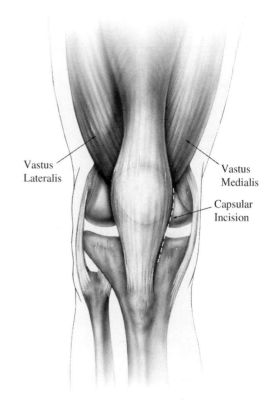

Fig. 28.7 The incision

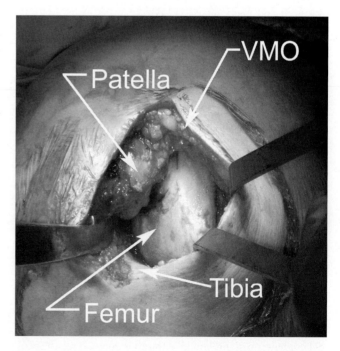

Fig. 28.8 The exposure in flexion. *VMO* vastus medialis oblique

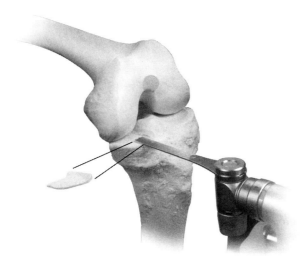

Fig. 28.9 Excise the anterior tibial boss

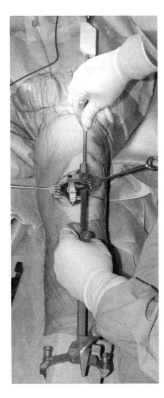

Fig. 28.10 Assemble the tensor device, connecting tower, and rods

With that done, align the tibial rod parallel to the tibia in both the AP and lateral planes and tighten the locking screws (Fig. 28.11). So doing determines the orientation but not yet the depth of the tibial cut. The femoral rod should now, in the uncorrected varus knee, project lateral to the marked femoral head. Manually correct the varus with a valgus stress until the soft tissue tension feels snug. Do not force the knee

beyond this point. The femoral rod typically still projects lateral to the femoral head, but only slightly (Fig. 28.12).

While maintaining this manual correction in extension, have an assistant turn the tensor screw to expand the spacer until contact is felt, implying that the space within the joint created with the manipulation is now filled with the spacing device. Release the manual stress to see that the correction is maintained and that the soft tissue tension is not excessive. If satisfied, position a collared screw in the proximal femoral hole and then two uncollared screws (posts) into the tibia.

Distal Femoral Cut

Remove the tower and rods, leaving the spacer and distal femoral cutting guide in place. Using an angled retractor medially and a skin retractor along the patella, resect the distal femur with the oscillating saw. The knee is in extension so be wary of soft tissue injury as the posterior extent of the cut is approached. Remove the femoral collared screw, retract the tensor, and slide the tensor off the retained tibial screws (posts) (Fig. 28.13).

Tibial Cuts

While still in extension so as to accommodate a small incision, position the tibial cutting block of choice (3, 5, or 7° slope) at the desired level (8, 10, 12, or 14 mm) and secure it with a Kocher clamp to each uncollared screw (post). Now flex the knee to 90° so as to relax and protect the posterior soft tissues. Manipulate the leg into valgus and external rotation and then position the retractors.

First, with the reciprocating saw blade just inside the notch in the sagittal plane, cut down to the cutting block. Leave the blade in place to serve as a visual and physical guide for the lateral extent of the ensuing cut. Now, with the oscillating saw, make the sloped cut of the tibial plateau between the protected cruciates and MCL (Fig. 28.14a, b).

Flexion and Extension Gaps

The femoral component's sizing and placement keys off the posterior condyle. Therefore, it is important to confirm that the yet-to-be-created flexion gap corresponds to the established extension gap before sizing the femoral component. This is done with the paired extension/flexion gap gauges. If at this time the space is found to be tight, before committing to the posterior condylar cut and its concomitant prosthetic width, open up the flexion gap by shaving off the necessary cartilage and bone from the posterior condyle. Now size the femur. It is easy to adjust the flexion gap before sizing and finishing the femoral cuts. It is difficult to do so afterward (Fig. 28.15a, b).

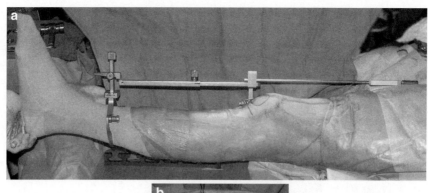

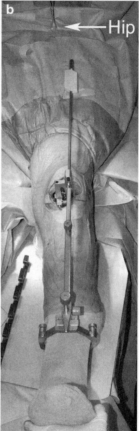

Fig. 28.11 The tibial rod is aligned parallel to the tibia in the (**a**) AP and (**b**) ML planes

First check the extension gap with an extension gap gauge. It is the thicker end that is equal to the composite width of a given femoral and tibial implant. Determine the one that is optimal in establishing the desired alignment and soft tissue balance. Presumably and usually this corresponds to the cut chosen for the tibia, that is, 8 or 10 mm as a rule. Whatever composite width is chosen, 8, 10, 12, or 14, be sure the flexion gap then accommodates those projected components by inserting the thinner end of the gauge, the width of which corresponds to the intended tibial component only. If the flexion gap is tight, unless the posterior reference point for the femoral guide is moved anteriorly, the implant when

implanted recreates the tight space. Thus, if tight, resect the cartilage and occasionally bone necessary to adequately open up the flexion space.

Anterior Femoral Marking

It is time now for sizing and positioning the femoral component. For that to be done accurately requires clear visualization of the entire cut distal surface of the femur. Doing so in flexion is compromised anteriorly by the tight quad and patella. However, while in extension and the quad relaxed,

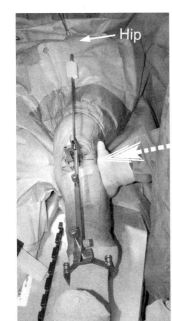

Fig. 28.12 Manually correct the alignment

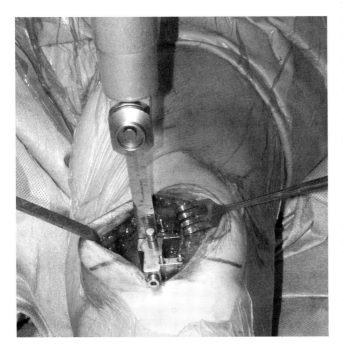

Fig. 28.13 Cut the distal femur

the entire cut surface is readily seen. Taking advantage of this clear view in extension, a mark can be made anteriorly on that cut distal surface that corresponds to where the femoral

finishing guide should go. Then, when the knee is next brought into flexion, only this mark need be seen, not the entire distal femoral cut surface. This reduces the need for a more extended division of the quad mechanism or the displacement of the patella (Fig. 28.16a, b).

Also, an advantage of marking the femur in extension for subsequent positioning of the finishing guide is the ability to center the anterior femoral component relative to the cut tibial surface. If the cuts and post holes for the femoral component are centered in extension and then next in flexion relative to the tibial cut surface, the components will be presumably centered upon one another throughout the arc of motion to, thus, avoid edge loading of the tibial plastic.

Femoral Finishing Guide Sizing and Positioning

Having marked the anterior femur with a Bovie or pen in extension, flex the knee to 90° and position the retractors. Choose the femoral finishing guide that, when keyed off the posterior condyle, has an anterior screw hole that corresponds to the mark. If in doubt as to which size fits best, choose the smaller size to avoid having the femoral implant extend beyond the cut femoral surface anteriorly where it might impinge on the patella.

Secure the guide anteriorly with a collared screw through the hole overlying the mark. With the knee still flexed, rotate the posterior aspect of the guide to a position that again centers it over the cut tibial surface. This typically is accomplished by lining up the notch side of the guide to the very edge of the notch side of the femoral cut surface, that is, rotate the guide to the extreme lateral edge of the femoral cut surface. With the guide secured posteriorly with one or two screws, the post holes are drilled, the chamfer cut is made, and then lastly, the posterior condyle. Remove the anterior screw and then the guide with its attached posterior condylar fragment (Fig. 28.17a–d).

With all cuts now made, visualization of the posterior aspect of the compartment is maximized. First, remove the remaining medial meniscus and then debride the posterior condyle with a curved osteotome to assure an unrestricting flexion recess.

Tibial Sizing and Finishing

Determine optimal coverage of the tibial cut surface with the sizing paddles. If in between sizes, cut away from the tibial spine the small amount necessary to accommodate the larger size. Impact that provisional plate into place and drill the holes. Impacting the plate will tend to push it posteriorly. Stabilizing the plate first with a short screw anteriorly can prevent this displacement (Fig. 28.18a, b).

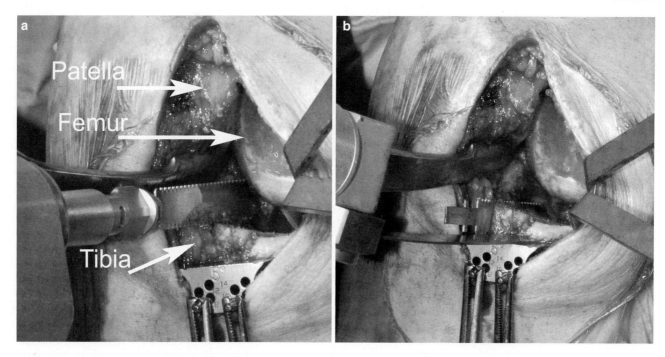

Fig. 28.14 (a) With the reciprocating saw just lateral to the medial condyle, cut down to the tibial cutting block. (b) Leave the blade in place and protect the MCL with retractors for the oscillating saw cut

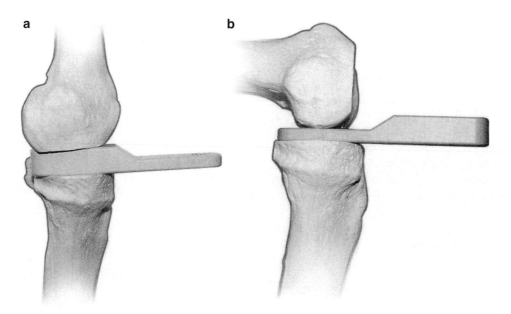

Fig. 28.15 (a) Extension and (b) flexion gauges

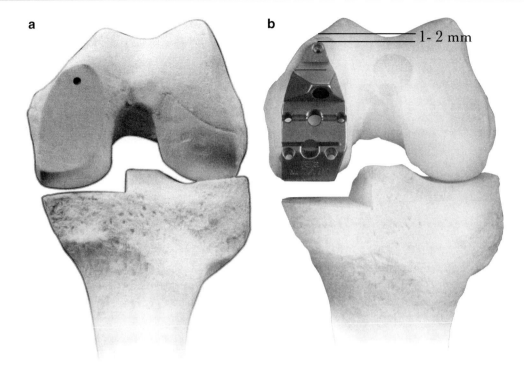

Fig. 28.16 (**a**) Mark the anterior femur at the (**b**) intended screw fixation site

Trialing and Cementing

The knee is flexed with the tibial plate in place. With a small incision and a patella that is not displaced, positioning of the trial femoral component, and later the prosthesis, is challenging. It is made easier by flexing the knee to 120° while maintaining a valgus and external rotational stress. With the femoral trial rotated away from the patella, place the longer posterior post into its hole in the femur and impact it slightly. Then slowly extend the knee until the patella is lax enough to allow the trial to be rotated into place beneath it. With the shorter anterior post aligned with its hole, impact the trial fully.

Flexing and stressing the knee once again, slip the plastic trial into place. In extension, the limb alignment should be noted. Of particular importance is to again check that the tissue balance is proper. For a given set of implants, it is thought that in both flexion and extension a valgus stress should produce approximately 2 mm of opening. A 2-mm-wide tension gauge is available. Do not accept a tight space. If all cuts

were made in the sequence described, that should not at this point be a problem. Nonetheless, check the tension carefully. Also, check to see that the femoral component tracks centrally over the tibial implant through its arc of motion and confirm that there is no trochlear impingement (Fig. 28.19a–d).

Having checked for debris, cleanse the cut bone surfaces with pulsatile lavage, dry, and then impact over cement the tibial implant with the knee in flexion. A valgus and external rotation stress to the leg improves viewing the extraction of excess cement using a small curved spatula.

For the femoral component, again flex the knee to 120° and position the femoral implant as previously described. With the posterior post positioned first, extend the knee until the shorter post can be rotated into place and then impacted fully. Remove all excess cement. Now insert the chosen plastic and prop the foot so as to maintain the knee in extension while the cement hardens. Insertion of a drain and closure of the wound can commence at this time (Fig. 28.20).

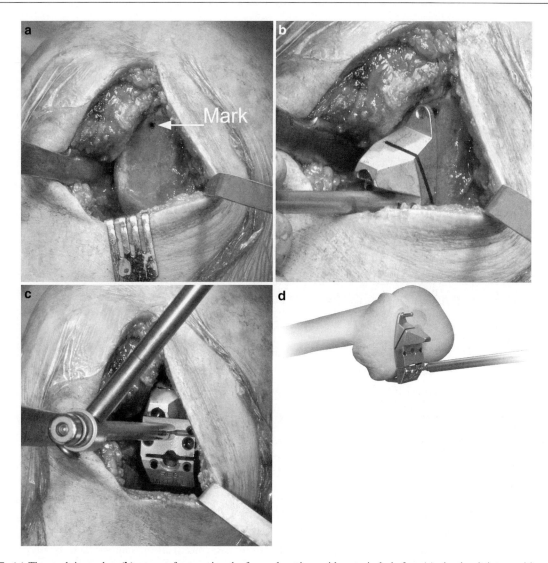

Fig. 28.17 (**a**) The mark is used as (**b**) a target for securing the femoral cutting guide anteriorly before (**c**) pivoting it into position posteriorly and (**d**) securing it with screws

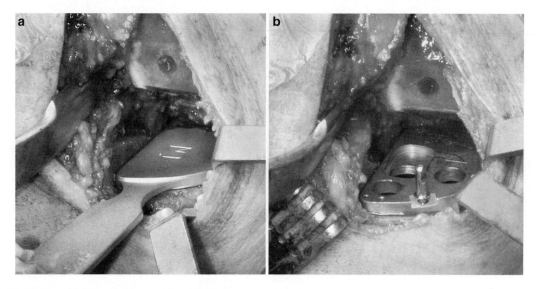

Fig. 28.18 (**a**) Size and (**b**) secure the provisional tibial plate

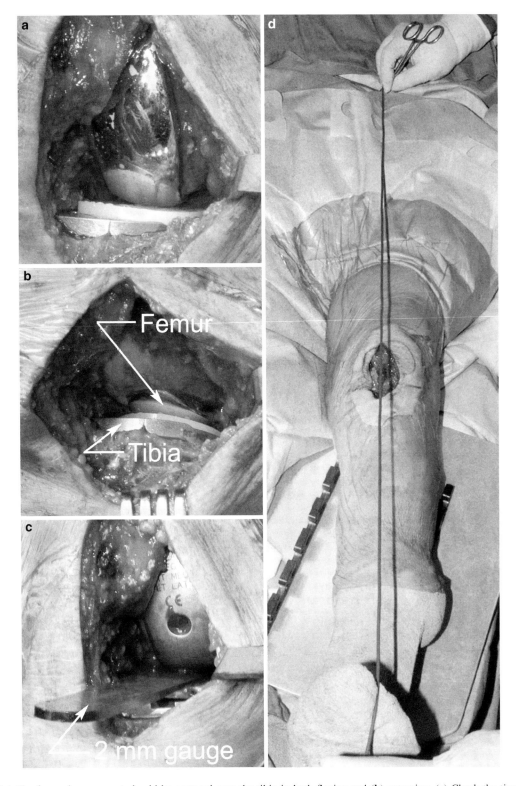

Fig. 28.19 (**a**) The femoral component should be centered over the tibia in both flexion and (**b**) extension. (**c**) Check the tissue tension and (**d**) the limb alignment

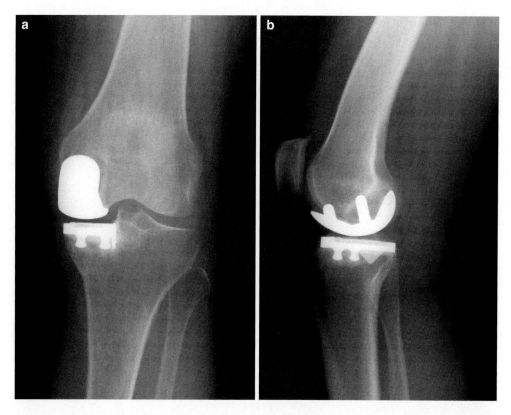

Fig. 28.20 Postoperative (**a**) AP and (**b**) lateral X-ray of an M/G unicompartmental knee

Conclusion

Implants such as the M/G unicompartmental prosthesis are known to work well for an intermediate time, at least. With improved materials and optimal designs, it is assumed that longer-term success can be achieved. Meanwhile, the challenge is to develop surgical techniques that will further diminish the morbidity of the implantation while enhancing the surgeon's ability to better align and balance the knee. The EM tensor technique using linked femoral and tibial cuts oriented after the alignment and soft tissue correction has been achieved with modestly sized EM instruments is consistent with those goals.

References

1. Caillouette JT. Fat embolism syndrome following the intramedullary alignment guide in total knee arthroplasty. Clin Orthop Relat Res 1990; 251: 198–199
2. Kolettis GT. Safety of one-stage bilateral total knee arthroplasty. Clin Orthop Relat Res 1994; 309: 102–109
3. Hasegawa Y, Opishi Y, Shimizu T. Unicompartmental knee arthroplasty for medial gonarthrosis: 5 to 9 years follow-up evaluation of 77 knees. Arch Orthop Trauma Surg [Germany] 1998; 117(4–5): 183–187
4. Murray DW, Goodfellow JW, O'Connor JJ. The Oxford medial unicompartmental arthroplasty: a ten-year survival study. J Bone Joint Surg (Br) 1998; 80(6): 983–989
5. Newman JW, Ackroyd DE, Shah NA. Unicompartmental or total knee replacement? Five-year results of a prospective, randomized trial of 102 osteoarthritic knees with unicompartmental arthritis. J Bone Joint Surg (Br) 1998; 80(5): 862–865
6. Tabor OB Jr, Tabor OB. Unicompartmental arthroplasty; a long-term follow-up study. J Arthroplasty 1998; 13(4): 373–379
7. Marmor L. Unicompartmental knee arthroplasty: ten to thirteen year follow-up study. Clin Orthop Relat Res 1988; 226: 14
8. Scott RD. Unicompartmental knee arthroplasty. Clin Orthop Relat Res 1991; 271: 96–100
9. Berger RA, Nedeff DD, Barden RM, et al. Unicompartmental knee arthroplasty: clinical experience at 6- to10-year follow up. Clin Orthop Relat Res 1999; 367: 50–60
10. Argenson JN, Chevrol-Benkeddache Y, Aubniac JM. Modern cemented metal-backed unicompartmental knee arthroplasty: a 3 to 10 year follow-up study. 68th annual Meeting of the American Academy of Orthopaedic Surgeons, 2001
11. Pennington DW, Swienckowski JJ, Lutes WB. Unicompartmental knee arthroplasty in patients sixty years of age or younger. J Bone Joint Surg 2003; 85A: 1968–1973

12. Laskin RS. Unicompartmental tibiofemoral resurfacing arthroplasty. J Bone Joint Surg 1978; 60: 182–185
13. Cartier P, Sanouiller JL, Dreisamer RP. Unicompartmental knee arthroplasty: 10-year minimum follow-up period. J Arthroplasty 1996; 11970: 782–788
14. Romanowski MR, Repicci JA. Technical aspects of medial versus lateral minimally invasive unicondylar arthroplasty. Orthopedics 2003; 26: 289–293

Suggested Readings

Philip Gavin. The History Place. http://www.historyplace.com. 4 July 1996
Scott Kurnin. 20th Century Timeline. About. http://www.history1900s.com. February 1997
Joanne Freeman. Timeline of the Civil War. http://www.memory.loc.gov/ammam/cwphtml/cwphone.html. 15 January 2000

Chapter 29
MIS Unicondylar Knee Arthroplasty with the Extramedullary Technique*

Giles R. Scuderi

Minimally invasive surgery (MIS) unicondylar knee arthroplasty has gained popularity over the recent years following the introduction of the limited approach by Repicci and Eberle.[1] Their limited approach was essentially a freehand technique that used limited instrumentation. Over the years there have been modifications in the surgical instruments in order to perform the procedure accurately and reproducibly through a MIS approach. The Miller Galante Unicondylar prosthesis (Zimmer, Warsaw, IN) introduced intramedullary instrumentation and most recently extramedullary instrumentation.[2] The smaller and reliable modified instruments clearly help in bone preparation and component position producing clinical results that are comparable with a conventional procedure.[3,4] Improved instrumentation allows the surgeon to operate through a minimally invasive arthrotomy, without everting the patella, and permits more accurate bone resection. It is the refinements in instrumentation that have contributed to successful clinical results.

General Principles

Alignment in unicondylar knee arthroplasty is determined by femoral and tibial bone resection, and not soft tissue release. Since soft tissue releases to correct deformity are not performed, if the varus or valgus deformity exceeds 15° or if there is a flexion contracture greater than 10°, a total knee arthroplasty should be considered. In unicondylar knee arthroplasty, overcorrection of the knee should be avoided, because this overloads the contralateral compartment and increases the potential for progression of the degenerative arthritis.

G.R. Scuderi (✉)
Director, Insall Scott Kelly Institute for Orthopaedics and Sports Medicine, Attending Orthopedic Surgeon, Assistant Clinical Professor of Orthopedic Surgery, North Shore-LIJ Health System, Albert Einstein College of Medicine, New York, NY, USA
e-mail: GScuderi@iskinstitute.com

*Adapted from Scuderi GR, Minimally invasive surgery for unicondylar knee arthroplasty: the extramedularly technique, in Scuderi GR, Tria AJ, Berger RA (eds.), *MIS Techniques in Orthopedics*, 2006, with kind permission of Springer Science + Business Media.

Reports have shown that slight undercorrection of the knee alignment is correlated with long-term survivorship.[5,6]

The advantage of extramedullary instrumentation in MIS is that it eliminates the need for violation of the femoral intramedullary canal. Extramedullary instruments are designed to provide a means of achieving precision in limb alignment. With the limb aligned in extension, the deformity may be passively corrected. By coupling an extramedullary femoral and tibial guide, the angle of resection for the distal femur and the proximal tibia can be determined, creating a parallel resection of the femur and tibia in extension. The linked cuts are perpendicular to the mechanical axis of the femur and tibia, respectively.

Approach

The skin incision is made with the knee in flexion and begins from the superior pole of the patella to 1–2 cm distal to the joint line. This straight incision is placed along the medial border of the patella for a medial unicondylar replacement. A limited medial parapatellar capsular arthrotomy is performed, extending from the lower border of the vastus medialis to a point just distal to the joint line along the proximal tibia. To aid visualization, the fat pad is excised along with the anterior horn of the medial meniscus. Subperisoteal dissection is then carried out along the proximal medial tibia, releasing the meniscal tibial attachment, but not releasing the medial collateral ligament. A curved retractor is then placed along the medial tibial border to protect the collateral ligament. Medial tibial and femoral osteophytes are removed along with any osteophytes along the femoral intercondylar notch. With the spacer block technique, the tibia is prepared first.[2]

For a lateral unicondylar replacement, the skin incision is made along the lateral border of the patella. The arthrotomy is a lateral capsular incision that extends from the superior pole of the patella, along the lateral border of the patella and patella tendon, and 1–2 cm distal to the joint line. The lateral fat pad can be excised to aid visualization. The meniscal tibial attachment is released and a curved retractor is placed along the lateral border of the tibia. Similar to a medial unicondylar replacement, the tibia will be prepared first.

G.R. Scuderi and A.J. Tria (eds.), *Minimally Invasive Surgery in Orthopedics*,
DOI 10.1007/978-0-387-76608-9_29, © Springer Science + Business Media, LLC 2010

Tibial Preparation

The tibia is resected with an extramedullary tibial cutting guide. The shaft of the resection guide is set parallel to the tibial shaft. The proximal cutting head is secured to the tibia and the depth and slope of resection is determined. A depth gauge is used so that 2–4 mm of bone is removed from the lowest point on the tibial plateau. Once the desired depth of resection is determined, a retractor is placed medially to protect the medial collateral ligament. With the knee flexed, the proximal tibia is resected (Fig. 29.1). Caution must be taken not to undercut the attachment of the anterior cruciate ligament and the lateral tibial plateau. With a reciprocating saw, the sagittal tibial cut is made in line with the medial wall of the intercondylar notch down to the level of the transverse cut. The resected tibial bone is then removed. The gap is checked with a spacer block to ensure that appropriate amount of bone has been resected and that the axial alignment is correct (Fig. 29.2). If the gap is too tight with the spacer block in place, additional bone should be resected from the proximal tibia. If the gap is too loose, a thicker spacer block, which correlates to a thicker tibial component, should be inserted.

Femoral Preparation

Following resection of the proximal tibia, the knee is brought into full extension and the 8-mm spacer block, or the appropriately sized spacer block as determined above, is inserted into the joint space. It should be fully inserted and sit flat on the resected tibia to ensure that the proper amount of distal femur will be resected (Fig. 29.3). If there is any difficulty inserting the 8-mm spacer block, then additional bone needs to resected from the proximal tibia. In contrast, if the 8-mm spacer block is too loose, then a thicker spacer block should be inserted.

With the appropriate spacer block in place and the knee in extension, the alignment tower is attached so that the position of the guide can be checked relative to the center of the femoral head (Fig. 29.4). The alignment tower is then removed and the distal femoral resection guide is attached to the spacer block (Fig. 29.5), which is then secured to the distal femur. The distal femur can be resected in full extension, but caution must be taken not to over cut the distal femur and have the saw blade extend beyond the posterior capsule and into the popliteal area. If desired, the femoral cut can be started in extension and finished in flexion. Once the distal femur is resected, the extension gap is checked with a spacer block and alignment rod (Fig. 29.6).

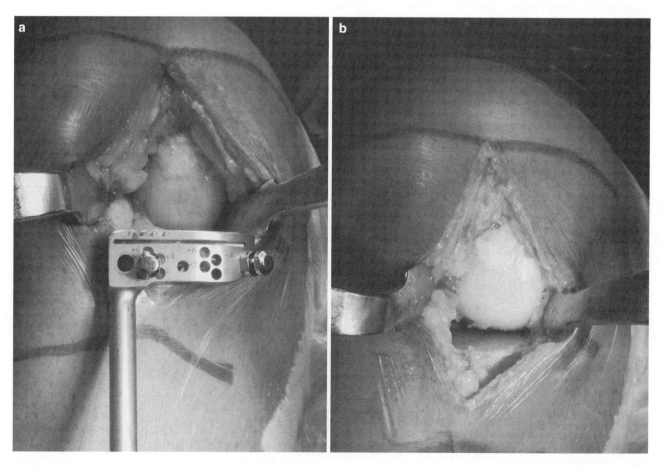

Fig. 29.1 Resection of the proximal tibia with the extramedullary guide (**a**); resected tibia (**b**)

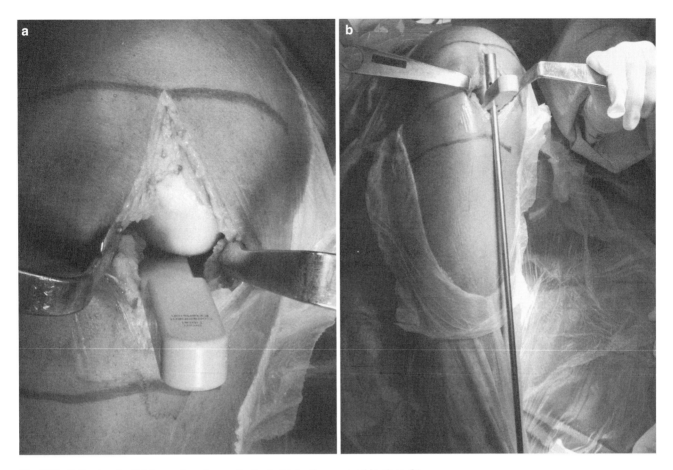

Fig. 29.2 Following the tibial resection, the gap is checked (**a**); alignment rod in place (**b**)

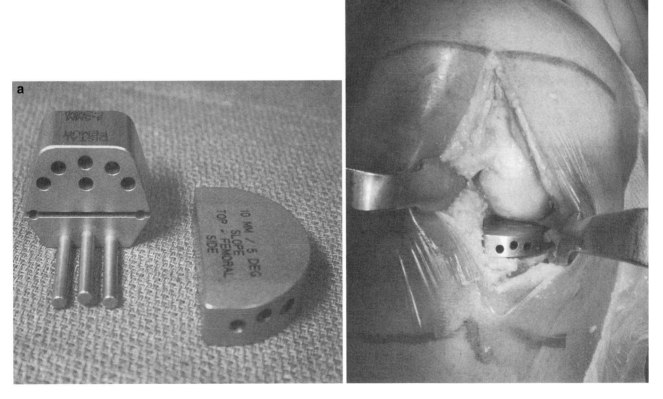

Fig. 29.3 The spacer block (**a**) is inserted into the joint on the resected tibia (**b**)

Fig. 29.4 The alignment tower is attached to the spacer block

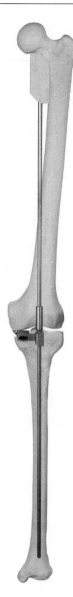

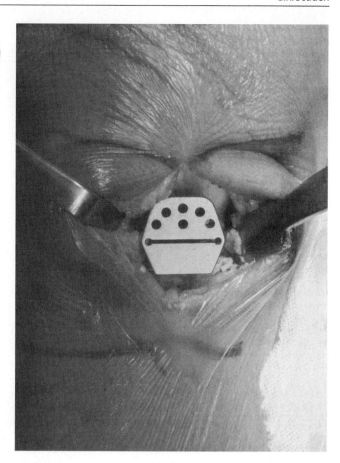

Fig. 29.5 The distal femoral resection guide is attached to the spacer block

a   b

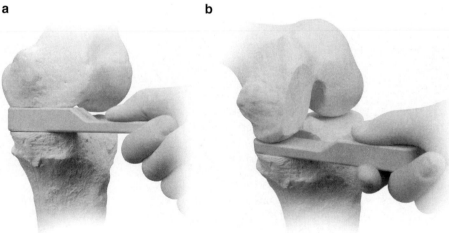

Fig. 29.6 The gaps are checked in extension (**a**) and flexion (**b**)

Finishing the Femur

Once the extension gap has been determined, the appropriate-sized femoral finishing guide is selected (Fig. 29.7). This guide rests on the flat surface of the distal femur and the posterior extension lies against the posterior condyles. To avoid oversizing the femoral component and causing impingement of the patellofemoral joint, there should be 1–2 mm of exposed bone along the anterior edge of the guide. If the femoral component appears to be in between sizes, it would be preferable to pick the smaller size. The femoral guide should also be rotationally set so that the posterior surface is parallel to the resected tibia. With the guide secured to the femur, the final cuts and lug holes are made. This completes the femoral preparation.

Finishing the Tibia

At this point, the remaining meniscus and osteophytes are removed. The appropriate-sized tibial template, which covers the entire surface without overhang, is selected (Fig. 29.8). The template is secured to the proximal tibia and the lug holes are drilled. The tibial template is left in place for the trial reduction.

Trial Reduction

With the knee in 90° of flexion and a retractor in the intercondylar notch to pull back the patella, the provisional femoral component is seated on the distal femur. A trial tibial articular surface is then placed on the tibial template. With all the provisional components in place, the knee is checked for range of motion and stability. Appropriate soft tissue tension is checked with the 2-mm tension gauge inserted between the femoral component and the tibial articulation (Fig. 29.9). In general, the correct thickness of the tibial prosthesis should allow for approximately 2 mm of joint laxity in full extension.

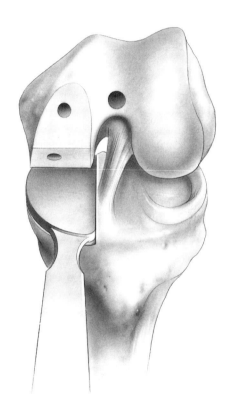

Fig. 29.8   The tibial template is placed on the resected tibia

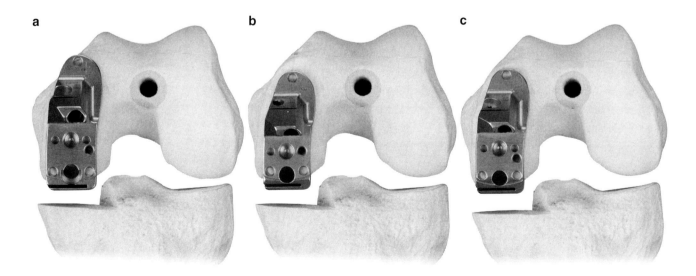

Fig. 29.7   (a–c) The correct femoral finishing guide is selected

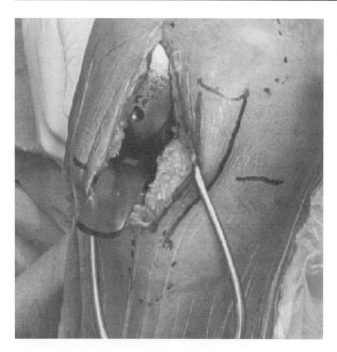

Fig. 29.9 With the provisional components in place, the 2-mm tension gauge is inserted in the joint

Final Components

The trial components are removed and the bone surfaces are cleansed with water pick lavage in an effort to remove blood and debris from the surfaces. In preparation for cementing, the bone is dried. The modular tibial component is cemented in place first. With the knee hyperflexed and externally rotated, a small amount of cement is placed on the exposed surface of the tibia. An additional amount of cement is placed on the undersurface of the tibial component. The final tibial component is then pressed into place and the excess cement is removed. To fully seat the tibial component, it is impacted into place and any extruded cement is removed.

With the knee in 90° of flexion, a retractor is placed in the intercondylar notch to hold the patella back so that the femur is exposed. A small amount of cement is placed on the distal femur and along the backside of the femoral component. The femoral component is impacted in place and all excess cement is removed. The modular tibial polyethylene articular surface is then inserted and a final check of motion and stability is performed.

With the final components in place (Fig. 29.10), the knee is irrigated with an antibiotic solution. The arthrotomy, subcutaneous layer and skin are closed in a routine fashion.

Summary

Minimally invasive unicondylar knee arthroplasty implanted with extramedullary instrumentation minimizes soft tissue dissection, does not violate the femoral intramedullary canal, and ensures accurate component positioning. Since the proximal tibial resection and the distal femoral resection are linked in extension, this coupled resection and desired soft tissue tension set limb alignment. The cuts are parallel and result in a preset gap that is calculated to match the thickness of the implants. Gap balancing reduces the need for recutting, will help preserve bone stock, and assures

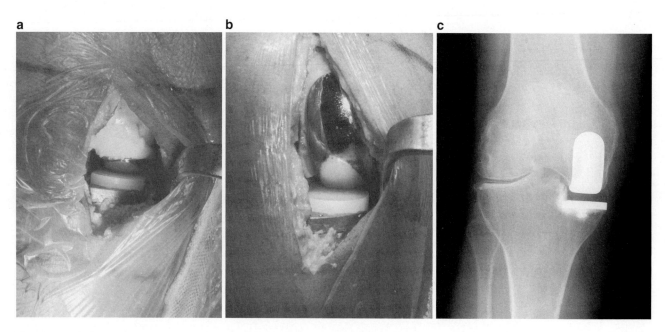

Fig. 29.10 The final components in place (**a**, **b**) with the resultant radiograph (**c**)

accurate component positioning. Final postoperative alignment is determined by the composite thickness of the components. Reliable instrumentation results in accurate bone resection and component position, which are necessary for a successful clinical outcome.

References

1. Repicci JA, Eberle RW. Minimally invasive surgical technique for unicondylar knee replacement. J South Orthop Assoc 1999; 8: 20–27

2. Zimmer monograph. The Zimmer unicompartmental high flex knee: intramedullary, spacer block option and extramedullary minimally invasive surgical techniques, 2004

3. Barnes CL, Scott RD. Unicondylar replacement. In: Scuderi GR, Tria AJ, eds Surgical Techniques in Total Knee Arthroplasty. Springer, New York, 2002, 106–111

4. Scuderi GR. Instrumentation for unicondylar knee replacement. In: Scuderi GR, Tria AJ, eds MIS of the Hip and the Knee: A Clinical Perspective. Springer, New York, 2004, 87–104

5. Berger RA, Nedeff DD, Barden RM, et al. Unicompartmental knee arthroplasty: clinical experience at 6- to 10- year follow-up. Clin Orthop 1999;367: 50–60

6. Cartier P, Sanouiller JL, Grelsamer RP. Unicompartmental knee arthroplasty: 10-year minimum follow-up period. J Arthroplasty 1996;11: 782–788

Chapter 30
MIS Arthroplasty with the UniSpacer*

Richard H. Hallock

Middle-age osteoarthritis of the knee remains a problem with many treatment options. It can be treated in its earlier stages with a combination of oral medication, intraarticular injection with cortisone or viscosupplementation, physical therapy, and arthroscopic debridement. Once the patient has reached a level of disability that is not responding to these less invasive treatment modalities, the patient and physician are both faced with the decision to choose a more invasive surgical option. The selection of the best surgical alternative will depend on many nonsurgical issues including the patient's age, weight, sex, activity level, and occupation. This decision will also be based on the extent of cartilage degeneration, as well as bony deformity. These options include high tibial osteotomy, uni-compartmental knee arthroplasty, total knee arthroplasty, and the UniSpacer. The final decision on which of these techniques is ultimately used will come down to patient and surgeon preference based on the individual set of circumstances.

The UniSpacer was designed on both very traditional orthopedic principles as well as some nontraditional orthopedic concepts.[1–5] It is a cobalt chrome metallic device that is inserted into the medial compartment of the knee. The bearing surfaces of the device have a metal on cartilage/bone interface on both the femoral and tibial surfaces. Metal on biologic interfaces have been used traditionally in orthopedics in hemiarthroplasty of the shoulder, hemiarthroplasty of the hip, and nonresurfaced patellae in total knee replacement. It serves as a self-centering shim, which replaces the missing articular and meniscal cartilage of the medial compartment.

As such, the thickness of the shim is determined by the amount of missing articular and meniscal cartilage within the constraints of the collateral and cruciate ligaments. The varus deformity will thus only be corrected back to the patient's premorbid knee alignment. This realignment will off load the medial compartment of the knee without over correcting the alignment and accelerating lateral compartment degeneration. What is different about this device from traditional arthroplasty is that it is neither fixed to the bony surfaces of the tibia or the femur, nor requires bone cuts or bone removal for implantation. The geometry of the device with its concave femoral surface and convex tibial surface allows it to function as a self-centering shim between the biological femoral and tibial surfaces of the patient. These nontraditional concepts avoid the traditional modes of arthroplasty failure including loosening, polyethylene wear, and malpositioning of components. As such, it can function either as a final arthroplasty or as a safe bridge procedure in younger patients, which does not alter the bony and ligamentous anatomy for a next-step procedure.

Preoperative Evaluation

The preoperative evaluation for the UniSpacer requires the same type of evaluation that would be necessary to perform a high tibial osteotomy, unicompartmental knee replacement, or total knee replacement. Routine X-ray evaluation should include anteroposterior (AP) erect views of the knee, which allow evaluation of the loss of joint space as well as the femoral tibial axis (Fig. 30.1). The surgeon should pay particular attention to medial subluxation of the femur relative to the tibia and deformity of the tibial plateau (Fig. 30.2).

Either of these two conditions would preclude the use of the UniSpacer. The lateral X-ray of the knee is necessary to view the relative position of the femoral condyle with respect to the tibia. Anterior translation of the tibia relative to the femur may indicate chronic anterior cruciate ligament insufficiency, which may also be a contraindication for the use of the UniSpacer (Fig. 30.3). The lateral view also demonstrates posterior femoral osteophytes. Large posterior femoral osteophytes can produce a flexion contracture greater than 5°, which is also a contraindication for the use of the UniSpacer. The skyline view is necessary to evaluate the patellofemoral joint. Any significant loss of joint space or osteophyte formation may also contraindicate the use of the UniSpacer, especially

R.H. Hallock (✉)
The Orthopedic Institute of Pennsylvania, 3399 Trindle Road, Camp Hill, PA, 17011, USA
e-mail: RHHALLOCK@aol.com

* Adapted from Hallock RH, MIS Arthroplasty with the UniSpacer, in Scuderi G, Tria A, Berger R (eds), *MIS Techniques in Orthopedics*, New York, Springer, 2006, with kind permission of Springer Science + Business Media, Inc.

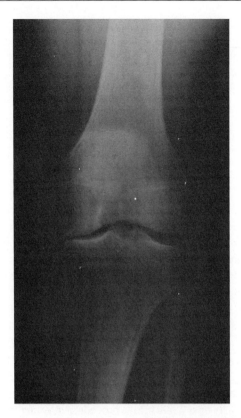

Fig. 30.1 Loss of medial joint space without deformation of the tibia

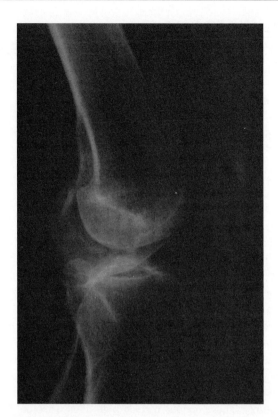

Fig. 30.3 A anterior subluxation of the tibia suggestive of chronic anterior cruciate ligament (ACL) deficiency

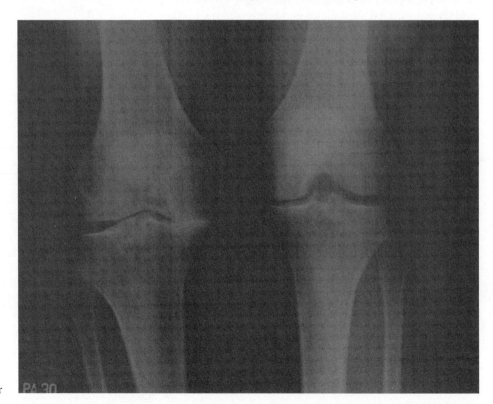

Fig. 30.2 Deformity of the tibia and medial subluxation of the femur

if the patient has symptoms, which can be confused medial joint pain. A magnetic resonance imaging (MRI) scan can also be useful in evaluating the status of the knee. Questions concerning the integrity of the anterior cruciate ligament as well as the status of the patella femoral joint can also be answered with an MRI scan.

Surgical Technique

Since the UniSpacer requires no bone cuts and has no fixation, the surgical technique is decidedly different than traditional arthroplasty. The surgical technique focuses on restoring the knee alignment through thorough joint debridement and implantation of an intraarticular shim. This will be broken down into steps including arthrotomy, osteophyte resection and anterior medial meniscectomy, chondroplasty, tweenplasty, sizing, insertion technique, fluoroscopy, and final implantation and closure.

Surgical Preparation

Preoperative antibiotic prophylaxis is utilized on all patients. The use of a thigh tourniquet is optional and left to surgeon preference. The arthroscopy portals and incision line can be infiltrated with local anesthetic with epinephrine to decrease intraoperative bleeding, especially if the patient does not have a tourniquet. The patient is placed in the supine position with the knee prepped and draped in a routine fashion.

Rigid leg holders should be avoided since they will inhibit the surgeon from placing the knee through a range of motion, and they will interfere with use of the fluoroscopy equipment later in the case.

Arthroscopy

Every patient who is considered for the UniSpacer should have an arthroscopy performed either at the time of surgery or during the previous 12 months. Inappropriate candidates can be deselected based on the extent of degeneration present at the time of the arthroscopy. The arthroscopy is also useful with some of the initial debridement necessary to proceed with insertion of the UniSpacer. An initial evaluation of the patellofemoral joint, lateral compartment including the lateral meniscus, as well as the cruciate ligament complex should be performed. Any significant degeneration in the patellofemoral compartment or the lateral compartment should result in deselection of the current UniSpacer candidate. Mild grade I to grade II chondromalacia of the patellofemoral joint and lateral compartment is acceptable. Any grade of chondromalacia worse than that degree of degeneration should lead to deselection of that patient for a UniSpacer. Since an intact lateral compartment, including an intact lateral meniscus, is critical when weight bearing is going to be shifted to that compartment, every patient should have an intact lateral meniscus as well as only mild chondromalacic changes involving the

lateral femoral condyle and lateral tibial plateau. It is very difficult to distinguish anteromedial knee pain originating from the medial compartment versus the patellofemoral joint. Any patient with significant degeneration involving the patella or femoral sulcus also should be deselected. The cruciate ligament complex also needs to be thoroughly examined.

Many of these patients have had previous arthrotomies for medial meniscectomy as a result of old injuries. When that occurs, the cruciate ligament complex should be examined for complete integrity of both the anterior and the posterior cruciate ligaments. Any patient with deficiency of either the anterior or posterior cruciate ligament will require either reconstruction of these ligaments or consideration of other treatment options. The most common reason for deselection of any UniSpacer candidate is evaluation of the medial compartment. Most UniSpacer candidates have bipolar degenerative disease involving both the femoral condyle and tibial plateau. If the patient has deformity of the tibial plateau subchondral bone plate resulting in remodeling of the medial edge of the tibial plateau, that patient should also be deselected. When this occurs, the tibial plateau has essentially a convex surface instead of the normal shallow, concave surface for the UniSpacer to translate on (Fig. 30.4). Any convex surface of the tibial plateau will inhibit normal translational and rotatory motion that is required for restoration of normal knee kinematics. If, after initial arthroscopic evaluation, the patient is considered to be a satisfactory candidate for utilization of the UniSpacer, several of the initial debridement steps can be performed arthroscopically. This includes resection of the posterior horn of the medial meniscus. The medial meniscus is usually degenerated in these patients, and completion of the posterior meniscectomy can be performed arthroscopically back to the junction of the red and white zones. Any residual leading

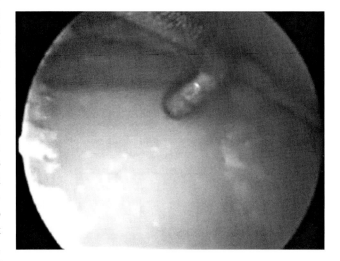

Fig. 30.4 Medial tibial bone loss, which cannot be contoured to create normal UniSpacer kinematics. The subchondral bone has been remodeled to create a convex surface

edge of the meniscus should be resected as this can result in translation of the UniSpacer over the leading edge of the meniscus. The residual boundary of the meniscus will act as a partial physical constraint. Once the posterior meniscectomy has been completed, the evaluation of the intercondylar osteophytes can proceed. It is not unusual for osteophytes to form in the intercondylar regions in these patients.

Osteophytes abrading the anterior cruciate ligament can cause degeneration of an intact anterior cruciate ligament and eventually result in incompetency. These osteophytes adjacent to the anterior cruciate ligament should be resected if visualized arthroscopically. The osteophytes on the lateral/posterior aspect of the medial femoral condyle can also be difficult to visualize after the arthroscopy has been performed. If that is the case, it is often easier to resect these osteophytes using the aid of the arthroscope. Again, the goal of osteophyte resection adjacent to the intercondylar notch is to restore normal cruciate ligament excursion in addition to removing any abnormal femoral anatomy that may cause aberrant UniSpacer motion.

Arthrotomy

The arthrotomy for insertion of the UniSpacer is very similar to the arthrotomy performed for insertion of a traditional unicompartmental arthroplasty. The incision usually extends from the mid patella down to the tibial joint line (Fig. 30.5). The subcutaneous tissue is undermined to allow a mobile view of the medial compartment. The medial retinaculum is incised from the superior pole of the patella down to the proximal tibia. The anteromedial corner of the knee is released, including transection of the anterolateral horn of the medial meniscus. Subperiosteal release of the proximal 2 cm of the tibia should be performed when it is necessary to resect osteophytes off of the medial aspect of the tibia (Fig. 30.6). This release is not necessary when there is only minimal medial tibial osteophyte formation present. The arthrotomy should allow visualization of the medial facet of the patella, intercondylar notch, medial femoral condyle, and medial tibial plateau when necessary. A small portion of the infrapatellar fat pad can be resected when visualization of the intercondylar notch or medial compartment is impaired with just the medial arthrotomy.

Osteophyte Resection and Anteromedial Meniscectomy

Following the arthrotomy, a complete debridement of medial compartment osteophytes is necessary to allow full excursion of the medial collateral and cruciate ligament complex.

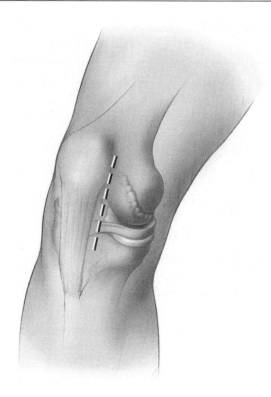

Fig. 30.5 A medial parapatellar incision from mid-patella to the tibial joint line (From Hallock RH, MIS arthroplasty with the UniSpacer. In: Scuderi G, Tria A, Berger R (eds.), *MIS Techniques in Orthopedics*, New York, Springer, 2006, with kind permission of Springer Science and Business Media, Inc.)

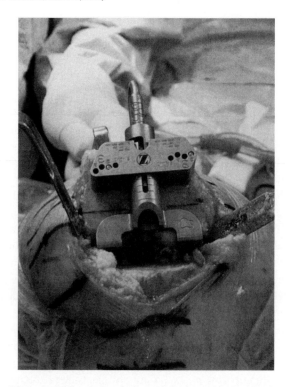

Fig. 30.6 A mobile window to the medial compartment with release of the anteromedial corner of the proximal tibia (From Hallock RH, MIS arthroplasty with the UniSpacer. In: Scuderi G, Tria A, Berger R (eds.), *MIS Techniques in Orthopedics*, New York, Springer, 2006, with kind permission of Springer Science and Business Media, Inc.)

Initially, any overhanging osteophytes adjacent to the medial aspect of the patella should be resected. Osteophytes are frequently present along the medial border of the patella. When the femoral tibial axis is corrected from varus to valgus alignment, these osteophytes can impinge on the medial aspect of the femoral sulcus. It is imperative to debride these osteophytes to avoid residual medial patellofemoral pain. Osteophytes are then resected completely from the anterior aspect of the femoral condyle to the posterior aspect of the femoral condyle. This can be performed usually using a rongeur. The osteophytes need to be resected down to the original borders of the femur.

A retractor is supplied with the instrumentation to allow resection of the posterior osteophyte formation on the femoral condyle (Fig. 30.7). This is most easily accomplished by placing the knee in the figure of four position with the knee flexed. An osteotome can be utilized to shear off the posterior osteophytes to restore the original bony contours. It is also imperative to resect any significant osteophyte formation along the medial border of the tibial plateau. When this occurs, it is necessary to release the deep fibers of the medial collateral ligament and meniscal tibial ligament along the proximal 2-cm region of the tibial plateau. Once this is released, osteophytes can easily be resected that overhang the medial border of the original tibial plateau. It is not unusual for the anterior and middle thirds of the medial meniscus to remain relatively intact in these patients. When this occurs, an open anteromedial meniscectomy should be performed at the level of the junction of the red and white zones to avoid any impingement of the UniSpacer on a residual leading edge of the meniscus. Leaving the red zone of the meniscus intact will create a stable border for the UniSpacer. The surgeon should be careful not to violate the superficial fibers of the medial collateral ligament during this procedure.

Chondroplasty

The degenerative surfaces of the femoral condyle and tibial plateau typically have irregular shapes created by variations in the thickness of the remaining articular cartilage. The tibial surface of the UniSpacer has a uniform, shallow convexity despite the size of the device. In an effort to create the most conformal surface that articulates against the UniSpacer, it is necessary to contour the patient's femoral condyle and tibial plateau. This femoral and tibial "sculpting" will ultimately create the best fit and sizing for the UniSpacer. The surgeon must, therefore, attempt to recreate the anatomic J-curve of the femoral condyle in addition to recreating the shallow dish curvature of the tibial plateau. Despite the fact that the UniSpacer will span cartilage defects on either of these surfaces, it is best to restore the most uniform surfaces, which, ultimately, distributes the load over a greater surface area

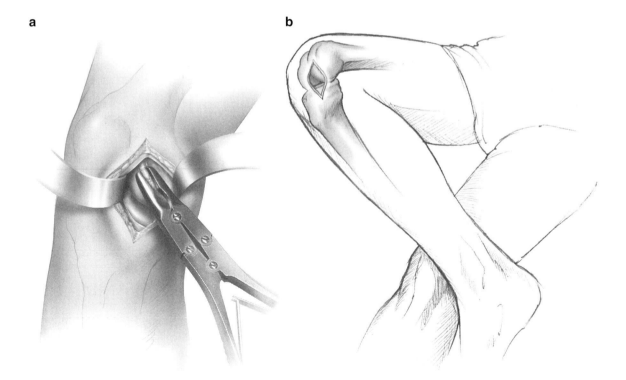

a **b**

Fig. 30.7 The Fig.-of-four position necessary to resect osteophytes from the posterior region of the medial femoral condyle (From Hallock RH, MIS arthroplasty with the UniSpacer. In: Scuderi G, Tria A, Berger R (eds.), *MIS Techniques in Orthopedics*, New York, Springer, 2006, with kind permission of Springer Science and Business Media, Inc.)

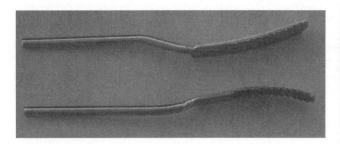

Fig. 30.8 The rasps are shown, which are available to contour the femoral and tibial surfaces to restore a smooth articular surface

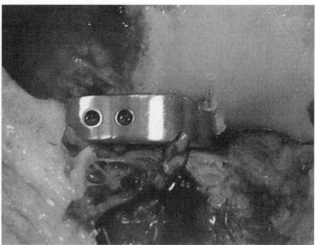

Fig. 30.9 A UniSpacer in position without a proper tweenplasty. Note the impingement on the femoral condyle (From Hallock RH, MIS arthroplasty with the UniSpacer. In: Scuderi G, Tria A, Berger R (eds.), *MIS Techniques in Orthopedics*, New York, Springer, 2006, with kind permission of Springer Science and Business Media, Inc.)

during loading. Convex and concave rasps are provided with the instrumentation that can be utilized to restore a "best fit" contour to the patient's biological surfaces. The rasps are utilized to smooth out divoted regions of the patient's articular surfaces in addition to restoring more uniform thickness to the remaining articular cartilage (Fig. 30.8). This process is necessary to create more stable kinematics for the UniSpacer during its normal translational/rotational motion. This often requires smoothing out ridges of articular cartilage that create an impediment to normal motion. Areas of full thickness articular cartilage may tend to exaggerate normal motion of the UniSpacer. This is most often seen on the posterior aspect of the femoral condyle where full thickness cartilage often remains. The concave rasp can be used to thin this remaining articular cartilage to avoid an exaggerated posterior translation of the device during flexion.

Although it is not necessary for the surgeon to create a fully conformal surface to the UniSpacer in extension, any attempt to do so will decrease the patient's recovery time. Increased conformity ultimately leads to distribution of medial compartment load over a greater surface area. This is confirmed when evaluating the clinical results that show improvement occurs not only during the first postoperative year, but also show improvement continues to occur during the second postoperative year.

Tweenplasty

There is one special area that needs to be addressed during the contouring procedure to allow normal anterior rotation of the UniSpacer in full extension. This area, the junction of Whitesides line and the superior aspect of the intercondylar notch, is critical in allowing normal anterior rotation of the UniSpacer in full extension. Since the UniSpacer is driven by the femoral condyle toward the femoral sulcus in full extension, this area needs to be recessed to allow normal rotational motion.

Full-thickness cartilage just above the intercondylar notch must be removed to allow the anterior flange of the device to "screw home" in full extension. If this cartilage is not removed, the UniSpacer will be driven out into an anteromedial position causing impingement and pain during full extension (Fig. 30.9). The degree of articular degeneration on the femoral surface of the patient will dictate how deep this recess needs to be. Most patients require removal of full-thickness articular cartilage in this zone.

Sizing

The UniSpacer comes in six different sizes with respect to length/width and four different thicknesses for each knee. Thus, both the left and right knee each have 24 different-sized implants. The AP length of the device remains proportional to the medial/lateral width of the device as the size increases and decreases. Thus the dimensions of the device increase and decrease proportionally relative to the size. Standard sets range in size between 38 mm in length and 58 mm in length. The device also comes in four varying thicknesses from 2 to 5 mm. Initially, the size of the device is estimated by measuring the AP length of the tibia.

The ultimate sizing, however, is determined by the remaining contour of the femoral condyle. The femoral surface of the UniSpacer must have a radius that is greater than or equal to the surface remaining on the contoured femoral condyle. In other words, the femoral condyle must fit the femoral surface of the UniSpacer without producing any edge loading anteriorly or posteriorly as this creates impingement and eventually may lead to pain or dislocation.

Sizing the Implant

The size of the implant that is ultimately chosen is based on length and thickness. The implant must restore the joint space of the medial compartment that corrects the axial alignment. There is a thickness gauge with the instrument set that can be used to help determine the appropriate thickness. The thickness gauge comes in four different thicknesses ranging from 2 to 5 mm, in 1-mm increments. This gauge is placed between the medial femoral condyle and tibial plateau in both flexion and extension. The correct thickness implant will retension the medial collateral ligament and anterior cruciate ligament while allowing full extension and maximum flexion. The thickness gauge gives the surgeon an initial trial size that may have to be modified after initial implant testing. The implant must ultimately be sized to fit the contour of the femoral condyle, however, the initial length measurement is taking from the AP dimension of the tibia. An arthroscopy probe is used to hook the posterior aspect of the tibial plateau and then mark the anterior aspect of the tibia using a hemostat (Fig. 30.10). There is a ruler with the instruments that can then be used to check the AP dimension off of the arthroscopy hook. This gives the surgeon an initial trial size with respect to length.

Once the initial measurements have been taken with respect to length and thickness, an implant trial is selected out of the set. The trial is placed on the insertion handle, and then implanted into the medial compartment. The final sizing is actually confirmed by evaluation of the conformity of the femoral surface of the UniSpacer to the femoral condyle. Once the implant is in place, the knee should be placed through a vigorous range of motion to ensure that the UniSpacer has both uniform translation and rotation during flexion and extension cycles. In extension, the UniSpacer should always translate and rotate toward the intercondylar notch, and demonstrate a small amount of anterior overhand off of the tibia. In flexion, the UniSpacer should rotate around the tibial spine, and translate posteriorly, and will frequently show posterior translation off of the tibia.

Insertion Technique

The insertion of both the UniSpacer trials as well as the final implant is often the most intimidating portion of the procedure to learn. Once this technique is mastered, however, it is relatively simple and reproducible. The handle of the testing device allows 360° of rotation, which allows the surgeon to choose the most optimal position of the handle to avoid impingement on the soft tissues during insertion. During the insertion, the trial is tucked into the medial compartment underneath the medial edge of the patella. With the knee flexed to approximately 45–60°, a valgus stress is applied to the knee and the UniSpacer is held against the femoral condyle with the testing handle. Using some posterior pressure on the handle in addition to a small wiggle, the knee is pulled into full extension and the UniSpacer will drop into the medial compartment. The surgeon must be careful to exert pressure that is directly posterior on the tibial plateau to allow the device to slide into position (Fig. 30.11). The most

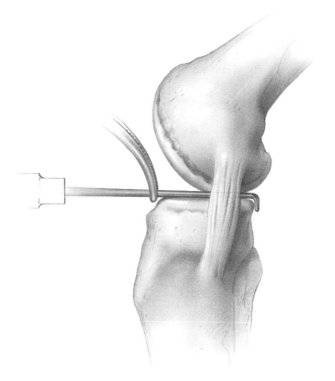

Fig. 30.10 The length initial measurement for the UniSpacer taken off the AP dimension of the tibial plateau (From Hallock RH, MIS arthroplasty with the UniSpacer. In: Scuderi G, Tria A, Berger R (eds.), *MIS Techniques in Orthopedics*, New York, Springer, 2006, with kind permission of Springer Science and Business Media, Inc.)

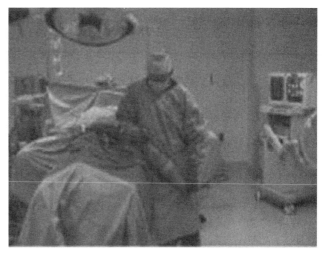

Fig. 30.11 Proper surgeon positioning for UniSpacer insertion (From Hallock RH, MIS arthroplasty with the UniSpacer. In: Scuderi G, Tria A, Berger R (eds.), *MIS Techniques in Orthopedics*, New York, Springer, 2006, with kind permission of Springer Science and Business Media, Inc.)

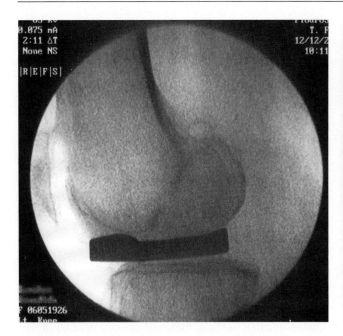

Fig. 30.12 Lateral fluoroscopy view with the knee extended. Note the anterior position of the UniSpacer on the tibial plateau

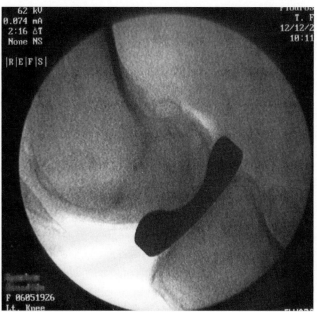

Fig. 30.13 A lateral fluoroscopy view with the knee flexed. Note the posterior translation of the UniSpacer on the tibial plateau. The UniSpacer follows the femoral condyle during femoral roll back

common error during this technique is improper insertion angle, which results in driving the UniSpacer into the tibial spine instead of into a posterior position on the tibial plateau. Once in position, the implant should center itself under the femoral condyle. To remove the trial implant from the knee, the reverse of this technique is performed. The knee is held in extension with a valgus stress applied to the knee. With the UniSpacer held against the femoral condyle, the knee is flexed. With that maneuver, the UniSpacer can easily be removed from the medial compartment.

Fluoroscopy

It is necessary to confirm correct implant sizing and motion using fluoroscopic guidance. Fluoroscopy allows the surgeon to check the size of the implant relative to the femoral condyle, again ensuring that the UniSpacer has the most anatomic fit to the femoral condyle without undersizing the implant. Fluoroscopy also allows the surgeon to view the motion of the device through normal range of motion. In the fully extended position, the UniSpacer should translate several millimeters anterior to the tibial plateau on the lateral view (Fig. 30.12). In flexion, the UniSpacer should translate to the posterior aspect of the tibia or extend several millimeters past the posterior aspect of the tibial plateau (Fig. 30.13). On the AP view in full extension, the UniSpacer should appear rotated with the anterior horn of the UniSpacer rotated centrally toward the tibial spine. As the surgeon becomes more comfortable with the technique, the fluoroscopy can be kept to a minimum.

Final Implantation and Closure

Once the optimum implant size has been selected, and fluoroscopy is completed, the final implant is inserted into the medial compartment. The handle of the insertion tool is slightly different than the testing tool. The implant is connected to the insertion handle using converging pins. These pins are more fragile than the large pin on the anterior aspect of the trial implants. The insertion technique, however, is basically the same. Once the final implant is in position, the surgeon should place the knee through a range of motion to confirm proper kinematics. The wound is closed in a standard fashion using heavier suture material in the deeper retinacular layer and the routine subcutaneous and skin closure preferred by the surgeon. Patients do not require immobilization unless the surgeon feels the patient would have improved initial ambulation with the extra support.

References

1. Hallock RH, Fell BM. Unicompartmental tibial hemiarthroplasty: early results of the UniSpacer knee. Clin Orthop Relat Res. 2003 Nov;(416):154–63
2. Hallock RH. The UniSpacer knee system: have we been there before? Orthopedics. 2003;26(9):953–4
3. Geier KA. UniSpacer for knee osteoarthritis. Orthop Nurs. 2003;22(5):369–70
4. Friedman MJ. UniSpacer. Arthroscopy. 2003 Dec;19(Suppl 1):120–1
5. Dressler K, Ellermann A. [UNISPACER - a new minimally-invasive therapeutic concept for the isolated medial knee joint disease]. Z Orthop Ihre Grenzgeb. 2004;142(2):131–3

Chapter 31
MIS Total Knee Arthroplasty with the Limited Medial Parapatellar Arthrotomy

Giles R. Scuderi

Minimally invasive (MIS) total knee arthroplasty (TKA) has become a popular procedure with surgeons using a variety of surgical exposures including the limited medial parapatellar arthrotomy, also known as the limited quadriceps-splitting approach; the midvastus approach; the subvastus approach; and the quadriceps-sparing approach.[1] The limited medial parapatellar arthrotomy is a versatile approach that can be easily converted to a traditional approach if necessary. Advantages of this technique include diminished postoperative morbidity, less postoperative pain, decreased blood loss, and an earlier functional recovery.[2–5] However, while limiting the exposure in MIS, the integrity of the TKA must not be compromised. Following specific guidelines in patient selection and surgical technique, the clinical outcome can be predictable.

MIS TKA is not for every patient or for every surgeon. Patient selection is critical and it has been observed that thin female patients with minimal deformity and good preoperative range of motion were ideal candidates for MIS TKA.[1,5] There is a gender bias with 71% of female subjects compared with 33% of male subjects being suitable candidates for the MIS TKA. Contributing to this gender difference is that male muscular patients with large femurs tended to be better served with a standard medial parapatellar arthrotomy. Furthermore, a broader femoral transepicondylar width dictates a longer skin incision and arthrotomy.[5] It has also been observed that when considering patients for a MIS TKA, they tend to be of shorter stature and lighter weight. When it comes to the variable of weight, realize that it is the distribution of the weight and the quality of the fat that are also contributing factors. While an obese patient with long thin legs, soft fat and elastic skin may be eligible for MIS TKA; short heavy legs with brawny skin are not ideal candidates. In the final analysis of female patients and weight it has been reported[5] that the average body mass index (BMI) was significantly smaller in the MIS group (<30 kg/mm^2).

The degree of deformity affects the extent of the surgical exposure. Knees with severe fixed angular deformities often require extensive soft tissue releases and may not be ideal for MIS TKA. Therefore, it is recommended that the MIS procedure be limited to knees with $<15°$ of varus or $<20°$ of valgus. Additionally, since the knee will have to be positioned into various angles of knee flexion during the procedure, it is recommended that the knee have an arc of motion of 90° and a flexion contracture $<10°$.[1,5] Preoperative radiographs can be used to determine the patella height and length of the patella tendon. Patella infera, as determined by the Insall Salvati ratio or Blackburn–Peel ratio, may pose technical difficulties in exposing the joint and laterally subluxing the patella. Therefore, if the patella tendon is short and patella infera is present, it is recommended that the arthrotomy be extended further into the quadriceps tendon, avoiding injury to the patella tendon or avulsion at the tibial tubercle.

The integrity of the skin must not be compromised and, for that reason, patients with rheumatoid or inflammatory arthritis must be approached with caution. Many of these patients have thin, friable skin that can easily tear, so it is better to control the length of the incision by sharp dissection and avoid an intraoperative traumatic injury. Additionally, it is not uncommon for a rheumatoid knee to have abundant hypertrophic inflammatory synovitis, which needs to be removed. In order to perform a complete synovectomy of all compartments, it is recommended that these knees be approached with a standard medial parapatellar arthrotomy. Finally, care must be taken not to place too much tension on the supporting structures in the presence of inflammatory arthritis, especially if associated with generalized osteopenia. Overzealous retraction may result in direct injury to the ligaments, avulsion injuries, or, worse, fracture. Therefore, for these cases, it is recommended that a traditional approach be performed.

Finally, when it comes to patient selection, there are several final variables that need to be considered, including hypertrophic osteoarthritis, prior surgical procedures, and complexity of the arthroplasty. In the presence of exuberant osteophyte formation around the femur, the osteophytes should be removed early during the exposure when performing

G.R. Scuderi (✉)
Insall Scott Kelly Institute, 210 East 64th Street, 4th Floor, New York, NY 10021, USA
e-mail: gscuderi@iskinstitute.com

a MIS approach. This enhances visualization of the joint and positioning of the retractors. Prior surgical procedures pose several problems, including incorporation of prior skin incisions, hardware removal, bone defects, loss of motion, and deformity. In dealing with complex cases that require bone grafting or component augmentation, an extensile approach should be employed. Following the recommendations detailed above, the ideal patient for a MIS TKA can be determined.

Surgical Technique

The limited medial parapatellar arthrotomy is the most versatile of the MIS approaches because it has evolved from a traditional approach performed by most surgeons.[6] The learning curve for this technique is short as surgeons gradually reduce the length of the skin incision and the arthrotomy into the quadriceps tendon in order to gain exposure of the knee joint. With lateral subluxation of the patella, instead of eversion, both the femur and tibia can be visualized without extending the arthrotomy high into the quadriceps tendon. Exposure and placement of the instrumentation does require placing the knee in various position of knee flexion through out the procedure, as well as careful placement of the retractors by the surgical assistant. Some key points are detailed in the following discussion.

The limb is prepped and draped free in the usual sterile fashion. The surgical assistants stabilize the leg with a sand bag placed at the foot of the table. Specialized leg-holding devices may be used but are not mandatory. A straight anterior midline incision is made in extension, extending from the superior aspect of the tibial tubercle to the superior

border of the patella. The skin incision is made as small as possible in every patient, but is extended as needed during the procedure to allow for adequate visualization and avoidance of excess skin tension. One intraoperative observation pertaining to the skin incision is the U sign and the V sign. If the skin is under a great deal of tension, the proximal and distal apex will form a U or possibly even flatten out (Fig. 31.1a). This may have a tendency to tear if put under further tension and should be lengthened. Skin under the appropriate tension should form a V at the apices (Fig. 31.1b).[6] Full-thickness medial and lateral flaps are created over the extensor mechanism. Release of the deep fascia proximally beneath the skin and superficial to the quadriceps tendon facilitates mobilization of the skin and enhances exposure. With the knee in flexion and due to the elasticity of the skin, the incision will stretch an average of 3.75 cm from extension to flexion.[5]

In an attempt to reduce intraoperative and postoperative bleeding, the quadriceps tendon, along the path of the arthrotomy and the medial retinaculum is injected with 1% lidocaine and epinephrine. This technique has shown a significant reduction in postoperative bleeding. In a comparison study, the average postoperative hemoglobin drop was 3.37 g/dL for the standard approach and 2.05 g/dL for the mini-incision with epinephrine injection.[7] The limited medial parapatellar arthrotomy is a shortened version of the traditional approach (Fig. 31.2). The arthrotomy is of a sufficient length to sublux the patella laterally over the lateral femoral condyle without eversion. In most cases, the incision into the quadriceps tendon extends 2–4 cm above the superior pole of the patella. If there is difficulty displacing the patella laterally or if the patella tendon is at risk of injury, the arthrotomy is extended proximally until adequate exposure can be achieved.

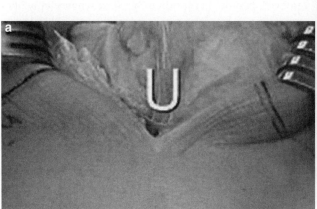
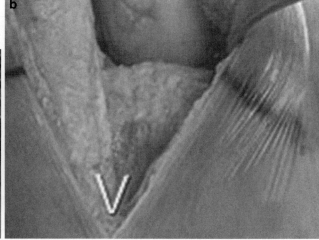

Fig. 31.1 (**a–c**) The skin incision under tension will form the U sign (**a**); minimal skin tension will form the V sign (**b**) (From Scuderi GR, Patient-based MIS TKA: for everything there is a season, OrthoSupersite, http://www.orthosupersite.com/view.asp?rID = 31438. Copyright © 2008 SLACK, Incorporated.)

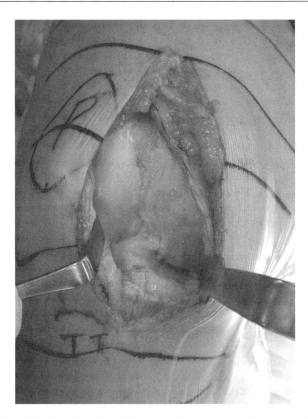

Fig. 31.2 The limited medial parapatellar arthrotomy (From Scuderi GR, Tria AJ, Jr., Minimal incision total knee arthroplasty. In: Scuderi GR, Tria AJ, Jr. (eds.), *MIS of the Hip and the Knee*. New York: Springer, 2004, with kind permission of Springer Science + Business Media, Inc.)

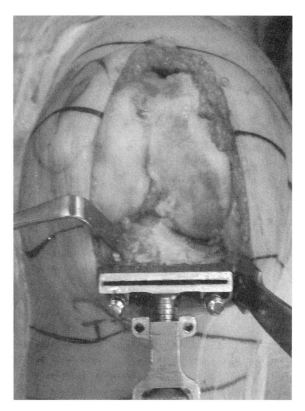

Fig. 31.3 The limited arthrotomy is actually a mobile window (From Scuderi GR, Tria AJ, Jr., Minimal incision total knee arthroplasty. In: Scuderi GR, Tria AJ, Jr. (eds.), *MIS of the Hip and the Knee*. New York: Springer, 2004, with kind permission of Springer Science + Business Media, Inc.)

Once the exposure is achieved, the bone preparation begins with the knee flexed at 90°, and retractors are placed both medially and laterally to help aid in exposure, avoid undue skin tension, and to protect the collateral ligaments and the patella tendon. In order to aid visualization and avoid undue tension to the skin, the surgical assistants are instructed in proper placement of retractors and positioning of the knee. This creates a mobile window of exposure (Fig. 31.3). With experience, it will become obvious that the bone preparation and resection is performed at different angles of knee flexion. In addition, as the bone is resected from the proximal tibia and distal femur, there is more flexibility to the soft tissue envelope and greater exposure is achieved.

For the limited medial parapatellar approach and other MIS approaches, smaller instruments have been developed. These smaller instruments, such as the modified 4-in-1 multi-referencing instruments (Zimmer, Warsaw, IN) are advantageous. Although the instrumentation has been modified, there is no difference in the surgical technique. However, since the instruments are reduced in size, care must be taken to make sure they are securely fixed to the bone. Screw fixation, in contrast to smooth nails, is more secure and is used

routinely. In addition, the saw blades are narrower to avoid impingement in the modified instruments.

The order of bone resection is dependent upon the surgeon's preference, but I recommend cutting the tibia first because the removal of bone from the proximal tibia will impact both the flexion and extension gap, thereby facilitating preparation of the femur. Tibial resection is accomplished with the assistance of an extramedullary guide that is side specific and medially biased (Fig. 31.4). The tibial guide is centered on the tibial tubercle and set at the appropriate depth and angle of resection. As mentioned earlier, the assistants are carefully protecting the supporting soft tissue structures during the bone resection.

Following resection of the proximal tibia and removal of the bone, attention is directed to the distal femur. An intramedullary femoral cutting guide is inserted into the distal femur, which is resected with the appropriate degree of valgus, as determined during the preoperative planning (Fig. 31.5). Once this is completed, the femur is sized and the rotational axis of the femur is determined. The femoral rotation can be set along the anteroposterior (AP) axis, the epicondylar axis, or a predetermined rotation based upon surgical preference. Sizing of the femur is based upon the

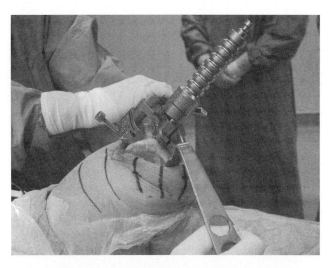

Fig. 31.4 The intramedullary tibial cutting guide is medially offset (From Scuderi GR, Tria AJ, Jr., Minimal incision total knee arthroplasty. In: Scuderi GR, Tria AJ, Jr. (eds.), *MIS of the Hip and the Knee*. New York: Springer, 2004, with kind permission of Springer Science + Business Media, Inc.)

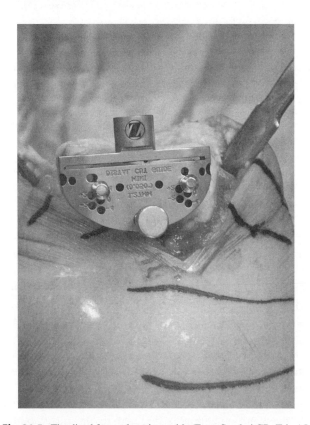

Fig. 31.5 The distal femoral cutting guide (From Scuderi GR, Tria AJ, Jr., Minimal incision total knee arthroplasty. In: Scuderi GR, Tria AJ, Jr. (eds.), *MIS of the Hip and the Knee*. New York: Springer, 2004, with kind permission of Springer Science + Business Media, Inc.)

surgeon's preference, the measured AP anatomy, and the type of prosthesis. When the AP dimension is in between sizes and a cruciate-retaining prosthesis is being implanted, the surgeon may downsize the prosthesis. In contrast, with a

posterior-stabilized prosthesis, the surgeon may upsize the component or pick the implant size that is closest to the measured anatomy. In either case, the chosen AP cutting block is secured in the appropriate degree of external rotation and the bone is resected (Fig. 31.6).

Once the femur and tibial bone are resected, laminar spreaders are used to distract the knee joint at 90° of flexion. Since it is my preference to implant a posterior-stabilized knee prosthesis, both cruciate ligaments along with the medial and lateral menisci are removed. For surgeons who prefer a posterior cruciate-retaining design, the mini-incision approach provides adequate exposure and the posterior cruciate ligament (PCL) can be preserved. Following removal of the menisci, cruciate ligaments and posterior osteophytes, the soft tissue balance is checked with a space block and alignment rod (Fig. 31.7). The collateral ligaments should be balanced. If there is any inequality, the proper soft tissue releases should be performed. The release for a residual varus deformity has been well described and it includes a subperiosteal elevation of the deep and superficial medial collateral ligament (MCL). This subperiosteal release of the MCL can be performed with the mini-incision approach, without excessive subcutaneous dissection along the proximal medial tibia. A lateral release for a valgus deformity can be performed through the medial arthrotomy. The "pie crust" technique selectively releases the arcuate ligament, the iliotibial band, and the lateral collateral ligament, with preservation of the popliteus tendon.

Once it is determined that the knee is appropriately balanced, the finishing cuts are performed on both the femur and tibia to allow testing with the provisional components. The knee is flexed to 90° and the bone is resected form the

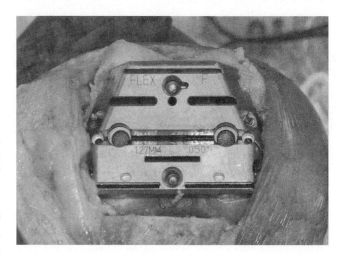

Fig. 31.6 The AP cutting guide

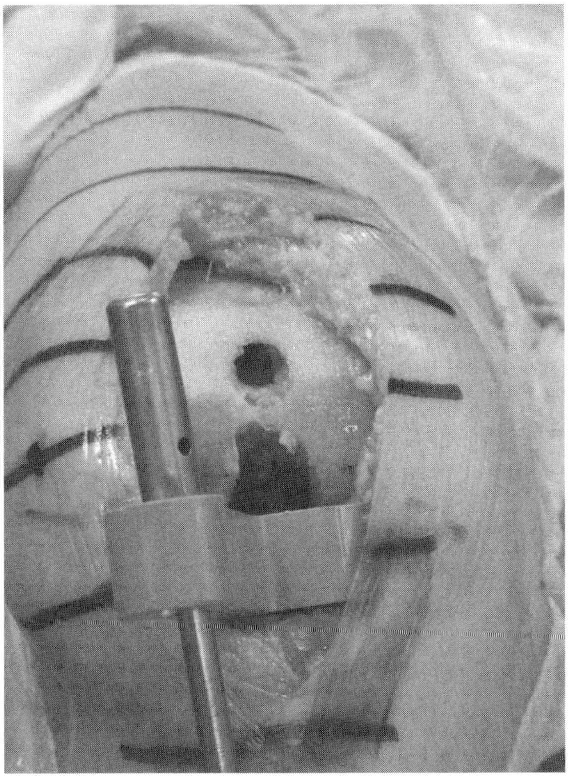

Fig. 31.7 The spacer block determines knee balance and alignment (From Scuderi GR, Tria AJ, Jr., Minimal incision total knee arthroplasty. In: Scuderi GR, Tria AJ, Jr. (eds.), *MIS of the Hip and the Knee*. New York: Springer, 2004, with kind permission of Springer Science + Business Media, Inc.)

femoral intercondylar notch to accommodate the posterior-stabilized femoral component. To gain exposure to the proximal tibial surface, the knee is hyperflexed and externally rotated. In this position, the femur falls beneath the extensor mechanism and does not interfere with visualization of the proximal tibia. The appropriately sized tibial template is positioned in the correct rotation and the tibia is prepared for the final component.

Patella preparation is performed after femoral and tibial resection. Following removal of the bone from the proximal tibia and distal femur, there is approximately a 20-mm gap, resulting in laxity of the soft tissue envelope, which allows easier manipulation of the patella during preparation. With the knee in either full extension or slight flexion, the patella is tilted. Following measurement of the patella thickness, using the appropriately sized reamer, the patella is resected to the appropriate depth. The three fixation holes are drilled and a trial button placed. The final thickness of the resurfaced patella is measured and compared with the original thickness.

Following all the bone preparation, the trial components are inserted. Since the provisional tibial component is inserted first, the knee is hyperflexed and externally rotated,

allowing the tibia to sublux forward through the arthrotomy. After the tibial tray is placed, the knee is then brought back to 90° of flexion, and, with distraction of the joint, the flexion space opens and the provisional femoral component is impacted onto the distal femur. The provisional tibial articular surface is then inserted. If there is difficulty gaining exposure and inserting the tibial articular surface, the knee is placed in mid-flexion, approximately 45–60°, and the articular surface is guided into place. Finally, the trial patellar button is placed. Patellar tracking can be assessed at this time. The incidence of lateral retinacular releases has not been impacted by this limited approach. I have reported a lateral release rate of 15% with both a mini-incision arthrotomy and the standard approach.[8] After the provisional components are tested and thought to result in excellent range of motion, stability, and patellar tracking, they are removed and the bone is prepared for cementation of the final components. The knee is copiously irrigated with pulsatile lavage and dried thoroughly. All patients receive a cemented modular fixed bearing posterior-stabilized knee prosthesis (NexGen LPS-Flex or LPS-Flex Gender Prosthesis, Zimmer, Warsaw, IN). Once the cement is of the appropriate viscosity, the knee is hyperflexed and externally rotated. Cement is placed on the proximal tibia and into the stem hole, and the tibial tray is impacted into place and any excess cement is removed. The knee is brought back to 90° of flexion. Cement is placed along the anterior and distal femur as well as on the posterior condyles of the implant. The femoral component is then impacted in place and all excess cement is removed. A careful inspection of the posterior recess and along the margins of the implant should confirm that there is no cement debris. A reduction is performed with a provisional tibial articular surface. The patella is cemented in place and held with the patellar clamp until the cement hardens. The knee is assessed for appropriate balance range of motion, and patellar tracking. If the results are satisfactory, the provisional tibial articular surface is removed and the final tibial polyethylene insert is locked in place. If there is difficulty inserting the final tibial polyethylene component, the knee can be placed in mid-flexion and, with a front-loading tibial tray, the polyethylene insert can be guided into place.

With the final components in place (Fig. 31.8), the tourniquet is released and any bleeding is addressed with electrocautery. The tourniquet is then reinflated for closure and the knee is copiously irrigated with an antibiotic solution. The arthrotomy is closed over a suction drain in an interrupted fashion using an absorbable suture. The deep tissues and the subcutaneous layer are closed with absorbable sutures and the skin is closed with staples. A light sterile dressing is applied and held in place with a compressive stocking.

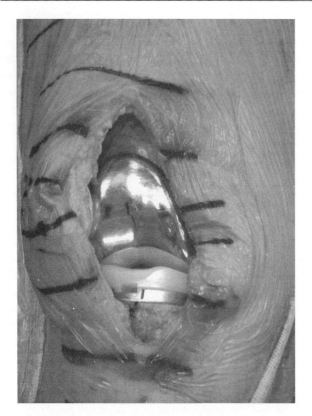

Fig. 31.8 The final components in place (From Scuderi GR, Tria AJ, Jr., Minimal incision total knee arthroplasty. In: Scuderi GR, Tria AJ, Jr. (eds.), *MIS of the Hip and the Knee*. New York: Springer, 2004, with kind permission of Springer Science + Business Media, Inc.)

Postoperative Management

Following surgery, pain management is achieved with either an indwelling epidural catheter for the first 24 h or a femoral nerve block. This is followed by intravenous patient controlled analgesia (PCA) under the direction of the pain service. Continuous passive motion (CPM) is initiated in the recovery room. Patients begin full weight-bearing ambulation and active range of motion exercises as soon as they are alert, stable, and able to follow the instructions of the physical therapists. Physical therapy is undertaken twice daily. Patients are discharged to either home or a rehabilitation center within 2–4 days depending on their progress with physiotherapy and their social situation. An integrated multidisciplinary postoperative clinical pathway is fundamental to patient satisfaction.[9]

Clinical Results

MIS TKA with a limited medial parapatellar arthrotomy is a technique with satisfactory results when the above key steps are followed. In a recently published comparison study,[5] the clinical outcome of a group of mini-incision TKA was compared with that of a group of knee arthrotomies performed with a standard approach. The amount of blood reinfused from the postoperative drain was less in the mini-incision group (mean 292 cc) compared with the group of knee arthrotomies performed with a standard approval (mean 683 cc). Postoperative day 3 hemoglobin measurements were similar between the groups. However, the mini-incision group had reduced transfusion requirements. Our current "bloodless surgery" protocol avoids a preoperative anemia by no longer collecting autologous blood preoperatively; checking the preoperative hemoglobin and using erythropoietin when indicated; and using a reinfusion drain in all patients. This protocol has significantly reduced our transfusion rate in unilateral TKA.[10]

The average length of hospital stay was similar in the two groups: 3.9 days for patients in the mini-incision group, and 4.2 days for patients in the standard group.[5] Thirty-eight percent of the patients in the mini-incision group were discharged directly to their homes compared with 24% of patients in the standard group. By postoperative day 3, the patients who had mini-incision procedures were walking an average 5.8 m further and climbing 1.2 more stair steps than patients who had standard procedures, but these differences were not significant. On postoperative day 3, the patients who had mini-incision procedures had better flexion than patients who had the standard procedures ($p = 0.014$), with an average 4° of difference. The average postoperative flexion for the mini-incision group on day 3 was 92° (range 48–120°), compared with an average of 88° in the standard arthrotomy group (range 69–105).

While one of the major concerns with the use of MIS TKA is that it will compromise the positioning of components, this has not been our experience. A radiographic analysis has revealed that the average alignment of the prosthesis and the overall limb alignment were consistent with previously published reports.[5,11] This is most likely due to the fact that the mini-incision approach is a familiar extensile approach permitting adequate visualization in the carefully selected patient without compromising the surgical accuracy. In addition, the procedure is performed with modified instruments, which are similar to prior instrumentation familiar to the surgeon.

Complications are avoided with meticulous surgical technique, and a review of our early experience has been previously reported.[5] In a group of mini-incision TKA, two patients had superficial erythema of the knee that resolved without sequelae; one patient with a varus deformity developed temporary common peroneal nerve palsy at the level of the proximal fibula, which resolved; and one patient had a traumatic patellar dislocation after a fall 12 weeks postoperatively, requiring a repair of the medial retinaculum. There were no skin or wound complications delaying the healing process. In the standard incision group, two patients had superficial erythema of the knee that resolved, one patient required manipulation under anesthesia at 5 weeks postoperatively, and one patient required arthroscopic lysis of adhesions in conjunction with manipulation at 22 weeks. Presently, the mini-incision approach is being used in the majority of my patients without any untoward effects, because I will gradually extend the skin incision and arthrotomy as needed in an effort to avoid complications.

Discussion

MIS TKA has gained popularity over the last several years and the limited medial parapatellar arthrotomy is part of the continuum of these modified approaches with limited access and visibility. The learning curve is short since the arthroplasty is performed with the same surgical technique using modified and smaller instruments that are more adaptable to the limited operative field. With a gradual shortening of the skin incision and medial parapatellar arthrotomy, a smaller and comfortable operative field will be obtained.

Others have reported a similar clinical experience with this approach. Coon and coworkers recently reported on their experience with MIS TKA using both the MIS mini-incision and the MIS quadriceps-sparing techniques.[3] They found a significantly shorter length of stay of 3.4 days versus 5.9 days for the traditional approach. Patients who had MIS had a lower transfusion requirement of 4% versus 34%. Looking at the early functional outcome, MIS patients walked three times farther on the third postoperative day (176 ft versus 58 ft) and had a better range of motion. This study also reported a potential cost reduction to the healthcare system as surgeons performing MIS improve their operative efficiency and further reduce the hospital length of stay.

The definition of success with MIS TKA is dependent upon the expectations of the surgeon, patient, and family. Patients have overwhelmingly become interested in the concept of MIS because of the anticipation of lower morbidity and a more rapid recovery. However, they need to realize that the clinical outcome is not solely dependent on the length of the incision. During preoperative counseling, patients are informed that they will receive the smallest incision possible to allow for proper placement of the prosthesis rather than guaranteed an incision of a specific length. Success is also multifactorial and dependent on appropriate blood loss management, effective pain control, a comprehensive physiotherapy program, and a supportive social services network.

Optimizing patient selection and paying specific attention to the operative details will ensure clinical success. Experience has demonstrated that there are certain patient characteristics that are better suited for MIS TKA. A shorter, thinner female patient with a lower BMI, a narrower femur, and better preoperative range of motion is better suited for MIS. Caution needs to be taken with patients who have rheumatoid arthritis or inflammatory arthritis, limited range of motion with severe fixed angular deformity, or prior surgery. Regarding the surgical technique, it is important to pay attention to the intraoperative details. The surgical procedure has not essentially changed from the standard techniques. The real difference is that the procedure is performed in an operative field with limited visibility. The addition of modified and smaller instruments has made it easier to access the joint with little or no damage to the extensor mechanism. Training of the surgical assistants to position the knee and retractors for specific surgical steps will greatly facilitate the operation. Finally, MIS TKA can easily be converted to a more extensile approach if there is any difficulty with exposure or positioning the instrumentation or the implants during the arthroplasty. TKA is historically a successful operation and the MIS technique should not compromise the outcome.

References

1. Scuderi GR, Tenholder M, Capeci C. Surgical approaches in mini-incision total knee arthroplasty. Clin Orthop Relat Res 428:61–67, 2004
2. Bonutti PM, Neal DJ, Kester MA. Minimal incision total knee arthroplasty using the suspended leg technique. Orthopedics 26:899–903, 2003
3. Coon TM, Tria AJ, Lavernia C, Randall L. The economics of minimally invasive total knee surgery. Semin Arthroplasty 16:235–238, 2005
4. Laskin RS. New techniques and concepts in total knee replacement. Clin Orthop Relat Res 416:151–153, 2003
5. Tenholder M, Clarke HD, Scuderi GR. Minimal incision total knee arthroplasty: the early clinical experience. Clin Orthop Relat Res 440:67–76, 2005
6. Scuderi GR. Minimally invasive total knee arthroplasty. Am J Orthop 7S:7–11, 2006
7. Kim R, Scuderi GR, Cushner F, et al. Use of lidocaine with epinephrine injection to reduce blood loss in MIS TKA. Proceedings of the 2007 Annual AAOS Meeting, San Diego, CA
8. Cook JL, Scuderi GR, Tenholder M. Incidence of lateral release in total knee arthroplasty in standard and mini approaches. Clin Orthop Relat Res 452:123–126, 2006
9. Scuderi GR. Pre-operative planning and peri-operative management for minimally invasive total knee arthroplasty. Am J Orthopedics 7S:4–6, 2006
10. Cushner FD, Lee GC, Scuderi GR, et al. Blood loss management in high risk patients undergoing total knee arthroplasty. J Knee Surg 19:249–253, 2006
11. Brassard MF, Insall JN, Scuderi GR, Colizza W. Does modularity affect clinical success? A comparison with a minimum 10-year follow-up. Clin Orthop Relat Res 388:26–32, 2001

Chapter 32
MIS TKA with a Subvastus Approach

Mark W. Pagnano

Performing minimally invasive (MIS) total knee arthroplasty (TKA) through a subvastus approach makes sense on an anatomic basis, on a scientific basis, and on a practical basis. Anatomically, the subvastus approach is the only approach that saves the entire quadriceps tendon insertion on the patella[1–5] (Fig. 32.1). Scientifically, the subvastus approach has been shown, in prospective randomized clinical trials, to be superior to the standard medial parapatellar arthrotomy and to the so-called quadriceps-sparing arthrotomy[3,6,7] (Table 32.1). Practically, MIS TKA with a subvastus approach is reliable, reproducible, and efficient and allows the MIS technique to be applied to a broad group of patients, not just a highly selected subgroup[8] (Table 32.2).

It is now accepted widely that the tenets of MIS TKA include a smaller skin incision, no eversion of the patella, minimal disruption of the suprapatellar pouch, and minimal disruption of the quadriceps tendon. To what degree any one of those factors contribute to improvements in postoperative function remains unclear. Our initial attempts at MIS TKA using the short medial arthrotomy (sometimes referred to as the quadriceps-sparing approach) and the mini-midvastus splitting approaches were frustrated by some substantial technical difficulties. We then modified the subvastus approach to the knee to meet the tenets of MIS TKA and found that it markedly facilitated MIS surgery and allowed MIS surgery to be applied to a broader group of patients. When coupled with instruments designed specifically for small-incision surgery, the modified subvastus approach is reliable, reproducible, and safe. Using a simple set of retractors, this procedure can be done without making any blind cuts or free-hand cuts, and that enhances surgical accuracy and patient safety.

Surgical Technique

The incision starts at the superior pole of the patella, ends at the top of the tibial tubercle, and typically measures 3.5 in. (8.8 cm) in extension. Surgeons should start with a traditional 6- to 8-in. incision and then shorten the incision length over time. The medial skin flap is elevated to clearly delineate the inferior border of the vastus medialis obliquus muscle (VMO). The fascia overlying the VMO is left intact because this helps maintain the integrity of the muscle belly itself throughout the case. The anatomy in this region is very consistent. The inferior edge of the VMO is always found more inferior and more medial than most surgeons anticipate. The muscle fibers of the VMO are oriented at a 50° angle and the VMO tendon always attaches to the midpole of the patella. It is very important to save this edge of tendon from the edge of muscle down to the midpole of the patella. That is where the retractor will rest so that the VMO muscle itself is protected throughout the case. The arthrotomy is made along the inferior edge of the VMO down to the midpole of the patella (do not be tempted to cheat this superiorly, because that will hinder, not help, the ultimate exposure) (Fig. 32.2). The proximal limb of the arthrotomy parallels the inferior edge of the VMO and is made at the same 50° angle relative to the long axis of the femur. At the midpole of the patella, the arthrotomy is directed straight distally along the medial border of the patellar tendon. A 90° bent-Hohmann retractor is placed in the lateral gutter and rests against the robust edge of VMO tendon that was preserved during the exposure. Surprisingly little force is needed to completely retract the patella into the lateral gutter. Any substantial medial or inferior osteophytes on the patella are debrided with a rongeur. The knee is then flexed to 90°, providing good exposure of both distal femoral condyles (Fig. 32.3). If the patella does not slide easily into the lateral gutter, typically it is because a portion of the medial patellofemoral ligament remains attached to the patella. That occurs if the proximal limb of the arthrotomy is made in too horizontal a fashion rather than at the 50° angle that parallels the VMO. By releasing that tight band of tissue, the patella will translate laterally without substantial difficulty.

The distal femur is cut with a modified intramedullary resection guide. Bringing the knee out to 60° of flexion better exposes the anterior portion of the distal femur. When a very small skin incision is used, the distal femur is cut one condyle at a time with the intramedullary portion of the cutting guide left in place for added stability. If a slightly longer skin

M.W. Pagnano (✉)
Department of Orthopedic Surgery, Mayo Clinic College of Medicine, Mayo Clinic, 200 First Street SW, Rochester, MN, 55905, USA
e-mail: Pagnano.mark@mayo.edu

G.R. Scuderi and A.J. Tria (eds.), *Minimally Invasive Surgery in Orthopedics*,
DOI 10.1007/978-0-387-76608-9_32, © Springer Science+Business Media, LLC 2010

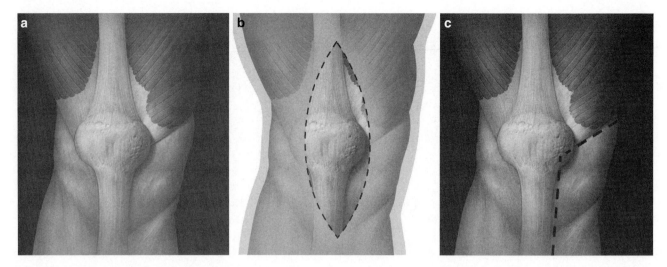

Fig. 32.1 Anatomy of the extensor mechanism. (**a**) The vastus medialis obliquus (VMO) tendon consistently inserts at the midpole of the patella at a 50° angle relative to the long axis of the femur. (**b**) When looking through a surgical incision, one could easily misidentify the most prominent part of the VMO (the point closest to the patella, akin to the bow of the ship) as the most inferior part of the VMO. Because that most prominent portion often lies close to the superior pole of the patella, some sur-geons might then mistakenly presume that the VMO inserts at the superior pole of the patella. Additional medial dissection will delineate the inferior border of the VMO, which is more inferior and more medial than most surgeons anticipate. (**c**) The arthrotomy for the subvastus exposure paral-lels the inferior border of the VMO, intersects the patella at the midpole, and then is turned straight distally to parallel the medial margin of the patellar tendon (Copyright Mayo Foundation, used with permission.)

Table 32.1 Prospective randomized trials of the subvastus approach in total knee arthroplasty

Authors	No. of patients randomized	Study variable	Key findings
Roysam and Oakley[7]	89	Subvastus versus medial parapatellar approach	1. Subvastus had earlier straight medial parapatellar leg raising; $p < 0.001$
			2. Subvastus used fewer narcotics week 1; $p < 0.001$
			3. Subvastus had greater knee flexion at 1 week; $p < 0.001$
Aglietti et al.[6]	60	Subvastus versus Zimmer quadriceps-sparing approach	1. Subvastus had earlier straight leg raising; $p = 0.004$
			2. Subvastus had better flexion at 10 days $p = 0.01$
			3. Subvastus had better flexion at 30 days; $p = 0.03$
Faure et al.[3]	20	Subvastus versus medial parapatellar approach	1. Subvastus had greater strength at 1 week and 1 month
			2. Subvastus had fewer lateral releases done
			3. Subvastus was preferred by patients 4:1

Table 32.2 Clinical results with the minimally invasive subvastus approach in 103 consecutive patients with osteoarthritis

Sex	Age (range)	Weight (range)	Operative time (range)	Functional outcomes mean
61 women; 42 men	66 years (40–90 years)	198 lbs (137–305 lbs)	58 min (35–115 min)	1. Hospital stay: 2.8 days
				2. Normal daily activities: 7 days
				3. No walker: 14 days
				4. No cane: 21 days
				5. Drive: 28 days
				6. Walk ½ mile: 42 days
				7. Flexion at 8 weeks: 116°

From Pagnano et al.[8]

incision is used, the distal cutting guide can be pinned in place and both condyles cut in a standard fashion.

The proximal tibia is cut next and, by doing that, more room is made for subsequently sizing and rotating the femoral component (the most difficult part of any MIS TKA). Three retractors are placed precisely to get good exposure of the entire surface of the tibia: a pickle-fork retractor posteriorly provides an anterior drawer and protects the neurovascular structures; and bent-Hohmann retractors medially and later-ally protect the collateral ligaments and define the perimeter of the tibial bone (Fig. 32.4). The tibial resection is done with an extramedullary guide optimized for small incision

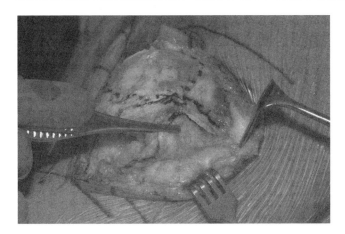

Fig. 32.2 The arthrotomy starts medially along the inferior border of the VMO and extends to the midpole of the patella at the same 50° angle as the muscle fibers of the VMO

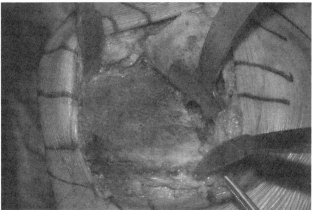

Fig. 32.4 After the distal femur has been cut, the tibia is prepared next, and that is done to provide more working room for subsequently sizing and rotating the femoral component (the most difficult part of any MIS TKA). Good exposure of the entire surface of the tibia is accomplished with three retractors placed precisely: a pickle-fork retractor posteriorly to provide an anterior drawer, and bent-Hohmann retractors medially and laterally to protect the collateral ligaments and define the perimeter of the tibial bone

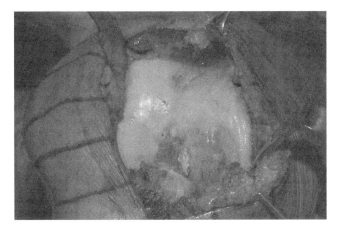

Fig. 32.3 With surprisingly little force, the patella is retracted completely into the lateral gutter. The knee is then flexed to 90° providing exposure of both condyles of the distal femur

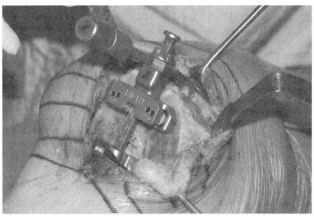

Fig. 32.5 The femoral sizing and rotation guide is designed to be pinned to the distal femur and is thin enough that the knee can subsequently be brought out to 60° of flexion to visualize the anterior femur for accurate sizing

surgery. The tibia is cut in one piece using a narrow but thick saw blade that fits the captured guide. The narrow blade is more maneuverable in the smaller guide and provides better tactile feedback for the surgeon to detect when the posterior and lateral tibial cortices have been cut.

The femoral sizing and rotation guide is thin enough to be pinned to the distal femur and then the knee can be brought out to 60° of flexion to visualize the anterior femur for accurate sizing (Fig. 32.5). At 60° of flexion, a retractor is placed anteriorly and the surgeon can see under direct vision that the femoral cortex will not be notched. Clearing some of the synovium overlying the anterior femoral cortex helps ensure that femoral sizing is accurate. The femoral finishing guide is adjusted medially or laterally. Femoral rotation is confirmed by referencing the surgeon's choice of the posterior condyles, Whiteside's line, or the transepicondylar axis, each of which can be defined with this subvastus approach. After the femoral and tibial cuts are made, the surgeon can carry out

final ligament releases and check flexion and extension gap balance in whatever fashion is desired.

Patellar preparation with this surgical approach is left until the end. Cutting the patella is not required for exposure and, by preparing the patella last, the risk of inadvertent damage to the cut surface of the patella is minimized. The patella cut is done freehand or with the surgeon's choice of cutting or reaming guides. When a patellar cutting guide is used, the trial components are removed because then the entire limb can shorten, taking tension off the extensor mechanism and allowing easier access to the patella for preparation.

The modular tibial tray is cemented first, then the femur, and finally the patella. The tibia is subluxed forward with the

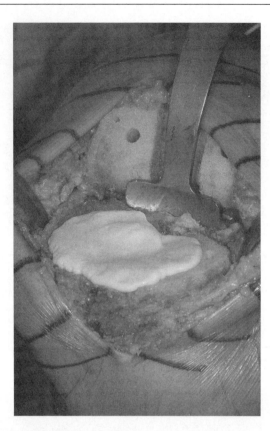

Fig. 32.6 Modular tibial components facilitate the cementing process and it is easiest to cement the tibia first. Excess cement is carefully removed, with particular attention given to the posterolateral corner of the knee

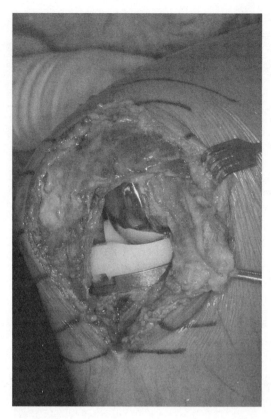

Fig. 32.7 With the final components in place, patellar tracking and range of motion are assessed

aid of the pickle-fork retractor and the medial and lateral margins of the tibia are exposed well with 90° bent-Hohmann retractors. Care is taken to remove excess cement from around the tibial base plate, particularly posterolaterally. The femur is exposed for cementing by placing bent-Hohmann retractors on the medial and lateral sides proximal to the collateral ligament insertions on the femur. A third retractor is placed under the VMO, where it overlies the anterior femur. Cement is applied to the entire undersurface of femoral implant prior to impaction. Special attention is paid to removing excess cement from the distal lateral surface of the femur because this area is difficult to see after the patella is cemented in place (Fig. 32.6). At this point, the real tibial insert can be placed or a trial insert can be used at the surgeon's discretion. The patella is cemented last. After the cement has hardened, the knee is put through a range of motion and final balancing and patellar tracking are assessed (Fig. 32.7).

The tourniquet is deflated so that any small bleeders in the subvastus space can be identified and coagulated. The closure of the arthrotomy starts by reapproximating the corner of capsule to the extensor mechanism at the midpole of the patella. Then three interrupted zero-Vicryl sutures are placed along the proximal limb of the arthrotomy (Fig. 32.8). These sutures can usually be placed deep to the VMO muscle itself and grasp either fibrous tissue or the synovium attached to

the distal or undersurface of the VMO instead of the muscle itself. These first four sutures are most easily placed with the knee in extension but are then tied with the knee at 90° of flexion to avoid overtightening the medial side and creating an iatrogenic patella baja postoperatively. A deep drain is placed in the knee joint and the distal/vertical limb of the arthrotomy is closed with multiple interrupted zero-Vicryl sutures placed with the knee in 90° of flexion. The skin is closed in layers. Staples are used, not a subcuticular suture. More tension is routinely placed on the skin during MIS TKA surgery than in standard open surgery, and our experience suggests the potential for wound-healing problems is magnified if the skin is handled multiple times as is the case with a running subcuticular closure.

Discussion

Minimally invasive total knee arthroplasty with a subvastus approach has proved reliable, reproducible, and efficient. The technique is amenable to stepwise surgeon learning and can be applied to a substantial range of patients who require total knee arthroplasty not just a selected subgroup. There are patients who are not good candidates for any MIS TKA

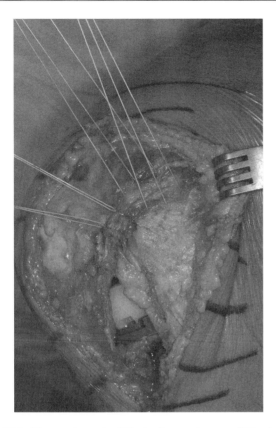

Fig. 32.8 The tourniquet should be let down and any small bleeders in the subvastus space should be cauterized. The closure is done by first reapproximating the corner of capsule at the midpole of the patella. Then three interrupted sutures are placed through the deep layer of synovium to close the knee joint itself. Those four sutures are tied with the knee at 90° of flexion to avoid creating iatrogenic patella baja

Surgeons should be aware that changes in surgical technique alone are unlikely to provide the dramatic early improvements in postoperative function that some surgeons have described after MIS TKA. Maximizing the early gains after surgery (minimal pain, early ambulation, rapid hospital discharge) typically requires a combination of advanced anesthetic techniques, a multimodal pain management program, a rapid rehabilitation protocol, and appropriate patient expectations. How much each of those contributes versus how much the surgical technique contributes to early functional improvement has not been determined scientifically.

procedure, including those with marked knee stiffness, fragile skin, or marked obesity. Similarly, any knee with patella baja will be markedly difficult with an MIS approach because subluxing the patella laterally often is not possible. In those cases, a traditional skin incision and more extensile exposure are in the interest of patient and surgeon alike.

References

1. Pagnano MW, Meneghini RM, Trousdale RT. Anatomy of the extensor mechanism in reference to quadriceps-sparing TKA. Clin Orthop Relat Res 2006 Nov, (452):102–105
2. Chang CH, Chen KH, Yang RS, Liu TK. Muscle torques in total knee arthroplasty with subvastus and parapatellar approaches. Clin Orthop Relat Res 2002, 398:189–195
3. Faure BT, Benjamin JB, Lindsey B, Volz RG, Schutte D. Comparison of the subvastus and paramedian surgical approaches in bilateral knee arthroplasty. J Arthroplasty 1993, 8(5):511–516
4. Gore DR, Sellinger DS, Gassner KJ, Glaeser ST. Subvastus approach for total knee arthroplasty. Orthopedics 2003, 26:33–35
5. Hoffman AA, Plaster RL, Murdock LE. Subvastus (southern) approach for primary total knee arthroplasty. Clin Orthop Relat Res 1991, 269:70–77
6. Aglietti P, Baldini A. A prospective, randomized study of the mini subvastus versus quad-sparing approaches for TKA. Presented at the Interim Meeting of the Knee Society. September 8, 2005, New York, NY
7. Roysam GS, Oakley MJ. Subvastus approach for total knee arthroplasty: a prospective, randomized, and observer-blinded trial. J Arthroplasty 2001, 16:454–457
8. Pagnano MW, Leone JM, Hanssen AD, Lewallen DG. Minimally invasive total knee arthroplasty with an optimized subvastus approach: a consecutive series of 103 patients. Presented at American Academy of Orthopaedic Surgeons Annual Meeting. 2005, Washington DC

Chapter 33
Mini-midvastus Total Knee Arthroplasty

Steven B. Haas, Samuel J. Macdessi, and Mary Ann Manitta

Total knee arthroplasty (TKA) is now considered a gold-standard treatment of advanced arthritis of the knee.[1-4] The early convalescence with standard surgical techniques however is longer than that of total hip arthroplasty, with significant pain and disability from the surgical insult delaying functional recovery. The traditional surgical approach for exposure in knee replacement remains the median parapatellar (MPP) approach. This was initially described by von Langenbeck in 1874 and then popularized by Insall in 1971.[5] Although this approach is the only true extensile approach, it incises the quadriceps tendon, which may delay functional recovery.

Both the midvastus[6] and subvastus[7] approaches have been described to minimize this trauma. The subvastus approach does not violate any portion of the vastus medialis obliquus (VMO) tendon, whereas the midvastus approach incises a small portion of this tendon, usually up to the superior pole of the patella. Technically, it is more difficult to expose the distal femur through the subvastus approach as preservation of the quadriceps attachment reduces proximal surgical visualization.

The midvastus approach is a compromise between the excellent exposure afforded by the MPP approach and the advantages provided by the subvastus approach. With this in mind, the authors developed a minimally invasive (MIS) TKA technique using a modification of the midvastus approach and have entitled it the "mini-midvastus approach." The fundamental principles of this technique are blunt and minimal splitting of the VMO, avoidance of patellar eversion, minimization of soft tissue violation, adequate visualization through the mobile window, and the use of smaller instrumentation. By adhering to these principles, we think that early patient recovery can be optimized without compromising the factors that contribute to long-term success.

Midvastus Approach

The midvastus approach was popularized by Engh[6,8] in an attempt to minimize violation of the quadriceps mechanism. It was thought that this approach would enhance patellofemoral stability, increase postoperative quadriceps control, and decrease scarring in the quadriceps mechanism should revision surgery be required.

The midvastus approach has been studied in several randomized trials comparing it with the MPP approach. Dalury and Jiranek[9] noted greater quadriceps strength at 6 weeks and earlier return of straight leg raise in a bilateral knee replacement study of 100 patients. In a similar but larger study of 100 patients, White et al.[10] also noted less pain at 8 days and 6 weeks in the midvastus group, a greater ability to straight leg raise at 8 days, and less patellar retinacular releases. Unilateral randomized trials have also verified these results. Maestro et al.[11] found a higher incidence of lateral release, loss of knee extension, and reduced range of motion with the MPP approach. Bathis et al.[12] reported early improvements in pain, early quadriceps strength, and proprioception with the midvastus approach. Parentis et al.[13] noted a trend for increased early functional recovery and significantly less blood loss in patients who had undergone a midvastus approach. Engh in 1997 found no difference in functional recovery, range of motion, or radiographic parameters in either group. Likewise, Keating et al.[14] found no difference in early functional recovery.

The midvastus approach may also influence patellar tracking by minimizing the amount of detachment of the VMO from the medial patella. This may decrease the need to perform a lateral release, which can increase postoperative morbidity, with increased lateral swelling and pain. Engh et al.[15] reported a lateral release rate of 3% in patients undergoing a midvastus approach compared with 50% using the MPP approach. White et al.[10] noted a 13% rate in the MPP approach compared with 8% in the midvastus approach which was statistically significant. Additionally, both Maestro et al.[11] and Parentis et al.[13] noted fewer lateral releases. Keating et al.[14] noted no differences in lateral release rates.

S.B. Haas(✉), S.J. Macdessi, and M.A. Manitta
Department of Orthopedic Surgery, Hospital for Special Surgery, Weill Medical College of Cornell University, 535 East 70th Street, New York, NY 10021, NY, USA
e-mail: haass@hss.edu

G.R. Scuderi and A.J. Tria (eds.), *Minimally Invasive Surgery in Orthopedics*, DOI 10.1007/978-0-387-76608-9_33, © Springer Science+Business Media, LLC 2010

Very little has been reported on postoperative patellar positioning using the midvastus approach. Ozkoc et al.[16] assessed time-dependent changes in patellar tracking in a randomized trial comparing the midvastus with the MPP approach. Although early tilt angles were similar, late patellar tilt was noted in the MPP group. Both early and late lateral subluxation and worse congruence angles were noted in the MPP group.

Anatomical Considerations with the Midvastus Approach

Cooper et al.[17] performed a cadaveric study assessing the neurovascular relationships in the midvastus approach. The perforating vessels were on average 8.8 cm from the patella. They recommend a safe distance for sharp muscle splitting to be 4.5 cm. If further exposure is necessary, the remaining muscle fibers can then be bluntly split to the level of the vastoadductor membrane and adductor magnus tendon without neurovascular injury.

Theoretically, concern exists of denervation of the distal portion of the VMO with the midvastus approach. Cooper et al.[17] noted extensive branching of the femoral nerve en route to the oblique portion of the muscle. Using the midvastus approach, the distal muscle segment could only be denervated by splitting the muscle fibers to the point of attachment to the vastoadductor membrane because the femoral nerve lies in a fascial tunnel just deep to this point.

Parentis et al.[13] found a 43% incidence of early VMO denervation on electromyographic testing when using the midvastus approach with the patella everted. They compared this with the MPP approach and found no muscle denervation changes in this group. A muscle split of approximately 10–15 cm was employed. Four of six cases with acute changes were distal to the muscle split. In patients with chronic changes, once again, five of six were in the distal portion of the muscle. One patient had acute and chronic changes both proximally and distally. Theoretically, patellar subluxation with greater stretch on the quadriceps mechanism may increase the risk of neuropraxia. Despite these electromyographic changes, there was a trend for superior functional recovery for up to 6 weeks in the midvastus group.

In a 5-year follow-up study of the same patient group, Kelly et al.[18] found that only two of the nine patients had persistent chronic abnormalities, with one having reinnervation changes and the other demonstrating ongoing denervation. Both of these cases were distal to the muscle split and both were performed by sharp dissection. All patients who had the muscle split performed bluntly had a normal electromyographic study. This raises the possibility of direct trauma to the nerve. No functional deficits were observed.

We recently performed a comparative study of 20 consecutive patients who had undergone a MIS-TKA using a midvastus

approach without patellar eversion.[19] Electromyographic analysis of the vastus medialis muscle above and below the muscle split was performed. Average time from surgery to electromyographic analysis was 3.9 months. Four patients (20%) demonstrated mildly abnormal polyphasic changes consistent with mild denervation only. Two were distal and two were proximal to the muscle split. At a similar follow-up interval, this was considerably less than that noted by Parentis et al. where the patella was everted.

The Mini-midvastus Modification

In 2001, the senior author (SBH) developed a modification to the midvastus approach where the patella is subluxed and not everted. This has been termed the mini-midvastus approach. Theoretically, this places less stress on the extensor mechanism, thereby minimizing the length of the muscle split required. By using the principles of the mobile window, downsized anatomically shaped instruments, and minimizing tibial subluxation, less splitting of the muscle is required.

Another potential advantage of the mini-midvastus approach is the need for smaller incisions. The incision with the traditional medial parapatellar approach is generally carried proximally to the end of the split in the quadriceps tendon. This is not necessary with the mini-midvastus technique. In fact, we have found that with improvements in instrumentation, a TKA can be safely and accurately performed through an 8.5–12 cm skin incision (Fig. 33.1).

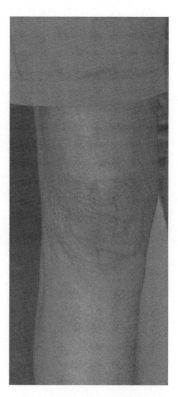

Fig. 33.1 Appearance of smaller incision used in MIS total knee replacement (TKR)

Preoperative Assessment

Several points are pertinent in the assessment of a potential candidate for MIS-TKA. Clinical examination should focus on the patient's size, knee range of motion, presence of scars, deformity of the extremity, and the limb's neurovascular status. Radiographs are interpreted for deformity, bone loss, presence of patellar baja and overall bone quality. All patients undergo a complete medical evaluation prior to their arthroplasty.

Although no absolute contraindications exist, certain patients are more amenable to undergo a MIS-TKA. Approximately 75% of patients have this approach whereas the remainder have a limited MPP approach performed with an identical technique. Relative contraindications include men with a substantial quadriceps muscle mass, significant obesity (body mass index [BMI] greater than 40) and the presence of severe coronal plane deformity. We also do not use a MIS-TKA technique with flexion contractures of more than 25°, passive flexion of less than 80°, or in patients with severe patellar baja or significant scarring of the quadriceps mechanism.

Instrumentation

Specialized instrumentation is critical in performing this procedure. Most systems today have made appropriate instrument modifications for a MIS-TKA to be performed. We use the Genesis II (Smith and Nephew, Memphis, TN) High-Flex posterior-stabilized or Journey (Smith and Nephew) systems.

To meet the demands of a mini-midvastus approach, cutting blocks and guides were made smaller with rounded edges to be accommodated through smaller incisions. Additionally, side-specific instruments have been developed so that the extensor mechanism does not impede placement of cutting blocks (Fig. 33.2). We also use a saw blade that is rigid with a narrow body that fans out at the distal tip to facilitate bone cuts.

The tibial guide has a side-specific medial wing that hugs the medial tibial plateau. The lateral wing was removed because it was impeded by the position of the patellar ligament. The lateral portion was never used to cut through, because iatrogenic laceration of the patellar ligament may result. This modification allows the lateral plateau to be cut from both anterior to posterior and medial to lateral.

Femoral instruments include a side-specific valgus alignment system in which the bulk of the guide can be placed medially where there is ample exposure (Fig. 33.3). The anterior femoral cutting guide, distal femoral cutting block, and the four-in-one finishing are narrower in the medial to lateral dimension and permit more freely angled cuts. The remainder of the instruments, including the anterior resection stylus, the distal resection stylus, the housing resection block (for posterior-stabilized knees), and the femoral sizing guide, have been downsized. Additionally, the anterior stylus is angled to allow placement under the skin when referencing the preliminary anterior cut.

Surgical Technique

Anesthesia

All patients receive epidural anesthesia, which is continued for 48 h. Patients also receive a Marcaine femoral nerve block, which we have found aids significantly in postoperative pain control. Intravenous cephazolin is our antibiotic of choice. Patients with significant allergies to penicillins are administered vancomycin.

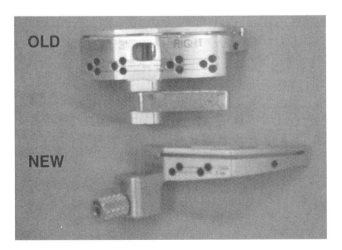

Fig. 33.2 *Top* – Standard Genesis II Tibial Cutting Block. *Bottom* – MIS Genesis II Tibial Cutting Block (Smith and Nephew)

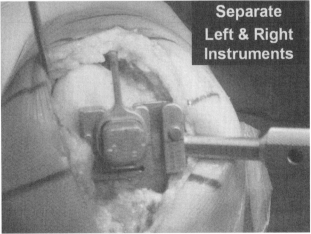

Fig. 33.3 Preparing a femur with a right-sided MIS valgus/rotation guide. The stylus is aligned with the AP axis line (Whiteside's line)

Patient Set-Up

An above-knee tourniquet is applied, with protection of the skin by wool. A sandbag is placed under the drapes at the level of the opposite ankle so that the knee can sit flexed at approximately 70–90°. The majority of the procedure is done in this position. Hyperflexion is sometimes required to prepare the proximal tibia and insert the definitive tibial tray. A lateral support is used so that the leg sits without being held by an assistant.

Exposure

Landmarks for the skin incision are the borders of the patella and the tibial tubercle. These are marked and then a longitudinal incision line is drawn at the junction of the middle and medial thirds of the patella. The incision extends from 1 cm above the superior pole of the patella to the proximal half of the tibial tubercle on its medial side. Our typical skin incision length is between 8.5 and 12 cm. However, we have no hesitation to extend this at any stage if there appears to be undue tension, especially at the distal apex of the incision.

A medial arthrotomy is performed. This extends from the superior pole of the patella to the level of the tibial tubercle. We leave a 5-mm cuff of tissue adjacent to the tubercle to aid in closure later on. The VMO is identified and an oblique split is made in the muscle in the line of its fibers at the level of the superior pole of the patella.

The first centimeter of the muscle split is started sharply but the remainder is performed bluntly with a finger, gently separating the muscle fibers. Performing the split completely by sharp dissection risks damaging the distal innervation of the vastus musculature. The muscle split generally is between 2 and 3 cm in length. The suprapatellar pouch is preserved except in cases of severe inflammatory disease.

With the knee extended, a subperiosteal dissection is carried around the medial pretibial border, releasing the meniscotibial attachments. The patella is then retracted laterally and a partial excision of the infrapatellar fat pad is performed. We also excise the medial fat pad at this stage. The tibial attachments of the anterior cruciate ligament and the anterior horn of the lateral meniscus are released. This allows placement of a thin bent Hohmann retractor laterally to sublux the patella. A small synovial window is made over the anterolateral femoral cortex to aid in our initial anterior femoral resection.

This is found more commonly in men and sometimes require initial patellar resection to assist in patellar subluxation. We caution against initial patellar resection in older, osteoporotic females because of the risk of Iatrogenic crushing of the patellar bone during lateral retraction.

Femoral Preparation

Femoral preparation is performed first to relax the extension space. This is done with the knee in 70° of flexion. Limiting knee flexion places the soft tissue window over the distal and anterior femur. Hyperflexion must be avoided because it not only tightens the extensor mechanism but also limits exposure. A thin, bent Hohmann retractor is placed laterally around the margin of the femoral condyle without excessive lateral traction to hold the patella subluxed.

The anteroposterior axis (Whiteside's line) is marked on the distal femur and is used as the major landmark for establishing component rotation. The posterior condylar axis is used as a secondary reference in varus knees, where it is most reproducible. The transepicondylar axis is more difficult to assess because it requires excessive retraction of the patella laterally.

A 9.5-mm drill is used to enter the femoral canal at a starting point in the notch just anterior to the posterior cruciate ligament insertion on the femur. The canal is then suctioned of its marrow contents to reduce fat embolization risk. An intramedullary alignment guide set at 5° of valgus relative to the anatomic axis is inserted. We only use posterior paddles for additional referencing if there is concern about rotational alignment. An anteroposterior (AP) stylus guide inserted over the rod is placed in line with the marking of the AP axis, and the block is pinned in place. An anterior referencing guide is then slid under the quadriceps mechanism touching the anterolateral femoral cortex, which usually represents the highest point.

The preliminary anterior resection guide is then pinned in place, and the preliminary cut is performed. We prefer to use an anterior resection first technique, so that later corrections in rotational or sagittal placement can be made if we are not satisfied with our initial position. Along with this, this cut relaxes the extensor mechanism prior to placement of the distal cutting guide and allows the guide to sit more evenly on a flat surface.

We then perform our distal femoral resection. Additional retraction is not required at this point because the guide's wedge shape usually retracts the proximal tissues adequately. The block is secured with two headed pins, the intramedullary rod is removed, and the distal resection is performed.

The femoral component size is then determined. The knee may require further flexion so that the posterior paddles can be passed behind the posterior condyles. If we are between sizes, we prefer to choose the smaller component size so as not to overtighten the flexion space. We then pin the appropriate four-in-one cutting guide in place, and once again assess our rotation. It is critical at this stage that a thin bent Hohmann retractor is placed deep to the medial collateral ligament (MCL) for protection. The femoral resection is performed in the following order: posterior condyles, posterior chamfer, anterior resection, and anterior chamfer.

Tibial Preparation

The proximal tibial resection is then performed (Fig. 33.4). We prefer extramedullary instrumentation however intramedullary rod alignment can be used with this technique. The knee is flexed to approximately 90°. Excessive external rotation, which is often utilized in the standard approach, must be avoided because this decreases visualization of the lateral compartment by rotating the lateral tibial plateau under the femur. A thin bent Hohmann retractor is then placed medially and laterally, to once again protect the MCL and the extensor mechanism. Any overhanging anteromedial osteophytes are removed at this stage with a rongeur so that the tibial resection guide can sit in direct contact with the margin of the tibia. The tibial guide is placed parallel to the tibial crest proximally. We also use the tibialis anterior tendon over the ankle and the second metatarsal as reference points distally. The posterior slope is then adjusted so that the alignment guide is parallel to the fibular shaft. We aim for an 11-mm resection off the intact side. The guide is then pinned in place. An Aufranc retractor is placed posteriorly in order to protect the posterior neurovascular structures without changing the position of the knee.

We then perform the proximal tibial resection. In order for the blade to be captured by the cutting guide, the saw must initially be angled at 45° aiming posteriorly. Once within the bone, the medial resection can be safely completed directing the blade in an anterior to posterior direction. We then direct the blade laterally to complete the resection. If we are in any doubt of the depth of the resection, we prefer to leave a small rim of bone. It is much safer to remove this later during the procedure as exposure increases, than to aim to remove the bone in one piece and cause an iatrogenic

injury to the ligaments or, less commonly, the neurovascular bundle. The alignment of our tibial cut is then rechecked using an alignment rod connected to a spacer block.

The knee is then placed in 90° of flexion. Using laminar spreaders, we assess the posterior condyles for any retained osteophytes (Fig. 33.5). These are removed with a curved osteotome and aid in reestablishing flexion capability. The meniscal remnants are excised at this stage along with the posterior cruciate ligament (if a posterior stabilized system is being used). We then place spacer blocks into both the flexion and extension spaces to ensure that we have obtained symmetrical spaces with adequate resection levels. Additionally, it is a useful tool to predict later soft tissue releases.

The knee is then flexed to 90–120° and an Aufranc retractor is once again placed posteriorly. This is the only time prior to component insertion that hyperflexion may be necessary. An appropriately sized tibial component is then pinned in place with one pin on the medial side. The proximal tibia is then reamed and broached to accept the definitive prosthesis. We then remove any overhanging tibial osteophytes, which are most commonly found posteromedially.

Final Preparation

Once we have confirmed that no further bone resection is required, we complete our femoral preparation. We place the posterior stabilized box cutter in place and mark the outline with a marking pen by drawing lines on the inner side of the resection box. We temporarily remove it to ensure adequate mediolateral positioning. We have found that lining

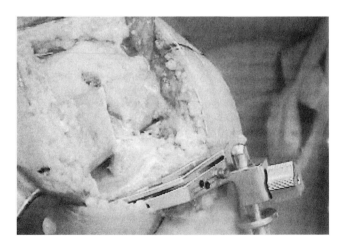

Fig. 33.4 Preparing a tibia with a MIS tibial cutting block (From Haas SB, Lehman AP, Manitta MA. Mini-midvastus total knee arthroplasty. In: Scuderi GR, Tria AJ Jr, Berger RA (eds.), MIS Techniques in Orthopedics, New York, Springer, 2006, with kind permission of Springer Science + Business Media, Inc.)

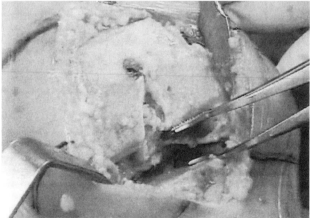

Fig. 33.5 A laminar spreader is placed after bone resection. Good visualization for resection of the meniscus and posterior cruciate ligament (PCL) and for posterior osteophyte removal (From Haas SB, Lehman AP, Manitta MA. Mini-midvastus total knee arthroplasty. In: Scuderi GR, Tria AJ Jr, Berger RA (eds.), MIS Techniques in Orthopedics, New York, Springer, 2006, with kind permission of Springer Science + Business Media, Inc.)

up the inside of the cutting box with the inner margin of the medial femoral condyle is a useful tool with this prosthesis. Overall, we aim for slight lateral position to optimize patellar tracking. Medial overhang should be avoided, because this is a cause of capsular pain. The guide is then pinned in place and the box is prepared.

If the patella is being resurfaced, it is usually done at this stage. It is easier to wait until both femoral and tibial cuts have been performed as the reduced tension on the extensor mechanism allows the patella to be more easily averted. The patella is then prepared for a trial component. Once the trial is in place, we chamfer the lateral margin with a saw to minimize lateral retinacular impingement.

The trial femoral component is then inserted. We then perform a trial reduction with a variety of inserts and assess for coronal plane stability with the knee in both extension and at 90° of flexion. Soft tissue releases are then performed until satisfactory balance is achieved. Patellofemoral tracking is then observed. If this is found to be suboptimal, it is rechecked with the tourniquet deflated to ensure that a lateral retinacular release is not required.

Component Insertion

We prefer the use of cemented implants; however, noncemented devices may be used. Prior to cementing, the bone surfaces are lavaged under pulsatile pressure to achieve a bloodless and dry bone bed. A bone plug is fashioned and impacted into the femoral hole of the intercondylar notch. Occasionally, sclerotic bone requires drilling with a 2.5-mm drill to enhance cement interdigitation.

The tibial component is inserted first. Exposure is obtained using an identical technique to that employed when inserting the trial component. The posterolateral overhang, which frequently occurs with symmetric tibial implants can lead to difficulty with implant insertion and cement removal. For this reason, we prefer to use an asymmetric tibial base plate to facilitate clearance of the femoral condyle during implantation and subsequent cement removal. Once the tibial component has been implanted, the femoral and patellar components are inserted along with a trial polyethylene insert.

Removal of cement from the posterior margins of the tibia can be aided by placing the knee in extension and applying traction prior to the femoral component implantation. A small curved curette can then be swept posteriorly along the margin of the tibial component to help remove any additional cement. On the femoral side, initial excessive proximal retraction should be avoided to remove cement when the component is being implanted at 90° of flexion. It is best to only remove the cement extruded into the intercondylar notch and the condylar margins at this stage. A trial liner is inserted and the knee is

then taken into extension. The mobile window will then easily deliver the anterior femoral cortex into view to remove the remaining extruded cement without the need for retraction.

The patellar component is then placed and clamped and the cement is allowed to harden. Any additional cement is removed at this stage. The definitive polyethylene insert is then inserted. If using a posterior-stabilized insert, the surgeon should begin insertion of the polyethylene in 90° of flexion. The knee should then be brought into extension to engage the locking mechanism. The poly liner is locked with the knee in 5–15° of flexion.

Closure

The tourniquet is deflated at this stage and bleeding is controlled. The knee is copiously lavaged with normal saline solution and two drains are inserted. The capsular layer is closed by placing 0-Vicryl sutures in to the VMO tendon and perimuscular fascia. Three to five sutures will usually suffice. The remainder of the arthrotomy and the subcutaneous tissues are closed with interrupted sutures as well. The authors prefer to use 0-Vicryl sutures for the capsular layer and deep fat and 3/0 Vicryl for the subcutaneous layers. Clips are used to oppose the skin edges.

Rehabilitation

All patients are started on a continuous passive motion (CPM) machine in the recovery room and flexion is increased as pain allows. Weight bearing is commenced on the first postoperative day. All patients receive Coumadin for thromboembolic prophylaxis and foot compressive devices are used until the patient is ambulating unassisted. A patient-controlled epidural is continued until the second postoperative day, when it is removed and the patient is placed on oral analgesics.

Results

The senior author (SBH) has performed over 750 MIS-TKAs using the mini-midvastus technique. It is now used in the majority of primary TKAs being performed. Our initial research[20] on this technique involved a comparative study of 40 TKAs performed using a standard technique with 40 MIS-TKAs using the mini-midvastus modification where the patella was subluxed but not everted. There were no preoperative differences in demographics, range of motion, Knee Society Scores, or function scores between the two groups.

Patients achieved return of motion faster in the MIS-TKA group. Mean flexion for the MIS-TKA group at 6 and 12 weeks was 114° (range 90–132°) and 122° (range 103–135°) respectively, compared with 95° (range 65–125°) and 110° (range 80–125°) for the control group. At 1 year, the MIS-TKA group retained higher mean flexion angles of 125° versus 116° in the control group. Knee Society Scores were also higher in the MIS-TKA group. There were no differences in radiographic alignment. Additionally, no infections, extensor mechanisms, or neurovascular complications occurred.

We recently performed a retrospective analysis of 335 consecutive patients (391 knees) who had underwent a MIS-TKA using the mini-midvastus approach from September 2001 to September 2004.[21] There were 248 women and 87 men. One third of patients had a BMI of between 30 and 39. The mean preoperative range of motion was 109°. The mean postoperative range of motion was 111° at 6 weeks, 121° at 3 months, and 125° at both 1 and 2 years. We observed no increased complication rate with this approach. There were no fractures, extensor mechanism complications, or neurovascular complications. Our infection rate was 0.5%.

Laskin et al.[22] performed a case-matched outcome study in patients undergoing MIS-TKA using a mini-midvastus approach compared with those having had a MPP approach. The surgeries on this occasion differed in that a cruciate-retaining condylar knee (Genesis II, Smith and Nephew) was used. Patients in the MIS-TKA group had lower pain scores and lower average total morphine sulfate usage when compared with the control arm. Mean flexion in the MIS-TKA group was greater at 6 weeks (115° vs. 110°). At 3 months, the groups had equalized with each other. No differences in limb alignment or stability were noted.

Laskin[23] also reviewed 100 consecutive patients undergoing the same MIS-TKA technique with a mean follow-up of 2.4 years. Patients were excluded from this technique if they had flexion of less than 80°, a flexion contracture of greater than 20°, prior open knee surgery, or rheumatoid arthritis. Weight, severity of deformity, or coronal plane instability was not a contraindication to this technique. The mean passive flexion measured 114° at 4 weeks and 122° at 2 years. Only one tibial component was malpositioned in 4° of varus in a man with a BMI of 40. No femoral components were malpositioned. It was concluded that the surgical approach was not applicable to patients with a BMI of greater than 40 or severe fixed valgus deformity.

Conclusion

The mini-midvastus approach appears to aid in early functional recovery with a more rapid return of motion and possibly a greater ultimate range of motion than the MPP approach.

The mini-midvastus approach provides results equal to or superior to those reported for the sub-vastus or "quadriceps-sparing" techniques; however, it gives the surgeon better visualization while limiting dissection of the quadriceps tendon.[24,25]

The use of smaller, well-designed instruments permits less surgical dissection while avoiding excessive soft tissue retraction. This avoids the need for patellar eversion, thereby reducing the length of the arthrotomy and skin incision. We have found this technique to enhance patient recovery, reduce pain, and improve cosmesis, without compromising the radiographic positioning of the implants or the clinical results.

References

1. Font-Rodriguez DE, Scuderi GR, Insall JN. Survivorship of cemented total knee arthroplasty. Clin Orthop Relat Res 1997; 345:79–86
2. Kelly MA, Clarke HD. Long-term results of posterior cruciate substituting total knee arthroplasty. Clin Orthop Relat Res 2002; 404:51–57
3. Pavone V, Boettner F, Fickert S, et al. Total condylar knee arthroplasty: a long-term follow-up. Clin Orthop Relat Res 2001;388:18–25
4. Ranawat CS, Flynn WF, Saddler S, et al. Long-term results of the total condylar knee arthroplasty: a 15-year survivorship study. Clin Orthop Relat Res 1993;286:94–102
5. Insall JN. A midline approach to the knee. J Bone Joint Surg 1971;53A:1584–1586
6. Engh GA, Holt BT, Parks NL. A midvastus muscle-splitting approach for total knee arthroplasty. J Arthroplasty 1997;12:322–331
7. Hofmann AA, Plaster RL, Murdock LE. Subvastus (southern) approach for primary total knee arthroplasty. Clin Orthop Relat Res 1991;269:70–77
8. Engh GA, Parks NL. Surgical technique of the midvastus arthrotomy. Clin Orthop Relat Res 1998;351:270–274
9. Dalury DF, Jiranek WA. A comparison of the midvastus and paramedian approaches for total knee arthroplasty. J Arthroplasty 1999;14:33–37
10. White RE, Allman JK, Trauger JA, et al. Clinical comparison of the midvastus and the median parapatellar surgical approaches. Clin Orthop Relat Res 1999;367:117–122
11. Maestro A, Suarez MA, Rodriguez L, et al. The midvastus surgical approach in total knee arthroplasty. Int Orthop Relat Res 2000;24:104–107
12. Bathis H, Perlick L, Blum C, et al. Midvastus approach in total knee arthroplasty: a randomized, double-blinded study on early rehabilitation. Knee Surg Sports Traumatol Arthrosc 2005;13: 545–550
13. Parentis MA, Rumi MN, Deol SG, et al. A comparison of the vastus-splitting and median parapatellar approaches in total knee arthroplasty. Clin Orthop Relat Res 1999;367:101–116
14. Keating EM, Faris PM, Meding JB, et al. Comparison of the midvastus muscle-splitting approach with the median parapatellar approach in total knee arthroplasty. J Arthroplasty 1999;14:29–32
15. Engh GA, Parks NL, Ammeen DJ. Influence of surgical approach on lateral retinacular releases in total knee arthroplasty. Clin Orthop Relat Res 1996;331:56–63
16. Ozkoc G, Hersekli MA, Akpinar S, et al. Time dependent changes in patellar tracking with medial parapatellar and midvastus approaches. Knee Surg Sports Traumatol Arthrosc. 2005;13:654–657

17. Cooper RE Jr, Trinidad G, Buck WR. Midvastus approach in total knee arthroplasty: a description and a cadaveric study determining the distance of the popliteal artery from the patellar margin of the incision. J Arthroplasty 1999;14:505–508

18. Kelly MJ, Rumi MN, Kothari M, et al. Comparison of the vastus-splitting and median parapatellar approaches for primary total knee arthroplasty: a prospective randomized study. J Bone Joint Surg 2006;88A:715–720

19. Macdessi SJ, Manitta MA, Wu A, Reichler B, Haas SB. Electromyographic analysis of the extensor mechanism following a mini-midvastus approach without patellar eversion. Unpublished data

20. Haas SB, Cook S, Beksac B. Minimally invasive total knee replacement through a mini midvastus approach: a comparative study. Clin Orthop Relat Res 2004;428:68–73

21. Haas SB, et al. Follow-up study of minimally invasive total knee replacement through a mini midvastus approach. Unpublished data

22. Laskin RS, Beksac B, Phongjunakorn A, et al. Minimally invasive total knee replacement through a mini-midvastus incision. Clin Orthop Relat Res 2004;428:74–81

23. Laskin RS. Minimally invasive total knee arthroplasty. The results justify its use. Clin Orthop Relat Res 2005;440:54–59

24. Tria AJ Jr, Coon TM. Minimally incision total knee arthroplasty: early experience. Clin Orthop Relat Res 2003;416:185–190

25. Boerger, TO, Agleitti, P, Mondanelli, N, Sensi, L. Mini-subvastus versus medial parapatellar approach in total knee arthroplasty. Clin Orthop Relat Res 2005;440:82–87

Chapter 34
Minimally Invasive Total Knee Arthroplasty

Suspended Leg Approach and Arthroscopic-Assisted Techniques

Peter Bonutti

Minimally invasive total knee arthroplasty (MIS TKA) was developed primarily due to patient demand for less pain, faster recovery, and, it was hoped, improved functional results. Traditional total knee arthroplasty (TKA) consisted of a technique of a supine patient, tourniquet, incision of 6–12 in., median parapatellar approach, everted patella, and dislocated tibiofemoral joint with large bulky instruments that may increase trauma to the soft tissue and prolong recovery.

We began developing MIS knee arthroplasty techniques in 1991 with the goal of reducing overall soft tissue trauma and sparing quadriceps mechanism. After instrumentation and techniques were developed, in 1999 we began performing MIS TKA on selected patients. Our goals were to (1) reduce incision size (12 cm or less); (2) avoid everting the patella; (3) use muscle-sparing techniques – vastus medialis oblique (VMO) snip (mini-midvastus); (4) use downsized instrumentation; and (5) make in situ bone cuts.

In 2001, we first presented our data and evolved into other muscle-sparing techniques.[1] In 2002, we developed the *suspended leg approach*, similar to arthroscopic surgery with the patient's leg hanging distracted by gravity, over the edge of the operating table. The goal was to develop a versatile approach allowing the surgeon to go from an arthroscopic procedure to a unicompartmental to TKA.[2]

In 2003, we began using MIS techniques with computer navigation. We then develop a direct lateral approach with Dr. Michael Mont.[3–5] In 2004, a mini-subvastus approach was developed for exposures.[6] We then used arthroscopic-assisted techniques for visualization of the joint, ligament balancing, and patellar tracking with quadriceps-sparing exposures.[7,8] In 2005, we utilized these techniques for revision TKA.[9] To date, we have performed nearly 2,000 MIS TKA procedures and are able to do this universally on all patients regardless of age, weight, or deformity.

There is no question that the MIS TKA technique is more difficult and results are only short term. To date, only one article reports a minimum of 2–4 year follow-up with a 97% success rate.[3] We have evaluated the pitfalls and complications of MIS TKA techniques[10] and found that although there is a significant learning curve, the complications once the technique is developed are no different than traditional TKA. This was confirmed in a prospective randomized multicenter clinical trial.[11]

Currently, MIS TKA has been classified primarily on the quadriceps exposure (Diagram 1,2): (1) VMO snip (mini-midvastus); (2) "quadriceps saving" (modification of median parapatellar); (3) mini-subvastus; and (4) direct lateral. In all these approaches, the patient is supine, usually with an adjustable leg holder. The incisions are usually shorter than 12 cm, the patella is not everted, and downsized instruments are utilized to make the bone cuts.

A novel approach, however, utilizing the leg in an arthroscopic position with the leg suspended – hanging over the edge of the table - with various MIS quadriceps exposures has been described.[2] This suspended leg technique has a number of advantages; (1) allowing gravity to distract the soft tissue; (2) enhancing exposure to the posterior joint; (3) allowing the surgeon to be in variable positions (sitting/standing); (4) controlling flexion/extension of the joint; and (5) optimizing patella tracking and soft tissue and ligament balancing both before and after capsular closure (arthroscopic assisted).

This novel approach does have a series of problems. It presents a new view for the reconstructive surgeon; therefore, issues such as patient position, retractor placement, and landmark assessment can be a challenge. Femoral position can be altered by rotating the leg in an adjustable leg support and evaluation of knee extension requires the surgeon to move from a sitting to a standing position. In addition, tibial implantation and cement pressurization require support of the lower extremity during implantation. However, despite these difficulties, the suspended leg approach has been used with quadriceps exposures, computer navigation, and arthroscopic assistance.

Historically, TKA has been performed with the patient supine and the leg in variable positions of flexion and extension.[7] As one progressively flexes and extends the joint, the posterior joint is compressed, which can limit soft tissue visualization,

P. Bonutti (✉)
Bonutti Clinic, 1303 West Evergreen Avenue, Effingham, IL, 62401, USA
e-mail: p@bonutti.net

G.R. Scuderi and A.J. Tria (eds.), *Minimally Invasive Surgery in Orthopedics*,
DOI 10.1007/978-0-387-76608-9_34, © Springer Science+Business Media, LLC 2010

posterior capsular exposure, and, more importantly, accurate ligament and soft tissue balancing.

Arthroscopic knee surgery traditionally is performed with the patient's leg in a leg holder and the joint distracted by gravity. This may enhance joint exposure, visualization, and soft tissue assessment. The surgeon is able to manipulate the extremity from flexion to extension with gravity for an accurate assessment of tissue and ligament balancing. This technique has been utilized in the UKA.[12] Our goal was to assess this suspended approach for TKA and arthroscopic-assisted arthroplasty. This versatile approach may allow different procedures going from arthroscopic to unicompartmental to TKA approach and allowing arthroscopic assistance for this continuum of surgical procedures.

Surgical Technique

The suspended leg approach was originally utilized for TKA in 2002 and was adopted from arthroscopic techniques and approaches. The leg is suspended in a leg holder or padded support (Fig. 34.1). The hip is generally flexed 10–20° and the knee is distracted by gravity and flexed to approximately 90°. This allows body weight and gravity to distract the joint and assess the true deformity, both soft tissue and bone. The soft tissue is stretched by gravity and the skin incision–mobile window can be controlled by variable flexion and extension.

Sterile technique for arthroplasty is critical. We utilize the technique where the patient's leg is sterilely draped directly to the surgeon and to the instrumentation table. The surgeon can be seated or standing and controlling flexion and extension of the joint, optimizing the surgical positioning of the patient's extremity (Fig. 34.2).

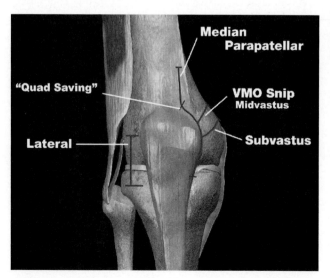

Fig. 34.1 Various quadriceps exposure from the median patellar, quadriceps saving, mini midvastus, mini subvastus, and direct lateral

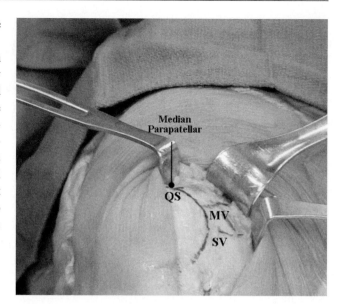

Fig. 34.2 Surgical picture showing the median parapatellar, quadriceps saving (QS), modification of median parapatellar, mini midvastus (MV), and mini subvastus (SV)

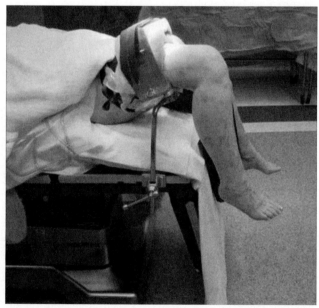

Fig. 34.3 Suspended leg technique. Uses an arthroscopic leg holder versus a padded bolster. The hip is flexed slightly and the knee is suspended with gravity

The suspended leg technique has been utilized with all of the described MIS muscle-sparing approaches. In all cases, the goal was the overall reduction of soft tissue trauma, avoiding everting the patella, use of downsized instrumentation, and in situ bone cuts (Figs. 34.3 and 34.4).

A well-trained assistant working with the surgeon is critical. Symbiotic utilization of retractors for exposure, progressively medially then laterally, and allowing a mobile window going from flexion and extension to enhance exposure are necessary.

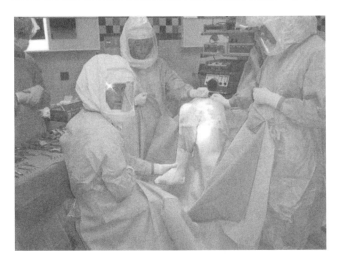

Fig. 34.4 Sterile surgical draping where the patient's leg is suspended and sterile surgical drapes are connected from the patient to the surgeon to the instrumentation table. This allows the surgeon to go from a seated to standing position and mobilize the lower extremity

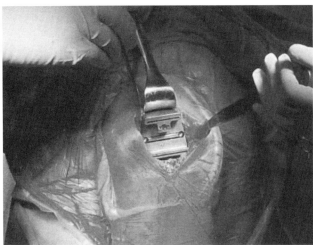

Fig. 34.6 Downsized 4-in-1 cutting instruments

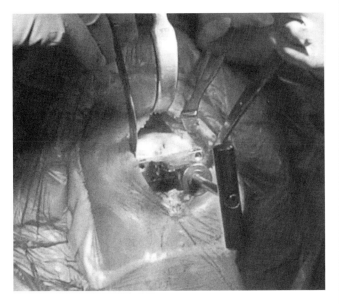

Fig. 34.5 The patella is retracted laterally and the quadriceps mechanism is elevated anteriorly to expose the distal femur

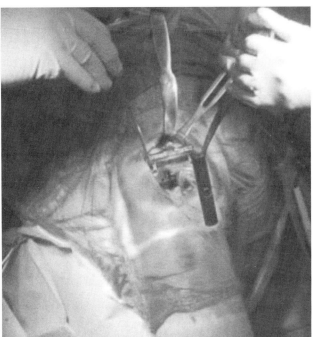

Fig. 34.7 Anterior referencing system

Downsized "soft tissue-friendly" instrumentation is critical. We use both anterior referencing instrumentation (Fig. 34.5) and posterior referencing (Fig. 34.6). Reducing the bulk of instrumentation allows one to decrease the overall soft tissue envelope required for exposure. This, coupled with the *mobile window*, allows improved visualization and can be further enhanced with arthroscopic assistance.

The suspended leg technique allows gravity to distract the joint, which can be further enhanced by manual distraction or stress medially to laterally to selectively enhance exposure to different segments of the joint (Fig. 34.7). This also enhances soft tissue balancing of the joint. Rather than the surgeon stressing the tibia against the femur to assess

tissue balancing, the patient's leg is flexed and distracted by gravity and can be gently rocked by one or two fingers medially and laterally to assess true ligament balancing (i.e., Rocker Test) (Figs. 34.8 and 34.9). This is physiologic, similar to a patient hanging their leg over the edge of a chair or bed to see if their knee clicks or makes noise in side-to-side motion. Appropriate ligament balancing by rocking the leg side to side and rotating with the suspended leg approach is a more a natural and physiologic test and can enhance true ligament balancing.

The patellofemoral joint can also be assessed in a similar fashion going from flexion to extension. We recommend deflating the tourniquet and, with the leg hanging, visualizing

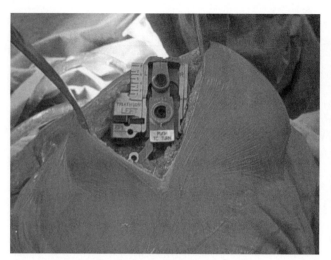

Fig. 34.8 MIS TKA with posterior referencing system

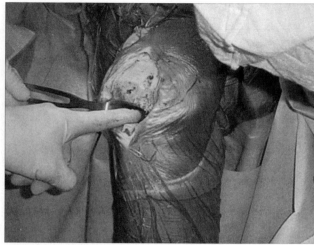

Fig. 34.9 Suspended leg with exposure to the posterior joint. Gravity distracts the joint, enhancing exposure to the posterior joint to improve visualization and access

a   b

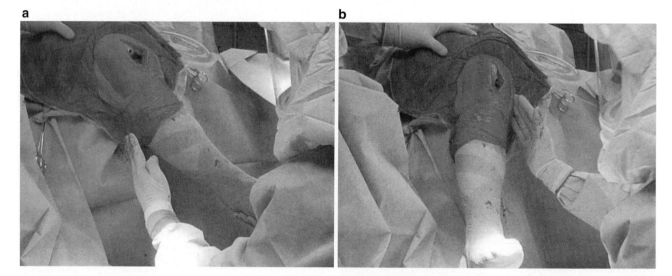

Fig. 34.10 Rocker test. The leg suspended and rocked gently medially and laterally to assess collateral ligament balancing once the trials are in position. One uses a single finger to slide the leg gently medially and laterally to assess ligament balancing with the leg suspended

the patellofemoral joint. This can be done both before and after capsular closure with arthroscopic assistance (Fig. 34.10).

The suspended leg approach has also allowed us to utilize arthroscopic assistance in all stages of the procedure (Fig. 34.11). Arthroscopy has a number of advantages and can address many of the difficulties of minimally invasive surgery. Arthroscopy delivers a light source, magnifies the view, allows the surgeon to see around angles (30°/70° arthroscopes), and allows visualization of the joint both before and after capsular closure. The suspended leg technique and arthroscopic assistance can be naturally linked, evolving from diagnostic surgery; ligament reconstruction; biological resurfacing; and arthroscopic-assisted arthroplasty. However, this approach requires further evaluation and new arthroscopic instrumentation (Figs. 34.12 and 34.13).

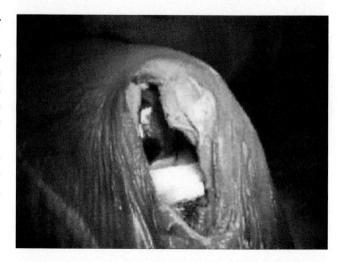

Fig. 34.11 Examination of patellofemoral tracking after implants are in position

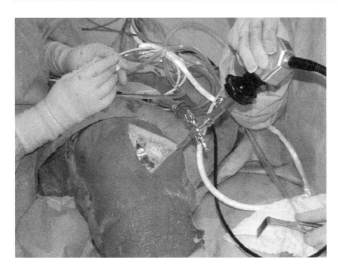

Fig. 34.12 Arthroscopic instruments utilized to examine the joint. Can be used "dry" (without fluid) with the capsule open or with fluid with the capsule closed

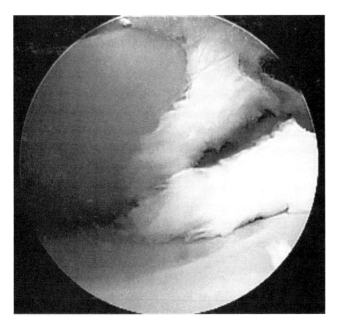

Fig. 34.13 Capsule closed and soft tissue impinging the lateral gutter. This is easily removed

Results

We performed a retrospective direct patient match study to assess: (1) standard TKA; (2) MIS TKA with a supine approach; and (3) MIS TKA with a suspended leg approach. This is a direct patient-matched study with a standard hospitalization and rehabilitation program. Sixteen patients (20 TKA) were in each group. The same surgeon, implant (Scorpio TKA, Stryker, Kalamazoo, MI), and rehabilitation protocol were utilized. There was a minimum 3-year follow-up. In group I, the standard technique utilized the 12- to 22-cm incision with an everted patella and median parapatellar approach with traditional instrumentation. In group II, the minimally invasive approach uses the patient supine in an adjustable leg holder with an incision of 6–11 cm, the patella was not everted, and the quadriceps-sparing technique – VMO snip (mini-midvastus) – was used. In group III, the MIS techniques were used with the suspended leg approach.

Clinical Data

Complications and radiographic analysis were similar in all three groups (Table 34.1). The patients who had MIS techniques, both suspended and supine, had faster recoveries and less postoperative pain. However, in the MIS suspended leg technique, there was a subtle improvement in ligament balancing and patellofemoral tracking observed by the surgeon. Although the sample size was small, there was a slight subjective patient preference for the MIS suspended leg approach.[13]

Table 34.1 Clinical data for study comparing standard TKA, MIS TKA with a supine approach, and MIS TKA with a suspended leg approach

	Group I	Group II	Group III
	Standard	MIS	Suspended leg
Clinical data			
Age (years)	75 (65–85)	72 (61–84)	71 (60–83)
Tourniquet time (min)	49 (39–61)	54 (50–62)	61 (56–67)
Knee Society Scores (KSS)			
Range of motion (ROM)			
Preoperative KSS	113 (92–122)	116 (92–125)	118 (86–128)
Postoperative KSS	42 (32–54)	41 (35–50)	42 (34–48)
	96 (80–100)	98 (88–100)	98 (82–100)
Radiographic analysis			
Femoral/tibial valgus	5.6° (2–10°)	5.2° (1–9°)	5.3° (2–9°)
Progressive lucent lines	0	0	0
Postoperative rehabilitation			
Cane 2 weeks	65%	16%	25%
Independent activity	8 weeks (4–16 weeks)	3 weeks (1–7 weeks)	3.5 weeks (2–7 weeks)
Complications			
Lateral release	2 patients	2 patients	1 patient
Manipulations	1 patient	1 patient	1 patient
Re-operation	1 patient— ROM (loss of extension)	0 patients	0 patients

Arthroscopic-Assisted Approach

In an additional study, 22 patients underwent the arthroscopic-assisted suspended leg approach.[14] In these patients, the arthroscopy was utilized to enhance visualization of the joint for soft tissue and bone removal, implant position, ligament balancing, and patellofemoral tracking both before and after capsular closure. In all patients, arthroscopy was useful to either remove impinging soft tissue, cement, bone fragments, or subtle ligament balancing and/or patellofemoral tracking issues after capsular closure (Fig. 34.14).

Combining the arthroscopic assistance with the suspended leg approach may overall enhance visualization and optimize many of the difficulties associated with MIS TKA techniques – reduced exposure and reduced visualization (Figs. 34.15–34.19).

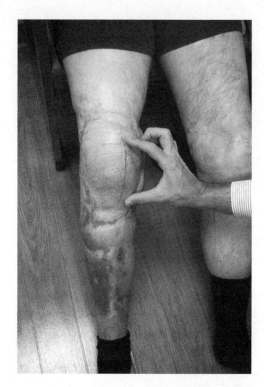

Fig. 34.16 Complex TKA case treated with suspended leg and arthroscopic assistance. The patient had substantial burns to the lower extremity and massive scarring. Suspended leg with MIS TKA approaches and arthroscopic assistance was utilized

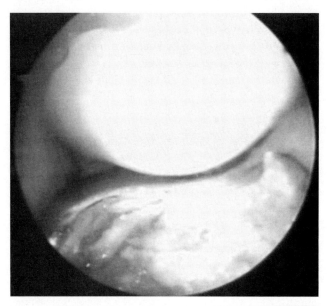

Fig. 34.14 Patellofemoral tracking after capsular closure, arthroscopically visualized

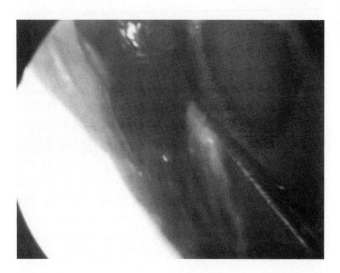

Fig. 34.15 Arthroscopic view of retained posterior cement using 70° scope – later removed

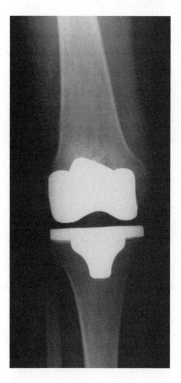

Fig. 34.17 Anteroposterior (AP) view of KM postoperatively

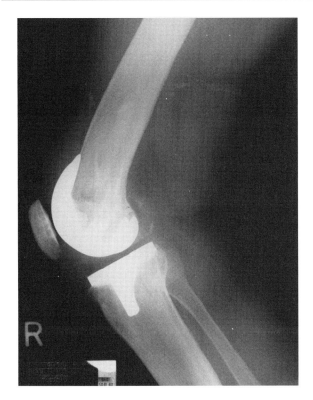

Fig. 34.18 Lateral view of KM postoperatively

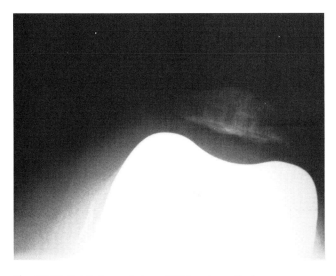

Fig. 34.19 Patellofemoral view of KM postoperatively

Conclusion

Although MIS technology is still in its early stages, we recommend an evolutionary approach to all minimally invasive techniques.[15] The surgeon should *evolve*, only change one variable at a time, first learning the downsized instrumentation, then gradually decreasing incision length, then developing muscle-sparing techniques, and then adopting in situ bone cuts.

Later, more complex techniques such as suspended leg approaches and arthroscopic assistance may by utilized. Computer navigation may enhance certain issues of alignment and implant position; it does not improve joint visualization, tissue and bone removal, and directly measured patellofemoral tracking ligament balancing. The combination of suspended leg technique, arthroscopic assistance, and computer navigation may optimize all aspects of MIS knee arthroplasty with a goal of improving results.[16] These, combined with future technologies including robotics/haptics for precision bone cuts, modular implants that require optimal implant position, and improved techniques, may afford high-demand patients a return to all functional activities. The goal is not only to improve overall implant survivorship, but to optimize patient satisfaction and functional activity, and even in the highest-demand patients, to give patients optimal surgical results. The suspended leg approach and arthroscopic assistance are two techniques that may enhance results for MIS TKA.

References

1. Bonutti P. Minimally Invasive TKR. First Series MIS TKA. Scientific Presentation. LaQuinta, CA, October 2001
2. Bonutti P, Neal D, Kester M. Minimal incision total knee arthroplasty using the suspended leg technique. Orthopedics 2003;26:899–903
3. Bonutti P, Mont M, McMahon M, et al. Minimally invasive total knee arthroplasty. J Bone Joint Surg Am 2004;86:26–32
4. Mont M, Stuchin S, Bonutti P, et al. Different surgical options for monocompartmental OA of the knee: HTO vs. UKA vs. TKA: indications, techniques, results, and controversies. Instr Course Lect 2004;53:265–283
5. Bezwada H, Mont M, Bonutti P, Chauhan S, et al. Minimally invasive lateral approach to total knee arthroplasty. In: Scuderi G, Tria A, Berger R (Eds.), *MIS Techniques in Orthopaedic Surgery*. Springer, New York, Chapter 21:339–348, 2006
6. Bonutti P. Surgical Techniques in Orthopedics. MIS TKA Mini-Subvastus Approach. Standing Room Only AAOS DVD 2005
7. Bonutti P. In: Hozack W, Krismer M, Nogler M, Bonutti P, Rachbauer F, Schaffer J, Donnelly W (Eds.), *Minimally Invasive Total Joint Arthroplasty*. Springer, New York, Chapters: 9.1:130 145; 28:284–288; 29:289–294, 2004
8. Bonutti PM. Minimally invasive total knee arthroplasty. OKU Hip and Knee Reconstruction 3, 8:81–91:01/2006
9. Bonutti P, Seyler TM, Kesler M, et al. Minimally invasive revision total knee arthroplasty. Clin Orthop Relat Res 2006;4469:69–75
10. Bonutti P. Minimally invasive total knee arthroplasty: pitfalls & complications. AAOS Presentation, 2006
11. Kolisek F, Mont M, Bonutti P. MIS TKA prospective randomized multicenter study. JOA, 2006
12. Epinette JA. Personal communication, 1997
13. Bonutti P. The use of the suspended leg minimally invasive technique for total knee arthroplasty. AAOS Presentation, 2005
14. Bonutti P. Arthroscopic assisted total knee arthroplasty. Poster Exhibit. AAOS, 2006
15. Bonutti P, Mont M, Kester M. Minimally invasive total knee arthroplasty: a 10 feature evolutionary approach. Orthop Clin North Am 2004;35:217–226
16. Bonutti P, Mont M. The future of high performance arthroplasty. Semin Arthroplasty, August 2006

Chapter 35
Quadriceps-Sparing Total Knee Arthroplasty

Rodney K. Alan and Alfred J. Tria

Much of the pioneering work for total knee arthroplasty (TKA) took place during the 1970s. For several years, the prosthesis and bearing surfaces were the major focus of efforts to improve the surgery. The result of this evolution is seen in the current success rate of modern TKA.[1–4]

During the same period in history, minimally invasive techniques in general surgery and other subspecialties of surgery were beginning to develop. This trend eventually influenced orthopedic surgeons to attempt minimally invasive arthroplasty. The logical first step for minimally invasive TKA was to begin with unicompartmental arthroplasty (UKA). The UKA implant was much smaller than the TKA implant. Repicci pioneered the concept of minimally invasive knee arthroplasty during the early 1990s. He demonstrated that UKA done through a small incision resulted in less blood loss, decreased morbidity, shorter hospitalization, and more rapid recovery.[5] Since his report, other authors have written articles to support the outcome of minimally invasive UKA. Argenson and Price reported decreased morbidity and accelerated rehabilitation with MIS UKA.[6,7] After the successful reports of MIS surgery in UKA, investigators began to search for ways to carry out minimally invasive TKA.

The first minimally invasive TKAs were attempted arthroscopically. Caspari, Whipple, and Goble made several attempts to complete the operative procedure with arthroscopic assistance but were unable to perfect the technique and never published any results. When the success of MIS UKA was reported, renewed interest in MIS TKA developed. Implants were modified, instrumentation was made smaller, and new techniques were established.

The development of the quadriceps-sparing TKA began in 2001. The first surgeries were completed in February of 2002 and an early report of the combined results was presented at the Knee Society annual meeting.[8] The paper showed that the arthroplasty was technically possible and reported some early complications. The complications included one transient peroneal nerve palsy, one hematoma, and one knee with decreased range of motion despite a manipulation under anesthesia.

The surgical approach for quadriceps-sparing TKA was not unique at the time it was developed. Many open meniscectomies were performed using the same arthrotomy, but the technique was new for TKA. The designers of the technique did not give the procedure a descriptive name; however, during the first year, the operative procedure began to be called the "quadriceps-sparing" technique. The name is not completely anatomically correct. The medial arthrotomy extends from the superior pole of the patella to 2 cm below the tibiofemoral joint line. The vastus medialis inserts along the medial side of the patella, and, in some cases, the muscle insertion is as low as the midpoint of the patella. Thus, the arthrotomy does divide the insertion in some cases; and, therefore, the technique is not always quadriceps sparing. With this proviso, the authors have continued to call the procedure "quadriceps sparing" because the name and the technique have become synonymous.

Other minimally invasive approaches have been described for TKA. Tenholder et al. used a minimally invasive medial parapatellar approach and reported that patients with this approach required fewer transfusions and achieved better flexion.[9] The subvastus approach avoids disruption of the quadriceps mechanism and may provide more rapid recover after TKA.[10–13] Boerger et al. reported less blood loss, less pain, greater motion, faster straight leg raising, but more complications with a minimally invasive subvastus TKA.[14]

A vastus-splitting approach has been described and used successfully in more than 420 minimally invasive TKAs by Bonutti et al.[15] Laskin reported that patients with an MIS midvastus approach required less analgesic drugs in the perioperative period, regained flexion faster, and achieved functional milestones more rapidly when compared with a matched group of patients with standard TKA.[16] Because there are different types of minimally invasive TKA techniques, it is difficult to compare one MIS procedure to another. The quadriceps-sparing procedure is the least invasive of the techniques. It is more difficult to perform and requires more of the surgeon and the patient.

R.K. Alan (✉) and A.J. Tria
Institute for Advanced Orthopaedic Study, The Orthopaedic Center of New Jersey, 1527 State Highway 27, Suite 1300, Somerset, NJ, USA
e-mail: Atriajrmd@aol.com

G.R. Scuderi and A.J. Tria (eds.), *Minimally Invasive Surgery in Orthopedics*,
DOI 10.1007/978-0-387-76608-9_35, © Springer Science+Business Media, LLC 2010

Defining Minimally Invasive

Minimally invasive surgery of the knee represents a spectrum of approaches and exposures. All of the skin incision lengths are shorter than the standard incision but the skin incision itself does not identify the MIS procedure. The ideal minimally invasive knee replacement should limit the skin incision, limit the disruption of the quadriceps mechanism, and avoid eversion of the patella while maintaining the quality and safety of standard TKA. In retrospect, it now appears that eversion of the patella is a central factor that may very well be the common defining point for the MIS procedures.[17]

Preoperative Evaluation

Patients must have radiographically confirmed symptomatic arthritis that has not responded to conservative measures. Age considerations do not differ for the quadriceps-sparing technique. Initially, the procedure was twice as long as the standard operation and the senior author deferred using the technique in patients older than the age of 80 years because of the increased anesthetic exposure. Now that the operative time is almost the same as the standard approach, this limitation has been somewhat relaxed.

The patient should be capable of performing the physical therapy regimen after the surgery and should understand the general goals of the MIS operation. The knee should have no significant previous arthrotomy or periarticular scarring because this makes the approach much more difficult. The clinical deformity should not exceed 15° in any given plane and the knee should have a minimum of 105° of motion. Obesity does play a role in the selection process but refers only to the local anatomy of the knee. If the circumference of the lower leg at the level of the knee is much smaller than the length of the thigh, the procedure will be much easier. The authors are trying to develop a meaningful ratio of these two measurements and it does appear that a three to one ratio (thigh length versus knee circumference) is ideal.

There are some factors that increase the difficulty of the surgical procedure but are not absolute contraindications. The rheumatoid knee is not ideal because the bone tends to be osteoporotic and may be injured at the time of the prosthetic insertion. Patella baja makes it difficult to retract the patella across the lateral femoral condyle. The vastus medialis may be very well developed in some muscular males and the insertion can be as low as the mid portion of the patella. When this occurs, it is difficult to retract the medial capsule. The largest femoral components from any design line will often require an extension of the capsular incision just to accommodate the prosthetic size.

The quadriceps-sparing technique is not meant for all knees. Strict criteria should certainly be observed at the initiation of the surgical approach so that the result will be rewarding both for the surgeon and the patient. The authors typically use the approach for 25–30% of all TKAs in a given year.

Surgical Technique

The patient is placed supine and an arterial tourniquet is applied to the upper thigh. A leg holder is used for the quadriceps-sparing technique because the bone cuts are made in varying positions of flexion and extension and the holder expedites the positioning (Fig. 35.1). A curvilinear skin incision is made from the superior pole of the patella to the tibial joint line just medial to the patella and patella tendon (Fig. 35.2). The arthrotomy is made in line with the skin incision beginning at the superomedial border of the patella, where the vastus medialis typically inserts, and ending 2 cm below the tibial joint line. Both the varus and valgus knee can be replaced through the medial arthrotomy; however, a lateral arthrotomy can also be used with elevation of the iliotibial band from Gerdy's tubercle posteriorly. The arthrotomy is not extended proximally into the quadriceps tendon, the vastus medialis, or the subvastus interval.

The extremity is brought into full extension and the patellar fat pad is excised. The patellar thickness is recorded and the MIS patellar guide is used to remove a measured amount of bone (Fig. 35.3). Alternately, the patella surface can be resected using a freehand technique; but the position of the patella is not typical and somewhat awkward. A metal protector is placed over the patellar surface for the remainder of the procedure (Fig. 35.4). Early patellar resection is not mandatory, but

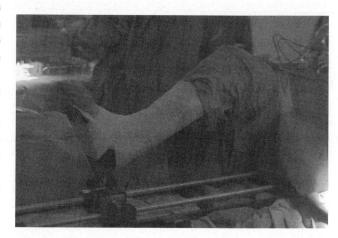

Fig. 35.1 The leg holder (Innovative Medical Products, Plainville, CT, USA) facilitates positioning of the knee throughout the range of motion

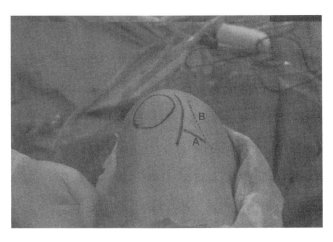

Fig. 35.2 The MIS incision. *"A"* is the tibiofemoral joint line and *"B"* is the outline of the medial femoral condyle

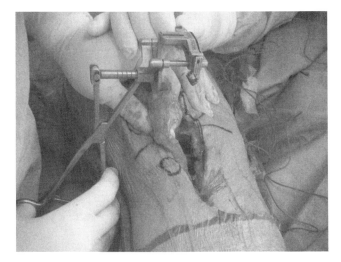

Fig. 35.3 The patellar clamp leaves a predetermined thickness for resurfacing (Zimmer Orthopedics, Warsaw, IN, USA)

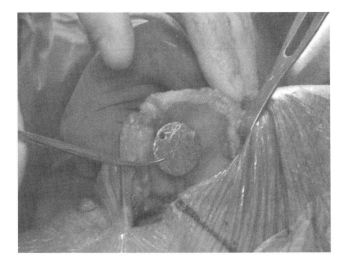

Fig. 35.4 The metal protector is centered on the cut surface of the patella

it increases the overall working room within the knee joint, thus making it easier for later steps in the procedure.

With the knee remaining in full extension, the anterior surface of the femur is cleared to permit subsequent sizing and positioning of the anterior femoral cut. The knee is flexed to 45°, and the anterior and posterior cruciate ligaments are resected from the intercondylar notch. The author's preference is a posterior cruciate-substituting knee replacement for both minimally invasive TKA and standard TKA. However, cruciate-substituting and cruciate-retaining knee replacements are both amenable to the quadriceps-sparing approach.[18]

The anteroposterior (AP) axis line of Whiteside's is drawn (Fig. 35.5) and an intramedullary rod is introduced into the femur through a hole just above the intercondylar notch. A modified intramedullary cutting guide is used to make the distal femoral cut in a medial to lateral direction. In order to complete the distal femoral cut, the intramedullary reference must be removed. The cutting guide remains secured to the medial aspect of the distal femur, and the resection is continued until the saw abuts the cutting guide. In patients with a small femur, the entire resection can be completed. In patients with large femurs, the cutting guide is removed, and the resection is completed by freehand technique, taking care not to violate the lateral capsule.

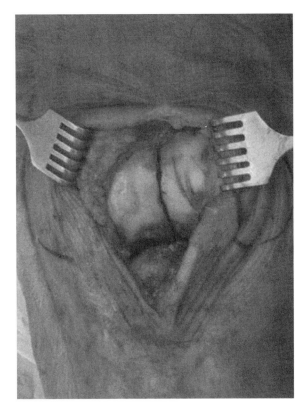

Fig. 35.5 Whiteside's line is drawn for rotational referencing for the femoral cuts

The proximal tibial cut is completed using a standard extramedullary cutting guide with the cutting attachment biased toward the medial side of the tibia (Fig. 35.6). The proximal tibial bone can usually be removed in a single piece. A spacer block can be inserted into the extension gap and the overall alignment and balance of the knee can be evaluated. Ligamentous releases can be completed at this juncture without difficulty because the bone resections leave approximately 20 mm of space in full extension.

The anterior aspect of the distal femur is cut using a guide that references the posterior femoral condyles and the antero-posterior axis (Fig. 35.7). A shelf is attached to the appropriate femoral finishing block and the shelf is set on the anterior femoral surface in full extension. The finishing block is centered on the distal femur and pinned in place (Fig. 35.8). The knee is flexed to 70° and the femoral finishing cuts and peg holes are completed. The flexion gap can now be compared with the extension gap and adjustments can be made in the standard fashion.

The proximal tibia finishing guide has two deployable posterior pins that reference the cortex of the tibia (Fig. 35.9). The tray is centered medial to lateral and rotated to reference the tibial tubercle, the femoral box cut, and the malleoli of the ankle. The broaching is completed in the standard fashion.

If the patella is resurfaced, the metal protector is removed and the pegs holes are completed.

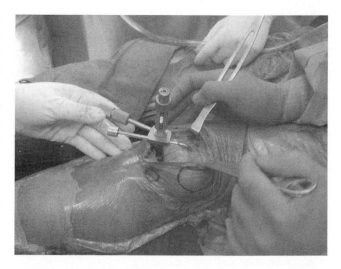

Fig. 35.7 The femoral cutting guide references the posterior femoral condyles and locates the site for the anterior cut

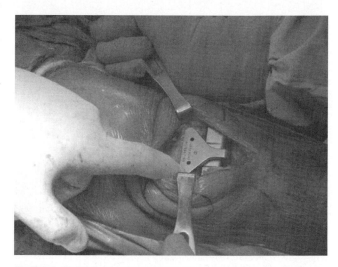

Fig. 35.8 The femoral finishing block is centered medial to lateral and pinned into position

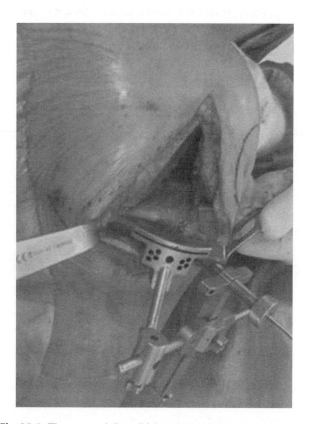

Fig. 35.6 The extramedullary tibial cutting guide is medially based

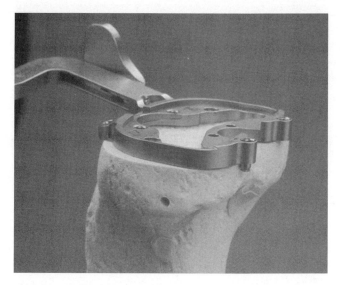

Fig. 35.9 Tibial cutting guide has deployable pins that can be used to hook the posterior cortex of the femur

The tibial tray, femoral component, polyethylene insert, and trial patella are inserted in order. Patellar tracking, ligament balance, range of motion, and overall knee alignment are confirmed and the surfaces are prepared for cementing. Palacos cement is preferred because of its prolonged "doughy" state. There are MIS tibial components now available with shortened intramedullary stems to facilitate insertion of the component (Fig. 35.10). While these are helpful, they are not absolutely necessary.

After cementing is completed and excess cement removed, the polyethylene insert is locked into position. The tourniquet is released and hemostasis is achieved by electrocautery. Surgical drains can be used if desired and closure is completed in the standard fashion.

Perioperative Management

The authors' postoperative management has evolved during the past 5 years. The original protocol shortened the hospital stay without making any other changes.[8] Minor changes have been made in the pain management but peripheral blocks have not been incorporated in our center because of the concern for muscle paralysis. The patients no longer donate

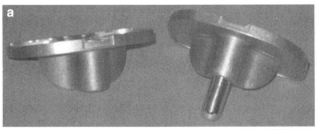
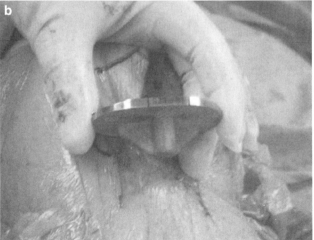

Fig. 35.10 (a) This MIS modular tibial component can be inserted with or without the pin (MIS tibia, Zimmer Orthopedics, Warsaw, IN, USA). (b) This MIS tibia is a single component with a shortened intramedullary stem (MIS tibia, Smith and Nephew, Memphis, TN, USA)

autologous blood and they can go home as soon as the first day after surgery. Full weight-bearing ambulation and range of motion exercises are routinely initiated within hours after the operation. Low molecular weight heparin (LMWH) is used for deep vein thrombosis (DVT) prophylaxis, and all patients undergo a Doppler study of both lower extremities before stopping the LMWH at 12–14 days after surgery.

Technical Pearls

Patient selection is important for the success of the procedure. The thinner patient, with a good range of motion, and some laxity of the joint is an ideal candidate.

Positioning the knee in varying degrees of flexion throughout the procedure is an important point that differentiates minimally invasive TKA from the standard TKA that is typically performed in full extension or 90° of flexion. The leg holder allows changing the position of the knee throughout the operation and does not require another assistant.

Initially, the quadriceps-sparing TKA required special instrumentation. The authors recognized the hesitation of surgeons to adopt radically different instruments and have now developed instruments that are modifications of standard existing designs (Fig. 35.11). The distal femoral cut can now be made from anterior to posterior. The femoral finishing block is a standard shape with an anterior shelf (Fig. 35.12). The tibial guide cuts more from anterior to posterior and the tibial trays can now be positioned on the cut surface without using posterior hooks.

There are some minimally invasive tibial components available that have an abbreviated intramedullary stem. The shorter stem does facilitate insertion of the component; however, as the authors have increased their experience with the MIS exposures, the need for the modified components

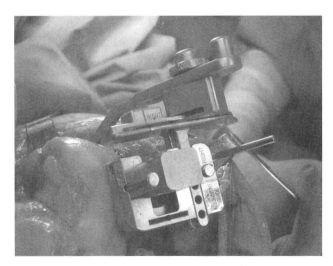

Fig. 35.11 The standard intramedullary guide has been downsized and the anterior cutting slot modified to fit into the smaller incision

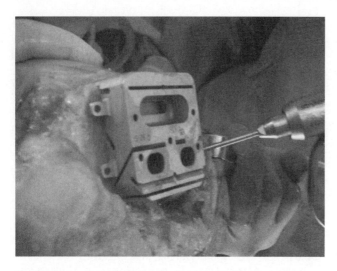

Fig. 35.12 A standard cutting block can be used with the edges cut down to fit into the smaller incision

decreases. The high-flex femoral component (Legacy High Flex, Zimmer, Warsaw, IN, USA) removes 2 mm of additional bone from the posterior aspect of the femur and this also increases some of the working space in the knee.

Results

The senior author has completed more than 500 quadriceps-sparing TKAs. The incisions have been extended on six occasions; four for implanting large femoral components, one for gaining additional exposure in an obese patient, and one for bleeding from the middle geniculate artery. The operative times have gradually decreased and the procedure is now routinely completely in less than 60 min. The blood loss is less than the standard TKA, the length of stay is less, and the pain is less. There is greater motion in the early postoperative period, but this difference diminishes over time. At a minimum of 2-year follow-up, patients with quadriceps-sparing TKA have more motion, but only by a few degrees. While this does not represent a clinically significant difference at this time, it does give a positive effect for future development.

The radiographic analysis of the results has shown that the quadriceps-sparing technique does have more outliers than the standard approach.[19] An outlier was defined as 4° or more outside the ideal alignment, size difference of 4 mm for a component, or 2 mm of femoral notching. There were 13 outliers in 32 MIS TKAs and 5 outliers in 38 standard TKAs. There was no statistical difference in coronal plane alignment between the two groups and, with 2–4 years of follow-up, there were no repeat surgeries or component failures in either group.

The results of quadriceps-sparing TKA have paralleled other investigators who have reported results of minimally invasive TKAs. Laskin et al. and Haas et al. have reported results of their minimally invasive TKA and found greater range of motion and excellent Knee Society scores at short-term follow-up.[16,20] With the quadriceps-sparing technique, there were no statistically significant differences in Knee Society scores when compared with standard TKA. The quadriceps-sparing group had slightly better scores, but the difference was neither clinically nor statistically different.

Summary

The impact of minimally invasive TKA continues to generate much discussion and controversy all over the world. Early results of the technique are encouraging, but long-term data is still lacking. Patient interest continues to be high and patients request the procedure because they look for less postoperative pain and earlier return to function. The quadriceps-sparing TKA addresses the patient's needs and desires. The technique does need to be further refined and the accuracy improved. The authors continued to address these issues. The instruments have been modified so that they are more user friendly; the postoperative management is constantly refined; and computer navigation has been incorporated to address the accuracy.

References

1. National Institutes of Health. NIH Consensus Statement on total knee replacement December 8–10, 2003. J Bone Joint Surg Am. 2004;86-A(6):1328–35
2. Ritter MA, Herbst SA, Keating EM, PM, Meding JB. Long-term survival analysis of a posterior cruciate-retaining total condylar total knee arthroplasty. Clin Orthop Relat Res. 1994 Dec;(309):136–45
3. Scott RD, Volatile TB. Twelve years' experience with posterior cruciate-retaining total knee arthroplasty. Clin Orthop Relat Res. 1986 Apr;(205):100–7
4. Stern S, Insall J. Posterior stabilized prosthesis. Results after follow-up of nine to twelve years. J Bone Joint Surg Am. 1992;74(7):980–6
5. Repicci JA, Eberle RW. Minimally invasive surgical technique for unicondylar knee arthroplasty. J South Orthop Assoc. 1999;8(1):20–7
6. Argenson JN, Flecher X. Minimally invasive unicompartmental knee arthroplasty. Knee. 2004;11(5):341–7
7. Price AJ, Webb J, Topf H, Dodd CA, Goodfellow JW, Murray DW; Oxford Hip and Knee Group. Rapid recovery after oxford unicompartmental arthroplasty through a short incision. J Arthroplasty. 2001;16(8):970–6
8. Tria AJ Jr, Coon TM. Minimal incision total knee arthroplasty: early experience. Clin Orthop Relat Res. 2003 Nov;(416):185–90
9. Tenholder M, Clarke HD, Scuderi GR. Minimal-incision total knee arthroplasty: the early clinical experience. Clin Orthop Relat Res. 2005 Nov;(440):67–76
10. Faure BT, Benjamin JB, Lindsey B, Volz RG, Schutte D. Comparison of the subvastus and paramedian surgical approaches in bilateral knee arthroplasty. J Arthroplasty. 1993;8(5):511–6

11. Hofmann AA, Plaster RL, Murdock LE. Subvastus (Southern) approach for primary total knee arthroplasty. Clin Orthop Relat Res. 1991 Aug;(269):70–7

12. Matsueda M, Gustilo, RB. Subvastus and medial parapatellar approaches in total knee arthroplasty. Clin Orthop Relat Res. 2000 Feb;(371):161–8

13. Roysam GS, Oakley MJ. Subvastus approach for total knee arthroplasty: a prospective, randomized, and observer-blinded trial. J Arthroplasty. 2001;16(4):454–7

14. Boerger TO, Aglietti P, Mondanelli N, Sensi L. Mini-subvastus versus medial parapatellar approach in total knee arthroplasty. Clin Orthop Relat Res. 2005 Nov;(440):82–7

15. Bonutti PM, Mont MA, Kester MA. Minimally invasive total knee arthroplasty: a 10-feature evolutionary approach. Orthop Clin North Am. 2004;35(2):217–26

16. Laskin RS, Beksac B, Phongjunakorn A, Pittors K, Davis J, Shim JC, Pavlov H, Petersen M. Minimally invasive total knee replace-ment through a mini-midvastus incision: an outcome study. Clin Orthop Relat Res. 2004 Nov;(428):74–81

17. Laskin RS. *Acquired patella baja after total knee replacement may be related to patellar tendon eversion.* Presented at the Annual Closed meeting of the Knee Society, September 29, 2006, Alexandria, VA

18. Berger RA, Sanders S, Gerlinger T, Della Valle C, Jacobs JJ, Rosenberg AG. Outpatient total knee arthroplasty with a mini-mally invasive technique. J Arthroplasty. 2005;20(7 Suppl 3): 33–8

19. Chen AF, Alan RK, Redziniak DE, Tria AJ Jr. Quadriceps sparing total knee replacement. The initial experience with results at two to four years. J Bone Joint Surg Br. 2006;88B(11): 1448–53

20. Haas SB, Cook S, Beksac B. Minimally invasive total knee replace-ment through a mini midvastus approach: a comparative study. Clin Orthop Relat Res. 2004 Nov;(428):68–73

Chapter 36
Minimally Invasive Quadriceps-Sparing Total Knee Replacement Preserving the Posterior Cruciate Ligament

Richard A. Berger and Aaron G. Rosenberg

Minimally invasive has been used to describe a wide spectrum of knee replacement procedures. This spectrum starts with a small skin incision with a standard incision into the capsular and the quadriceps muscle and includes patellar eversion. The spectrum currently ends with a small skin incision with a minimal capsular incision without quadriceps muscle violation and no patellar eversion. This is currently called the quadriceps-sparing or capsular-only approach.

Whatever the definition used, minimally invasive knee replacement can be done and has been shown to be beneficial to patients by minimizing surgical trauma, pain, and recovery.[1–10] All of the varied minimally invasive techniques share common elements of reducing the trauma necessary for exposure, component alignment, soft tissue balance, and component fixation. Ultimately, these benefits of minimally invasive knee replacement result in a more satisfied patient.

Additionally, to achieve potential rapid recovery that a minimally invasive technique can offer, the entire traditional perioperative pathway needs to be expedited. By combining one of these minimally invasive total knee replacement techniques with new pathways that expedite the entire recovery process, rapid recovery is not only possible, but outpatient total knee replacement is both possible and is currently being performed at our hospital daily.[1–3]

Wherever approach you ultimately choose, minimally invasive knee replacement has to adhere to the basic principles of knee replacement: proper alignment, proper balance, and good fixation. In addition, any new technique should not increase the complication rate compared with traditional knee replacement and must not compromise the outcome or longevity of a traditional knee replacement.

Indications

The limited mobility of the patella and extensor mechanism, the inability to evert the patella, and the inability to anteriorly dislocate the tibia in hyperflexion that result from the small retinacular arthrotomy make this approach the most challenging of all of the minimally invasive total knee approaches. However, with proper experience, the quadriceps-sparing approach can be used in almost all patients undergoing traditional total knee replacement. The approach allows for the exposure, proper resections, proper ligamentous balancing, and component insertion in most patients undergoing primary total knee arthroplasty (TKA).

The initial attempts at the quadriceps-sparing approach should be restricted to the easiest cases; thin female patients with good range of motions and lax tissues. Patients with patella alta and minimal varus-valgus deformity are also easier cases for learning the technique. As with all new approach in orthopedics, there is a learning curve to this quadriceps-sparing approach. Alternative positioning and retraction using the mobile window to gain appropriate exposure is key. The more of the procedure that can be done in extension, the easier it is to mobilize the patella and extensor mechanism. Once a surgeon has gained sufficient experience and comfort with the procedure, then the management of cases that are more difficult is possible: heavy male patients with poor range of motion and stiff tissues. In addition, cases with patellar baja and severe varus–valgus deformities are also possible. In our experience, even patients with moderate to severe deformities are candidates for the quadriceps-sparing approach.

The type and size of the component also influence the difficulty of the technique. Due the small arthrotomy and the inability to mobilize the extensor mechanism in flexion, this approach is more difficult in patients with larger femoral components. The inability to sublux the tibia makes it is extremely difficult to use a monoblock tibia or large-stemmed tibial components. This approach is easiest for primary knee arthroplasty using a low-profile tibial component or a modular tibial component.

R.A. Berger (✉) and A.G. Rosenberg
Department of Orthopedic Surgery, Rush-Presbyterian-St. Luke's Medical Center, 1725 West Harrison Street, Suite 1063, Chicago, IL 60612, USA
e-mail: r.a.berger@sbcglobal.net

G.R. Scuderi and A.J. Tria (eds.), *Minimally Invasive Surgery in Orthopedics*, DOI 10.1007/978-0-387-76608-9_36, © Springer Science+Business Media, LLC 2010

Lastly, this minimally invasive approach can be increased to gain exposure in a stepwise fashion if difficulties are encountered. A very low threshold for lengthening the arthrotomy should be maintained at all times, especially while learning minimally invasive approaches. The quadriceps-sparing arthrotomy may be easily extended in a stepwise fashion, into a medial parapatellar arthrotomy or into the midvastus or subvastus interval. Therefore, there are easy methods to increase exposure should intraoperative difficulty arise.

Patient Positioning

Unlike traditional approaches where the majority of the procedure is done in flexion, the quadriceps-sparing approach requires more of the procedure to be performed in relative extension. Furthermore, this approach, as with most minimally invasive approaches, requires constantly flexing and extending the knee to gain the best exposure for each step; small changes in the flexion of the knee result in large changes in exposure. Furthermore, while performing a femoral preparation with the approach, which is normally done in hyperflexion in traditional TKA, the knee should be extended as much as possible without interference with the cutting block. Therefore, a leg holder that will accommodate variations in positioning for incremental changes in knee flexion is very helpful.

As with a traditional TKA, the patient is positioned supine, with a bump under the ischium to tilt the pelvis and allow the knee to stay vertical during the surgery. The extremity is prepared and draped in standard fashion, including the incorporation of a leg holder to allow for incremental positioning of the flexed extremity. A thigh tourniquet is helpful to limit blood loss. Lastly, although this technique for total knee replacement can be done with one assistant, two assistants make the procedure much easier for the surgeon. However, care should be taken to ensure that the two assistants are not applying traction to both sides of the incision at once, which would potentially injure the tissue and inhibit the exposure.

Exposure

Proper positioning of the incision is important for maximal exposure. With the knee at 70° flexion, the medial patellar border, joint line, and tibial tuberosity are usually easy to palpate. A curvilinear incision that begins at the superomedial patella and ends at the medial edge of the tibial tuberosity is drawn (Fig. 36.1). Throughout its course, the incision curves; at its midpoint, it is 1 cm medial patella.

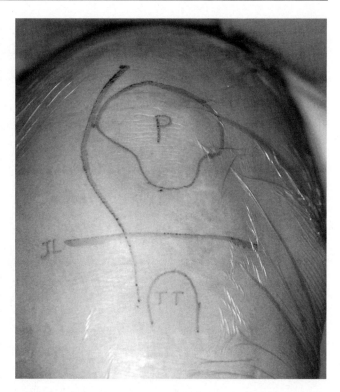

Fig. 36.1 Skin incision for the minimally invasive, quadriceps-sparing, total knee arthroplasty. *P* patella; *JL* joint line; *TT* tibial tubercle

After the incision is made through the skin and subcutaneous tissue, a self-retractor is placed. Two curved joint retractors are placed at the superior and medial edge of the incision, revealing the distal extent of the vastus medialis oblique (VMO), which is seen in the superior medial aspect of the incision. At this point, the entire extent of the joint capsule from the superior pole of the patella down to the medial edge of the tibial tubercle is exposed.

The borders of the patella, the distal extent of the VMO, and the medial border of the tibial tubercle is identified. The distal VMO insertion varies, with lower insertions on muscular patients and male patients. An arthrotomy is made from the superior pole of the patella, extending along the medial border of the patella, to the medial aspect of the tibial tubercle, avoiding the patellar tendon (Fig. 36.2). The arthrotomy is extended distally to 1 cm inferior to the tibial plateau. Care is taken to leave enough retinaculum between the arthrotomy and VMO to prevent tearing of the arthrotomy into the VMO. The exposure is aided in some patients, especially in muscular males, by back cutting the retinaculum 1–2 cm. This is done distal to the VMO, approximately 1/2 cm distal to the edge of the VMO. This back cut should not extend more than 2 cm. If this back cut is made, the inferior medial retinaculum is tagged with a stitch, which helps as a retractor.

With the arthrotomy completed, blunt dissection is used to define the plane between the medial retinaculum and

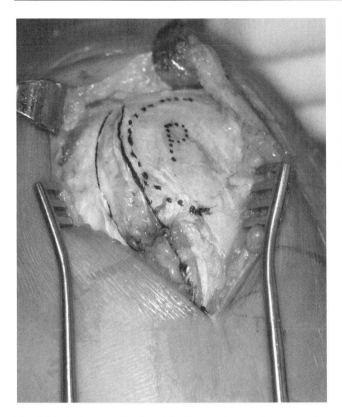

Fig. 36.2 Arthrotomy for the minimally invasive, quadriceps-sparing total knee arthroplasty

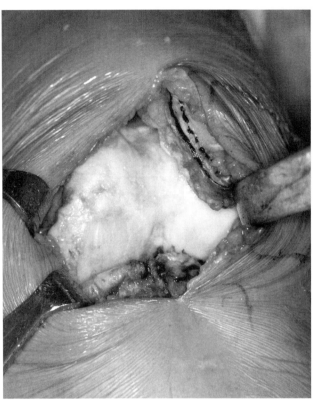

Fig. 36.3 Initial exposure of the knee showing the distal femoral condyle

synovium. Then a portion of the superior medial synovium is excised, thus providing excellent exposure to the medial condyle. A retractor is positioned around the medial condyle, and it retracts the medial collateral ligament (MCL) and medial retinaculum. The anterior insertion of the medial meniscus is then detached. This then exposes the medial femoral condyle. As with a traditional exposure, the deep MCL is released from the proximal medial tibial plateau. This release may be extended with a curved osteotome to achieve the appropriate ligamentous release. Finally, the leg can be extended and externally rotated to extend the medial release posteriorly. In this position, the medial osteophytes on the tibial plateau are removed.

With the knee in extension, using blunt dissection, the space between the fat pad and patellar tendon is developed and a knee joint retractor is placed in the plane. Scissors are used to extend this plane and resect the attachments of the fat pad to the patella and tibia, thus excising a large portion of the fat pad. The knee is then flexed to 70°. A retractor exposes the medial femoral condyle and the medial osteophytes on the femoral condyle are removed. Finally, the anterior cruciate ligament (ACL) and meniscal attachments are incised to mobilize the tibia, which also facilitates the tibial cut. With the knee flexed to 70°, a double-pronged Hohmann retractor is placed over the lateral femoral condyle that gently retracts the patella laterally (Fig. 36.3).

Distal Femoral Resection

During a conventional total knee replacement, the distal femoral cut is made from anterior to posterior. This step is traditionally aided by hyperflexion of the knee. However, the quadriceps-sparing approach requires this step to be performed in less flexion, usually approximately 70–80°. In this position, the distal cut must be made from the medial side, cutting from medial to lateral; this avoids the extensor mechanism. More than 70–80° of flexion tightens the extensor mechanism, making this resection more difficult.

A double-pronged Hohmann retractor is placed over the lateral femoral condyle and gently retracts the patella laterally, exposing the intercondylar notch (Fig. 36.3). In this position, with the intercondylar notch exposed, an 8-mm hole is made with a drill in the axis of the femoral canal (Fig. 36.4).

Through this hole, the distal femoral cutting guide will be inserted into the femoral canal. The cutting guide is chosen to match the difference between the mechanical axis and anatomic axis. In this case, a 5° distal femoral guide is chosen. Prior to inserting, the L-shaped cutting guide is attached to the distal femoral cutting guide. Then the intermedullary rod is inserted into the distal femoral canal and the flat plate is seated against the medial femoral condyle. This will resect 10 mm of bone from the medial condyle plate at the specific valgus angle. The L-shaped cutting slot is seated against the medial and superior edge of the medial femoral condyle. This is done at approximately 70–80° of flexion. This cutting guide is designed to avoid the intact quadriceps tendon, cutting the distal femur from the medial aspect of the knee. The guide must be seated against the medial femoral condyle. Retraction of the medial soft tissue facilitates insertion (Fig. 36.5).

The distal femoral cutting guide is secured against the medial condyle with threaded screw pins. The orthogonal orientations of the screws hold the cutting block securely and prevent angular change during the cutting of the distal femur.

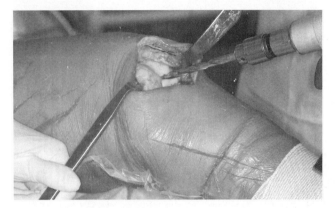

Fig. 36.4 Drill the intramedullary hole for the distal femur. Extending the knee slightly relaxes the extensor mechanism, facilitating the process

The distal condyles are resected using an oscillating saw from medial to lateral; first the medial condyle is resected then the lateral condyle is resected. The medial condyle is resected using the "L" shaped guide from anterior to posterior. The very posterior aspect of the distal lateral condyle can then resected with the intramedullary rod in place. The cut is made as shown in Fig. 36.5. The central and anterior portion of the distal lateral femoral condyle cannot be resected until the intramedullary rod is removed. At this point, the L-shaped cutting block is detached from the intramedullary rod and the rod is removed. With the L-shaped cutting block remaining pinned to the medial femoral condyle, the central aspects of the lateral condyle can then resected (Fig. 36.5). During this step, care is taken not to cut the lateral retinaculum; this is aided by cutting from anterior to posterior and retractor may be placed over the lateral knee to protect the lateral retinaculum as the lateral femoral condyle is resected. After the L-shaped cutting block is removed the anterior aspect of the distal lateral condyle is resected with the knee in extension with a reciprocating saw. The knee in extension allows better expose the lateral condyle so it can be resected and removed.

Preparing the Patella

The patella cannot be everted. However, after the distal femoral condyles are removed, the knee is placed in slight

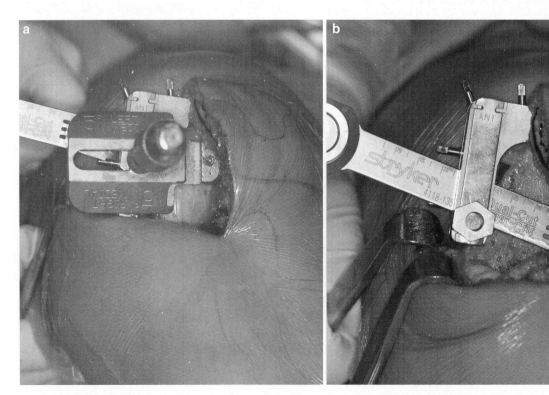

Fig. 36.5 Cutting the distal femur. (**a**) Distal femoral cutting guide in place. After the medial condyle resected, the posterior distal lateral femur is cut obliquely from the anterior medial side. (**b**) L-shaped cutting block as a guide for the central portion of the lateral distal femoral

hyperextension. This hyperextension allows the patellar to be tilted between 45° and 90° from the coronal axis. This is the reason that the patella is resected after the distal femoral condyles. In addition, the unresected patella prevents the patella from unintentional damage during the distal femoral resection.

In this position, one towel clip is placed on the superior pole and one towel clip is placed on the inferior poles of the patella. These two clips allow the patella to be tilted between 45° and 90°. This is adequate exposure for the patellar resection (Fig. 36.6). Patellar eversion is not needed to resect the patella. The patellar thickness is measured with a caliper and the patella is resected to recreate the patellar thickness with the implant in place. The patellar component size is chosen to cover the resected surface of the patella without overhanging. The patellar bone is then prepared with drill holes. Lastly, a patellar protector is placed on the resected surface to prevent damage to the soft cancellous bone of the patella with subsequent retractors (Fig. 36.6).

Preparing the Tibia

The tibia is resected with the knee in relative extension. A small bolster is placed under the proximal tibia, positioning the knee in approximately 15° of flexion (Fig. 36.7). This position takes tension off the extensor mechanism and allows visualization and access to the proximal tibia. This position facilitates placement of the tibial cutting guide beneath the patellar tendon into the proximal tibia. The tibial cutting guide is positioned just proximal to the tibial tubercle, along the medial tibial tubercle. With the overall alignment and slope of the tibial guide set, the guide is set to achieve the correct level of tibial plateau resection. A retractor is placed on the medial plateau to protect the medial collateral ligament and a second retractor is used to retract the patellar tendon laterally (Fig. 36.7). Then, an oscillating saw is used to resect the proximal tibia. While most of the resection in completed under direct visualization, care must be taken resecting the posterolateral tibia where either a retractor or

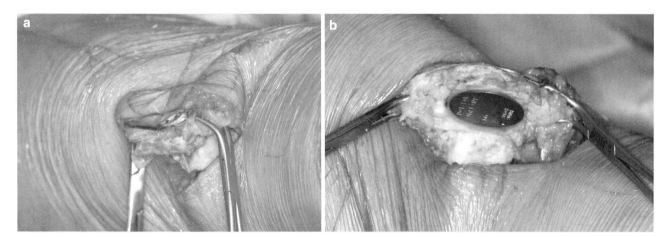

Fig. 36.6   Resecting the patella. (**a**) Distal femur in extension. The patella is seen and resected. (**b**) A patellar protector is placed

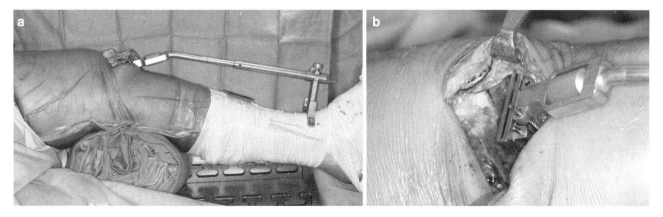

Fig. 36.7   Tibial resection. (**a**) Positioning for the tibial cut with a bolster. (**b**) The extended position relaxes the extensor mechanism and retractors protect the soft tissue

tactile sense can be used to avoid cutting through the posterior-lateral capsule and injuring posterolateral structures.

After resection, the medial edge of the tibial resection is grasped with a Kocher. The Kocher is used externally to rotate the fragment as the proximal attachments are sequentially released. With the ACL and meniscal attachments divided, the tibial fragment is easily removed. After the tibial fragment is removed, the leg is placed into full extension. A laminar spreader is then used in the extension space to expose the menisci. In this position, the menisci are easily seen and completely resected (Fig. 36.8). Any additional soft tissue releases to balance the knee can be easily accomplished in this extended position where both the lateral and medial structures are easily seen (Fig. 36.8). Lastly, a spacer block is used in extension to gauge the extension gap and to assess the soft tissue balancing.

Completing the Femur

Completion of the femur requires the knee to be positioned in 80–90° of flexion. A double-pronged Hohmann retractor is placed over the medial femoral condyle and another is placed over the lateral femoral condyle; this exposes the femur. The final femoral sizing guide is then positioned on the distal femur with the two skids placed under the posterior condyles (Fig. 36.9). This sets rotation at 3° external to the posterior condyles. This position usually coincides with Whitesides' line in varus knees; however, in valgus knees, the posterior condyles will internally rotate the guide. Therefore, in valgus knees, the guide must be externally

rotated from the femoral condyles to align with Whitesides' line. After the guide is positioned, it is fixed to the distal femur with two pins. The knee is then placed in extension

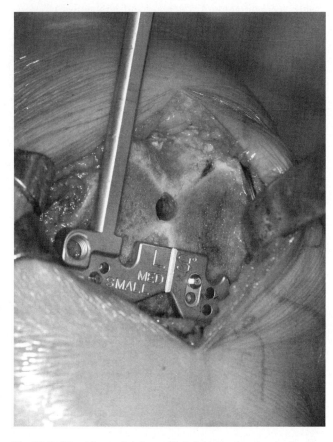

Fig. 36.9 Distal femoral sizing guide is initially placed under the femoral condyle in flexion. This is aligned with *Whitesides line*

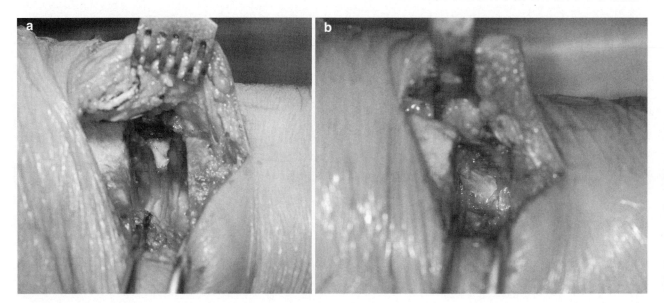

Fig. 36.8 (**a**) The lateral menisci is seen well in full extension. (**b**) After the menisci are removed, the lateral structures are easily visualized and can be subsequently released

and the femoral sizing guide is then attached to the anterior sizing rod. The anterior referencing finger is placed on the anterior lateral surface of the anterior femur, and adjusted to avoid anterior femoral notching (Fig. 36.10). The size of the femur is read from the femoral sizing guide. Usually, when between sizes, the smaller size is chosen for cruciate-retaining knees while the larger size is chosen for the posterior-stabilized knees (Fig. 36.10). The anterior reference finger is removed. With the knee flexed to 80–90°, the drill guide is positioned in the slot where the anterior reference finger was removed. With this guide, two drill holes are placed in the distal femur, which creates the reference for the final femoral finishing guide.

With the knee still flexed to 80–90°, the proper femoral finishing guide is then placed under the patella on the distal femur. Two pins are placed through the femoral finishing guide in the drill holes in the distal femur. The knee is then positioned in full extension and the femoral finishing guide is then positioned centrally on the femur. In this extended position, both the lateral and medial edges of the femoral condyles are easily seen. In extension, a medial screw pin is used to fix the guide to the femur. The knee is then flexed to 40° so that the lateral screw can be placed. Retractors are then positioned around the collateral ligaments. The femoral finishing guide is used to complete the final femoral cuts (Fig. 36.11). The femoral finishing guide is then removed and the resected femoral cuts are removed (Fig. 36.12).

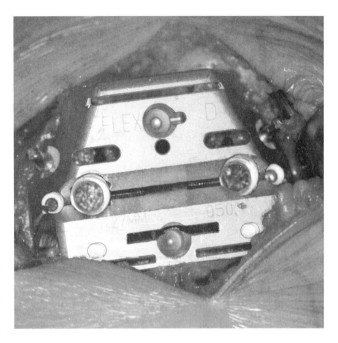

Fig. 36.11 Femoral finishing guide on the distal femur

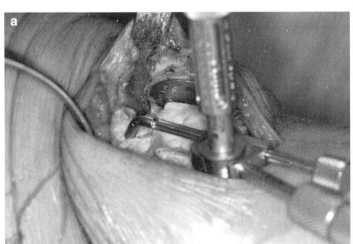

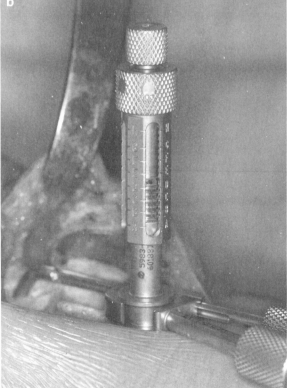

Fig. 36.10 Distal femoral sizing guide. (**a**) Anterior view after attachment of the anterior referencing arm. (**b**) Sizing guide is shown. The sizing shown here is between "*D*" and "*E*." In this cruciate-retaining TKA, a size "*D*" is chosen

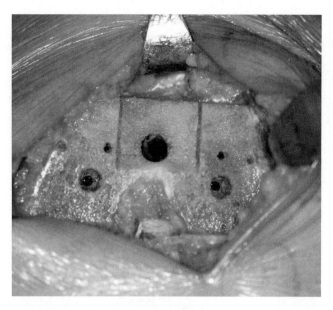

Fig. 36.12 The distal femur finished

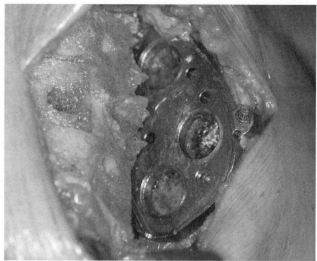

Fig. 36.13 Preparation of the tibia for the four-pegged component

Testing the Components

First the knee is placed in extension with retractors around the tibia. The tibia is sized in extension where the entire surface can be seen. Then the knee is placed in 90° of flexion, with Hohmann retractors positioned over the medial and lateral femoral condyles. The femoral trial component is then positioned between these retractors and maneuvered onto the distal femur. Care is taken to align the femoral trial with the lug holes before final seating of the trial. The knee is again extended to take tension off the extensor mechanism and the tibial trial is positioned with the tibial insert. Stability and range of motion is then assessed and any adjustments are made, as with a standard technique. The trial tibial tray is then pinned in place with the knee in extension. The tibial insert is removed in extension and the knee is flexed to remove the trial femoral component. In this flexed positioned, the tibia is prepared for the four-pegged tibial component by drilling the four pegs (Fig. 36.13).

Fixation of Final Components

A cemented or porous ingrowth femoral component may be used. The tibial and patellar components are fixed with cement. In extension, the tibia is irrigated and a layer of cement is placed on the tibial plateau with an angled nozzle cement gun and cement is also placed on the back of the tibial component. The tibial component is then placed on the tibial plateau (Fig. 36.14). The component is compressed against the tibia, starting posterior-laterally and progressing

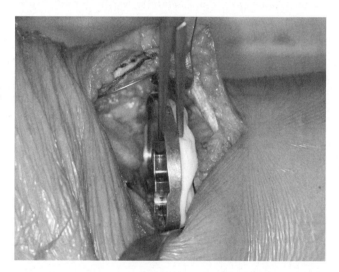

Fig. 36.14 Cementing of the tibial component in extension. This allows the tibia to be completely visualized and excess cement removed

anterior-medially; this extrudes cement anterior-medially, where it is easy to remove. A spacer block is used to place pressure on the tibial component in extension while extruded cement is removed from the posterior and peripheral component with a series of cement removal curettes. The cement on the tibia is allowed to fully cure to avoid tibial component shift during femoral component placement.

If a cemented femur is used, meticulous removal of cement must be completed. A porous ingrowth femoral component obviates cement removal. The knee is placed in 90° of flexion with Hohmann retractors positioned over the medial and lateral femoral condyles. The femoral component is then positioned between these retractors and maneuvered onto the distal femur. Care is taken to align the femoral

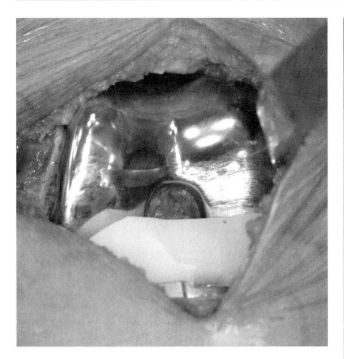

Fig. 36.15 Final components in place

component with the lug holes before final seating of the component. The knee is again extended to take tension off the extensor mechanism and a polyethylene spacer is inserted into place with the knee at 15° of flexion with traction on the tibia (Fig. 36.15). Finally, the patella is cemented with second batch of cement. Stability and range of motion is then assessed and any adjustments are made as with a standard technique.

Wound Closure

The knee is irrigated and a drain is placed. The retinaculum is closed with #1 Vicryl sutures. The deep layer of adipose and the dermis are closed with 2-0 Vicryl. A running 3-0 Monocryl and Dermabond are used to close and seal the skin (Fig. 36.16).

Conclusion

TKA with the quadriceps-sparing approach avoids violation of the quadriceps tendon, VMO fibers, and subvastus interval. In addition, since the interval remains in the retinaculum, the incision cannot self-extend with retraction as the subvastus and midvastus approaches. Furthermore, along with rapid perioperative recovery protocols,[2] patients usually ambulate with minimal assistance and are discharged to home later on the same day of surgery.[3]

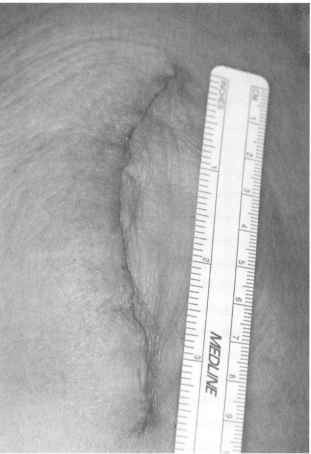

Fig. 36.16 Skin after wound closure is complete

This minimally invasive approach to total knee replacement is very safe. Furthermore, this approach potential can be easily extended into a medial parapatellar or midvastus approach if needed. Converse to the traditional approach to total knee replacement, where the hyperflexion of the knee increases exposure, extension improves exposure in this quadriceps-sparing approach. Lastly, this technique cannot be completed with traditional cutting guides; proper retractors and cutting guides are necessary to complete each step in this procedure.

References

1. Berger RA, Deirmengian CA, Della Valle CJ, Paprosky WG, Jacobs JJ, Rosenberg AG. A technique for minimally invasive, quadriceps-sparing total knee arthroplasty. *J Knee Surg*, 19(1): 63–70, 2006
2. Berger RA, Sanders S, D'Ambrogio E, Buchheit K, Deirmengian C, Paprosky W, Della Valle CJ, Rosenberg AG. Minimally invasive quadriceps-sparing TKA: results of a comprehensive pathway for outpatient TKA. *J Knee Surg*, 19(2): 145–148, 2006

3. Berger RA, Sanders S, Gerlinger T, Della Valle C, Jacobs JJ, Rosenberg AG. Outpatient total knee arthroplasty with a minimally invasive technique. *J Arthroplasty*, 20(6 Suppl 3): 33–38, 2005
4. Bonutti PM, Mont MA, McMahon M, Ragland PS, Kester M. Minimally invasive total knee arthroplasty. *J Bone Joint Surg Am*, 86-A(Suppl 2): 26–32, 2004
5. Goble EM, Justin DF. Minimally invasive total knee replacement: principles and technique. *Orthop Clin North Am*, 35(2): 235–245, 2004
6. Hofmann AA, Plaster RL, Murdock LE. Subvastus (Southern) approach for primary total knee arthroplasty. *Clin Orthop Relat Res*, (269): 70–77, 1991
7. Laskin RS. Minimally invasive total knee replacement using a mini-mid vastus incision technique and results. *Surg Technol Int*, 13: 231–238, 2004
8. Laskin RS, Beksac B, Phongjunakorn A, Pittors K, Davis J, Shim JC, Pavlov H, Petersen M. Minimally invasive total knee replacement through a mini-midvastus incision: an outcome study. *Clin Orthop Relat Res*, (428): 74–81, 2004
9. Tria AJ, Jr. Minimally invasive total knee arthroplasty: the importance of instrumentation. *Orthop Clin North Am*, 35(2): 227–234, 2004
10. Tria AJ, Jr, Coon TM. Minimal incision total knee arthroplasty: early experience. *Clin Orthop Relat Res*, (416): 185–190, 2003

Chapter 37
Bi-unicompartmental Knee Protheses

Sergio Romagnoli, Francesco Verde, Eddie Bibbiani, Nicolò Castelnuovo, and F. d'Amario

In the past few years, with the introduction of minimally invasive surgery (MIS) and based on excellent unicompartmental prosthesis (UKR) long-term results, we are experiencing a renewed interest in single or associate compartmental substitutions of the knee compared with anterior cruciate ligament (ACL). The UKR prosthesis is used in tissue-sparing surgeries (TSS).[1] TSS is a surgical philosophy that mandates a maximum respect for tissues and for anatomy and biomechanics. The aim of TSS is to reduce aggressive local and general surgical procedures, and thereby to optimize the patient's postoperative course and functional recovery. The surgical access routes in TSS are chosen with respect to the soft tissues, cartilaginous tissue, and bones. Surgical incision of the skin, a soft tissue, is minimized as much as possible while still permitting the intervention and the correct implantation of the prosthesis. The surgery is performed with care taken for the blood vessels and nerves, but also for the musculotendinous apparatus and the capsuloligamentous system.

The use of unicompartmental prostheses in the knee, especially those that require only minimal bone removal, represent a fundamental use for TSS. These unicompartmental prostheses have led, almost automatically, to the use of small, conservative access routes. Even more than in the hip, unicompartmental knee prostheses require careful insertion into the complex biomechanical and kinematic situation of the knee, especially when bi-unicompartmental prostheses are used. In this case, the tissue-sparing principal that the prosthesis does not substitute for the joint but integrates with it is especially apparent. In fact, when implanting a UKR, it is wrong to correct the joint biomechanics that caused the pathology; instead, one simply substitutes the part that degenerated due to the disease.

Bicompartmental prosthesis was introduced in the 1970s by Marmor, Gunston, and Lubinus.[2,3] The surgical technique is based on the substitution of the two femorotibial compartments using two femoral and two tibial independent components preserving the tibial eminentia and the ACL. With the term *bicompartmental*, we mean a surgical procedure that substitutes one only of the tibiofemoral compartments in association with the patellofemoral (PF) compartment. Actually, the improved screening technique and treatment of knee arthritis enable more young patients to consider prosthetic surgery. In these cases, minimally invasive conservative solutions are sought that can guarantee maximum results to patients with high-level expectations.

Epidemiology

In the treatment of bicompartmental arthritis, the presence of a functional ACL represents the basis of the surgical indication. In the last 1,000 bi-tricompartmental implants performed at the Centro di Chirurgia Protesica at the Istituto Ortopedico Galeazzi in Milano, we have observed that, in 35.1% of the cases, the patients had an intact ACL, while in 15.7% of cases, the ACL appeared slightly degenerated but still functioning, and finally, in 49.2% of cases, the ACL could not be observed intraoperatively. We studied the relationship between the ACL and its mechanical function in a long-term survivorship study of bicompartmental prosthesis and in the Allegretto (Zimmer) unicompartmental prosthesis with 10–15 years of follow-up.[4–12] This article and several other long-term survivorship studies of unicompartmental prosthesis[6–16] show that anteroposterior (AP) long-term stability remains unchanged. This shows that the ACL has the ability to maintain the same mechanical function over the course of years. As a matter of fact, in our studies on 124 patients treated with unicompartmental prosthesis, we had only one case of failure due to ACL deficiency.

If we consider age as a selective criteria, we observe that in 1,000 cases of knee prosthesis performed, 7.6% of patients were younger than 55 years of age while 25.8% were aged between 55 and 65 years, 39.5% were aged between 65 and 75 years, and 27.1% were older than 75 years of age. Therefore, 33.4% of patients were younger than 65 years of

S. Romagnoli (✉), F. Verde, E. Bibbiani, N. Castelnuovo, and F. d'Amario
Centro Chirurgia Protesica, Istituto Ortopedico "R. Galeazzi", 20161 Via R. Galeazzi 4, Milano, Italy
e-mail: sergio.romagnoli@grupposandonato.it

G.R. Scuderi and A.J. Tria (eds.), *Minimally Invasive Surgery in Orthopedics*, DOI 10.1007/978-0-387-76608-9_37, © Springer Science+Business Media, LLC 2010

age. Thirty-five percent of these patients had an intact ACL and were potential users of cruciate-retaining prostheses.

Indications

This surgery is indicated for patients with bilateral femorotibial degeneration but with an asymptomatic patella, with cruciate ligament integrity, flexum deformity <5°, varus-valgus deformity <15°, and range of motion (ROM) >80° (Fig. 37.1).[8,9,13]

Radiographic evaluation is based on AP, lateral, and sky view projections that show a femorotibial degeneration higher than grade I on Ahlback scale and a PF involvement lower than grade II. Furthermore, on a long weight-bearing AP X-ray view, we can calculate the mechanical axis of the limb, highlighting the correct range of tolerated deformity. Magnetic resonance imaging (MRI) can highlight both an ACL instability or deficiency and a PF degeneration. The knee must be stable clinically, and only a minimal laxity due to cartilaginous degeneration is tolerated. We can usually observe clinical signs, such as pain while walking and climbing stairs and effusion. Age and weight are not a limit, but this solution is especially suitable in active patients younger than 65 years of age and with a body mass index (BMI) < 32. Bi-Uni is, in fact, suitable in young patients with high functional expectations. As previously mentioned, the main limits of this implantation selection are ACL and PF integrity. In the first case, when a femorotibial bicompartmental degeneration defines a correct indication for a Bi-Uni implant, but the absence of ACL is a clear limitation, only then can we consider an ACL reconstruction.

A secondary degeneration of PF joint with chronic anterior pain is something to keep in mind when selecting patients. Evaluation criteria are symptoms, X-ray evaluation of alignment and overload, and the intraoperative evidence of grade III or IV chondromalacia. Symptoms, only if accompanied by other parameters, which can be X-ray or intraoperative observation, are a clear limit to the indication. Bi-UKR can sometimes be the result of a UKR revision due to degeneration and the pain of the untreated femorotibial compartment. In this case, the implant of a UKR in the other degenerated compartment of the same knee results in a Bi-UKR. Obviously, in this case, the previous implant must be stable, and the only contraindications are polyethylene (PE) wear and ACL deficiency (Fig. 37.2). Absolute contraindications to the Bi-UKR are ligaments instability, severe axial deformity >15°, flexum deformity >5°, and compartmental bone stock defect >12 mm.

Surgical Technique

Bi-UKR uses the same surgical technique as UKR applied to both the medial and lateral compartments. We can choose between two different approaches: a double mini skin incision or an isolated medial parapatellar approach. The first choice relies on a parapatellar medial, 4- to 6-cm mini skin incision and a mini lateral parapatellar incision of 6–8 cm, depending on the individual case. Usually, we start in the medial compartment with a tibia-first technique; once we have positioned the trials, we proceed with cutting the lateral compartment. This gives us the perception of the stability we want to reach. The second choice, which we prefer, is based

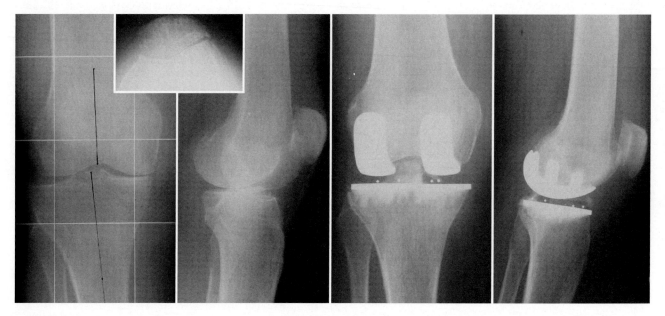

Fig. 37.1 Bicompartmental knee arthritis with asymptomatic and not degenerated PF joint (56-year-old woman)

on a minimally invasive parapatellar medial incision of 8–10 cm. In this case, a mini-midvastus incision allows patella subluxation, creating a good exposition of both the medial and lateral compartments. Once the compartments are exposed, surface bone cuts are performed with the tibia-first technique. Tibial cuts are performed using a minimally invasive tibial guide at the same time in the two compartments. Vertical cuts have to be between 15 and 20° oblique on the AP axis of the medial compartment and 10–15° in the lateral,

respecting the ACL.[9] The horizontal cut must respect the height and obliquity of the joint line, reproducing the perpendicular cut more on the proximal epiphysary axis than on the diaphysary axis (Fig. 37.3).

The obliquity of the joint line varies depending on the varus or valgus morphotype and so allows us to avoid the need for a release. In the sagittal plane, the tibial cut must reproduce the preoperative slope and respect posterior cruciate ligament (PCL) integrity. On the femoral side, we perform the

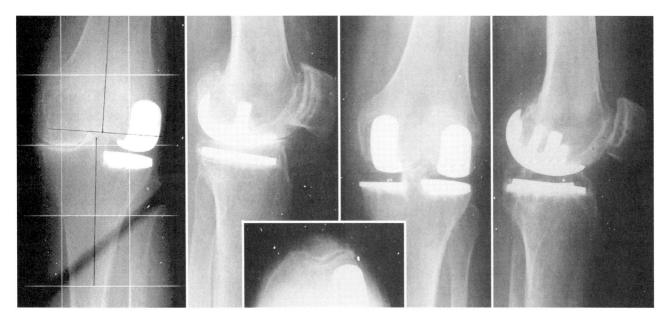

Fig. 37.2 Medial UKR, compatible with the existing UKR (16 years follow-up), due to medial compartment degeneration

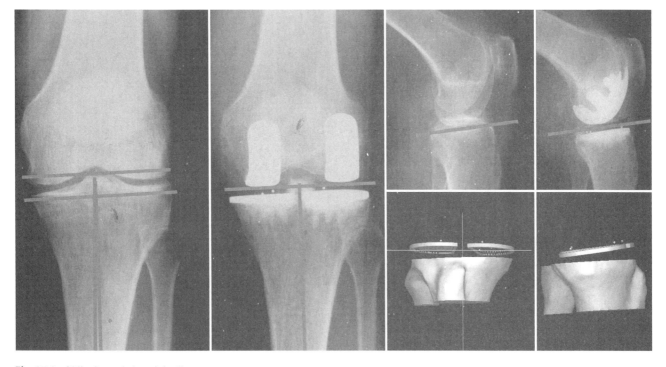

Fig. 37.3 Obliquity and slope joint line respect

distal cut in extension and the posterior cut in flexion using a tensor guide that calibrates the same amount of resections, creating a balanced flexion-extension gap (Fig. 37.4).

First, the distal cut in extension creates the perception of the stability we want to reach, adjusting the tensor to avoid overcorrection and release. Subsequently, the flexion cut is calibrated on the same quantity and tension in order to obtain balance. The same thickness of the prosthesis to be implanted needs to be removed (2 mm), 2–3 mm of bone from the medial femoral condyle and 1–2 mm from the lateral, depending on the axis correction needed. Femoral components are often lateralized to obtain a femorotibial centralization in flexion-extension (Fig. 37.5). Once we have assessed the stability with the trials, we prepare the bone for cementing (Fig. 37.6).

In well-selected cases of young patients in whom the only limit to Bi-UKR is the absence of the ACL, we can perform a reconstruction procedure (Fig. 37.7). Currently, we prefer using hamstrings to avoid complications caused by patellar tendons. In this case, tibial fixation is done right before femoral cementing. In young patients, in whom PF joints are

symptomatic, together with grade II-III chondromalacia observed intraoperatively, we use a bicondylar femoral component with an ACL-retention design. Actually, a cruciate-retaining total knee arthroplasty (TKA) is another interesting solution, but is more invasive (Fig. 37.8).

Complications

Bicompartmental implant failure may be caused by intraoperative complications or it may occur over time. Intraoperative complications include incorrect positioning of components, tibial eminentia fracture, incorrect ligament balancing, and cementation mistakes. In the case of tibial eminentia fracture during surgery, this can be stabilized with one or two divergent cortical screws that have to be fixed before cementation[9–13] (Fig. 37.9).

Long-term follow-up in cases treated with eminentia fixation have never shown secondary loosening of the

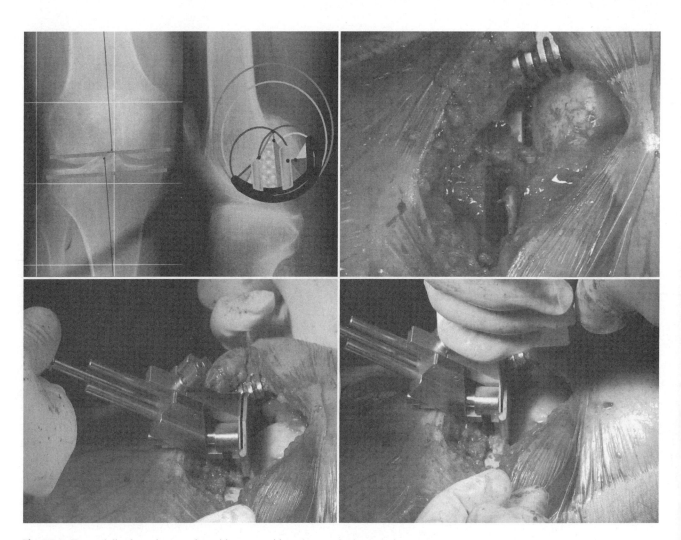

Fig. 37.4 Femoral distal curt in extension with tensor guide and spacer in the opposite compartment

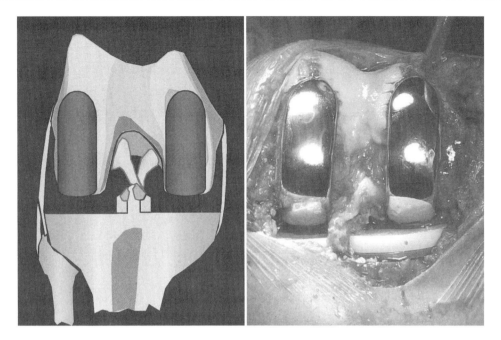

Fig. 37.5 Component lateralization

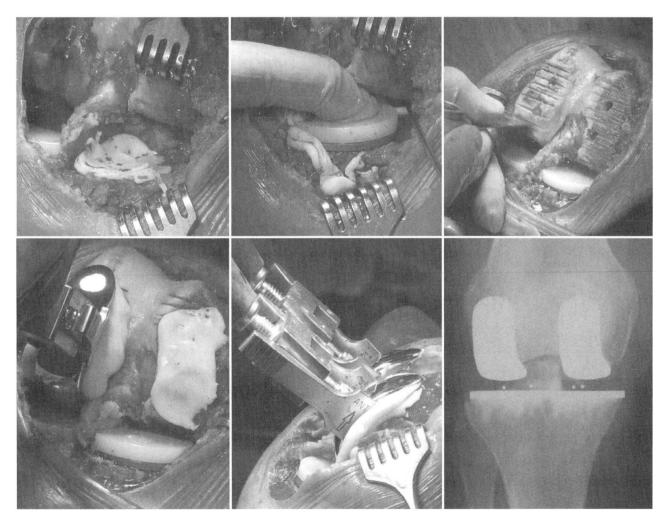

Fig. 37.6 Surgical technique and cementation of tibia and femur. We start with lateral tibial compartment cementation

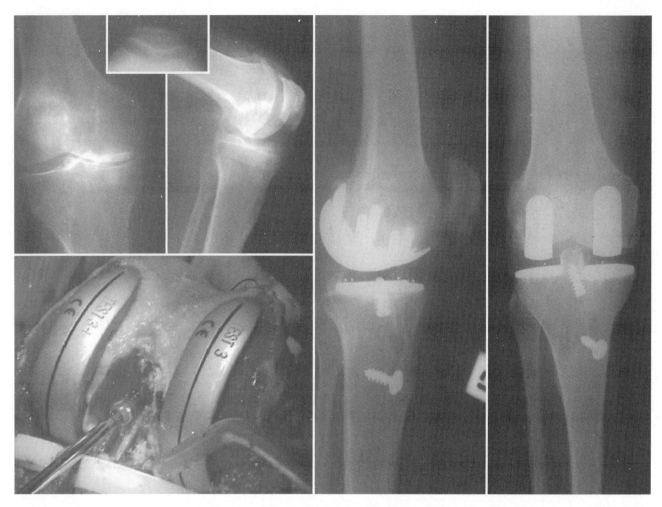

Fig. 37.7 A 53-year-old man with a bilateral meniscectomy and ACL rupture sequelae. A BTB reconstruction procedure was performed in 1998

intercondylar spine. Complications that occurred over the course of time included PF joint degeneration or secondary ligament degeneration, component loosening, or PE wear. Finally, septic loosening has the same incidence as in other prosthetic procedures.

Bicompartmental Arthritis

Knee arthritis often involves only one of the two femorotibial compartments, along with symptomatic PF joint degeneration. Among our patients, this represents only 15% of knee arthritis, whereas 5% have isolated bicompartmental femorotibial involvement. Treatment of bicompartmental arthritis involves a lateral or medial UKR to treat arthritis and correct the axial deformity and the use of a PF prosthesis.[14] This combined use widens indications and reduces limits to a UKR and isolated PF prosthesis. This procedure is suitable in cases of borderline UKR indications with femorotibial compartmental arthritis and symptomatic patella and in cases of borderline indications for PF prosthesis due to isolated PF arthritis with

3° mechanical axis deviation and initial femorotibial unicompartmental involvement. In our experience, two kinds of bicompartmental arthritis exist, femorotibial and PF. In the first case, an initial PF joint pathology is associated with an axial limb deviation, with varus or valgus morphotype and secondary femorotibial arthritis. In the second case, the pathology initially concerns one of the two femorotibial compartments with a varus or valgus morphotype involving the secondary PF joint. The isolated use of the isolated PF prosthesis is an uncommon procedure with few references in the literature and even rarer is the combined use with a UKR. The advantages of a bicompartmental implant, UKR plus PF, are cruciate preservation, respect for rotational axis, bone stock preservation, patellar height and tracking, normal joint kinematic reproduction, and morphotype respect. Selection criteria are the same as for UKR in which the PF joint is degenerated (Fig. 37.10).

The surgical approach is the same as in UKR, medial in varus or lateral in valgus, but 2–3 cm longer.[4,8,10,12] Usually, the procedure starts with UKR steps, the tibia-first technique, and a distal femoral cut in extension. Once stability has been tested with trials, continue with the preparation of the implant

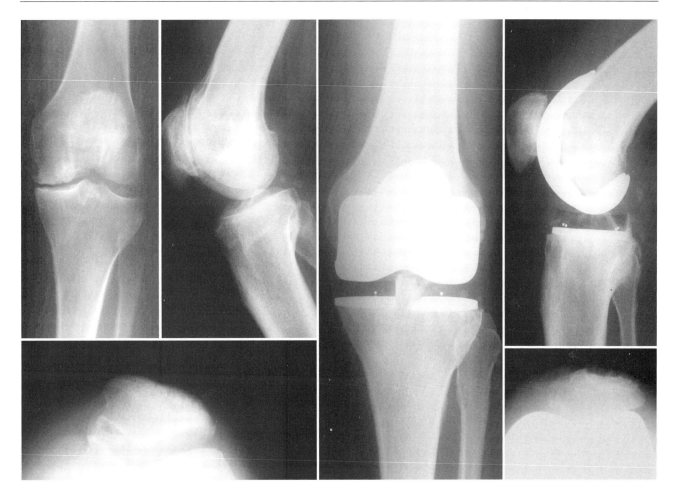

Fig. 37.8 Bi-UKR with total femur (NexGen CR, Zimmer) in the case of symptomatic PF degeneration

surface for the PF prosthesis, first the femoral trochlea and then the patella. It is important to keep a distance of >3 mm between the two prosthetic components. Our objective is to respect the femoral surfaces rotational axis and trochlear depth, avoiding excessive tension on the patella. Trials implanted must highlight perfect PF tracking without patellar clunk and tilting in the area of the component transition.

Biomechanics

Preserving both cruciate ligaments in unicondylar knee arthroplasty provides more normal knee mechanic function, and it contributes to enhanced patient function as shown in our study in 2001.[11] Preserving both cruciate ligaments with total knee arthroplasty should provide functional benefit if compared with arthroplasty, which sacrifices one or both cruciate ligaments. We have compared knee kinematics in patients with well-functioning cruciate-preserving medial unicondylar and bi-unicondylar arthroplasty to determine if knee motions were different.

Material and Methods

Twelve consenting patients with seven medial unicondylar and five bi-unicondylar arthroplasties participated in this Institutional Review Board-approved study (Table 37.1). Patients were recruited for participation based on combined Knee Society scores greater than 195[17] at a minimum of 8 months after surgery, who returned to high levels of activity after arthroplasty, had high satisfaction with the procedure and outcome, and had a willingness to drive up to 4 h to participate in the study. All patients had surgery by a single surgeon (SR) using a cemented metal-backed fixed-bearing tibial baseplate and a cemented cobalt-chrome femoral prosthesis (Allegretto, Centerpulse Orthopedics Ltd., Winterthur, Switzerland). The surgical technique fully maintained both cruciate ligaments and replicated as closely as possible the normal articular surfaces and posterior slope of each tibial plateau. Tibial prostheses were implanted in 2–3° varus with respect to the tibial mechanical axis. Femoral prostheses were positioned perpendicular to the tibial implants with resurfacing bone preparation. The medial and lateral femoral components were lateralized slightly to maintain contact on

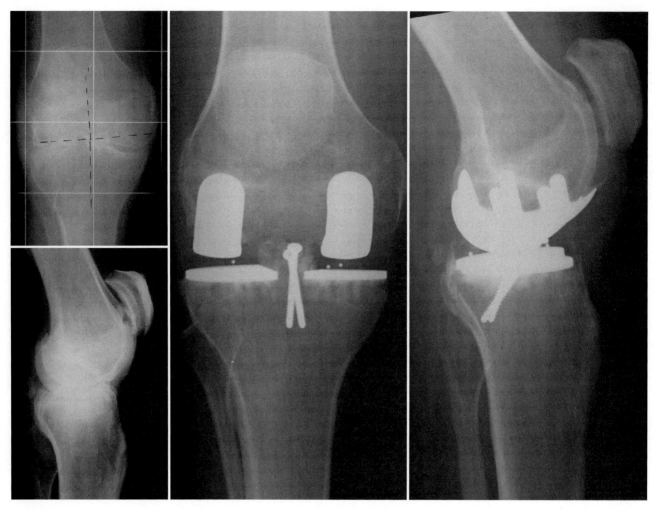

Fig. 37.9 Fixation of intraoperative tibial eminentia fracture with two divergent cortical screws

the center of the tibial bearing surface with flexion and endorotation/exorotation. Patients' knee motions were recorded using lateral fluoroscopy during treadmill gait at 1 m/s, single limb stepping up and down on a 25-cm stair, maximum flexion in a lunge with the foot placed on the 25-cm step, maximum flexion kneeling on a padded stool, and weight-bearing straight-leg stance.

Image matching-based measurements of knee arthroplasty kinematics typically use surface models of the implanted metal components. Since the tibial components of this unicondylar system had only a thin metal wafer base and two small beads within the PE, it was determined that a shape model incorporating implant and bone geometry would permit better measurement sensitivity and robustness for large out-of-plane motions. The three-dimensional position and orientation of the proximal and distal knee segments was determined using a toolbox of model-based shape-matching techniques, including previously reported techniques,[24] manual matching, and automated matching using nonlinear least-squares (modified Levenberg-Marquardt) techniques (Fig. 37.11).

Three thousand two hundred and eleven fluoroscopic images, an average of 268 images per knee, were analyzed. The results of this shape-matching process have standard errors of approximately 0.5–1.0° for rotations and 0.5–1.0 mm for translations in the sagittal plane.[18] Joint kinematics were determined from the three-dimensional pose of each knee component using Cardan/Euler angles.[19] The anterior/posterior locations of tibiofemoral contact were computed, independently for each implanted compartment, by transforming the joint pose into a reference system parallel to the transverse plane of the flat tibial component and finding the lowest point on the femoral component. For the stair, kneeling, and lunge activities, kinematics were expressed relative to the joint pose in straight-leg weight-bearing stance. For gait, the kinematics were expressed relative to the joint pose at heel-strike. Kneeling and lunge data were compared using t-tests. For the stair and gait data, an average curve for each knee was created from four trials of data. These average curves were then combined to create group averages.

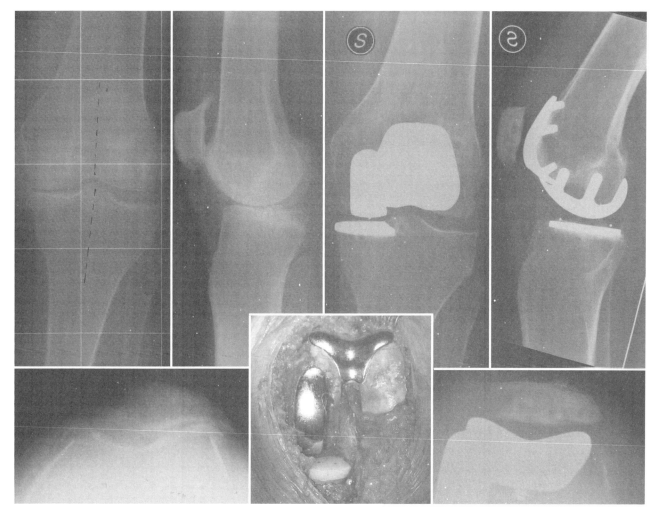

Fig. 37.10 Bicompartmental arthritis (medial compartment plus PF) and solution with a combined PF + UKR implant

Table 37.1 Characteristics of knee replacement patients.

Sex	Age (year)	Weight (kg)	Right knee	Right follow-up (months)	Left knee	Left follow-up (months)	Lifestyle
M	42	75	Healthy		Bi-Uni	26	Sports
F	55	65	Bi-Uni	18	Healthy		Active
F	60	80	Bi-Uni[a]	8	Uni	9	Long walk
M	73	78	Uni	10	Uni	10	Long walk
M	73	75	Bi-Uni	21	Healthy		Sports
M	74	72	Uni	21	Uni	21	Sports
F	79	74	Uni	15	Uni	22	Long walk
M	79	65	Uni[b]		Bi-uni	36	Active

From Romagnoli et al.[11]
[a]Total knee replacement femoral component used with bi-unicondylar tibial components
[b]Well-functioning unicondylar knee, but no computed tomography (CT) data to permit inclusion in study

Results

Maximum knee flexion in kneeling and lunge was an average of 10° greater ($P > 0.22$) for unicondylar knees at 135°/133° (Table 37.2). Average tibial internal rotation was greater in the unicondylar knees for kneeling ($P = 0.18$) and lunge ($P = 0.06$) activities. None of these differences was statistically significant. Posterior translation of the medial condyle averaged 2 mm or less for both types of knees in the lunge and kneeling activities. Posterior translation of the lateral condyle in the bi-unicondylar knees averaged 4 mm for the lunge and kneeling activities. Both groups of knees

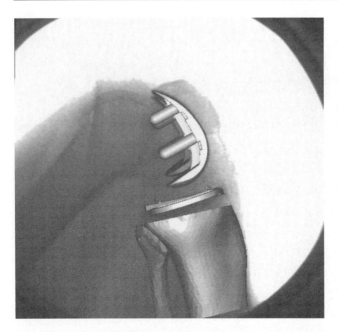

Fig. 37.11 Three-dimensional pose measurements for the femur and tibia/fibula segments were accomplished by projecting the shape models onto the digitized and distortion-corrected fluoroscopic images. The model pose was varied until the projected shapes matched those in the image

Discussion

Well-done contemporary knee arthroplasty provides excellent 10-year outcomes almost without regard to the particular philosophy or implant type used. In this context, the focus for improvement shifts to patients' functional abilities and limitations. Contemporary unicondylar knee arthroplasty is widely acknowledged to provide more normal postoperative function compared with total knee arthroplasty, and it is assumed that retaining both cruciate ligaments contributes to this functional advantage. It is natural, therefore, to ask whether bi-unicondylar knee arthroplasty might provide similar knee kinematics and function. This study attempts to answer that question for a highly selected small group of active patients with excellent outcomes. This selected group of unicondylar and bi-unicondylar knees showed average maximum flexion that was equivalent to or better than has been previously reported for knee arthroplasty in Western patients.[20–23] These knees prove that excellent flexion can be achieved with these techniques, but it is likely that the mean maximum flexion would be less for a more broadly representative group of patients. Kinematics in both groups varied substantially between knees for the deep flexion activities, so that no statistically significant differences could be demonstrated (Table 37.2). Posterior translation of the medial condyle with flexion was observed in both knee groups for the stair activity, 3.5 mm for the unicondylar and 5 mm for the bi-unicondylar knees. This finding is consistent with prior studies of anterior cruciate ligament-retaining total knee arthroplasty,[24,25] but the translations were greater than reported in studies of medial unicondylar knee arthroplasty[26] or the healthy knee[23,27] for quasistatic activities. It was particularly surprising in the bi-unicondylar knees that the medial and lateral condyles translated posteriorly the same amount in early flexion (0–40°), again contrasting with reports for normal knee kinematics during quasistatic activities.[23,28] The unicondylar knees showed less than 2 mm AP translation of the medial condyle during the stance phase of gait. The bi-unicondylar knees showed more than 5 mm posterior translation of the medial condyle just after heel-strike, indicating greater dynamic laxity. Two factors likely contributed to increased medial condylar sliding. First, these knees had greater flexion in early stance phase, so the knees were in a position of increased passive laxity.[28]

showed tibial internal rotation with flexion during the stair activity (Fig. 37.12).

The unicondylar knees showed greater tibial rotation for flexion from 20 to 80° ($P < 0.01$). For 0–30° flexion during the stair activity, the medial condyle translated posterior 3.5 ± 2.5 mm in unicondylar knees and 4.7 ± 1.9 mm in bi-unicondylar knees ($P = 0.035$). Lateral condyle posterior translation was 5.0 ± 2.3 mm in bi-unicondylar knees for 0–30° flexion. The bi-unicondylar knees showed greater knee flexion from heel-strike to midstance phase than the unicondylar knees ($P < 0.01$), but similar flexion from late stance through swing phase (Fig. 37.13a). The bi-unicondylar knees showed greater tibial external rotation throughout stance phase ($P < 0.01$; Fig. 37.13b), which correlates closely to greater posterior translation of the medial condyle in early to mid stance phase ($P < 0.01$, Fig. 37.13c). Lateral condylar AP translations in the bi-unicondylar knees were similar in pattern, but smaller in magnitude, compared with the medial condylar translations (Fig. 37.13d).

Table 37.2 Knee kinematics in deep flexion kneeling and lunge postures (mean ± 1 standard deviation, range in parentheses).

	Kneeling		Lunge	
Parameter	Uni	Bi-Uni	Uni	Bi-Uni
Flexion (degrees)	135 ± 14 (114–150)	123 ± 14 (108–136)	133 ± 15 (111–150)	124 ± 12 (107–135)
Axial rotation (degrees)	9.0 ± 6 (3–19)	3 ± 7 (−3–13)	12.0 ± 7 (−1–19)	4 ± 6 (−2–12)
Medial rollback (mm)	2 ± 5 (−5–11)	0 ± 5 (−6–5)	2 ± 4 (−2–11)	1 ± 5 (−6–6)
Lateral rollback (mm)		4 ± 9 (−4–16)		3 ± 9 (−6–16)

From Romagnoli et al.[11]

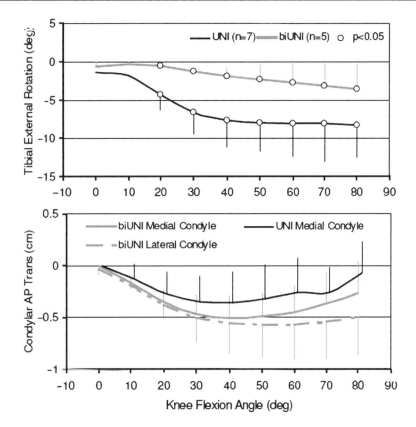

Fig. 37.12 The pattern of tibial rotation (mean ± 1 standard deviation) for Uni and Bi-Uni knees differed ($P < 0.001$) during the stair activity (*top*). Medial condyle AP translations also differed ($P = 0.035$), but there were no statistically significant differences for specific flexion ranges (*bottom*). AP translations for the medial and lateral condyles of the Bi-Uni knees were the same from 0 to 40° flexion. The *white circles* indicate where there is a significant pair-wise difference between the two data series (From Romagnoli et al.[11] with kind permission of Springer Science + Business Media.)

Second, the bi-unicondylar knees had bicompartmental disease preoperatively and no longer maintained the normal laxity of the lateral compartment after arthroplasty. As a result, the pattern of motion during gait in the bi-unicondylar knees was closer to motions reported for fixed-bearing total knee replacements in identical tests.[28,29] As reported by others and confirmed in this study, preserving both cruciate ligaments in knee arthroplasty maintains some basic features of normal knee kinematics, including posterior translation of the femoral condyles and tibial internal rotation with flexion. These motions were most evident during the stair activity for the unicondylar and bi-unicondylar knees. As one might expect, the dynamic laxity of the knee increased when both tibiofemoral compartments were replaced, which was most apparent during gait. In conclusion, the kinematics of unicondylar and bi-unicondylar knee arthroplasty share common features, but differ in ways that are consistent with bicompartmental preoperative disease and loss of the normal lateral compartment in the bi-unicondylar knees. Despite kinematic differences compared with unicondylar knees, bi-unicondylar arthroplasty can provide functional outcomes similar to unicondylar knees in appropriately selected patients.

Results

We started our experience in 1990 and until now, the percentage of Bi-UKR has been modified each year. However, from 1990 to 2006, the percentage of Bi-UKR was 2.3%, while from July 2002 to 2006 it was 4.8%; however, if we consider only patients younger than 55 years, from 1990 to 2006 the percentage was 14.6%. This confirms that this surgical option is strongly indicated in young active patients. The UKR + PF, bicompartmental implants, performed from 2003 to 2005 represent 8% of our knee implants. This surgical technique, which seems new, is actually the result of 15 years of experience, during which, the indications were restricted to isolated PF knee arthritis and to surgical treatment of unicompartmental knee arthroplasty for chronic anterior knee pain due to secondary PF degeneration. In 2006 we revised our three main types of implants related to ACL: Bi-UKR with two femoral and tibial independent components, Bi-UKR with two tibial components and a total femoral component and ACL retaining, and bicompartmental UKR + PF (we have always used Allegretto, Zimmer unicompartmental prosthesis, with tibia Sulmesh and minimum PE thickness of

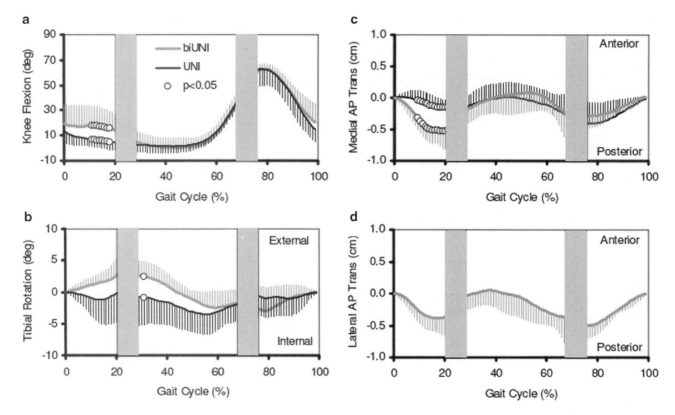

Fig. 37.13 Knee kinematics during gait differed between the Uni and Bi-Uni knees (mean ± 1 standard deviation). The Bi-Uni knees showed greater flexion in early stance, but similar flexion in late stance and swing (**a**). Bi-Uni knees showed greater tibial external rotation during stance (**b**). Bi-Uni knees showed significantly greater posterior translations of the medial condyle in early stance (**c**), and a similar pattern of AP motion for the lateral condyle (**d**). The two *gray regions* on each graph indicate gaps in the fluoroscopic data, when the contralateral knee occludes the view, which are filled by interpolation. The *white circles* indicate where there is a significant pair-wise difference between the two data series (From Romagnoli et al.[11] with kind permission of Springer Science + Business Media.)

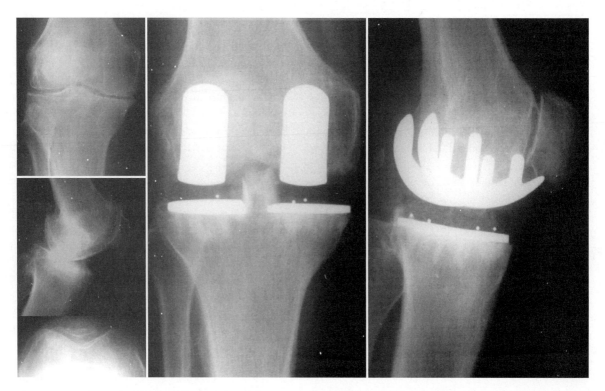

Fig. 37.14 Radiographs showing 12-year follow-up after Bi-Uni

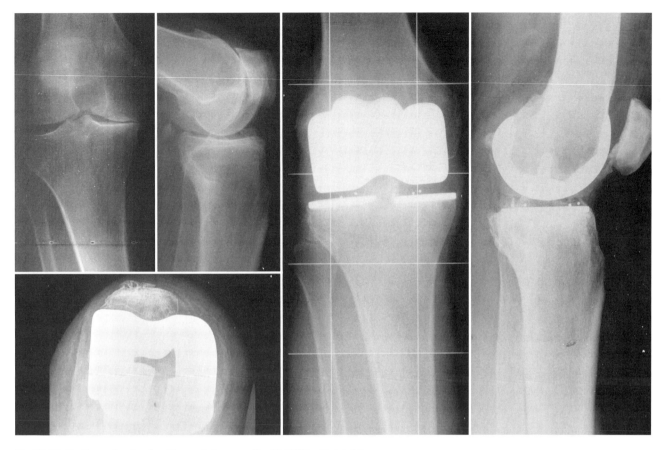

Fig.37.15 Radiographs showing 11-year follow-up after Bi-UKR with total femur

6 mm). From 1990 to 2005, we performed 148 Bi-UKR and 103 with two independent tibial components and that were total femur and ACL retaining (Fig. 37.14). We have studied 129 Bi-UKR consecutive cases with independent femoral components implanted between 1990 and 2005 with a 1- to 15-year follow-up. This study has proved a medium ROM of 126°. In this series, we had three failures, one caused by acquired ligament instability, another caused by PF degeneration, and the last one for chronic anterior knee pain.

We have also studied 91 consecutive cases of prosthesis with tibia bicompartmental and total femur implanted between 1990 and 2003 with 2- to 11-year follow-up. In this series, the average ROM was 116° and we had one failure due to ligament instability. In 88 cases of bicompartmental prosthesis (UKR + PF) 3 years after the indication extension, we had only one case of failure due to patellar tilt related to prosthetic design, which we eventually abandoned, and revision with a primary total knee implant (Fig. 37.15).

Conclusion

The cruciate-retaining knee bicompartmental arthroplasties, even if not common, seem to offer a high level functionality and a joint kinematic that presents essential features similar to a normal knee and a survivor rate comparable to TKA. Bi-UKR has shown an average range of motion of 126°, higher than the average standard total knee replacement (TKR). Bi-UKR with total femur has never used a resurfaced patella, but despite this has never shown PF long-term complications. UKR + PF represent the technique's further expansion with good prospects for the future.

References

1. Pipino F (2006) Tissue sparing surgery (T.S.S.) in hip and knee arthroplasty. J Orthop Traumatol 7:33–35
2. Gunston FH (1971) Polycentric knee arthroplasty. Prosthetic simulation of normal knee movement. J Bone Joint Surg Br 53(2):272–277
3. Marmor L (1973) The modular knee. Clin Orthop Relat Res 94:242–248
4. Romagnoli S, Verde F, Eberle RW (2006) 10-year minimum follow-up of medial unicompartmental knee arthroplasty with the allegretto prosthesis. Presented at AAOS, Chicago 2006, San Francisco 2007; exhibit SE41, Poster P203
5. Romagnoli S (1996) The unicompartmental knee prosthesis and the rotatory gonarthrosis kinematic. In: *Current Concept in Primary and Revision, Total Knee Arthroplasty*, edited by John N. Insall, W. Norman Scott, Giles R. Scuderi, Lippincott-Raven Publishers, Philadelphia
6. Cartier P, Sanouiller JL, Grelsamer RP (1996) Unicompartmental knee arthroplasty surgery. 10 years minimum follow-up period. J Arthroplasty 11(7):782–788

7. Romagnoli S, Grappiolo G, Ursino N, Broch C (2000) Dexa evaluation of bone remodelling in the proximal tibial after unicompartmental prosthesis. Traumalinc 2:2 Pabst Science Publishers

8. Romagnoli S, Grappiolo G, Camera A (1998) Indicazioni e limiti delle protesi monocompartimentali, Il Ginocchio, Anno XIV, vol. 18

9. Romagnoli S, Camera A, Bertolotti M, Arnaldi E (2000) La protesi Bimonocompartimentale con rispetto ricostruzione del LCA, Il Ginocchio, Anno XIV, vol. 19, anno

10. Romagnoli S, Camera A, Bertolotti M (2000) Deformità rotatoria e protesi monocompartimentale, Il Ginocchio, Anno XVI, vol. 19

11. Romagnoli S, Banks SA, Fregly BJ, Boniforti F, Reinschmidt C (2005) Comparing in vivo kinematics of unicondylar and bi-unicondylar knee replacement. Knee Surg Sports Traumatol Arthrosc 13(7):551–6

12. Romagnoli S (2004) Allegretto: Protesi Monocompartimentale di ginocchio. Pronews, Anno 2 – numero 1, Marzo

13. "Die unicondylare Schlittenprothese – (Unicompartmental Knee Arthroplasty). Klaus Buckup Herausgeber, Steinkopff Darmstadt 2005

14. "Bi-Unikondylare Schlittenprothese" S. Romagnoli, F. Verde

15. Romagnoli S., Verde F., Damario F., Castelnuovo N (2006) La protesi femoro-rotulea. Archivio di Ortopedia e Traumatologia 117(1)-

16. Chassin EP, Mikosz RP, Andriacchi TP, Rosenberg AG (1996) Functional analysis of cemented medial unicompartmental knee arthroplasty. J Arthroplasty 11(5):553–559

17. Banks SA, Hodge WA (1996) Accurate measurement of three-dimensional knee replacement kinematics using single-plane fluoroscopy. IEEE Trans Biomed Eng 43(6):638–649

18. Tupling S, Pierrynowski M (1987) Use of Cardan angles to locate rigid bodies in three-dimensional space. Med Biol Eng Comput 25(5):527–532

19. Scott RD, Cobb AG, McQueary FG, Thornhill TS (1991) Unicompartmental knee arthroplasty. Eight- to 12-year follow-up evaluation with survivorship analysis. Clin Orthop Relat Res (271):96–100

20. Cloutier JM, Sabouret P, Deghrar A (1999) Total knee arthroplasty with retention of both cruciate ligaments. A nine to eleven-year follow-up study. J Bone Joint Surg 81-A(5):697–702

21. Stiehl JB, Komistek RD, Cloutier JM, Dennis DA (2000) The cruciate ligaments in total knee arthroplasty: a kinematic analysis of 2 total knee arthroplasties. J Arthroplasty 15(5):545–550

22. Iwaki H, Pinskerova V, Freeman MAR (2000) Tibio-femoral movement 1: the shapes and relative movements of the femur and tibia in the unloaded cadaver knee. J Bone Joint Surg 82-B: 1189–1195

23. Hill PF, Vedi V, Williams A, Iwaki H, Pinskerova V, Freeman MAR (2000) Tibiofemoral movement 2: the loaded and unloaded living knee studied by MRI. J Bone Joint Surg 82-B:1196–1198

24. Komistek RD, Allain J, Anderson DT, Dennis DA, Goutallier D (2002) In vivo kinematics for subjects with and without an anterior cruciate ligament. Clin Orthop Relat Res (404):315–325

25. Insall JN, Dorr LD, Scott RD, Scott WN (1989) Rationale of the Knee Society clinical rating system. Clin Orthop Relat Res (248):13–14

26. Goodfellow JW, O'Connor J (1986) Clinical results of the Oxford knee. Surface arthroplasty of the tibiofemoral joint with a meniscal bearing prosthesis. Clin Orthop Relat Res (205):21–42

27. Blankevoort L, Huiskes R, de Lange A (1988) The envelope of passive knee joint motion. J Biomech 21(9):705–720

28. Banks SA, Markovich GD, Hodge WA (1997) The mechanics of knee replacements during gait. In vivo fluoroscopic analysis of two designs. Am J Knee Surg 10(4):261–267

29. Banks SA, Hodge WA (2004) 2003 Hap Paul Award Paper of the International Society for Technology in Arthroplasty: design and activity dependence of kinematics in fixed and mobile bearing knee arthroplasties. J Arthroplasty 19(7):809–816

Chapter 38
MIS Patellofemoral Arthroplasty

Jess H. Lonner

The prevalence of isolated patellofemoral arthritis is high, occurring in as many as 11% of men and 24% of women older than the age of 55 years with symptomatic osteoarthritis of the knee in one study.[1] Symptomatic patellofemoral chondromalacia occurs with even greater frequency and is a very common reason for presentation for orthopedic evaluation, particularly in women between the ages of 30 and 50 years. This gender predilection is undoubtedly related to the often subtle patellar malalignment and dysplasia that is common in women. The patellofemoral cartilage is also at risk for direct traumatic injury, considering its vulnerable location in the body.

Patellofemoral arthroplasty is an attractive option for the treatment of debilitating isolated patellofemoral arthritis and diffuse grade IV patellofemoral chondromalacia. The traditional surgical alternatives, long recognized for their shortcomings, are losing ground to this increasingly more popular treatment method. The pain relief resulting from patellofemoral arthroplasty is superior to other patellofemoral-specific treatment strategies, like patellectomy and tibial tubercle-unloading procedures. Additionally, enthusiasm for patellofemoral arthroplasty continues to increase as newer designs with improved features emerge, surgical indications are refined, and techniques and instrumentation improve. Furthermore, revision to total knee arthroplasty is not compromised after patellofemoral arthroplasty, making it a reasonable intermediate procedure in young and middle-aged patients with isolated patellofemoral arthritis.[2]

Selecting an implant of sound design is important to optimize the ultimate results, but surgical technique, namely accurate implantation of the components and balancing the soft tissues, is paramount. The success of minimally invasive approaches to total and unicompartmental arthroplasty is creating a natural intrigue with their potential application to patellofemoral arthroplasty. It is important, however, since this is a newer treatment alternative for most, to first familiarize

oneself with the nuances of the procedure through a more extensile approach, and then reduce the incision length and arthrotomy more gradually. Until recently, designs and implant systems either required completely free-handed techniques, or instruments were so large and bulky that extensile incisions and arthrotomies were necessary (Fig. 38.1). Now, particularly because of refinements in instrumentation, instrumented minimally invasive surgery (MIS) will soon be possible in patellofemoral arthroplasty.

This chapter discusses the role of patellofemoral arthroplasty for isolated patellofemoral arthritis, describes a free-handed, uninstrumented MIS surgical technique, and reviews the results of the procedure (independent of surgical approach).

Indications and Contraindications

Patellofemoral arthroplasty may be considered in the treatment algorithm for patients with localized patellofemoral osteoarthrosis, posttraumatic arthrosis, or grade IV bipolar (involving both the patella and the trochlea) or unipolar (involving either the patella or the trochlea) chondromalacia. Oftentimes, patients will have had arthroscopic procedures and these do not preclude the opportunity for patellofemoral arthroplasty. Microfracture, autologous osteochondral transplantation plug(s), and autologous chondrocyte implantation, generally less effective in the patellofemoral compartment than in the weight bearing surfaces of the femoral condyles, are not uncommon prior to patellofemoral arthroplasty and if unsuccessful can easily be converted to patellofemoral arthroplasty.

Patellofemoral arthroplasty is appropriate for patellofemoral arthritis in the presence of dysplasia; it should be avoided in patients with considerable patellar maltracking or malalignment, unless these conditions are corrected preoperatively. Slight patellar tilt or trochlear dysplasia are not contraindications for this procedure; in such cases, a lateral retinacular release may be necessary at the time of arthroplasty.[3–5] Excessive Q angles should be corrected with tibial tubercle realignment before or simultaneous with patellofemoral arthroplasty. The procedure should not be performed in patients with inflammatory arthritis or chondrocalcinosis involving the menisci or tibiofemoral

J.H. Lonner (✉)
Knee Replacement Surgery, Orthopaedic Research, Booth Bartolozzi Balderston Orthopaedics, Pennsylvania Hospital, 800 Spruce Street, Philadelphia PA, 19107, USA
e-mail: lonnerj@pahosp.com

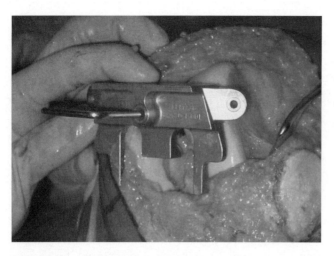

Fig. 38.1 Intraoperative photograph showing large cutting block that precludes MIS surgery

chondral surfaces, nor should it be offered to patients with diffuse pain.[3–5] Tibiofemoral arthrosis or diffuse grade III or IV chondromalacia are contraindications to patellofemoral arthroplasty, although recent work suggests a role for concomitant patellofemoral arthroplasty and biological condylar resurfacing when there is focal grade IV chondromalacia on the weight-bearing condylar surfaces noted in addition to the patellofemoral wear.[6]

Patellofemoral arthroplasty is most effective in patients younger than 55 years with isolated anterior compartment arthrosis,[3–5] and less predictable in elderly patients, who may be better off undergoing total knee arthroplasty.

Clinical Evaluation

History and Physical Examination

Taking a detailed history and performing a thorough physical examination of the patient under consideration for patellofemoral arthroplasty are necessary to corroborate that the pain is, in fact, localized to the anterior compartment of the knee, and that it emanates from the patellofemoral chondral surfaces and not from soft tissues (such as the patellar or quadriceps tendons or pes anserinus bursa) or other remote sites, such as the lumbar spine or ipsilateral hip.

The history should include questions about whether there was prior trauma to the knee and its mechanism, patellar dislocation, or other patellofemoral "problems." A history of recurrent atraumatic patellar dislocations may suggest considerable malalignment. Pain should characteristically be directly retropatellar, or just lateral or medial to the patella, and is often exacerbated by activities that load the patellofemoral compartment, such as stair climbing and descent,

ambulating on hills, standing from a seated position, sitting with the knee flexed, and squatting. Medial or lateral joint line pain is not typical in truly isolated patellofemoral arthritis. A description of anterior crepitus is common.

The physical examination will often note pain on patella inhibition and compression, patellofemoral crepitus, and retropatellar knee pain with active and passive flexion. The presence of medial or lateral tibiofemoral joint line tenderness is concerning for the possibility of more diffuse chondral disease (even in the presence of relatively normal radiographs) and may be a contraindication to patellofemoral arthroplasty. Patellar tracking and the Q angle must be assessed, since maltracking and malalignment can compromise the outcomes after patellofemoral arthroplasty.

Imaging Studies

Standing anteroposterior and midflexion posteroanterior radiographs are critical to identify tibiofemoral arthritis. Supine coronal radiographs should be avoided because they may underestimate the presence or extent of tibiofemoral disease. Mild squaring-off of the femoral condyles and even small marginal osteophytes are not contraindications for patellofemoral arthroplasty if the patient has no tibiofemoral pain with activities and on physical exam, and if there is less than grade III chondral degeneration noted during arthroscopy or arthrotomy. Lateral X-ray results occasionally demonstrate patellofemoral osteophytes, but, particularly in younger patients, there may be minimal radiographic joint space narrowing and osteophytes; the lateral X-ray results can show whether there is patella alta or baja. Axial radiographs will demonstrate the position of the patella within the trochlear groove and the extent of arthritis, but, again, the radiographs may underestimate the extent of patellofemoral cartilage damage. Often subchondral sclerosis and facet "flattening" may be the only radiographic clues (Fig. 38.2a–c). Computed tomographic (CT) scan and magnetic resonance imaging (MRI) are not necessary for evaluating patellofemoral arthrosis, although they can be useful for evaluating patellar instability. Photographs from prior arthroscopic treatment will provide valuable information regarding the extent of anterior compartment arthrosis and the status of the tibiofemoral articular cartilage and menisci.

Surgical Technique

Like all procedures, first developing a comfort level and proficiency with a procedure and instrumentation through a more extensile arthrotomy is absolutely paramount before

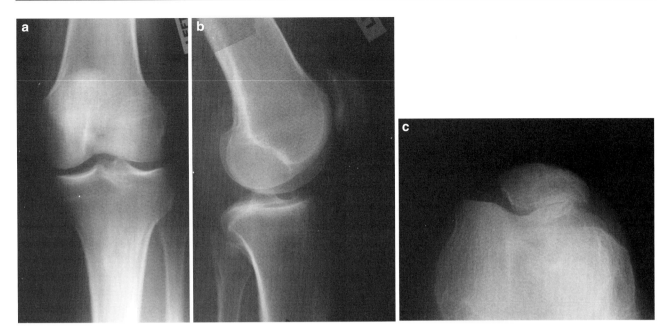

Fig. 38.2 (**a–c**) Weight-bearing anteroposterior, lateral, and axial radiographs demonstrating advanced patellofemoral arthrosis with sparing of the tibiofemoral compartments

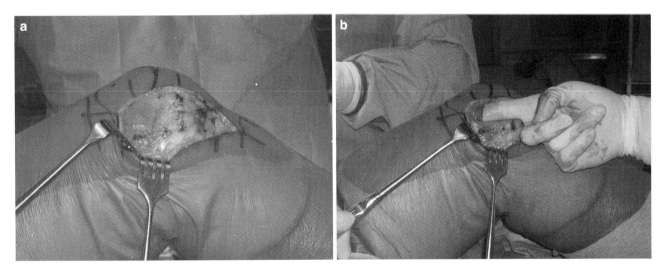

Fig. 38.3 (**a**, **b**) Defining the inferior border of the vastus medialis for a mini-subvastus approach

transitioning to minimally invasive techniques. Patellofemoral arthroplasty is unforgiving; errors in alignment and soft tissue balancing can be deleterious to the outcomes. To be clear, no surgeon should struggle with a minimally invasive approach at the expense of ensuring that the critical tenets of patellofemoral arthroplasty are fulfilled – namely, component alignment, soft tissue balance, and implant fixation. Additionally, even at present, instrumentation for patellofemoral arthroplasty has not been MIS compatible. Cutting blocks, when available, are bulky and cannot be used through less invasive arthrotomies (Fig. 38.1). Free-hand techniques, however, are more amenable to MIS approaches, but carry a risk of inaccuracy. Newer designs and instrumentation will be intended to be MIS compatible (Zimmer, Warsaw, IN).

Considering the need for exposure and preparation of the anterior surface of the femur and retropatellar surface, a small or moderate incision in the quadriceps tendon or muscle is often prudent, even advisable, particularly initially in one's early clinical experience with this procedure. As one's comfort level expands and proficiency with this procedure improves, and as newer instrumentation becomes available, a mini-subvastus approach can be utilized (Figs. 38.3a, b). The natural evolution in terms of surgical arthrotomy for patellofemoral arthrotomy should involve a standard medial parapatellar arthrotomy, followed by a standard midvastus or subvastus approach, and thereafter, mini arthrotomies can be pursued. I commonly use the gamut of MIS arthrotomies, including a mini-parapatellar limited quadriceps incision, mini-midvastus, or mini-subvastus, depending on several features, such as the presence of patellar tilt or subluxation (in those cases I try to use the mini-subvastus or mini-midvastus approach to optimize patellar tracking), the level of insertion of the vastus medialis obliquus on the patella (with distal insertions, I prefer a mini-parapatellar quadriceps incision or mini-midvastus incision), and the bulk and mass of the quadriceps muscle.

At its most conservative, the skin incision will extend from the medial aspect of the proximal edge of the patella (in flexion) to the joint line, just medial and proximal to the tibial tubercle (Fig. 38.4). As with all MIS approaches to the knee, the incision should be lengthened liberally if the skin edges become compromised or if there is unnecessary technical difficulty arising from the small incision or arthrotomy. During arthrotomy, it is essential to avoid cutting normal articular cartilage or the menisci. Before proceeding with patellofemoral arthroplasty, carefully inspect the entire joint to make sure the tibiofemoral compartments are free of gross cartilage degeneration.

With MIS approaches to patellofemoral arthroplasty, most of the procedure is performed with the knee either in full extension (patellar preparation), or alternating between 0 and 60° of flexion for trochlear preparation, depending on whether the anterior or posterior part of the trochlea is being prepared, respectively. My preference is to resect the articular surface of the patella before preparing the trochlea to help develop the anterior space of the knee and allow better exposure of the trochlea. This is generally done with the patella subluxed laterally and everted to 90° (Fig. 38.5a–c). The objective of patella resurfacing is to restore the original patella thickness and medialize the component. The exposed cut surface of the lateral patella that is not covered by the patellar prosthesis should be beveled or removed to reduce the potentially painful articulation on the trochlear prosthesis

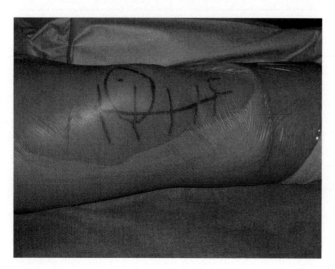

Fig. 38.4 Typical skin incision for MIS approach to patellofemoral arthroplasty

in extension and midflexion, and on the lateral femoral condyle in deeper flexion (Fig. 38.6). It is important to avoid crushing the cut surface of the patella with the lateral retractor during trochlear preparation.

The trochlear component should be externally rotated parallel to the epicondylar axis to enhance patellar tracking;[4,5] however, when using MIS approaches, palpation of the epicondyles is very difficult, if not impossible. Using a line perpendicular to the anteroposterior axis (which is a line drawn from the nadir of the trochlear sulcus anteriorly to the apex of the intercondylar notch posteriorly) is an accurate surrogate and my guide for component rotation in all cases unless there is profound trochlear dysplasia (Fig. 38.7). A cut is made flush with the anterior surface of the femoral cortex, avoiding notching (Figs. 38.8 and 38.9). The trochlear component should maximize coverage of the trochlea, without extending beyond the medial-lateral femoral margins anteriorly, encroaching on the weight-bearing surfaces of the tibiofemoral articulations, or overhanging into the intercondylar notch. Osteophytes bordering the intercondylar notch should be removed so that they do not impinge on the resurfaced patella or the tibia. The trochlear component edges should be flush with or recessed approximately 1 mm from the adjacent articular cartilage at the transition with the femoral condyles (Figs. 38.10 and 38.11).

Assessment of patellar tracking is performed with the trial components in place, paying particular attention to identify patellar tilt, subluxation, or catching of the components (Fig. 38.12). Patellar tilt and mild subluxation usually can be addressed successfully by performing a lateral retinacular release, unless there is considerable extensor mechanism malalignment, which needs to be addressed with either tibial tubercle realignment (if the Q angle is excessive) or a proximal realignment. In the absence of a high Q angle, patellar maltracking with the trials in place is concerning for the possibility of component malposition. The components can then be cemented into place, removing extruded cement while it cures (Fig. 38.13a–c).

Postoperative Management

Various strategies for preemptive analgesia can be employed and these are outlined elsewhere in this book. The postoperative care is similar to that after total knee arthroplasty. A continuous passive motion machine is started immediately after surgery and used for the duration of hospitalization (average, 2 or 3 days); however, while this may accelerate early return of flexion, it is not as critical as active patient participation in flexion exercises. Isometrics and range of motion exercises are started immediately. Immediate full weight bearing is permitted, initially with the support of crutches and then a

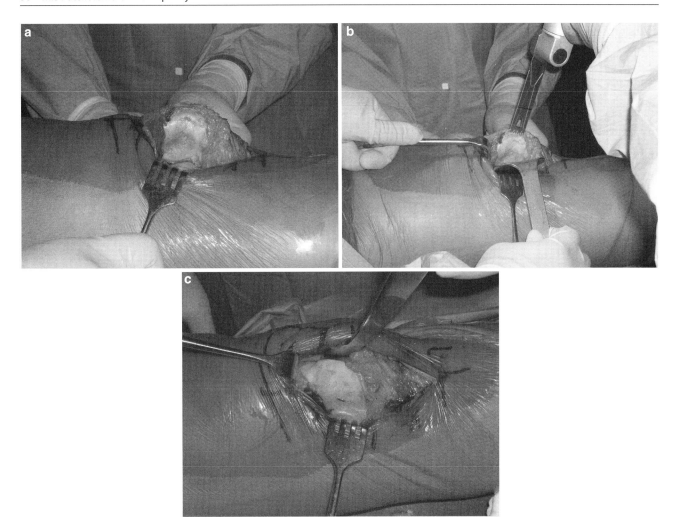

Fig. 38.5 (a–c) Patella preparation is performed with knee fully extended, and patella held vertically for resection. After patella preparation, exposure of the anterior femur is easier with the patella effectively reduced in size and subluxed laterally

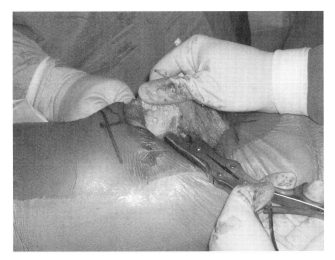

Fig. 38.6 The uncapped lateral edge of the patella is removed to prevent bony impingement

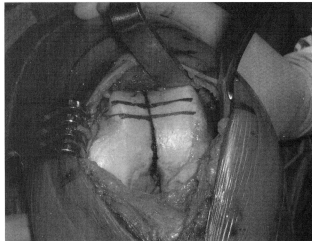

Fig. 38.7 It is the anteroposterior axis and lines perpendicular to it are marked

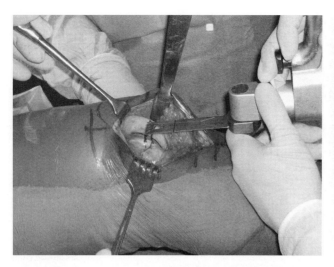

Fig. 38.8 Free-hand resection of the anterior femur, perpendicular to the anteroposterior axis, performed with the knee in approximately 30° of flexion

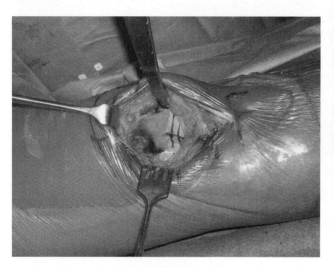

Fig. 38.9 Trochlear resection flush with the anterior surface of the femur

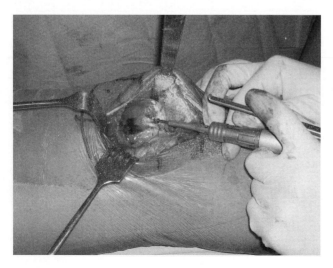

Fig. 38.10 Free-hand preparation of the distal bed for the trochlear component

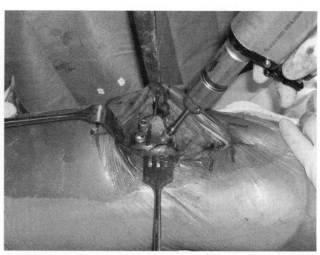

Fig. 38.11 Edges of the template are flush with the transition with the femoral condyles

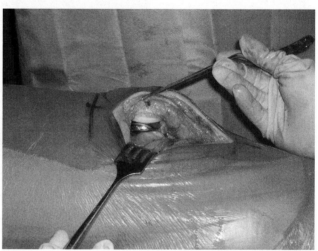

Fig. 38.12 Patellar tracking is assessed

cane until there is adequate recovery of quadriceps strength. Depending on the extent of preoperative quadriceps atrophy, adequate recovery of quadriceps strength can vary; in some extreme cases, it can take 6 months or longer. Thromboembolism prophylaxis is utilized for 4–6 weeks. Twenty-four hours of perioperative antibiotics is advisable, and appropriate precautions regarding antibiotic prophylaxis for dental procedures or other interventions should follow standard recommendations of the American Academy of Orthopaedic Surgeons.[7]

Clinical Results

No studies have focused specifically on how the surgical approach impacts the results of patellofemoral arthroplasty. Nonetheless, drawing from the experience of MIS total knee

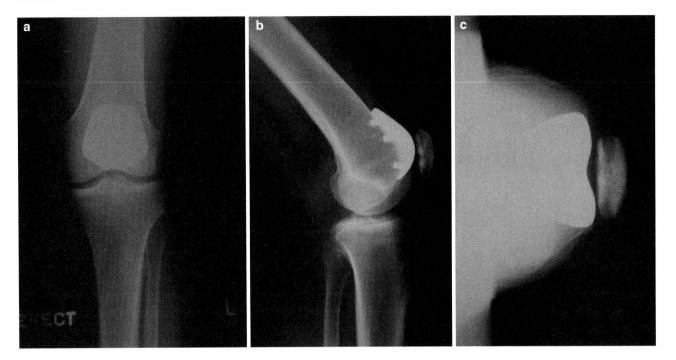

Fig. 38.13 (a–c) Postoperative radiographs

arthroplasty (TKA) and unicondylar knee arthroplasty (UKA), we would expect that the various MIS techniques will accelerate recovery and reduce early postoperative pain compared with standard approaches in patellofemoral arthroplasty.

Most series have reported good and excellent results in roughly 85% of cases, although there have been some outliers (Table 38.1), and the reported results in some series have been confounded by the inclusion of patients who had simultaneous patellofemoral and unicompartmental tibiofemoral arthroplasty or osteotomy, without distinguishing the clinical outcomes of those with isolated patellofemoral arthroplasties.[8–12]

Results of patellofemoral arthroplasty are impacted by component position and alignment, soft tissue balance, quadriceps angle and patellofemoral alignment, implant design, indications for surgery, and presence and extent of tibiofemoral chondromalacia. Patellar instability, resulting from soft tissue imbalance, component malposition, or extensor mechanism malalignment, is the major source of short- and mid-term failure in patellofemoral arthroplasty, and a prominent source of residual anterior knee pain.[5,9,13–16] Improved designs have substantially reduced the incidence of patellofemoral complications.[5] In the reported series, less than 1% of patellofemoral arthroplasties have failed because of loosening or wear of the implants, although follow-up in most series has averaged less than 7 years.[5,9,13–18]

One series has highlighted how the trochlear shape can impact the incidence of patellofemoral-related problems.[5] Thirty consecutive patellofemoral arthroplasties using one implant were compared with 25 consecutive patellofemoral arthroplasties using another implant. Patients in each group had similar demographic characteristics and preoperative range of motion and knee scores. Overall, satisfactory results were noted in 84% of patellofemoral arthroplasties, but the incidence of patellofemoral dysfunction, including subluxation, catching, and substantial pain was 17% with one prosthesis and less than 4% with the other.[5]

The design characteristics of the trochlear component geometry that impact patellofemoral mechanics and tracking include the sagittal radius of curvature, the proximal extension of the anterior flange, the width of the anterior surface of the implant, and the degree of constraint. Trochlear implants with an obtuse radius of curvature commonly end up malpositioned, with the implant flexed and offset proximally from the anterior surface of the femoral cortex or extending off the bone in the intercondylar region of the knee. The former problem can often result in patellar snapping, clunking, and maltracking in the initial 30° of flexion as the distal edge of the patellar implant transitions over the proximal edge of the trochlear implant; the latter causes similar mechanical symptoms as the knee is extended from deep flexion, if the proximal edge of the patellar component impinges on the prominent distal edge of the trochlear component, or it can cause impingement on the tibia or anterior cruciate ligament (ACL) in extension. Trochlear components with a radius of curvature that mates better with most distal femora have a lesser tendency to have these problems. Broader anterior surfaces allow more freedom for patellar excursion and tracking than narrow implants. Implants with

Table 38.1 Clinical results of MIS patellofemoral arthroplasty

Series	Implant	Number of PFAs	Age (years)	Diagnosis	Duration of follow-up	Percentage of good/excellent results
Blazina[13]	Richards types I and II	57	39 (range, 19–81)	NA	2 years (range, 8–42 months)	NA
Arciero[8]	Richards type II (14); CFS-Wright (11)	25	62 (range, 33–86)	OA (25); malalignment or instability (14)	5.3 years (range, 3–9 years)	85%
Cartier[9]	Richards types II and III	72	65 (range, 23–89)	Dysplasia/grade IV chondromalacia (29); PTA (3); chondrocalcinosis (5)	4 years (range, 2–12 years)	85%
Argenson[10]	Autocentric	66	57 (range, 19–82)	Dysplasia or dislocation (22); PTA (20); OA (24)	5.5 years (range, 2–10 years)	84%
Krajca[20]	Richards types I and II	16	64 (range, 42–84)	Primary OA (10); PTA (2); recurrent dislocation (1)	5.8 years (range, 2–18 years)	88%
Tauro[15]	Lubinus	62	66 (range, 50–87)	PTA (2); primary OA (74)	7.5 years (range 5–10 years)	45%
deWinter[14]	Richards type II	26	59 (range, 22–90)	Primary OA (17); malalignment (8); PTA (1)	11 years (range, 1–20 years)	76%
Ackroyd[16]	Avon	306	62 (range, 34–92)	Primary OA (187); dysplasia (12); subluxation/dislocation (41); PTA (5); other (4)	NA	NA
Smith[17]	Lubinus	45	72 (range, 42–86)	Primary OA (44); PTA (1)	4 years (range, 6 months–7.5 years)	69%
Kooijman[19]	Richards type II	45	50 (range, 20–77)	OA (45)	17 years (range, 15–21 years)	86%
Lonner[5]	Lubinus	30	38 (range, 34–51)	Primary OA (26); PTA (4); s/p tibial tubercle realignment (10)	4 years (range, 2–6 years)	84%
Lonner[5]	Avon trochlea; Nexgen patella	25	44 (range, 28–59)	Primary OA (25); s/p realignment (2)	6 months (range, 1 month–1 year)	96%
Merchant[18]	LCS	15	49 (range, 30–81)	Subluxation/dislocation (12); PTA (2); osteochondritis dissecans (1)	3.75 years (range, 2.25–5.5 years)	93%
Cartier[11]	Richards types II and III	59	60 (range, 36–81)	Primary OA (7); dysplasia/subluxation (41); grade IV chondromalacia (4); PTA (3); s/p realignment (13)	10 years (range, 6–16 years)	72%

PFA patellofemoral arthroplasty, *NA* not applicable, *OA* osteoarthritis, *PTA* posttraumatic arthrosis, *LCS* low contact stress

limited proximal extension on the anterior femur are susceptible to patellar prosthesis snapping and catching at the point of transition from the anterior femoral surface in full extension onto the trochlear prosthesis at approximately 10–30° of flexion; again, this is hastened if the trochlear component is flexed or offset anteriorly. This is less likely with a trochlear prosthesis that extends further proximally because the patellar component articulates entirely with the trochlear component in extension. The problem may be compounded by the degree of trochlear constraint (manifest by the sulcus angle) in the axial plane. An increased degree of freedom within the trochlear groove is more forgiving in extension than those implants with lower sulcus angles, and less likely to cause wear of the patellar component or dynamic tracking problems.

Several studies have reported the long-term outcomes after patellofemoral arthroplasty. Tibiofemoral degeneration is the most common reason for late "failures" of patellofemoral arthroplasties. Kooijman et al. reported that after a mean of 15.6 years (range, 10–21 years), 25% of 45 patellofemoral arthroplasties required secondary surgeries for progressive tibiofemoral arthritis, including two proximal tibial osteotomies and ten total knee arthroplasties. In other words, 75%

of the implants studied were still functioning well into the second decade after implantation. Of those patellofemoral implants that were still in place, 86% were considered successful.[19] Cartier et al. performed an analysis of 59 patellofemoral arthroplasties from a cohort of 117.[11] A large number had previous or concomitant surgeries, including tibial tubercle realignment procedures or soft tissue surgeries for patellofemoral maltracking. At a mean follow-up of 10 years (range, 6–16 years), 47 knees were pain free and 12 had moderate or severe pain, primarily from tibiofemoral arthritis, but also from lateral patellar subluxation in one knee and trochlear soft tissue impingement in two. Stair ambulation was considered normal in 91% of patients. Knee Society knee scores were excellent (77%), fair (14%), and poor (9%); Knee Society function scores were excellent (72%), fair (19%), and poor (9%). No cases of patellar or trochlear loosening were identified. Patellar snapping was observed in 2% of cases. Substantial polyethylene wear was present in one case and moderate in five. There were two drop off points on the survivorship curve: an early one, at 3 years, related to inappropriate indications for the surgery, and another in the ninth and tenth years, corresponding to the development of symptomatic tibiofemoral osteoarthritis. The authors reported a survivorship of 75% at 11 years.[11]

In a series by Argenson et al., the best results were achieved after patellofemoral arthroplasty performed for posttraumatic arthritis (resulting from patella fracture) or patellar subluxation and dysplasia, and the least favorable in those with primary degenerative arthritis. The development of tibiofemoral arthritis was the most frequent cause of failure.[10,12] In 66 patellofemoral arthroplasties in patients with a mean age of 57 years (range, 21–82 years) and with a mean follow-up of 16.2 years (range, 12–20 years), there were 14 concomitant procedures, including 9 tibiofemoral osteotomies and 5 distal patellar realignments. While most patients had substantial and sustained pain relief, 25% were revised to TKA for tibiofemoral arthritis (at a mean of 7.3 years after patellofemoral arthroplasty), 14% for aseptic trochlear component loosening (at a mean of 4.5 years after patellofemoral arthroplasty; 38% of which were uncemented designs), and 5% for infection. In those who retained their patellofemoral arthroplasties at most recent follow-up, Knee Society knee and function scores improved from 53 (range, 43–70) to 79 (range, 60–100), and 41 (range, 10–80) to 81 (range, 40–100), respectively. The cumulative 16-year survivorship was 58%, but the authors continue to advocate for the procedure as an intermediate stage before TKA in the absence of tibiofemoral arthritis or coronal plane malalignment.[12]

Summary

Patellofemoral arthroplasty can be an effective treatment for patellofemoral arthritis resulting from primary osteoarthrosis, dysplasia, or posttraumatic arthrosis in young and middle-aged patients who have normal patellofemoral alignment without considerable maltracking or subluxation. The results of patellofemoral arthroplasty can be impacted by the design features of the trochlear component, the presence of uncorrectable patellar instability or malalignment, implant malposition (potentially hastened by particular designs), and tibiofemoral chondromalacia or arthrosis. Evolving designs can reduce considerably the incidence of patellofemoral dysfunction, leaving progressive tibiofemoral arthritis as the primary potential failure mechanisms of patellofemoral arthroplasty. If the early patellofemoral failures are excluded, the short-term failure rate is reduced.

As with all knee procedures, MIS techniques can be applied to patellofemoral arthroplasty, but only after the procedure has been performed effectively and accurately through more extensile approaches. MIS may be particularly effective in this patient cohort, which often has significant preoperative quadriceps atrophy associated with the advanced patellofemoral arthritis, because minimizing trauma to the extensor mechanism during surgery may reduce the problem of iatrogenic postoperative quadriceps atrophy. The surgical approach should not negatively impact the outcome of patellofemoral arthroplasty because of errors in implantation or fixation, but instead should facilitate the experience, accelerate the recovery, and not impact the long-term outcomes. That is what MIS, done well, can provide.

References

1. McAlindon RE, Snow S, Cooper C, Dieppe PA. Radiographic patterns of osteoarthritis of the knee joint in the community: The importance of the patellofemoral joint. Ann Rheum Dis 51:844–849, 1992
2. Lonner JH, Jasko JG, Booth RE. Revision of a failed patellofemoral arthroplasty to a total knee arthroplasty. J Bone Joint Surg (Am) 88:2337–2342, 2006
3. Lonner JH. Patellofemoral arthroplasty. Semin Arthroplasty 11:234–240, 2000
4. Lonner JH. Patellofemoral arthroplasty. Tech Knee Surg 2:144–152, 2003
5. Lonner JH. Patellofemoral arthroplasty: pros, cons, design considerations. Clin Orthop Relat Res (428):158–165, 2004
6. Lonner JH, Mehta S, Jasko JG. Ipsilateral patellofemoral arthroplasty and femoral condylar osteochondral autograft. J Arthroplasty (in press)
7. Hanssen AD, Osmon DR, Nelson CL. Prevention of deep periprosthetic joint infection. J Bone Joint Surg 78A:458–471, 1996
8. Arciero R, Toomey H: Patellofemoral arthroplasty. A three to nine year follow-up study. Clin Orthop Relat Res (236):60–71, 1988
9. Cartier P, Sanouiller JL, Grelsamer R. Patellofemoral arthroplasty. J Arthroplasty 5:49–55, 1990
10. Argenson JN, Guillaume JM, Aubaniac JM. Is there a place for patellofemoral arthroplasty? Clin Orthop Relat Res (321):162–167, 1995
11. Cartier P, Sanouiller JL, Khefacha A. Long-term results with the first patellofemoral prosthesis. Clin Orthop Relat Res (436):47–54, 2005
12. Argenson JN, Flecher X, Parratte S, Aubaniac JM. Patellofemoral arthroplasty: an update. Clin Orthop Relat Res (440):50–53, 2005
13. Blazina ME, Fox JM, Del Pizzo W, Broukhim B, Ivey FM. Patellofemoral replacement. Clin Orthop Relat Res (144):98–102, 1979
14. deWinter WE, Feith R, van Loon CJ. The Richards type II patellofemoral arthroplasty: 26 cases followed for 1–20 years. Acta Orthop Scand 72:487–490, 2001
15. Tauro B, Ackroyd CE, Newman JH, Shah NA. The Lubinus patellofemoral arthroplasty. A five to ten year prospective study. J Bone Joint Surg 83B:696–701, 2001
16. Ackroyd CE, Newman JH, Webb JM, Eldridge JDJ. The Avon patellofemoral arthroplasty. Two to five year results. Proceedings of the American Academy of Orthopaedic Surgeons. New Orleans, LA, February 2003
17. Smith AM, Peckett WRC, Butler-Manuel PA, Venu KM, d'Arey JC. Treatment of patellofemoral arthritis using the Lubinus patellofemoral arthroplasty. A retrospective review. Knee 9:27–30, 2002
18. Merchant AC. Early results with a total patellofemoral joint replacement arthroplasty prosthesis. J Arthroplasty 19:829–836, 2004
19. Kooijman HJ, Driessen APPM, van Horn JR. Long-term results of patellofemoral arthroplasty. J Bone Joint Surg 85-B:836–840, 2003
20. Krajca-Radcliffe JB, Coker TP. Patellofemoral arthroplasty. A 2 to 18 year follow up study. Clin Orthop Relat Res 330:143–151, 1996

Chapter 39
Round Table Discussion of MIS Total Knee Arthroplasty

Giles R. Scuderi: Minimally invasive surgery (MIS) total knee arthroplasty (TKA) has become a popular surgical technique. Surgeons are performing the procedure through smaller skin incisions and limited arthrotomies. Yet this is not a technique for all patients and all surgeons. I have gathered a group of experts who will share their experiences. This panel includes Mark Pagnano, Steven Haas, Richard Berger, Alfred Tria, and Peter Bonutti. Let us start this discussion with patient selection. My own experience has shown that MIS total knee arthroplasty is more applicable to a thin female patient with minimal deformity and good preoperative range of motion. Mark, is there a way of determining who is an ideal candidate for a minimally invasive total knee?

Mark Pagnano: For me, the easiest patient is the elderly female patient who is slightly overweight and has moderate angular deformity with a reasonable range of motion. The patient who is somewhat overweight has some of that adipose tissue distributed within the muscle and that makes the muscle and soft tissue easier to mobilize during surgery. A moderate angular deformity allows me to do some ligamentous release early in the case and that facilitates both visualization and the placement of retractors under direct vision to protect the collateral ligaments and the posterior neurovascular structures. A small flexion contracture is of no concern but I like to see at least 100° of flexion. Finally, the ideal patient will require tibial and femoral implant sizes that are in the small to medium size range; the largest implants often have a dimension that approaches the skin incision size and those are difficult to maneuver into place gracefully.

Giles R. Scuderi: With these variables in mind, Steve, which patients are better served with a more traditional approach?

Steve Haas: It is generally much easier to perform MIS total knee arthroplasty in female patients. Large muscular men are the most difficult. Men that are heavier than 210 to 220 pounds will receive a larger arthrotomy extending into the quadriceps and a proportionally larger incision. It is, however, not necessary to evert the patella in these patients. Patients with severe deformities, particularly flexion contractures greater than 20–25°, require a standard medial parapatellar

arthrotomy. Additionally stiff patients with flexion less than 80° are not good candidates for MIS TKA.

Giles R. Scuderi: Rich, Mark, and Steve have nicely outlined the patient factors, but what about the surgeon? What are your recommendations for the surgeons beginning to learn this technique?

Rich Berger: Fortunately, minimally invasive total knee arthroplasty is perfectly situated for a stepwise approach to getting started. I recommend first becoming accustomed to your minimally invasive instruments using whichever approach you are most familiar with – for most, this will be a medial parapatellar approach. Then as you become facile with the instruments, begin making a smaller arthrotomy without everting the patella. If you experience difficulty during a case, simply extend the arthrotomy. With more experience, further reduce the arthrotomy, eventually using a capsular-only incision (such as Fred will address) or explore other approaches such as a mini-midvastus or mini-subvastus, both of which give you more exposure than the capsular-only incision. However, both the mini-midvastus and mini-subvastus will self-extend as you stress the tissues; thus, becoming closer to standard midvastus or standard subvastus. While this self-extension aids exposure, it is difficult to control and will hinder the patient's recovery. I believe that the limited medial parapatellar and the capsular only incision does not self-extend; you control exactly how much exposure you have by the length of the capsular incision.

Giles R. Scuderi: Rich, I agree with you, that is why I prefer a limited medial parapatellar arthrotomy that can be lengthened as I need to gain exposure. It is an approach with which I have a great deal of experience and feel the most comfortable and believe can be used in the vast majority of case. I also use instruments that are similar to my traditional instruments. The only difference is that they are reduced in size to fit within the limited arthrotomy. Now, Fred, in contrast, you are doing your cases through a quadriceps-sparing approach. How difficult is that? Did you not have to change the way you do the knee?

Fred Tria: Initially, we had to change the surgical technique quite a bit to accommodate the limited incision for the quadriceps-sparing approach. We resected the patellar surface

G.R. Scuderi and A.J. Tria (eds.), *Minimally Invasive Surgery in Orthopedics*,
DOI 10.1007/978-0-387-76608-9_39, © Springer Science + Business Media, LLC 2010

first to increase the overall space in the knee. The distal femoral cut was made from the medial side, as was the proximal tibial resection. The finishing blocks for the femur were cut down and the alignment guides for the block were unique. We used grasping hooks on the posterior aspect of the tibial finishing plates and modified the tibial tray by decreasing the length of the intramedullary stem. Our accuracy was not as good as the standard arthrotomy and we looked for a way to simplify the technique. Now, we use instruments that are more standard that allow the surgeon to cut from anterior to posterior with improved methods for exposure of the bone. We hope that these efforts in combination with navigation will show improvement in the overall accuracy.

Giles R. Scuderi: But, Fred, you know it is a struggle to work through such a very limited arthrotomy and I am always concerned that I may not be seeing enough of the joint to accurately cut the femur and tibia and then get the implant into the joint. Yet, I do applaud your efforts to preserve the integrity of the extensor mechanism. Steve, you use the midvastus approach, do you think it has an advantage over the quadriceps-sparing technique?

Steve Haas: I believe it is easier to gain adequate exposure to the knee with a mini-midvastus approach compared with a "quad-sparing" technique. There is much better access to the front of the femur, and it is much easier to expose the tibia for tibial component insertion. The "quad-sparing" technique also stretches the vastus medialis oblique (VMO) to a much greater extent than the mini-midvastus approach. Clinical results have been equal for the two approaches and I believe the learning curve for the mini-midvastus approach is shorter.

Giles R. Scuderi: Steve, I must say, when I have used the midvastus approach, the fascia would split proximally until the vastus medialis is released. Have you seen this and do you think it really matters?

Steve Haas: While the VMO can spread further in a midvastus approach, our studies indicate that there is less spreading with the "mini" midvastus approach than the standard midvastus approach. Even with a standard midvastus approach with greater splitting, long-term studies have shown no persistent electromyogram (EMG) changes from this muscle splitting. Generally, the amount splitting with the mini-midvastus approach is less than 2–3 cm, and we have not seen any splits greater than 4 cm.

Giles R. Scuderi: Peter, You also use a midvastus approach, do you have anything to add?

Peter Bonutti: I have used numerous approaches, the mini-midvastus, mini-subvastus, and direct lateral approach. We have performed prospective randomized studies using isokinetic analysis and have found that the mini-midvastus approach seems to have less pain postoperatively, but via isokinetic analysis, the subvastus approach appears to have faster quadriceps recovery. Currently, we have evolved from a mini-midvastus and now use a modified mini-subvastus approach and are able to do this universally in all patients. Using the mini-subvastus approach, it is more difficult to obtain exposure to the femur, but use of this approach may allow slightly faster recovery of the quadriceps mechanism.

Giles R. Scuderi: Peter, I agree and think those are great comments. But I do need to ask Mark, with the subvastus approach, you suggest that this is also a quadriceps-sparing approach, do you think it is easier then the midvastus approach? I have found that if the vastus medialis is bulky it is difficult to laterally sublux the patella.

Mark Pagnano: The key to visualization with the MIS subvastus approach is to understand that the inferior fibers of the vastus medialis insert at a 50° angle relative to the long axis of the femur and that the tendon of the vastus medialis extends all the way to the mid-pole of the patella. One must preserve that triangular extension of tendon down to the mid-pole because that is where your retractor will rest when you translate the patella into the lateral gutter. By preserving that triangular portion of tendon above the mid-pole you gain two benefits: first the retractor will always rest against a robust edge of tendon so the vastus medialis itself does not become cut, split, or macerated and, second, you gain a geometric advantage so that as you retract the patella laterally the vastus medialis drapes over the anterior femur and not over the distal femur. When surgeons have difficulty translating the patella laterally it is usually because the approach into the subvastus space has been made too horizontally. A horizontal capsular incision often results in a portion of the medial patellofemoral ligament remaining intact and that will limit lateral translation of the patella. Instead, the capsular incision into the subvastus interval should parallel the inferior fibers of the vastus medialis and that means extending it at a 50° angle from inferior to superior starting at the mid-pole of the patella.

Giles R. Scuderi: Rich, it seems as I listen to my colleagues, the real issue is whether the extensor mechanism is partially released or not and the whether or not the patella is laterally subluxed. Does it really matter and is there a significant difference in the clinical outcome?

Rich Berger: Ideally, there should be little difference in the approaches if all approaches used very small instruments, did not evert the patella under tension, did not stress the surrounding tissues, and did not dislocate the knee. Any approach, done mostly in extension with minimal retraction of the extensor mechanism, should similarly benefit our patients. Unfortunately, most instruments are still too large and are used in flexion where retractors stress the extensor mechanism. In this environment, I believe that the approaches that can self-extend (midvastus and subvastus) do extend significantly under the skin. Therefore, the mini-midvastus and mini-subvastus become close to a standard midvastus and standard subvastus; these standard approaches clearly are not as beneficial to the patients as approaches that limit the detachment of the quadriceps.

I have done a significant number of cases with each of the four approaches discussed here. I believe, the more exposure you have, the more trauma you are causing for the patient; therefore, some struggle is necessary to help your patient recover more rapidly postoperatively. From this experience, I have found that the capsularly only exposure cause the least trauma and has the best results in my hands; however, it also affords the least exposure.

Giles R. Scuderi: I would like to summarize the surgical approaches by saying that there are several techniques to perform the total knee arthroplasty, but it is important that the surgeon know his options and not compromise the clinical outcome. In choosing an approach, there must be an option for extending the exposure in order to gain full exposure. Now let's talk about specific issues and start with correction of fixed deformities. Fred, how do you manage the fixed varus deformity with a MIS quadriceps-sparing technique?

Fred Tria: The varus deformity is not difficult to correct with the quadriceps-sparing approach because the dissection is right in the operative field on the medial side of the knee. The deep medial collateral ligament is always released as part of the initial exposure and the posterior medial capsule is also visible with this early release. The insertion of the semimembranosus can be exposed by externally rotating the tibia with the knee flexed approximately 30°. The superficial medial collateral ligament can be released by using a periosteal elevator beneath the ligament and tapping the instrument distally along the medial tibial metaphysis beneath the insertion of the pes anserinus. If a complete release is necessary, the insertion of the medial collateral over the fascia of the soleus muscle can be released with a knife along the posterior medial corner of the tibia. A complete release with the quadriceps-sparing approach would rarely be necessary because we limit the indications to a knee that has no more than 10° of fixed varus deformity. The valgus deformity can be approached with the quadriceps-sparing technique but it is slightly more difficult because all of the releases are on the opposite side of the joint. We do not recommend a lateral arthrotomy approach for the quadriceps-sparing technique.

Giles R. Scuderi: I would agree. Mark, what about a fixed valgus deformity, can you correct it with the subvastus approach and, if so, how do you do it?

Mark Pagnano: The fixed valgus deformity is easily addressed with the subvastus technique. A contemporary method of dealing with the valgus deformity is the so-called pie-crusting or multiple puncture technique. The initial bone cuts are performed on the tibia and the femur and a spacer block is placed in the extension space and then in the flexion space to determine the relative symmetry between the medial and lateral sides. When the lateral side is found to be tight, we bring the leg into extension and place a laminar spreader

in the extension space. In full extension, there is no substantial tension on the extensor mechanism and the subvastus approach affords an unobstructed view of the extension space. The surgeon can then palpate the lateral-sided structures including the iliotibial band, the fibular collateral ligament, the posterolateral capsule, and the popliteus tendon and decide which structure is tightest. Multiple small punctures are then made in the tightest structure with a #15 blade, using care not to plunge toward the peroneal nerve in the posterolateral corner. If release of one structure is insufficient to balance the lateral side with the medial side, then sequential multiple puncture release of the next tightest structure is carried out until a rectangular extension gap is obtained.

Giles R. Scuderi: Peter, how about ligament balancing with the suspended leg technique? Do you find it easier to correct deformities and do you have any comments about femoral component rotation?

Peter Bonutti: The suspended leg technique has a number of advantages. The procedure is performed with the knee primarily in flexion, distracted by gravity. This may enhance exposure to the distal femur. One needs to use caution on femoral rotation with the suspended leg approach as the extremity may be rotated with use of the retractors because the extremity is free to rotate. Gravity for distraction can enhance exposure and, by applying torsional stress and variably flexing and extending the joint with the surgeon in a seated position, it can enhance exposure to the joint and may assist in true ligament balancing.

Giles R. Scuderi: I think all of you have clearing reinforced the point that the surgical principles have not changed with the MIS approaches. I do find however that the placement of the components is sometimes difficult and, for that reason, I put the tibia in first, followed by the femoral component, and then the tibial polyethylene. If I am unable to sublux the tibia forward, I insert the tibial polyethylene in mid flexion, approximately 60–70°. This is easy with a front-loading tibial tray. Fred, how do you do it with the quadriceps-sparing approach?

Fred Tria: We also insert the tibial tray first and prefer the MIS type tibia with a more limited intramedullary stem. Initially, we were inserting the tray into the knee with the knee in almost full extension. Now, with more experience in the exposure, we have been able to sublux the tibia forward in approximately 80° of flexion and place the tray on the top of the cut surface. This permits more accurate tray placement and easier cement removal. The components are cemented with separately mixed batches to allow time for each step. The femur is inserted with a holder attached to it and with the knee flexed approximately 70°. The polyethylene is inserted with the knee flexed approximately 30° with the front-loading design. The patella does not have to be resurfaced but we do so in all of our cases. This is performed as the last step, with the knee in full extension, using some of the remaining cement from the femoral prosthesis.

Giles R. Scuderi: As you all are aware, I prefer a posterior stabilized implant for all my cases and find it easier to perform a minimally invasive approach with this implant design because once you release the anterior cruciate ligament (ACL) and posterior cruciate ligament (PCL), both the flexion and extension gaps open up and it is easier to manipulate the knee and insert the components and balance the knee. Rich, how about with a cruciate-retaining knee design, do you find a difference?

Rich Berger: I have used both cruciate-retaining and cruciate-substituting designs in MIS total knee approaches; I see no clear advantage of one design over the other for minimally invasive approaches. I have found that retaining the cruciate ligament makes the exposure slightly more difficult and the bone cuts slightly harder to make. However, without a femoral box and without a keel on the tibial component (a four-peg tibial design), component placement is slightly easier in a cruciate-retaining design. Conversely, in the cruciate-substituting designs, the exposure is slightly better when the PCL is released and the bone cuts are easier to make, however, as you mentioned above, final component placement is harder due to the femoral box and the tibial keel. (The advent of the mini keel tibial component and the modular tibial component has made component placement in a cruciate-substituting designs easier, but still more difficult than a cruciate-retaining design.) Since there is no clear advantage of one design over the other, I would stronger recommend that the surgeon stay with the design they are most familiar with when moving to minimally invasive total knee techniques.

Giles R. Scuderi: How about cement versus cementless fixation? Rich, aren't you doing cementless knees?

Rich Berger: Even in large standard incisions, removing all the excess cement is difficult. Retained cement, acting as a third body, is one of the most significant causes of wear in our retrieval study of well-functioning total knees. Smaller incisions make it more difficult to properly cement components and remove excess cement. Therefore, I believe that the use of cementless knees will increase in the near future, just as cementless fixation for total hips has evolved to be the major form of fixation. Personally, I do many hybrid total knees (cementless femoral fixation). I believe that as cementless fixation improves, especially with trabecular metal, that I will do more cementless femoral and tibial fixation. I am not sure if I will ever feel comfortable using cementless patella fixation.

Giles R. Scuderi: With the evolution of MIS TKA, came improved clinical pathways, especially pain management. I am now using preemptive analgesics, regional blocks, and improved postoperative pain management techniques, which, along with a team approach with rehabilitation and nursing, has improved patient satisfaction and reduced the length of stay. Mark, I know that you have a specific pain management protocol. Can you share with us your experience?

Mark Pagnano: We have found that effective postoperative pain management markedly improves patient satisfaction, decreases hospital stays, and facilitates discharge to home instead of to rehabilitation or nursing centers. The emphasis has been to use a comprehensive multimodal approach and to be preemptive. By using multiple modalities, you can often stay below the threshold for side effects and, by staying ahead of the pain, these patients end up using less opioid medication. The focus of our approach is to eliminate the use of parenteral opioid medication altogether. Preoperatively patients are given a COX-II anti-inflammatory, acetaminophen, and a sustained-release oral opioid. Intraoperatively, patients have a femoral nerve block done and an indwelling catheter is left for the first two nights after surgery. Patients also have a single shot sciatic nerve block because the femoral block alone fails to address posterior knee pain after surgery. A short-acting spinal anesthetic and intravenous sedation is used during the total knee surgery. Postoperatively patients are given medication on a schedule in an effort to stay ahead of the pain: a sustained-release oral opioid (OxyContin) is given twice daily for the first 2 days, acetaminophen is given three times daily, Celebrex is given twice daily and oxycodone is available on an as-needed basis for breakthrough pain. Patients can ambulate toe-touch weightbearing on day 1 even with the femoral nerve catheter in place. Thus, physical therapy does not need to be delayed, but patients can not put full weight on the leg until the femoral nerve catheter has been pulled. With this protocol, the pain scores on a verbal analog scale routinely are zero to two throughout the entire 2- or 3-day hospitalization and patients are discharged on acetaminophen, the COX-II anti-inflammatory, and a short-acting oral opioid.

Giles R. Scuderi: Rich, I am fascinated that you are now able to perform MIS total knee arthroplasty as an ambulatory procedure? How do you do it?

Rich Berger: Outpatient total knee replacement is a comprehensive approach to the patient. This includes the surgery, perioperative anesthesia and pain management, preoperative patient education, and rapid rehabilitation protocols. Clearly, starting with a minimally invasive surgical technique, done without detecting or cutting into the quadriceps is imperative. I do the procedure mostly in extension, without patella eversion, with little tension on the surrounding tissues. This technique allows less perioperative anesthesia and pain medications. The combination of less soft tissue injury with less medication allows patients to ambulate with only a cane or no assistive device within a few hours after the procedure in most patients. With little pain and little functional deficits, most of my patients choose to go home the day of surgery. My perioperative pathways and pain management protocol is similar to what Mark discussed above. However, without releasing the vastus off the intramuscular septum, without dislocating the knee, and without stressing the extensor mechanism, almost all of my capsular-only incision total knee replacement patients go home the day of surgery.

Giles R. Scuderi: Peter, how about deep vein thrombosis (DVT) prophylaxis and anticoagulation with a rapid recovery protocol? What is your current practice?

Peter Bonutti: I think anticoagulation is an important issue. Many surgeons who use rapid recovery do not use postoperative anticoagulation. In our limited study, we have found a substantive difference between those patients who utilize anticoagulation (Coumadin, Lovenox, Heparin) versus those patients who use aspirin and pulsatile stockings. The patients who use aspirin and pulsatile stockings clearly recover faster and have less postoperative pain, so this may be an important adjunct factor. The faster recovery and immediate range of motion (ROM) and weightbearing may decrease the risk for DVT and this needs to be evaluated because clearly there is a substantial difference in recovery between these two groups.

Giles R. Scuderi: Well, I want to thank all of you for sharing with me your tips and pearls in performing MIS total knee arthroplasty. This has been a very insightful and enlightening discussion. While the surgical technique has drifted toward smaller incisions and limited arthrotomies, the well-established principles of total knee arthroplasty have not changed. Adequate exposure is needed to appropriately correct deformities and balance the knee, restore alignment, and secure component fixation. These principles must not be compromised in favor of a smaller incision. It also appears that it is not the surgical technique alone, but the newer clinical pathways that have influenced clinical outcomes.

Section IV
The Foot and Ankle

Chapter 40
Percutaneous Repair of Acute Rupture of the Achilles Tendon

Jonathan Young, Murali K. Sayana, and Nicola Maffulli

The Achilles tendon is the strongest tendon in the human body, with a tensile strength on the order of 50–100 N/mm^2.[1] Despite this, the Achilles tendon is the most commonly ruptured tendon in the human body.[2,3] Rupture commonly occurs in middle-aged men who play sports occasionally. There is possibly a link with a sedentary lifestyle.[3] The aetiopathogenesis of Achilles tendon ruptures is still unknown, but histological evidence of degeneration is relatively common.[2]

Anatomy

The tendinous portions of the gastrocnemius and soleus muscles merge to form the Achilles tendon.[2] The gastrocnemius tendon emerges as a broad aponeurosis at the distal margin of the muscle bellies, whereas the soleus tendon begins as a band proximally on the posterior surface of the soleus muscle. Distally, the Achilles tendon becomes progressively rounded in cross section until approximately 4 cm from its calcaneus insertion, where it flattens out prior to inserting into the proximal calcaneal tuberosity.[4]

The calcaneal insertion is specialised. It is composed of an attachment of the tendon, a layer of hyaline cartilage, and an area of bone not covered by periosteum. There is a subcutaneous bursa between the tendon and the skin and a retrocalcaneal bursa between the tendon and the calcaneus.[5]

Diagnosis

There is often a history of an audible snap at the back of the heel followed by pain and an inability to weight bear on the affected side. A palpable gap is often present (Fig. 40.1). The diagnosis is also aided with the Simmonds and Matles clinical tests.[6,7] For the Simmonds test, the examiner gently squeezes the patient's calf muscles with the palm of the examiner's hand. If the Achilles tendon is intact, the ankle plantarflexes (Fig. 40.2). If the Achilles tendon is torn, the ankle remains still, or plantarflexes minimally (Fig. 40.3). The Matles' test involves asking patients to lie prone, and to flex both knees to 90°. If the injured foot falls into neutral or dorsiflexion, a ruptured Achilles tendon is diagnosed (Fig. 40.4).

Both tests are performed on the injured and uninjured sides for comparison. If there is uncertainty about the diagnosis, imaging can be considered, although it is not routine in our practice, because the imaging does not add to the management of the injury. Ultrasound[8] or magnetic resonance imaging (MRI) scans[9] help confirm the diagnosis. Ultrasonography will reveal an acoustic vacuum between the tendon edges. Magnetic resonance imaging will reveal generalised high signal intensity on T2-weighted images. On T1-weighted images, the rupture will appear as a disruption of the signal within the tendon substance.

Management

The management options of acute ruptures of the Achilles tendon can be divided into two broad categories: conservative or operative. Operative methods can be divided into open or percutaneous techniques. There is still ongoing debate regarding what type of management is best.[2] This depends on the patient' condition, age, and level of fitness.

Conservative Management

Wallace et al.[10] reported excellent results with conservative management using a hard cast for 1 month before switching

J. Young, N. Maffulli (✉), and M.K. Sayana
Queen Mary University of London, Centre for Sports and Exercise Medicine, Barts and the London School of Medicine and Dentistry, Mile End Hospital, 275 Bancroft Road, London E1 4DG, UK
e-mail: n.maffulli@qmul.ac.uk

G.R. Scuderi and A.J. Tria (eds.), *Minimally Invasive Surgery in Orthopedics*,
DOI 10.1007/978-0-387-76608-9_40, © Springer Science+Business Media, LLC 2010

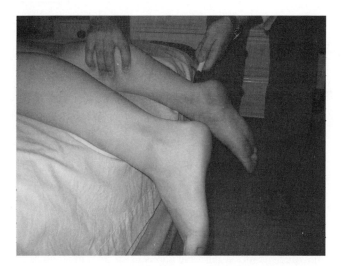

Fig. 40.1 Simmond's test: plantar flexion of the left foot with an intact Achilleser

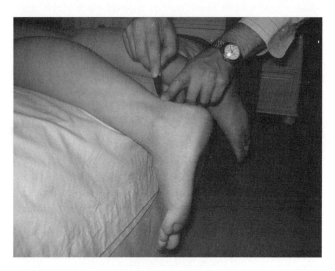

Fig. 40.2 Palpable gap, illustrated with finger

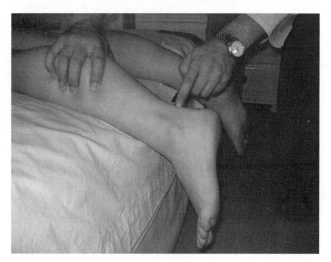

Fig. 40.3 Simmond's test: no plantar flexion on calf squeeze of the right foot due to a ruptured Achilles tendon

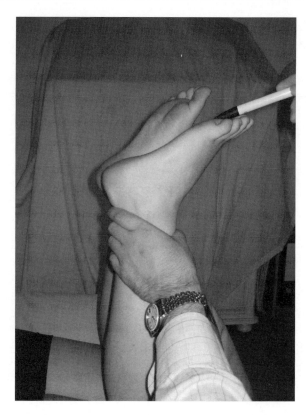

Fig. 40.4 Matles test, showing a ruptured right Achilles tendon

conservative management of rupture. Lo et al.[16] reported an overall re-rupture rate of 2.8% for operatively managed and 11.7% for non-operatively managed patients ($P < 0.001$).

Open Repair

Surgical management significantly reduces the risk of Achilles tendon re-rupture, but can increase the risk of infection when compared with conservative management.[17] Arner and Lindholm[18] reported a 24% complication rate in 86 operative repairs including one death from pulmonary embolism. Lo et al.[16] reported that open repair induces 20 times more minor to moderate complications than conservative management, but there were no significant differences between open surgical and conservative management regarding major complications.

Open repair can be performed in a variety of ways using simple end to end repairs (Bunnell/Kessler), or more complex techniques with fascial reinforcement or tendon grafts.[19,20] There is no evidence that, in fresh ruptures, one suture method is superior to others. There is some evidence that primary augmentation with local reinforcement or tendon grafts prolongs operating times, and induces a greater rate of complications. There is no significant evidence to support more complex primary repairs in acute Achilles tendon ruptures.[21] The results of open repair vary markedly.[18,22] These differences are likely to be multifactorial, and may well result from subtle variations in technique, degree of experience of the operating surgeon, the type of suture material used, and the location of incision.

Percutaneous Repair

Percutaneous repair[23] is a compromise between open surgery and conservative management. The aim of this procedure is to provide a better functional outcome than conservative treatment, with a similar functional outcome to that of open repair. Percutaneous repair also aims to decrease the problems of wound healing and skin breakdown associated with open repair. The early reports outlined an increased risk of re-rupture and of damage to the sural nerve, a potential downside to the procedure. Ma and Griffith[23] pioneered the technique with an excellent success rate with no re-ruptures and two minor complications. Some studies have demonstrated that the rate of re-rupture after percutaneous repair is higher than that after open operative procedures,[24,25] although these studies are now dated, and do not compare like with like.

More recent studies comparing open and percutaneous repair show that the two repair techniques produce similar outcomes. For example, Lim et al.[26] advocate percutaneous repair when comparing it with open techniques, concluding that percutaneous repair had a lower infection rate and was more cosmetically acceptable. The functional results comparing the open technique with the percutaneous technique showed no significant difference. Cretnik at al.[27] further expanded on the benefits of percutaneous repair and the controversy regarding the optimal treatment of fresh total Achilles tendon ruptures. A cohort study compared the results of percutaneous and open Achilles tendon repair. The results of 132 consecutive patients with acute complete Achilles tendon rupture who were operated on exclusively with modified percutaneous repair under local anaesthesia and followed up for at least 2 years were compared with the results of 105 consecutive patients who underwent open repair under general or spinal anesthesia in the same period. There were significantly fewer major complications in the group of percutaneous repairs in comparison with the group of open repairs ($P = 0.03$), and a lower total number of complications ($P = 0.013$). The study did report slightly more re-ruptures and sural nerve complications following percutaneous repairs, but no statistically significant difference. Functional assessment with the American Orthopaedic Foot and Ankle Society scale and the Holz score did not show any statistically significant difference.

Several percutaneous repair techniques have been described.[23,28–31] Ma and Griffith[23] described a technique of percutaneous repair of the Achilles tendon using six stab incisions over the tendon in 18 patients. The suture was passed through the stab incisions, and crisscrossed through the tendon. They reported one incidence of sensory disturbance and one patient with sural nerve entrapment.

Webb and Bannister[28] described a percutaneous technique that reduced the potential risk to the sural nerve by placing the proximal of the incisions to the medial side, away from the sural nerve. McClelland and Maffulli[31] described a percutaneous technique of repair of ruptured Achilles tendons similar to that described by Webb and Bannister,[28] but using a Kessler-type suture. We now perform percutaneous repair of Achilles tendon rupture using a minimally invasive procedure with five small incisions, four of which are 1-cm long, and the fifth, 2-cm long.

Pre-operative Planning

Once the diagnosis is made, the patient needs a full assessment regarding their general health and co-morbidities, their pre-operative functional status should also be noted.

The affected limb should be examined with regard to skin quality and also neurovascular status. Particular attention should be made to the possible pre-operative involvement of the sural nerve. Appropriate blood tests, electrocardiography (ECG) and chest X-ray (CXR) may also be required if the patient has a relevant co-morbidity. Deep vein thrombosis (DVT) prophylaxis may be necessary. An equinus backslab may be used pre-operatively for comfort. Once assessed and surgically worked up for the operating theatre, the patient will require valid written consent, ideally obtained by the operating surgeon. Sural nerve damage, re-rupture, infection, and impaired function should be discussed with the patient.

Operative Technique

Local anaesthetic infiltration is used. A 50:50 mixture of 20 ml of 1% lignocaine hydrochloride (Antigen Pharmaceuticals Ltd, Roscrea, Ireland) and 5 mg/ml of Chirocaine (Abbot Laboratories Ltd, Berkshire, England) is instilled into an area of between 8 and 10 cm around the ruptured Achilles tendon. The patient is placed prone, and a pillow is placed beneath the anterior aspect of the ankles to allow the feet to hang free. The operating table is angled down 20° cranially to reduce venous pooling in the feet and ankles.

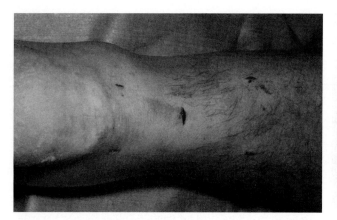

Fig. 40.5 The five stab incisions over the ruptured Achilles tendon

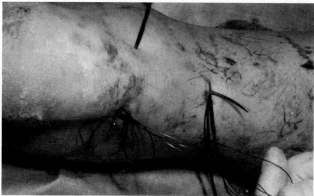

Fig. 40.6 Needle reintroduced into the medial distal stab incision through a different entry point in the tendon and passed longitudinally and proximally through the tendon, directed towards the middle incision and out through the ruptured tendon end

The affected leg is prepped. A calf tourniquet is used and inflated to 250 mmHg.

Five stab incisions are made over the Achilles tendon (Fig. 40.5). The first is directly over the palpable defect, and is approximately 2 cm in a transverse direction. A small piece of tendon from the rupture site is removed and sent for histological examination. The other incisions are approximately 4 cm proximal and 4 cm distal to the first incision. The proximal incisions are vertical 1-cm stab incisions on the medial and lateral aspect of the Achilles tendon. We advocate blunt dissection with a small haemostat directly onto the Achilles tendon, and therefore avoid damaging the sural nerve, which crosses the lateral border of the Achilles tendon approximately 10 cm proximal to its insertion into the calcaneus.[32]

A small haemostat is used to free the tendon sheath from the overlying subcutaneous tissue. A 1 Maxon (Tyco Healthcare UK Ltd) double-strand suture on a long curved needle is passed transversely through the lateral distal stab incision passing through the substance of the tendon and out through the medial distal stab incision. The needle is then reintroduced into the medial distal stab incision through a different entry point in the tendon and passed longitudinally and proximally through the tendon, to lock the tendon, and is directed towards the middle incision and out through the ruptured tendon end (Fig. 40.6).

The suture that is still protruding from the lateral distal stab incision is re-threaded onto the needle and reintroduced via the lateral distal stab incision into the tendon substance. It is passed longitudinally and proximally through the tendon to exit from the middle incision (Fig. 40.7). Traction is applied to the suture to ensure a satisfactory grip within the tendon (Fig. 40.8). If the suture pulls through, the procedure is repeated. The same procedure is carried out for the proximal half of the ruptured tendon. The sutures are then tied with the ankle in maximum plantar flexion (Fig. 40.9). The transverse skin wound is closed with subcuticular 3/0 Biosyn (Tyco Healthcare UK Ltd) sutures. The longitudinal stab wounds are juxtaposed, and closed with Steri-Strips. A non-adherent

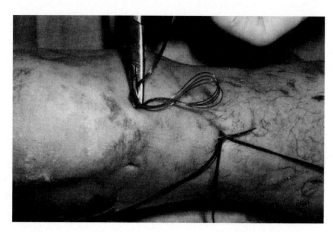

Fig. 40.7 The suture protruding from the lateral distal stab incision is re-threaded onto the needle and reintroduced via the lateral distal stab incision into the tendon substance. It is passed longitudinally and proximally through the tendon to exit from the middle incision

dressing is applied. A full Plaster of Paris cast is applied in the operating theatre with the ankle in maximum equinus. The cast is split on both the medial and lateral sides to allow for swelling (Fig. 40.10).

Complications

Haematomas can lead to infection and wound breakdown especially in light of the tenuous blood supply to the Achilles tendon.[31] This is very infrequent given the small incisions used. Sural nerve damage can cause altered dermatomal sensation or a painful neuroma. Patients can experience anaesthesia of the lateral aspect of the foot, and some report difficulty with shoes as a result of this.[33] This can be avoided with blunt dissection directly onto the Achilles tendon using a blunt haemostat. The placement of the skin incision is such,

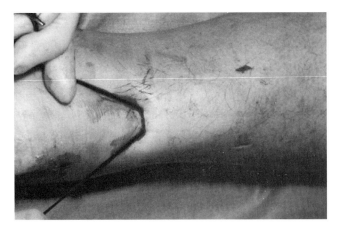

Fig. 40.8 Traction is applied to the suture to ensure a satisfactory grip within the tendon

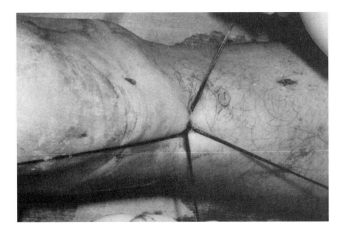

Fig. 40.9 The sutures are tied with the ankle in maximum plantar flexion

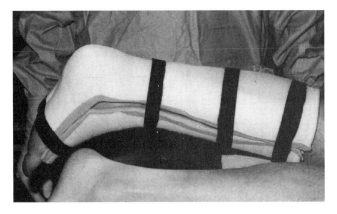

Fig. 40.10 A full plaster of Paris cast is applied in the operating theatre with the ankle in maximum equinus. The cast is split on both the medial and lateral sides to allow for swelling

however, that the sutures are distant from the sural nerve. The tenuous blood supply of the Achilles tendon increases the chance of wound infection. This is a recognised complication of the open approach, and is reduced with percutaneous techniques.[26,31]

Re-rupture is a documented complication.[24,25] The use of modern suture materials with a number of intra-tendinous threads comparable to that used in open repairs minimises this complication. More recent studies comparing the two repair techniques show similar results, with no difference in re-rupture rate between percutaneous and open repair,[26] but a significantly higher rate of infective wound complications using open repair.[26] DVT should also be considered because the patient will be in a plaster cast. DVT should therefore be looked for when the patient is re-examined routinely out of the cast, and appropriate management administered if suspected.[33] Early post-operative rehabilitation aims to reduce this risk.

Post-operative Management

The operated leg is elevated immediately post-op. If the neurovascular status of the limb is acceptable, and after assessment by a physiotherapist making sure the patient is safe and the patient is comfortable in their cast, patients can be discharged. The full cast is retained for 2 weeks, and the patient is able to weight bear as comfort allows. During the period in the cast, patients are advised to perform gentle isometric contractions of the gastro-soleus complex, and elevate the limb when at rest.

At this time, patients are reviewed in outpatient clinic where the wounds are inspected. An anterior splint is worn with the foot plantarflexed for a further 4 weeks. During this period, patients are advised to mobilise partial weight bearing initially, increasing to weight bearing as able by 4 weeks. In addition, patients are encouraged to invert and evert the foot and to plantar flex it against resistance on a regular basis. The splint is then removed, and physiotherapy follow-up for gentle mobilisation is arranged. Light exercise can be started 2 weeks after cast removal. Patients should be fully weight bearing by that time.

References

1. Viidik A. Tensile strength properties of Achilles tendon systems in trained and untrained rabbits. Acta Orthop Scand 1962; 10: 261–272
2. Maffulli N. Rupture of the Achilles tendon. J Bone Joint Surg Am 1999; 81: 1019–1036

3. Jozsa L, Kvist M, Balint BJ, Reffy A, Jarvinen M, Lehto M, Barzo M. The role of recreational sport activity in Achilles tendon rupture. A clinical, pathoanatomical, and sociological study of 292 cases. Am J Sports Med 1989; 17(3): 338–343

4. Cummins EJ, Anson BJ, Carr BW, Wright RR. The structure of the calcaneal tendon (of Achilles) in relation to orthopaedic surgery. With additional observations on the planatris muscle. Surg Gynecol Obstet 1946; 83: 107–116

5. Rufai A, Ralphs JR, Benjamin M. Structure and histopathology of the insertional region of the human Achilles tendon. J Orthop Res 1995; 13(4): 585–593

6. Simmonds FA. The diagnosis of the ruptured Achilles tendon. Practitioner 1957; 179: 56–58

7. Matles AL. Rupture of the tendo Achilles. Another diagnostic test. Bull Hosp Joint Dis 1975; 36: 48–51

8. Maffulli N, Dymond NP, Capasso G. Ultrasonographic findings in subcutaneous rupture of Achilles tendon. J Sports Med Phys Fitness 1989; 29(4): 365–368

9. Kabbani YM, Mayer DP. Magnetic resonance imaging of tendon pathology about the foot and ankle. Part I. Achilles tendon. J Am Podiatr Med Ass 1993; 83: 418–420

10. Wallace RG, Traynor IE, Kernohan WG, Eames MH. Combined conservative and orthotic management of acute ruptures of the Achilles tendon. J Bone Joint Surg Am 2004; 86: 1198–1202

11. Persson A, Wredmark T. The treatment of total ruptures of the Achilles tendon by plaster immobilisation. Int Orthop 1979; 3: 149–152

12. Moller M, Movin T, Granhed H, Lind K, Faxen E, Karlsson J. Acute rupture of tendon Achillis. A prospective randomised study of comparison between surgical and non-surgical treatment. J Bone Joint Surg Br 2001; 83(6): 843–848

13. Bohnsack M, Ruhmann O, Kirsch L, Wirth CJ. Surgical shortening of the Achilles tendon for correction of elongation following healed conservatively treated Achilles tendon rupture. Z Orthop Ihre Grenzgeb 2000; 138: 501–505

14. Soma C, Mandelbaum B. Repair of acute Achilles tendon ruptures. Orthop Clin North Am 1976; 7: 241–246

15. Wong J, Barrass V, Maffulli N. Quantitative review of operative and nonoperative management of Achilles tendon ruptures. Am J Sports Med 2002; 30: 565–575

16. Lo IK, Kirkley A, Nonweiler B, Kumbhare DA. Operative versus nonoperative treatment of acute Achilles tendon ruptures: a quantitative review. Clin J Sport Med 1997; 7: 207–211

17. Bhandari M, Guyatt GH, Siddiqui F, Morrow F, Busse J, Leighton RK, Sprague S, Schemitsch EH. Treatment of acute Achilles tendon ruptures: a systematic overview and metaanalysis. Clin Orthop Relat Res 2002; Jul(400): 190–200

18. Arner O, Lindholm A. Subcutaneous rupture of the Achilles tendon. A study of 92 cases. Acta Chir Scand 1959; 116(239): 1–5

19. Bosworth D. Repair of defects in the tendo Achilles. J Bone Joint Surg Am 1956; 38: 111–114

20. Lynn T. Repair of torn Achilles tendon, using the plantaris tendon as a reinforcing membrane. J Bone Joint Surg Am 1966; 48: 268–272

21. Jessing P, Hansen E. Surgical treatment of 102 tendo Achilles ruptures – suture or tenoplasty? Acta Chir Scand 1975; 141: 370–377

22. Soldatis J, Goodfellow D, Wilber J. End to end operative repair of Achilles tendon rupture. Am J Sports Med 1997; 25: 90–95

23. Ma GWC, Griffith TG. Percutaneous repair of acute closed ruptures Achilles tendon. A new technique. Clin Orthop Relat Res 1977; Oct(128): 247–255

24. Aracil J, Lozano J, Torro V, Escriba I. Percutaneous suture of Achilles tendon ruptures. Foot Ankle 1992; 13: 350–351

25. Bradley J, Tibone J. Percutaneous and open surgical repairs of Achilles tendon ruptures. A comparitive study. Am J Sports Med 1990; 18: 188–195

26. Lim J, Dalal R, Waseem M. Percutaneous vs. open repair of the ruptured Achilles tendon – a prospective randomized controlled study. Foot Ankle Int 2001; 22(7): 559–568

27. Cretnik A, Kosanovic M, Smrkolj V. Percutaneous versus open repair of the ruptured Achilles tendon: a comparative study. Am J Sports Med 2005; 33(9): 1369–1379

28. Webb JM, Bannister GC. Percutaneous repair of the ruptured tendo Achillis. J Bone Joint Surg Br 1999; 81(5): 877–880

29. Gorschewsky O, Vogel U, Schweizer A, van Laar B. Percutaneous tenodesis of the Achilles tendon. A new surgical method for the treatment of acute Achilles tendon rupture through percutaneous tenodesis. Injury 1999; 30(5): 315–321

30. Cretnik A, Zlajpah L, Smrkolj V, Kosanovic M. The strength of percutaneous methods of repair of the Achilles tendon: a biomechanical study. Med Sci Sports Exerc 2000; 32(1): 16–20

31. McClelland D, Maffulli N. Percutaneous repair of ruptured Achilles tendon. J R Coll Surg Edinb 2002; 41: 613–618

32. Webb J, Moorjani N, Radford M. Anatomy of the sural nerve and its relation to the Achilles tendon. Foot Ankle Int 2000; 21(6): 475–477

33. Young JS, Kumta SM, Maffulli N. Achilles tendon rupture and tendinopathy: management of complications. Foot Ankle Clin 2005; 10(2): 371–382

Chapter 41
Endoscopic Gastrocnemius Recession

Amol Saxena and Christopher W. DiGiovanni

Percutaneous techniques are becoming popular for treating many musculoskeletal conditions. Those developed for endoscopic carpal tunnel and plantar fascial release are currently among the most common. The reported benefits of endoscopic surgery include smaller incisions and shorter postoperative recovery time.[1–3] Visualization with an endoscope may also decrease perioperative complications from scarring such as incisional irritation or neuritis, although the overall safety of these interventions has yet to be determined. An endoscopic means of gastrocnemius recession (EGR) has recently been popularized for correction of ankle equinus contracture as an alternative to formal open gastrocnemius release (OGR) or Achilles tendon lengthening.[4–21] The OGR remains today's gold standard for aponeurotic lengthening because of its proven record as a safe, rapid, and effective procedure. This open "slide," however, can involve a large unsightly incision, which is particularly unpopular with young women, and can be associated with sural nerve scarring and neuritis.[11,14, 15,19, 22] The EGR, an alternative percutaneous approach, has been sought in an effort to avoid those problems, but it has a significant learning curve, can be associated with poor visualization, and is somewhat instrument dependent.[14,17] In consideration of its potential advantages and drawbacks, the authors have tried over the last several years to develop a safe and reliable endoscopic technique for gastrocnemius recession.

Gastrocnemius recession has been used successfully for over a century to correct ankle contracture, originally described to treat neurologically impaired individuals.[16] More recent data suggesting the presence of isolated gastrocnemius tightness in otherwise healthy patients, however, has popularized more widespread use of OGR in the United States and Europe during the past decade. EGR was first introduced as a treatment alternative in 2002.[13, 21] Its purported benefits over the standard open means of gastrocnemius release included a smaller incision, a potentially faster recovery, and the versatility of being performed in any patient position. While its recent interest has emerged primarily in response to complications from the open technique, to date, its advantages remain promising but incompletely substantiated.[14]

Early results of the endoscopic procedure appear comparable to the open technique regarding improvement of ankle dorsiflexion.[5, 10–12, 14, 20] Using an endoscopic technique, Saxena and Widtfeldt obtained an average 15° immediate improvement in postoperative dorsiflexion, which remained at 12.6° after 1-year follow-up of 18 cases.[14] Pinney et al. reported an 18° dorsiflexion increase sustained 2 months after open Strayer procedure.[11] DiDomenico et al. reported their results on 31 procedures of EGR and noted an improvement of 18° with the knee extended.[5] Trevino et al. did not report the amount of dorsiflexion achieved with their endoscopic results, noting only "significant improvement in ankle dorsiflexion."[20] All three of these studies dealt with nonspastic equinus. A recent European study reported on 18 procedures on patients with cerebral palsy who exhibited neurological equinus.[12] These authors were also able to achieve total dorsiflexion improvement of almost 20 degree after using the endoscopic technique. Interestingly, despite available data, the amount of equinus correction actually required for gastrocnemius recession to be successful in impacting long-term outcome in these patients remains unknown. In fact, although many (including these authors) think that such equinus correction remedies varying pathologies of the foot, even the relationship between isolated gastrocnemius release and functional improvement remains obscure. For example, as of today, the mere definition of pathological equinus has only recently been more closely studied.

Historically, functional ankle joint dorsiflexion has been defined as 10° with the knee extended and more than 10° with the knee flexed (the Silverskiold maneuver).[23] Values below these have been somewhat arbitrarily defined as "equinus contracture." In 2002, DiGiovanni et al. studied ankle dorsiflexion in nonneurologically impaired populations of individuals

A. Saxena and C.W. DiGiovanni (✉)
Division of Foot and Ankle, Department of Orthopedic Surgery,
Brown University Medical School, Rhode Island Hospital, 1287 North
Main Street, Providence, RI, 02904 USA
e-mail: Christopher_Digiovanni@Brown.EDU

G.R. Scuderi and A.J. Tria (eds.), *Minimally Invasive Surgery in Orthopedics*,
DOI 10.1007/978-0-387-76608-9_41, © Springer Science+Business Media, LLC 2010

who were either asymptomatic controls or patients with symptomatic midfoot and/or forefoot complaints.[24] They concluded that 5° of ankle dorsiflexion with the knee extended and 10° with the knee flexed represented reasonably normal values, and suggested that values less than these should be considered evidence of gastrocnemius or Achilles contracture, respectively. They also found a statistically significant association between those individuals who met the criteria for gastrocnemius equinus and an increased incidence of painful midfoot and forefoot pathology. Another study contended that 0° of ankle dorsiflexion with the knee in extension could be "normal" in asymptomatic, adolescent athletes.[25] Based on this data, we consider patients candidates for gastrocnemius recession when their ankle dorsiflexion is less than 5° with the knee extended and they exhibit signs or symptoms of chronic foot overload or inflammation. Common examples would be posterior tibial tendon insufficiency, diabetic forefoot ulceration or Charcot arthropathy, stress fractures, metatarsalgia, Morton's foot deformity, plantar fasciitis, and insertional Achilles tendonitis, although we think this contracture may potentially play a role in many other biomechanical and functional pathologies of the foot as well. Alternative potential indications for performing an open or endoscopic gastrocnemius recession include patients with symptomatic ankle contracture or those who necessitate midfoot (Lisfranc) reconstruction/arthrodesis, calcaneal osteotomy for hindfoot realignment, or subtalar arthroereisis (Table 41.1). Whether performed openly or endoscopically, however, the procedure is not meant to take the place of an Achilles lengthening when indicated based on the Silverskiold test. Gastrocnemius recession should also be used cautiously in athletes.

The EGR procedure is typically performed supine under general anesthesia. It can also be performed prone in the event the patient requires such positioning during their foot/ankle surgery. Spinal or local anesthesia may be considered an option for patients who are not good candidates for or do not desire general anesthesia, but we have less experience with this method under such circumstances. Incision placement has been clarified by a recent anatomic study by Tashjian et al.[22] Ideal sites are determined by locating the inferior extension of the medial gastrocnemius muscle belly as well as identifying the midpole of the fibular shaft. These landmarks provide useful keys to optimal aponeurotic release. Knowledge of the neurovascular anatomy is mandatory, par-

ticularly the sural and saphenous structures. The great saphenous vein and the saphenous nerve should be anterior to a medially based incision, which is ideally placed in the midaxial line. This incision is made adjacent to edge of the medial gastrocnemius aponeurosis, typically 9–12 cm proximal to the medial malleolus, and is 1–1.5 cm long (Fig. 41.1). Once the superficial posterior compartment fascia is opened, a fascial elevator is used to create a pathway between subcutaneous fat and gastrocnemius fascia, in a medial to lateral direction. Care is taken to remain directly posterior to (on top of) the gastrocnemius aponeurosis, a characteristically glistening white structure. An endoscopic cannula with a blunt obturator is then placed through the medial incision and carefully advanced laterally. The obturator can then be removed for insertion of a 4.0-mm, 30° endoscope through the cannula. The gastrocnemius tendon (Fig. 41.2) is visual-

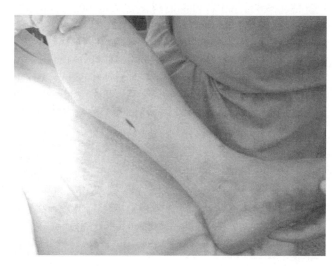

Fig. 41.1 Medial incision placement

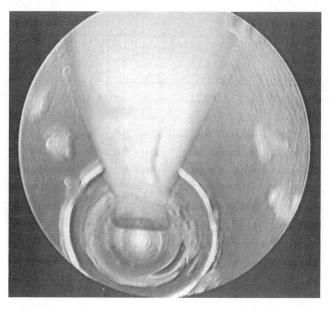

Fig. 41.2 Endoscopic view of gastrocnemius

Table 41.1 Indications for endoscopic gastrocnemius recession

1. Gastrocnemius equinus/tightness: (ankle dorsiflexion
   <5° with the knee in extension)
2. Nonspastic and nonbony deformity and
   Asymmetric posttraumatic symptomatic contracture and/or
   Calcaneal osteotomy and/or Hindfoot realignment and/or
   Subtalar arthroereisis and/or
   Midfoot arthrodesis and/or
   Noninfected forefoot ulcers/derangement

ized anteriorly, and the endoscope subsequently advanced toward the lateral aspect of the leg where the subcutaneous tissue appears yellow. The endoscope and cannula are rotated posteriorly and then retrograded back medially approximately 1 cm to locate the sural nerve. Pinney et al. found that the sural nerve can lay directly behind this aponeurosis less than 25% of the time, but is more often outside of the field of view, and equally common interior and exterior to the superficial posterior compartment fascia at this level. Regardless, care must be taken to ensure that the nerve does not exist between cannula and the site of aponeurotic release. Based on the findings of Tashjian et al., the sural nerve has been shown to course approximately 1.2 cm or 20% medial to the lateral gastrocnemius border at the myotendinous junction.[19] Their study did report one sural nerve transection with this EGR approach in the cadaveric setting, and the nerve was seen in only one third of the specimens evaluated endoscopically.[19, 22] Webb et al. also showed the sural nerve to cross the proximal portion of the Achilles tendon from the lateral side.[26] If possible, it is always advantageous to document that the nerve is located posterior to the cannula, and thereby protected by it (Fig. 41.3) Pinney et al. have also shown in their study on the Strayer technique that the nerve can often be adherent to the gastrocnemius aponeurosis.[11] Such situations may require modification or even abandonment of the endoscopic technique in lieu of a more formal, open procedure. Transillumination of the lateral aspect of the leg allows the surgeon to carefully make a cutdown incision over the cannula and insert a narrow-tipped suction device, which also helps avoid possible portal neuromas (Fig. 41.4). The use of suction improves visualization due to the moisture from the subcutaneous fat during transection of the gastrocnemius. Occasionally, serial swabbing with a cotton tip applicator is also helpful to clean the lens of the endoscope and its cannula.

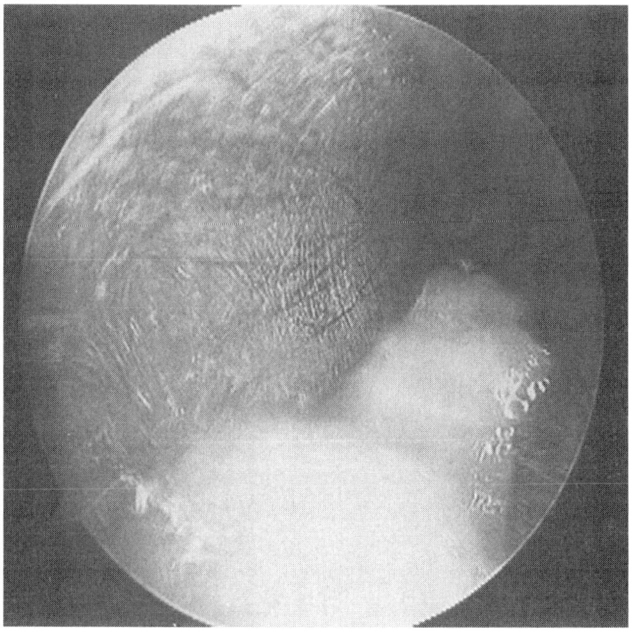

Once anatomy has been properly and safely defined, the endoscope is temporarily removed and a cannulated knife is introduced as part of the camera, stabilized over the endoscope (Fig. 41.5). This assembly is designed to transect the tendon while pushing the blade located forward in its position immediately ahead of the camera, and can be done through only the medial portal. Alternatively, a separate independent "hook-blade" can be used, which is useful in cases when the sural nerve or numerous venous structures are located in the vicinity of the proposed transection. This latter technique requires two portals and a separate knife blade/handle, which is pulled from the far end toward itself during transaction, using the camera to follow the release.

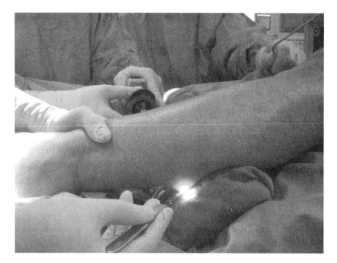

Fig. 41.4 Creation of lateral portal

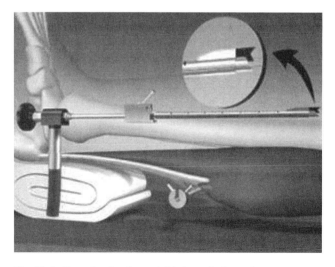

Fig. 41.3 Endoscopic view of sural nerve with the endoscope and cannula rotated posteriorly 180°

Fig. 41.5 Cannulated endoscopic blade applied to endoscope

We have identified no specific advantage with either technique, and in either case the foot must remain forcibly dorsiflexed to tension the thick gastrocnemius aponeurosis and permit clean transection. Clamping the medial and lateral margins of the aponeurosis through each portal with a Kocher clamp may also facilitate this process, but requires slightly larger incisions. This adjunct technique can be useful because the gastrocnemius rests more curvilinear rather than straight when viewed in the coronal plane. Thus, the straight, rigid endoscope is sometimes ineffective at releasing the very medial and lateral edges of the tendon as they course more anteriorly away from the endoscope/cannula. As the gastrocnemius is transected with either blade construct, the soleus muscle belly should become visible anteriorly (Fig. 41.6). Ideally, the fascia of the soleus is not violated. If this occurs, the resultant bleeding can obscure visualization. Although typically only superficial, however, unfortunately this is sometimes unavoidable, and under such circumstances suction from the lateral portal can be helpful. While this inadvertent violation of the soleus fascia/muscle has not been of any identifiable clinical consequence in our experience, it still represents a potential risk and undesirable pitfall of this procedure. If the neurovascular structures limit advancement of the cannulated knife, one can transect the aponeurosis from either portal with various endoscopic blades. The hook blade can be used from the lateral portal to complete the transection.

After complete transaction of the tendon, ankle dorsiflexion improvement should be noted of at least 10–15°. Anything short of this suggests either the need for an Achilles lengthening or incomplete resection of the gastrocnemius. Recent research by Barouk et al. suggests that most if not almost all of the dorsiflexion correction is obtained by release of the medial as opposed to the lateral gastrocnemius aponeurosis.[27] This is in keeping with our own observations. Once instruments are removed, the medial incision is explored for the plantaris tendon, which is then also transected. In our experience, leaving this tendon behind intact can result in medial-sided discomfort as a result of its bowstringing while under dorsiflexion tension. Surgical sites are thereafter irrigated and 5 mL of 0.5% bupivacaine are introduced into the portals. Incisions are closed with one or two 3-0 nylon sutures, which remain for 2 weeks postoperatively. Oral muscle relaxants, along with dorsiflexion night splinting, can be useful in the postoperative setting to maintain release and minimize muscle cramping. If EGR is performed as an isolated procedure, patients are maintained in a below-knee walking boot for 4–6 weeks, during the latter half of which, it is only required at night and patients are allowed ambulation as tolerated during waking hours. When more extensive foot or ankle procedures are concomitantly performed, they generally dictate postoperative immobilization and weightbearing status. During the first few months of recovery, self-massage of the transection region and portals is recommended. Physical therapy after surgery is also encouraged, and can be helpful to improve gait and decrease fibrosis. The ability to single-leg "heel-raise" can occur as soon 6 weeks post-EGR.[14]

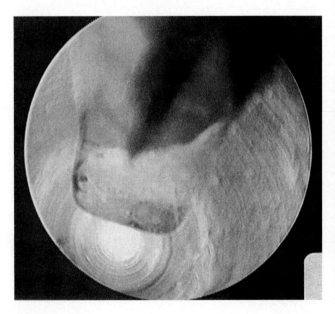

Fig. 41.6 Endoscopic view of gastrocnemius transection with soleus muscle above

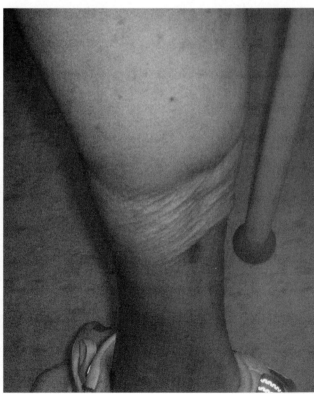

Fig. 41.7 "Tenting" or soleus adherence to subcutaneous tissue

Table 41.2 Other authors' results of endoscopic gastrocnemius recession

Author	Comment	Net improvement in ankle dorsiflexion	Nerve transection	Lateral dysesthesia	Hematoma	Calcaneal gait	Poor cosmesis
Tashjian et al.[19, 22]	Cadaveric	NS	1	NA	NA	NA	NA
Saxena and Widtfeldt[14]	18 cases	12.6°	None	3	NS	NS	1
Trevino et al.[20]	31 cases	NS	None	NS	NS	NS	NS
DiDomenico et al.[5]	31 cases	18°	None	NS	1	3	NS
Poul et al.[12]	18 cases with cerebral palsy	20°	NS	NS	0	NS	NS
Saxena and Widtfeldt[15]	54 cases	14.8°	None	6/54 (11%)	1	1	6/54 (11%)

NS not studied; *NA* not applicable

The EGR procedure represents an evolving percutaneous technique that has the potential to minimize postoperative scar formation and maximize recovery after gastrocnemius recession. Caution must be exercised in recommending this technique, however, because its long-term outcome and relative complication rate as compared with the traditional open technique remain unknown. The most common adverse event noted postoperatively with this approach appears to be transient lateral foot dysesthesia. In our experience, this is most likely due to traction neuritis of the sural nerve, which we have also seen with the open procedure after obtaining an acute increase in ankle dorsiflexion.[5, 15] However, this is typically a benign and self-limiting problem. Based on cadaveric experimentation, sural nerve laceration and/or incomplete gastrocnemius release may prove to be significant risks of this procedure as compared with the open approach, primarily due to impaired visualization. Other potential complications of EGR yet to be fully defined include hematoma, adherence/tenting, push-off weakness, and calcaneus deformity (Fig. 41.7). The procedure is also highly equipment dependent, requiring significantly greater amounts of instrumentation as compared with the standard release. Unfortunately, this equipment is often not otherwise required for most foot/ankle procedures that might be required at the time of gastrocnemius recession, and thus this need represents an added burden to both surgeon and operating room personnel. With experience, the total time required for the EGR approaches that for the OGR.

Experience with the EGR technique remains in its infancy. Few studies have been published on any advantages, disadvantages, or comparative results of EGR. While the procedure may hold promise in terms of minimizing incisional issues and maximizing recovery times after isolated gastrocnemius recession, its use should be considered cautiously, and more thorough evaluation is mandatory before EGR can be safely advocated for general use (Table 41.2). With increased experience, however, we think the EGR may eventually become a safe and preferable means of gastrocnemius recession. To date, however, the open technique remains the gold standard and should still be considered the most efficient, reliable, and user-friendly means of gastrocnemius recession.

References

1. Leversedge F, Casey P, Seiler J, Xerogeanes J. Endoscopically assisted fasciotomy: description of technique and in-vitro assessment of lower-leg compartment decompression. Am J Sports Med 30(2): 272–278, 2002
2. Mirza E, King E. Newer techniques of carpal tunnel release. Orthop Clin North Am 27: 355–371, 1996
3. Saxena A. Uniportal endoscopic plantar fasciotomy: a prospective study on athletic patients. Foot Ankle Int 25(12): 882–889, 2004
4. Armstrong D, Stacpoole-Shea S, Nguyen H, Harkless L. Lengthening of the achilles tendon in diabetic patients who are at high risk for ulceration of the foot. J Bone Joint Surg 81A(4): 535–538, 1999
5. DiDomenico L, Adams H, Garehar, D. Endoscopic gastrocnemius recession for the treatment of gastrocnemius equinus. J Am Podiatr Med Assoc 95(4): 410–413, 2005
6. Hansen ST. Midfoot arthrodesis In: Wulker N, Stephens M, Cracchiolo A (eds.) Atlas of Foot and Ankle Surgery. St. Louis, MO, Mosby, p. 154, 1998
7. Hansen ST: Tendon transfers and muscle balancing techniques. Achilles tendon lengthening. In: Hansen S (ed.) Functional Reconstruction of the Foot and Ankle. Lippincott Williams & Wilkins, Baltimore, MD, pp. 415–421, 2000
8. Laborde J. Tendon lengthenings for forefoot ulcers. Wounds 17(5): 122–130, 2005
9. Mueller M, Sinacore D, Hastings M, Johnson J. The effect of Achilles tendon lengthening on neuropathic plantar ulcers: a randomized clinical trial. J Bone Joint Surg 85-A(8): 1436–45, 2003
10. Pinney S, Sangeorzan B, Hansen ST. Surgical anatomy of the gastrocnemius recession (Strayer procedure) Foot Ankle Int 25(4): 247–250, 2004
11. Pinney SJ, Hansen ST, Sangeorzan BJ. The effect on ankle dorsiflexion of gastrocnemius recession. Foot Ankle Int 23(1): 26–29, 2002
12. Poul J, Tuma J, Bajerova J. Video-assisted tenotomy of the triceps muscle of the calf in cerebral palsy patients. Acta Chir Orthop Traumatol Cech 72(3): 170–172, 2005
13. Saxena A. Endoscopic gastrocnemius tenotomy. J Foot Ankle Surg 41(1): 57–58, 2002
14. Saxena A, Widtfeldt A. Endoscopic gastrocnemius recession: a preliminary report on 18 cases. J Foot Ankle Surg 43(5): 302–306, 2004
15. Saxena A, Gollwitzer H, DiDomenico L, Widtfeldt A, Die endoskopische Verlängerungsoperation des Musculus gastrocnemius zur Behandlung des Gastrocnemius equinus (German) Z Orthop Unfall 145:1–6, 2007
16. Saxena A, DiGiovanni C. Ankle equinus and the athlete. In: Maffulli N, Almekinders M (eds.) The Achilles Tendon. Springer, New York, 2006
17. Sgarlato TE. Medial gastrocnemius tenotomy to assist in body posture balancing. J Foot Ankle Surg 37(6): 546–547, 1998

18. Takao M, Ochi M, Shu N, Uchio Y, Naito K, Tobita M, Matsusaki M, Kawasaki K. A case of superficial peroneal nerve injury during ankle arthroscopy. Arthroscopy 17(4): 403–404, 2001

19. Tashjian RZ, Appel AJ, Banerjee R, DiGiovanni CW. Anatomic study of the gastrocnemius-soleus junction and its relationship to the sural nerve. Foot Ankle Int 24: 473–476, 2003

20. Trevino S, Gibbs M, Panchbhavi V. Evaluation of results of endoscopic gastrocnemius recession. Foot Ankle Int 26(5): 35–364, 2005

21. Trevino S, Panchbhavi V. Technique of endoscopic gastrocnemius recession: cadaveric study. Foot Ankle Surg 8: 45–47, 2002

22. Tashjian R, Appel A, Banerjee R, DiGiovanni C. Endoscopic gastrocnemius recession: evaluation in a cadaver model. Foot Ankle Int 24: 607–613, 2003

23. Silverskiold N. Reduction of the uncrossed two-joints muscles of the leg to one-joint muscles in spastic conditions. Acta Chir Scand 56: 315–30, 1924

24. DiGiovanni C, Kuo R, Tejwani N, Price R, Hansen T, Cziernecki J, Sangeorzan B. Isolated gastrocnemius tightness. J Bone Joint Surg 84A(6): 962–970, 2002

25. Saxena A, Kim W. Ankle dorsiflexion in adolescent athletes. J Am Podiatr Assoc 93(4): 312–314, 2003

26. Webb J, Moonjani N, Radford M. Anatomy of the sural nerve and its relation to the Achilles tendon. Foot Ankle Int 21(6): 475–477, 2000

27. Barouk L, Barouk P. Techniques, results and comparison between the medial and lateral proximal gastrocnemius release. Presented at the International Spring Meeting, French Foot Society. Toulouse, France June 8–10, 2006

Chapter 42
Percutaneous Reduction and Internal Fixation of the Lisfranc Fracture-Dislocation

Anish R. Kadakia and Mark S. Myerson

The success of minimally invasive percutaneous reduction and fixation of tarsometatarsal or Lisfranc injuries lies in understanding the appropriate injury pattern for this method of treatment. The eponym *Lisfranc dislocation* is derived from injuries sustained to cavalry troops in the Napoleonic era. These were associated with significant vascular and soft tissue injury, as they were treated with an amputation through the tarsometatarsal joints by Lisfranc, Napoleon's surgeon. Although the injuries secondary to equestrian activity have declined, the injury pattern is commonly associated with high-energy motor vehicle accidents, falls, and crushing injuries to the foot.[1-4] These mechanisms typically involve significant bony and soft tissue injury that rarely can be managed by closed methods (Fig. 42.1). Percutaneous fixation is most amenable in those patients with low-energy mechanisms, particularly in the athletic and elderly populations involving primarily a ligamentous injury (Fig. 42.2).

Mechanism of Injury

The indirect mechanism associated with the low-energy injury typically results from an axial longitudinal force with rotation on a plantar flexed foot.[5,6] The plantar flexed position of the foot placed the weaker dorsal ligamentous restraints on tension, resulting in their failure allowing further displacement and rupture of the plantar ligamentous restraints or metatarsal base fracture.[1,6,7] This type of injury may not produce the obvious clinical picture associated with direct high-energy injuries of severe swelling, deformity, inability to bear weight, and neurovascular compromise.[8] Typical presentation includes swelling throughout the midfoot that improves after 1 week and therefore delayed presentations may not appear to have a significant injury upon visual examination.[5] Persistent pain and tenderness across the midfoot that is aggravated with stress testing of the tarsometatarsal joints is indicative of this injury pattern.[9]

A.R. Kadakia and M.S. Myerson (✉)
Foot and Ankle Institute, Mercy Medical Center, 301 St. Paul Pl, 21202, Baltimore, MD, USA
e-mail: mark4feet@aol.com

Radiographic Evaluation

The radiographic series for a suspected Lisfranc injury should include anteroposterior (AP), lateral, and 30° internal oblique views of both feet. Additionally, external oblique views in both 10° and 20° have demonstrated efficacy in delineating the amount of displacement in the transverse plane.[9] In order to stress the midfoot and demonstrate the injury radiographically, the X-rays should be performed with as much weight-bearing as possible. Occasionally, weight bearing is too difficult for the patient, therefore, if the non-weight-bearing X-ray results are normal, repeat weight-bearing views should be performed at 10–14 days.[6] Stress radiographs can be performed to diagnosis the instability, however, they should be performed under anesthesia to prevent a false negative finding. The foot is stressed with pronation combined with abduction to detect subtle diastasis or angulation.[5,6,10] Coss et al.[11] have shown in a cadaveric model that disruption of the dorsal and Lisfranc ligamentous restraints resulted in a radiographic instability pattern consistently noted on abduction stress examination, verifying the utility of the clinical examination.

The anatomic relationships of the tarsometatarsal joints have consistent radiographic appearances, deviations from these patterns are consistent with injury.[12] The medial border of the second metatarsal is in colinearity with the medial border of the middle cuneiform on the AP radiographic exam along with the first intermetatarsal space and the space between the medial and middle cuneiforms (Fig. 42.3a, b). The lateral border of the third metatarsal is colinear with the lateral border of the lateral cuneiform on the internal oblique radiograph. In addition, the medial border of the fourth metatarsal is colinear with the medial border of the cuboid. Subtle radiographic findings include minor angulation or displacement of the first metatarsal (Fig. 42.4). Myerson et al.[3] described the "fleck sign," a small avulsion fracture of either the medial cuneiform or the base of the second metatarsal, which is diagnostic of a Lisfranc disruption. Careful review of the radiographs should be performed so that Lisfranc variants with intercuneiform instability are not overlooked (Fig. 42.5).

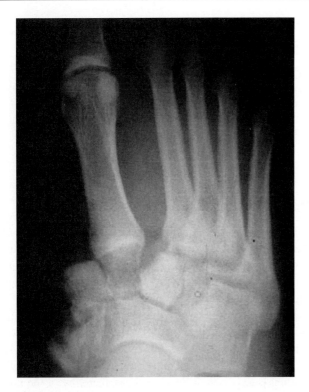

Fig. 42.1 An AP radiograph of a direct injury mechanism with significant displacement and bony comminution that is not amenable to percutaneous treatment

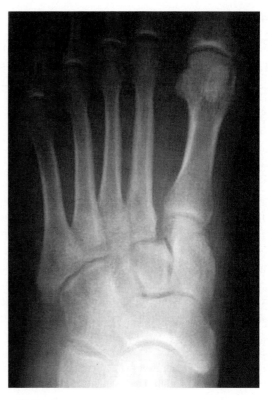

Fig. 42.2 An AP radiograph of a pure ligamentous injury that is ideally treated by percutaneous methods

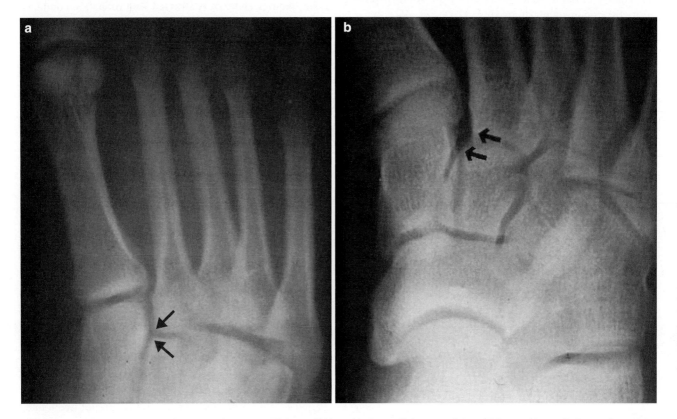

Fig. 42.3 (a) Note that the base of the second metatarsal is in continuity with the medial aspect of the middle cuneiform. (b) In a patient with a Lisfranc injury, note the lateral displacement of the second metatarsal in relation to the medial aspect of the middle cuneiform

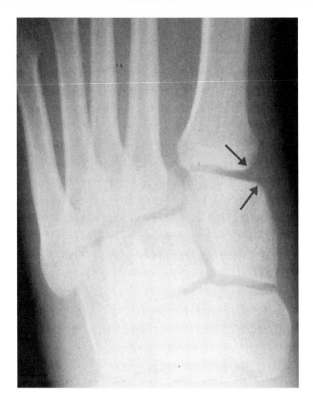

Fig. 42.4 An AP radiograph demonstrating lateral translation of the first metatarsal consistent with a Lisfranc injury

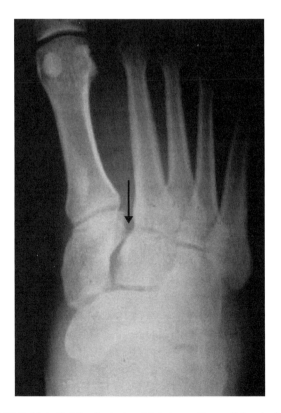

Fig. 42.5 Note that the diastasis exists between the medial and middle cuneiforms, consistent with a Lisfranc injury, despite the normal relationship between the second metatarsal and the middle cuneiform

Classification

Multiple classification systems exist to describe the injury to this joint complex.[2,3,13] The use of the columnar classification developed by Myerson[6,10,14] divides the midfoot based on the respective motion segments. The medial column includes the first tarsometatarsal and the medial cuneiform-navicular joints (Fig. 42.6a). The middle column includes the second and third tarsometatarsal, intercuneiform, and the naviculo-cuneiform joints (between the middle and lateral cuneiforms) (Fig. 42.6b). The lateral column includes the articulations between the fourth and fifth metatarsals and the cuboid (Fig. 42.6c). This system of classification has prognostic implications based on the motion of the midfoot. The medial and middle columns have minimal motion (3.5 mm and 0.6 mm, respectively) and do not tolerate incongruity, suffering the highest incidence of posttraumatic arthritis.[14,15]

Nunley and Vertullo have proposed a classification system to define the midfoot sprain typically seen in athletes.[16] Stage 1 is consistent with pain at the Lisfranc joint without any evidence of diastasis on weight-bearing radiographs. Stage 2 involved 1–5 mm of diastasis between the first and second metatarsal on the AP radiograph, with evidence of lateral arch collapse. Stage 3 is greater than 5 mm of diastasis and loss of midfoot arch height. Patients with Stage 1 injuries were successfully treated with a non-operative treatment protocol that included an initial 6 weeks of a non-weight-bearing fiberglass cast.

Treatment

Although recent literature may suggest that primary arthrodesis offers improved scores at a mean of 42.5 months of follow-up in ligamentous injuries over reduction and internal fixation, the longer-term complications of early arthrodesis may diminish these early results.[17] Therefore, treatment should consist of reduction and internal fixation of Lisfranc injuries and Stage 2 and 3 midfoot sprains via either percutaneous or open approaches. Non-operative treatment of these injuries is inappropriate as greater than 2 mm of displacement or 15° of angulation is associated with a poor outcome.[3]

Surgical Technique

The use of a percutaneous technique requires a thorough understanding of the anatomy of the tarsometatarsal joints and their appearance under fluoroscopy. The undertaking of a percutaneous approach should not be performed unless the surgeon is capable of performing an open reduction, as, on occasion, soft tissue or bony fragment interposition may prevent an anatomic reduction using closed methods.

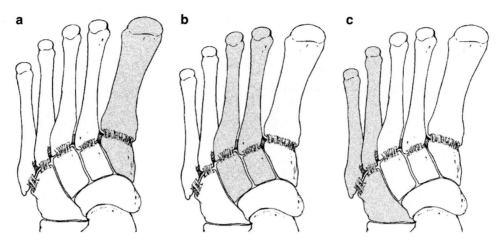

Fig. 42.6 The medial (**a**), middle (**b**), and lateral columns (**c**) are depicted

Initial attention must be performed to obtaining an anatomic reduction prior to any attempts at fixation. Longitudinal traction is required to reduce the tarsometatarsal joints and utilization of gauze rolls secured around the phalanges is a powerful aid in reduction (Fig. 42.7). Initial attention is paid to the medial column, which provides a stable post to which the middle column is reduced. The reduction maneuver involves grasping the hallux firmly and placing a medial- or lateral-directed force to the base of the metatarsal to reduce the deformity. Once an anatomic reduction is achieved, provisional fixation is achieved with a guidewire for a cannulated screw (Fig. 42.8a, b). A large bone clamp facilitates reduction of the second metatarsal into the mortise (Fig. 42.9a, b). If persistent diastasis remains despite adjustment of the clamp, then conversion to an open reduction should be performed. Typically, this realigns the third and fourth metatarsals into an anatomic position. A partially threaded screw is then placed obliquely from the medial cuneiform to the base of the second metatarsal. Stability of the lateral column is assessed fluoroscopically and, if persistent instability exists, stabilization is performed with either a 1.6-mm K-wire or screw fixation (Fig. 42.10a, b). If K-wire fixation is utilized for the lateral column, subcutaneous placement is important to prevent infection and premature removal.

Postoperative Rehabilitation

Initial immobilization is a below knee posterior plaster splint to decrease swelling and enhance wound healing. Early mobilization and range of motion is encouraged and rigid fixation with screws is important to prevent loss of reduction. Removal of the splint at 2 weeks is followed by placement into a

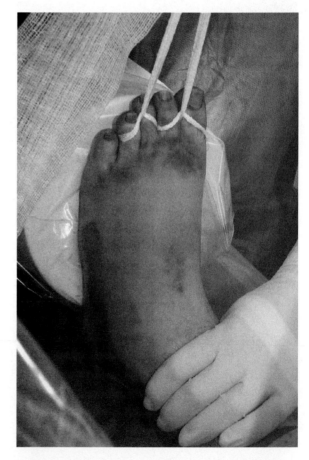

Fig. 42.7 Use of the gauze roll to create phalangeal slings to provide longitudinal traction and aid in closed reduction of the deformity

removable boot, although non-weight bearing is continued for 8 weeks. Patients are allowed to begin range of motion and strengthening in a pool at 4 weeks and stationary biking is allowed at 6 weeks. Full weight bearing is allowed at 12

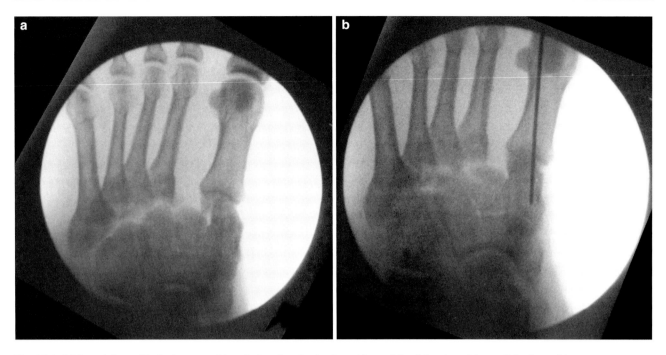

Fig. 42.8 Lisfranc injury with displacement (**a**) and after closed reduction with provisional fixation of the medial column (**b**)

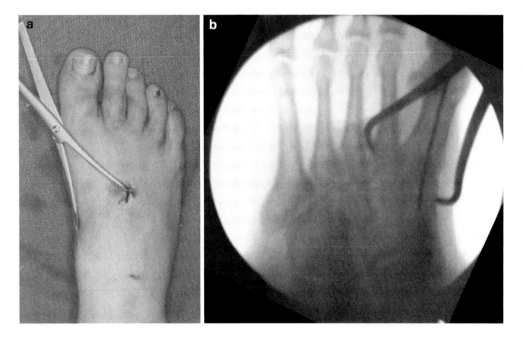

Fig. 42.9 Clinical (**a**) and fluoroscopic (**b**) depicting the use the bone clamp to reduce the base of the second metatarsal into the mortise

weeks, with conversion to an athletic shoe with an orthotic. Hardware removal is typically performed at 4 months, after which aggressive rehabilitation is performed under the direction of a therapist. Single plane running is initiated at 20 weeks and cutting sports are allowed at 24 weeks.

Summary

Disruptions of the tarsometatarsal joints can lead to significant disability if misdiagnosed and undertreated. Detailed review of weight-bearing radiographs of the affected extremity

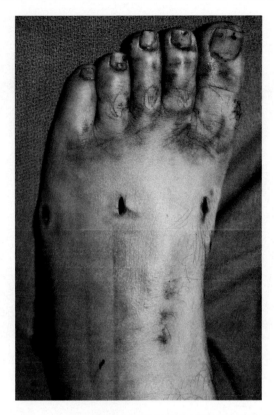

Fig. 42.10 Final view of the foot after closed reduction and fixation

and a thorough understanding of the normal anatomic landmarks will consistently lead the clinician to diagnosis of even subtle injuries to the midfoot. Percutaneous treatment of these injuries is ideal as it avoids the risk of wound complications and morbidity associated with extensile incisions. However, if any question of malreduction exists, conversion to an open reduction must be performed.

References

1. Myerson M. Tarsometatarsal arthrodesis: technique and results of treatment after injury. Foot Ankle Clin 1996;1:73–83.
2. Hardcastle P, Reschauer R, Kutscha-Lissberg E, Schoffmann W. Injuries to the tarsometatarsal joint. Incidence, classification and treatment. J Bone Joint Surg Br 1982;64B(3):349–56.
3. Myerson M, Fisher R, Burgess A, Kenzora J. Fracture dislocations of the tarsometatarsal joints: end results correlated with pathology and treatment. Foot Ankle 1986;6(5):225–42.
4. Gossens M, De Stoop N. Lisfranc fracture dislocations: etiology, radiology, and results of treatment. A review of 20 cases. Clin Orthop Relat Res 1983;176:154–62.
5. Curtis M, Myerson M, Szura B. Tarsometatarsal joint injuries in the athlete. Am J Sports Med 1993;21:497–502.
6. Chiodo C, Myerson M. Developments and advances in the diagnosis and treatment of injuries to the tarsometatarsal joint. Orthop Clin North Am 2001;32(1):11–20.
7. Buzzard B, Briggs P. Surgical management of acute tarsometatarsal fracture dislocation in the adult. Clin Orthop Relat Res 1998;353:125–33.
8. Aronow M. Treatment of the missed Lisfranc injury. Foot Ankle Clin N Am 2006;11:127–42.
9. Myerson M. The diagnosis and treatment of injuries to the Lisfranc joint complex. Orthop Clin North Am 1989;20:655–64.
10. Myerson M. The diagnosis and treatment of injury to the tarsometatarsal joint complex. J Bone Joint Surg (Br) 1999;81-B:756–63.
11. Coss H, Manos R, Buoncristiani A, Mills W. Abduction stress AP weightbearing radiography of purely ligamentous injury in the tarsometatarsal joint. Foot Ankle Int 1998;19(8):537–41.
12. Stein R. Radiological aspects of the tarsometatarsal joints. Foot Ankle 1983;3:286–9.
13. Quenu E, Kuss G. Etude sur les luxations du metatarse. Reb Chir Paris 1909;39(281).
14. Komenda G, Myerson M, Biddinger K. Results of arthrodesis of the tarsometatarsal joints after traumatic injury. J Bone Joint Surg Am 1996;78:1665–76.
15. Ouzounian T, Shereff M. In vitro determination of midfoot motion. Foot Ankle 1989;10:140–6.
16. Nunley J, Vertullo C. Classification, investigation, and management of midfoot sprains. Lisfranc injuries in the athlete. Am J Sports Med 2002;30(6):871–8.
17. Ly T, Coetzee J. Treatment of the primarily ligamentous Lisfranc joint injuries: primary arthrodesis compared with open reduction and internal fixation. J Bone Joint Surg Am 2006;88-A(3):514–20.

Chapter 43
Arthroscopic Repair of Chronic Ankle Instability

Peter B. Maurus and Gregory C. Berlet

Lateral ankle ligament sprains are some of the most common injuries encountered in the orthopedic office, occurring in an estimated 1/10,000 persons per day.[1] These injuries can be seen in as many as 40% of all sports injuries.[2] While the majority of acute ankle sprains heal reliably with activity modification and physical therapy/ankle rehabilitation, approximately 29–42% of patients experience chronic functional ankle instability.[3] Functional lateral instability, as introduced by Freeman et al., describes a subjective complaint of giving way in the ankle joint.[4] Tropp's work further described this condition as motion beyond voluntary control, but not exceeding the physiologic range of motion.[5] Mechanical instability is motion beyond the normal physiologic limits of the ankle joint. This is manifested as excessive anterolateral ankle laxity.

The anterior talofibular ligament (ATFL) is the most commonly injured ligament during ankle sprains. Although described as mainly limiting anterior translation in relative plantarflexion, it serves as the primary restraint to inversion and translation at all angles of ankle flexion.[6,7] During an inversion ankle sprain, the anterolateral capsule is typically injured first, followed by the ATFL, the calcaneofibular ligament (CFL), and the posterior talofibular ligament (PTFL). Persistent failure (repeated giving way) of this lateral ligament complex is an indication for surgical stabilization of the ankle.

There are multiple surgical options for stabilization of the chronically unstable ankle, both anatomic and nonanatomic. Nonanatomic lateral ligament stabilizations are characterized by reconstruction with tendon grafts to recreate the lateral ligament complex. These techniques risk overconstraining the ankle joint and are not isometric in their kinematic effect on the ankle joint. Thus, they should be reserved for revisions or unique clinical situations.

Anatomic procedures maintain the natural ligament insertion points, but alter the tension on the native ligamentous structures. Isometry is not disturbed and overconstraint is rarely seen. Anatomic reconstructions include the modified Brostrom lateral ligament reconstruction and thermal capsular modification. Open techniques are not discussed in this chapter.

Whether an open or arthroscopic approach to treating instability is chosen, arthroscopy can and should be an important adjunct to the surgical treatment of ankle instability. Arthroscopy allows for a minimally invasive evaluation of the ankle joint and the ability to treat intraarticular pathology at the time of lateral ligament reconstruction. In the 1993 study by Taga et al. of 31 ankles, chondral lesions were found in 89% of the freshly injured ankles and 95% of the ankles with chronic injuries.[8] Hintermann et al. noted cartilage damage in 66% of ankles scoped prior to ligament reconstructions.[9] Komenda and Ferkel found that 93% of 51 ankles had intraarticular abnormalities including loose bodies, synovitis, osteochondral lesions of the talus, ossicles, osteophytes, adhesions, and chondromalacia.[10] Takao et al. studied 72 patients with residual ankle disability lasting more than 2 months after injury and illustrated intraarticular pathology at the time of arthroscopy in 14 patients that was not identified on any clinical or radiologic testing.[11]

Thermal-Assisted Capsular Modification

Thermal-assisted capsular modification for chronic lateral ankle instability was introduced recently.[12,13] This technique has been successful in treating shoulder instability and early results in the ankle are encouraging. The concept is based on the fact that thermal energy between 65°C and 70°C shrinks collagen, which comprises more than 90% of joint capsules, ligaments, and tendons (TACS). Thermal energy may be applied using electrical energy (monopolar or bipolar) or laser energy.

Factors such as tissue properties themselves or variables related to the energy source (including the density, application

G.C. Berlet (✉)
Chief Foot and Ankle Ohio State University, Orthopedic Foot and Ankle Centre, Columbus Ohio
e-mail: Gberlet@aol.com

time, and concentration area) determine the amount of energy delivered to the tissue.[14] *Pulsing* the energy can minimize tissue damage and control depth of penetration. In the authors' experience, electrical energy is more reliable and we have had success with the Mitek (Vapr TC; Mitek Products, Division of Ethicon, Somerville, NJ) or Arthrocare (CAPSure, ArthroCare Corporation, Austin, TX) devices.

Our decision to use thermal capsular modification for lateral ligament reconstruction is influenced by the patient's body habitus, activity pattern, and degree of ligament injury. Indications include patients with moderate build, intraligament stretching (not avulsed from bone), generalized ligamentous laxity with functional ankle instability, a commitment to adhere to the postoperative rehabilitation protocol, and no previous ankle ligament reconstructive surgery. Contraindications include muscle weakness, tendon tears and instability, subtalar instability, and tibiofibular joint instability.

Preoperatively, each patient undergoes a focused physical examination assessing ankle instability, muscle weakness, tendon tears and tendon instability, proprioceptive disorders, subtalar instability, and tibiofibular joint instability. Radiographs of the affected ankle are obtained and magnetic resonance imaging (MRI) should be performed if peroneal tears and chondral injuries of the talus are suspected.

Technique

After sterile preparation and draping of the ankle, a noninvasive ankle distractor strap is applied (Acufex, Smith & Nephew, Memphis, TN). Anteromedial and anterolateral portals are established. The surgeon should then perform a complete arthroscopic examination and treat any pathology encountered (e.g., synovitis, osteochondral defects) accordingly. Impingement lesions in the anterolateral gutter are encountered frequently and should be debrided aggressively with an arthroscopic trimmer to allow adequate exposure of the anterolateral gutter. The capsule should be preserved for use in the thermal procedure to follow.

Once visualization of the anterolateral capsule and distal fibula is confirmed, introduce a thermal control wand through the lateral portal and release the distraction device once the thermal wand is in position. The ATFL can be identified consistently.[15] With the maximum temperature set at 65°C (with the thermal feed backward or on level 2 with the Arthrocare system), the tissue of the anterolateral capsule (just distal and anterior to the distal fibula) and ATFL can be treated with the thermal wand by using a painting technique starting deep in the lateral gutter and working anteriorly, avoiding repetitive treatment of a specific location. Thermal treatment is below the equator of the lateral arthroscopy portal to avoid creating an iatrogenic impingement lesion. The treated capsule will show a blushing after treatment. Surgeons familiar with shoulder thermal modification will note that there is a visual contraction of the shoulder capsule that occurs while working in the inferior glenohumeral pouch. There is much less visual confirmation of contraction in the ankle. After adequate exposure to the thermal effects of the wand, the arthroscopic instrumentation can be removed. The ankle should be held in slight dorsiflexion and eversion as the portals are closed with suture and a well-padded posterior/gutter splint (with cooling pack) is applied to the operative extremity.

Results

Between February 1999 and December 2001, the authors performed 42 arthroscopic thermal-assisted capsular modifications of the anterolateral capsule and the ATFL.[16] The AOFAS hindfoot scores improved significantly: scores averaged 29.57 preoperatively (standard deviation [SD] 15.6) and improved to 55.36 (SD 13.56) at an average follow-up of 14.1 months ($p < 0.001$).

One patient had skin breakdown over the calf where the ankle distracter strap had been, which resolved with conservative wound care. There were no infections.

Postoperatively, patients undergo physical examinations at 3-week intervals. Patients wear a non-weightbearing cast for the first 3 weeks, followed by a weightbearing cast for 3 weeks, and then a weightbearing boot walker for 3 weeks. Physical therapy ankle rehabilitation begins 9 weeks postoperatively.

Favorable outcomes using thermal stabilization have been reported, however, no prospective studies have been published reporting the use of thermal modification for ankle instability.[12,17–19]

The authors think that select patients with chronic lateral instability who have failed a course of conservative treatment are good candidates for arthroscopic thermal capsular and ATFL shrinkage. Longer follow-up will be necessary to determine whether the ankle will remain stable over time. Longer-term follow-up will determine how the outcomes compare with traditional surgical methods (i.e., modified Brostrom repair).

Thermal-assisted capsular modification has potential limitations. While the ATFL is easily visualized during arthroscopy, the CFL is not accessible. Therefore, the CFL cannot be addressed arthroscopically. Moreover, the extensor retinaculum, which is used in the open modified Brostrom procedure is not an intraarticular structure and cannot be incorporated into the repair. Both the CFL and the extensor retinaculum can be important restraints to medial talar tilt on varus stress. Perhaps a *hybrid* procedure that involves arthroscopic evaluation and treatment of the ATFL in conjunction with a mini-open approach to either the CFL or extensor retinaculum would be able to address the entire lateral ligament complex.

On the Horizon

As arthroscopists become more comfortable with arthroscopic knot tying techniques and new orthopedic implants are developed, we may see more novel ideas emerge. Early work is proceeding on a suture-based capsular ATFL imbrication technique. No published results are yet available.

References

1. Trevino SG, Davis P, Hecht PJ. Management of acute and chronic lateral ligament of the ankle. Orthop Clin North Am 1994;25:1–16
2. Holmer P, Sondergaard L, Konradsen L, Nielsen PT, Jorgensen LN. Epidemiology of sprains in the lateral ankle and foot. Foot Ankle Int 1994;15:72–74
3. Berlet GC, Anderson RB Davis WH. Chronic lateral ankle instability. Foot Ankle Clin 1999;4:(4): 713–728
4. Freeman MAR. Instability of the foot after injuries to the lateral ligament of the ankle. J Bone Joint Surg 1965;47B:669–676
5. Tropp H, Ekstrand J, Gillquist J. Stabilometry in functional instability of the ankle and its value in predicting injury. Med Sci Sports Exerc. 1984;16:64–66
6. Colville MR, Marder RA, Boyle JJ, Zaring B. Strain measurement in lateral ankle ligaments. Am J Sports Med 1990;18:196–200
7. Johnson EE, Markolf KL. The contribution of the anterior talofibular ligament to ankle laxity. J Bone Joint Surg 1983;65:81–88
8. Taga I, Shino K, Inoue M, Nakata K, Maeda A. Articular cartilage lesions in ankles with lateral ligament injury. An arthroscopic study. Am J Sports Med 1993;21(1):120–126
9. Hintermann B, Boss A, Schafer D. Arthroscopic findings in patients with chronic ankle instability. Am J Sports Med 2002;30(3): 402–409
10. Komenda GA, Ferkel RD. Arthroscopic findings associated with the unstable ankle. Foot Ankle Int 1999;20(11):708–713
11. Takao M, Uchio Y, Naito K, Fukazawa I, Ochi M. Arthroscopic assessment for intra-articular disorders in residual ankle disability after sprain. Am J Sports Med 2005;33(5):686–692 (Epub 2005 Feb 16)
12. Ryan AH, Lee TH, Berlet GC. Arthroscopic thermal assisted capsular shrinkage in anterolateral ankle instability: a retrospective review of 13 patients. AOFAS Annual Summer Meeting, Vail, CO, July 2000
13. Myers JB, Lephart SM, Bradley JP, et al. Proprioception following thermal capsulorrhaphy. AAOS Annual Meeting, San Francisco, CA, 2001
14. Arnoczky SP, Aksan A. Thermal modification of connective tissues: basic science considerations and clinical implications. J Am Acad Orthop Surg 2000;8:305–13
15. Leyes M, Hersch J, Sferra J. Arthroscopic identification of the anterior talofibular ligament. AOSSM, Orlando, FL, July 2002
16. Berlet GC, Saar WE, Ryan A, et al. Thermal-assisted capsular modification for functional ankle instability. Foot Ankle Clin 2002;7:567–76
17. Orecchio A. "Running Start," Study reports heat shrinkage technique for ankle instability. Biomechanics April 2000, 14–15
18. Berlet GC, Raissi A, Lee TH. Thermal capsular modification for chronic lateral ankle instability, AOFAS Annual Summer Meeting, Traverse City, MI, July 2002
19. Fanton GS. Thermal ankle stabilization – clinical Update 2002. AOSSM Annual Meeting, Orlando, FL, July 2002

Chapter 44
Arthroscopic Subtalar Arthrodesis: Indications and Technique

Dominic S. Carreira and Pierce Scranton

The subtalar joint is an important joint, playing a major role in eversion and inversion of the foot as it transmits and dissipates forces applied to the calcaneus proximally. Arthrosis of the subtalar joint may be a significant source of pain and dysfunction. It may have a rheumatoid, inflammatory, post-traumatic, or degenerative etiology. In patients with painful subtalar arthrosis with or without progressive deformity, arthrodesis is an accepted form of salvage.[1] If the arthritic subtalar joint is well aligned, a simple subtalar arthrodesis without the use of bone graft has been shown to be effective. Mann and Baumgarten reported a high rate of success by denuding the posterior facet articular surface, *feathering* the bony surface, and using internal fixation.[2] This and other open techniques for subtalar arthrodesis may be significantly painful and may require hospitalization for pain control.

In an effort to decrease potential morbidity and reduce costs, alternative techniques have been introduced. Arthroscopic procedures have demonstrated decreased morbidity in a variety of joints. The theoretic advantages include smaller incisions, less blood loss, less pain, and a shorter rehabilitation time.

The indications for arthroscopy of the subtalar joint are similar to those for open procedures, including removal of loose bodies, evaluation of chondral and osteochondral fractures, excision of intraarticular adhesions, and arthrodesis. If one chooses to perform an arthroscopic-assisted arthrodesis, relative contraindications include significant deformity, bone loss, severe edema, and poor vascularity. An absolute contraindication is infection.

A retrospective comparison study has been reported between arthroscopic and open procedures. This nonrandomized study of in situ, isolated subtalar arthrodesis compared open treatment with autogenous bone graft versus arthroscopic treatment using injectable morphogenic protein-enhanced grafts.[3] Eight patients were treated by open arthrodesis and five patients were treated arthroscopically. During

follow-up, in each group, one AO screw required removal. There was one diabetic patient who was treated open and who was the sole patient requiring an additional procedure (revision bone grafting) to achieve fusion. Tourniquet time averaged 5 min longer in the arthroscopic group (63 vs. 58 min). Average savings in the arthroscopy group was related to the length of stay (approximately $600/day at the time of that report).

In a study of arthroscopic fusions, Tasto et al. reported on 24 patients with an average follow-up of 31 months.[4] All 24 patients had a successful fusion with an average time to union of 8.9 weeks. Tasto et al. cited additional advantages of preservation of the blood supply to the hindfoot joints and a low complication rate.

In a report of open isolated subtalar arthrodesis, Easley and Myerson reported on 148 patients.[5] The union rate was 84%. Complications reported included prominent hardware (20%), sural nerve injury (9%), infection (3%), lateral impingement (10%), and malalignment of the hindfoot (6%). Of the 30 nonunions, all had 2 mm or more of avascular bone noted at the time of the procedure.

The routine use of supplementary bone graft is not always necessary for isolated subtalar fusions as reported by Mann and Baumgarten[2] and Mangone et al.[6] Its use is dependant on the amount of deformity and bone stock, and may be indicated in cases of poliomyelitis, spastic cerebral palsy, or posttraumatic calcaneal fracture care.[68] Further, Thordarson and Kuehn were not able to demonstrate a superior union rate with the use of Grafton putty or Orthoblast compared with historical controls or between one another.[9]

The use of pulsed electromagnetic fields at the time of hindfoot arthrodesis was studied in 64 consecutive patients.[10] All patients who underwent open elective triple/subtalar arthrodesis were randomized into control and pulsed electromagnetic field study (PES) groups. Subjects in the PES group were treated and an electromagnetic field was applied for 12 h per day with its application over the cast. All joint fusions, as evaluated by radiographic union, occurred over less time in the study group. For subtalar arthrodesis, the average time was 14.5 weeks in 33 primary subtalar arthrodeses with 4 nonunions. In the study group, the average time was 12.9

D.S. Carreira and P. Scranton (✉)
Orthopedics International, 12333 NE 130 Lane, 400, Kirkland,
WA 98034, USA
e-mail: piercescranton@hotmail.com

G.R. Scuderi and A.J. Tria (eds.), *Minimally Invasive Surgery in Orthopedics*,
DOI 10.1007/978-0-387-76608-9_44, © Springer Science+Business Media, LLC 2010

weeks to fusion, with no nonunions. Of note, the average cost was $3,000 and most insurance companies did not cover the cost in a primary arthrodeses.

Anatomy

The subtalar joint is divided by the sinus tarsi and tarsal canal into an anterior and posterior part. The tarsal canal is formed by a sulcus on the undersurface of the talus and the superior surface of the calcaneus, and laterally this opening is termed the sinus tarsi. The borders of the tarsal canal include the anterior portion of the posterior subtalar joint capsule, which forms the posterior border of the canal. The anterior boundary is the posterior portion of the talocalcaneal navicular joint capsule. The contents of the tarsal canal include the cervical ligament, the interosseous talocalcaneal ligament, the medial part of the inferior extensor retinaculum, vessels, and fatty tissue.

The anterior part of the subtalar joint is formed by the anterior and medial joint facet, the talonavicular joint, and the spring ligament. There is usually no communication between the anterior and posterior parts of the subtalar joint because of the thick interosseous ligament, which fills the tarsal canal.

The posterior portion of the subtalar joint is very close to the posterior ankle joint. As the talus tapers posteriorly, the posterior talofibular ligament is just proximal to the posterior subtalar joint line. The axis of the posterior joint facet is directed 40° laterally in relation to the longitudinal axis of the foot. The calcaneal surface is shaped in a convex fashion, whereas the talar joint surface is concave. The lateral joint capsule is reinforced by the calcaneofibular and the talocalcaneal ligaments. The capsule contains a posterior pouch and a small lateral recess.

The ligamentous support of the subtalar joint has been divided into three layers.[11] The superficial layer consists of the lateral root of the inferior extensor retinaculum, the lateral talocalcaneal ligament, the calcaneofibular ligament, the posterior talocalcaneal ligament, and the medial talocalcaneal ligament. The intermediate layer consists of the intermediate root of the inferior extensor retinaculum and the cervical ligament. The deep layer consists of the medial root of the inferior extensor retinaculum and the interosseous talocalcaneal ligament.

Portal Anatomy

Parisien described an anterior and posterior portal. Frey and coworkers described the middle portal. Mekhail described the medial portal, and Ferkel described the accessory anterolateral and posterolateral portals. One must maintain enough separation between portals to prevent instrument crowding.

The posterior portal (named the posterolateral portal by Ferkel) is approached from the lateral side. It has the greatest risk of causing sural nerve injury. The lesser saphenous vein, peroneal tendons, and Achilles tendon can also be injured with posterior portal placement. The sural nerve is typically located 2 cm posterior and 2 cm inferior to the lateral malleolus. After making a superficial small skin incision, a hemostat should be used to spread through the subcutaneous tissue down to the level of the capsule. The trocar is angled upward and in a slightly anterior direction (Fig. 44.1).

In a study by Frey[12] describing portal anatomy and safety, the portal is located, on average, 25 mm (range, 20–28 mm) posterior and 6 mm (range, 0–10 mm) proximal to the tip of the fibula, behind the saphenous vein and nerve and anterior to the Achilles tendon. In seven of ten dissection cases, the posterior portal was located posterior to the sural nerve, and in two cases it was anterior. One sural nerve was transected, and in another case, a small transection of the lesser saphenous vein was made. The peroneal tendon sheath was located on average 11 mm anterior to the portal and the Achilles tendon an average of 15 mm posterior to the portal.

For the anterior portal (named the anterolateral portal by Ferkel), the point of entry is 2 cm anterior and 1 cm distal to the tip of the lateral malleolus. The trocar is angled slightly upward and approximately 40° posterior.[13] In the study by Frey et al.,[14] this portal was located an average of 28 mm (range, 23–35 mm) anterior to the tip of the fibula. Structures at risk with placement of this portal include the dorsal intermediate cutaneous branch of the superficial peroneal nerve, the dorsolateral cutaneous branch of the sural nerve, the peroneus tertius tendon, and a small branch of the lesser saphenous vein. The dorsal intermediate cutaneous branch of the superficial peroneal nerve is located an average of 17 mm (range, 0–28 mm) anterior to the portal (Fig. 44.1).

The accessory anterolateral portal is usually slightly anterior and superior to the anterior portal. This portal is best made under direct visualization from either the posterior or anterior portal. The accessory posterolateral portal is made lateral to the posterior portal, using caution to avoid the abovementioned structures and under direct visualization.

The middle portal is approximately 1 cm anterior to the tip of the fibula, directly over the sinus tarsi.[14] It places no structures at risk and is therefore relatively safe.

Mekhail et al.[15] described the establishment of a medial portal. A blunt-ended trocar is placed into the sinus tarsi and is pushed through the tarsal canal in a posteromedial and slightly cephalad direction. While the ankle is in equinus and the foot is inverted in order to relax the posteromedial neurovascular bundle and slightly displace it posteriorly, the trocar is advanced to exit the skin medially and is angled approximately 45° to the lateral border of the foot. The portal entry lies

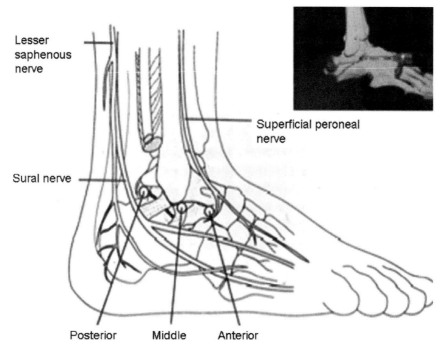

Fig. 44.1 Subtalar arthroscopy portal placement and relationship to verves (From Frey CC, DiGiovanni C. Gross and arthroscopic anatomy of the foot In: Guhl JF, Parisien MD, Boyton JS (eds.) Foot and Ankle Arthroscopy, 2004, with kind permission of Springer Science + Business Media.)

along a line between the medial malleolus and the medial calcaneal tubercle, at the point where the anterosuperior ¾ meets the posteroinferior ¼. Improved visualization was described of the posteromedial and anterolateral aspects of the posterior subtalar joint. The authors also warned that in feet with significant adipose tissue or edema, the portal would be situated more posteriorly and therefore in closer approximation to the neurovascular bundle. The indications for use of this portal are rare.

The best combination for portal access to the cartilage of the posterior facet involves placement of the arthroscope through the anterior portal and instrumentation through the posterior portal.[16] This allows for direct visualization and instrumentation of nearly the entire posterior facet, the posterior aspect of the interosseous ligament, the lateral capsule and its small recess, and the posterior pouch.

Instrumentation through the anterior portal allows for improved visualization of the lateral aspect of the posterior facet. Access to the anterior and lateral compartments of the posterior facet, as well as structures of the extraarticular sinus tarsi, is best obtained by placing the arthroscope in the anterior portal and the instrumentation through the middle portal.

Arthroscopic Technique

For patient positioning, the preferred technique is to place the patient supine with a bolster under the ipsilateral buttock.

Other options for positioning include the lateral decubitus or 90° flexion at the knee. The procedure can be performed with the patient under general or regional anesthesia. A sciatic nerve block can provide additional prolonged postoperative anesthesia. Relaxation is critical and therefore local anesthesia is not recommended. A tourniquet is applied and used as necessary. Distraction is applied with invasive or noninvasive instrumentation. Tasto has reported the use of a lamina spreader in sinus tarsi to allow for easier introduction of instrumentation.[17] We prefer the use of AO distraction pins, which are inserted manually and confirmed fluoroscopically. The calcaneal pin is inserted from the lateral side, just posterior to the vascular triangle. The threaded tip engages the opposite medial cortex without penetrating it. The talar pin is inserted across the neck of the talus just anterior to the anterior talofibular ligament insertion. The AO distractor then is attached and gradual distraction applied (Fig. 44.2).

The superficial anatomy is outlined: the fibula, sinus tarsi, and anterior, middle, and posterior portals. An 18-gauge needle may be used to distend the joint and check for backflow. Care should be taken to ensure the ankle joint has not been entered by checking for distension about the ankle joint. A number 11 blade is used to initiate the portals. As the distraction progresses, the borders of the cervical and interosseous ligaments increase in tension and are sequentially cut using the number 11 blade. A 30°, 2.7-mm or 4.0-mm arthroscope (depending on patient size) is then introduced through the anterior portal. A 70° scope also may be quite useful to look around corners for further visualization. Gravity is usually sufficient to fill the joint with fluid and an arthroscopic pump usually is not usually necessary. A shaver is introduced through the middle portal and obscuring synovial debris is removed. A number of sizes of shaver-type blades may be used, including 1.9 mm, 2.0 mm, 2.9 mm, and 4.0 mm.

The primary fusion is performed at the posterior facet, which makes up most of the area of the subtalar joint. The middle facet is also debrided and fused after resecting the contents of the sinus tarsi. Fusion of the anterior facet requires extensive ligamentous resection and is generally avoided. A 4-mm burr is used to abrade the bone to ensure a good bleeding base of bone.

A cannulated pin is driven from the anteromedial shoulder of the talar neck until the pin protrudes from the superior talar surface of the posterior facet (Fig. 44.3). Keep the pin away from the anterior ankle joint so that the screw does not impinge and interfere with ankle dorsiflexion. Once the position is confirmed, the guide pin is backed away from the joint surface and the 4-mm burr is reintroduced. A bone slurry is then generated by burring both sides of the joint, keeping the suction turned off (Fig. 44.4). If bone graft is used, the arthroscope only is then removed and 5 mL of osteoinductive gel is injected through the arthroscopic sheath. The obturator is used as a plunger to push the gel into place.

The distractor is removed and the joint is held reduced (0–5° valgus, neutral in the sagittal and axial planes) by compressing the talar and calcaneal pins. The cannulated talar pin is driven across the subtalar joint and into the calcaneus. The cannulated screw is then driven across and confirmed fluoroscopically (Fig. 44.5). An alternative method is to drive one or more screws up from the calcaneus into the talus. Closure is performed with 4–0 nylon sutures. Compression dressings are applied along with a posterior splint.

Postoperative Rehabilitation

Patients are seen in follow-up at 7–14 days for a wound check, and then placed either in a cast or boot walker. They are placed on crutches nonweightbearing for 6 weeks and then are placed in a boot walker for 6 weeks. If there is radiographic evidence of union, a good intermediate transition shoe is an aerobics shoe that has good arch support and a slight rocker-bottomed sole. If there is doubt regarding the completeness of the arthrodesis, the patient may be recasted for another 4–6 weeks.

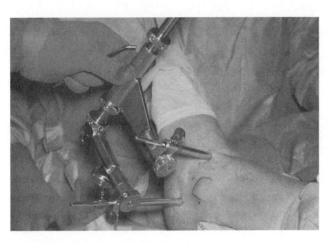

Fig. 44.2 Setup of AO distractor for subtalar arthrodesis

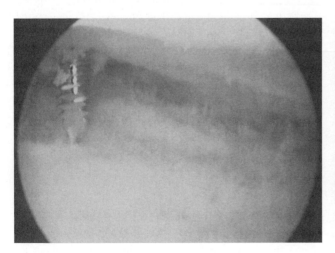

Fig. 44.3 Intraarticular view of posterior facet demonstrating adequate pin placement

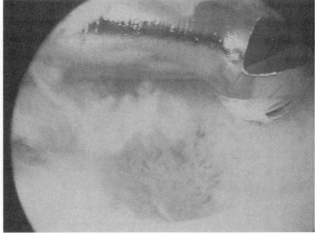

Fig. 44.4 A 4-mm burr at the posterior facet demonstrating creation of bone slurry

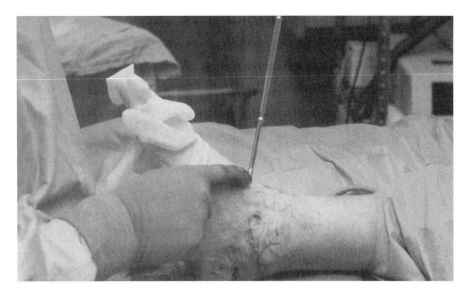

Fig. 44.5 Insertion of cannulated screw

References

1. Scranton PE. Results of arthrodesis of the tarsus: talocalcaneal, midtarsal, and subtalar joints. Foot Ankle Int 12:156–164, 1991
2. Mann RA, Baumgarten M. Subtalar fusion for isolated subtalar disorders. Clin Orthop Relat Res 226:260–265, 1988
3. Scranton PE. Comparison of open isolated subtalar arthrodesis with autogenous bone graft versus outpatient arthroscopic subtalar arthrodesis using injectable bone morphogenic protein-enhanced graft. Foot Ankle Int 20(3):162–165, 1999
4. Tasto JP, Frey C, Laimans P, et al. Arthroscopic ankle arthrodesis. Instr Course Lect 49:259–280, 2000
5. Easley ME, Trnka H-J, Schon LC, et al. Isolated subtalar arthrodesis. J Bone Joint Surg 82A:613–624, 2000
6. Mangone PG, Fleming LL, Fleming SS, Hedrick MR, Seiler JG III, Bailey E. Treatment of acquired adult planovalgus deformities with subtalar fusion. Clin Orthop Relat Res, 341:106–112, 1997
7. Grice DS. An extra-articular arthrodesis of the subastragalar joint for correction of paralytic feet in children. J Bone Joint Surg 34A:927–930, 1952
8. Scranton PE, McMaster JH, Kelly E. Dynamic fibular function: a new concept. Clin Orthop Relat Res 118:76–82, 1976
9. Thordarson DB, Kuehn S. Use of demineralized bone matrix in ankle/hindfoot fusion. Foot Ankle Int 24(7):557–60, 2003
10. Dhawan SK, Conti SF, Towers J, Abidi NA, Vogt M. The effect of pulsed electromagnetic fields on hindfoot arthrodesis: a prospective study. J Foot Ankle Surg 43(2):93–96, 2004
11. Harper MC. The lateral ligamentous supports of the subtalar joint. Foot Ankle Int 12:354, 1991
12. Frey C, Gasser S, Feder K. Arthroscopy of the subtalar joint. Foot Ankle Int 15:424–428, 1994
13. Parisien JS (ed.). Arthroscopic Surgery. New York, McGraw-Hill, 1988
14. Frey C, Gasser S, Feder K. Arthroscopy of the subtalar joint. Foot Ankle Int 15:424–428, 1994
15. Mekhail AO, Heck BE, Ebraheim NA, et al. Arthroscopy of the subtalar joint: establishing a medial portal. Foot Ankle Int 16: 427–431, 1995
16. Frey C. Subtalar arthroscopy. In: Myerson MS (ed.) Foot and Ankle Disorders. Philadelphia, PA, Saunders, 1999, pp. 1494–1501
17. Tasto JP. Subtalar arthrodesis. Presented at the Arthroscopy Association of North America, Orlando, FL. February, 1995

Chapter 45
Minimally Invasive Ankle Arthrodesis

Jamal Ahmad and Steven M. Raikin

The ankle joint is a constrained mortise and tenon-type joint consisting of the distal tibial plafond and fibula articulating with the dome of the talus. Arthritis of the ankle can result in pain, joint incongruence, decreased motion, and functional disability. The most common etiology of ankle arthritis is posttraumatic, which includes cartilaginous injury and ligamentous insufficiency.[1] Other less common causes of arthritis include the inflammatory arthritides, osteonecrosis, infection, and Charcot neuroarthropathy.[2]

To date, the ankle remains one of the few major extremity joints in which arthrodesis is the gold standard surgical treatment for advanced arthritis that has failed nonoperative management. Open ankle arthrodesis was first described by Albert in 1879.[3] Fusion through an open arthrotomy has received numerous modifications since that time, but remains a widely used technique for surgical exposure. Currently, the most common surgical exposure for open ankle arthrodesis is the lateral transfibular approach. Upon osteotomy, the distal fibula can be used either as bone graft or as a lateral strut to increase the stability of the arthrodesis construct. Preparations of the distal tibia and talar dome through these open techniques include either "dome" cuts or flat cuts. Dome cuts allow for minimal loss of height, but do not offer much in terms of angular correction. Straight, flat cuts allow for correction of significant deformity, but can result in loss of joint height.

However, ankle arthrodesis through an open arthrotomy is not without its shortcomings. Skin slough, wound dehiscence, and wound infection may occur with a sizable wound at the ankle. As the distal fibula and syndesmotic ligaments are removed during the open fusion, the ankle's mortise and lateral stability are lost. This is undesirable should the arthrodesis be taken down and later converted to an ankle arthroplasty. Greisberg et al. recently showed that patients who received a distal fibula resection with their fusion had a more complicated postoperative course in terms of pain and loosening following conversion to arthroplasty than patients in whom the fibula was spared for their fusion.[4] Distal fibular osteotomy also often sacrifices the peroneal artery, which may affect healing of the ankle fusion and wound. At the ankle, the peroneal artery gives rise to the artery of the tarsal sinus to supply the lateral one eighth to one fourth of the talus. The artery of the tarsal sinus then links to the artery of the tarsal canal at the tarsal canal to form the artery of the tarsal sling. This artery enters the talar neck inferiorly to supply it and the remainder of the bone in a distal-to-proximal direction. Without the peroneal artery, the blood supply to the ankle fusion may not be optimal. Additionally, open ankle fusion techniques typically involve a high degree of soft tissue stripping, which can damage the extraosseous blood supply of the fusion site. When the blood supply is compromised in some manner, the quality and time to union may be deleteriously affected. Finally, there is concern that, after resection of the distal fibula during the approach to the ankle joint, the peroneal tendons will lose their biomechanical fulcrum around which they act during eversion of the hindfoot.

To avoid these shortcomings of open ankle arthrodesis, the technique of arthroscopic fusion was proposed.[5-7] For this procedure, a standard two or three portal ankle arthroscopy is performed. With the joint distracted, the articular cartilage and subchondral bone is removed with curettes and mechanical burrs. Two or three percutaneous cannulated cancellous screws are then placed across the ankle under fluoroscopic guidance to achieve fusion. Since first being described in 1983, several authors have reported their experience.[5] Ogilvie-Harris et al. presented an 89% union rate among 19 arthroscopic fusions with a mean time to union of 10.5 weeks.[8] Zvijac et al. reported a 95% union rate among 21 arthroscopic fusions with an average time to fusion of 8.9 weeks.[9] Myerson and Quill retrospectively compared arthroscopic with open arthrodesis in 33 patients.[10] The arthroscopic group showed 100% union at a mean of 8.7 weeks while the open population displayed a 94% union rate at a prolonged mean of 14.5 weeks after surgery. However, patients who had more deformity or osteonecrosis were

J. Ahmad and S.M. Raikin (✉)
Departments of Orthopaedic Surgery,
Rothman Institute and Thomas Jefferson University Hospital,
925 Chestnut Street, Philadelphia, PA 19107, USA
e-mail: steven.raikin@rothmaninstitute.com

selectively placed in the open population due to the study's inherent retrospective nature. In one of the largest studies to date, Winson et al. described a 7.6% nonunion rate in 105 arthroscopic ankle arthrodeses, with 20% of patients describing their results as fair or poor.[11] In the literature to date, arthroscopic ankle arthrodesis has been mainly reserved for patients with minimal deformity.

However, this technique of arthroscopic ankle arthrodesis is not without its own shortcomings. The technique itself is technically demanding and has a steep learning curve.[1] Because a burr is used to prepare the distal tibia and talar dome surfaces, there is a genuine concern of thermal injury to the bony surfaces, which can increase the risk of nonunion.[12]

To combine the advantages of the open and arthroscopic ankle fusion methods while limiting their respective disadvantages, a minimally invasive or "mini-open" technique was detailed in 1996.[1,12] The advantages of this newer procedure are as follows: (1) decreased incision sizes to minimize morbidity, which include the risks of skin slough, wound dehiscence, and postoperative infection; (2) distal fibula preservation, which is preferred should the fusion later be converted to an arthroplasty; (3) preservation of the peroneal artery; (4) elimination of burrs to prepare bony surfaces, which could otherwise cause thermal necrosis; and (5) decreased time to union.

Indications

The primary indication for minimally invasive ankle arthrodesis is pain and dysfunction from severe ankle arthritis that has failed conservative treatment. Such nonoperative modalities may include nonsteroidal anti-inflammatory medications (NSAIDs), soft-laced ankle gauntlets, and motion-limiting braces. However, this specific technique of ankle arthrodesis is best reserved for patients with minimal or absent deformity of the ankle.[1,12] An additional theoretical advantage is the younger patient who is not a candidate for ankle arthroplasty on the basis of their age, but who wishes to potentially pursue this option in the future.

Contraindications

The following factors are relative contraindications for performing minimally invasive ankle arthrodesis: (1) significant ankle deformity or subluxation; (2) bone loss at the ankle; and (3) osteonecrosis involving a significant portion of the talus or distal tibia. This is because it is difficult to address the above conditions through a minimally invasive technique.

Correcting a significant ankle deformity usually necessitates correction via bony cuts at the tibial plafond and the talar dome, combined with more extensive soft tissue release and rebalancing that is not possible with small incisions. Ankles that display significant bone loss, osteonecrosis, and collapse often require thorough debridement of pathologic bone and supplementation with structural bone graft. Such situations are best suited for an open ankle arthrodesis via a transfibular approach.

Preoperative Planning

Weightbearing radiographs of the ankle in the anteroposterior (AP), lateral, and mortise plane are critical to planning a minimally invasive ankle arthrodesis (Fig. 45.1). Weightbearing films allow for more accurate evaluation of malalignment and loss of joint space. As stated earlier, ankles that exhibit minimal radiographic deformity on weightbearing remain best suited for minimally invasive fusion techniques. Characteristic radiographic findings of ankle arthritis are decreased joint space, subchondral sclerosis, subchondral cysts, osteophytes, loose bodies, and malalignment.[13]

A complete and informed discussion with the patient should be undertaken to prepare the patient for realistic

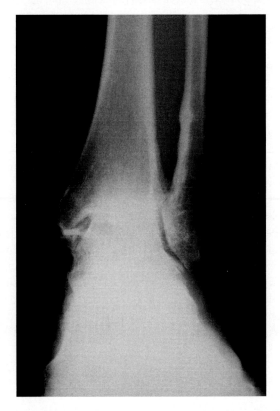

Fig. 45.1 AP radiograph of a severely arthritic ankle without significant varus or valgus deformity

postoperative expectations. Patients should be informed that the risks of minimally invasive ankle fusion include but are not limited to bleeding, infection, nerve injury, and non-union. Patients should also be advised about the potentials to require prolonged weightbearing restrictions and accommodative footwear postoperatively.

Operative Procedure

The patient is administered a general or spinal anesthetic for the operation supplemented with a regional nerve block for postoperative pain control. The patient is positioned supine with a bump underneath the ipsilateral hip rotating the pelvis to bring the foot into a straight upright position, aligning the tibial tubercle with the web space between the first and second toes. A radiolucent table is used to facilitate fluoroscopy assistance throughout surgery. A "mini image" dose radiation fluoroscopy device is usually adequate for visualization in this procedure. A pneumatic tourniquet is applied to the proximal calf and inflated to 250 mmHg after exsanguination during the procedure. Surgical drapes are applied to leave the foot, ankle, and leg distal to the tourniquet exposed in the surgical field. Preoperative prophylactic antibiotics are routinely indicated for this procedure, prior to tourniquet inflation.

Technique

Two 2-cm vertical incisions are utilized for this technique. These incisions are centered over the standard portal sites for ankle arthroscopy. An 18-gauge needle should be inserted into the joint at each proposed incision site to confirm the appropriate level of the incision and that adequate access to the ankle can be achieved. The anteromedial incision is made immediately medial to the tibialis anterior tendon, between the tendon and the notch of the medial malleolus. Care must be taken with this incision to avoid injury to a branch of the saphenous nerve, which could result in painful neuroma formation. The anterolateral incision is made in the space between the lateral border of the peroneus tertius tendon and the anterior border of the fibular. Special care should be taken not to injure the lateral cutaneous branch of the superficial peroneal nerve, which should be identified and retracted medially with the peroneus tertius tendon (Fig. 45.2). Through both incisions, blunt dissection is continued down to the ankle joint capsule, which is incised longitudinally to expose the joint. Subperiosteal dissection around the anterior aspect of the ankle is performed with an elevator to optimize joint exposure. Anterior ankle osteophytes are removed with a sharp chisel to enhance visualization of the joint. The joint

is then denuded of articular cartilage through one of the incisions while distraction is maintained via the other incision. Upon proper exposure of the ankle joint, a laminar spreader is placed in one of the incisions to distract the joint (Fig. 45.3). Proper insertion of the laminar spreader within the joint is crucial so as not to excessively plantarflex the ankle. With the joint distracted, a sharp chisel and/or angled curette is placed

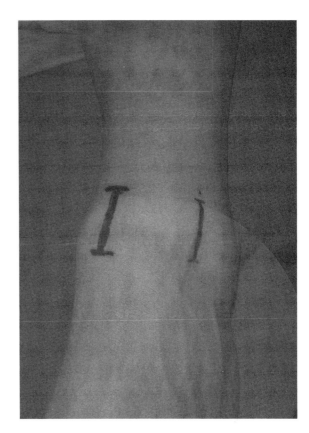

Fig. 45.2 Incision sites marked out for the minimally invasive ankle arthrodesis

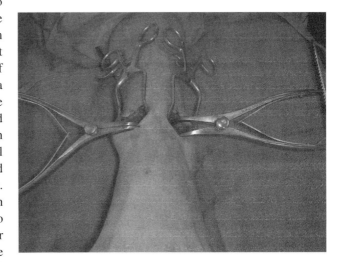

Fig. 45.3 Incisions are extended through the retinaculum to expose the ankle joint

in the other incision and used to remove cartilage through the other incision (Fig. 45.4a, b). Enough cartilage is removed from the distal tibia and talar dome to penetrate through the subchondral plate and observe bleeding cancellous bone from each surface. This layer of resection is typically 1–2 mm. Once one side (medial or lateral) of the ankle joint is devoid of cartilage, the laminar spreader is switched to the other incision. The chisel and curettes are placed in their corresponding alternate incision to remove cartilage from the other side of the ankle. Great care must be utilized to ensure that the medial and lateral gutters are adequately debrided to allow the ankle joint to be appropriately aligned for the arthrodesis (Fig. 45.5). It is our recommendation that no power saws or burrs be utilized to limit potential thermal necrosis of the bone, which may lead to nonunion of the arthrodesis. All of the resected bone and cartilage is removed utilizing a rongeur. Once all of the cartilage has been removed from the ankle, the joint is copiously irrigated with saline to remove loose bodies and bone shavings.

To date, there is a general lack of consensus regarding the use of bone autograft or allograft during minimally invasive ankle arthrodesis. The senior author routinely enhances this arthrodesis with autogenous cancellous bone graft.[1] This is harvested from the lateral aspect of the calcaneal body.[14]

The ankle is then held in an appropriate position for fusion, which is checked fluoroscopically. The ankle is fused in 5° of valgus, 0° of dorsiflexion, and 10° of external rotation.[15] This position is optimal as it results in a plantigrade foot and maximal functional results.[16] Note that it may be tempting for the surgeon to fuse a female's ankle in slight plantarflexion such that she may wear shoes with raised heels. However, this should be avoided for two reasons. The first is that fusing the ankle in equinus increases the stress and risk of developing secondary arthritis at the transverse tarsal joints. In addition, this ankle position causes genu recurvatum while walking without a raised heeled shoe.[17,18] Provided that there is no hindfoot or midfoot arthritis,

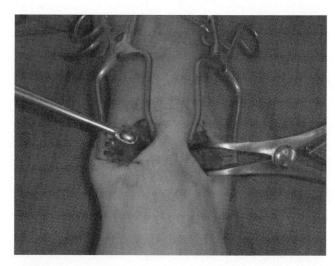

Fig. 45.5 With one side of the ankle joint distracted, the gutter of the opposite side is debrided

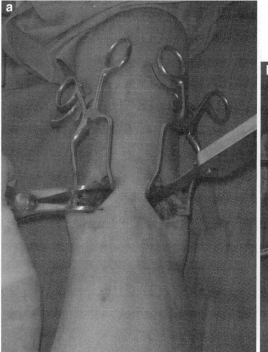

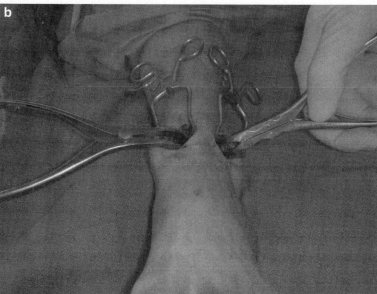

Fig. 45.4 (**a, b**) One side of the ankle joint is distracted with a laminar spreader while the other side is debrided with a rongeur and/or chisel

compensatory motion after ankle arthrodesis often allows for walking in as much as a 2-in. heel.

Once an optimal alignment is obtained, guide pins for screw fixation are inserted under fluoroscopic guidance. The ankle arthrodesis is held with three 7.3-mm (or 6.5-mm) short-threaded cannulated cancellous screws. Using three screws to achieve an ankle arthrodesis has been shown biomechanically to impart the greatest amount of rigidity to the fusion.[19–21] A method of using three screws involves the following technique of two crossing screws and a third posterior to anterior (PA) "home run" screw.[1,22] The first guidewire is placed percutaneously from the medial distal tibia to the lateral talar body. The second guidewire is placed percutaneously from the anterolateral distal tibia to the medial talar body. Both wires are placed crossing each other. This configuration of the two screws has shown increased rigidity in laboratory tests.[12,23] The positions of these wires are checked under fluoroscopy to confirm they have sufficient purchase of distal tibia and talus and that they do not penetrate the subtalar joint (Fig. 45.6). Once wire positioning is deemed acceptable, the length of both is measured. The two guidewires are overdrilled and a 7.3-mm (or 6.5-mm) short-threaded cannulated cancellous

screw for each are inserted over them (Fig. 45.7). Typically, screws selected for use are 5–10 mm shorter than the measured length of their respective guidewires. This allows for compression of the ankle fusion during screw fixation without the screws themselves violating the subtalar joint. After placement of these two screws, the guidewires are removed. While screw length is determined by the size of the individual patient's bone size, these two screws are usually approximately 50 mm in length.

A third guidewire is then placed from the posterior distal tibia, just lateral to the Achilles tendon, into the neck and head of the talus. The position of this wire is assessed under fluoroscopy to confirm that it has adequate purchase of distal tibia and talar neck and that it does not penetrate the talonavicular joint. Once wire positioning is deemed acceptable, its length is measured. The guidewire is overdrilled and a 7.3-mm short-threaded cannulated cancellous screw is inserted over it. Akin to the first two screws, the third screw selected for use is 5 mm shorter than the measured length of the guidewire. This allows for compression of the ankle fusion during screw fixation without the screw violating the talonavicular joint. Again, while variable, dependent on individual bone size, this screw is usually approximately 65 mm in length. After screw placement, the guidewire is removed. For any of the three screws, adding a washer may improve compression in osteopenic bone. Final fluoroscopy

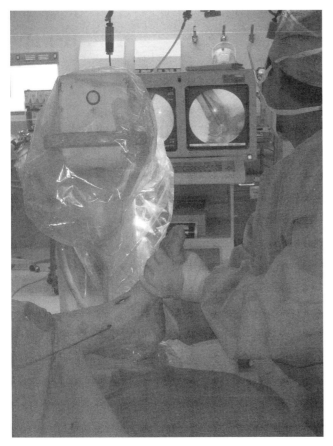

Fig. 45.6 Correct position of the arthrodesis is confirmed under fluoroscopy

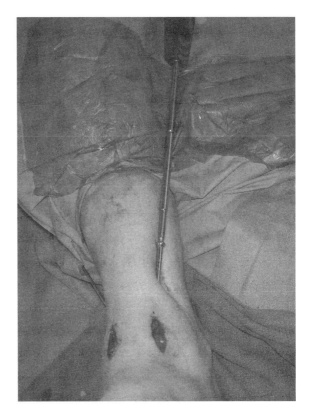

Fig. 45.7 Screws to achieve fusion are placed percutaneously

is performed to confirm proper alignment of the ankle fusion and screw placement. When performing this procedure we routinely leave preexisting hardware in place unless it blocks the reduction of the joint or the placement of one of the arthrodesis screws.

All wounds are closed in a routine fashion. The ankle retinaculum is closed with interrupted 0 Vicryl suture. The subcutaneous tissue of all three wounds is closed with interrupted 2.0 Vicryl suture. The skin of all of the wounds is closed with a skin stapler.

The wounds are then dressed in sterile fashion. Sterile Xeroform, gauze, and Webril are applied to the wounds in a layered fashion. At this point, the tourniquet is deflated and the sterile drapes are removed. Immediately after surgery and application of the dressing, the patient is placed in a non-weightbearing posterior and "U" coaptation plaster splint.

Postoperative Care

The initial postoperative splint remains intact for 2 weeks. At 2 weeks postoperatively, the splint is removed and the patient is placed in a nonweightbearing short leg cast for 4 weeks.

Typically, at 6 weeks postoperatively, radiographs start to show bony union across the fusion. So long as this is the case, the cast is removed and the patient is placed into a fracture boot to allow for progressive weightbearing. Currently, there is no uniform postoperative weightbearing regimen for patients following a minimally invasive ankle fusion. The senior author instructs patients to begin 25–50% weightbearing in the boot at 6 weeks postoperatively so long as there is radiographic evidence of bony consolidation. The patient may then apply an additional 25% of weight in the boot every 2 weeks as comfort allows. Thus, patients should be fully weightbearing on the ankle arthrodesis in the boot by 12 weeks postoperatively. Once the patient is fully weightbearing in the boot without discomfort, and radiographs show adequate fusion of the arthrodesis (Fig. 45.8), the patient may gradually wean out of the fracture boot and return to their previous level of activity. Footwear modifications such as a rocker-bottom sole with a solid ankle cushioned heel (SACH) may help patients to resume a more normal gait.

After minimally invasive ankle arthrodesis, patients should be provided with conservative guidelines regarding postoperative activity level. Bicycle riding, swimming, and other low-impact activities are encouraged for aerobic exercise. Patients may return to playing golf at 9–12 months postoperatively. Jogging and running are discouraged after ankle arthrodesis. The repetitive high-impact loading of the ankle fusion can irritate and place additional load upon the knee, hindfoot, and midfoot.

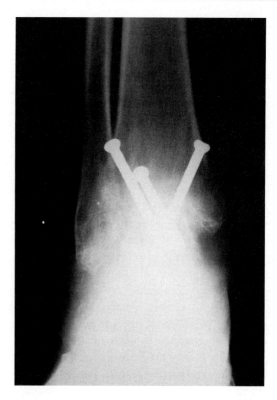

Fig. 45.8 Radiograph of a patient with a completely healed ankle arthrodesis done through a minimally invasive technique

Published Results

To date, very little published data exists for the mini-open ankle arthrodesis. Myerson et al. described the procedure and published their results in two separate studies.[12] In the same paper where the technique was first described and the compromise of vascularity with the fibular resection was studied, Miller et al. reported on 32 ankles undergoing the mini-arthrotomy technique.[24] They described a 96.8% union rate in 32 ankles, with two delayed unions. Their average time to union was 8 weeks, with a range of 6–22 weeks. Paremain et al. separately reported a union rate of 100% at a mean time of 6 weeks (range, 3 to 15 weeks) in 15 ankles undergoing this minimally invasive technique of arthrodesis.[12]

No specific studies have been published on takedown of the mini-open ankle arthrodesis for conversion to total ankle arthroplasty. However, Greisberg et al. did report on conversion of 23 open ankle arthrodeses to arthroplasty.[4] They reported 3 of 19 patients who were available for follow-up finally choosing to undergo below-knee amputation for recalcitrant pain, but the remaining 16 patients improved their AOFAS ankle hindfoot score from an average of 42 points to an average of 68 points out of 100. They did comment that all patients who had undergone a distal fibular resection as part of their initial arthrodesis had complicated courses after arthroplasty. This supports the theory that the mini-open fibular preserving technique may result in superior arthroplasty conversion results in the future.

Senior Author's Experience

The senior author (SMR) has performed 16 minimally invasive ankle arthrodeses in 16 ankles, with longer than 12 months follow-up. Patients' ages ranged from 28 to 52 years (average 24.1 years), with ten male patients six female patients. The right and left ankle were equally involved, with eight cases each. The most common underlying diagnosis was posttraumatic arthritis, which was present in 14 (87%) patients, with one patient having a history of juvenile rheumatoid arthritis (JRA) and one patient with talar osteonecrosis secondary to steroid use for asthma. All patients had minimal or no deformity at the ankle joint without significant bone loss or collapse. Postoperative follow-up averaged 37.5 months, with the range being from 15 to 68 months. The rate of union in this population was 100%. Mean time to union was 11.4 weeks after surgery, with the range being from 10 to 16 weeks. When asked if they were satisfied with their postoperative outcome, all of the patients (100%) stated they would have their respective procedure done identically unless an arthroplasty could be done as an alternative. There were no observed postoperative complications such as wound infections, nerve injuries, or delayed healing. Of incidental note, none of these patients were involved in the workers compensation system, litigation, or secondary gain related to their injuries. To date, none of these fusions have been attempted to be taken down and converted to an ankle arthroplasty.

References

1. Raikin S. Arthrodesis of the ankle: arthroscopic, mini-open, and open techniques. Foot Ankle Clin North Am 8: 347–359, 2003
2. Coughlin M. Arthritides. In: Coughlin M (ed.) Surgery of the foot and ankle. St. Louis: Mosby; pp. 560–650, 1999
3. Albert E. Beitrage zur operativen chiurgie. Zur resection des kniegelenkes. Wien Med Press 20: 705–708, 1879
4. Greisberg J, Assal M, Flueckiger G, Hansen, ST. Takedown of ankle fusion and conversion to total ankle replacement. Clin Orthop Relat Res 424: 80–88, 2004
5. Schneider D. Arthroscopic ankle fusion. Arth Video J 3, 1983
6. Morgan C. Arthroscopic tibio-talar arthrodesis. Jefferson Orthop J 16: 50–52, 1987
7. Myerson M, Allon S. Arthroscopic ankle arthrodesis. Contemp Orthop 19: 21–27, 1989
8. Ogilvie-Harris D, Lieberman I, Fitsialos D. Arthroscopically assisted arthrodesis for osteoarthrotic ankles. J Bone Joint Surg 75A: 1167–1173, 1993
9. Zvijac J, Lemak L, Schurhoff M, Hechtman K, Uribe J. Analysis of arthroscopically assisted ankle arthrodesis. Arthroscopy 18(1): 70–75, 2002
10. Myerson M, Quill G. Ankle arthrodesis: a comparison of an arthroscopic and an open method of treatment. Clin Orthop Relat Res 268: 84–95, 1991
11. Winson IG, Robinson DE, Allen PE. Arthroscopic ankle arthrodesis. J Bone Joint Surg Br 87(3): 343–347, 2005
12. Paremain G, Miller S, Myerson M. Ankle arthrodesis: results after the miniarthrotomy technique. Foot Ankle Int 17(5): 247–252, 1996
13. Demetriades L, Strauss E, Gallina J. Osteoarthritis of the ankle. Clin Orthop Relat Res 349: 48–57, 1998
14. Raikin SM, Brislin K. Local bone graft harvested from the distal tibia or calcaneus for surgery of the foot and ankle. Foot Ankle Int 26(6): 449–453, 2005
15. Buck P, Morrey BF, Chao EY. The optimum position of arthrodesis of the ankle. A gait study of the knee and ankle. J Bone Joint Surg 69A: 1052–1062, 1987
16. Mann R, Van Manen J, Wapner K, et al. Ankle fusion. Clin Orthop Relat Res 268: 49–55, 1991
17. King H, Watkins T Jr, Samuelson K. Analysis of foot position in ankle arthrodesis and its influence on gait. Foot Ankle 1: 44–49, 1980
18. Wu W, Su F, Cheng Y, et al. Gait analysis after ankle arthrodesis. Gait Posture 11: 54–61, 2000
19. Dohm M, Benjamin J, Harrison J, et al. A biomechanical evaluation of three forms of internal fixation used in ankle arthrodesis. Foot Ankle Int 15: 297–300, 1994
20. Ogilvie-Harris D, Fitsialos D, Hedman T. Arthrodesis of the ankle. A comparison of two versus three screw fixation in a crossed configuration. Clin Orthop Relat Res 304: 195–199, 1994
21. Verkelst M, Mulier J, Hoogmartens M, et al. Arthrodesis of the ankle joint with complete removal of the distal part of the fibula: experience with the transfibular approach and three different types of fixation. Clin Orthop Relat Res 118: 93–99, 1976
22. Holt E, Hansen S, Mayo K, et al. Ankle arthrodesis using internal screw fixation. Clin Orthop Relat Res 268: 21–28, 1991
23. Nasson S, Shuff C, Palmer D, et al. Biomechanical comparison of ankle arthrodesis techniques: crossed screws vs. blade plate. Foot Ankle Int 22: 575–580, 2001
24. Miller SD, Paremain GP, Myerson MS. The miniarthrotomy technique of ankle arthrodesis: a cadaver study of operative vascular compromise and early clinical results. Orthopedics 1996 19(5): 425–430

Chapter 46
Arthroscopic Ankle Arthrodesis

C. Christopher Stroud

The benefits of minimally invasive surgery have received significant attention in the lay press as well as in scientific meetings. Often patients will ask whether such a "minimalistic" approach is available for treatment of their specific problem. While ankle fusion has long been treated via an open approach with generally excellent results,[1,2] there has been a push to perform this procedure through smaller incisions. While the extended lateral approach to the ankle has been the norm in the past, we have seen the evolution of the "mini-open" procedure as a technique used in a significant proportion of these procedures today.[3] Following this line of thinking, the arthroscopic approach has been used in performing arthro-desis procedures of the ankle and foot. However, with the use of these novel techniques, it is incumbent on us, as the treating physicians, to ensure surgical results that equate or surpass these historical results.

The benefits of a standard arthroscopic procedure are clear and well documented in the literature. Less perioperative pain experienced by the patient, smaller and more cosmetically appealing incisions, less surgical dissection, and a procedure that can be performed as an outpatient are clear advantages. What remains to be seen are the definite indications for the procedure, including the extent of deformity and bone loss that can be handled with the arthroscopic approach. It also should be noted that this "lesser" approach does not reduce the time to healing or to fusion. This chapter focuses on the surgical technique for those appropriately selected patients who will undergo an arthroscopic ankle arthrodesis.

Indications

Arthrosis of the ankle is generally uncommon, despite the ankle being a major weight-bearing joint.[4] Posttraumatic causes are the most common etiology, followed by primary osteoarthrosis, osteonecrosis, inflammatory arthropathy, and neuropathic causes. Patients typically present with complaints of pain globally about the ankle, usually of insidious onset. Potential causes for ankle pain should be investigated and include a history of trauma, instability, or systemic illnesses such as diabetes or other inflammatory or autoimmune diseases. The pain is usually described as a dull ache while sedentary and at times a sharp pain with weightbearing and pivoting. Patients may note a "grind" or a "click" with activity or movement. On examination, swelling is often present and tenderness is noted about a portion of, or the entire ankle joint itself. The presence of a deformity should be noted. Examination of limb alignment is particularly important, paying close attention the knee and hindfoot. Any deformity about the knee should be investigated with mechanical axis, weightbearing radiographs, and symptoms associated with the knee sought. Range of motion of the ankle, hindfoot, and midfoot should be recorded, noting any restriction of movement. The patient's neurovascular status is also assessed.

Radiographs consisting of weightbearing anteroposterior (AP), lateral, and mortise views of the ankle and foot are required (Fig. 46.1). These X-rays should be examined for the degree of arthrosis and the presence of osteophytes, cystic changes, and deformity. An anterior tibiotalar osteophyte of significant size will make the initial arthroscopic approach more difficult. If a bone defect is noted, the judgment will have to be made whether this defect is contributing to any ankle deformity and whether a grafting procedure will need to be performed. While smaller cystic defects are common and can be dealt with arthroscopically, larger defects that need to be filled with autograft or those that occur on the tibial side probably are best dealt with in an open fashion. There are no clear guidelines as to when an arthroscopic procedure should be abandoned in favor of the open approach but roughly a defect 30% or larger of the talar or tibial surface is best handle with direct visualization, i.e., a traditional open approach.[5] Additionally radiographs should be examined for any deformity that is present. If the deformity if extraarticular, consideration should be given to a supramalleolar or calcaneal osteotomy. If the deformity occurs at the ankle joint, then the decision becomes one of judgment. If the patient has a correctable ankle, that is, it can be placed in a plantigrade position passively, then one can proceed

C.C. Stroud (✉)
Department of Surgery, William Beaumont Hospital-Troy, 44199 DeQuindre, Suite 250, Troy, MI, 48085, USA
e-mail: stroudmdrn@aol.com

G.R. Scuderi and A.J. Tria (eds.), *Minimally Invasive Surgery in Orthopedics*,
DOI 10.1007/978-0-387-76608-9_46, © Springer Science+Business Media, LLC 2010

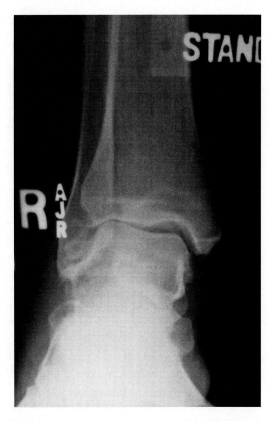

Fig. 46.1 AP radiograph of a patient with symptomatic right ankle arthrosis noting joint space narrowing and a slight valgus deformity. This minimal deformity is amenable to an arthroscopic arthrodesis

with an arthroscopic approach. If the deformity is rigid and exceeds 10–15°, the arthroscopic procedure should be abandoned in favor of the open approach.[5] This is especially true if there is a bony defect preset.

A patient who presents with ongoing complaints of ankle pain as a result of arthrosis should initially be treated with conservative measures. These include the use of oral analgesics or anti-inflammatories and limitations or modulations in their activities. It is difficult to totally restrict normal activities, but patients will often find it helpful to note that fewer weight-bearing activities can reduce their symptoms. Use of a pool or a stationary bike can often help the active patient stay healthy yet reduce the load on their symptomatic ankle. Proper footwear is important as well. This would include a soft-soled tennis type shoe and perhaps an accommodative orthotic that would lessen pain about the ankle. There are a multitude of braces available ranging from a lace-up ankle brace to an ankle foot orthosis or a custom semi-rigid ankle gauntlet type brace, all in order to diminish the pressure and load that the ankle bears. Judicious use a steroid injection can, at times, offer some temporary relief to the symptomatic ankle.

The patient that has failed these conservative measures and that has radiographic evidence of advanced arthrosis is a candidate for an arthrodesis procedure. The benefits of such

a procedure include the elimination or significant reduction in pain, and the ability to increase their normal activities of daily living. Potential disadvantages of an arthrodesis procedure include loss of motion of one segment of the ankle/foot complex. This may, with time, transfer stress to other areas of the foot and ankle, namely the subtalar joint complex, which may in turn become symptomatic at a future date. Other disadvantages include limb shortening, chronic swelling, and a limp. Overall, however, the results have been extremely satisfactory to patients in long-term follow-up studies to date.

The arthroscopic ankle fusion can offer the advantages noted above, but with less perioperative pain, less surgical dissection, and can be done as an outpatient procedure. The downside of this approach includes the demanding surgical technique and its relatively steep learning curve. One must be very patient and extremely facile with arthroscopic instrumentation in order to take on this procedure.

Contraindications

Arthroscopic arthrodesis is contraindicated in the presence of infection, or in the neuropathic joint. Relative contraindications include severe bony deformity in which tibiotalar alignment exceeds 15° or there is greater than 1 cm of translation in the sagittal plane. Bony defects or significant osteonecrosis greater than 30% of the talar or tibial area are also difficult to treat arthroscopically.

Technique

The patient is brought to the operative suite and placed supine on the table. Preoperative prophylactic antibiotics are administered within 1 h of incision time. A general anesthetic coupled with a paralyzing agent is useful for complete muscle relaxation. Otherwise a spinal, or regional, anesthetic is used. A thigh tourniquet is placed. The patients' leg is placed in an angled thigh holder, which elevates the leg and ankle off the table (Fig. 46.2). One should ensure that there is adequate clearance under the foot and ankle for maneuvering instrumentation during the case (Table 46.1). The limb is then prepped and draped. At this point, a commercially available ankle distractor can be used (Fig. 46.3). The ankle strap is attached to a sterile side post attached directly to the table. This can obviate the use of an assistant for distraction purposes. The limb is exsanguinated and the thigh tourniquet inflated.

A standard anteromedial portal is made with a #15-blade scalpel. This portal lies immediately medial to the tibialis anterior tendon (Fig. 46.4). The skin is incised and the soft

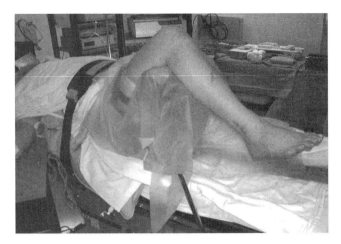

Fig. 46.2 A well-padded leg holder is placed under the thigh to suspend the ankle with room for instrumentation from the posterola-teral portal

Table 46.1 Instruments required for arthroscopic ankle arthrodesis

Thigh holder
Ankle distractor
30/70°, 2.7-mm, short arthroscope
Short, straight, and angled curettes
Short, straight, and angled open curettes
Arthroscopic elevator
Motorized shaver/burr

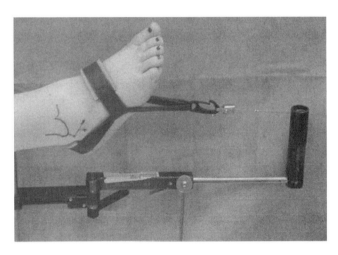

Fig. 46.3 A commercially available ankle distractor is available for autodistraction purposes

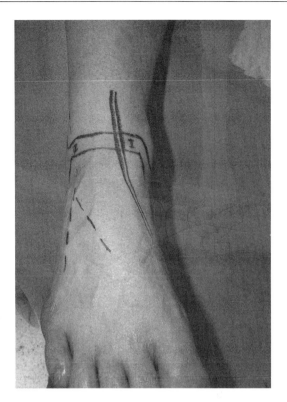

Fig. 46.4 The landmarks are noted on the anterior aspect of the ankle. Note the anteromedial portal just medial to the tibialis anterior tendon. The anterolateral portal lies just lateral to the peroneus tertius tendon and usually lies adjacent to the superficial branch of the peroneal nerve, visible just under the skin in most patients

tissues are spread down to the capsule with a mosquito clamp. The blunt obturator is angled approximately 30° laterally and the ankle joint is entered. Inflow can be accomplished through the scope or through a separate posterolateral portal. Gravity inflow can be used or alternatively the pump is usually set at 40 mmHg. At this point, often there is significant scarring and adhesions present precluding adequate visualization. The anterolateral portal is then established using a 23-gauge needle placed just lateral to the peroneus tertius muscle. Care is taken to avoid the branch of the superficial peroneal nerve, which often can be visualized just under the skin (Fig. 46.5). Proper placement of this portal is crucial. The needle should be visualized from inside the ankle and moved around, simulating instrument placement. The skin about the anterolateral ankle is then incised and the soft tissues are again spread down to the capsule. A larger blunt obturator will dilate the portal for future instrument passage (Fig. 46.6).

At this point, the anterior tibial osteophyte should be taken down with a motorized shaver or a burr. Care should be taken to point the instruments toward the ankle joint itself and not anteriorly, because significant bleeding can occur with disruption of the anterior neurovascular structure, obscuring visualization. An arthroscopic elevator, often found in the shoulder arthroscopic instruments, can be useful to elevate a capsule that is scarred down to the anterior aspect of the joint. An aggressive removal of anterior osteophytes, from the tibiofibular joint to the notch of Hardy is often required as one often under appreciates the extent of these spurs noted on preoperative radiographs. Extreme care and patience are required at this point of the procedure, because careful debridement at this point can make the remainder of the case significantly less difficult.

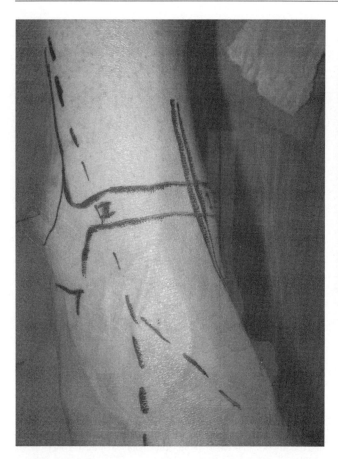

Fig. 46.5 A close up of the anterolateral portal lies adjacent to the superficial peroneal nerve branch

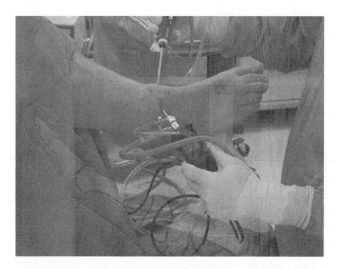

Fig. 46.6 The ankle joint is suspended allowing enough clearance for instrumentation

Next, the lateral gutter is debrided (Fig. 46.7). Curettes are used progressing from posterior to anterior, alternating with the shaver to remove extraneous debris and osteophytes. One should then be able to visualize the inferior fibula and anterior talofibular ligament. The portals are switched and a

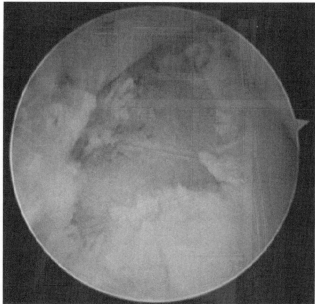

Fig. 46.7 The lateral ankle gutter often has significant scarring and cartilaginous debris, which needs to be cleared during the procedure

debridement of the medial ankle gutter is accomplished in a similar fashion. Again it can be helpful to use a posterolateral portal for inflow purposes in order to avoid *clogging* of the arthroscope or shaver with suction/irrigation. Once the debridement has been performed, which again often takes a significant amount of time, the remaining articular cartilage about the tibiotalar joint is removed. Open, curved curettes are useful for this step. Progressing posterior to anterior and from lateral to medial, on both sides of the joint, in a stepwise fashion is helpful. The portals are again switched and the cartilage removed from medial to lateral. The curettes are placed through the posterolateral portal and the posterior cartilage is removed. Any cystic defects are thoroughly debrided with a curette and shaver to remove fibrous tissue. The decision is then made as to whether a bone grafting procedure will need to be performed concurrently.

Once the damaged cartilage has been removed and the ankle joint lavaged, a motorized egg-shaped burr is used to remove 1–2 mm of sclerotic bone to a bleeding surface. This is done in the stepwise fashion noted above. The inflow can be turned off at this point to ensure an adequate amount of resection. If necessary, a 1.6-mm K wire can be used to create small perforations in the tibia and talus bone to act as channels for future vascular ingress and aid in healing. Use of the MICRO VECTOR drill guide (Smith & Nephew, Andover, MA) can aid in placement of this wire if done via a transtibial approach.

Once the joint has been debrided, guide wires from a large fragment cannulated screw set are placed. Through a 1-cm incision placed approximately 3–4 cm proximal to the joint line, one wire is placed medially and advanced just to the

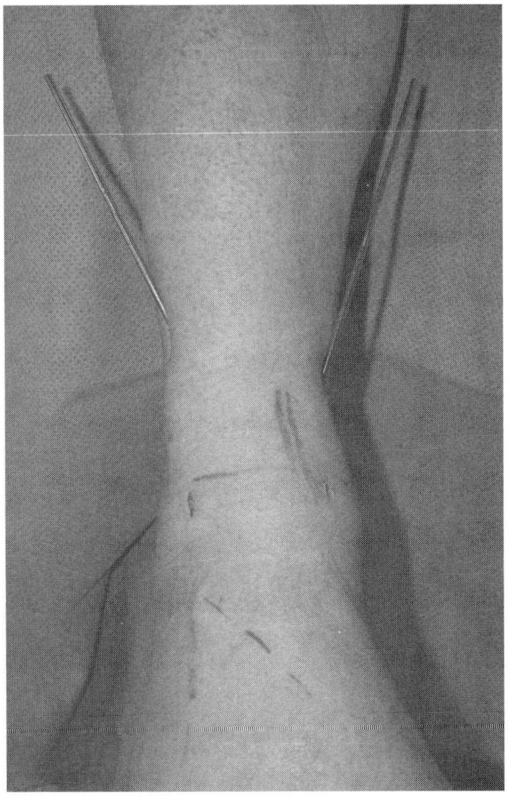

Fig. 46.8 Once the articular cartilage has been removed, two guide-wires are placed percutaneously, with the ankle in the proper position

articular surface. This wire should be aimed centrally or slightly posteriorly. A second wire is placed either through the fibula to the joint surface, or from the lateral tibia, aiming slightly anteriorly (Fig. 46.8). There is debate about the number of screws required and their placement. Most authors recommend at least a minimum of two screws with satisfactory purchase and placement. A third wire is preferred and is placed through an incision posteriorly, just lateral to the Achilles tendon, approximately 4 cm proximal to the joint line. This guidewire is advanced just to the articular surface aiming down the neck of the talus, slightly medially. The instruments are removed and the joint reduced. Reduction should be confirmed clinically in the appropriate position. That is, neutral in the sagittal plane, and neutral to 5° valgus in the coronal plane, with external rotation equivalent to the contralateral side (roughly 10°). At this point, inspection of the position of the hindfoot and limb alignment should be performed. The tibial crest should be in line with the second metatarsal and the hindfoot should be in slight valgus. One should not attempt to correct an extraarticular malalignment with compensation through the ankle joint. Rather, a calcaneal or supramalleolar osteotomy should be performed at this time.

Mini C-arm fluoroscopic views in the AP, oblique, and lateral planes are obtained. If any incongruency exists at this point, the instruments are reinserted and the surfaces smoothed. If at this point, alignment cannot be obtained, then the incisions should be extended and a formal "mini-open" procedure performed.

If the alignment is satisfactory, the joint is held reduced by an assistant and the pins are advanced. Again, proper length of the pins and alignment is confirmed fluoroscopically, taking care to avoid violation of the subtalar joint complex. Once confirmed, the 6.5- or 7.3-mm cannulated screws are placed. Excellent fixation should be accomplished. Final radiographs are then obtained again.

The portals are reapproximated with nylon sutures and a padded dressing with posterior and U-shaped splints are applied. A popliteal nerve block applied at this time (or pre-operatively) is helpful in postoperative analgesia.

The patient is instructed to elevate and ice the limb and remain nonweightbearing until the first postoperative visit at 10 days. At that time, the limb can be placed in a cast or a removable boot brace. The patient remains nonweightbearing for 6–8 weeks time and can begin weight bearing when swelling has resided and there are signs of radiographic consolidation (Fig. 46.9a, b).

Literature Review

Since the year 2000, the number of published reports noting the results of arthroscopic ankle arthrodesis has doubled. This highlights the push toward minimally invasive surgery advocated both by physicians experienced in this arena as well as the lay public. But are the results comparable to the traditional open experience, which as noted, has a long and reasonably satisfactory track record? While the nonunion rate of the traditional open procedure has been reported to occur in up to 41% of patients, recent reports note the nonunion rate to be in the 1–5% range.[1] Other disadvantages of the open approach include the significant soft tissue stripping required for the procedure as well as the discomfort associated with such an approach.

Myerson and Quill[6] retrospectively compared open versus arthroscopic arthrodesis in 33 patients. They noted a shortened time to fusion in the arthroscopic group (8.7 weeks) versus the open procedure (14.5 weeks). Additionally the fusion rate as well as the complication rate was similar in the two groups. O'Brien et al.[7] also retrospectively reviewed a group of patients who underwent an arthroscopic fusion procedure, noting similar fusion rates between the two groups. Both studies noted a shortened hospital stay in the arthroscopic group, but limitations included being retrospective in nature with a bias toward more difficult cases, i.e., those with more deformity, undergoing the open procedure.

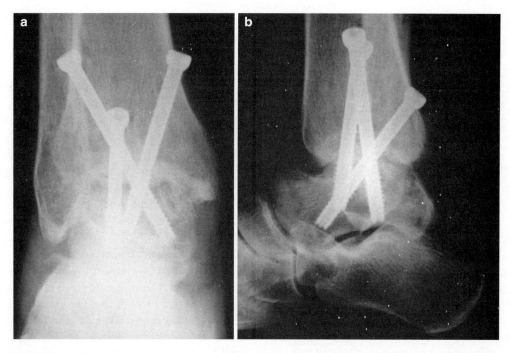

Fig. 46.9 (a) Final AP radiograph showing consolidation of the tibiotalar fusion site at 8 weeks. (b) Final lateral radiograph showing proper position of the screws placed during the arthroscopic procedure

Ferkel and Hewitt[8] reported on 35 patients who underwent the procedure at their institution, with a follow-up averaging 72 months. They noted the average time to fusion of 11.8 weeks and three delayed unions, with one requiring revision surgery. The most common complication was prominent hardware with 11 patients requiring screw removal. They noted 83% excellent or good results using a consistent (Mazur) scoring system. Glick et al.,[5] in a retrospective multicentered study, noted a 97% fusion rate at an 8-year follow-up study on 35 arthroscopic arthrodeses. Eighty-six percent of their patients were rated as good or excellent. Deformity greater than 15° and/or 1 cm of translation presented significant difficulties in achieving a good result.

While older literature reports noted prolonged union rates with a significant nonunion percentage in groups of patients treated with an arthroscopic approach to ankle fusion,[9–11] most recent reports have noted fusion rates of 90–95% with healing times between 8 and 12 weeks.[12–20] Complication rates appear to be similar to the open procedure, with nonunion, infection, prominent hardware, and thromboembolic event, among the most events noted.[10] The rate of radiographic hindfoot arthrosis has been reported to be high in the follow-up of patients with an ankle arthrodesis.[2] However, Winson et al.[16] have shown that this condition is probably present preoperatively in a significant number of patients, but that most do not need specific treatment for this condition at the index procedure.

Conclusion

As has been shown, the arthroscopic technique can be utilized in the arthrodesis of the ankle,[21–26] albeit with a reasonably steep learning curve. The results appear to be at least equivalent to the standard open procedure with the benefits of less perioperative pain and shorter hospitalization times. This procedure, similar to arthroscopic shoulder techniques, should increase in popularity in the future.

References

1. Monroe MT, Beals TC, Manoli A. Clinical outcome of arthrodesis of the ankle using rigid internal fixation with cancellous screws. Foot Ankle Int 20:227–231, 1999
2. Coester LM, Saltzman CL, Leupold J, Pontarelli W. Long-term results following ankle arthrodesis for post-traumatic arthritis. J Bone Joint Surg 83-A:219–228, 2001
3. Paremain GD, Miller SD, Myerson MS. Ankle arthrodesis: results after the miniarthrotomy technique. Foot Ankle Int 17:247–252, 1996
4. Schon LC, Ouzounian TJ. The ankle. In: Jahss MH (ed.). Disorders of the Foot and Ankle, Vol. 2, Edition 2. Philadelphia, WB Saunders, pp. 1417–1460, 1991
5. Glick JM, Morgan CD, Myerson MS, Sampson TG, Mann JA. Ankle arthrodesis using an arthroscopic method: long-term follow-up of 34 cases. Arthroscopy 12(4):428–434, 1996
6. Myerson MS, Quill G. Ankle arthrodesis. A comparison of an arthroscopic and an open method of treatment. Clin Orthop Relat Res 268:84–95, 1991

7. O'Brien TS, Hart TS, Shereff MJ, Stone J, Johnson J. Open versus arthroscopic ankle arthrodesis: a comparative study. Foot Ankle Int 20(6):368–374, 1999

8. Ferkel RD, Hewitt M. Long-term results of arthroscopic ankle arthrodesis. Foot Ankle Int 26(4):275–280, 2005

9. Dent CM, Patil M, Fairclough JA. Arthroscopic ankle arthrodesis. J Bone Joint Surg 75-B(5):830–832, 1993

10. Crosby LA, Yee TC, Formanek TS, Fitzgibbons TC. Complications following arthroscopic ankle arthrodesis. Foot Ankle Int 17(6):340–342, 1996

11. DeVriese L, Dereymaeker G, Fabry G. Arthroscopic ankle arthrodesis preliminary report. Acta Arthop Belg 60(4):389–392, 1994

12. Ogilvie-Harris DJ, Lieberman I, Fitsialos D. Arthroscopically assisted arthrodesis for osteoarthrotic ankles. J Bone Joint Surg 75-A(8): 1167–1174, 1993

13. Kats J, van Kampen A, de Waal-Malefijt MC. Improvement in technique for arthroscopic ankle fusion: results in 15 patients. Knee Surg Sports Traumatol Arthrosc 11:46–49, 2003

14. Turan I, Wredmark T, Felländer-Tsai L. Arthroscopic ankle arthrodesis in rheumatoid arthritis. Clin Orthop Relat Res 320:110–114, 1995

15. Zvijac JE, Lemak L, Schurhoff MR, Hechtman K, Uribe J. Analysis of arthroscopically ankle arthrodesis. Arthroscopy 18(1):70–75, 2002

16. Winson IG, Robinson DE, Allen PE. Arthroscopic ankle arthrodesis. J Bone Joint Surg 87-B(3):343–347, 2005

17. Cameron SE, Ullrich P. Arthroscopic arthrodesis of the ankle joint. Arthroscopy 16(1):21–26, 2000

18. Fisher RL, Ryan WR, Dugdale TW, Zimmermann GA. Arthroscopic ankle fusion. Conn Med 61(10):643–646, 1997

19. Corso SJ, Zimmer TJ. Technique and clinical evaluation of arthroscopic ankle arthrodesis. Arthroscopy 11(5):585–590, 1995

20. Fleiss DJ. Arthroscopic arthrodesis of the ankle joint. Arthroscopy 16(7)::788, 2000

21. Wasserman LR, Saltzman CL, Amendola A. Minimally invasive ankle reconstruction: current scope and indications. Orthop Clin North Am 35:247–253, 2004

22. Raikin SM. Arthrodesis of the ankle: arthroscopic, mini-open, and open techniques. Foot Ankle Clin 8(2):347–359, 2003

23. Stroud CC. Arthroscopic arthrodesis of the ankle, subtalar, and first metatarsophalangeal joint. Foot Ankle Clin 7(1):135–146, 2002

24. Tasto JP, Frey C, Laimans P, Morgan CD, Mason RJ, Stone JW. Arthroscopic ankle arthrodesis. Instr Course Lect 49:259–280, 2000

25. Fitzgibbons TC. Arthroscopic ankle debridement and fusion: indications, techniques, and results. Instr Course Lect 48:243–248, 1999

26. Stone JW. Arthroscopic ankle arthrodesis. Foot Ankle Clin 11(2): 361–368, 2006

Chapter 47
Endoscopic Calcaneoplasty

P.A.J. de Leeuw and C. Niek van Dijk

The first case of a patient with posterior heel pain, caused by hypertrophy of the posterosuperior part of the calcaneus in combination with wearing rigid low-back shoes, was described by Haglund in 1928.[1] Nowadays in Haglund's disease, we describe a clinical situation of tenderness and pain of the posterolateral aspect of the calcaneus. On physical examination, a bony prominence can be palpated at this location. This entity is described by a variety of different names such as "pump-bump,"[2] cucumber heel,[3] winter heel,[4] etc. In Haglund's syndrome, the retrocalcaneal bursa is inflamed and therefore swelled, sometimes in combination with insertional tendinopathy of the Achilles tendon. The syndrome is caused by repetitive impingement between the anterior aspect of the Achilles tendon and the enlarged posterosuperior aspect of the calcaneus. The patient typically describes the onset of pain when starting walking after a period of rest. Operative treatment consists of removal of the inflamed retrocalcaneal bursa and resection of the bony calcaneal prominence.

A distinction between Haglund's disease and other pathologic conditions of the posterior aspect of the heel, most importantly Achilles tendinitis, must be made. Achilles tendon pathology can be divided in insertional and noninsertional problems.[5,6] Noninsertional pathology can be divided into tendinopathy, paratendinopathy, or a combination of both. Symptoms typically occur 4–6 cm proximal of the insertion to the calcaneus. Insertional tendinopathy is defined as a tendinopathy of the tendon at its insertion. The pain is most frequently located in the midline at the insertion into the calcaneus. Coexistence with retrocalcaneal bursitis is known. In retrocalcaneal bursitis, as part of Haglund's syndrome, pain can be reproduced by palpating laterally and medially of the Achilles tendon at the level of the posterosuperior calcaneal prominence. With dorsiflexion of the ankle, the anterior part of the tendon impinges against the posterosuperior rim of the calcaneus, leading to retrocalcaneal bursitis.

In the cavus foot, the calcaneus is not only varus, but is also more vertical, which results in a more prominent projection posteriorly.[7]

Multiple treatments have been described to treat chronic retrocalcaneal bursitis. Conservative treatment of retrocalcaneal bursitis includes avoidance of tight shoe heel counters, nonsteroidal anti-inflammatory drugs, activity modification, the use of padding, physiotherapy, and a single injection with corticosteroids into the retrocalcaneal space. If the conservative treatment fails, there are basically two distinct operative methods and one endoscopic surgical treatment. The open operative alternatives include resection of the posterosuperior part of the calcaneus or a calcaneal wedge osteotomy. Complications include skin breakdown, tenderness around the operative scar, ugly operative scars, and altered sensation around the heel.[8–12] Complications that are more serious include Achilles tendon avulsions and calcaneal (stress) fractures.[10,12,13] Also recurrent persistent pain secondary to an inadequate amount of bone resected and stiffness of the Achilles tendon resulting in decreased dorsiflexion have been reported.[14] Wound-healing problems have been described in 30% of the patients treated with open procedures.[15]

Endoscopic treatment offers the advantages that are related to any minimal invasive surgical procedure, such as a low morbidity, excellent scar healing, functional aftertreatment, short recovery time, and quick sports consumption as compared with open surgical approaches. In this article we describe the technique of endoscopic calcaneoplasty and will compare the results of this minimal invasive technique[16] with those reported for the open surgical techniques.

Indication Endoscopic Calcaneoplasty

Patient complaints include pain at rest, when standing, (uphill) walking, running, and walking on hard surfaces. X-ray shows hypertrophy of the posterosuperior aspect of the calcaneus (Fig. 47.1). If conservative treatment fails, endoscopic surgery is indicated.

P.A.J. de Leeuw and C.N. van Dijk (✉)
Department of Orthopaedic Surgery, Academic Medical Centre,
University of Amsterdam, Amsterdam,
The Netherlands
e-mail: m.lammerts@amc.uva.nl

G.R. Scuderi and A.J. Tria (eds.), *Minimally Invasive Surgery in Orthopedics*,
DOI 10.1007/978-0-387-76608-9_47, © Springer Science + Business Media, LLC 2010

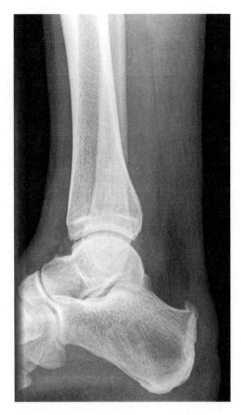

Fig. 47.1 Lateral X-ray of a right ankle in a patient with persistent posterior heel pain showing a hypertrophic posterosuperior calcaneal aspect (Haglund's syndrome)

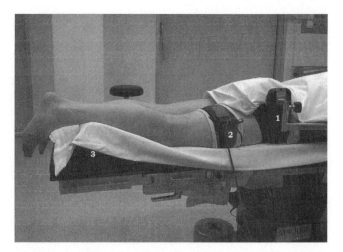

Fig. 47.2 For an endoscopic calcaneoplasty, the patient is placed in the prone position with a support in the hip (*1*), a tourniquet around the upper leg (*2*), and a small support is placed under the lower leg (*3*), making it possible to move the ankle freely

Surgical Technique

The operation is performed with the patient in the prone position under general or regional anaesthesia. The involved leg is marked by the patient with an arrow to avoid wrong-side surgery. The feet are positioned just at the edge of the operation table. The involved leg is slightly elevated by placing a small support under the lower leg (Fig. 47.2). The position of the foot is in plantarflexion through gravity. Dorsiflexion of the foot can be controlled by leaning into the plantarflexed foot with the surgeon's body, thereby still having both hands free to manipulate the arthroscope and instruments. Prior to the surgery, important anatomical structures are marked. These include the medial and lateral border of the Achilles tendon and the calcaneus. The lateral portal is situated just lateral of the Achilles tendon at the level of the superior aspect of the calcaneus. This portal is created first as a small vertical incision through the skin only. The retrocalcaneal space is penetrated by a blunt trocar. A 4.5-mm arthroscopic shaft with an inclination angle of 30° is introduced (Fig. 47.3a, b). Irrigation is performed by gravity flow or pressured flow at 100 mmHg. A 70° arthroscope can also be useful but is seldom necessary. Under direct vision, a

spinal needle is introduced just medial to the Achilles tendon, again at the level of the superior aspect of the calcaneus, to locate the medial portal (Fig. 47.4a, b). After having made the medial portal by a vertical stab incision, a 5.5-mm bonecutter shaver (Dyonics Bonecutter, Smith & Nephew, Andover, MA, USA) is introduced and visualized by the arthroscope. The inflamed retrocalcaneal bursa is removed first (Fig. 47.5a, b). Next, the superior surface of the calcaneus is visualized and its fibrous layer and periosteum are stripped off. During the resection of the bursa and the fibrous layer and periosteum of the superior aspect of the calcaneus, the full radius resector is facing the bone to avoid damage to the Achilles tendon. When the foot is brought into full dorsiflexion, impingement between the posterosuperior calcaneal edge and the Achilles tendon can be detected. The foot is subsequently brought into plantarflexion and now the posterosuperior calcaneal rim is removed. This bone is quite soft and can be removed by the aggressive synovial full radius resector or bonecutter. A burr is not needed at this point. The portals are used interchangeably for both the arthroscope and the resector, in order to remove the entire bony prominence. It is important to remove enough bone at the posteromedial and lateral corner (Fig. 47.6a, b). These edges have to be rounded off by moving the synovial resector beyond the posterior edge onto the lateral respectively medial wall of the calcaneus. The Achilles tendon is protected throughout the entire procedure by keeping the closed end of the resector against the tendon. With the foot in the fully plantarflexed position, the insertion of the Achilles tendon can be visualized. The bonecutter is placed on the insertion against the calcaneus to smoothen this part of the calcaneus. Finally, the resector is introduced to clean up loose debris and to smooth

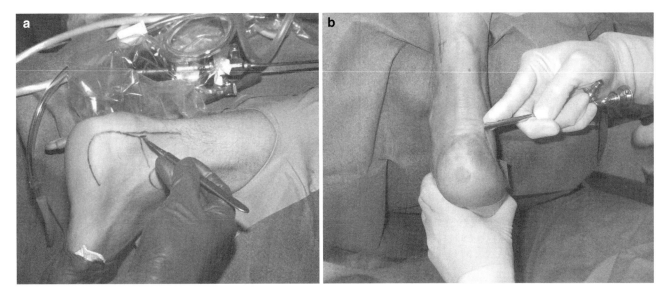

Fig. 47.3 (a) The lateral portal is situated just lateral of the Achilles tendon at the level of the superior border of the calcaneus. The important landmarks are indicated. (b) The portal is made by a vertical skin incision followed by introduction of a 4.5-mm arthroscopic shaft with an inclination angle of 30°

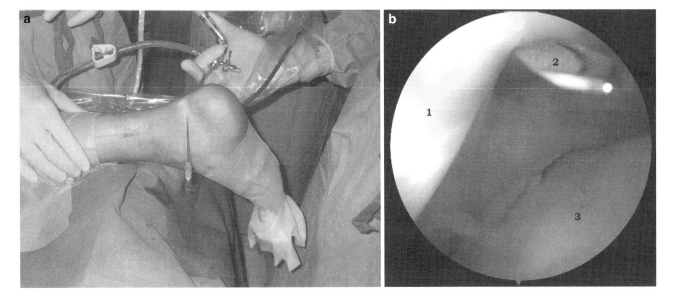

Fig. 47.4 (a) The exact position of medial portal is determined with a spinal needle that approximately needs to be introduced just medial of the Achilles tendon at the superior level of the calcaneus. (b) Under direct endoscopic view, the location of the spinal needle (at the location of medial portal) is checked. *1* Achilles tendon; *2* spinal needle; *3* calcaneus

possible rough edges (Fig. 47.6c). To prevent sinus formation, at the end of the procedure, the skin incisions are sutured with 3.0 Ethilon. The incisions and surrounding skin are injected with 10 ml of a 0.5% bupivacaine/morphine solution. A sterile compressive dressing is applied (Klinigrip, Medeco BV, Oud Bijerland, The Netherlands). Postoperatively, the patient is allowed weight bearing as tolerated and is instructed to elevate the foot when not walking. The dressing is removed 3 days postoperatively and the patient is allowed to shower. The patient is encouraged to perform active range of motion exercises for at least three times a day for 10 min each. The patient is allowed to return to regular footwear as soon as this is tolerated. Two weeks postoperatively, the stitches are removed. An X-ray is made to ensure that sufficient bone has been excised (Fig. 47.6d). With satisfaction of the surgeon and patient, no further outpatient department contact is necessary. Patients with limited range of motion are directed to a physiotherapist.

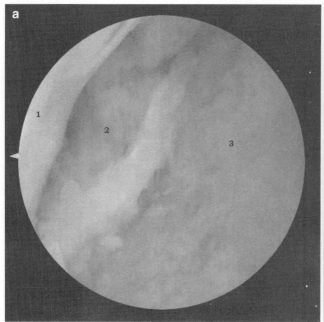
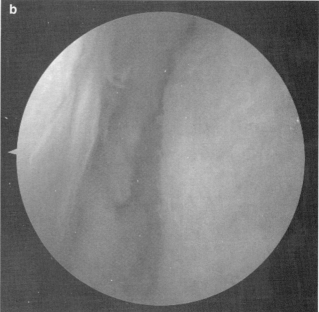

Fig. 47.5 (**a**) Endoscopic picture of the right ankle with the arthroscope in the posterolateral portal showing the inflamed retrocalcaneal bursa (*1* Achilles tendon; *2* inflamed retrocalcaneal bursa; *3* superior border calcaneus after partial resection). (**b**) Endoscopic picture after complete removal of the inflamed retrocalcaneal bursa with the full radius resector

Patient Outcomes

Between 1995 and 2000 in the Academic Medical Centre in Amsterdam, we performed 39 procedures in 36 patients. The average age was 35.0 years (range 16–50 years). Patients had a painful swelling of the soft tissue of the posterior heel, medial and lateral of the Achilles tendon on physical examination, without pain on palpation of the tendon itself. Conservative treatment for at least 6 months did not relieve the symptoms. The X-rays showed a superior calcaneal angle of more than 75°. The mean follow-up was 4.5 years (range 2–7.5 years). There were no surgical complications except from one patient who experienced an area of hypoaesthesia over the heel pad. Postoperatively, there were no infections, no sore or ugly scars, and all patients were happy with their small incisions. Except for two patients, all patients were improved. The Ogilvie-Harris score[17] for fair results was rated by 4 patients, 6 rated good, and 24 had an excellent result. Work and sports resumption took place at an average of 5 weeks (range 10 days–6 months) and 11 weeks (range 6 weeks to 6 months), respectively.

Discussion

Conservative therapy for retrocalcaneal bursitis includes a single cortisone injection in the retrocalcaneal bursa.[14,18,19] Repeated injections are not advised because these can weaken the tendon with the potential danger of a rupture. The aim of operative treatment for retrocalcaneal bursitis, after failure of the conservative treatment, is preventing impingement between the Achilles tendon and os calcis. This can be accomplished by means of removal of the inflamed retrocalcaneal bursa followed by either resection of the posterosuperior calcaneal rim or by means of a closing wedge osteotomy. Posterosuperior calcaneal resection can be performed via a posterolateral or posteromedial incision or via a combination of both.[8,11,20]

Endoscopic calcaneoplasty offers a good, minimal invasive, alternative to open surgery. Surgeons familiar with the endoscopic approach tend to favour this procedure, because it has better visualization as compared with the open procedure. Due to an inappropriate visualization of the Achilles tendon during the open procedure, weakening or even rupture of the tendon have been reported.[10,13] Full recovery time after the open resection can take as long as 2 years.[21] Our patient series shows a high percentage of good to excellent results based on the Ogilvie-Harris score. These results are comparable with the reports of Morag et al.[22] and Jerosch and Nasef.[23] Morag et al. treated four patients with endoscopic calcaneoplasty and after an average follow-up of 2 years (range 1–3.5 years) no complications, pain, decrease in range of motion, or disability were reported.[22] In the report of Jerosch and Nasef in 2003, ten patients were treated with the endoscopic calcaneoplasty approach and after a mean follow-up of 5.2 months (range 2–12 months); three patients rated good results and seven excellent, based on the Ogilvie-Harris score.

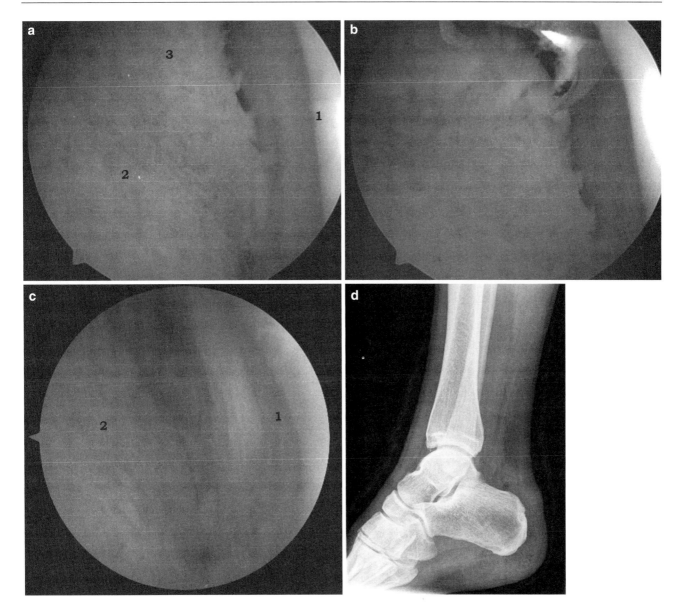

Fig. 47.6 (a) Endoscopic picture of the right ankle with the arthroscope in the posteromedial portal. Via the posteromedial portal, part of the bony prominence has been removed by means of a full radius resector (2). After switching portals, the bony prominence is now visualized (3) (1 Achilles tendon). (b) Shaver on top of the remaining bony promi-nence. The closed end of the resector is facing the Achilles tendon. (c) Situation after total resection of the bony prominence. (d) Postoperative lateral X-ray showing the result of the endoscopic calcaneoplasty oper-ation of the patient presented in Fig. 47.1

There were no intraoperative or postoperative complications. Full recovery lasted 2–5 weeks, except for two patients who did not follow the study protocol advising no weight bearing immediately after the surgery.[23]

The advantage of the endoscopic procedure over the open procedure are the small incisions, avoiding the complications such a wound dehiscence, painful and/or ugly scars, and nerve entrapment within the scar, as was described for the open procedure by Huber et al.[9] He found a considerable amount of residual complaints in 32 clinically and radiologically examined patients treated by resection of the posterosuperior calcaneal prominence for Haglund's exostoses at a mean follow-up of 18.6 years (range 2–41 years). Fourteen of the 32 patients had soft tissue problems including excessive scar formation and persistent swelling. In eight patients, not enough bone was excised and two had new bone formation, both resulting in persistent painful swelling. The function of the Achilles tendon was disturbed in eight patients.[9]

There is no consensus regarding the ideal surgical approach, medial, lateral, or both.[8,11,24] Jones and James performed ten partial calcaneal ostectomies for retrocalcaneal bursitis followed by a short walking cast and rehabilitation period for aftertreatment. All patients were back to their desired level of activity within 6 months.[24] Angermann operated on 40 heels for the same indication using the posterolateral approach in 32 patients. Postoperatively, 29 patients were allowed immediate weight bearing. Complications consisted of one superficial heel infection, one haematoma, and two patients with delayed skin healing. At an average follow-up of 6 years (range 1–12 years) 50% of the patients were cured, 20% improved, 20 remained unchanged, and in 10% the preoperative symptoms worsened.[8] The rate of poor results in this study corresponds to the results of Taylor, who reported 36% poor results after the same type of surgery.[25] Pauker et al. operated 28 heels in 22 patients with Haglund's disease. All patients received a walking cast for 4 weeks followed by mobilization exercises for aftertreatment. At a mean follow-up of 13 years in 19 patients (range 3–20 years), 15 had a good result, 2 fair, and 2 poor. The authors advocate using one incision, because many patients have complaints of tenderness over the operative scar up to 1 year postoperatively, which might be exaggerated by a more extensive approach.[11] In a study of Schepsis et al., 24 patients with retrocalcaneal bursitis 6 (25%) had a fair result requiring reoperation.[26] In the study of Schneider, 49 heels were operated from a consecutive group of 36 patients with a mean follow-up of 4.7 years (range 1–11 years). Early complications were reported in four cases (haematomas and a superficial infection) and late complications resulting in revision surgery in three cases. Seven patients noted some improvement, one patient described no change, and seven patients reported worsening of their symptoms after surgery.[27] Brunner et al. operated on 39 heels from 36 patients and reported at an average follow-up of 51 months, with an average improvement of the AOFAS score of 32 points as compared with the mean preoperative score. Recovery time took up from 6 months to 2 years. Six of the 36 patients reported persistent posterior heel pain after surgery.[21]

Because no consensus exists whether Haglund's deformity needs to be treated by endoscopy or by an open procedure, comparative studies were done. Leitze et al. compared the endoscopic approach ($n = 30$; 22 months follow-up) with the open surgical technique ($n = 17$; 42 months follow-up). The endoscopic approach revealed 19 excellent, 5 good, 3 fair, and 3 poor results, which was numerically but not significantly better than the open surgical procedure. The recovery time was identical, nevertheless the operation time and the amounts of complications and scar tissue favorite the endoscopic approach.[28] In the recent study of Lohrer et al., a comparison was made between the endoscopic and open resection for Haglund's disease. In this anatomic study, nine cadaver feet were operated on by means of open surgery and six were operated on with endoscopic calcaneoplasty. After the procedure, the feet were dissected to determine the amount of damage after surgery. Comparable amounts of damage were found for the sural nerve, the plantaris tendon, and the medial column of the Achilles tendon.[29] Since this is an anatomic study, no data could be gathered regarding recovery

time and scar healing, which seems to be the advantage points of the endoscopic procedure. In addition, the cadaver feet could have been stiffer as compared with patients, which makes the endoscopic approach more difficult to perform.

In summary, whether the operation is performed by endoscopic or open surgery, enough bone has to be removed to prevent impingement between the calcaneus and Achilles tendon. The endoscopic calcaneoplasty has demonstrated to show several advantages including low morbidity, functional aftertreatment, outpatient treatment, excellent scar healing, a short recovery time, and quick sports resumption as compared with the results for the open technique.

References

1. Haglund P. Beitrag zur Klinik der Achillessehne. Zeitschr Orthop Chir 1928; 49:49–58
2. Dickinson PH, Coutts MB, Woodward EP, Handler D. Tendo Achillis bursitis. Report of twenty-one cases. J Bone Joint Surg Am 1966; 48(1):77–81
3. Fowler A., Philip JF. Abnormalities of the calcaneus as a cause of painful heel: Its diagnosis and operative treatment. Br J Surg 1945; 32:494–498
4. NISBET NW. Tendo Achillis bursitis (winter heel). Br Med J 1954; 2(4901):1394–1395
5. Clain MR, Baxter DE. Achilles tendinitis. Foot Ankle 1992; 13(8):482–487
6. Saltzman CL, Tearse DS. Achilles tendon injuries. J Am Acad Orthop Surg 1998; 6(5):316–325
7. Fuglsang F, Torup D. Bursitis retrocalcanearis. Acta Orthop Scand 1961; 30:315–323
8. Angermann P. Chronic retrocalcaneal bursitis treated by resection of the calcaneus. Foot Ankle 1990; 10(5):285–287
9. Huber HM, Waldis M. [The Haglund exostosis - a surgical indication and a minor intervention?]. Z Orthop Ihre Grenzgeb 1989; 127(3):286–290
10. Miller AE, Vogel TA. Haglund's deformity and the Keck and Kelly osteotomy: a retrospective analysis. J Foot Surg 1989; 28(1):23–29
11. Pauker M, Katz K, Yosipovitch Z. Calcaneal ostectomy for Haglund disease. J Foot Surg 1992; 31(6):588–589
12. Leach RE, DiIorio E, Harney RA. Pathologic hindfoot conditions in the athlete. Clin Orthop Relat Res 1983; (177):116–121
13. Le TA, Joseph PM. Common exostectomies of the rearfoot. Clin Podiatr Med Surg 1991; 8(3):601–623
14. Nesse E, Finsen V. Poor results after resection for Haglund's heel. Analysis of 35 heels in 23 patients after 3 years. Acta Orthop Scand 1994; 65(1):107–109
15. Segesser B, Goesele A, Renggli P. [The Achilles tendon in sports]. Orthopade 1995; 24(3):252–267
16. van Dijk CN, van Dyk GE, Scholten PE, Kort NP. Endoscopic calcaneoplasty. Am J Sports Med 2001; 29(2):185–189
17. Ogilvie-Harris DJ, Mahomed N, Demaziere A. Anterior impingement of the ankle treated by arthroscopic removal of bony spurs. J Bone Joint Surg Br 1993; 75(3):437–440
18. Myerson MS, McGarvey W. Disorders of the Achilles tendon insertion and Achilles tendinitis. Instr Course Lect 1999; 48:211–218
19. Subotnick SI, Block AJ. Retrocalcaneal problems. Clin Podiatr Med Surg 1990; 7(2):323–332
20. Kolodziej P, Glisson RR, Nunley JA. Risk of avulsion of the Achilles tendon after partial excision for treatment of insertional

tendonitis and Haglund's deformity: a biomechanical study. Foot Ankle Int 1999; 20(7):433–437

21. Brunner J, Anderson J, O'Malley M, Bohne W, Deland J, Kennedy J. Physician and patient based outcomes following surgical resection of Haglund's deformity. Acta Orthop Belg 2005; 71(6): 718–723

22. Morag G, Maman E, Arbel R. Endoscopic treatment of hindfoot pathology. Arthroscopy 2003; 19(2):E13

23. Jerosch J, Nasef NM. Endoscopic calcaneoplasty – rationale, surgical technique, and early results: a preliminary report. Knee Surg Sports Traumatol Arthrosc 2003; 11(3):190–195

24. Jones DC, James SL. Partial calcaneal ostectomy for retrocalcaneal bursitis. Am J Sports Med 1984; 12(1):72–73

25. Taylor GJ. Prominence of the calcaneus: is operation justified? J Bone Joint Surg Br 1986; 68(3):467–470

26. Schepsis AA, Wagner C, Leach RE. Surgical management of Achilles tendon overuse injuries. A long-term follow-up study. Am J Sports Med 1994; 22(5):611–619

27. Schneider W, Niehus W, Knahr K. Haglund's syndrome: disappointing results following surgery – a clinical and radiographic analysis. Foot Ankle Int 2000; 21(1):26–30

28. Leitze Z, Sella EJ, Aversa JM. Endoscopic decompression of the retrocalcaneal space. J Bone Joint Surg Am 2003; 85-A(8):1488–1496

29. Lohrer H, Nauck T, Dorn NV, Konerding MA. Comparison of endoscopic and open resection for haglund tuberosity in a cadaver study. Foot Ankle Int 2006; 27(6):445–450

Chapter 48
Arthroscopy of the First Metatarsophalangeal Joint

Nicholas Savva and Terry Saxby

Attempts to arthroscope small joints in the 1930s failed due to the disparity in size between the arthroscope and joint. In 1968, a new light-emitting material known as Selfoc was developed jointly by the Nippon Sheet Glass Company, Osaka and the Nippon Electrical Company, Tokyo. In 1970, the Selfoc arthroscope was developed for arthroscopy of small joints by Watanabe using a Selfoc glass rod. The gauge of the scope was 1.7 mm and the outer diameter of the sheath was 2 mm. The first report of arthroscopy of the first metatarsophalangeal (MTP) joint was by Watanabe reporting on five cases in his book titled *Atlas of Arthroscopy* published in 1972.[1]

Anatomy

The first MTP joint is a ball and socket joint, which gains little support from its shallow articulation. The major stabilising elements are the capsule and the medial and lateral collateral ligaments. Abductor and adductor hallucis and the short flexor and extensor tendons contribute to stability. Most of the stabilizing structures are on the plantar aspect making the dorsum the obvious choice for portal placement. The dominant landmark on the dorsum is the extensor hallucis longus (EHL) (Fig. 48.1).

The metatarsal head has the central crista on its plantar surface. Both tendons of flexor hallucis brevis contain a sesamoid bone, which sit either side of the crista. The tendons then go on to insert into the base of the proximal phalanx as well as sending fibres to the thick plantar plate. The flexor hallucis longus is both superficial to the plantar plate and between the two heads of the flexor hallucis brevis as it passes distally to insert into the distal phalanx.

Structures most at risk during arthroscopy are cutaneous nerves, principally the dorsomedial branch of superficial peroneal, which provides much of sensation of hallux. It passes 6–18 mm medial to the EHL at the level of the joint.[2] The plantar aspect is supplied by the digital nerves, which are branches of the medial plantar nerve. These lie just plantar to the collateral ligaments and superficial to the transverse metatarsal ligament on the lateral side.

Arthroscopic Anatomy

Ferkel has described a systematic sequential examination of the MTP joint starting laterally and progressing medially.[3] He developed a 13-point examination through the dorsolateral portal. The structures of the plantar surface, including the sesamoids as well as the centre of the metatarsal head may be better visualised through the dorsomedial or direct medial portal.

1. Lateral gutter
2. Lateral corner of metatarsal head
3. Central portion of metatarsal head
4. Medial corner of metatarsal head
5. Medial gutter
6. Medial capsular reflection
7. Central bare area
8. Lateral capsular reflection
9. Medial portion of proximal phalanx
10. Central portion of proximal phalanx
11. Lateral portion of proximal phalanx
12. Medial sesamoids
13. Lateral sesamoid

Indications

Plain radiographs, bone scans, and computed tomography (CT) scans are all useful investigations in the diagnosis of first MTP joint pathology. Magnetic resonance imaging (MRI) of the first MTP joint has improved considerably in the last 10 years, rendering diagnostic arthroscopy almost obsolete. However, a diagnostic arthroscopy may be performed if persistent pain, swelling, stiffness, and locking or grinding symptoms continue despite conservative treatment.

N. Savva and T. Saxby (✉)
Foot and Ankle Surgery, Brisbane Private Hospital, 259 Wickham Terrace, BrisbaneQLD 4000, Australia

G.R. Scuderi and A.J. Tria (eds.), *Minimally Invasive Surgery in Orthopedics*,
DOI 10.1007/978-0-387-76608-9_48, © Springer Science + Business Media, LLC 2010

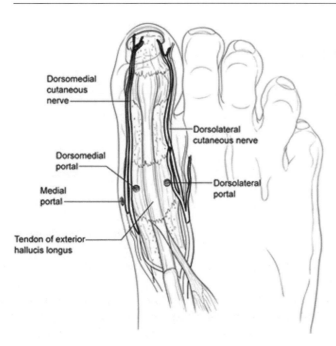

Fig. 48.1 Dorsal view of portals. Note the relative position of portals to the extensor hallucis longus tendon and the neurovascular structures

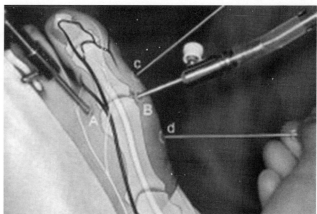

Fig. 48.2 The 1.9-mm 30° arthroscope and finger trap

Portals

Three portals are commonly used to visualise the joint (Fig. 48.1). The dorsomedial portal is placed just medial to the tendon of EHL at the level of the joint. This is placed close to the tendon to avoid injury to the dorsomedial branch of the superficial peroneal nerve. The dorsolateral portal is placed just lateral to the tendon of EHL and the medial portal, midway between the dorsal and plantar aspects of the joint. This can be done under direct vision if necessary.

Technique

Arthroscopy of the first MTP joint can be carried out under general, spinal, epidural, or local anaesthesia. The patient is placed supine on the operating table and with skin preparation applied to the level of the knee with standard draping. Distraction is helpful to allow full visualisation, although manual traction has been reported as being adequate to visualise the whole joint. A sterile finger trap is applied to the great toe and a pulley system rigged over the shoulder traction system. Two to three kilograms of traction is usually ample to allow full visualisation of the joint (Fig. 48.3). A 23-gauge needle is inserted into the joint just medial to the tendon of EHL at the level of the joint. The joint is then distended with normal saline. A second needle is then placed into the joint just lateral to the tendon of EHL at the level of the joint. When free flow has been established (Fig. 48.4), longitudinal incisions are made through the skin only using a #15 blade. Small artery forceps are then used to spread soft tissues and identify the capsule. This minimises risk of injury to neurovascular structures, in particular, the dorsomedial cutaneous nerve close to the dorsomedial portal. The capsule is penetrated through either portal using a 2-mm cannula with a blunt-tipped obturator and the arthroscope is introduced. A 2-mm probe is inserted

Therapeutic indications include treatment of chondromalacia, synovitis, osteochondral lesions, osteophytes, loose bodies, and arthrofibrosis. More recently, cheilectomy has been described for hallux rigidus.[4] The technique of arthroscopically assisted arthrodesis has also been described, although it was noted to be time consuming and technically difficult.[5,6] Arthroscopic excision of the medial and lateral sesamoids has also been described but may require extra portals or a small arthrotomy.[7–9]

Equipment

Because of the small size of the joint, a small arthroscope is required (Fig. 48.2). Ideally, a short 1.9-mm arthroscope with a 30° oblique viewing lens is used. Great care should be taken because this is a very fragile instrument. If this is not available, a 2.7-mm scope is acceptable but much more difficult to manoeuvre.

    Shoulder traction system
    Thigh tourniquet
    Sterile finger trap
    1.9-mm 30° arthroscope
    Small joint shaver system
    2-mm probe
    2-mm curette
    Small joint grasper
    Two 23-gauge needles
    10-cc syringe

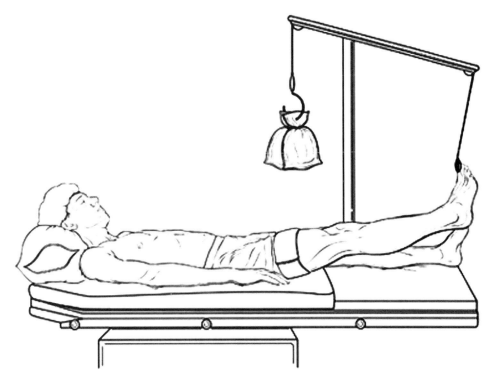

Fig. 48.3 Patient on an operating table with a tourniquet in place and great toe suspended from finger trap. A suspension gantry is fixed to the opposite side of the operating table

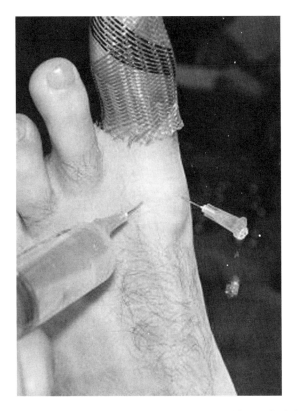

Fig. 48.4 Two 23-gauge needles, correctly placed intraarticularly, demonstrated by the free flow of normal saline

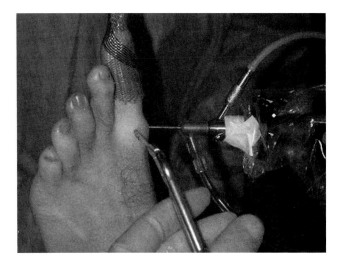

Fig. 48.5 Arthroscope and instrument successfully placed into the joint

through the other dorsal portal. The medial portal can be made under direct vision to ensure correct placement, which is helpful to view the plantar structures and also to avoid injury to the digital nerve. Arthroscope and instruments are swapped around the portals during the procedure to aid visualisation and allow access to pathology (Fig. 48.5).

After the procedure is completed, the joint is washed out, instilled with local anaesthetic, and the wounds closed with 4-0 nylon sutures. A bulky dressing is applied. Postoperatively, the patient is encouraged to elevate the limb to reduce swelling and the risk of infection. Patients are allowed to mobilise in a stiff-soled shoe until approximately 10 days, when the wound is reviewed and sutures removed. Mobilisation then depends upon the pathology treated. If a fusion has been undertaken, then the patient is mobilised in the shoe for a further 4–5 weeks, otherwise range of motion and strengthening exercises are started as comfort allows.

Results

The first report of arthroscopy of the first MTP joint was by Watanabe reporting on five cases in his book titled *Atlas of Arthroscopy* published in 1972.[1] The results of the first series of 22 arthroscopies of the first MTP joint were reported by Watanabe in his book *Equipment and Procedures of Small Joint Arthroscopy* published in 1986.[10] In the same year, Yovich and McIlwraith reported arthroscopic debridement of osteochondral defects in the MTP joint of the horse.[11] In 1988, Bartlett described debridement of an osteochondral lesion of the first MTP joint in an adolescent that allowed return to sport and complete resolution of symptoms at 1 year.[12] Since these first reports, there have been four case series reported and numerous case reports.

In his book titled *Arthroscopic Surgery: The Foot and Ankle* published in 1996, Ferkel described the technique and indications of first MTP joint arthroscopy.[3] He also reported on 22 patients who underwent the procedure with follow-up at a mean of 54 months. The following pathologies were identified.

Degenerative joint disease	5
Arthrofibrosis	4
Synovitis	3
Osteophytes	3
Osteochondral lesions of the metatarsal	3
Loose bodies	2
Chondromalacia	2

Good results were found in 73% of patients, with the remainder going on to arthrodesis. For most patients who had a limited movement preoperatively, the range of motion was improved by surgery. There were no specific complications.

In 1987, Iqbal and Chana reported on 15 patients, with a mean follow-up of 9.4 months, who underwent arthroscopic cheilectomy for hallux rigidus.[4] All patients were at least satisfied with the outcome with complete resolution of pain in two thirds of the patients. Return to nonathletic activity at an average of 3.7 weeks shows an advantage over the open technique, but a mean postoperative range of movement of 47.6° is less than might be expected after an open procedure. In some cases, an inferomedial portal was required to fully access the osteophyte. It was also noted that distraction was not beneficial because this tightened the dorsal capsule over the osteophyte, making its excision more difficult. There were no complications in this series.

In 1998, van Dijk et al. published their review of 25 first MTP joint arthroscopies at a mean of 2 years.[9] Twelve procedures were performed for dorsal impingement with removal of the dorsal osteophyte arthroscopically, of which eight had a good or excellent result. Three of four patients treated for osteochondritis dissecans by debridement of the lesion and removal of loose bodies had good or excellent results. Treatment of hallux rigidus by debridement of osteophytes was less successful. Five patients had sesamoid pathology warranting excision, of which, three gained good or excellent results. Two extra portals were necessary, one proximal and in the medial midline and one in the first dorsal web space. Two patients had the lateral sesamoid removed arthroscopically but a small separate incision was required to remove the medial sesamoids in three patients. Overall in this series, one patient suffered transient loss of sensation on the medial aspect of the hallux and one other patient on the lateral side, which continued to follow-up.

In the author's series of 12 arthroscopies in 11 patients, 6 patients had suffered an injury.[13] In six patients, there was no radiological abnormality detected on plain radiography but isotope, CT, and MRI bone scans were helpful in some cases. The true diagnosis was only established at arthroscopy in some cases. At arthroscopy, seven joints were noted to have synovitis, including one case of pigmented villonodular synovitis (PVNS). A chondral lesion was noted in four cases and an osteochondral lesion of the metatarsal head was found in four joints (Figs. 48.6 and 48.7). There was one dorsal osteophyte, one proximal phalangeal cyst, one loose body, and one meniscoid lesion (Fig. 48.8). The latter lesion was thought to be a condensation of fibrous tissue akin to the soft tissue lesion in the ankle described by Wolin et al.[14] All pathologies were dealt with arthroscopically at the time. In three cases, a small arthrotomy was required to complete the surgical procedure. In one case, early on in the series, an arthrotomy was performed to exclude other pathology, none was found. On another occasion, an arthrotomy was performed due to equipment failure and on another to complete an extensive synovectomy. Apart from a minor wound infection, there were no complications relating to surgery. At a mean of 19.3 months, all patients had minimal or no pain with an increased range of movement. The one patient who had residual stiffness was known to have degenerative joint disease and had fractured a dorsal osteophyte.

Arthroscopy of the first MTP joint has a small but well-defined role in the armamentarium of the foot surgeon. It is indicated in patients with persistent pain, swelling, stiffness,

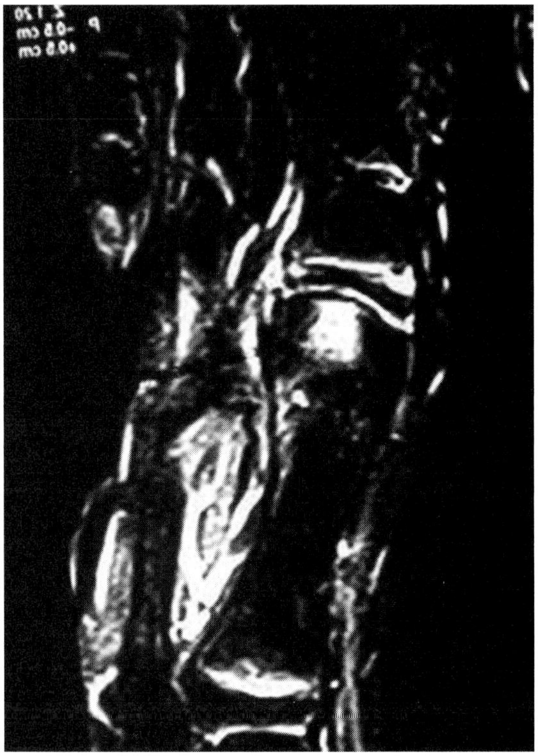

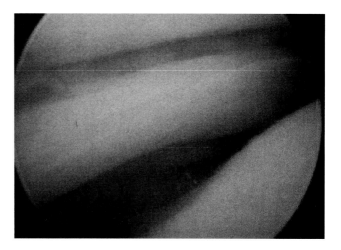

Fig. 48.8 Meniscoid lesion (From Davies and Saxby,[13] by permission of J Bone Joint Surg (Br).)

the open procedure. Dealing with sesamoid pathology is also technically demanding and may require extra portals.

References

1. Watanabe M, Takeda S, Ikeuchi H. Atlas of Arthroscopy, 2nd edition. Igakui-Shoin, Tokyo, 1969
2. Solan MC, Lemon M, Bendall PS. The surgical anatomy of the dorsomedial cutaneous nerve of the hallux. J Bone Joint Surg Br 2001; 83B: 250–252
3. Ferkel RD. Arthroscopic Surgery. The Foot and Ankle. Lippincott-Raven, Philidelphia. 1996
4. Iqbal MJ, Chana GS. Arthroscopic cheilectomy for hallux rigidus. J Arthrosc Relat Surg 1998; 14: 307–310
5. Perez Carro L, Busta Vallina B. Arthroscopic-assisted first metatarsophalangeal joint arthrodesis. J Arthrosc Relat Surg 1999; 15: 215–217
6. Stroud CC. Arthroscopic arthrodesis of the ankle, subtalar, and first metatarsophalangeal joint. Foot Ankle Clin N Am 2002; 7: 135–146
7. Chan PK, Lui TH. Arthroscopic fibular sesamoidectomy in the management of the sesamoid osteomyelitis. Knee Surg Sports Traumatol Arthrosc 2005; 14: 1–4
8. Perez Carro L, Escevarria Llata JI, Martinez Agueros JA. Arthroscopic medial bipartite sesamoidectomy of the great toe. J Arthrosc Relat Surg 1999; 15: 321–323
9. van Dijk CN, Veenstra KM, Nuesch BC. Arthroscopic surgery of the metatarsophalangeal first joint. J Arthrosc Relat Surg 1998; 14: 851–855
10. Watanabe M, Ito K, Fuji S. Equipment and procedures of small joint arthroscopy. In: Watanabe M (ed.) Arthroscopy of Small Joints. Igakui-Shoin, Tokyo. 1986
11. Yovich JV, McIlwraith CW. Arthroscopic surgery for osteochondral fractures of the proximal phalanx o the metacarpophalangeal and metatarsophalangeal fetlock) joints in horses. J Am Vet Med Assoc 1986; 188: 273–279
12. Bartlett DH. Arthroscopic management of osteochondritis of the first metatarsal head. Arthroscopy 1988; 4: 51–54
13. Davies MS, Saxby TS. Arthrosopy of the first metatarsophalangeal joint. J Bone Joint Surg Br 1999; 81B: 203–206
14. Wolin J, Glassman F, Sideman S. Internal derangement of the talofibular component of the ankle. Surg Gynaecol Obstet 1950; 91: 193–200

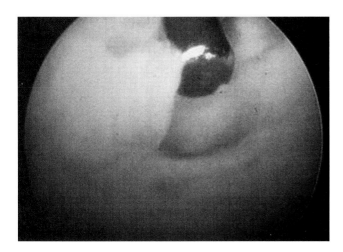

Fig. 48.6 MRI scan of an osteochondral lesion of the metatarsal head

Fig. 48.7 Intraoperative photograph of an osteochondral lesion of the metatarsal head (From Davies and Saxby,[13] by permission of J Bone Joint Surg (Br).)

and locking or grinding symptoms despite conservative measures and in whom the diagnosis is not clear. It can be used to treat multiple pathologies including chondromalacia, synovitis, osteochondral lesions, osteophytes, loose bodies, and arthrofibrosis, particularly in those whose symptoms do not warrant arthrodesis or arthroplasty. Arthroscopic arthrodesis and cheilectomy for hallux rigidus have been demonstrated to be effective but technically demanding procedures, but have yet to demonstrate any significant advantage over

Chapter 49
Arthroscopic Management of Disorders of the First Metatarsal–Phalangeal Joint

A.C. Stroïnk and C.N. van Dijk

Arthroscopic surgery is one of the basic types of procedures in orthopaedic surgery. In the 1980s, there was a drift toward performing arthroscopic procedures on smaller joints.[1-4] Although nowadays arthroscopic surgery of the knee, shoulder, elbow, ankle, and wrist have become routine procedures, arthroscopy of the first metatarsophalangeal (MTP-I) joint has received scant attention[5] and has scarcely been reported in articles. Watanabe[1] was the first to describe an arthroscopic procedure of the big toe in 1986. In 1999, Frey et al.[6] reported that arthroscopic surgery of the MTP-I was still a developing procedure with a grey area for application. We published our first 27 MTP-I joint arthroscopic procedures in 1998, and, in a further publication, we reported the most important indications: osteochondral defect, dorsal impingement, and infectious arthritis.[7] Currently, we lack evidence based on long-term follow-up studies on arthroscopic surgery of the MTP-I joint. After all these years, the procedure is still considered investigational. Although the arthroscopic procedure of the MTP-I joint is technically feasible and amenable for arthroscopy, the procedure is dependent on the skills of the surgeon. In this chapter, we describe the basic anatomy of the joint, the indication, the arthroscopic procedure, and the outcome.

Anatomy

Marked variations occur in the skin and the subcutaneous tissue of the foot. The skin on the dorsal side is less sensitive and much thinner in comparison with the plantar side. The majority of the stability of the MTP-I joint is obtained by the soft tissues surrounding the joint, such as the capsule, the ligaments, and the musculotendinous structures. A minor stability contribution is obtained from the shallow ball of the distal metatarsal head and the socket form of the proximal

phalanx.[6] From the dorsal view of the joint, the extensor hallucis longus tendon divides the joint into a medial and a lateral part. The medial part of the joint is innervated by branches of the superficial peroneal nerve and the lateral part of the joint by the deep peroneal nerve. The medial side of the great toe is innervated by the terminal branches of the saphenous nerve. The plantar blood supply is from the medial and lateral plantar artery, which are branches of the posterior tibial artery. They form anastomoses with the vessels from the dorsal side, which have their origin from the dorsalis pedis artery.

The MTP-I joint has two sesamoid bones at the plantar side, which are situated on the medial and lateral side of the flexor hallucis brevis tendon. The fibres of this tendon are subsequently attached to the plantar plate and the proximal part of the proximal phalanx. The superficial tendon of the hallucis longus tendon is situated between the two tendons of the flexor hallucis brevis.

Indications

Along with the development of the arthroscopic technique and the instrumentation of the arthroscopic equipment, it is important to understand the relative advantage of the arthroscopic surgery of the MTP-I joint; meanwhile, it should be kept in mind that arthroscopic surgery is a patient-centred procedure.

Open surgery of the first metatarsophalangeal joint can result in restriction of range of motion, prolonged swelling, poor wound healing, and difficulties finding footwear.[6] The arthroscopic approach results in a good intraarticular visualization, minimal surgical joint trauma, and minimal soft tissue dissection, with excellent cosmetic and functional results.[7,8] Another advantage of the arthroscopic procedure is a faster rehabilitation to sports and work. The indications of the arthroscopic procedure of the MTP-I joint are listed in Table 49.1. For pathology of the medial sesamoid bone, the arthroscopic procedure of the MTP-I joint does not have any great advantages compared with the more conservative techniques.

A.C. Stroïnk and C.N. van Dijk (✉)
Department of Orthopaedic Surgery, Academic Medical Center,
University of Amsterdam, Amsterdam,
The Netherlands
e-mail: m.lammerts@amc.uva.nl

G.R. Scuderi and A.J. Tria (eds.), *Minimally Invasive Surgery in Orthopedics*,
DOI 10.1007/978-0-387-76608-9_49, © Springer Science+Business Media, LLC 2010

Table 49.1 Indications for arthroscopy of the MTP-I joint.

Dorsal osteophytes
    Hallux limitus
    Hallux rigidus
Osteochondritis dissecans/chondromalacia
    Corpora libera
    Impingement syndrome
Pathology of the sesamoid bone
Inflammation/infection
    Arthritis
    Synovitis
Diagnostic procedure

Operative Technique

The arthroscopic procedure can be performed under spinal, general, or regional anaesthesia, using a tourniquet at the homolateral thigh. The patient is placed in the operating room in the supine position with the heel resting on the edge of the operation table.[7] To improve the joint space and to give the best direction of traction, a sterile finger trap is placed on the first toe and connected to the belt of the surgeon (Fig. 49.1).

For the majority of procedures, enough working space is created with two main portals; a dorsolateral portal and a dorsomedial portal, these accessory portals are placed at the level of the joint line on either side of the extensor hallucis longus tendon.[7]

A complete overview of the first metatarsophalangeal joint is attained by the insertion of two extra portals, the true medial portal and the proximal plantar portal, which are placed at the joint line midway between the dorsal and plantar side of the foot. The proximal plantar portal is placed 4 cm proximal to the joint line in between the flexor hallucis brevis and the flexor hallucis longus (Fig. 49.2).

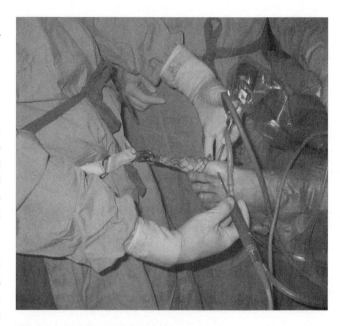

Fig. 49.1 Position during surgery

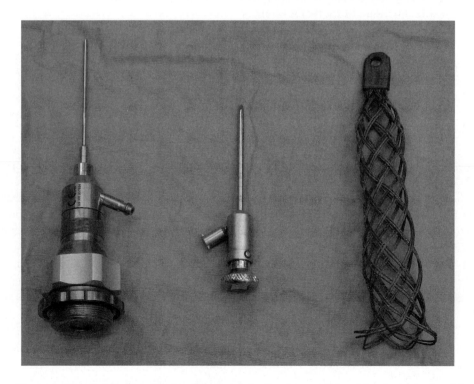

Fig. 49.2 Insertion of the two main portals (**a**, **b**) and the two extra portals (**c**, **d**). **a** dorsomedial portal; **b** dorsolateral portal; **c** true medial portal; **d** proximal plantar

The operation starts by placing the dorsomedial portal, just medial from the extensor hallucis longus tendon. Before placing the portals, a 4-mm longitudinal, through the skin only, stab incision is made. To prevent neurovascular injury, especially of the medial dorsal cutaneous branch of the superficial peroneal nerve, the subcutaneous layer is divided by a haemostat until the capsule is identified.

The 2.7-mm shaft with blunt trocar is introduced into the joint, followed by the 2.7-mm arthroscope with a 30° inclination angle. The joint is distended with saline. The clarity can be enhanced by a high-flow system of normal saline. After achieving visualisation of the joint, the remaining portals can be introduced by using a spinal needle under direct vision.

The working instruments are situated in the dorsomedial portal and the arthroscopic examination is performed through the dorsolateral portal. The nine major areas that should be inspected are the lateral and medial gutter; the lateral and medial corner and the central portion of the metatarsal head; the medial, central, and lateral portion of the proximal phalanx; and the medial sesamoid bone. For inspection of the lateral sesamoid bone, the two additional portals are necessary. A basic list of required instruments is listed in Table 49.2.

A dorsal osteophyte of the metatarsal head is best visualized by bringing the MTP-I joint into dorsal flexion. Subsequently, they can be removed, working from distal to proximal and from medial to lateral, by the abrader, shaver, or a small acromionizer. To improve the range of motion, up to one third of the articular surface can be eliminated.[6] Before removing the osteophyte, the finger trap should be unstressed to prevent the capsule from pulling against the osteophyte.[6]

In case of a large osteophyte, it is recommended to convert the operation to an open cheilectomy.

The arthroscopic cheilectomy can be performed through the two main portals. In the presentation of osteochondritis dissecans or a corpora libra, the defect is curetted and debrided until a bleeding surface is exposed; subsequently, the loose fragments are removed (Fig. 49.3). When the lateral sesamoid bone needs to be resected, the two additional portals, as described above, are mandatory.

In case of an infection of the MTP-I joint, the arthroscopic procedure allows differentiation between arthritis, synovitis, and osteitis; material for culture should be collected. The infected synovia will be treated by a shaver or a whisker. When arthritis is present, drainage through the system should be performed, whereupon the joint should be rinsed with saline.

Table 49.2 List of required equipment for arthroscopy of the first metatarsophalangeal joint.

2.7-mm arthroscope (30°)
Blunt trocar
Blade (No. 11)
Haemostat
Mosquito clamp
Shaver system
Acromionizer
Spinal needle
Thigh/ankle tourniquet
Sterile finger trap
Belt
Saline

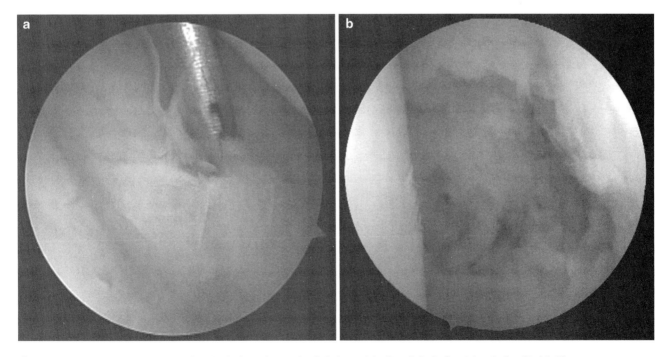

Fig. 49.3 Osteochondritis dissecans of the basis from the proximal phalanx of the first digit. Before (**a**) and after (**b**) debridement

A diagnostic arthroscopic procedure of the MTP-I joint is indicated in the following situations: presentation of recurrent inflammatory symptoms, with locking complaints, which have failed to respond to any conservative treatment;[6] or appearance of swelling, persistent pain, and a reduced range of motion without any improvement after conservative treatment in patients who are classified as "too good" for arthrodesis or arthroplasty.[5]

After the procedure, the small portal wounds are closed with 4/0 nylon sutures, which can be removed 10–14 days after the operation. To prevent formation of fistula, a bulky dressing is placed for 4–7 days and the patient is given two elbow crutches. Normal shoe wearing is resumed as comfort and swelling allows.[5] After removing a dorsal osteophyte, the patient starts flexion–extension exercises immediately after the operation, and weight bearing is permitted 5 days after surgery.[6] After debridement of the joint, the range of motion exercises are started 5 days after the operation and the patient is allowed full weight bearing 14 days after the intervention.

Complications

Similar to other arthroscopic operations, the arthroscopic procedure of the MTP-I joint can be complicated by an infection or a fistula formation. However, the most specific complication is a (transient) loss of sensation on the medial or lateral side of the first toe, induced by neurapraxia or compression of the peroneus profundus nerve.[5]

Results

We performed 27 arthroscopic procedures,[7,9] concluding that the main diagnosis for this procedure are: osteochondritis dissecans, infectious arthritis, dorsal impingement syndrome, and removal of pathologic sesamoid bone. For patients with a dorsal impingement syndrome, the arthroscopic procedure gives good relief of symptoms and increased range of motion.

In 1998, Iqbal et al.[10] compared 15 patients with an arthroscopic cheilectomy with previous results from the open procedure. Their main outcomes were the recurrence rate of exostosis, which was 10% in the open procedure, compared with none in their arthroscopic cheilectomy series.

Compared with the arthrotomy, an arthroscopic approach provides a better assessment of the intraarticular conditions of the MTP-I joint.[8] However, the open procedure causes more extensive soft tissue dissection and disruption of ligamentous and tendinous structures around the sesamoid bones, which may result in hallux varus and cock-up deformity.[8]

Other chief advantages of the arthroscopic procedure is the shorter revalidation period with a faster resumption of sports and work;[9,10] excision methods appear to allow a shorter hospitalisation, less postoperative pain and stiffness, and a better cosmetic result.[7]

Discussion

Arthroscopy of the MTP-I gives an excellent view of the joint. The main indications are treatment of osteochondritis dissecans, removal of loose bodies, and removal of dorsal osteophytes in cases of dorsal impingement syndrome. Intraarticular evaluation in patients with persistent pain and swelling despite conservative therapy is another indication for performing a diagnostic procedure (recurrent inflammatory symptoms and locking complaints, failure of conservative treatment; persistent swelling and reduced range of motion).[5]

MTP-I arthroscopy has not yet had the attention it deserves; when performed for the correct indication, it is just as rewarding as for the ankle, knee, and shoulder joints. Technically, the procedure is limited only by the skills of the surgeon, the pathology, and the available instrumentation. As a result of the smaller operation incisions with a smaller chance of scar fibrosis, the range of motion in the MTP-I joint is less affected by the procedure. Thus the MTP-I arthroscopy has an added value, especially for athletes and dancers whose performances are dependent on their range of motion from their great toe.[9]

References

1. Watanabe M, Ito K, Fuji. Equipment and procedures of small join arthroscopy. In: Watanbe M, editor. Arthroscopy of small joints. New York: Igaku-Shoin, 1986
2. Lundeen R. Arthroscopic approaches to the joints of the foot. J Am Podiatr Med Assoc 1987; 77:41–55
3. Richard O, Lundeen R. Review of diagnostic arthroscopy of the foot and ankle. J Foot Surg 1987; 26:33–36
4. Bartlett M. Arthroscopic management of osteochondritis dissecans of the first metatarsal head. Arthroscopy 1988;4:51–54
5. Davies M, Saxby T. Arthroscopy of the first metatarsophalangeal joint. J Bone Joint Surg 1999;81-B:203–06
6. Frey C, Van Dijk C. Arthroscopy of the great toe. AAOS Instr Course Lect 1999;48:343–346
7. Van Dijk C. Arthroscopy of the first metatarsophalangeal joint. In: James F, Serge Parisien J, Melbourne D, eds. Foot and ankle arthroscopy. New York: Springer, 2004:207–14
8. Chan K, Lui T. Arthroscopic fibular sesamoidectomy in the management of the sesamoid osteomyelitis. Knee Surg Sports Traumatol Arthrosc 2006;14:664–67
9. Van Dijk C, Kirsten M, Veenstra M. Arthroscopic surgery of the metatarsophalangeal first joint. Arthroscopy 1998;14:851–55
10. Iqbal M, Gursharan S, Chana F. Arthroscopic cheilectomy for hallux rigidus. Arthroscopy 1998;14:307–10

Chapter 50
Endoscopic Plantar Fasciotomy

Steven L. Shapiro

Plantar fasciitis is the most common cause of heel pain in adults. The predominant symptom is pain in the plantar region of the foot when initiating walking. The etiology is a degenerative tear of part of the fascial origin from the calcaneus, followed by a tendinosis-type reaction.

Anatomy

The plantar fascia is a ligament with longitudinal fibers attaching to the calcaneal tuberosity. The normal medial band is the thickest, measuring up to 3 mm. The central and lateral bands measure 1–2 mm in thickness.[1] Distally, the plantar fascia divides into five slips, one for each toe. The plantar fascia provides support to the arch. As the toes extend during the stance phase of gait, the plantar fascia is tightened by a windlass mechanism, resulting in elevation of the longitudinal arch, inversion of the hindfoot, and external rotation of the leg. Endoscopically, the pertinent anatomy is the abductor hallucis muscle medially, then the plantar fascia. After fasciotomy, the flexor digitorum brevis comes into view as well as the medial intermuscular septum.

Pathogenesis

Specimens of plantar fascia obtained during surgery reveal a spectrum of changes including degeneration of fibrous tissue to fibroblastic proliferation. The fascia is usually markedly thickened and gritty. These pathologic changes are more consistent with fasciosis than fasciitis, but fasciitis remains the accepted description in literature.

S.L. Shapiro
Savannah Orthopaedic Foot and Ankle Center, 6715 Forest Park Drive, Savannah, GA 31406, USA
e-mail: savannahfoot@bellsouth.net
e-mail: bblackburn@savannahfoot.com

Natural History

The typical patient is an adult who complains of plantar heel pain aggravated by activity and relieved by rest. Start-up pain when initiating walking is common. Strain of the plantar fascia can result from prolonged standing, running, or jumping. Excessive pronation is a common mechanical cause. The rigid cavus foot type can also predispose to plantar fasciitis. Obesity is present in up to 70% of patients. Plantar fasciitis is common among runners and ballet dancers. About 15% of cases are bilateral. Women are affected more than men.

Physical Findings

Localized tenderness over the calcaneal tuberosity is the most common physical finding. Pain is usually medial, but occasionally lateral. Rarely, pain may be located distally and this condition is called distal plantar fasciitis. Frequently, there may be soft tissue swelling of the plantar medial heel. Careful comparison with the contralateral heel is essential to observe this finding (Fig. 50.1).

Imaging

X-rays are ordered routinely in patients with plantar heel pain. Plantar calcaneal spurs occur in up to 50% of patients but are not thought to cause heel pain. Stress fractures, unicameral bone cysts, and giant cell tumors can usually be seen on plain films. Bone scans are rarely necessary but are positive in up to 95% of cases of plantar fasciitis. Magnetic resonance imaging (MRI) can be used in questionable cases and elegantly demonstrates thickening of the plantar fascia, and rules out soft tissue and bone tumors, subtalar arthritis, and stress fractures. Ultrasound is cost-effective and easily measures the thickness of the plantar fascia, documenting plantar fasciitis when thickness exceeds 3 mm (Fig. 50.2).

G.R. Scuderi and A.J. Tria (eds.), *Minimally Invasive Surgery in Orthopedics*,
DOI 10.1007/978-0-387-76608-9_50, © Springer Science+Business Media, LLC 2010

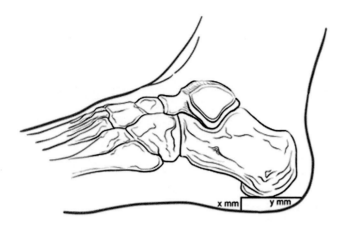

Fig. 50.1 Diagram of preoperative nonweightbearing lateral X-ray demonstrating the appropriate measurements to identify the location of the medial portal incision

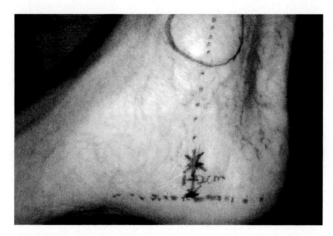

Fig. 50.2 Photograph of a second method to determine the placement of the medial incision. The incision is made along a line that bisects the medial malleolus 1–2 cm superior to the junction of keratinized and nonkeratinized skin

Differential Diagnosis

Plantar fascia rupture generally occurs acutely following vigorous physical activity. There may be visible ecchymosis in the arch. MRI or ultrasound confirms the diagnosis.

Tarsal tunnel syndrome occurs with compression of theT posterior tibial nerve, which can cause numbness, and pain in the heel, sole, or toes. A positive percussion test is elicited and electromyogram (EMG) and nerve conduction study results are positive in 50% of cases.

Stress fractures may sometimes be diagnosed on plain film, but can always be diagnosed on MRI.

Neoplasms can be visualized on plain film at times. MRI is diagnostic. Pain is typically constant and nocturnal.

In *infection*, pain is often constant. There may be swelling, redness, or fluctuance. Plain films, MRI, and/or Ceretec Scan can be diagnostic. Laboratory results may show increased

erythrocyte sedimentation rate (ESR), C-reactive protein (CRP), or white blood cell count (WBC).

Painful heel pad syndrome occurs most often in runners, and is thought to result from disruption of fibrous septae of the heel pad.

Heel pad atrophy occurs in the elderly, and is usually not characterized by morning pain.

Inflammatory arthritis is usually bilateral and diffuse in nature. It may be associated with positive results for rheumatoid arthritis (RA), HLA, B27, and increased ESR.

Nonsurgical Management

Conservative management includes rest, ice, nonsteroidal anti-inflammatory drugs (NSAIDs), plantar fascia and Achilles tendon stretching, silicone heel pads, prefabricated and custom orthoses, night splints, CAM walkers, casts, physical therapy, athletic shoes, judicious use of steroid injections, and shockwave therapy. Ninety-five percent of patients will respond to conservative management. Surgery is indicated after 6–12 months of no improvement with conservative treatment.

Surgical Management

Plantar fasciotomy is indicated in the small percentage of patients who fail to respond to conservative treatment. Although open techniques have yielded good results, endoscopic plantar fasciotomy (EPF) offers several important advantages: (1) minimal soft tissue dissection; (2) excellent visualization of the plantar fascia; (3) precision in transecting only the medial one third to one half of the plantar fascia; (4) minimal postoperative pain with early return to full weightbearing status; and (5) earlier return to activities and work.

Preoperative Planning

Nonweightbearing lateral X-rays of the affected foot are performed. A point just anterior and inferior to the calcaneal tubercle is marked and measurements are made to the inferior and posterior skin lines.[2] These measurements are used to help select the incision site.

Positioning and Anesthesia

The patient is positioned supine with a bump under the buttock of the affected side to provide external rotation of the limb.

The operative foot is then elevated on a foot prop, with a tourniquet in place at the distal calf. The limb is prepped and draped in this position. One gram of Ancef is administered. Anesthesia may be regional or general. Ankle block or popliteal nerve block is used with general anesthesia or intravenous sedation. The procedure is performed on an outpatient basis.

Equipment

The equipment required includes the Instratek Endotrac System (Houston, TX), consisting of a plantar fascia elevator, cannula and obturator, probe, nondisposable knife handles, and disposable hook and triangle knives. A 4-mm 30° short arthroscope is used. Finally, several Q-tips lightly fluffed with a Bovie scratch pad will be needed (Fig. 50.3).

Surgical Technique

The foot is prepped and draped on the foot prop and then exsanguinated with an Esmarch bandage. The tourniquet is inflated at the distal calf to 250 mmHg. An 8-mm vertical incision is made just anterior and plantar to the medial tubercle of the calcaneus. The measurements from the nonweight-bearing lateral X-ray are used as a guide. Another good landmark is the medial malleolus. The incision can be placed on a line dropped from the midpoint of the medial malleolus or the junction of the middle and posterior third of the medial malleolus. Portal placement is critical to the success of the procedure.

The incision is deepened with blunt tenotomy scissors. Next, the plantar fascia elevator is placed through the incision and swept from medial to lateral just plantar to the plantar fascia. The obturator and cannula are then passed through this pathway and brought out through a lateral incision overlying the tip of the obturator. The obturator is then removed from the cannula and the cannula is cleared of fat with Q-tips. The cannula should be perpendicular to the long axis of the foot (Fig. 50.4).

The 4-mm 30° scope is then brought into the medial portal. The abductor hallucis muscle is visualized medially and then the plantar fascia is visualized. The probe is passed from the lateral portal and advanced medially to palpate the medial band of the plantar fascia. The probe is removed and the triangle knife is then advanced to the medial band. The foot is dorsiflexed to place tension on the plantar fascia. With a controlled motion, the triangle knife is pulled across the medial band of the plantar fascia. Several passes are often necessary to completely divide this band. The flexor digitorum brevis muscle belly should be visible after the medial band is divided. The fasciotomy is complete when the medial intermuscular septum is visualized. The amount of fascia divided is usually 14 mm, which can be measured off markings on the probe. The hook knife can be used to cut the fascia, but the triangle knife can be more easily manipulated with less likelihood of cutting into the muscle. After performing a partial fasciotomy, the scope is moved into the lateral portal to check to see if any bands of fascia remain uncut.

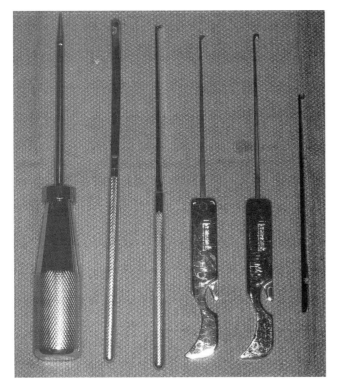

Fig. 50.3 The Instratek Endotrac system for endoscopic plantar fasciotomy. From left to right: (*1*) obturator with cannula, (*2*) plantar fascia elevator, (*3*) probe, (*4*) disposable triangle knife with nondisposable handle, (*5*) disposable hook knife with nondisposable handle, (*6*) disposable triangle knife without handle

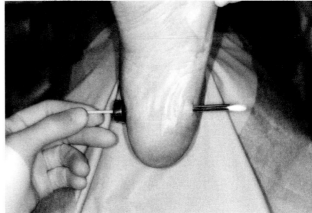

Fig. 50.4 Clearing fat from the cannula with a fluffed Q-tip to allow good visualization of the plantar fascia

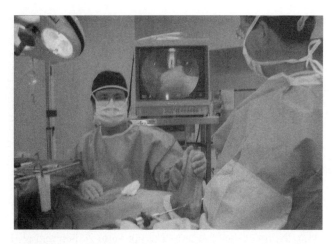

Fig. 50.5 Intraoperative set-up with foot draped on the foot prop, and the monitor on the same side as the foot, the scope placed in the cannula through the medial portal, and the probe through lateral portal. The plantar fascia is visualized on the monitor with the probe palpating the fascia

The triangle knife can be passed through the medial portal to cut these bands. The two-portal system allows this versatility, which is lacking in the single-portal system.

The wound is irrigated through the cannula. The trochar is reinserted and the trochar and cannula are removed together. The incisions are closed with 4-0 nylon suture. A light dressing and posterior splint are applied. Prints and/or CD of before and after fasciotomy are made (Fig. 50.5).

Postoperative Care

Ice and elevation are recommended for 48–72 h postoperatively. Minimal postoperative pain medication is required. Sutures are removed at 1 week postoperatively and a CAM walker, weight bearing as tolerated, is applied and used for 3 weeks to minimize the risk of lateral column pain. Most patients can resume normal activities at 6 weeks and vigorous athletic activities at 12 weeks postoperatively.

Outcomes

All published literature on EPF reports greater than 90% success with shorter recovery times than traditional open surgery.[1-7] My experience mirrors the literature with no infections or nerve damage and only four cases of lateral column pain in more than 400 procedures in the last 11 years. The success rate of EPF is significantly higher than extracorporeal shockwave treatment. In addition, EPF is reimbursed by all insurance companies, whereas shockwave procedures still have erratic insurance reimbursement.

EPF is minimally invasive with a simple, easy-to-learn surgical technique. The equipment is minimal and cost-effective. The incision is 8 mm compared with open procedures, where the incision is at least 4 cm and, with some more extensile approaches, as long as 10 cm.

Surgeons with prior arthroscopic experience should find EPF to be a straightforward procedure to master. DVDs and technique guides are readily available through Instratek. Training courses with cadavers are also given through the Orthopaedic Learning Center or Instratek. After ten cases, the surgeon should feel confident with this procedure. With experience, the average surgery time should be 10–15 min.

Complications

Lateral column pain and arch pain have been the most common complications reported in up to 3–5% of cases. Immobilization in a CAM walker for 4 weeks and limiting the division of the plantar fascia to the medial and central bands should reduce this complication even further. The Instratek System has single and double lines etched into the cannula to guide the surgeon to limit the plantar fasciotomy to 14 mm. The probe also has 1-cm markings. The disposable knives can also be marked with a marking pen to 14 mm. Finally, using the intermuscular septum as a guide for where to stop the fasciotomy is probably the best anatomic reference to indicate where the central band ends and the lateral band begins.

Infection rates are extremely low with EPF. I have had just one superficial wound infection (in a diabetic patient) in more than 400 cases. Injury to the medial and lateral plantar nerves is discussed extensively, but rarely reported. Cadaver studies reveal a reasonable safe zone as long as the incision is appropriate. One case of pseudoaneurysm of the lateral plantar artery and one case of a cuneiform stress fracture have been reported. With appropriate technique and postoperative immobilization, these complications should be rare.

Perils and Pitfalls

Performing the procedure on a prep stand or prop and ensuring that the foot and ankle are stable is vital to the smooth operation of this procedure. U-shaped padded foot-prepping devices that attach to the side of the operating room table are ideal. We also use the Lift-A-Limb foot prop, which cradles the limb and is an excellent device.

The placement of the incision is critical. The ideal placement is 1.5–2.0 cm superior to the junction of keratinized and nonkeratinized skin on a plumb line from the midpoint of the medial malleolus. Fluffed Q-tips and a defogging liquid to apply to the tip of the scope allow good visualization (Fig. 50.6).

Maintaining tension on the plantar fascia while cutting is key. The triangle knife is usually more predictable than the hook knife. Staying in the center of cannula and not skiving are important elements of technique. Although it is possible for the surgeon to hold the scope in one hand and the knife in the other hand, it is usually easier to have the assistant hold the scope and dorsiflex the foot, while the surgeon makes precise and controlled cuts with both hands on the knife, if necessary (Fig. 50.7).

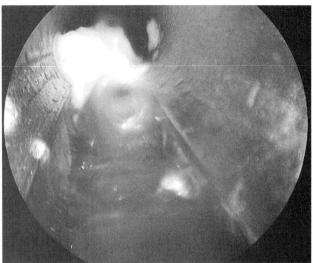

Fig. 50.8 Flexor digitorum brevis muscle seen after endoscopic plantar fasciotomy. Note that the central and lateral bands remain intact

In some cases, the central band is incredibly thick and gritty. Several passes of the triangle knife may be needed. Using the hook knife as well in such cases may be helpful. Remember also to clearly see the complete separation of the plantar fascia with the flexor digitorum brevis muscle plainly visible. Failure of EPF is usually due to incomplete or inadequate division of the plantar fascia (Fig. 50.8).

Other causes of failure include portal placement that is too proximal. It is difficult to release the fascia so proximally, directly off the calcaneus. Finally, misdiagnosis may lead to a poor result. Careful evaluation of the patient to rule out other etiologies in the differential diagnosis (described in detail previously) should be performed preoperatively.

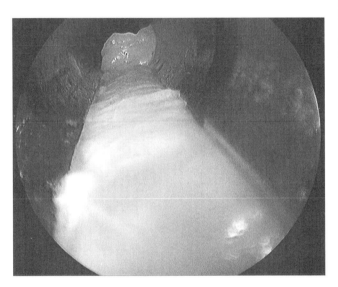

Fig. 50.6 Plantar fascia prior to fasciotomy as seen through a cannula

References

1. Barrett SL, Day SV. Endoscopic plantar fasciotomy: preliminary studies with cadaveric specimen. J Foot Surg. 1991 30: 170–172.
2. Barrett SL, Day SV. Endoscopic plantar fasciotomy two portal endoscopic surgical techniques – clinical results of 65 procedures. J Foot Surg. 2004 32: 248–256.
3. Buchbinder R. Clinical practice. Plantar fasciitis. N Engl J Med. 2004 350(21): 2159–2166.
4. Hofmeister EP, Elliott MJ, Juliano PJ. Endoscopic plantar fascia release: an anatomic study. Foot Ankle Int. 1995 16(H): 719–723.
5. Hogan KA, Weber D, Shereff M. Endoscopic plantar fascia release. Foot Ankle Int. 2004 25 (12): 875–881.
6. Sabir N, Debirlenk S, Yagzi B, Karabulut N, Cubukus S. Clinical utility of sonography in diagnosing plantar fasciitis. J Ultrasound Med. 2005 24 (8); 1041–1048.
7. Saxena A. Uniportal endoscopic plantar fasciotomy: a prospective study on athletic patients. Foot Ankle Int. 2004 25 (12): 882–889.

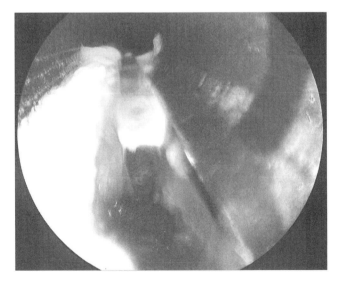

Fig. 50.7 Endoscopic plantar fasciotomy performed with a triangle knife as seen through a cannula

Chapter 51
Uniportal Endoscopic Decompression of the Interdigital Nerve for Morton's Neuroma

Steven L. Shapiro

Morton's neuroma represents a nerve entrapment syndrome in which the intermetatarsal nerve in the second and/or third webspace becomes compressed by the intermetatarsal ligament, enlarges, and undergoes perineural fibrosis.[1-4]

The most recent literature attributes Morton's neuroma to nerve entrapment, which has been confirmed by electron microscopy. Perineural fibrosis is seen at the level of nerve compression.

Endoscopic Anatomy

The most important soft tissue structure is the transverse intermetatarsal ligament (TIML). The TIML is a continuation of the plantar plates. This structure becomes taut during the late midstance and push-off phases of gait. The TIML should be well visualized. It measures 10–15 mm in length and 2–3 mm in thickness.[1]

The lumbrical tendon will be located on the plantar lateral aspect of the TIML. It is the most likely structure to be severed during endoscopic decompression of the intermetatarsal nerve, but with proper identification it can be spared. Inadvertent severing of the lumbrical tendon, however, has not resulted in any adverse sequelae. The plantar interossei muscles are superior to the TIML in the second, third, and fourth intermetatarsal spaces.

The intermetatarsal nerve is plantar to the TIML and should not be visualized during endoscopic division of the TIML; the nerve, however, may be seen by rotating the cannula 180° to the 6 o'clock position. This will be discussed in the Surgical Technique section.

Pathogenesis

The clinical symptoms of this condition were first described by Durlacher in 1845 and later by Morton in 1876. It is Morton's name that has remained linked to this condition.

Natural History

The symptoms of Morton's neuroma are dull, aching pain in the ball of the foot, often radiating into the second, third, and/or fourth toes. This may be associated with tingling, burning, or numbness. This may occur gradually over several months or progress more acutely. Overuse activities, and compression by narrow-toed shoes and high heels have been implicated. Seventy-five percent of patients are women. The average age of onset is 54 years.[5] Occasionally, trauma can result in formation of an interdigital neuroma. Pain is sometimes relieved by removing the shoe.

Physical Findings

Classic findings include localized tenderness in the second and/or third webspace. Subtle swelling may be present in the affected webspaces. The two adjacent toes may be slightly separated. Mulder's click (a palpable snap) may be elicited in the affected webspace. Finally, the metatarsal compression test may be positive. This is performed by grasping and squeezing the patient's forefoot with the examiner's hand. The results of this maneuver are positive if it reproduces the patient's symptoms.

Imaging

Plain films should routinely be performed to rule out other pathologies. If the diagnosis or correct webspace is in doubt, sonographic imaging can be performed with a high degree of

S.L. Shapiro
Savannah Orthopaedic Foot and Ankle Center, 6715 Forest Park Drive, Savannah, GA, 31406 USA
e-mail: savannahfoot@bellsouth.net
e-mail: bblackburn@savannahfoot.com

G.R. Scuderi and A.J. Tria (eds.), *Minimally Invasive Surgery in Orthopedics*,
DOI 10.1007/978-0-387-76608-9_51, © Springer Science+Business Media, LLC 2010

accuracy in experienced hands. MRI is not operator dependent, but yields a large percentage of false negatives and positives and is also much more costly. On ultrasound, a neuroma appears as a hypoechoic oval mass in the interspace at the level of the metatarsal heads. The size of the neuroma can be measured.[5]

Differential Diagnosis

Differential diagnosis should include metatarsal stress fracture, Frieberg's disease (avascular necrosis [AVN] of the metatarsal head), synovitis, intermetatarsal bursitis, metatarsophalangeal (MTP) synovitis, peripheral neuropathy, lumbar radiculopathy, tarsal tunnel syndrome, vascular claudication, and spinal stenosis.

Nonsurgical Management

Conservative treatment may include metatarsal pads, orthotics, shoes with a wide toebox, steroid injections, and, more recently, alcohol injections. In my experience, conservative treatment has been successful in approximately 70% of patients.

Surgical Management

Preoperative Planning

Surgery is indicated when conservative treatment has failed to relieve pain after 6 months. All patients should have plain films preoperatively. Preoperative ultrasound is valuable if available. Otherwise, the surgeon should determine which webspace is most tender. Diagnostic lidocaine injection may also pinpoint the appropriate webspace. If both the second and third webspaces are symptomatic, consider endoscopy on both spaces.

Positioning and Anesthesia

The patient should be positioned supine. A bump under the buttock and thigh is used when the leg is externally rotated. The toes should extend just beyond the end of the operating room (OR) table with the heel firmly resting on the table. Anesthesia may be general or regional (popliteal or ankle block). Local anesthesia should be avoided because it may distort the endoscopic anatomy.

Prophylaxis and Equipment

Prophylactic intravenous antibiotics are given when the patient comes to the OR. An ankle tourniquet inflated to 250 mmHg is routinely used. Equipment required includes the AM Surgical set and a 30° 4-mm scope. The AM Surgical system includes an elevator, slotted cannula and obturator, locking device, and disposable knife blade.

Surgical Technique

The advantage of division of the TIML without excision of the interdigital neuroma is that there is no loss of sensation or possible formation of a stump neuroma, which is a very difficult problem to treat. Barrett and Pignetti introduced endoscopic decompression of the intermetatarsal nerve, which offers several advantages including a smaller incision, faster postoperative recovery, and reduced incidence of hematoma and infection.[1] Although Barrett reported good and excellent results in 88% of patients, the original technique was difficult with a steep learning curve. He has since modified his technique, changing from two portals to a single portal.

Presented here is a single-portal technique using the AM Surgical system originally designed by Dr. Ather Mirza for endoscopic carpal tunnel release. I have adapted the instrumentation for uniportal endoscopic decompression of the intermetatarsal nerve (UDIN) (Fig. 51.1). The following is a step-by-step guide to the procedure (Fig. 51.2).[6]

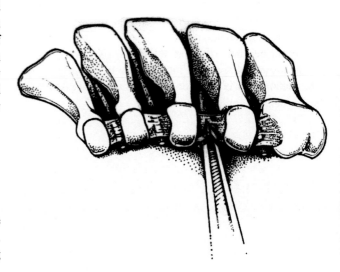

Fig. 51.1 Illustration of surgical technique for UDIN. The cannula is in the interspace just plantar to the TIML and dorsal to the intermetatarsal (interdigital) nerve. The TIML is being transected from distal to proximal (Courtesy of A.M. Surgical, Inc., Smithtown, NY.)

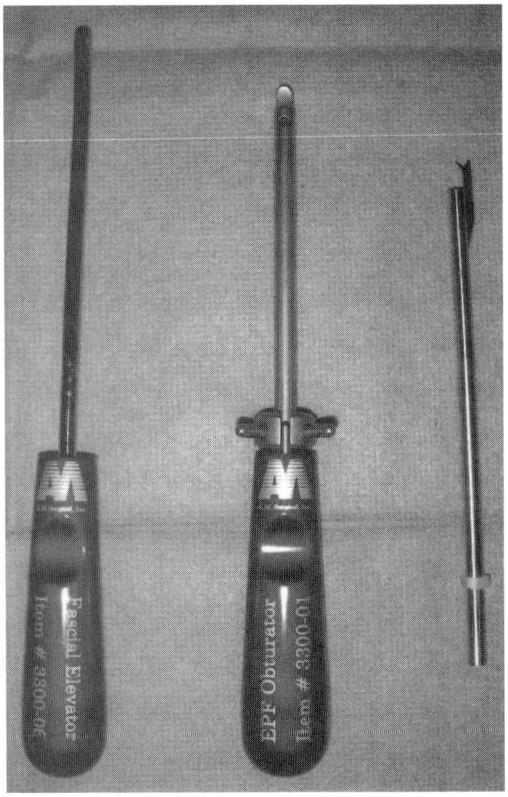

Fig. 51.2 Instrumentation. From left to right: elevator, cannula and obturator, and disposable knife

1. Make a 1-cm vertical incision in the appropriate webspace.
2. Spread the subcutaneous tissue gently with blunt Steven's scissor.
3. Use the AM Surgical elevator to palpate and separate the TIML from the surrounding soft tissues. Scrape the elevator both dorsal and plantar to the TIML.
4. Place the slotted cannula/obturator through the same path just plantar to and scraping against the TIML. The slot should face dorsally at the 12 o'clock position.
5. Remove the obturator from the cannula.
6. Remove any fat or fluid from the cannula with absorbent cotton tip applicators.
7. Insert a short 4-mm 30° scope into the cannula.
8. Visualize the entire TIML by advancing the scope. The ligament is dense and white. The lumbrical tendon can often be seen just lateral to the TIML.
9. The intermetatarsal nerve can be visualized by rotating the cannula 180° so that the slot is facing plantar at 6 o'clock. The nerve can often be seen unless obscured by fat. It is often thickened distally, tapers, and becomes normal proximally.
10. Return the cannula back to the 12 o'clock position.
11. Remove the scope from the cannula.
12. Slide the disposable endoscopic knife onto the locking device with the lever in the open position.

13. Insert the knife and locking device assembly into the scope and advance the knife blade until it nearly touches the lens. The blade should also be parallel to the lens. Push the lever of the locking device forward until finger tight.
14. Advance the scope and knife assembly through the cannula. Visualize the knife blade transecting the TIML from distal to proximal. While cutting the TIML, maintain the cannula tight against the ligament. Place more tension on the TIML by placing a finger of the nondominant hand between the adjacent metatarsal necks.
15. Withdraw the scope and knife assembly and remove the knife from the scope. Reinsert the scope to confirm complete transection of the TIML. The divided edge of the ligament can be observed to further separate by applying manual digital pressure between the adjacent metatarsal heads.
16. Irrigate the wound through the cannula.
17. Remove the cannula and insert the elevator into the wound and palpate the interspace. The taut TIML should no longer be palpable.
18. Deflate the tourniquet; irrigate and close the wound with one or two interrupted mattress sutures. Apply a soft compression dressing and postoperative shoe.
19. If the surgeon chooses to perform a neurectomy in cases in which the nerve is very large and bulbous, the incision can be extended proximally 1–2 cm and neurectomy can be performed in routine fashion (Figs. 51.3–51.6).

Postoperative Care

Ice and elevation are recommended for the first 48–72 h. Weightbearing as tolerated is permitted in a surgical shoe. Crutches or a walker are provided as needed. Sutures are removed in 12–14 days. A comfortable shoe or sandal may then be worn. Vigorous activities such as running or racket sports should be avoided for 4–6 weeks. Patient should be advised that complete resolution of symptoms may take up to 4 months.

Outcomes

Barrett reported 88% good and excellent results in more than 40 patients.[1] In my first 24 patients, there were 82% good and excellent results at 6 months postoperatively.

Complications

In the first 50 patients, there have been no infections. Two wound dehiscences occurred that healed uneventfully. The

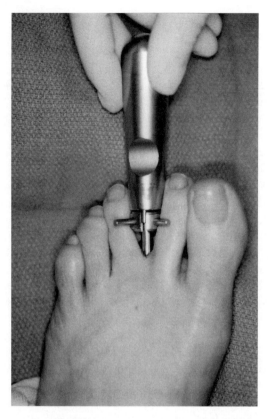

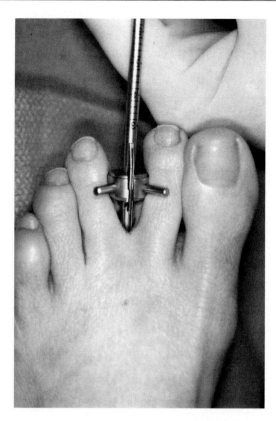

Fig. 51.3 Intraoperative view of insertion of the cannula and obturator into the second webspace, notch at 12 o'clock, positioned to view the TIML

Fig. 51.4 (**a**) Endoscopic view of TIML. (**b**) Normal interdigital nerve. (**c**) Thickened interdigital nerve (neuroma)

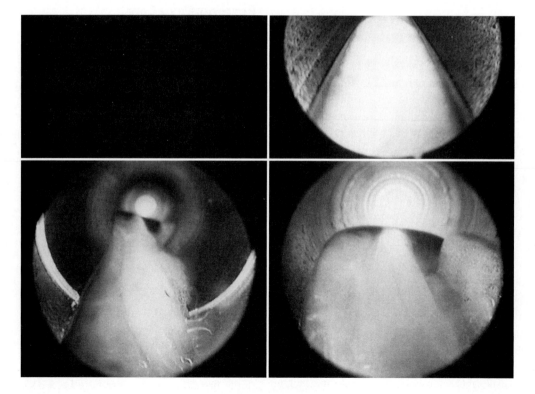

Fig. 51.5 Intraoperative view of knife mounted to scope in position in cannula ready to enter second webspace and transect the TIML

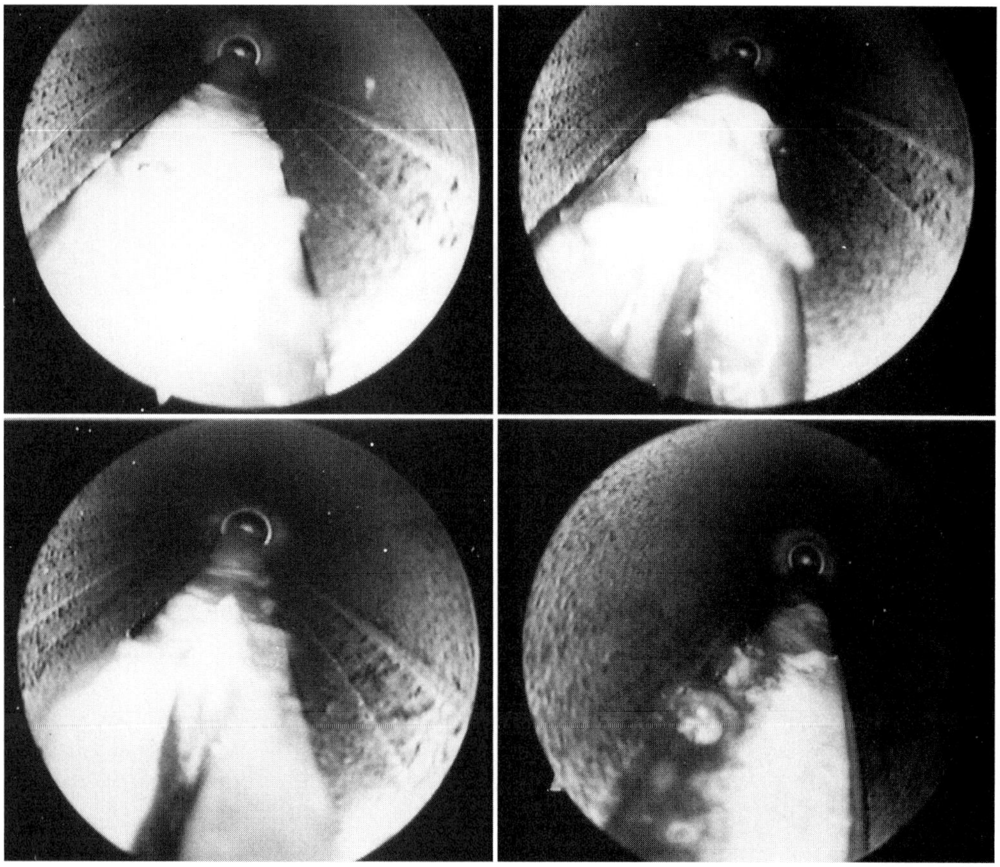

Fig. 51.6 (**a**) Endoscopic view of TIML. (**b**, **c**) Endoscopic views of knife blade transecting the TIML. (**d**) Endoscopic view after release of TIML

postoperative protocol was then changed from suture removal at 10 days postoperative to 14 days postoperative. No further dehiscences have occurred.

Perils and Pitfalls

The key to the procedure is isolating and separating the TIML from the soft tissues. Developing these tissue planes with the elevator is the critical step. Everything else follows. Hugging the TIML with the cannula while cutting is very important. If unable to visualize the TIML, abort the procedure and perform the procedure open.

References

1. Barrett, SL, Pignetti, TT. Endoscopic decompression for routine neuroma: preliminary study with cadaveric specimen: early clinical results. J Foot Ankle Surg 1994;33(5):503–8
2. Dellon, AL. Treatment of Morton's neuroma as a nerve compression; the role for neurolysis. J Am Podiatr Med Assoc 1992;82: 399–402
3. Gauthier, G. Thomas Morton's disease: a nerve entrapment syndrome. A new surgical technique. Clin Orthop Relat Res 1979; 142: 90–2
4. Graham, CE, Graham, DM. Morton's neuroma: a microscopic evaluation. Foot Ankle 1984; 5:150–3
5. Shapiro, PS, Shapiro, SL. Sonographic evaluation of interdigital neuroma. Foot Ankle 1995; 16:10, 604–606
6. Shapiro, S.L. Endoscopic decompression of the intermetatarsal nerve for Morton's neuroma. Foot Ankle Clin N Am 2004; 9: 297–304

Chapter 52
Percutaneous Z Tendon Achilles Lengthening

Bradley M. Lamm and Dror Paley

Achilles tendon lengthening is a delicate procedure whereby the risk of over lengthening (creating calcaneus), rupture, and weakening of the gastrocnemius-soleus muscle is devastating. The Silfverskiöld test is clinically performed to differentiate gastrocnemius equinus from gastrocnemius-soleus equinus. Many surgical techniques have been developed to treat negative results of the Silfverskiöld test. The authors prefer a gastrocnemius-soleus recession in order to preserve muscle strength. However, when a large amount of equinus deformity is present, an Achilles tendon lengthening is performed in order to achieve an adequate amount of length.1 The authors present a percutaneous technique for Achilles tendon lengthening.2

Surgical Technique

A longitudinal percutaneous incision is made centrally and just proximal to the Achilles tendon insertion into the calcaneus. This incision is deepened through the Achilles tendon. A Smillie knife is inserted into the split beneath the Achilles tendon sheath and pushed approximately 4 cm proximally. A second percutaneous longitudinal central tendon incision is made over the tip of the Smillie knife. Then each half of the tendon is cut transversely at the level of the incisions, being careful not to injure the tendon sheath. Dorsiflexion of the foot in conjunction with making these transverse cuts allows for the tendon to slide on itself. When a varus hindfoot is present, cut distal medial and proximal lateral. When a valgus hindfoot is present, cut distal lateral and proximal medial. The Achilles tendon fibers spiral distally; therefore, be careful to ensure a complete Z lengthening. In addition, do not cut the tendon sheath. Dorsiflex the foot and observe the tendon lengthening within the sheath, which therefore does not need to be repaired. Because this technique maintains the Achilles tendon sheath, the Thompson's test produces normal plantarflexion. The ankle is then immobilized for 3 weeks postoperatively (Figs. 52.1a–e–52.5).

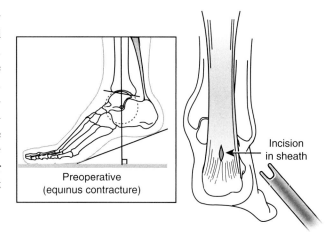

Fig. 52.1 Percutaneous Z tendon Achilles lengthening for correction of equinus. Make a central distal incision through the skin and the Achilles tendon, creating a short split through the tendon longitudinally (From Paley D: *Principles of Deformity Correction.* rev ed, 2005, with kind permission of Springer Science + Business Media.)

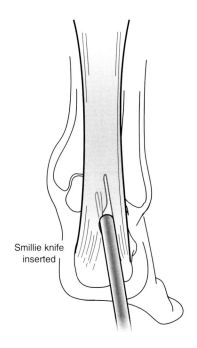

Fig. 52.2 Insert the Smillie knife into the short split (From Paley D: *Principles of Deformity Correction.* rev ed, 2005, with kind permission of Springer Science + Business Media.)

B.M. Lamm (✉) and D. Paley
Rubin Institute for Advanced Orthopedics, Sinai Hospital of
Baltimore, 2401 West Belvedere Avenue, Baltimore, MD 21215, USA
e-mail: blamm@lifebridgehealth.org

G.R. Scuderi and A.J. Tria (eds.), *Minimally Invasive Surgery in Orthopedics,*
DOI 10.1007/978-0-387-76608-9_52, © Springer Science + Business Media, LLC 2010

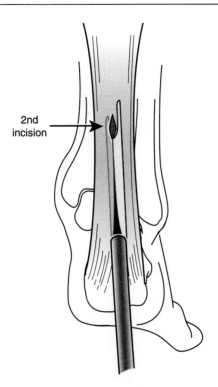

Fig. 52.3 Push the Smillie knife proximally for at least 4 cm and, at the tip of the knife, make a second central longitudinal skin incision (From Paley D: *Principles of Deformity Correction*. rev ed, 2005, with kind permission of Springer Science + Business Media.)

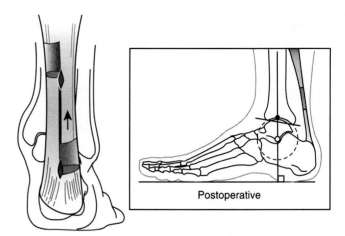

Fig. 52.5 When dorsiflexion of the foot is performed, the tendon sides on itself but maintains tension within the intact sheath. Note the plantigrade foot position (From Paley D: *Principles of Deformity Correction*. rev ed, 2005, with kind permission of Springer Science + Business Media.)

References

1. Lamm BM, Paley D, Herzenberg JE. Gastrocnemius soleus recession: a simpler, more limited approach. J Am Podiatr Med Assoc 95:18–25, 2005
2. Paley D. *Principles of Deformity Correction*. 2nd edition, Springer, Berlin, 2003.

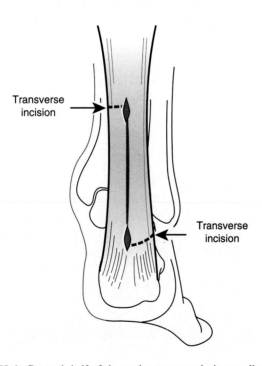

Fig. 52.4 Cut each half of the tendon transversely in one direction proximally and the other direction distally, creating a Z lengthening. The direction of release proximal and distal is performed occurring to the patient's heel position (valgus or varus). Do not cut the tendon sheath (From Paley D: *Principles of Deformity Correction*. rev ed, 2005, with kind permission of Springer Science + Business Media.)

Chapter 53
Percutaneous Distraction Osteogenesis for Treatment of Brachymetatarsia

Bradley M. Lamm, Dror Paley, and John E. Herzenberg

A short metatarsal can be acquired or congenital in origin.[1] A congenitally short metatarsal or brachymetatarsia presents unilaterally or bilaterally, typically involving the fourth metatarsal (Figs. 53.1 and 53.2). Congenitally short metatarsals can occur in isolation or in association with systemic syndromes, endocrinopathies, and dysplasias. Syndactyly or polydactyly can occur in combination with congenitally short metatarsals. The cause of brachymetatarsia is thought to be premature closure of the metatarsal epiphyseal growth plate (Fig. 53.3). Acquired short metatarsals are caused by trauma, infection, tumor, Freiberg disease, radiation, and surgery. In addition, acquired short metatarsals can be associated with skeletal and systemic abnormalities (sickle cell anemia, multiple epiphyseal dysplasia, multiple hereditary osteochondromas, and juvenile rheumatoid arthritis). Surgically induced (iatrogenic) shortening of metatarsals are caused by transphyseal fixation, osteotomies of the metatarsals, and internal or external fixation producing a growth arrest or synostoses between metatarsals. A failed bunionectomy or overly aggressive first metatarsal cuneiform arthrodesis also can result in an acquired short first metatarsal.[1,2]

Patients with brachymetatarsia exhibit a dorsally displaced toe, toe dysplasia, short phalanges, transfer metatarsalgia, cosmetic concerns, and painful corns and calluses. These patients have difficulty wearing shoes because of the high riding toe on the dorsum of the foot, which produces plantar metatarsal head calluses and dorsal digital corns.[1,3] Surgery to lengthen the short metatarsal can improve cosmesis and shoe wearing and can decrease the pain associated with this deformity.

Acute and gradual lengthening surgical techniques have been described for correction of brachymetatarsia. Acute lengthening of a short metatarsal with autogenous bone grafting was first described in 1969 by McGlamry and Cooper.[4] Since then, many other techniques for acute lengthening

(one-stage) have been reported and include interposition of synthetic materials, allograft, and step-cut or oblique osteotomy with distraction and internal fixation.[5-8] Some authors have performed shortening of adjacent metatarsals or proximal phalanxes so as to decrease the amount of metatarsal lengthening needed.[9-11]

Gradual lengthening with external fixation (distraction osteogenesis) is preferred for lengthening more than 1 cm.[1] With gradual lengthening, the rate of postoperative lengthening can be adjusted, the patient can bear weight during treatment, and the patient can have input regarding the final length. Gradual lengthening reduces the risk of neurovascular compromise compared with acute lengthening, which can cause severe soft tissue stretch.[1,2] Gradual lengthening of short metatarsals has been performed with subsequent interpositional bone graft[12,13] and with distraction osteogenesis alone.[14-16] Various types of external fixation devices (mini-Hoffman, Ilizarov semicircular, and monolateral fixators) have been used to achieve metatarsal lengthening.[17-20]

The metatarsal phalangeal joint (MTPJ) is at risk for subluxation during gradual lengthening of a metatarsal.[21,22] With greater amounts of lengthening, the joint is more susceptible to subluxation. The subluxation forces decrease with distance from the osteotomy to the joint. Soft tissue rebalancing of the digit and pinning of the MTPJ are important adjunctive steps to maintain the MTPJ reduced during lengthening. Traditionally, a separate Kirschner wire is used to stabilize the MTPJ.[2] However, this pin can easily become dislodged during the lengthy treatment time. By connecting the digital pin to the external fixation device, this pin is incorporated into the apparatus to form a more stable ray construct. At the time of surgery, it might be necessary to perform a release of the dorsal toe contracture to allow for appropriate toe realignment to pin the digit. Pinning the digit to the metatarsal head stabilizes the MTPJ throughout the lengthening. Attaching the pin to the external fixator ensures that this important stabilizing pin will not dislodge. Other potential complications result from inadequate restoration of the metatarsal parabola in the transverse plane. Creating a plantigrade metatarsal head in the sagittal plane provides the necessary realignment for normal pedal function.

B.M. Lamm (✉), D. Paley, and J.E. Herzenberg
Rubin Institute for Advanced Orthopedics, Sinai Hospital of Baltimore, 2401 West Belvedere Avenue, Baltimore, MD 21215, USA
e-mail: blamm@lifebridgehealth.org

G.R. Scuderi and A.J. Tria (eds.), *Minimally Invasive Surgery in Orthopedics*,
DOI 10.1007/978-0-387-76608-9_53, © Springer Science+Business Media, LLC 2010

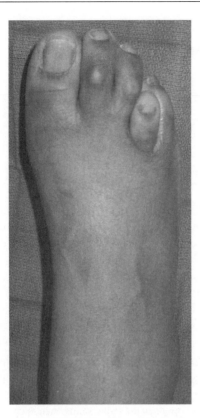

Fig. 53.1 Anteroposterior clinical photograph of a congenitally short fourth metatarsal. Note the underlapping fifth toe

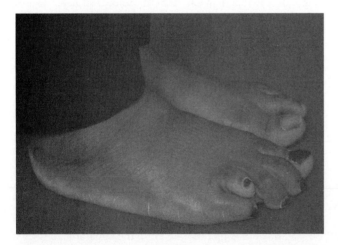

Fig. 53.2 Lateral clinical photograph of a congenitally short fourth metatarsal. Note the dorsal displacement and flexion deformity at the MTPJ of the fourth digit

We present our percutaneous metatarsal lengthening technique to prevent MTPJ subluxation during metatarsal lengthening. In addition, we present a systematic technique to ensure the proper plane and vector of metatarsal lengthening to maintain anatomic sagittal and transverse plane alignment, respectively.

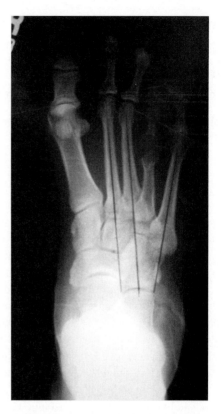

Fig. 53.3 Anteroposterior view radiograph of a congenitally short fourth metatarsal. The metatarsal length is abnormal, with the fourth metatarsal being short of the line formed by drawing the metatarsal parabola angle. Note the slight medial bowing of the short metatarsal. The transverse plane deviation of the adjacent digits converging toward the short metatarsal can be observed

Surgical Technique

A systematic percutaneous technique to ensure the proper plane and direction of metatarsal lengthening is outlined. Position the patient supine on the radiolucent table with a bump under the left hemisacrum to obtain a foot forward position. Based on the reducibility of the MTPJ contracture, digital surgery (partial or complete MTPJ release with or without arthroplasty or arthrodesis of the proximal interphalangeal joint) should be performed to realign the digit before the metatarsal lengthening procedure is begun. A partial MTPJ release (dorsal capsulotomy) should be performed when the digit is reducible. It is not recommended to perform an arthroplasty or arthrodesis because this will result in shortening of an already short ray. In some cases, it might be necessary to release the dorsal MTPJ capsule or rarely lengthen the combined extensor tendon of the toe. After the appropriate MTPJ release is performed, the toe is pinned with a 0.062-in.-diameter Kirschner wire in the realigned position. Under fluoroscopic guidance, the wire is inserted from the tip of the toe across the MTPJ, stopping at the distal external fixation pins. Preoperative planning with a four-pin

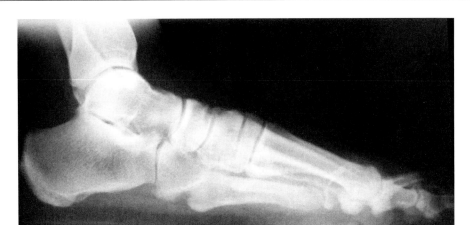

Fig. 53.4 Lateral view radiograph of a congenitally short fourth metatarsal. Note the extension c e-mail: bradankle@yahoo.com ontracture of the toe and increased fourth metatarsal declination at the level of the distal metaphyseal-diaphyseal junction (region of the growth plate). The dorsal cortex of the short metatarsal is parallel to the adjacent metatarsals

Orthofix Mini-M100 external fixator (Verona, Italy) determines the initial spread and locations of the pins. Insert the half-pins percutaneously, under fluoroscopic control, bicortical and perpendicular to the shaft of the metatarsal.

The first half-pin is placed at the distal-most region of the metaphyseal-diaphyseal junction. A 1.8-mm wire works well to predrill the hole, under fluoroscopic control, perpendicular to the metatarsal on the lateral view. Remove the wire and insert a 3.0- to 2.5-mm tapered half-pin, typically measuring 60 mm in total length and 20 mm of thread length (Fig. 53.4). Because the fixator is mounted perpendicular to this first pin, the first pin determines the plane of lengthening. It is important that the plane of metatarsal lengthening be such that the final position of the metatarsal head is located at the appropriate level in the sagittal plane.

Set the monorail mini external fixator so that the half-pin clamps are at the smallest distance apart, minimizing the pin spread. This ensures maximum lengthening capability and that all of the half-pins are maintained within the short metatarsal. If the metatarsal is very short, it might be necessary for the most proximal half-pin to be placed in the tarsus (cuboid) spanning the Lisfranc joint. Insert the second half-pin, the most proximal of the four half-pins, proximally in the base of the metatarsal, parallel to the first pin and just distal to the adjacent metatarsal cuboid joint. A 1.8-mm wire works well to predrill the hole for half-pin placement and is bent distally, under fluoroscopic guidance, to check the direction of lengthening (Fig. 53.5). This second half-pin establishes the direction of metatarsal lengthening (two fixed points determine a line) and is important because it determines the final position of the metatarsal head in the transverse plane (Fig. 53.6). Also, this second (most proximal) half-pin determines the position of the most proximal half-pin cluster and thus indirectly determines the osteotomy level. Therefore, the more

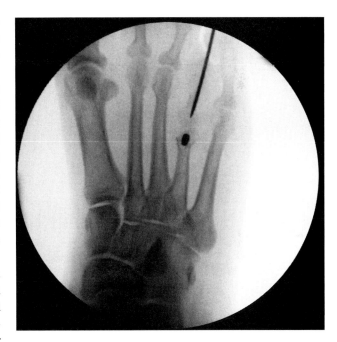

Fig. 53.5 Fluoroscopic anteroposterior view showing that the first pin is placed at the distal most region of the metatarsal metaphyseal-diaphyseal junction. This half-pin is inserted in the center of the metatarsal (bicortical) and perpendicular to the longitudinal bisection of the metatarsal (sagittal plane axis) on the lateral view. The placement of this pin defines the sagittal plane of metatarsal lengthening

proximal this second pin is placed, the more metaphyseal the osteotomy level is. Diaphyseal osteotomy requires a longer consolidation phase. According to the preoperative plan, two half-pins are placed in the distal end of the metatarsal and two in the base of the fourth metatarsal adjacent to the metatarsal cuboid joint (Fig. 53.7). Make a percutaneous incision (5 mm in length) lateral to the short metatarsal at the proximal metaphyseal-diaphyseal junction between the two half-pin clusters.

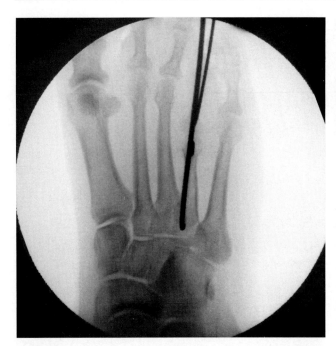

Fig. 53.6 Fluoroscopic anteroposterior view showing that the second pin is placed at the most proximal region of the metatarsal. Similar to the first half-pin, it is inserted perpendicular to the sagittal plane axis of the metatarsal on the lateral view (parallel to the first pin). In addition, the exact medial/lateral position of this second half-pin defines the direction or vector of metatarsal lengthening (two points define a line). This second pin defines the vector of metatarsal lengthening and thus the final position of the metatarsal head, compared with the adjacent metatarsal heads in the transverse plane

Use a small hemostat to dissect down to the metatarsal, and with a perio-steal elevator, gently lift the dorsal and plantar periosteum. To begin the osteotomy, a 1.5-mm wire is used to drill multiple orthogonal holes into the metatarsal under fluoroscopic control. The level of the osteotomy is just distal to the most distal of the proximal half-pin clusters; care needs to be taken not to extend the osteotomy into the half-pin. A small osteotome is then used to complete the osteotomy without producing excessive osteotomy displacement, which can tear the periosteum (Figs. 53.8 and 53.9). The osteotomy is then reduced with the use of fluoroscopy and the Orthofix Mini-M100 external fixator, which is applied and tightened. Next, the toe Kirschner wire is bent 90° outside the skin and again 90° over the dorsum of the toe. A third 90° bend is needed to attach it with an end clamp to the external fixator. It is necessary to have the screw distraction end of the fixator proximal and the tapped end of the fixator distally oriented (Figs. 53.10 and 53.11). Traditionally, a separate Kirschner wire is used to stabilize the MTPJ.[2] However, the pin can easily become dislodged during the lengthy treatment time. By connecting the digital pin to the external fixation device, the pin is incorporated into the apparatus to form a more stable construct. Note that the digital pin is attached to the moving

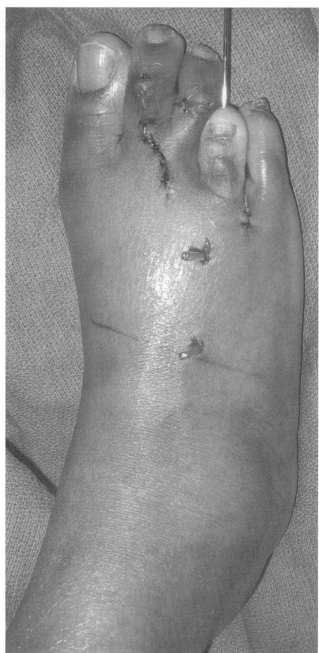

Fig. 53.7 Clinical photograph showing the parallelism of the most distal and proximal half-pins in the fourth metatarsal. Note that the second and third hammertoes have been corrected. To correct the dorsal contracture of the fourth toe, a dorsal capsulotomy was performed through a percutaneous dorsal lateral incision and pinning was then performed. The 0.062-in. Kirschner wire is advanced across the MTPJ after all the half-pins are placed

segment of the external fixator. The percutaneous osteotomy incision is closed and a compressive dressing applied along with toe dressings. Begin distraction after 5 days, at a rate of 0.25 mm twice per day. When the bone is at the final length and fully consolidated, the frame is removed (Figs. 53.12–53.18).

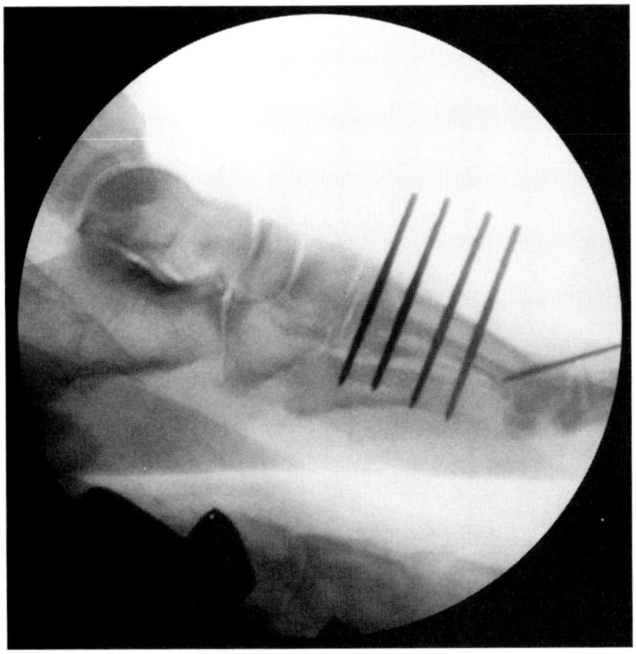

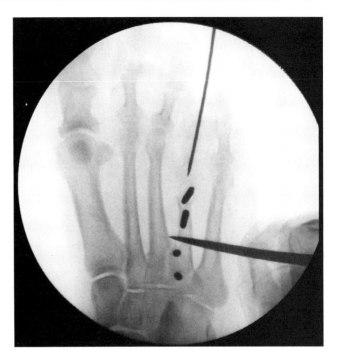

Fig. 53.8 Fluoroscopic lateral view confirms that all four half-pins are parallel to each other and perpendicular to the longitudinal axis of the fourth metatarsal

Fig. 53.10 Intraoperative fluoroscopy is used to ensure completion of the osteotomy

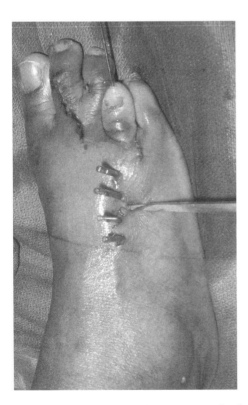

Fig. 53.9 Intraoperative photograph of the percutaneous fourth metatarsal osteotomy. A percutaneous dorsal lateral incision is made, and, under fluoroscopic guidance, a 1.5-mm wire is used to drill multiple orthogonal holes into the metatarsal at the level of metaphyseal-diaphyseal junction. A small osteotome is then used to complete the osteotomy

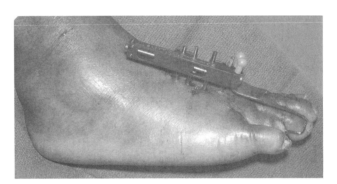

Fig. 53.11 Immediate postoperative lateral view clinical photograph showing parallel half-pins and the fourth digit pinned in a reduced position. The 0.062-in. diameter Kirschner wire is then bent to attach it with an end clamp into the distal aspect of the external fixator

Discussion

Preoperative planning is important to identify the amount of metatarsal length necessary to reestablish the metatarsal parabola. For example, if the amount of metatarsal length needed to reestablish the metatarsal parabola is 20 mm, the amount of time required to obtain this length would be approximately 45 days, based on the latency period of 5 days and the desired distraction rate of 0.5 mm per day. This is useful information to discuss with the patient preoperatively. The rate of distraction might need to be adjusted during the

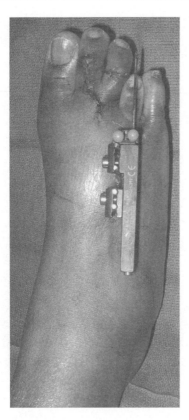

Fig. 53.12 Immediate postoperative anteroposterior view clinical photograph showing that the tapped end of the external fixator should be oriented distally to allow for attachment of the digital Kirschner wire. Note that the lengthening end of the external fixator is oriented toward the patient

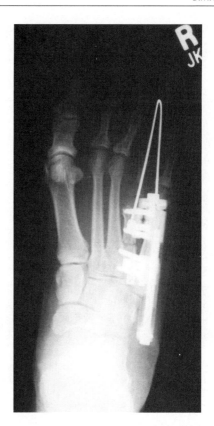

Fig. 53.13 Postoperative anterop\osterior view radiograph showing the fixator in place. The distraction begins after 5 days, at a rate of 0.25 mm twice per day

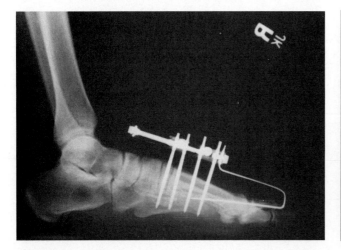

Fig. 53.14 Postoperative lateral view radiograph showing the fixator in place. Note that the pinning of the MTPJ prevents joint subluxation. This method of attaching the digital pin to the fixator prevents dislodgment of the pin during the lengthening and consolidation phases of treatment

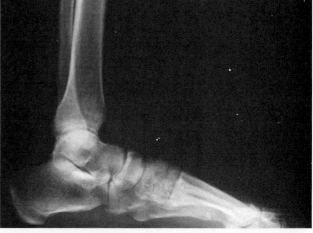

Fig. 53.15 Lateral view radiograph, obtained with the patient in a weight-bearing position after removal of the fixator, showing healed regenerated bone with accurate sagittal plane alignment

postoperative period; therefore, appropriate patient education is important. The consolidation period varies depending on a multitude of factors (location of osteotomy, age of patient, whether the patient smokes, rate of lengthening, and amount of lengthening) but typically ranges from 2 to 4 months. Therefore, the prediction of needed metatarsal length provides a time line for the patient's total length of treatment (lengthening phase and consolidation phase).

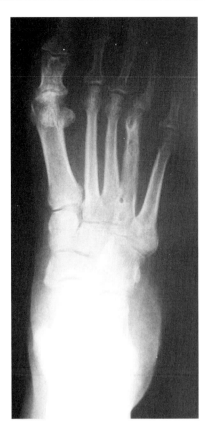

Fig. 53.16 Anteroposterior view radiograph, obtained with the patient in a weight-bearing position after removal of the fixator, showing healed regenerated bone with accurate transverse plane alignment and proper length restoration

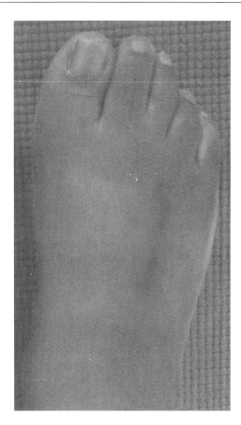

Fig. 53.17 Anteroposterior clinical photograph, obtained with the patient in a weight-bearing position at final follow-up, showing correction of the second and third hammertoes and proper length restoration of the fourth digit

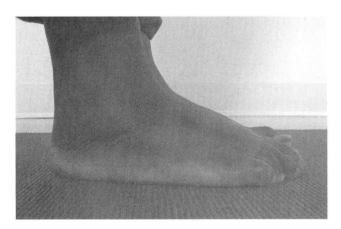

Fig. 53.18 Lateral clinical photograph, obtained with the patient in a weight-bearing position at final follow-up, showing accurate sagittal plane alignment of the second, third, and fourth digits

ment. Because the fixator is mounted perpendicular to the first half-pin, this half-pin ensures the correct plane for bone lengthening. Almost no room for error exists in transverse placement because of the narrow nature of the bone. It is important that the plane of metatarsal lengthening be such that the final position of the metatarsal head is located at the appropriate level in the sagittal plane. The second half-pin determines the direction or vector of lengthening (two fixed points define a line). Little room for error exists because the fifth and third metatarsals are located a set distance apart in the transverse plane. It is important that the vector of metatarsal lengthening be such that the final position of the metatarsal head is located at the appropriate level in the transverse plane.

Conclusion

Intraoperatively, applying four half-pins that are perpendicular to the mid-diaphyseal axis of that metatarsal and parallel to each other is important for accurate sagittal and transverse plane lengthening and thus for the final align-

Therefore, accurate placement of the most distal half-pin and the most proximal half-pin defines the plane and direction of lengthening in both the sagittal and transverse planes, respectively. The technique of a percutaneous minimally invasive osteotomy in the metaphyseal region of the metatarsal is essential for successful formation of regenerate bone. Pinning of the toe across the MTPJ is important to minimize digital subluxation and digital flexion contracture during lengthening. In addition, our technique of connecting the digital wire to the external fixator prevents dislodgment of this wire during treatment. Currently, the senior author (B.M.L.) has modified the technique to further prevent stiffness of the metatarsophalangeal joint after treatment. Pinning across the MTPJ has been shown to produce stiffness regardless of the length of time the pin is maintained. Therefore, piggybacking or adding a second fixator to span the MTPJ provides joint distraction and digital realignment thereby protecting the joint. This modification has shown excellent short-term results and maintains MTPJ position and flexibility (Fig. 53.19). Preoperative consultation should include the time prediction for both the lengthening and consolidation phases and a cosmetic discussion of toe length (phalanges also can be short in cases of congenitally short metatarsals) and forefoot width (after lengthening, patients might feel as if the forefoot is wider). Routine biweekly follow-up is critical during the lengthening phase to avoid complications such as under lengthening and over lengthening of the metatarsal, premature consolidation, nonunion, and malunion.

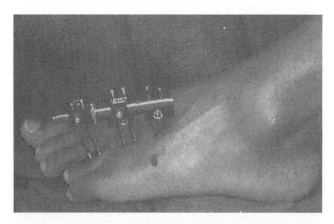

Fig. 53.19 Clinical photograph obtained immediately after surgery shows the senior author's (B.M.L.) modified technique to prevent postoperative MTPJ stiffness. Note the parallelism of the half-pins in the fourth metatarsal and toe. The fourth toe was manually reduced (without MTPJ release) and was maintained in a neutral position with the second fixator. The distal most external fixator (Penning minifixator, Orthofix, Inc., Mckinney, TX) across the MTPJ provides distraction, prevents joint subluxation during lengthening, and maximizes postoperative joint flexibility. In addition, the small percutaneous metatarsal osteotomy incision is seen laterally

Acknowledgments I thank Alvien Lee for expertise and assistance with the photography.

References

1. Davidson RS. Metatarsal lengthening. Foot Ankle Clin 6:499–518, 2001
2. Levine SE, Davidson RS, Dormans JP, Drummond DS. Distraction osteogenesis for congenitally short lesser metatarsals. Foot Ankle Int 16:196–200, 1995
3. Root ML, Orien WP, Weed JH. Normal and abnormal function of the foot. Clinical Biomechanics, Vol 2. Los Angeles: Clinical Biomechanics Corp. 455, 1977
4. McGlamry ED, Cooper CT. Brachymetatarsia: a surgical treatment. J Am Podiatry Assoc 59:259–264, 1969
5. Choudhury SN, Kitaoka HB, Peterson HA. Metatarsal lengthening: case report and review of the literature. Foot Ankle Int 18:739–745, 1997
6. Page JC, Dockery GL, Vance CE. Brachymetatarsia with brachymesodactyly. J Foot Surg 22:104–107, 1983
7. Mah KK, Beegle TR, Falknor DW. A correction for short fourth metatarsal. J Am Podiatry Assoc 73:196–200, 1983
8. Handelman RB, Perlman MD, Coleman WB. Brachymetatarsia: a review of the literature and case report. J Am Podiatr Med Assoc 76:413–416, 1986
9. Kim HT, Lee SH, Yoo CI, Kang JH, Suh JT. The management of brachymetatarsia. J Bone Joint Surg 85B:683–690, 2003
10. Kaplan EG, Kaplan GS. Metatarsal lengthening by use of autogenous bone graft and internal wire compression fixation: a preliminary report. J Foot Surg 17:60–66, 1978
11. Biggs EW, Brahm TB, Efron BL. Surgical correction of congenital hypoplastic metatarsals. J Am Podiatry Assoc 69:241–244, 1979
12. Martin DE, Kalish SR. Brachymetatarsia: a new surgical approach. J Am Podiatr Med Assoc 81:10–17, 1991
13. Urbaniak JR, Richardson WJ. Diaphyseal lengthening for shortness of the toe. Foot Ankle 5:251–256, 1985
14. Saxby T, Nunley JA. Metatarsal lengthening by distraction osteogenesis: a report of two cases. Foot Ankle 13:536–539, 1992
15. Magnan B, Bragantini A, Regis D, Bartolozzi P. Metatarsal lengthening by callotasis during the growth phase. J Bone Joint Surg 77B:602–607, 1995
16. Wakisaka T, Yasui N, Kojimoto H, Takasu M, Shimomura Y. A case of short metatarsal bones lengthened by callus distraction. Acta Orthop Scand 59:194–196, 1988
17. Skirving AP, Newman JH. Elongation of the first metatarsal. J Pediatr Orthop 3:508–510, 1983
18. Steedman JT, Peterson HA. Brachymetatarsia of the first metatarsal treated by surgical lengthening. J Pediatr Orthop 12:780–785, 1992
19. Masada K, Fujita S, Fuji T, Ohno H. Complications following metatarsal lengthening by callus distraction for bracthymetatarsia. J Pediatr Orthop 19:394–397, 1999
20. Herzenberg JE, Paley D. Ilizarov applications in foot and ankle surgery. Adv Orthop Surg 16:162–174, 1992
21. Baek GH, Chung MS. The treatment of congenital brachymetatarsia by one-stage lengthening. J Bone Joint Surg 80B:1040–1044, 1998
22. Kawashima T, Yamada A, Ueda K, Harii K. Treatment of brachymetatarsia by callus distraction (callotasis). Ann Plast Surg 32:191–199, 1994

Chapter 54
Minimally Invasive Realignment Surgery for the Charcot Foot

Bradley M. Lamm and Dror Paley

The aftermath of Charcot, joint subluxation and loss of the bone quality, produces abnormal osseous prominences, which are potential areas for ulceration. Due to the deformed pedal position, the muscle-tendon balance is altered and the resultant aberrant weight-bearing forces increase the risk for ulceration. If ulcers are present, osteomyelitis can ensue, thus, if ulcers are present, they should be eradicated. The best treatment results are achieved when treatment is initiated during the early stages of Charcot neuroarthropathy.

The goal of treatment in the acute Charcot neuroarthropathy is to stabilize the condition. The traditional treatment is total contact casting for immobilizing. However, non-weight bearing in a total contact cast produces osteopenia of the ipsilateral foot and increased weight-bearing forces on the contralateral foot. These resulting sequelae can make it difficult for sequent surgery and can lead to ulceration and Charcot neuroarthropathy in the contralateral foot. Maintaining non-weight-bearing status is difficult for this patient population for multiple reasons (e.g., muscle atrophy, obesity, diminished proprioception).

The goal of treatment in the chronic Charcot neuroarthropathy is to perform Achilles tendon lengthening, ostectomy, débridement, osteotomy, arthrodesis, and open reduction with internal fixation. Acute correction via open reduction with rigid internal fixation or plantar plating are frequently used for reconstruction.[1] In addtion, acute correction via open reduction with application of static external fixation has been reported.[2] A recently described method for treating acute Charcot neuroarthropathy is to apply a static external fixator, which acts like a cast by immobilizing the affected joints and bones.[3] A new minimally invasive gradual correction method with the use of external fixation is presented.[4,5]

Clinical Evaluation

Charcot deformities of the foot and ankle are observed at isolated or multiple anatomic locations at various stages (Eichenholtz stages 0, 1, 2, 3) with varying degrees of severity.[6,7] Plantar ulcers correlate to the anatomic location of the Charcot neuroarthropathy. For example, medial column ulcers of the foot are generally associated with Charcot neuroarthropathy of the tarsometatarsal region and correlate with a medial column collapse. Tarsometatarsal Charcot deformities are typically stable due to the interlocking anatomy and are successfully treated conservatively or with a limited surgical approach (ostectomy or acute wedge resection with stabilization).[8,9] However, lateral column ulcers are associated with a midfoot Charcot deformity, which typically is not stable. Instability of the lateral column leads to recurrent ulcers, therefore conservative treatment generally fails and surgical reconstruction often becomes necessary.[10,11] Catanzariti et al.[10] suggested that patients with lateral column Charcot deformity require a more complex surgical reconstruction.

Radiographs of the Charcot foot and ankle can be difficult to decipher; the bones of the hindfoot and midfoot are superimposed because of the subluxation/dislocation of these joints. In addition, bone fragmentation and proliferation of new bone during the early and late stages of Charcot neuroarthropathy, respectively, add to the complexity of radiographic interpretation. Radiographs that show the patient during weight bearing should be obtained in all planes to more easily locate the Charcot deformity. Axial view radiographs are helpful to evaluate hindfoot and ankle deformity.[12]

Minimally Invasive Gradual Charcot Foot Reconstruction

The goals of surgical intervention for the Charcot foot and ankle are to restore alignment and stability, prevent amputation, prepare for a shoe or brace, and allow the patient to be

B.M. Lamm(✉) and D. Paley
Rubin Institute for Advanced Orthopedics, Sinai Hospital of
Baltimore, 2401 West Belvedere Avenue, Baltimore, MD 21215, USA
e-mail: blamm@lifebridgehealth.org

G.R. Scuderi and A.J. Tria (eds.), *Minimally Invasive Surgery in Orthopedics*,
DOI 10.1007/978-0-387-76608-9_54, © Springer Science+Business Media, LLC 2010

ambulatory. Historically, open reduction with internal fixation was the mainstay for treatment of Charcot foot deformities. Large open incisions were made to remove the excess bone and to reduce the fragmented or dislocated bone. In addition, screw fixation or plantar plating was traditionally performed in an attempt to stabilize the Charcot joint. These invasive surgical procedures typically resulted in a nonanatomic correction (e.g., shortening of the foot or incomplete deformity correction) and occasionally resulted in neurovascular compromise, incision-healing problems, infection, and the use of casts or boots for non-weight-bearing patients. Although performing open reduction has disadvantages, in cases of tarsometatarsal Charcot deformity, it is advantageous. Typically, Charcot neuroarthropathy of the tarsometatarsal joints is associated with mild to moderate deformities because the tarsometatarsal joints are structurally interlocked. Acute realignment achieved by performing a wedge resection and applying internal fixation produces a stable foot.

Gradual deformity correction with external fixation is preferred for large deformity reductions of the dislocated Charcot joint(s). Correction with external fixation allows for gradual, accurate realignment of the dislocated/subluxated Charcot joints. One advantage of using an Ilizarov apparatus to gradually correct the deformity is that the technique is minimally invasive, especially for patients with multiple previous incisions. Gradual correction also allows for anatomic correction without loss of foot length or bone mass. External fixation allows for partial weight bearing and limits neurovascular compromise because the correction occurs slowly over a period of time.

A stable or coalesced foot with Charcot deformity will require an osteotomy for correction of the deformity. The osteotomy can be performed by using the percutaneous Gigli saw technique. Midfoot osteotomies can be performed across three levels (i.e., talar neck and calcaneal neck, cubonavicular osseous level, and cuneocuboid osseous level. Performing a proximal osteotomy across multiple metatarsals is best avoided because of the disturbance of the interossei, the risk of neurovascular injury, and the multiple bones that require stabilization.[11]

For an unstable or an incompletely coalesced Charcot foot, correction can be obtained through gradual distraction. Despite the radiographic appearance of coalescence, the majority of Charcot deformities can undergo distraction without ostectomy to realign the pedal anatomy. This first stage consists of osseous realignment is achieved with an external fixator utilizing ligamentotaxis. After realignment, the correction is maintained by creating an osseous fusion with rigid intramedullary metatarsal screws that are inserted percutaneously. This two-stage correction is a new technique that was developed by the senior author (DP). The distraction restores the osseous anatomy and allows for ulcer healing.

Surgical Technique

The first stage consists of osseous realignment achieved by performing ligamentotaxis. A Taylor Spatial Frame (TSF) forefoot 6 × 6 butt frame construct is applied and provides gradual relocation of the forefoot on the hindfoot. The distal tibia, talus, and calcaneus are fixed with two U-plates joined and first mounted orthogonal to the tibia in both the anteroposterior and lateral planes. The U-plate is affixed to the tibia with one lateromedial 1.8-mm wire and two to three other points of fixation (combination of smooth wires or half-pins). For additional stability, a second distal tibial ring can be added, creating a distal tibial fixation block. It is essential to fix the hindfoot in a neutral position; an Achilles tendon lengthening typically is required to achieve a neutral hindfoot position. We prefer performing percutaneous Z-lengthening of the Achilles tendon. With the hindfoot manually held in a neutral position, the U-plate is fixed to the calcaneus with two crossing 1.8-mm wires. A 1.8-mm medial-lateral talar neck wire also is inserted and fixed to the U-plate. Next, two 1.8-mm stirrup wires are inserted through the osseous segment just proximal and distal to the Charcot joint(s). Stirrup wires are bent 90° just outside the skin to extend and attach but are not tensioned to their respective external fixation rings distant from the point of fixation. These stirrup wires capture osseous segments that are far from an external fixation ring, thereby providing accurate and precise Charcot joint distraction. A full external fixation ring is then mounted to the forefoot with two 1.8-mm crossing metatarsal wires and the aforementioned distal stirrup wire. Digital pinning often is required whereby the digital wires (1.5 or 1.8 mm) are attached to the forefoot ring. Finally, the six TSF struts are placed and final radiographs obtained (anteroposterior and lateral views of the foot to include the tibia). Orthogonal anteroposterior and lateral view fluoroscopic images are obtained of the reference ring; the images provide the mounting parameters that are needed for the computer planning. The choice of which ring (distal or proximal) to use as the reference ring is per the surgeon's preference; typically, a distal reference is chosen for foot deformity correction. Superimposition of the reference ring on the final films is critical for accurate postoperative computer deformity planning (www.spatialframe.com). TSF planning is critical to fully comprehend before attempting this procedure. In summary, the surgeon enters the deformity and mounting parameters into an Internet-based software that produces a daily schedule for the patient to perform adjustments on each of the six struts. The rate and duration of the patient's schedule is controlled by the surgeon's data entry. The patient is clinically and radiographically followed in the office weekly or biweekly.

Creative frame construction is required because of the small pedal anatomy, which renders it difficult to apply external fixation. When applying the forefoot 6 × 6 butt frame, it is important to mount the U-plate on the hindfoot and the full ring on the forefoot as posteriorly and anteriorly as possible, respectively. The greatest distance of forefoot and hindfoot ring separation is critical to accommodate the TSF struts. Bone segment fixation is important; otherwise, failure of osteotomy separation or incomplete anatomic reduction occurs. Small wire fixation is preferred in the foot because of the size and consistency of the bones. When treating a patient with neuropathy, construction of extremely stable constructs is of great importance. External fixation for Charcot deformity correction should include a distal tibial ring with a closed foot ring.

After gradual distraction with the TSF has realigned the anatomy of the foot, the second stage is performed. In the second stage, the external fixator is removed while simultaneously performing minimally invasive arthrodesis of the affected joints with percutaneous insertion of internal fixation. Gradual distraction for realignment of the dislocated Charcot joint(s) is obtained in approximately 1–2 months. Before frame removal, small transverse incisions (2–3 cm in length) overlying the appropriate joint(s) are made to perform cartilage removal and joint preparation for arthrodesis. Minimally invasive arthrodesis is easily preformed because the Charcot joint(s) are already distracted. Under fluoroscopic guidance, the guidewires for the large-diameter cannulated screws are inserted percutaneously through the plantar skin incision into the metatarsal head by dorsiflexing the metatarsophalangeal joint. After the lateral and medial column guidewires are inserted to maintain the corrected foot position, the frame is removed and the foot is re-prepped. Typically, three large-diameter cannulated intramedullary metatarsal screws are inserted: medial and lateral column partially threaded screws for compression of the arthrodesis site and one central fully threaded screw for additional stabilization. These screws span the entire length of the metatarsals to the calcaneus and talus, provide compression across the minimally invasive arthrodesis site, and stabilize the adjacent joints. The intramedullary metatarsal screws cross an unaffected joint, the Lisfranc joint, thereby protecting the Lisfranc joint from experiencing a future Charcot event. The minimally invasive incisions are then closed, and a well-padded U and L splint is applied. Before hospital discharge (length of hospital stay ranges from 1 to 4 days), the patient's operative splint and dressing are removed and a short leg cast applied. A non-weight-bearing short leg cast is maintained for 2–3 months, and then gradual progression to weight bearing is achieved. Thus, the entire treatment is completed in 4–5 months (Figs. 54.1–54.8).

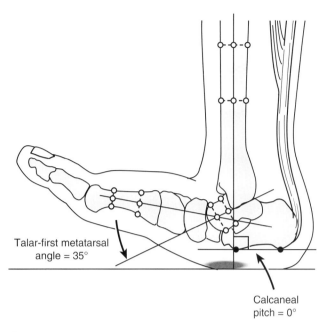

Fig. 54.1 Illustration of a midfoot (midtarsal joint) Charcot neuroarthropathy with equinus deformity (Eichenholtz stage II or III, with ulceration). Lateral view shows equinus (calcaneal pitch, 0°) and rocker bottom (talar-first metatarsal angle, 35°) (From Paley,[11] with kind permission of Springer Science + Business Media.)

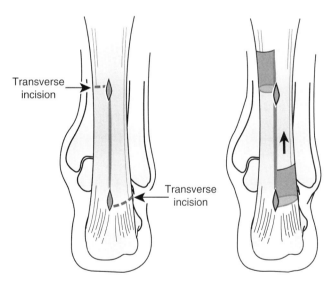

Fig. 54.2 Percutaneous Achilles tendon Z-lengthening is performed to acutely correct the equinus deformity (*Inset*, modified from Paley,[11] with kind permission of Springer Science + Business Media.)

Conclusion

We have used this gradual distraction technique during the past 5 years and have achieved good to excellent success. Our short-term results are promising considering that neither recurrent ulceration nor deep infections have occurred. The advantages of our method when compared with the resection and plating method reported by Schon et al.[1] or the resection and external fixation method reported by Cooper[13] are

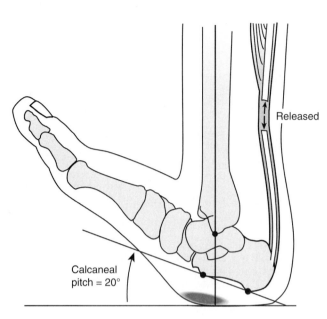

Fig. 54.3 After tendon Achilles lengthening, the calcaneal pitch is restored to 20°. Note the resultant forefoot position (From Paley,[11] with kind permission of Springer Science + Business Media.)

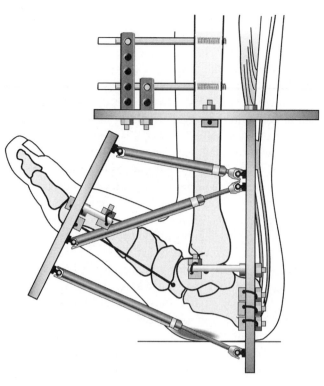

Fig. 54.5 The forefoot ring is mounted perpendicular to the longitudinal axis of the metatarsals. Note that this ring is mounted as distal as possible in order to allow adequate space between the forefoot and hindfoot ring for strut placement (From Paley,[11] with kind permission of Springer Science + Business Media.)

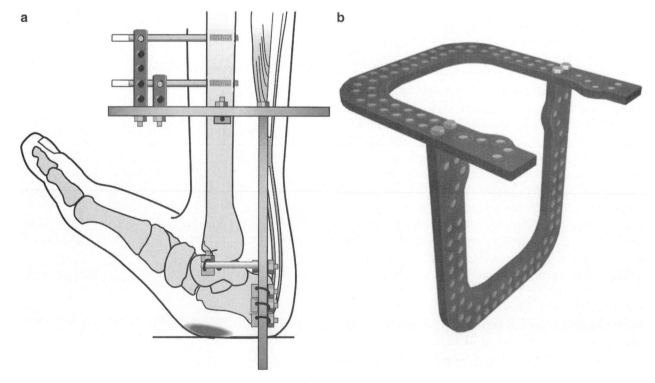

Fig. 54.4 (**a**) The hindfoot and ankle are then fixed in the corrected position with the Taylor spatial frame (TSF) (forefoot 6 × 6 butt). Note the stirrup wires placed adjacent (just distal and proximal) to the midtarsal joint to ensure focused distraction at the Charcot joint. (**b**) A three-dimensional illustration of two joined U-plates that form the posterior construct for the forefoot 6 × 6 butt frame (From Paley,[11] with kind permission of Springer Science + Business Media.)

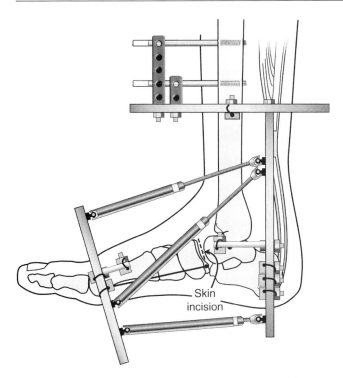

Fig. 54.6 Gradual distraction (5–15 mm) and realignment of the forefoot to the hindfoot are performed with the external fixator. Just before fixator removal, a minimally invasive fusion of the midtarsal joint is performed through a vertical incision. The plantar ulcer is now healed (From Paley,[11] with kind permission of Springer Science + Business Media.)

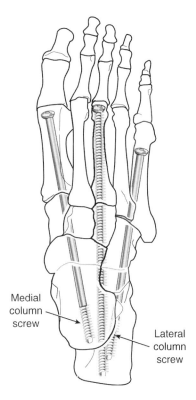

Fig. 54.8 Anteroposterior view shows a third fully threaded screw inserted to increase midfoot stability. Note the accurate anatomic reduction, fusion of the involved Charcot joint (in this example the midtarsal joint), protection of the adjacent Lisfranc joints (stability via screw fixation), ridged internal stability, restoration of foot length, healed ulceration, and preservation of the subtalar and ankle joints (From Paley,[11] with kind permission of Springer Science + Business Media.)

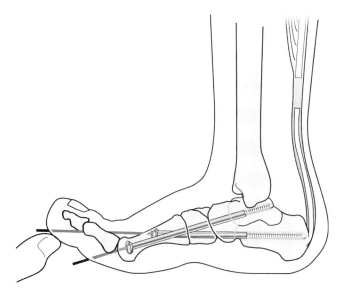

Fig. 54.7 After inserting the percutaneous guidewires for the large-diameter cannulated screws, the fixator is removed. Then, partially threaded intramedullary metatarsal cannulated screws are inserted beneath the metatarsal head percutaneously to compress both the medial and lateral columns of the foot to ensure fusion of the midtarsal joint (From Paley,[11] with kind permission of Springer Science + Business Media.)

preservation of foot length, soft tissue, and osseous anatomy, and cosmesis. Furthermore, our method is much less invasive.

Acknowledgments I thank Joy Marlowe, BSA, for her excellent illustrative artwork.

References

1. Schon LC, Easley ME, Weinfeld SB. Charcot neuroarthropathy of the foot and ankle. Clin Orthop Relat Res 349:116–131, 1998
2. Jolly GP, Zgonis T, Polyzois V. External fixation in the management of Charcot neuroarthropathy. Clin Podiatr Med Surg 20:741–756, 2003
3. Wang JC, Le AW, Tsukuda RK. A new technique for Charcot's foot reconstruction. J Am Podiatr Med Assoc 92:429–436, 2002
4. Frykberg RG, ed. The High Risk Foot in Diabetes Mellitus. New York, NY: Churchill Livingstone, 1991
5. Trepman E, Nihal A, Pinzur MS. Current topics review: Charcot neuroarthropathy of the foot and ankle. Foot Ankle Int 26:46–63, 2005
6. Eichenholtz SN. Charcot Joints. Springfield, IL: C. C. Thomas, 1966

7. Shibata T, Tada K, Hashizume C. The results of arthrodesis of the ankle for leprotic neuroarthropathy. J Bone Joint Surg 72A:749–756, 1990

8. Brodsky JW, Rouse AM. Exostectomy for symptomatic bony prominences in diabetic Charcot feet. Clin Orthop Relat Res 296:21–26, 1993

9. Simon SR, Tejwani SG, Wilson DL, Santner TJ, Denniston NL. Arthrodesis as an early alternative to nonoperative management of Charcot arthropathy of the diabetic foot. J Bone Joint Surg 82A:939–950, 2000

10. Catanzariti AR, Mendicino R, Haverstock B. Ostectomy for diabetic neuroarthropathy involving the midfoot. J Foot Ankle Surg 39:291–300, 2000

11. Paley D. Principles of Deformity Correction, Rev ed. Berlin: Springer; 2005

12. Lamm BM, Paley D. Deformity correction planning for hindfoot, ankle, and lower limb. Clin Podiatr Med Surg North Am 21:305–326, 2004

13. Cooper PS. Application of external fixators for management of Charcot deformities of the foot and ankle. Foot Ankle Clin 7:207–254, 2002

Chapter 55
Percutaneous Supramalleolar Osteotomy Using the Ilizarov/Taylor Spatial Frame

S. Robert Rozbruch

The supramalleolar osteotomy (SMO) can be used to reposition the ankle and foot by correcting deformity about the ankle. Indications for this procedure include malunion of fracture, stiff nonunion, malunion of ankle fusion, arthrosis of the ankle with talar tilt, growth arrest deformity, and congenital or developmental deformity.[1,2]

The SMO can be performed in isolation or can be combined with other procedures such as ankle distraction, ankle fusion, or simultaneous lengthening. In general, SMO can be performed with acute or gradual correction, internal or external fixation, and closing, opening, or neutral wedge technique. While a mild to moderate valgus deformity of the ankle can be corrected with a traditional open surgery using a medial closing wedge technique, acute correction, and internal fixation, this technique has limitations and drawbacks. These include the need for open surgery and implantation of hardware, deformity correction limitations, and no postoperative adjustability.

SMO can be performed using a percutaneous technique in conjunction with an Ilizarov/Taylor Spatial Frame (TSF) (Smith and Nephew, Memphis, TN). The circular frame is percutaneously mounted to match the complete deformity (coronal, sagittal, and axial planes). Then the SMO of the tibia is percutaneously performed. Acute and/or gradual correction can be accomplished by moving the frame-bone complex. All aspects of the deformity can be corrected and there is postoperative adjustability. There is no implantation of internal fixation, making this an attractive option if there is a history of infection. When skin is compromised and the soft tissue envelope is a concern, this technique is advantageous because it avoids open incisions and bulky subcutaneous hardware. Complex deformities in an oblique plane and combined with rotational deformity can be efficiently approached in this manner. Excellent frame stability generally allows the patient to weight bear as tolerated.

S.R. Rozbruch (✉)
Limb Lengthening and Deformity Service, Hospital for Special Surgery, New York, NY, 10021, USA
Associate Professor of Clinical Orthopaedic Surgery, Weill Medical College of Cornell University, 535 East 70th Street, New York, NY, 10021, USA
e-mail: RozbruchSR@hss.edu

This chapter addresses the clinical indications, preoperative assessment, surgical technique, and postoperative care for the technique of percutaneous SMO using the Ilizarov/TSF.

Clinical Indications

Malunion of Fracture

Malunion of a tibia fracture in the distal third of the leg will cause abnormal force transmission across the ankle and lead to posttraumatic arthrosis.[1,3,4] While valgus deformities are more easily compensated through inversion of the subtalar joint, the deformity will lead to wear of the ankle joint. A varus deformity is functionally debilitating to the patient because there is limited ability to compensate with hindfoot eversion. Recurvatum deformity leads to uncovering of the talus and compensatory ankle equines contracture. Procurvatum deformity limits dorsiflexion of the ankle and leads to anterior ankle impingement.[4] Oblique plane deformities and rotation and translation deformities are common in malunions.

A malunion of the mid-distal third of the leg that is composed of varus and translation may have a center of rotation and angulation (CORA)[4,5] or apex of deformity in the supramalleolar region. The SMO becomes a convenient way to correct this because the supramalleolar bone is metaphyseal, previously uninjured, and has better healing potential than the actual site of the nonunion (Fig. 55.1).

The goal is to correct the deformity in both the coronal and sagittal planes. The goal is to achieve a lateral distal tibial angle (LDTA) of 90° (Fig. 55.2a) and an anterior distal tibial angle (ADTA) of 80°[4,5] (Fig. 55.2b). The use of the Ilizarov/TSF is particularly useful for a gradual correction of a simple or large oblique plane deformity.[6-8]

Associated symptomatic arthritis may be addressed as well. Ankle distraction[9] (Fig. 55.3) or ankle fusion (Fig. 55.4) can be performed distal to the SMO with the addition of another level of treatment.

G.R. Scuderi and A.J. Tria (eds.), *Minimally Invasive Surgery in Orthopedics*,
DOI 10.1007/978-0-387-76608-9_55, © Springer Science+Business Media, LLC 2010

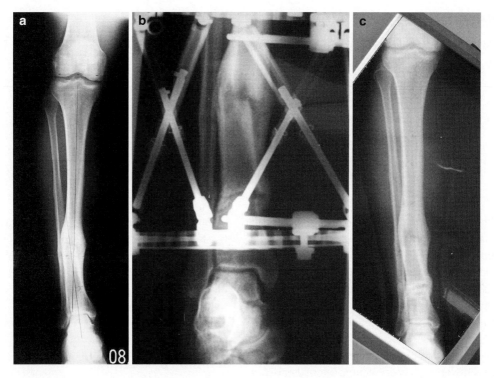

Fig. 55.1 A 35-year-old man with 15-year-old malunion of the tibia who presents with ankle pain and varus deformity. (**a**) Preoperative AP radiograph showing varus deformity at the mid-distal third of the tibia. The apex of the deformity was located in the supramalleolar region because of the translation at the malunion site. (**b**) AP radiograph at end of distraction of the SMO correction. (**c**) One-year follow-up AP radiograph showing a good restoration of the tibial axis

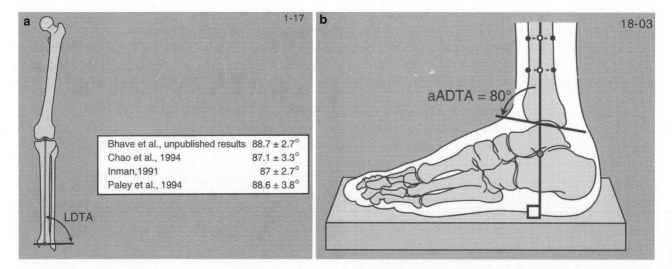

Fig. 55.2 (**a**) Normal lateral distal tibial angle (LDTA) (**b**) Normal anterior distal tibial angle (ADTA) (From Scuderi GR, Tria AJ Jr, Berger RA (eds.), MIS Techniques in Orthopedics. New York: Springer, 2006, with kind permission of Springer Science + Business Media, Inc.)

Stiff Nonunion

The same deformity types mentioned in malunions will be seen in this group. An excellent application of gradual correction is for a hypertrophic stiff nonunion with deformity.[8,10,11] This type of nonunion has fibrocartilage tissue in the nonunion site that has the biologic capacity for bony union. It lacks stability and axial alignment. Gradual distraction of this type of nonunion to achieve normal alignment results in bone formation. The nonunion acts like regenerate and bony healing occurs. Modest lengthening of no more than 1.5 cm should be done through the nonunion. If additional lengthening is needed, a second osteotomy for lengthening is performed. Several studies have confirmed Ilizarov's success with this technique.[1,6,8] The principle advantages are not having to open the nonunion site in the face of poor skin and

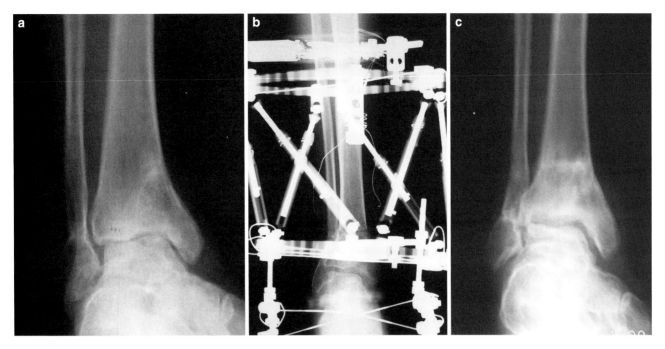

Fig. 55.3 A 20-year-old woman with posttraumatic arthrosis of the ankle. (**a**) Preoperative AP radiograph showing varus tilt of the talus and extensive medial cartilage loss. (**b**) After SMO to put talus in neutral and ankle distraction. (**c**) Two-year follow-up showing normal alignment and improved joint space

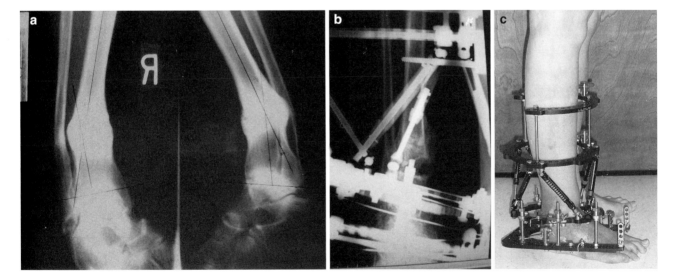

Fig. 55.4 A 50-year-old woman with a malunion of the distal tibia and advanced ankle arthrosis. (**a**) Preoperative AP and lateral radiograph showing varus and recurvatum deformity with arthrosis of the ankle. (**b, c**) AP radiograph and side view showing an ankle arthrodesis and simultaneous gradual correction of the deformity with a TSF

widened callus and gaining length through an opening wedge correction. This is particularly beneficial to the region above the ankle where the soft tissue envelope is often compromised. This technique is not useful for mobile atrophic nonunions and less applicable to infected nonunions.

Malunion of Ankle Fusion

An ankle fusion that is malpositioned can be corrected through an SMO.[10–12] In this case, the osteotomy can be done very distally because wire penetration into the ankle joint is not a concern. One can correct all deformities including anterior translation (Fig. 55.5). If some lengthening is needed, it may be done through the same osteotomy or through an osteotomy in the proximal tibia.

Ankle Arthrosis with Deformity

Ankle arthrosis may be associated with an angular deformity of the distal tibia.[13] Tilt of the talus may develop with joint space narrowing on one particular side of the ankle joint. In this situation, the SMO may be used to achieve a neutral talus relative to the axis of the tibia.[2,14,15] This can be combined with an ankle distraction[9,10] (Fig. 55.3).

Ankle and Foot Deformity

A combined deformity consisting of ankle valgus with foot planovalgus and forefoot abduction can be seen in rheumatoid arthritis, as an example (Fig. 55.6). An SMO can be used to correct (and even overcorrect to a small degree) the ankle valgus. In addition, internal rotation at the SMO can be used to compensate for some of the planovalgus and forefoot abduction.[14,16] Correction of a foot deformity above the ankle is very powerful in that it effects a large translation change to

the foot. One is limited by the desire to avoid an oblique ankle joint line. In cases of ankle fusion or correction of ankle fusion, obliquity of the ankle fusion mass is not a significant problem.

Growth Arrest Deformity

Asymmetric damage to the distal tibial growth plate can occur from trauma or infection. This will lead to deformity and shortening of the leg. The distal tibial growth plate contributes 40% of the tibial growth (Fig. 55.7).

Congenital and Developmental Deformity

Neuromuscular

Asymmetric muscle pull can lead to deformity at the ankle.[17] This is seen in Charcot–Marie–Tooth (CMT) disease with first equinovarus of the foot and later talar tilt, which further increases the varus deformity. This pattern can also be seen after nerve injury. Valgus deformities have been observed in myelomeningocele.[18,19] External rotation deformities have been observed in patients with cerebral palsy[20] and sacral agenesis.

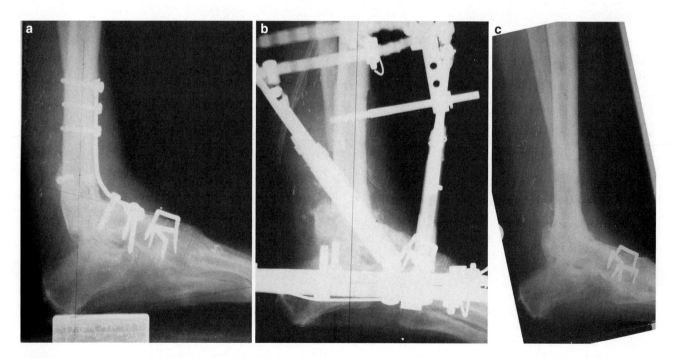

Fig. 55.5 A 40-year-old woman with malunion of ankle fusion. (**a**) Lateral radiograph showing anterior translation deformity. (**b**) After correction with an SMO and gradual correction with a TSF. (**c**) One-year follow-up

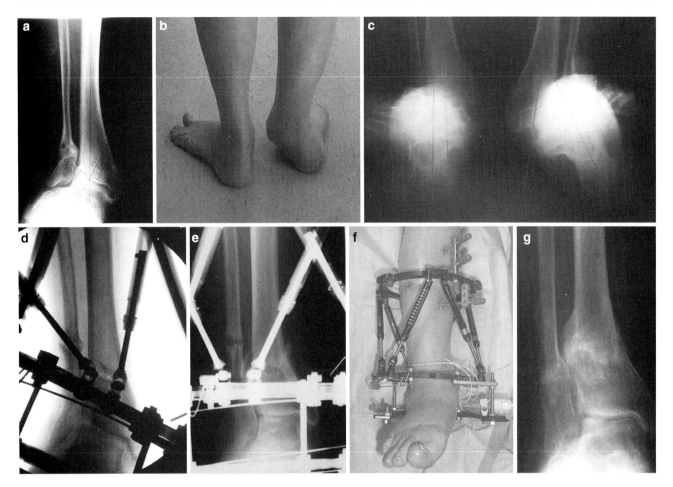

Fig. 55.6 A 77-year-old woman with rheumatoid arthritis who has an ankle/foot deformity. (**a**) Preoperative AP radiograph showing valgus ankle deformity. (**b**) Back view showing ankle/hindfoot valgus and forefoot abduction. (**c**) Saltzman view illustrating the deformity. Note that the apex of deformity is in the supramalleolar region. (**d**) After SMO and application of frame to match the deformity. (**e**, **f**) After the distraction phase, showing correction of the deformity. (**g**) One year later, showing a healed osteotomy

Fibrous Dysplasia and Ollier's Disease

These tumor-like conditions are associated with deformity. This seems to occur when the lesions affect the growth plate. Deformities of the ankle related to growth disturbance at the distal tibial physis can be corrected with an SMO. When an osteotomy is performed through Ollier's bone, new normal bone will grow.

Achondroplasia

In addition to varus deformities of the proximal tibiae, there are often varus deformities of the distal tibiae as well. Double-level tibial osteotomies including an SMO may be done to correct all deformities and to divide a large lengthening between two sites.

Preoperative Assessment

Clinical Evaluation

In the history, one should obtain information about the type of bony and soft tissue injury, surgical procedures performed, history of infection, and the use of antibiotics. High-energy injuries and open fractures have a higher risk for infection. Information about back pain, perceived leg length discrepancy (LLD), use of a shoe lift, and deformity should be elicited from the patient. The presence of deformity will often lead to the patient's report of a feeling of increased pressure on the medial or lateral part of the foot with a valgus or varus deformity, respectively. A short leg will often lead to complaints of low back pain and contralateral hip pain. If antibiotics are being used to suppress an infected nonunion, an attempt should be made to discontinue these for 6 weeks prior to surgery in order to obtain reliable intraoperative cul-

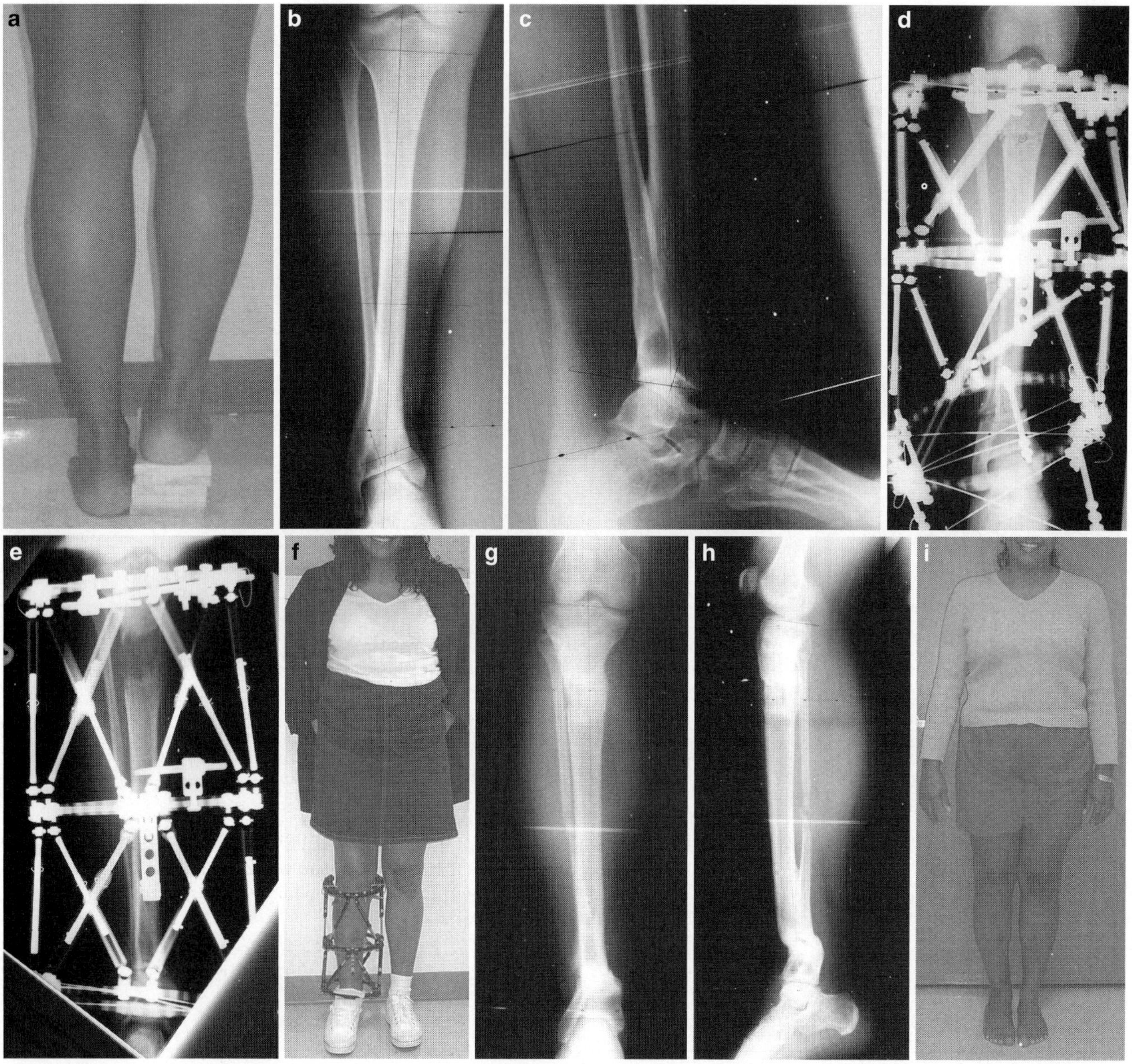

Fig. 55.7 A 25-year-old woman with posttraumatic growth arrest of the distal tibia. (**a**) Back view showing that an LLD of 6-cm ankle varus is compensated by mobile hindfoot eversion. (**b**) Preoperative AP radiograph showing the varus deformity. (**c**) Lateral radiograph showing a procurvatum deformity. The apex of the deformity is periarticular. (**d**) Postoperative radiograph showing nondisplaced SMO and proximal tibial osteotomy. (**e**) After distraction, showing a proximal tibial lengthening and distal tibia correction. (**f**) Standing front view at end of distraction. (**g**, **h**) AP and lateral radiographs 1 year later, showing healed osteotomies. Note the intentional medial and posterior translation of the distal fragment because the osteotomy site was away from the apex of deformity. (**i**) Standing front view showing equal leg lengths and correction of deformity

ture samples. Discontinuation of antibiotics must be done with caution and careful observation, particularly in compromised patients like those with diabetes or on immunosuppressive medications. The current amount of pain, the use of narcotics, and the ability to ambulate with or without support should be noted.

On physical examination, one should look for deformity and LLD with the patient standing still and walking. The inability to bear weight suggests an unstable nonunion. The view from the back is helpful for seeing coronal plane deformity.

LLD is evaluated by using blocks under the short leg and by examining the level of the iliac crests. The view from the side is helpful for observing sagittal plane deformity, and equines contracture. The combination of recurvatum deformity above the ankle and equines contracture of the ankle will lead to a foot translated forward position with an extension moment on the knee. Range of motion of the ankle, subtalar, forefoot, and toes should be recorded. Rigid compensation for ankle deformity through the subtalar joint is an important factor. This typically occurs when there is long-standing ankle deformity. If this is present, it must be taken into account when correcting the ankle. The condition of the soft tissue envelope, especially previous surgical wounds and flaps, and neurovascular findings should be recorded. This includes the posterior tibial and dorsalis pedis pulses, foot sensation, and dorsiflexion and plantarflexion motor function of the ankle and toes.

Rotational deformity is best assessed on clinical exam with the patient in the prone position. *Thigh-foot axis* (TFA) is used to assess rotational deformity of the tibia. Rotational profile of the femur is used to assess rotational deformity in the femur. Computed tomographic (CT) scan can also be used for this purpose. CT scan cuts at the proximal femur, distal femur, proximal tibia, and distal tibia allow analysis of rotational deformity.[4,10]

Radiographic Assessment

Radiographs should include anteroposterior (AP), lateral, and mortise views of the ankle, Saltzman's view of both feet, (Fig. 55.8) and a 51″ bipedal erect leg X-ray including the hips to ankles with blocks under the short leg to level the pelvis. LLD as well a limb alignment can be measured from a standing bipedal 51″ radiograph. The short leg is placed on blocks to level the pelvis and the height of the blocks is recorded.[4,5] This can be done with the patient using crutches if necessary. These radiographs yield crucial information about LLD, deformity, presence of hardware, arthritis, and bony union. A supine scanogram can also be used to measure length discrepancy but this is not useful for alignment analysis. CT scan and magnetic resonance imaging (MRI) can be

used for further evaluation as needed. The CT scan can be helpful in getting more information about bony union. The MRI can be helpful for obtaining information about the condition of cartilage in the ankle and subtalar joints and the presence of infection. Nuclear medicine studies can also be used, but we have not found them to be very helpful in this evaluation.

Laboratory studies including white blood cell count, erythrocyte sedimentation rate, and C-reactive protein can be helpful for diagnosing the presence of infection. Selective lidocaine injections into the ankle and subtalar joints may be helpful for diagnosing the dominant source of pain.

Surgical Planning

The proximal tibial axis is represented with an antegrade mid-diaphyseal tibial line. The coronal plane distal tibial axis is represented with a perpendicular line to the ankle joint drawn retrograde (normal LDTA is 90°) (see Fig. 55.2a). The intersection of these lines is the apex of deformity (Fig. 55.9). In the sagittal plane, the distal tibial axis is drawn 80° to the lateral joint line (remember that normal ADTA is 80°) (see Fig. 55.2b). The intersection of these lines is the apex of deformity. The rotational deformity is assessed from the TFA done on physical examination. If the osteotomy is at the level of the CORA, then no translation is needed. If the osteotomy is done at a level that is different from the CORA, then translation at the osteotomy site will be needed to fully correct the deformity[4,5] (Fig. 55.10).

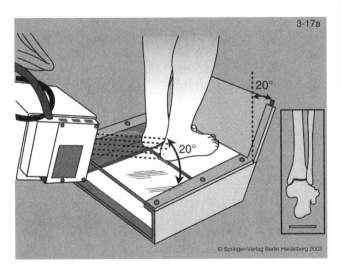

Fig. 55.8 Saltzman view schematic diagram (From Scuderi GR, Tria AJ Jr, Berger RA (eds.), MIS Techniques in Orthopedics. New York: Springer, 2006, with kind permission of Springer Science + Business Media, Inc.)

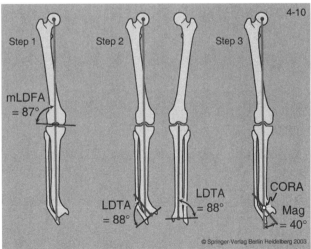

Fig. 55.9 (**a**) Correction of varus can cause injury to the posterior tibial nerve with stretch and needed medial translation. (**b**) Correction of procurvatum can cause injury to the posterior tibial nerve with stretch and needed posterior translation (From Scuderi GR, Tria AJ Jr, Berger RA (eds.), MIS Techniques in Orthopedics. New York: Springer, 2006, with kind permission of Springer Science + Business Media, Inc.)

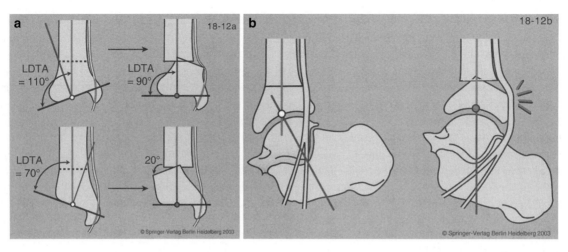

Fig. 55.10 Mechanical axis planning for SMO (From Scuderi GR, Tria AJ Jr, Berger RA (eds.), MIS Techniques in Orthopedics. New York: Springer, 2006, with kind permission of Springer Science + Business Media, Inc.)

Treatment Principles

Features of the Ilizarov Method

The Ilizarov method is particularly useful for addressing the full spectrum of posttraumatic ankle pathology. Listed below are versatile features of the Ilizarov method.[7,9–12,21]

1. Avoid internal fixation in the presence or history of infection
2. Allows a minimal incision technique in setting of poor soft tissue
3. Utilizes acute and/or gradual correction of deformity
4. Utilizes opening wedge correction, avoiding the need for bone resection
5. Useful for large deformity correction
6. Postoperative adjustability for compression or correction
7. Simultaneous lengthening is possible for optimization of LLD
8. Allows multiple-level treatment (a modular approach)
9. Weight bearing and ankle range of motion are encouraged.

Acute Versus Gradual Correction

One can employ either acute or gradual correction of a nonunion or malunion.[1,8] Acute corrections can be performed in conjunction with all methods of fixation including plates[19,22], intramedullary (IM) nails, and external fixation frames. Gradual correction requires the use of specialized frames. The personality of the problems helps guide the surgeon toward the best method. For example, a distal tibial malunion with 15° valgus deformity and 2 cm shortening is best handled with an osteotomy to gradually correct the angular

deformity and lengthen the bone with a specialized frame. The Ilizarov method is utilized to gradually correct the complete deformity with distraction osteogenesis. One may choose to perform the deformity correction and lengthening at one level if bone regeneration potential is good. Alternatively, one may choose to perform a double level osteotomy - one level at the CORA[5] for deformity correction, and one level for lengthening in the proximal tibia metaphysis (see Fig. 55.7). Gradual correction achieves treatment of shortening and carries less risk of posterior tibial nerve stretch neuropraxia than if attempted with an acute correction (Fig. 55.10).

The use of plates and IM nails requires an acute correction of angular and translational deformity. Acute corrections are particularly useful for modest deformity correction, mobile atrophic nonunions that are opened and bone grafted, and small bone defects that can be acutely shortened. The principle advantage of acute correction is earlier bone contact for healing and a simpler fixation construct. Acute corrections are generally better tolerated in the femur and humerus and less well tolerated in the tibia and ankle, related to issues of neurovascular insult.

Gradual correction with a specialized frame is useful for large deformity correction[11,21,23], associated limb lengthening, bone transport to treat segmental defects,[24] and for stiff hypertrophic nonunion repair.[8] Gradual correction employs the principle of *distraction osteogenesis* commonly referred to as the *Ilizarov method*.[12,25] Bone and soft tissue is gradually distracted at a rate of approximately 1 mm per day in divided increments. Bone growth in the distraction gap is called *regenerate*. The interval between osteotomy and the start of lengthening is called the *latency phase* and is usually 7–10 days. The correction and lengthening is called the *distraction phase*. The *consolidation phase* is the time from the end of distraction until bony union.[25] This phase is most variable and is most affected by patient factors such as age and health. If the *structure at risk* (SAR) is a nerve, such as the peroneal nerve for a proximal tibia valgus deformity or the posterior tibial nerve for an equinovarus deformity of the ankle (Fig. 55.9), gradual correction may be the safer option. The correction can be planned so that the SAR is stretched slowly. If nerve symptoms do occur, the correction can be slowed or stopped. Nerve release can be employed in select situations based on the response to gradual correction.[4]

Surgical Technique

Wire and Pin Configuration

Tensioned skinny wires and half-pins lend approximately the same stability to the frame. The proximal ring or ring block is secured with three or four points of fixation. We typically use one skinny wire (1.8-mm wire for adults) as a reference wire from anterolateral to posteromedial for purposes of mounting the ring. Additional fixation is secured with half-pins. Six-millimeter hydroxy-coated pins are our first choice for adult patients. These are inserted after drilling a 4.8-mm tract.[7]

The distal tibial ring is usually secured with two or three skinny wires (tensioned to 130 kg) and a half-pin. The reference wire is placed in the tibia alone parallel to the ankle. Next, a fibula-tibia wire is inserted posterolateral to anteromedial to reinforce the syndesmosis and prevent fibula migration. A posteromedial to anterolateral wire can also be added. Finally, an anteromedial (medial to the tibialis anterior tendon) to posterolateral 6-mm half-pin is used to add stability in the sagittal plane. Fixation may be extended across the ankle to the foot if additional stability of the distal segment is needed.

Taylor Spatial Frame

Terminology

Rings are placed on either side of the defect site and the anticipated lengthening site(s) (Fig. 55.10). The rings can be placed independently to optimally fit the leg. This is called the *rings first method*. One ring is chosen as the *reference ring* for each level of movement, and it is important that this ring be placed orthogonal to the axis of the tibia. Mounting parameters are defined by the center of the reference ring and this defines the point in space where the deformity correction will occur. It is important to maintain enough distance between rings so that the struts can fit properly. In this frame, one is limited by the shortest length of strut. The advantages

of this frame are that the application is easier and the fit on the leg is better when using the *rings first method*. In addition, residual deformity at the lengthening and docking sites can be addressed by using the same frame to correct angulation and translation simultaneously in the coronal, sagittal, and axial planes without major frame modification. This minimizes angular deformity at the lengthening sites.[6,7]

One ring is chosen to be the *reference ring*. The "virtual hinge" around which the correction occurs is defined by the origin and corresponding point (CP). The *origin* is a point chosen on the edge of one bone segment at the defect site. A *corresponding point* on the other bone segment is chosen with the goal of reducing the CP to the origin. *Mounting parameters* define the location of the origin relative to the reference ring. Mounting parameters are defined by the spatial relationship between the center of the reference ring and the origin in the coronal, sagittal, and axial planes. This defines a virtual hinge around which the deformity correction will occur. TSF struts are used to connect the rings across the deformity.

Deformity Parameters

There are six deformity parameters that will describe the relationship between the proximal segment and the distal segment (the reference segment has the origin and the moving segment has the corresponding point) (Fig. 55.11a, b). Deformity parameters consist of an angulation and a translation in the coronal, sagittal, and axial planes. In the coronal plane, the angulation is varus or valgus and the translation is medial or lateral. In the sagittal plane, the angulation is apex anterior or apex posterior and the translation is anterior or posterior. In the axial plane, the angulation is internal or external rotation and the translation is short or long.

Mounting Parameters

Because the TSF enables correction around a virtual hinge, one must communicate its location (origin) to the computer program (Fig. 55.11c). A grid projected from the reference ring allows one to specify the location of the origin. The location of the origin relative to the center of the reference ring in the coronal, sagittal, and axial planes is recorded. For example, the center of the reference ring may be 10 mm lateral, 25 mm posterior, and 35 mm distal to the origin.

Structure at Risk

The speed of the correction is determined by the surgeon by choosing a structure that he or she wants to move at a determined rate (Fig. 55.11d). Typically, a structure in the concavity of the deformity is the SAR. For example, if we are correcting a varus deformity, the SAR may be the medial cortex of the tibia or the posterior tibial nerve. If we are correcting a valgus, recurvatum deformity, the SAR will be the anterolateral surface of the tibia. We usually move the SAR at 1 mm per day[25], although, this can be varied.

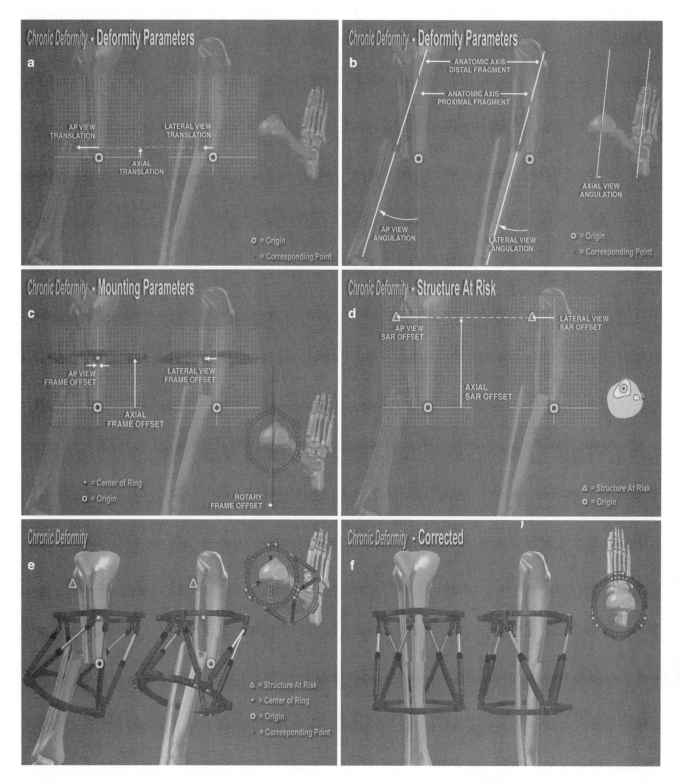

Fig. 55.11 Taylor Spatial Frame concept and language. (**a**) Measurement of translation deformity parameters. (**b**) Measurement of angulation deformity parameters. (**c**) Measurement of mounting parameters. (**d**) Structure at risk relative to origin. (**e**) Before correction. (**f**) After correction

Fibula Osteotomy

Osteotomy of the fibula is usually performed with the use of a tourniquet at the beginning of the procedure prior to frame application. A lateral exposure is a simple and safe way to approach the fibula. It is best to locate the osteotomy at or near the apex of deformity, although osteotomy at exactly the same level of the tibia is avoided. This is done to avoid formation of a synostosis.

The shape of osteotomy may be transverse or oblique. When correcting valgus deformity gradually, a transverse osteotomy is done that will be gradually distracted and the gap will fill in with regenerate. When correcting varus deformity, the fibula will need to shorten.[3,21,26] This is accomplished with either fibula resection or an oblique osteotomy where the fragments can overlap.

Supramalleolar Tibial Osteotomy

After the frame has been mounted on the intact bone, the tibial osteotomy is performed. The strut connections between the rings are recorded and then removed. Through a 1-cm skin incision, medial to the tibialis anterior tendon and approximately 1 cm proximal to the distal tibial pins, the SMO is performed. The fluoroscopy is positioned to obtain a lateral Xray of the distal tibia. A multiple drill hole osteotomy technique is used. This entails three passes of the drill along the planned osteotomy line. The SMO is then completed by passing the osteotome across the medial cortex, lateral cortex, and through the bone center to crack the posterior cortex. Rotation of the osteotome and ultimately rotation of the rings completes the osteotomy.[4] Alternatively, a Gigli saw technique can be used to perform the SMO.

Extension Across the Ankle

If there is an ankle contracture, then a foot ring is placed and gradual correction can be done simultaneously. Hinges are placed at the axis of the ankle as in the situation of an ankle distraction. A pulling rod can be placed anterior or a pushing rod posterior to motor the correction (Fig. 55.12).

Proximal Tibial Osteotomy

If there is shortening of the tibia, this can be addressed at the same time as the deformity correction at the apex of the deformity. An osteotomy at the proximal tibia for lengthening can be done if the bone-healing potential at the apex of deformity is not optimal (see Fig. 55.7).

Postoperative Care

Patients are admitted to the hospital for 2–3 days. Nonsteroidal anti-inflammatory medications are avoided in all osteotomy patients for fear of adverse affects on bone formation. The patients receive intravenous antibiotics for 24 h and are then switched to oral antibiotics. The patients are discharged on oral antibiotics for 10 days and oral pain medication. Patients return to the office 10 days postoperatively where sutures are removed and they are educated on how to perform strut adjustments. Patients are seen every 2 weeks during this adjustment period and then once monthly during the consolidation period.

Deformity Correction

Correction of the deformity begins after a latency period of 7–10 days. The web-based Smith and Nephew program is used to generate a daily schedule for strut adjustments that the patient will perform at home. The computer requires the input of basic information including the side, the deformity parameters, the size of the rings and length of struts used, the mounting parameters measured during frame application, and rate of daily adjustment. Additionally, a SAR is selected and entered into the program to assure the correct speed of gradual correction. For valgus producing osteotomy, the structures at risk are the medial soft tissues because they are in the concavity of the correction and will be stretched the greatest distance. Using this information, a clear and simplified prescription is created for the patient to follow every day. We prescribe that struts 1 and 2 be turned in the morning, struts 3 and 4 in the afternoon, and struts 5 and 6 in the evening for a total movement of 1 mm per day. The duration of the adjustment phase depends on the amount of correction needed and is typically between 14 and 28 days. The length of time in the frame is approximately 3 months.

Pain Management

Transdermal wires and pins can be irritating, and we encourage patients to use appropriate oral pain medications. This is especially true during the adjustment period. Once the correction is complete, the frame is no longer moving, and the pain level decreases. Severe or atypical pain merits an evaluated for infection or deep vein thrombosis (DVT).

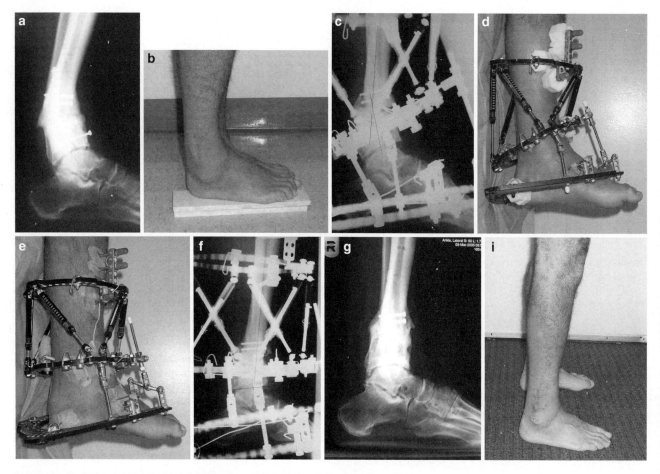

Fig. 55.12 A 48-year-old man with deformity after pilon fracture. (**a**) Preoperative lateral X-ray showing a recurvatum malunion combined with an ankle equines contracture. (**b**) Side view showing foot forward position. (**c, d**) Postoperative X-ray and clinical photo showing the frame matching the deformity at the two levels of correction. (**e, f**) After correction of the two levels of deformity. (**g, h**) Two years later, the patient has minimal pain

Pin Care

The dressings are removed on postoperative day 2. Nurses teach proper daily pin care consisting of a mixture of half normal saline and half hydrogen peroxide applied to the pin sites with sterile cotton swabs. Pins and wires are covered with Xeroform dressings at the skin. Patients are allowed to begin showering on the fourth postoperative day. They are instructed to wash the frame and pin sites with antibacterial soap as an adjuvant form of pin care. Problematic smooth wires can be removed in the office without anesthetic. This is particularly done after the distraction phase or if a wire is painful and infected.

Rehabilitation

Ilizarov stressed the importance of early physical conditioning in conjunction with the application of circular fixators.

Early motion increases blood flow to the lower extremity, prevents joint stiffness, and shortens recovery time.[25] Physical therapy assists with weight bearing as tolerated ambulation and range of motion exercises for the knee and ankle joints. Crutches are typically needed for the first 4–6 weeks after surgery. Occupational therapy provides a custom neutral foot splint to prevent equines posturing during sleep. Patients are encouraged to attend outpatient physical therapy where they continue with their rehabilitation programs.

Frame Removal

Fixators are removed when patients are ambulating without pain or the use of an assistive device and when callus is seen on three cortices around the osteotomy site. This is typically 3 months after the index surgery. We prefer to remove the frames in the operating room. The removal of HA coated pin can be painful and is best done under sedation. We choose to curette and irrigated all half pins sites in an effort to keep pin tracts clean. Transfixation wire sites are not debrided unless there is concern over a specific site. At the time of frame removal, bony union and maturation of the regenerate may be evaluated with a routine X-ray or a stress test under C-arm fluoroscopy. If there is a real concern about bony union, then the struts are removed and the rings manually compressed and distracted, looking for motion at the osteotomy site. A lack of consolidation will require replacement of the struts and prolonging the time in the frame. Once the fixator is removed, patients are placed into a short leg cast for 2 weeks. They are allowed 50% partial weight bearing for 2 weeks then progress to full weight bearing thereafter, first in a cam walker boot and then in a regular shoe.

Complications

Pin Infection

Pin-site infection is a common complication that we encounter when using external fixation. Pin infections are marked by erythema, increasing pain, and drainage around the pin or wire. The vast majority of these infections respond well to more aggressive local pin care and oral antibiotics. If the infection does not resolve quickly, then broader spectrum antibiotics are added or the pin or wire is removed. More advanced infections are treated with removal of the pin or wire and local bone debridement in the operating room, and intravenous antibiotics as needed. Loose pins and wires are removed and the pin sites debrided even in the absence of infection.

Premature Consolidation

Incomplete corticotomy can complicate SMO. A circumferential division of the tibial cortex may be assured by rotating the proximal and distal rings in opposite directions and witnessing uninhibited motion through the corticotomy site. Other methods have been described, including acute distraction and angulation at the osteotomy site, but these techniques are more disruptive to the periosteum and not recommended.

True premature consolidation of the osteotomy is rare in the adult patient. Once the osteotomy is performed, there is a latency period of 7–10 days before any correction is attempted. If the latency period is prolonged, then the osteotomy site will consolidate prematurely. Similarly, if the correction is carried out too slowly, the osteotomy site may heal, preventing further correction.

Patient Related

The success of any gradual correction system is founded in the patients' abilities to participate in their own care. Patients are responsible for performing their own strut adjustment three times daily at the outset of treatment. The TSF has simplified this process through color coordination and a precise numbering system. Even so, patients have made strut adjustment errors. These mistakes are usually quickly acknowledged and remedied. Patients need to be seen frequently (every 10–14 days) during the adjustment period to avoid errors.

Nonunion

Osseous nonunion can complicate any osteotomy procedure. Causes may include inadequate fixation, lack of weight bearing, smoking and other causes of poor blood flow to the extremity, patient comorbidities, too rapid a correction, poor osteotomy technique, and an osteotomy through diaphyseal bone. Nonunions are treated aggressively with a variety of methods including compression across the osteotomy site, percutaneous periosteal and endosteal stimulation, and additional points of fixation. Nonunions are rare when using the TSF technique. In fact, when there is impaired healing, this specialized frame provides ideal circumstances for effective treatment.

Nerve Injury

Direct injury to the nerve can occur during surgery from pin or wire insertion during the osteotomy. A more common mechanism is stretch injury that occurs during distraction. This is discussed above in the section "Acute Versus Gradual Correction."

Deep Vein Thrombosis

Deep vein thrombosis is always a concern with surgery of the lower extremity. Treatment is aimed at prevention. Patients are launched into early rehabilitation programs emphasizing immediate mobility to avoid venous stasis. There is no restriction to movement at the ankle, knee, or hip, and frame stability allows comfortable weight bearing early in the postoperative period. While in the hospital, patients receive subcutaneous low molecular weight heparin. Upon discharge, patients start a 1-month course of aspirin

(ASA) despite concerns about its effects on bone healing. With this regimen, we have not had any cases of DVT or pulmonary embolism.

References

1. Pugh K, Rozbruch SR. Nonunions and malunions. In: Baumgaertner MR, Tornetta P (eds.) Orthopaedic Knowledge Update Trauma 3. Rosemont, IL: American Academy of Orthopaedic Surgeons, 2005, pp. 115–130
2. Stamatis ED, Myerson MS. Supramalleolar osteotomy: indications and technique. Foot Ankle Clin 2003; 8(2):317–333
3. Graehl PM, Hersh MR, Heckman JD. Supramalleolar osteotomy for the treatment of symptomatic tibial malunion. J Orthop Trauma 1987; 1(4):281–292
4. Paley D. Principles of Deformity Correction, 1st ed. Berlin: Springer, 2005
5. Paley D, Herzenberg JE, Tetsworth K, McKie J, Bhave A. Deformity planning for frontal and sagittal plane corrective osteotomies. Orthop Clin North Am 1994; 25(3):425–465
6. Feldman DS, Shin SS, Madan S, Koval KJ. Correction of tibial malunion and nonunion with six-axis analysis deformity correction using the Taylor Spatial Frame. J Orthop Trauma 2003; 17(8):549–554
7. Fragomen A, Ilizarov S, Blyakher A, Rozbruch SR. Proximal tibial osteotomy for medial compartment osteoarthritis of the knee using the Taylor Spatial Frame. Tech Knee Surg 2005; 4(3):175–183
8. Rozbruch SR, Helfet DL, Blyakher A. Distraction of hypertrophic nonunion of tibia with deformity using Ilizarov/Taylor Spatial Frame. Report of two cases. Arch Orthop Trauma Surg 2002; 122(5):295–298
9. Inda JI, Blyakher A, O'Malley MJ, Rozbruch SR. Distraction arthroplasty for the ankle using the Ilizarov Frame. Tech Foot Ankle Surg 2003; 2(4):249–253
10. Rozbruch SR. Post-traumatic reconstruction of the ankle using the Ilizarov method. J Hosp Spec Surg 2005; 1:68–88
11. Shtarker H, Volpin G, Stolero J, Kaushansky A, Samchukov M. Correction of combined angular and rotational deformities by the Ilizarov method. Clin Orthop Relat Res 2002 Sep; (402):184–195
12. Paley D. The correction of complex foot deformities using Ilizarov's distraction osteotomies. Clin Orthop Relat Res 1993 Aug; (293):97–111
13. Pearce MS, Smith MA, Savidge GF. Supramalleolar tibial osteotomy for haemophilic arthropathy of the ankle. J Bone Joint Surg Br 1994; 76(6):947–950
14. Benthien RA, Myerson MS. Supramalleolar osteotomy for ankle deformity and arthritis. Foot Ankle Clin 2004; 9(3):475–487, viii
15. Stamatis ED, Cooper PS, Myerson MS. Supramalleolar osteotomy for the treatment of distal tibial angular deformities and arthritis of the ankle joint. Foot Ankle Int 2003; 24(10):754–764
16. Sen C, Kocaoglu M, Eralp L, Cinar M. Correction of ankle and hindfoot deformities by supramalleolar osteotomy. Foot Ankle Int 2003; 24(1):22–28
17. Fraser RK, Menelaus MB. The management of tibial torsion in patients with spina bifida. J Bone Joint Surg Br 1993; 75(3):495–497
18. Abraham E, Lubicky JP, Songer MN, Millar EA. Supramalleolar osteotomy for ankle valgus in myelomeningocele. J Pediatr Orthop 1996; 16(6):774–781
19. Selber P, Filho ER, Dallalana R, Pirpiris M, Nattrass GR, Graham HK. Supramalleolar derotation osteotomy of the tibia, with T plate fixation. Technique and results in patients with neuromuscular disease. J Bone Joint Surg Br 2004; 86(8):1170–1175
20. Inan M, Ferri-de Baros F, Chan G, Dabney K, Miller F. Correction of rotational deformity of the tibia in cerebral palsy by percutaneous supramalleolar osteotomy. J Bone Joint Surg Br 2005; 87(10):1411–1415
21. Rozbruch SR, Blyakher A, Haas SB, Hotchkiss R. Correction of large bilateral tibia vara with the Ilizarov method. J Knee Surg 2003; 16(1):34–37
22. Best A, Daniels TR. Supramalleolar tibial osteotomy secured with the Puddu plate. Orthopedics 2006; 29(6):537–540
23. Mangone PG. Distal tibial osteotomies for the treatment of foot and ankle disorders. Foot Ankle Clin 2001; 6(3):583–597
24. Rozbruch SR, Weitzman AM, Watson JT, Freudigman P, Katz H, V, Ilizarov S. Simultaneous treatment of tibial bone and soft-tissue defects with the Ilizarov method. J Orthop Trauma 2006; 20(3):197–205
25. Ilizarov GA. Clinical application of the tension-stress effect for limb lengthening. Clin Orthop Relat Res 1990 Jan; (250):8–26
26. Mendicino RW, Catanzariti AR, Reeves CL. Percutaneous supramalleolar osteotomy for distal tibial (near articular) ankle deformities. J Am Podiatr Med Assoc 2005; 95(1):72–84

Chapter 56
Hallux Valgus Surgery: The Minimally Invasive Bunion Correction

Sandro Giannini, Roberto Bevoni, Francesca Vannini, and Matteo Cadossi

Historical Perspective

The main goal of surgical correction of hallux valgus is the morphologic and functional rebalance of the first ray, correcting all other characteristics of the deformity.[1] Historically, distal metatarsal osteotomies have been indicted in cases of mild or moderate deformity with an intermetatarsal angle as large as 15°. Using certain osteotomies, it is possible to correct intermetatarsal angles as large as 20°. Distal osteotomies may also be used to correct deformities characterized by deviation of the distal metatarsal articular angle (DMAA) or to address concomitant stiffness.[2] Since the first operation published by Revenrdin[3] in 1881, many authors have reported their experience using different operations, each of them characterized by different indications, approaches, designs, and fixation.[4–12] Several comparative studies have been reported comparing radiographic and clinical results among many different techniques, and a review of the literature reveals the satisfaction with all operations to be in the upper 80% level or higher.[2, 13] In 1983, New (personal communication) reported a percutaneous technique for hallux valgus correction. This technique was then reported by Bosh et al.,[14] who perform a Hohmann-type[4] osteotomy fixed by only one K-wire, as described by Lamprecht and Kramer[15] in 1982, and, more recently, Magnan et al.[16] reported a description of his experience. These percutaneous operations reduce the surgical trauma because they are performed without large incisions and soft tissue procedures. They require, on the other hand, the use of particular instrumentation, such as Lindemann's osteotrite, manipulators, or dislocators. Furthermore, with these percutaneous techniques, the correction is performed blindly, and the intraoperative use of fluoroscopy is needed. The minimally invasive bunion correction used by us is not a new technique[17, 18] because it uses an osteotomy and a stabilization method already reported by other authors,

making the surgical technique usable in accordance with current concepts in hallux valgus surgery.

Our technique, in fact, consists of a linear distal osteotomy at the metatarsal neck level, as described by Hohmann,[4] Wilson,[6] and Magerl,[9] which is performed through a small medial incision and is stabilized using only one K-wire, as reported by Lamprecht and Kramer[15] and Bosh et al.[14] The characteristics of this technique can be summarized with the abbreviation SERI (simple, effective, rapid, inexpensive). This technique is simple and can be easily repeated, without removal of the eminence and without lateral release. It is minimally invasive and is performed under direct vision and without radiations. The technique is effective because, using different inclinations of the bone cut and different displacements of the head (lateral, dorsal, plantar, medial tilt, or rotation), it is possible to correct the pathoanatomy of each deformity. The surgical time spent is approximately 5 min. This can be reached after an adequate learning curve and permits obtaining a surgical time saving of 12 min compared with the most commonly used techniques (i.e., scarf). Finally, the technique is inexpensive because no particular instrumentation is needed, the hardware is only one K-wire for stabilization, a short surgical time is spent, and fewer complications are reported.

Indications and Contraindications

The SERI technique is indicated to correct mild to moderate reducible deformity when the hallux valgus angle is as large as 40° and the intermetatarsal angle is as large as 20°. The operation is indicated if the metatarsophalangeal joint is either incongruent or congruent, or with modification of the DMAA, and if mild degenerative arthritis is present. The technique is indicated even in cases of recurrent deformity. Specific contraindications of the SERI technique are patients older than 75 years, severe deformity with the intermetatarsal angle larger than 20°, severe degenerative arthritis or stiffness of the metatarsophalangeal joint, and severe instability of the cuneometatarsal or metatarsophalangeal joint.

S. Giannini (✉), R. Bevoni, F. Vannini, and M. Cadossi
School of Orthopaedics at Instituto Ortopedico Rizzoli,
Bologna University, Via GC Pupilli 1, 40136, Bologna, Italy
e-mail: sandro.giannini@ior.it

G.R. Scuderi and A.J. Tria (eds.), *Minimally Invasive Surgery in Orthopedics*,
DOI 10.1007/978-0-387-76608-9_56, © Springer Science+Business Media, LLC 2010

Preoperative Planning

The preoperative plan includes acquiring a complete history of the patient, and a physical and radiographic examination. The patient's complaints of pain, limitation in the use of footwear, and cosmetic concerns should be considered. Moreover, the severity of the prominent medial eminence and the hallux valgus deformity, as well as the great toe mobility at the metatarsophalangeal joint and the reducibility of the deformity should be evaluated. The latter is tested by pushing laterally the metatarsal head with one hand, and simultaneously pushing the great toe medially with the other hand. Stability of the metatarsophalangeal and cuneometatarsal joints must be assessed. Combined rotational deformity of the great toe or callosities under the first or second and third metatarsal heads must be considered, as well as any associated deformities of the lesser toes.

A standard radiographic examination, including anteroposterior and lateral weight-bearing views of the forefoot, allows the assessment of the arthritis and congruency of the joint; measurement of the hallux valgus angle, intermetatarsal angle, DMAA, and metatarsal and the digital formula. Therefore, planning of the operation is performed in terms of the obliquity of the bone cut, the extent of the medial-lateral or dorsal-plantar dislocation of the metatarsal head, and the correction of the DMAA.

As with any other technique, during bunion correction, the main concern is the ability to perform precisely and surgically what has been planned preoperatively. To facilitate this, we developed software that, beginning with a scanned, standard weight-bearing anteroposterior view, is able to simulate the correction needed, considering any anatomic variables of each patient. The software is able to state the precise amount of the bone cut inclination and the dislocation of the metatarsal head (Fig. 56.1).

Technique

Before surgery, the patient's foot or feet are scrubbed using disinfectant soap. The operation is usually performed using local or block anaesthesia and 7.5 mg ropivacaine hydrochlorate monohydrate. An Esmarch bandage is used at the ankle level. The patient is placed in the supine position. The foot is kept extrarotated, and the lateral edge is placed on the operating table. Normally, with this technique, soft tissue release is not needed because attenuation is achieved with the lateral offset of the metatarsal head itself. If a slight stiffness of the metatarsophalangeal joint is present, manual stretching of the adductor hallucis is performed, forcing the big toe into a varus position.

A 1-cm medial incision is made just proximal to the medial eminence through the skin, subcutaneous tissue, and down to the bone (Fig. 56.2a). The soft tissues are separated dorsally and plantarly, and they are divaricated using two retractors that are 5 mm in width (Fig. 56.2b). The medial wall of the metatarsal neck is now evident, and a complete

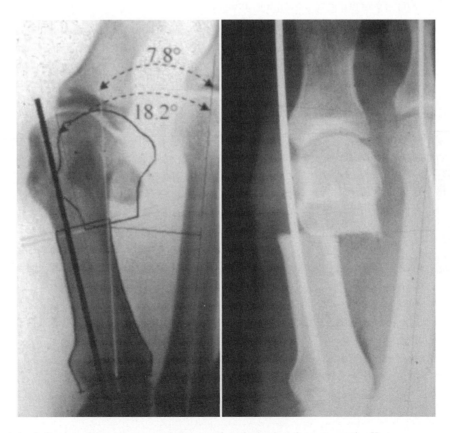

Fig. 56.1 The computerized planning of the osteotomy and the correction obtained on the postoperative X-rays

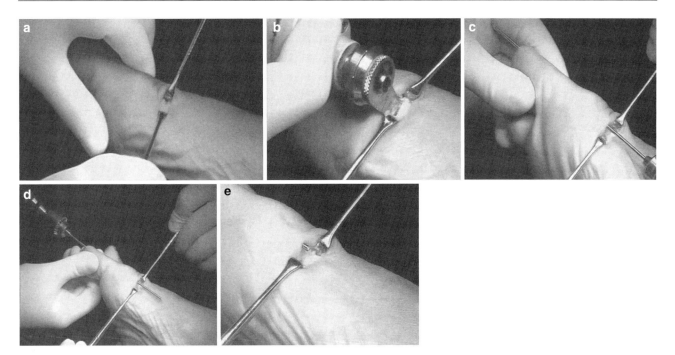

Fig. 56.2 Surgical technique: the skin incision is approximately 1 cm in length. The soft tissues are separated and divaricated by two retractors 5 mm in width (**a**). The metatarsal osteotomy performed by a standard saw (**b**).The insertion of a 2-mm K-wire in the soft tissue of the great toe along the long axis in a proximal-distal direction (**c**). The K-wire is retracted (**d**) up to the proximal end reaching the osteotomy line (**e**)

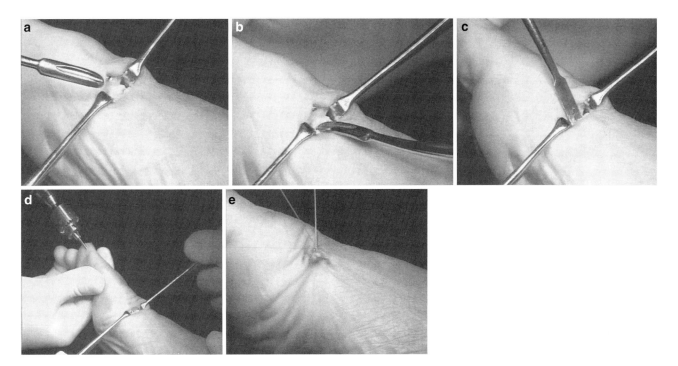

Fig. 56.3 Surgical technique: the grooved small lever (**a**). The correction of the deformity prizing the osteotomy and moving the metatarsal head as necessary (**b**, **c**). The osteotomy is stabilized by inserting the K-wire into the diaphyseal channel in a distal-proximal direction (**d**). The skin is sutured using only one 3–0 reabsorbable stitch (**e**)

osteotomy is performed using a standard pneumatic saw with a 9.5 × 25 × 0.4-mm blade (Hall Surgical Linvatec Corporation, Largo, FL, USA; Fig. 56.2c). With a small osteotome, the head is mobilized. A 2-mm K-wire is inserted, using a normal drill passing through the incision, into the soft tissue adjacent to the bone in a proximal to distal direction along the longitudinal axis of the great toe (Fig. 56.2d). The K-wire exits at the medial area of the tip of the toe close to the nail, is retaken by the drill (Fig. 56.2e), and is retracted up to the proximal end, reaching the osteotomy line (Fig. 56.2f). Using a small, grooved lever (Fig. 56.3a) to prize the osteotomy, the correction is obtained by moving the metatarsal head depending on the pathoanatomy of the deformity (Fig. 56.3b, c). Stabilization of the correction is obtained by inserting the K-wire into the diaphyseal channel in a distal to proximal direction until its proximal end reaches the metatarsal base (Fig. 56.3d). A slight varus position (approximately 10°) of the toe is necessary and is obtained by forcing the toe after K-wire stabilization. If the proximal stump of the osteotomy is prominent medially, a small wedge of bone is removed. The skin is sutured with one 3–0 reabsorbable stitch (Fig. 56.3e). The distal extremity of the K-wire is curved and cut out of the tip of the toe (Fig. 56.4). This technique can be performed bilaterally or combined with the correction of any other associated deformity of the forefoot or hind foot during the same surgical session. The key points of the technique are the inclinations of the osteotomy in the medial-lateral and dorsal-plantar directions, the displacement of the head

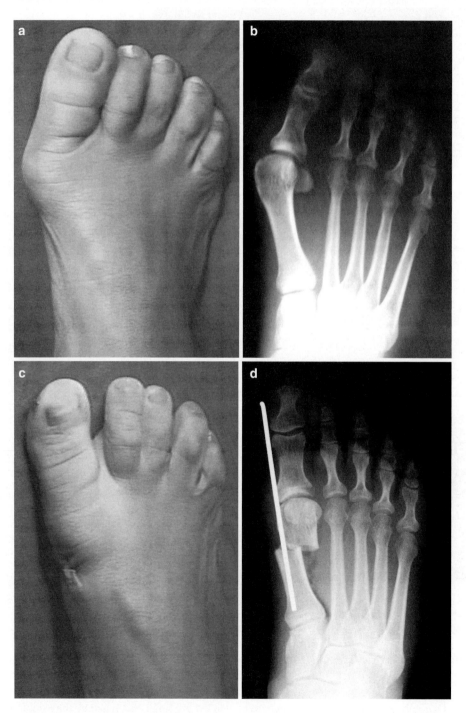

Fig. 56.4 Illustrative case preoperative (**a**, **b**) and postoperative (**c**, **d**)

vin the medial-lateral and dorsal-plantar directions, and the rotation of the metatarsal head and its medial tilt according to the correction of the DMAA. The inclination of the osteotomy in the medial-lateral direction is perpendicular to the foot axis (i.e., to the long axis of the second metatarsal bone) if the length of the first metatarsal bone must be maintained (Fig. 56.5a). The osteotomy is inclined in a distal to proximal

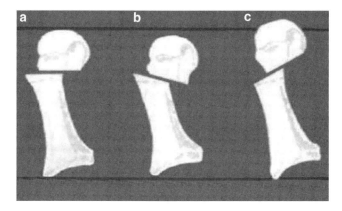

Fig. 56.5 Outline showing the different inclination of the bone cut and dislocation of the metatarsal head allowed by this technique in a medio-lateral direction, perpendicular to the long axis of the second metatarsal bone (foot longitudinal axis) (**a**), proximally inclined (**b**), and distally inclined (**c**)

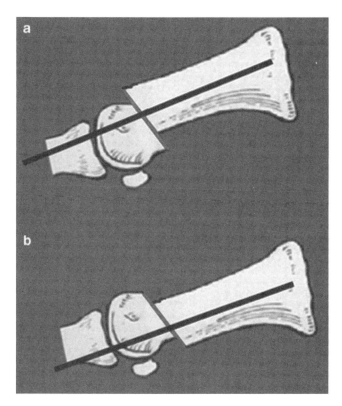

Fig. 56.6 Outline showing the inclination of the osteotomy in a dorso-plantar direction (15° in distal-proximal way) and the plantar (**a**) or dorsal (**b**) dislocation of the metatarsal head. The different position of the K-wire related to the metatarsal head and toe is evident

direction up to 25° if shortening of the metatarsal bone or decompression of the metatarsophalangeal joint is necessary in case of mild arthritis (Fig. 56.5b). More rarely, if a lengthening of the first metatarsal bone is necessary (i.e., if the first metatarsal bone is shorter than the second or if laxity of the metatarsophalangeal joint is present), the osteotomy is inclined in a proximal to distal direction as much as 15° (Fig. 56.5c). In a dorsal-plantar direction, the osteotomy is normally inclined approximately 15° in a distal to proximal direction to control the dorsal dislocation of the metatarsal head under weight bearing (Fig. 56.6). The adjustment of the medial-lateral dislocation of the metatarsal head is performed by introducing the K-wire more or less superficially with regard to the medial eminence. The adjustment of the plantar dislocation of the metatarsal head, and more rarely of the dorsal dislocation, is obtained by introducing the K-wire in the upper (Fig. 56.6a) or more rarely in the lower (Fig. 56.6b) site, with regard to the long axis of the metatarsal head (Fig. 56.7). If shortening of the metatarsal bone is needed, normally, it is necessary to dislocate the metatarsal head in the plantar direction by several millimeters according to the extent of the shortening performed.

If pronation of the first metatarsal bone is present, the correction is obtained with a derotation of the big toe up to the neutral position (Fig. 56.8). To correct the DMAA, the K-wire is introduced into the soft tissue obliquely in a medial to lateral direction by as many degrees as necessary to obtain the correction (Fig. 56.9).

Results

Results regarding our first consecutive 54 feet in 37 patients (17 bilateral; 34 female patients, 3 male patients; mean age, 48 years; range, 10–70 years) are reported with a mean follow-up of 36 months (range, 22–52 months). The clinical evaluation was carried out postoperatively using the American Orthopaedic Foot and Ankle Society score. The radiographic evaluation preoperatively and postoperatively was carried out considering the hallux valgus angle, intermetatarsal angle, and DMAA measurements. All patients except four (7.4%) declared their satisfaction with the result. Postoperatively, the mean score obtained was 81 points: 35 feet (64.8%) were considered excellent, 10 (18.5%) were good, 5 (9.2%) were fair, and 4 (7.4%) were considered poor. All of the osteotomies healed well, with callus evidence after an average of 3 months. All of the metatarsal bones remo-delled themselves over time (Fig. 56.10), even in cases with marked offset at the osteotomy (several millimetres of bony contact). In our experience, the healing of the osteo-tomy and remodelling capability of the metatarsal bone are not related to the offset at the osteotomy, but it is preferable to obtain a bony contact not less than one third of the metatarsal section.

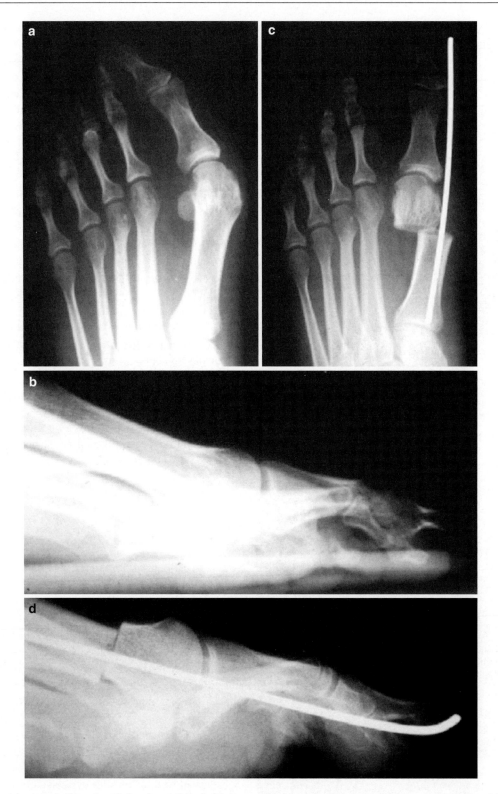

Fig. 56.7 Illustrative case: hallux valgus deformity combined with first metatarsal overloading (**a**, **b**). Postoperative X-ray in which the combined dorsal and lateral dislocation of the metatarsal head is evident (**c**, **d**)

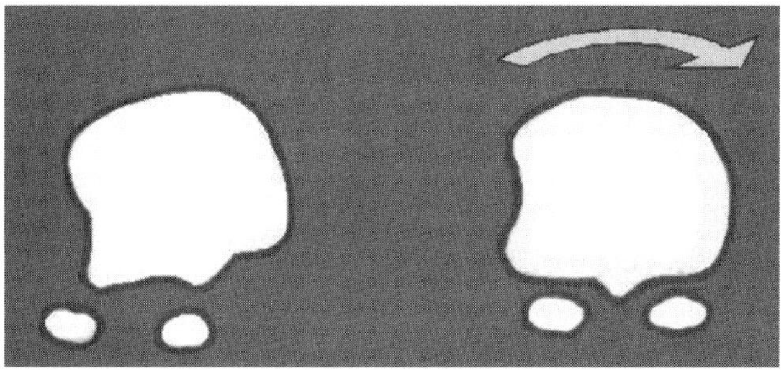

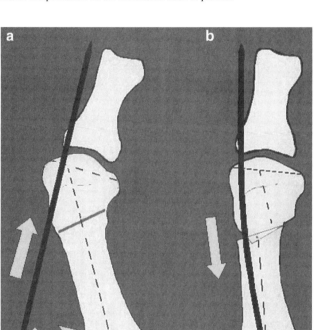

Fig. 56.8 Outline showing the derotation of the metatarsal head to assess the pronation of the metatarsal bone if present

Fig. 56.9 Outline showing the correction of the distal metatarsal articular angle (DMAA). The K-wire is inserted into the soft tissue with a mediolateral inclination according to the correction of the DMAA. (**a**). After the medial tilting of the head, the K-wire is introduced in a distal-proximal direction into the diaphysis (**b**)

Complications

No severe complications, such as avascular necrosis of the metatarsal head or nonunion of the osteotomy, have been reported. In five feet (9.2%), the radiographic healing

of the osteotomy occurred more than 4 months after surgery. Three feet (5.5%) underwent a skin inflammatory reaction around the K-wire outlet at the tip of the great toe, and one patient sustained a deep vein thrombosis. All fair and poor results are the results of an incorrect indication, such as severe arthritis, or incorrect surgical technique with an incomplete correction. Transfer metatarsalgia with plantar callosities under the second and third metatarsal head are reported in the four feet (7.4%) considered poor.

Postoperative Management

After the operation, a gauze compression dressing is applied and a control radiograph (anteroposterior and oblique views) is acquired to confirm the placement of the osteotomy and the correction of any characteristics of the deformity. Ambulation is allowed immediately using "talus" shoes, and foot elevation is advised when the patient is at rest. K-wire fixation resulting from wire bending on insertion produces a very stable and elastic stabilization, maintaining the same position obtained during surgery, and favouring early healing of the osteotomy combined with early weight bearing (Fig. 56.11). After 1 month, the dressing, the suture, and the K-wire are removed. Passive and active exercises such as cycling and swimming are advised, and wearing comfortable, normal shoes, and gradually returning to former footwear is recommended. As a general rule, postoperative swelling does not linger for more than 1 month.

Conclusions

This minimally invasive technique enables surgeons to treat approximately 80– 90% of all hallux valgus deformities without removal of the eminence and without open lateral release, performing only a manipulation of the big toe, with more than 90% excellent and good results after the learning curve. This technique is simple, and is performed under direct vision and without radiation. It is inexpensive because no particular instrumentation is needed, a short surgical time is spent, and fewer complications are reported.

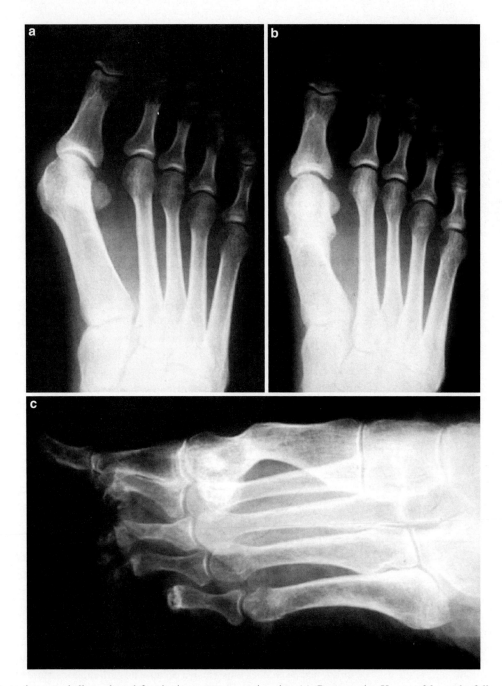

Fig. 56.10 Illustrative case: hallux valgus deformity in an anteroposterior view (**a**). Postoperative X-ray at 36-months follow-up. Good bone remodelling is evident (**b**, **c**)

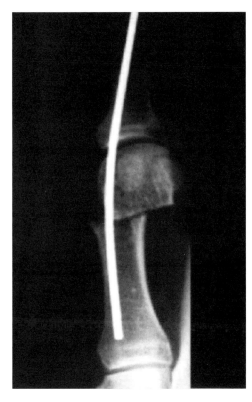

Fig. 56.11 The very stable and elastic stabilization produced by the bent K-wire, combined with early weight bearing, favours an early healing of the osteotomy

References

1. Giannini S, Ceccarelli F, Mosca M, et al. Algoritmo nel trattamento chirurgico dell'alluce valgo. In: Malerba F, Dragonetti L, Giannini S (eds.), Progressi in medicina e chirurgia del piede, "L'alluce valgo." Bologna: Aulo Gaggi, 1997:155–65

2. Chang JT. Distal metaphyseal osteotomies in hallux abducto valgus surgery. In: Banks AS, Downey MS, Martin DE, et-alet al.et-al (eds.), McGlamry's comprehensive textbook of foot and ankle surgery. Philadelphia: Lippincott, 2001:505–27

3. Revenrdin J. De la deviation en dehors du gros orteil (hallux valgus. Vulg. "oignon" "bunions" "ballen") et de son traitment chirurgical. Trans Int Med Congr 1881;2:406–12

4. Hohmann G. Symptomatische oder Physiologische Behandlung des Hallux Valgus? Munch Med Wochenschr 1921;33:1042–5

5. Mitchell CL, Fleming JL, Allen R, et al. Osteotomy bunionectomy for hallux valgus. J Bone Joint Surg Am 1958;40:41–60

6. Wilson JN. Oblique displacement osteotomy for hallux valgus. J Bone Joint Surg Br 1963;45:552–6

7. Austin DW, Leventen EO. A new osteotomy for hallux valgus: a horizontally directed "V" displacement osteotomy of the metatarsal head for hallux valgus and primus varus. Clin Orthop Relat Res 1981 Jun;157:25–30

8. Youngswick FD. Modifications of the Austin bunionectomy for treatment of metatarsus primus elevatus associated with hallux limitus. J Foot Surg 1982;21:114–6

9. Magerl F. Stabile osteotomien zur Behandlung des Hallux valgus und Metatrsale varum. Orthopade 1982;11:170–80

10. Kalish SR, Spector JE. The Kalish osteotomy: a review and retrospective analysis of 265 cases. J Am Podiatr Med Assoc 1994;84: 237–49

11. Lair PO, Sirvers SH, Somdhal J. Two Reverdin-Laird osteotomy modifications for correction of hallux abducto valgus. J Am Podiatr Med Assoc 1988;78:403–5

12. Elleby DH, Barry LD, Helfman DN. The long plantar wing distal metaphyseal osteotomy. J Am Podiatr Med Assoc 1992;82:501–6

13. Grace DL. Metatarsal osteotomy: which operation? J Foot Surg 1987;36:46–50

14. Bosh P, Markowski H, Rannicher V. Technik und erste Ergebnisse der subkutanen distalen Metatarsale -I- Osteotomie. Orthopaedische Praxis 1990;26:51–6

15. Lamprecht E, Kramer J. Die Metatarsale -I- Osteotomie nach Behandlung des Hallux valgus. Orhopaedische Praxis 1982;8: 636–45

16. Magnan B, Bortolazzi R, Samaila E, Pezze L, Rossi N, Bartolozzi P. Percutaneous distal metatarsal osteotomy for correction of hallux valgus. Surgical technique. J Bone Joint Surg Am 2006;88 Suppl 1 Pt 1:135–48

17. Giannini S. Indications, techniques and results of minimal incision bunion surgery. Presented at the 32nd Annual Meeting of the American Orthopaedic. Foot and Ankle Society February 16, 2002, Dallas, Texas, USA

18. Giannini S, Ceccarelli F, Bevoni R, Vannini F. Hallux valgus surgery: the minimally invasive bunion correction (S.E.R.I.) Tech Foot Ankle Surg 2003;2(1):11–20,

Chapter 57
Minimally Invasive Closed Reduction and Internal Fixation of Calcaneal Fractures

J. Chris Coetzee and Fernando A. Pena

Calcaneal fractures are the most common fractures in the foot, but treatment protocols vary significantly depending upon surgeon and institute preference. As far back as 1984, Yuang-Zhang et al.[1] published an approach where they combined manual manipulation of the heel with "percutaneous poking" of the fracture fragments. In 2001, Omoto et al.[2] published their results after just manual manipulation of the heel after a calcaneus fracture. Their results are difficult to interpret because no standardized outcome tool is included on their results.

Buckley et al. showed that without stratification of the groups, the functional results after nonoperative care of displaced intraarticular calcaneal fractures were equivalent to those after operative care.[3] This paper confirmed that not all calcaneal fractures are created equal, and that one should have very specific guidelines on how and when to surgically treat a fracture. With this in mind, there is a subgroup of calcaneal fractures that are best treated with minimally invasive techniques.

The initial indication for percutaneous fixation of calcaneal fractures was a compromise when risks of formal open reduction were moderately high and likely result of nonoperative treatment would be predictably poor, as in the following examples in Figs. 57.1 and 57.2. At the present time, those criteria still hold true, but there are certain fractures that are probably preferentially treated with percutaneous fixation.

Indications

The following fractures lend themselves perfectly to minimally invasive treatment: two-part tongue-type fractures (Essex-Lopresti); two-part joint depression-type fractures; and fracture dislocations with simple joint injury (no more than two-part injuries).

J.C. Coetzee (✉) and F.A. Pena
Minnesota Sports Medicine and Twin Cities Orthopedics,
775 Prairie Center Drive # 250, Eden Prairie, MN, 55344, USA
e-mail: jcc@ocpamn.com

Surgical Technique

Prerequisites

- Percutaneous reduction and limited internal fixation must be performed early, ideally within 3–5 days of the injury. After that time, it will be increasingly difficult, if not impossible to manipulate the fragments.
- Anesthesia must provide complete muscular relaxation. A general anesthetic is preferred.
- Employ indirect reduction techniques; a very good fluoroscope is essential to adequately visualize the reduction.

The patient is placed in a lateral or semilateral position on a beanbag to allow easy and direct access to the lateral aspect of the calcaneus. A semilateral position is preferred. That position allows the surgeon to externally and internally rotate the leg to allow proper fluoroscopy views to evaluate reduction and K-wire placement. The usual sterile prepping and draping is done. A tourniquet is not routinely used. In fact, if the procedure is done very early, it is probably advisable not to use a tourniquet. This might further compromise the blood supply to the skin.

Tongue Type Essex-Lopresti Fracture

Two or three nonthreaded guide wires for 3.5- or 4.5-mm cannulated screws are inserted. One or two into the posterior (tuberosity) fragment, and one in the posterior, plantar fragment. The guide wires should not cross the fracture plain at this point (Fig. 57.3). This is followed by inserting a Steinmann pin from medial to lateral through the posterior, plantar fragment. This will help to dislodge the fracture fragment with longitudinal traction on the pin. A threaded pin or "joystick" is then inserted into the tuberosity fragment. This pin should be somewhat parallel to the fracture plain, and should be deep enough to be close to the hard subchondral bone of the subtalar joint. It will be used to lever the tuberosity fragment in place while the assistant applies traction on the Steinmann pin (Figs. 57.4, 57.5, and 57.6).

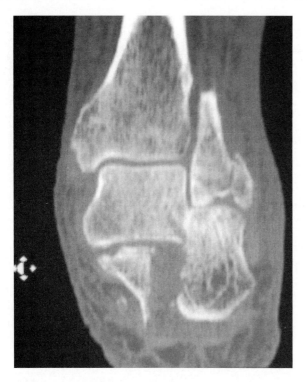

Fig. 57.1 A 53-year-old construction worker who fell off a roof. He smokes a pack of cigarettes a day. Note the lateral dislocation of the calcaneus with impaction and impingement of the distal fibula

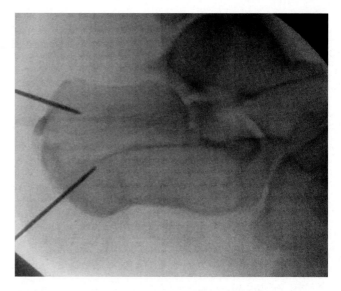

Fig. 57.3 Initial K-wire placement for reduction of a Saunders II fracture with the posterior tuberosity rotated and impacted

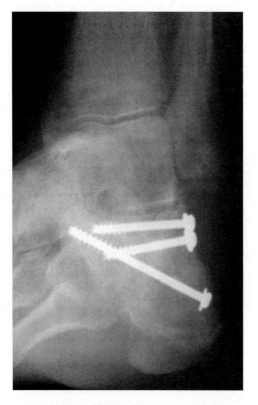

Fig. 57.2 One year after a percutaneous reduction and fixation of the calcaneal fracture dislocation

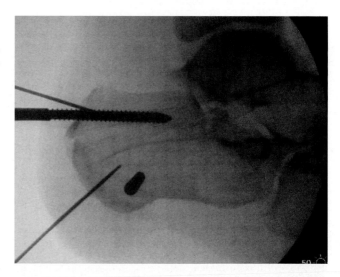

Fig. 57.4 Placement of the Steinmann pin for traction is done from medial to lateral through the plantar aspect of the calcaneus. Placing the screw from the medial aspect limits potential tibial nerve and vascular injuries. The "joystick" for reducing the tuberosity and posterior facet is placed from the posterior aspect just lateral to the Achilles tendon and should be in the lateral (rotated) portion of the posterior facet and tuberosity

Saunders Type 2b

In this situation, the pin from medial to lateral through the posterior tuberosity is most important. Significant traction is usually required to disimpact the fragments. Two guide wires are then inserted from lateral into the lateral wall fragment of the posterior facet. While the assistant applies longitudinal traction on the Steinmann pin, the two wires are used as

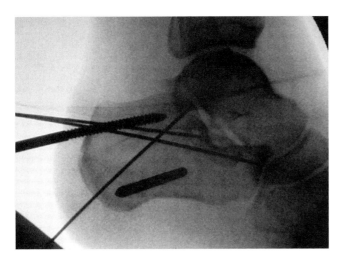

Fig. 57.5 The posterior facet is reduced under fluoroscopy by manipulating the fragments with the joystick while pulling on the transverse Steinman pin that allows disimpaction of the fragments. The guide wires are advanced to cross and immobilize the fragments. A cannulated drill is then used to overdrill, and followed by screw placement

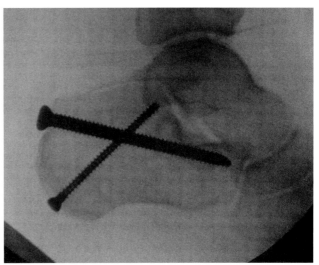

Fig. 57.6 Final screw placement, with good reduction of the joint

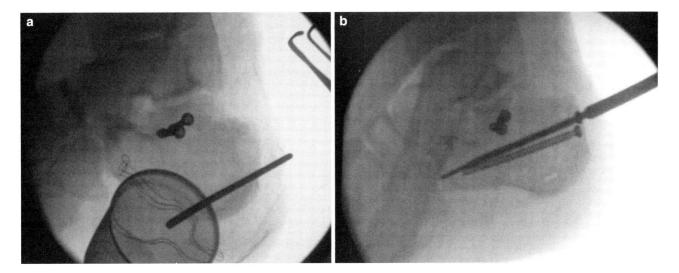

Fig. 57.7 (a) Reduction of the posterior facet with the traction pin still in place. (b) After securing the posterior facet fragment, the calcaneal tuberosity is further immobilized by two screws from posterior both sides of the Achilles to the anterior part of the calcaneus

joysticks to reduce the lateral wall to the stable medial portion of the posterior facet. It is especially important to also tilt the fragment out of its "plantar flexed" position. The longitudinal traction could either be done manually, or a Buehler clamp can be applied. I personally find manual traction more reliable because one can apply more traction on one side if the reduction requires that. The guide wires are then advanced into the medial stable portion of the subtalar joint and sustentaculum tali, overdrilled, and short thread cancellous compression screws are inserted (Fig. 57.7a).

Complications

In our own series of 57 patients since 2000, the perioperative complications included three patients with sural nerve injury symptoms, and only one minor wound complication. There were no major wound problems. The sural nerve, however, is at risk of being injured because it is not exposed and protected.

We speculate that the long-term complications will be mainly caused by the fact that one seldom gets a true anatomic reduction with an indirect technique. At a minimum of 2-year follow-up, however, there was not any significant increase in subtalar degenerative joint disease (DJD) or other issues compared with the formal open reduction and internal fixation (ORIF) group.

Discussion

With the minimally invasive technique, the surgeon must be theoretically willing to accept less than an anatomic reduction. Even so, the reported literature shows very satisfactory results with this method. There is no report in the literature comparing a no treatment group with a conventional ORIF group with a percutaneous fixation group.

Forgon[4] reported on a series of 265 cases with 89.8% good and excellent results and 10.2% moderate or poor results. Complications included 4.1% loss of reduction, 3.7% wound-healing problems, and 2% failure of technique.

Schildbauer and Sangeorzan[5] published a technical tip to improve distraction of the calcaneus tuberosity through percutaneous means. Placement of a fully threaded screw through the calcaneus tuberosity, in a similar fashion to the one placed for a subtalar fusion, will provide distraction of the calcaneus tuberosity when the screw is turned forward while being stopped from progressing by placing a hard instrument against the plantar aspect of the posterior talar facet. By turning the screw, the calcaneus tuberosity can only be transported posteriorly and distally through the threads of the screw. This is a minimally invasive way to accomplish a large amount of distraction that otherwise would require large forces to be applied.

Tornetta[6] published his series of 46 patients who underwent percutaneous reduction and internal fixation (PRIF) of the calcaneus for a tongue-type fracture (Sanders 2C) and Sanders 2B. Only six fractures (three type 2B and three type 2C fractures) could not be successfully reduced. At an average follow-up of 3.4 years, 50% of patients had excellent results and 35% had good results. No patient required another surgical intervention. Early discomfort and drainage from the use of K-wires led the surgeon to substitute the use of K-wires with screws at the time of fixation. The final recommendation of the author is to emphasize the need for a preoperative discussion with the patient regarding the possibility of having to either abort the procedure or convert to an ORIF if a satisfactory reduction cannot be accomplished.

In 2002, Gavlik et al.[7] published their series of 15 calcaneus fractures after PRIF. All fractures were classified as Sanders 2. Fractures were reduced with arthroscopic assistance and subsequently fixed with permanent osteosynthesis after anatomic reduction was accomplished. No complications were reported. The AOFAS score of 10 of the 15 patients at an average of 14 months was 93.7 out of 100. Eighty percent of patients were reported as having no complaints during activities of daily living (ADLs) and work-related activities. All patients used normal footwear and no orthotic devices. Their most outstanding recommendation relates to the use of an arthroscopically assisted technique. They report a 25% incidence of not recognized malreduction of the posterior facet fragments while being examined under fluoroscopy. For those cases, the use of subtalar arthroscopy will help to avoid a step off of the posterior facet fragments.

In 2004, Nehme et al.[8] published the results of 15 fractures treated by arthroscopic- and fluoroscopic-assisted PRIF. The type of fractures included on their series were mixed (Sanders 2B), vertical (Sanders 2A), and horizontal (according to the Utheza classification). After administration of the AOFAS outcome tool, the average score at 20 months from the time of injury was 94.5 out of 100. No signs of osteoarthritis could be observed on the last radiographs. Postoperative motion of the subtalar joint was within 80% of the healthy side. The authors point out the moderate steepness of the learning curve and the obligation of converting to an ORIF if the reduction obtained is not satisfactory.

In 2004, Rammelt et al.[9] reviewed their experience with PRIF of calcaneus fractures. Their first recommendation is to address the fracture as early as possible to avoid bony consolidation and therefore the subsequent difficulties to closely manipulate the fragments. Their limit is 14 days from the time of injury. They also emphasize the importance of patient selection and fracture pattern because there is a direct correlation with the final outcome. The fractures eligible for PRIF were tongue type (Sanders 2C), and Sanders type 2A and 2B. The indications for the remaining fracture types are more dependent on the surgeon's experience. They mentioned an alternative to PRIF for the less skillful surgeon that consists of application of an external fixator in a triangular fashion with points of fixation at the talus, calcaneus, and cuboid. The goal is to maintain the proper alignment but mostly the relative position of the hindfoot bones to each other to improve joint mechanics and muscle strength. They discourage the routine use of a trans-subtalar pin and recommend only thinking about that option with severe contraindications for ORIF or/and when dealing with an extremely unstable fracture pattern. They recommend the use of arthroscopically assisted reduction for the Sanders 2A and 2B, but not so much for the type 2C. The scope is placed along the posterior or anterolateral portal. For the Sanders 2C, they prefer to rely more on high-definition fluoroscopic examination. Finally, any remaining lack of reduction (beyond 2 mm) should be converted to ORIF because the final outcome will be improved.

One can therefore summarize that, in selected cases, closed reduction and percutaneous internal fixation provides a good option of treatment for calcaneal fractures. It might also be possible to avoid the "high" rate of complications seen with ORIF, and at the same time, improve on the poor outcome of nonoperatively treated calcaneus fractures.

References

1. Ma Y, Chen Z, Qu K, et al. Os calcis fracture treated by percutaneous poking reduction and internal fixation. Chinese Med J 1984; 97:105–110
2. Omoto H Nakamura K. Method for manual reduction of displaced intra-articular fractured of the calcaneus: technique, indications and limitations. Foot Ankle Int 2001;22:874–879
3. Buckley R, Tough S, McCormack R, et al. Operative compared with nonoperative treatment of displaced intra-articular calcaneal fractures: a prospective, randomized, controlled multicenter trial. J Bone Joint Surg Am 2002;84-A:1733–1744
4. Forgon M. Closed reduction and percutaneous osteosynthesis: technique and results in 265 calcaneus fractures. In: Tscherne H, Schatzker J, (eds.) *Major fractures of the pilon, the talus and the calcaneus.* New York, Springer, 1993, pp. 207–213
5. Schildhauer TA, Sangeorzan BJ. Push screw for indirect reduction of severe joint depression-type calcaneal fractures. J Orthop Trauma 2002;16:422–424
6. Tornetta P. Percutaneous treatment of calcaneal fractures. Clin Orthop Relat Res 2000;375:91–96
7. Gavlik JM, Rammelt S Zwipp H. Percutaneous, arthroscopically-assisted osteosynthesis of calcaneus fractures. Arch Orthop Trauma Surg 2002;122:424–428
8. Nehme A, Chaminade B, Chiron P, et al. [Percutaneous fluoroscopic and arthroscopic controlled screw fixation of posterior facet fractures of the calcaneus]. Rev Chir Orthop Reparatrice Appar Mot 2004;90:256–264
9. Rammelt S, Amlang M, Barthel Z. Minimally-invasive treatment of calcaneal fractures. Injury 2004;35:S-B55-S-B63

Chapter 58
Minimally Invasive ORIF of Calcaneal Fractures

Juha Jaakkola and James B. Carr

Calcaneal fracture fixation can be performed using multiple approaches, methods, and implants. There is no consensus regarding the best approach or method of fixation. Moreover, the end result of calcaneal fractures is unsatisfactory in many cases. Some authors have questioned the necessity of operative intervention, arguing that the risk of surgery may not exceed the benefit it may provide.[1] A procedure that reduces the risk while still providing a benefit over nonoperative treatment would appear to be a reasonable compromise.

Described approaches include use of a lateral approach (Kocher approach[2-5] or extensile lateral[6-12]), a medial approach,[13-16] and a medial and lateral combined approach.[17-19] The extensile lateral approach is currently popular because it provides excellent exposure to the calcaneus, minimizes peroneal tendonitis, and preserves the sural nerve.[7,20] However, an association with an elevated rate of soft tissue complications, that include amputation, have raised concerns.[6,8,21]

In this chapter, we discuss a technique using lateral and medial approaches to the calcaneus through small (mini) incisions. This approach limits surgical dissection, therefore preserving biology. Since exposure is limited, an excellent understanding of the fracture anatomy is essential. The patho-anatomy of calcaneal fractures and how it relates to the reduction technique will consequently be addressed. The technique also utilizes low-profile Synthes mini-fragment plates and screws to reduce the soft tissue tension and implant bulk.

Review of the Literature

The lateral approach was initially described in 1948 by Ivar Palmer.[5] He described a curved 6-cm incision made beneath the lateral malleolus. Unlike the extensile lateral approach, it does not lift up a large soft tissue flap. Reduction of the

fracture was subsequently performed with a downward traction via a transfixion wire through the tuberosity and aided by an elevator to lever the fragments through the lateral incision. However, he did not use internal fixation, rather he placed a block of iliac crest to maintain reduction of the posterior facet fragments. He reported that 23 patients treated with this technique all had "favorable" results and returned to work 4–8 months after surgery.[5]

Subsequent authors have described the use of this lateral approach in combination with internal fixation with variable results.[2-4,22,23] The largest series have been reported by Letrounel[4] and Bézes et al.[2] Letrounel[4] reported 99 cases with 56% good to excellent results with no or occasional pain after longer than 2 years follow-up. Bézes et al.[2] reported 257 cases with 85% good to excellent results with a 2.7% infection rate at a 3-year average follow-up.

McReynolds[16] has reported that he first began using the medial approach for open reduction and fixation of calcaneal fractures in 1958. This technique has been adopted by later authors,[17-19] but the most extensive experience has been reported by Burdeaux.[13-15] Burdeaux[13,14,15] advocated the use of a medial incision because it addresses the sustentacular or superomedial spike, which he thought was the key to reduction. He stated that once the medial wall of the calcaneus was restored, "the length and height of the calcaneus are automatically restored"; the other fragments are then reduced to the sustentacular fragment.[15] Reduction using is performed by pulling the tuberosity fragment downward, backward, and medially to the sustentacular fragment.[15] Once reduced, the interlocking of the bone and the tension of the soft tissues stabilizes the fracture. Burdeaux stabilized the medial wall with a staple[15] or a Steinmann pin.[13]

Burdeaux recommended reduction of the lateral fragments with the use of an elevator passed through the medial fracture line and direct digital pressure on the lateral side.[14,15] When reduction of the lateral fragments is unsuccessful, a lateral incision above the peroneal tendons is added. This is more common with joint depression fractures than tongue-type fractures.[13,15] His other indications for the lateral approach include fractures treated more than 2–3 weeks after injury, severely comminuted fractures, fracture dislocations, and displaced fractures of the calcaneocuboid joint.[14]

J. Jaakkola (✉) and J.B. Carr
Southeastern Orthopedic Center, Staff Physician, 210 East DeRenne Avenue, Savannah GA, 31405, USAMailing 101 Washington Avenue, Savannah GA, 31405, USA
e-mail: juhajaakkola@yahoo.com

G.R. Scuderi and A.J. Tria (eds.), *Minimally Invasive Surgery in Orthopedics*,
DOI 10.1007/978-0-387-76608-9_58, © Springer Science+Business Media, LLC 2010

Burdeaux reported a series of 61 calcaneal fractures in which 77% were reduced with a single medial incision and 14 fractures (23%) required an additional lateral incision.[13] Using this technique, he reported 75% good to excellent results at a 4.4-year average follow-up. Similarly McReynolds reported 64% good to excellent, 18% good-minus, and 18% fair to poor results in a series of 51 calcaneal fractures.[16] Lateral displacement was treated by bimanual compression of the heel, all cases were approached only from the medial side.[16]

Romash[24] also reported a series of cases based on the technique described by McReynolds and Burdeaux. He also began with a medial incision and then would add a lateral incision if the posterior facet was not reduced after fixation of the medial spike. He reported 20 cases of displaced intra-articular calcaneal fractures, of which 8 cases (40%) were treated with a single medial incision and 12 cases (60%) required a combined approach.[24] Using this technique, Romash observed that all of the patients were standing and wearing shoes within 6 months, had subtalar ranges of motion at least 60% of the contralateral side, and 70% of the patients were able to return to a preinjury level of activity at an average follow-up longer than 2 years.[24]

Although similar to the previously described approaches, Stephenson initially approached the fracture from the lateral side through an incision similar to Palmer.[19] If the medial wall was not aligned after reduction of the posterior facet, lateral wall, and the tuberosity fragment, then a medial incision was added. Stephenson was able to obtain an average restoration of the tuber-joint angle of 86% in 22 patients treated with this technique; 7 of 22 patients required a medial incision.[19] The average subtalar range of motion was 75% of normal, and he obtained a good result in 77% and a fair result in 4% of the 22 patients.

Johnson and Gebhardt also supported the use of a combined approach when a fracture cannot be reduced by a single approach.[21] They reported nine cases treated with a medial and extensile lateral combined approach. The fractures were approached medially and fixation of the medial wall was achieved with a staple. A lateral extensile incision was subsequently used for reduction of the posterior facet and lateral wall. The authors claimed that medial fixation provided enough stability that lateral fixation could be performed with multiple lag screws or limited plate fixation (3.5-, 2.7-, 2.0-mm plates). Using this technique, the authors were able to obtain a reduction of Böhler's and Gissane's angle within 1° of the contralateral foot. Results were good in six and fair in three patients.

Carr and Scherl reported good results using a combined approach in 38 cases at the OTA annual meeting in 1998.[17] Their description of exposing and reducing all major fragments prior to fixation forms the basis of the ensuing technique.

Fixation

Definitive internal fixation of calcaneal fractures has been performed using various combinations of 2.7-, 3.5-, or 6.5-mm screws,[18,19,25–28] staples,[19] K-wires and Steinmann pins,[14,22,25] small fragment plates,[2,3,7,9,10,29] mini-fragment plates,[12,18] and specialty plates.[4,10,11,30,31] Proponents of smaller implants suggest that they may reduce wound necrosis and peroneal tendon irritation, and that they are amendable to contouring and placement.[12,18,29] In a large study of 120 displaced intraarticular calcaneal fractures fixed with 3.5-mm screws and AO anterior cervical H-plates, Sanders et al. reported an 18% incidence of peroneal tendonitis requiring hardware removal.[9] In comparison, Tornetta reported only two cases (6%) of peroneal irritation, which did not require hardware removal, when using mini-fragment plates and screws.[12] In Tornetta's series of 35 cases, 91% had an anatomic reduction and there were no cases of loss of hardware fixation or loosening.

In addition to clinical studies, biomechanical studies have suggested that the smaller implants provide adequate strength of fixation. Carr et al. compared the biomechanical strength of a flattened 1/3 tubular plate to a thicker 3.5-mm reconstruction plate in a cadaver calcaneal fracture model.[29] They reported no statistical difference between the two in cyclic loading or load to failure testing. They hypothesized that the results were attributed bone-to-bone contact obtained by an anatomic reduction of the fracture.

Arthroscopy

The use of arthroscopy has been described for use in the evaluation of reduction for various different fractures. Authors have found arthroscopy to be useful in conjunction with reduction and fixation of distal radius fractures,[32,33] tibial plateau fractures,[34] and ankle fractures.[35] Its use has also been described for the evaluation of reduction of calcaneal fractures.[27,36] Rammelt et al. reported the use of open subtalar arthroscopy to evaluate fracture reduction in 59 cases of displaced intraarticular calcaneus fractures during surgery.[27] Open reduction was performed using an extensile lateral approach and temporary fixation was performed with K-wires. Then the adequacy of posterior facet reduction was assessed with open subtalar arthroscopy prior to definitive fixation. A minor 1- to 2-mm stepoff was identified in 13 (22%) of the cases and reduction was repeated prior to definitive fixation. The same article described 28 patients evaluated with subtalar arthroscopy while undergoing hardware removal 1 year after fixation of a displaced intraarticular calcaneus fracture.[27] The authors found 23.7% of the patients had steps of 2 mm or more and associated full-thickness articular damage. The authors concluded that the existence of a strong correlation between the functional result and the condition of the posterior facet and that open arthroscopy is superior to fluoroscopic imaging.

Pathoanatomy

An understanding of the anatomy of the calcaneus and the pathoanatomy of calcaneal fractures are especially important when using small incision techniques. Since the exposure is limited and fracture reduction is in part indirect, fracture anatomy and imaging studies play a crucial role in this technique.

The articular anatomy of the calcaneus consists of four articulating facets, the posterior, middle, anterior, and cuboid facets. The three articular facets occupying the superior surface (posterior, middle, and anterior facets) all lie at different angles to one another. Between the middle and anterior facets lies the strong ligamentous complex comprised of the talocalcaneal and cervical ligaments.[37,38] Relative to the talus, the center of the calcaneus is slightly lateral to the center of the talus.

The mechanism of the calcaneal fracture has been previously described.[5,15,39,40] At the time of impact, a shear stress on the subtalar joint fractures the calcaneus into medial and lateral portions. This longitudinal or sagittal split occurs within the subtalar joint more laterally if the foot is in valgus and more medially if it is in varus at the time of injury.[40] This primary fracture line runs longitudinally and often includes the cuboid and anterior facets. If this longitudinal fracture line runs posteriorly the length of the tuberosity, a tongue-type fracture as described by Essex-Lopresti is created; and if it does not, a joint depression fracture pattern occurs.[14,40] Multiple longitudinal fracture lines can also occur, which accounts for comminuted Sanders type 3 and 4 fracture patterns.[20] The medial (or superomedial) fragment containing the strong talocalcaneal ligaments remains attached to the talus and moves downward and medially, leaving the tuberosity fragment forward and lateral.[14] The talus then recoils upward with the superomedial fragment and leaves the lateral fragment imbedded in the body of the calcaneus producing and intraarticular stepoff. A second primary fracture line, created by the talar process, runs in the coronal plane to divide the calcaneus into anterior and posterior fragments. This fracture line extends laterally to create an inverted "Y" pattern and accounts for lateral wall outward displacement (i.e., blow out).[40] It can also course medially to divide the superomedial fragment in half. The end effect is that the calcaneus is widened and shortened and the articular surface has a stepoff.

The fracture fragments produced by this mechanism include the superomedial fragment, anterolateral fragment, posterior facet, and the tuberosity fragment (Fig. 58.1). The superomedial fragment is attached to the talus as previously described. The anterolateral fragment displaces superiorly. The posterior

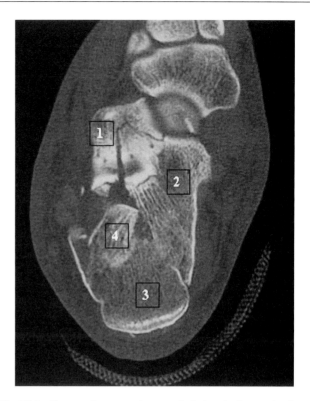

Fig. 58.1 Computed tomography scan depicting the four major fragments produced by a displaced intraarticular calcaneal fracture. (1) Anterolateral fragment; (2) superomedial fragment; (3) tuberosity; (4) posterior facet fragment

facet is fractured into two, three, or multiple fragments. The tuberosity fragment is translated laterally, tilted into varus or valgus, and has migrated up in between the superomedial fragment and the posterior facet fragment. It is the restoration of the tuberosity fragment to its original length that is most critical during reduction.

Technique

Preoperative Planning

Patient evaluation begins with thorough history and a physical examination. Although the mini-open technique reduces the risk of wound complications, the vascular status and skin condition must be addressed preoperatively. Severe peripheral vascular disease and an elevated medical or cardiac risk may be prohibitive for a surgical procedure. The physical examination must assess for associated injuries, the presence of a compartment syndrome, and skin condition of the extremity. Associated injuries have been reported in up to 25% of cases[1] and may preclude surgery or modify the approach. The skin must be assessed for the presence of fracture blisters. Previous studies have suggested that skin blistering, especially blisters with bloody fluid, may increase wound infections.[41] If fracture blisters are very large or cover the area for the surgical approach, surgery should be delayed until they have resolved.

The patient should also be evaluated using plain radiographs. Plain radiographs should include an axial (Harris), dorsoplantar, lateral, and oblique view of the foot. In addition, biplanar computed tomographic (CT) scanning is imperative when using mini-open techniques. CT scans will provide detailed information regarding the pathoanatomy of the fracture and will aid in facilitating the reduction.

Timing

Surgery should be performed within the first week or when the soft tissue condition of the foot and the medical condition of the patient allows. If surgery cannot be performed within 2–3 weeks after injury, then an extensile lateral technique or conservative treatment should be considered. Three to five working days are typically required to obtain the appropriate imaging and schedule operative time.

Surgery

Surgery should be performed with the patient under general anesthesia with muscular relaxation. The patient is placed on the operative table in the supine position with a bump placed under the ipsilateral hip to compensate for the external rotation of the extremity. A tourniquet is placed on the thigh and will be inflated prior to incision. Equipment needed for the procedure includes a 1.9-mm arthroscope and arthroscopy tower, a large C-arm fluoroscope, Steinmann pins and traction bows, an AO mini-fragment set with extra long screws, a number 15 scalpel, a Jocher elevator, a ball spike pusher, and a drill system.

Surgery typically begins with the lateral approach, but it can also be initiated from the medial side. Irrespective of the initial approach, the reduction of the calcaneal fracture should follow a systematic order (Fig. 58.2). Reduction should first assess the superomedial fragment, which, when reduced, will restore the height, length, and width of the calcaneus. Occasionally the superomedial fragment is relatively well reduced preoperatively, or it may be reducible from the lateral side with a Jocher elevator and calcaneal traction. If the medial wall is reduced, a medial incision may not be necessary.

The lateral approach starts with a 4- to 5-cm incision made 1 cm distal to the lateral malleolus and carried in line with the fourth metatarsal base (Fig. 58.3). The incision is carried down with sharp or blunt scissor dissection. Care must be observed because the peroneal tendons are more laterally and proximally displaced by the fractured calcaneus than normally encountered. The tendons are identified and plantarly retracted. The peroneal tendon sheath and lateral soft tissue is elevated off of the lateral wall of the calcaneus using a Cobb elevator. Proximal dissection is performed using a 15 blade scalpel to release the calcaneofibular ligament from its calcaneal attachment, and the posterior facet of the calcaneus should be identifiable. A thin threaded Steinmann pin is then drilled medial to lateral through the posterior aspect of the

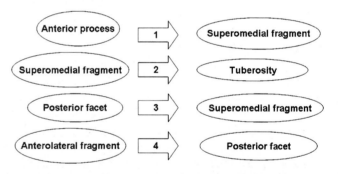

Fig. 58.2 Sequence for reduction of displaced intraarticular calcaneal fractures.

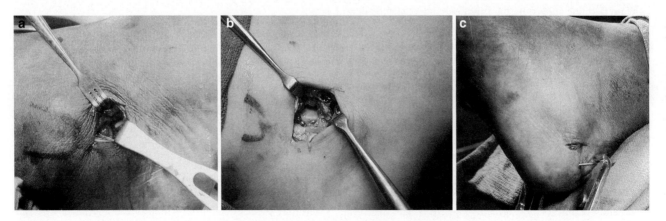

Fig. 58.3 Illustrative cases showing typical lateral (**a** and **b**) and medial (**c**) incisions. Typical lateral plate and subarticular screw positions are also demonstrated (**b**)

calcaneal tuberosity and attached to a tensioned traction bow. Traction is then pulled to visualize the posterior facet.

A medial approach is usually necessary to reduce the superomedial fragment. The incision is made vertically approximately 2–3 cm distal to the posterior edge of the heel, beginning at the edge of the plantar and dorsal skin (Fig. 58.3). The approach is completed using blunt dissection down to bone. The medial calcaneal sensory nerve branch, which lies immediately below the flexor retinaculum, should be identified and protected. A blunt elevator or hemostat is then passed distally and proximally to elevate the soft tissues off of the medial tuberosity and superomedial fragment. The major neurovascular bundle is located within the soft tissue flap anterior to the incision and is protected with a small retractor. A four- or five-hole 2.7-mm mini-fragment plate can be placed along the superomedial spike and used as an anti-glide plate. If the superomedial fragment is not reducible with traction and manipulation, an anterior process fracture fragment may be preventing reduction. This fracture may be recognized on preoperative CT scans and should be addressed by reduction from the lateral aspect with a leverage "shoehorn" maneuver.[42] Once reduced, it is provisionally pinned with a K-wire from the anterior process into the superomedial fragment. If recognized, the surgeon should address this relationship first.

Once the medial wall has been reduced and fixed, the posterior facet is reduced by elevating the lateral fragment up to the superomedial fragment. Placing an elevator under the fragment, and derotating it up should achieve reduction. A carefully applied ball spike pusher can assist with this reduction. While it is easy to get a close facet reduction, it is difficult to get an exact reduction. The arthroscope best displays the anterior portion of the facet, while the C-arm best visualizes the posterior portion. After provisional pinning with K-wires, the reduction should be assessed with arthroscopy and fluoroscopic imaging. Definitive fixation is performed with 2.0- or 2.7-mm screws placed subchondrally and directed toward the sustentaculum. The anterolateral fragment is addressed by derotating it medially and plantarly. A 2.0- or 2.7-mm mini-fragment plate is used to fix the anterolateral fragment and can be extended across the lateral wall fragment to the tuberosity fragment (Fig. 58.4).

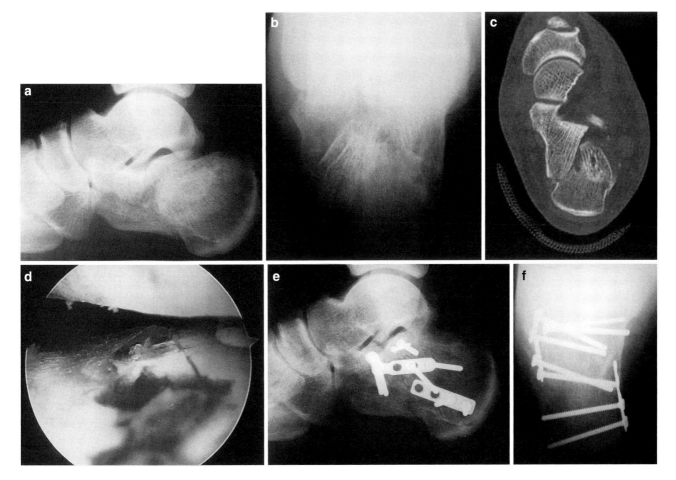

Fig. 58.4 A clinical example of a medial lateral approach used for a joint depression fracture (Sanders type 2). Preoperative radiographs (**a** and **b**) and a CT scan (**c**) show depression of Böhler's angle and an intraarticular stepoff. Postoperative arthroscopic image (**d**) and radiographs (**e** and **f**) showing correction of intraarticular stepoff and restoration of Böhler's angle

After the reduction and fixation, wound closure is completed with absorbable subcutaneous sutures and nylon skin sutures. The foot is protected in a bulky splint for 2 weeks. At 2 weeks, the wounds are assessed, radiographs are obtained, and the patient is placed into a nonweightbearing cast for another month. At 6-week follow-up, gentle range of motion exercises are instituted and the foot is placed into an off-the-shelf boot walker nonweightbearing. At 10 week follow-up, if radiographs are stable, partial weightbearing advancing to full weightbearing is initiated. The boot walker is discontinued and a slow progressive increase in activity is introduced at 12–14 weeks.

Conclusion

A combined medial and lateral approach using small incisions and low-profile mini-fragment AO plates and screws is an effective technique for addressing most displaced intraarticular calcaneal fractures. The technique may reduce the incidence of soft tissue complications reported using extensile lateral techniques, reduce the tendon irritation from using more bulky implants, and improve range of motion (Fig. 58.5). However, limited-exposure techniques also require a thorough understanding of the fracture pathoanatomy and the methods for its reduction. Experienced surgeons should be able to utilize this technique, especially in conjunction with previous training in calcaneal fracture treatment and when utilizing it initially on less complex fracture patterns.

References

1. Buckley R, Tough S, McCormack R, Pate G, Leighton R, Petrie D, Galpin R. Operative compared with nonoperative treatment of displaced intra-articular calcaneal fractures. A prospective, randomized, controlled multicenter trial. J Bone Joint Surg Am 2002; 84(A):1733–1744
2. Bézes H, Massart PL, Delvaux D, Fourquet J, Tazi F. The operative treatment of intraarticular calcaneal fractures. Indications, technique and results in 257 cases. Clin Orthop Relat Res 1993; 290: 55–59
3. Gupta A, Ghalambor N, Nihal A, Trepman E. The modified Palmer lateral approach for calcaneal fractures: wound healing and postoperative computed topographic evaluation of fracture reduction. Foot Ankle Int 2003; 24:744–753
4. Letrounel E. Open treatment of acute calcaneal fractures. Clin Orthop Relat Res. 1993; 290:60–67
5. Palmer I. The mechanism and treatment of fractures of the calcaneus: open reduction with the use of cancellous grafts. J Bone Joint Surg 1948; 30(A):2–8

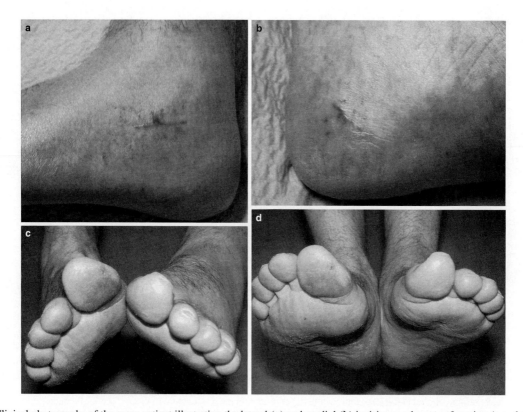

Fig. 58.5 Clinical photographs of the same patient illustrating the lateral (**a**) and medial (**b**) incisions and range of motion (**c** and **d**) at 6-month postoperative follow-up

6. Abidi N, Dhawan S, Gruen G, Vogt M, Conti S. Wound-healing risk factors after open reduction and internal fixation of calcaneal fractures. Foot Ankle Int 1998; 19:856–861

7. Benirschke S, Sangeorzan B. Extensive intraarticular fractures of the foot: surgical management of calcaneal fractures. Clin Orthop Relat Res 1993; 290: 128–134

8. Folk J, Starr A, Early J. Early wound complications of operative treatment of calcaneus fractures: analysis of 190 fractures. J Orthop Trauma 1999; 13:369–372

9. Sanders R, Fortin P, DiPasquale T, Walling A. Operative treatment in 120 displaced intraarticular calcaneal fractures: results using a prognostic computed tomography scan classification. Clin Orthop Relat Res 1993; 290:87–95

10. Thordarson D, Krieger L. Operative vs. nonoperative treatment of intra-articular fractures of the calcaneus: a prospective randomized trial. Foot Ankle Int 1996; 17:2–9

11. Thordarson D, Latteier M. Open reduction and internal fixation of calcaneal fractures with a low profile titanium calcaneal perimeter plate. Foot Ankle Int 2003; 24:217–221

12. Tornetta P. Open reduction and internal fixation of the calcaneus using minifragment plates. J Orthop Trauma. 1996; 10:63–67

13. Burdeaux B. Fractures of the calcaneus: open reduction and internal fixation from the medial side a 21-year prospective study. Foot Ankle Int 1997; 18:685–692

14. Burdeaux B. The medial approach for calcaneal fractures. Clin Orthop Relat Res 1993; 290:97–107

15. Burdeaux B. Reduction of calcaneal fractures by the McReynolds medial approach technique and its experimental basis. Clin Orthop Relat Res 1983; 177:87–103

16. McReynolds I. The case for operative treatment of fractures of the os calcis. In: Leach RE, Hoaglund FT, Riseborough EJ (eds.) Controversies in Orthopaedic Surgery. Philadelphia, WB Saunders, 1982, pp. 232–254

17. Carr J, Scherl J. Small incision approach for intraarticular calcaneal fractures. Presented at *Orthopaedic Trauma Association Annual Meeting*; 1998; Toronto, ON, Canada

18. Johnson E, Gebhardt J. Surgical management of calcaneal fractures using bilateral incisions and minimal internal fixation. Clin Orthop Relat Res 1993; 290:117–124

19. Stephenson J. Surgical treatment of displaced intraarticular fractures of the calcaneus: a combined lateral and medial approach. Clin Orthop Relat Res 1993; 290: 68–75

20. Sanders R. Displaced intra-articular fractures of the calcaneus. J Bone Joint Surg 2000; 82(A):225–250

21. Koski A, Koukkanen H, Tukiainen E. Postoperative wound complications after internal fixation of closed calcaneal fractures: a retrospective analysis of 126 consecutive patients with 148 fractures. Scand J Surg 2005; 94:243–245

22. Ebraheim N, Elgafy H, Sabry F, Freih M, Abou-Chakra I. Sinus tarsi approach with trans-articular fixation for displaced intra-articular fractures of the calcaneus. Foot Ankle Int 2000; 21:105–113

23. Wiley W, Norberg J, Klonk C, Alexander I. "Smile" incision: an approach for open reduction and internal fixation of calcaneal fractures. Foot Ankle Int 2005; 26:590–592

24. Romash M. Calcaneal fractures: three-dimensional treatment. Foot Ankle Int 1988; 8:180–197

25. Fernandez D, Koella C. Combined percutaneous and "minimal" internal fixation for displaced articular fractures of the calcaneus. Clin Orthop Relat Res 1993; 290: 108–116

26. Levine D, Helfet D. An introduction of the minimally invasive osteosynthesis of intra-articular calcaneal fractures. Injury 2001; 32: S-A51–S-A54

27. Rammelt S, Gavlik J, Barthel S, Zwipp H. The value of subtalar arthroscopy in the management of intra-articular calcaneus fractures. Foot Ankle Int 2002; 23: 906–916

28. Tornetta P. Percutaneous treatment of calcaneal fractures. Clin Orthop Relat Res 2000; 375: 91–96

29. Carr J, Tigges R, Wayne J, Earll M. Internal fixation of experimental calcaneal fractures: a biomechanical analysis of two fixation methods. J Orthop Trauma 1997; 11:425–429

30. Raymakers J, Dekkers G, Brink P. Results after operative treatment of intra-articular calcaneal fractures with a minimum follow-up of 2 years. Injury 1998; 29:593–599

31. Zwipp H, Tscherne H, Therman H, Weber T. Osteosynthesis of displance intraarticular fractures of the calcaneus. Results in 123 cases. Clin Orthop Relat Res 1993, 290.76–86

32. Edwards C2nd, Haraszti C, McGillivary G, Gutow A. Intraarticular distal radius fractures: arthroscopic assessment of assessment of radiographically assisted reduction. J Hand Surg (Am) 2001; 26: 1036–1041

33. Geissler W. Intra-articular distal radius fractures: the role of arthroscopy? Hand Clin. 2005; 21:407–416

34. Lubowitz J, Elson W, Guttmann D. Part I: arthroscopic management of tibial plateau fractures. Arthroscopy 2004; 20:1063–1070

35. Ono A, Nishikawa S, Nagao A, Irie T, Sasaki M, Kouno T. Arthroscopically assisted treatment of ankle fractures: arthroscopic findings and surgical outcomes. Arthroscopy 2004; 20:627–631

36. Rammelt S, Amlang M, Barthel S, Zwipp H. Minimally-invasive treatment of calcaneal fractures. Injury 2004; 35:S-B55–63

37. Hall R, Shereff M. Anatomy of the calcaneus. Clin Orthop Relat Res 1993; 290: 27–35

38. Sarrafian S. Biomechanics of the subtalar joint complex. Clin Orthop Relat Res. 1993; 290:17–26

39. Carr J. Mechanism and pathoanatomy of the intraarticular calcaneal fracture. Clin Orthop Relat Res 1993; 290:36–40

40. Carr J, Hamilton J, Bear L. Experimental intra-articular calcaneal fractures: anatomic basis for a new classification. Foot Ankle Int 1989; 10: 81–87

41. Giordano C, Koval K, Zuckerman J, Desai P. Fracture blisters. Clin Orthop Relat Res 1994; 307: 214–221

42. Carr J. Surgical treatment of intra-articular calcaneal fractures. A review of small incision approaches. J Orthop Trauma 2005; 19:109–117

Chapter 59
Minimal Dual-Incision ORIF of the Calcaneus

Michael M. Romash

The treatment of calcaneal fractures continues to evolve. In the past 25 years, a great deal of information about the mechanism of injury, the fracture patterns, and treatment have been *rediscovered*, confirmed, and instituted. This progress has established the principles that are applied in open reduction and internal fixation (ORIF) of these fractures. The techniques by which these principles are applied continue to advance and change. What was done through a large exposure can be done with smaller incisions and less tissue disruption without diminishing the end result. The dual-incision approach to the heel fracture is an example of this change.

Mechanism of Injury

The calcaneus fails when it is suddenly axially loaded.[1-5] The tuberosity of the calcaneus is lateral to the axis of the leg. When the fracturing force is applied, a shear stress occurs in the bone. The plane of this stress is directed obliquely from superior lateral to inferior medial, anterior lateral to posterior medial (Fig. 59.1). The calcaneus fractures along this plane producing the primary fracture line. The tuberosity displaces laterally, proximally, and angles into some varus. (A patient described this as a shifting of tectonic plates when his fracture was discussed with him.) While this is occurring, the lateral aspect of the posterior facet impacts the talus. This drives this portion of the posterior facet down into the calcaneus. It rotates forward while it is pushed down. If the facet fractures within the posterior limit of the subtalar joint, it is a *joint depression* fracture. If this fragment continues back and exits through the tuberosity, it is a *tongue* fracture. The anterior body of

the talus then continues to drive into the calcaneus at the angle of Gissane, causing another fracture involving the anterior calcaneus (Fig. 59.2).

These fractures produce four major fragments, the sustentacular fragment, the tuberosity fragment, the posterior lateral fragment, and the anterior fragment. These major fragments may further comminute into smaller fragments. The number of smaller fragments in the posterior facet correlates with the success of treatment.

The sustentacular fragment is referred to as the constant fragment. This stays in its anatomic position relative to the talus. During reduction, all fragments are reduced to the sustentacular fragment.

Principles of Reduction

The displacements and angulations described above must be reversed. Motion of the hindfoot complex depends upon the smoothness of the articular surfaces of the calcaneus and the three-dimensional (3D) spatial relationships that result between the talus, calcaneus, and cuboid due to the proper shape length and height of the calcaneus. Carr[2] has described the concept of the medial and lateral columns of the calcaneus. It is necessary to reconstruct both columns.

Disimpaction of the fragments must be accomplished. Then reduction of the tuberosity to the sustentaculum reestablishes the medial wall of the calcaneus. This establishes the height by reconstructing the medial column. The posterior lateral facet fragment can then be elevated, derotated, and fixed to the sustentacular fragment. After this is accomplished, the lateral wall can be molded into its anatomic position.

In the process of derotating the posterior facet fragment, its anterior margin provides the landmarks for the reduction of the anterior lateral fragment to the remainder of the construct, thus reestablishing the length of the lateral column. The articular surface of the anterior process may then be reduced (Fig. 59.3).

M.M. Romash (✉)
Orthopedic Foot and Ankle Center of Hampton Roads, Chesapeake Regional Medical Center, 100 Wimbledon Square, 736 North Battlefield Blvd, Chesapeake, VA, 23320, USA
e-mail: orthofoot@cox.net

G.R. Scuderi and A.J. Tria (eds.), *Minimally Invasive Surgery in Orthopedics*,
DOI 10.1007/978-0-387-76608-9_59, © Springer Science+Business Media, LLC 2010

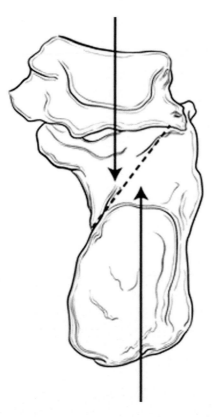

Fig. 59.1 Axial load causes internal oblique shear stress along plane of primary fracture line

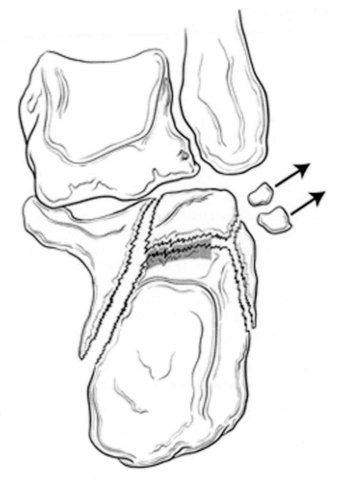

Fig. 59.2 Resultant secondary fractures in the posterior aspect of the heel

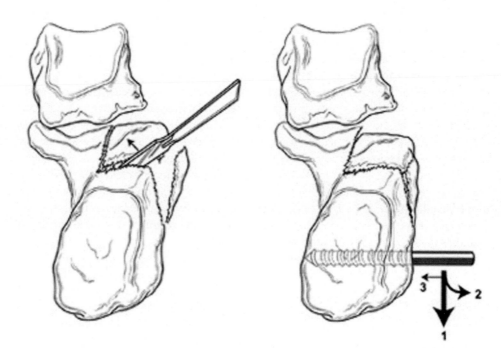

Fig. 59.3 Reduction of the tuberosity to the sustentaculum. Reduction of the posterior lateral fragment to the tuberosity

Preoperative Assessment

The medical history must be obtained. Specifically, a history of smoking, diabetes, neuropathy, and vascular disease must be sought. These presence of these conditions may effect the decision-making process. These are relative contraindications to surgery, but do not exclude surgical intervention.

The standard physical examination parameters are to be observed. These are the evaluation of the vascular and neurological status of the foot. The possibility of compartment syndrome must be considered. Specific findings to look for are skin "tenting" over boney prominences and fracture blisters.[6,7] Skin tented over the posterior prominence of a tongue-type fracture or the spike of bone that marks the inferior margin of the sustentacular fragment carry the risk of skin necrosis. If this situation exists, a reduction must be accomplished quickly to relieve the tenting.

X-ray assessment is mandatory. Plane films include the axial heel view, lateral view, Broden's oblique view, and anteroposterior (AP) view of the foot.[8–10] A lateral view of the uninjured foot is recommended. What appears to be a minimally displaced fracture can be shown to have significant displacement when compared with the healthy heel. Measure Bohler's angle of the injured as well as the uninjured heel (Figs. 59.4–59.7).[11,12]

Computed tomographic (CT) examination provides the best evaluation of the fracture.[3] Axial, coronal, sagittal, and 3D volumetric reconstructions of the heel provide the surgeon with a blueprint of the internal and external architecture of the fracture.[13] The 3D volumetric reconstruction is particularly helpful because it shows the surgeon what will be seen through the portal of exposure during the procedure[9] (Figs. 59.8–59.12).

Timing of Surgery

Unless there is tenting of the skin or another forcing factor, the ORIF is not performed immediately. These patients often are referred a few days after their injury. The foot is often

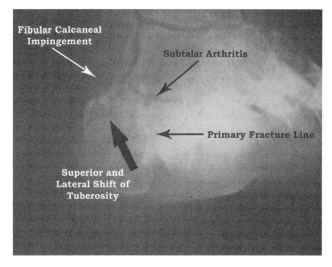

Fig. 59.5 Broden's view of an acute fracture, primary fracture line, shift of tuberosity, and intraarticular component

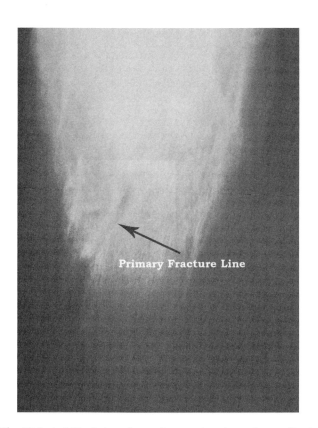

Fig. 59.4 Axial heel view of acute fracture, the primary fracture line is apparent

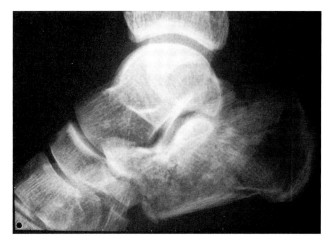

Fig. 59.6 Lateral view demonstrating loss of Bohler's angle and depression of the subtalar facet

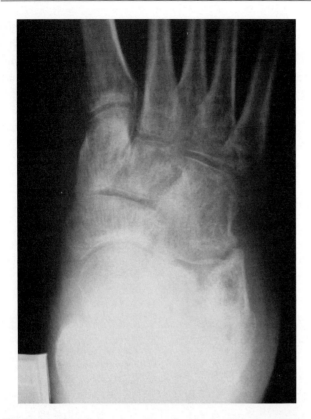

Fig. 59.7 AP view demonstrating calcaneocuboid involvement in a primary fracture of an anterolateral fragment

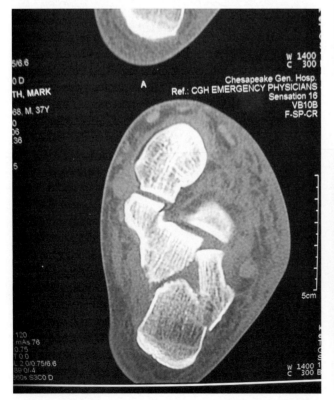

Fig. 59.8 Semicoronal CT scan clearly shows fracture pattern and displacement

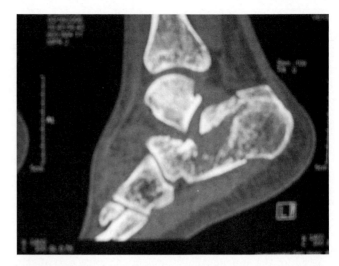

Fig. 59.9 Sagittal CT of acute fracture

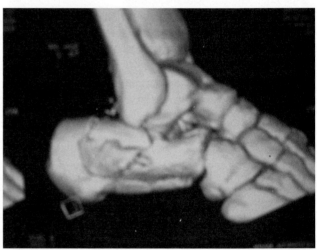

Fig. 59.10 3D volumetric CT, lateral side showing joint depression and lateral wall injury

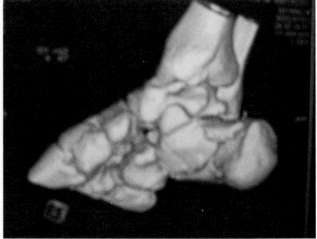

Fig. 59.11 3D volumetric CT, medial side showing displacement of tuberosity, sustentacular fragment, and "shingle" effect medially

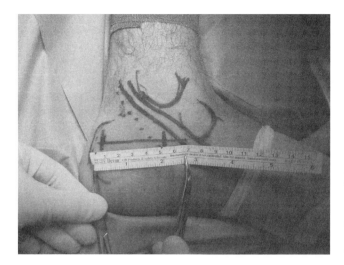

Fig. 59.12 Medial incision

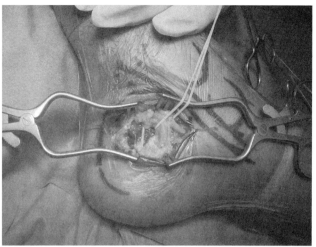

Fig. 59.13 Exposure of the neurovascular bundle medially

swollen and fracture blisters may be present. I advise waiting until the swelling has diminished and the skin wrinkles are visible. This is the positive wrinkle sign. Blisters may be unroofed and sterilely dressed. Be aware that the blisters often signal significant underlying soft tissue injury.

Technique of Small Dual-Incision ORIF

Patient Positioning

The patient is placed in the supine position with a bolster under the hip on the involved side. An elevated workstation for the foot is created under the drapes from pads. A radiolucent operating table is mandatory and the patient's foot should be placed close to the end of the table so that an intraoperative axial heel view can be seen with the fluoroscope.

Exposure

Medial and lateral exposure of the fracture will be accomplished. The order of exposure is not critical and may be dictated by the preoperative assessment of the fracture. The area requiring the most disimpaction should be approached first. This exposure is much as described by Ian McReynolds.[1, 14]

The medial incision is three to four fingerbreadths below the medial malleolus, parallel to the sole centered over the tuberosity fragment. The anterior aspect of the incision just crosses the neurovascular bundle area (Fig. 59.12). Dissect through the abductor hallucis. The fascia under the muscle will be encountered and sectioned. This is entering the tarsal tunnel through the "side door." The neurovascular bundle

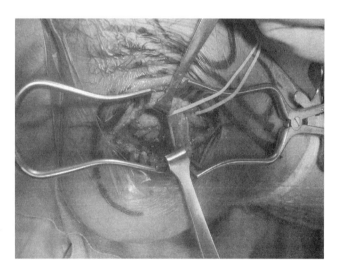

Fig. 59.14 Medial wall of the calcaneus exposed

will be in the anterior aspect of the wound. The neurovascular bundle is mobilized superiorly and inferiorly and generally retracted toward the toes (Fig. 59.13). The short flexors may then be elevated from the medial wall of the calcaneus using a small key elevator. It is important to have a good visual image and orientation to the fracture pattern at this point. The 3D volumetric reconstruction CT scan is quite helpful. The tuberosity fragment shifts lateral and superiorly. The sustentacular fragment then overlays the medial wall of the tuberosity much as roofing shingles overlay each other. The medial wall of the sustentacular fragment may be encountered initially. The surgeon must be aware of this, and be prepared to expose the tuberosity more plantarly and define any Z collapse or minor fragments that may be present (Fig. 59.14).

The lateral incision starts just below the tip of the fibula and extends forward in the line between fourth and fifth ray to the calcaneocuboid joint (Fig. 59.15). The peroneal ten-

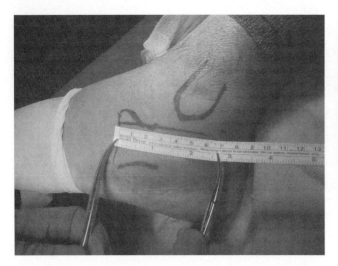

Fig. 59.15 Lateral incision

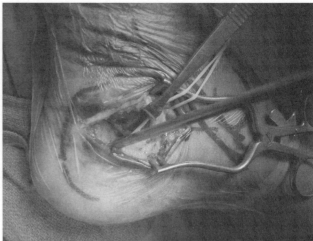

Fig. 59.17 Steinman pin placed through the tuberosity fragment from the medial side

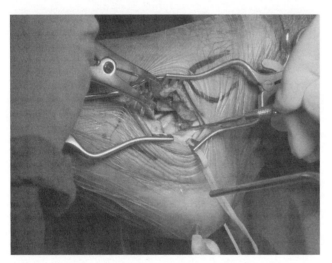

Fig. 59.16 Lateral exposure through the sinus tarsi

dons (often displaced) are mobilized. The extensor digitorum brevis is mobilized with the extensor retinaculum. The sinus tarsi region is cleared and the subtalar joint opened. The includes incision of the anterior as well as the lateral capsular structures. The lateral wall of the calcaneus in the area of the incision is exposed. The view into the subtalar joint is enhanced by placing a baby Inge lamina spreader in the sinus tarsi. At this juncture, the lateral and dorsal aspect of the anterior calcaneus is exposed (Fig. 59.16).

The Reduction

Disimpaction

The fragments have been impacted into each other by the injuring force; therefore, the first task is to mobilize them to

permit the reduction. Through the medial incision, a large Steinmann pin is placed through the tuberosity fragment from medial to lateral. This is best placed toward the posterior and plantar margin of the fragment (this keeps the area for fixation clear). This pin protrudes 2–3 in. out the lateral side of the heel. A joker elevator, ¼-in. curved Lambotte osteotome, or other instrument is insinuated along the primary fracture plane and in conjunction with pressure on these instruments lifting the posterior lateral facet fragment (blindly), rocking the tuberosity with the Steinman pin and placing traction on the Steinman pin, the tuberosity may be freed (Fig. 59.17). If progress toward this end is not apparent, the lateral incision is used and, through the lateral wall (there is often some comminution here), a boney trapdoor is used to allow a joker elevator to be placed under the depressed and rotated posterior lateral facet fragment to lift and derotate it. The primary fracture plane may also be disimpacted obliquely across the calcaneus from here.

Reduction and Fixation

I usually rebuild/reduce the heel medially first. The patient is placed in a figure four position. The tip of the Steinman pin that protrudes through the lateral heel is supported on towels placed on the contralateral tibia (Fig. 59.18). This provides a pivot point and reaction point to help with the reduction. This pivot is placed laterally away from the heel. As the medial lever arm of the pin is pulled plantarly and posteriorly, motion about this distant hinge point guides the tuberosity out of varus and translates it into proper position. This is the same principle of the offset hinge used in external fixators to effect angular and translational correction. The reaction force pushes the tuberosity medially, accomplishing the reduction (Figs. 59.19–59.22).

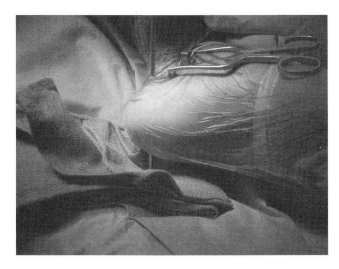

Fig. 59.18 Steinman pin through to the lateral side acting as the point of application of reduction force and the pivot point

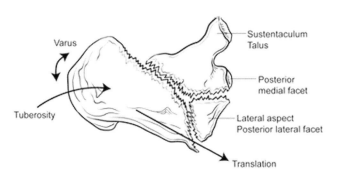

Fig. 59.19 Diagram of initial deformity as viewed with the patient's leg in a figure four position, lateral side down

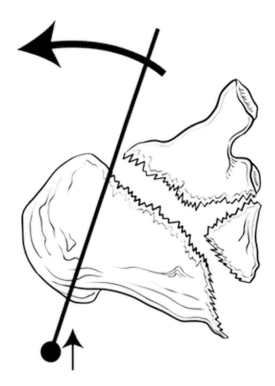

Fig. 59.21 Diagram of the mechanics of the tuberosity reduction maneuver. The point of the Steinman pin acts as the point of application for a medial directed vector of reduction force. The lateral position of the point acts as an offset hinge to permit correction of varus and translational displacement

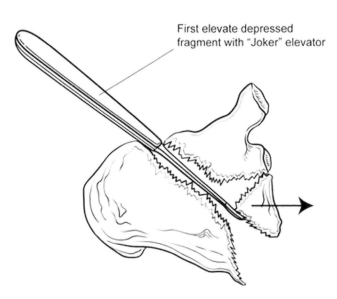

Fig. 59.20 Diagram of the disimpaction of fragments through medial entry point to primary fracture plane and posterolateral fragment

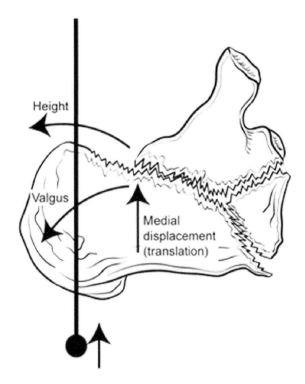

Fig. 59.22 Diagram of position after reduction

Once disimpaction and reduction have been accomplished (Fig. 59.23), fixation may be delayed until the posterior facet reduction and internal fixation have been accomplished. I usually choose this sequence.

Alternatively, medial fixation can now be introduced. Staples or a hindfoot plate (Ascension) may be used. If staples are used, one or two 3/32 Steinman pin bone staples of appropriate width to bridge the fracture site (there may be a segment of intercalary comminuted fragments) from the tuberosity fragment to the sustentacular fragment are placed. These do not compress the fracture; rather, they maintain the height and position of the reduction. Predrill the holes for the staples. Use a 3/32 Steinman pin or drill bit for this. Impact the staples only half way (50%) so that they do not interfere with any lateral fragments (Fig. 59.24). The staples will be seated fully at the completion of the procedure.

If a hindfoot plate is used, the hindfoot plate is "turned over" so that the convex side curve of the plate lays on the concave surface of the medial calcaneus. Further contouring of the plate is done with a bending vise grip. Temporary fixation can be accomplished with short screws. The short screws will not interfere with manipulation of the posterior lateral fragment and will be replaced by appropriate-length screws at the end of the procedure (Fig. 59.24a).

Now address the lateral side. Introduce a baby Inge lamina spreader in the sinus tarsi and use it to lengthen the calcaneus and push the anterior lateral fragment forward. The posterior facet is elevated and derotated, reducing it to the sustentacular fragment. This can be observed anteriorly and posteriorly (Fig. 59.25). Ensure that the posterior aspect of the facet is not *over reduced*, i.e., elevated higher than the medial side. Temporary fixation is done with 0.62-in. K wires from lateral to medial (Fig. 59.26). As the wires are placed, aim slightly plantarly as the joint falls away medially. What appears to be a *transverse shot* may pierce the subchondral bone and go intraarticularly. Usually a significant lateral wall

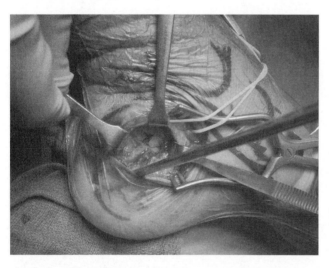

Fig. 59.23 Medial wall reduction after the described maneuver

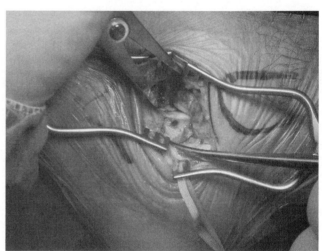

Fig. 59.25 Lateral reduction

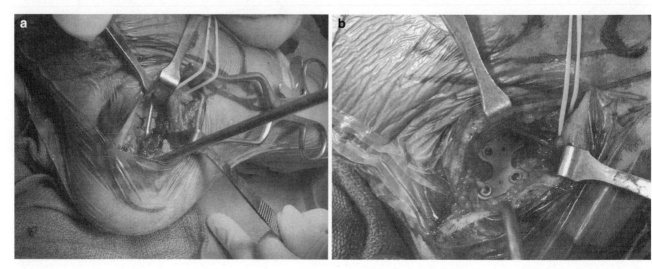

Fig. 59.24 (**a**) Placement of initial medial staple. (**b**) Medial hindfoot plate

surface is present on the posterior lateral facet fragment. This is often buried behind other fragments of the lateral wall that have been displaced laterally. It is this area of the bone that it is of good quality and best able accept the fixation. The lamina spreader is then eased and the anterior fragment reduced to the posterior fragment.

Intraoperative X-rays are then taken. Use a good quality C-arm fluoroscope. Image the foot in three or four views: axial heel, Broden's oblique view,[10] lateral view, and AP foot view. The AP foot view will show the calcaneocuboid joint and may not be needed routinely. The other three views are needed in all cases. The axial heel view shows the medial wall reduction, and Broden's view shows the subtalar joint and permits assessment of the joint surface reduction. The lateral view allows assessment of the height of the heel and the orientation of the medial plate or staple fixation.

If the position is proper, lateral fixation is continued. Cancellous bone graft may be placed under the posterior facet

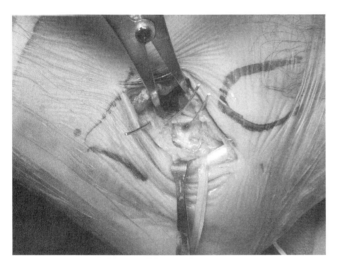

Fig. 59.26   K wires temporarily fixing the lateral reduction

at the surgeon's discretion. This is done before applying the plate. The "mini calc" plate (Ascension) or anterolateral plate (Synthes, Paoli, PA) is applied. Some shaping of the plate at its distal flange is usually necessary to conform it to the anterior calcaneus. Bending the proximal plate is not always necessary because it will conform to the bone. Locking or nonlocking 3.5-mm screws are used with the mini calc plate, 4.0-mm cancellous screws are used with the Synthes anterolateral plate. The most lateral fragments can be over drilled. The plate is designed to lay along the good quality bone of the posterior facet just inferior to the joint, cross the fracture at the angle of Gissane, and then engage the anterior fragment. It serves as a "washer" laterally, allowing compression from lateral to medial. It keeps the posterior facet and construct elevated and reduced to the anterior fragment (Figs. 59.27 and 59.28).

The medial plate is now applied. A hindfoot plate (Ascension) is turned over so that the convex side curve of the plate lays on the concave surface of the medial calcaneus. Further contouring of the plate is done with a bending vise grip. Temporary fixation can be accomplished with short screws. The short screws will not interfere with manipulation of the posterior lateral fragment and will be replaced by appropriate length screws at the end of the procedure. If staples are used, they are now fully seated (Fig. 59.29a, b).

Final X-rays are made (Figs. 59.30–59.32). The wounds are closed in layers. The muscle over the neurovascular structures on the medial side is approximated. The skin may be closed with simple or running suture (Figs. 59.33 and 59.34).

Special Situations

A Sander's three- or four-fracture pattern usually requires more work to reduce the facet fragments. I have found success by reducing the mid fragment to the sustentaculum with 0.45-in. K wires. These wires are placed from lateral to medial, exiting

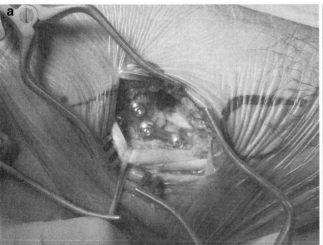
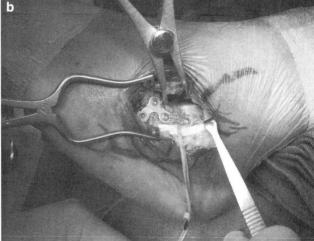

Fig. 59.27   (**a, b**) Anterolateral plate applied

the skin on the medial side. They are then withdrawn from the medial side until the wire just disappears into the minor fragment. The lateral portion of the posterior facet is then reduced to the construct, held with K wires, and the procedure goes on as described above. After final fixation has been placed, these K wires are removed from the medial side.

It is possible to use this fixation pattern and do a primary subtalar arthrodesis if desired in the case of a destroyed joint. If the

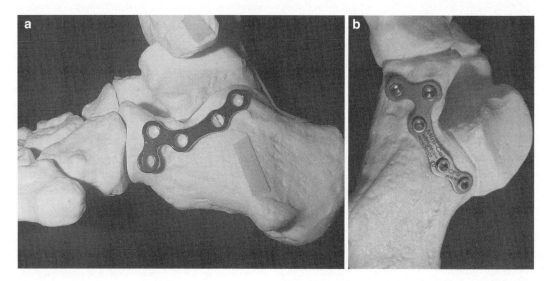

Fig. 59.28 (**a**, **b**) Anterolateral plate on sawbones model

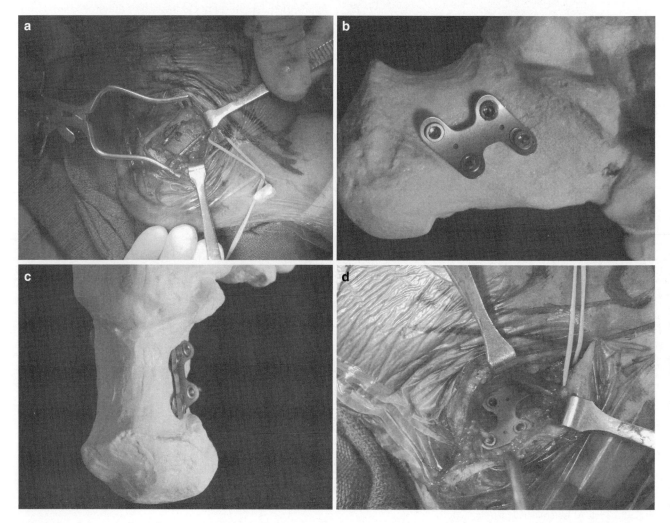

Fig. 59.29 (**a**) Medial staples impacted, final fixation. (**b**, **c**) Hindfoot plate on sawbones model. (**d**) Hindfoot plate fixed to medial wall

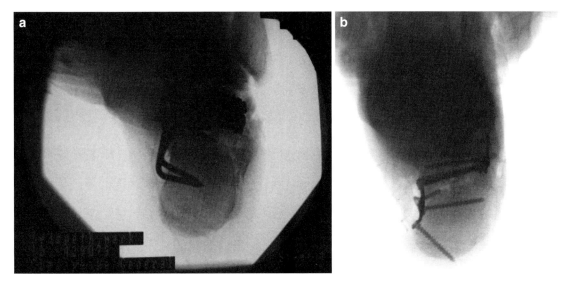

Fig. 59.30 (**a**) Intraoperative axial heel view after ORIF. (**b**) Intraoperative axial after ORIF with mini calc and medial hindfoot plate

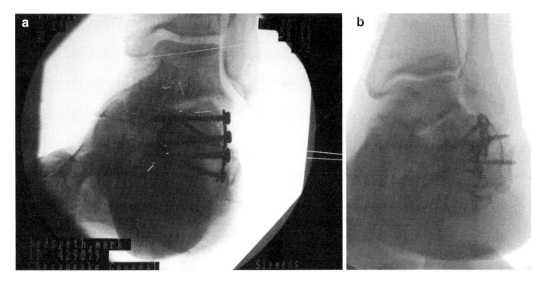

Fig. 59.31 (**a**) Intraoperative Broden's view after ORIF. (**b**) Intraoperative Broden's view after ORIF with mini calc and medial hindfoot plate

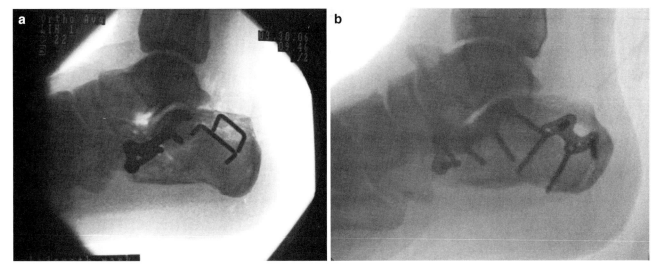

Fig. 59.32 (**a**) Intraoperative lateral view after ORIF. (**b**) Intraoperative lateral view after ORIF with mini calc and medial hindfoot plate

medial "zone of injury" has caused considerable change in the muscle layer with noted discoloration and unhealthy appearance, more advanced treatment may be necessary. This is seen and may be anticipated if there has been blistering of the skin in the area.[6, 7] We have had success by excising the questionable tissue and performing an abductor hallucis flap with a split thickness skin graft (STSG) to close and cover the medial side[15] (Fig. 59.35).

Postoperative Management

The foot is placed in a well-padded short leg cast with an A-V impulse bladder under the cast.[16] The foot is in a neutral position. The cast is bivalved within the first 24 h. Anticipate blood staining on the cast. This dressing is changed 3–7 days postoperatively. A new cast is applied. Sutures are removed 14 days postoperatively. The foot is held in a cast with the patient non-weightbearing (NWB) for 6 weeks. The cast is then exchanged for a fracture boot and the patient encouraged to perform non-weightbearing active and passive motions of the ankle and subtalar complex (Figs. 59.36 and 59.37).

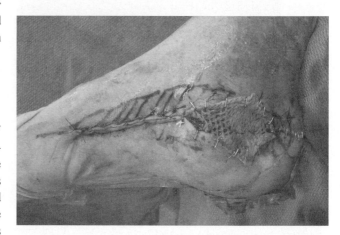

Fig. 59.35 Extended medial incision for abductor hallucis flap

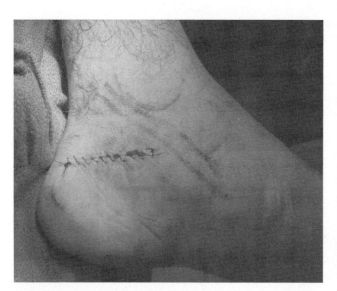

Fig. 59.33 Medial wound closed

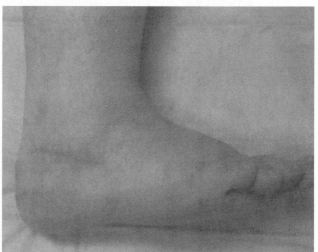

Fig. 59.36 Healed lateral incision

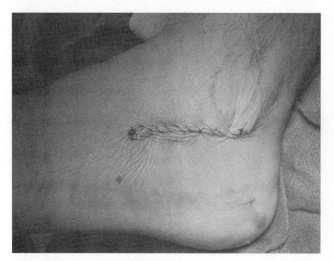

Fig. 59.34 Lateral wound closed

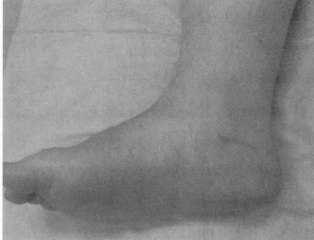

Fig. 59.37 Healed medial incision

At 8 weeks postoperatively, weightbearing is encouraged. Progression from the fracture boot to a postoperative shoe with rubber or gel heel cup helps this transition. Physical therapy is initiated. This includes calf-strengthening exercises, ankle and subtalar range of motion exercises, and a balance board program. As the patient progresses, exercise bicycle, ski machine, and elliptical trainer use are encouraged. Improvement plateaus approximately 4 months postoperatively. Maximum improvement can be expected at a year from surgery.

Results

One hundred and twenty-nine fractures have been treated in this fashion from 1996 to 2008. The results have been encouraging. Reduction has been accomplished in all cases. Wound problems have been minimal and limited to delayed wound healing in four cases. This occurred with smokers. There have been no sloughs of flaps.

There was one deep infection in a poly traumatized patient who had initial stabilization of the Sander' four-fracture dislocation by a Steinman pin placed percutaneously through the plantar heel into the talus before being referred. He was treated by ORIF with subtalar arthrodesis. He responded to wound café to include wound vacuum and parenteral antibiotics.

One patient, a heavy recalcitrant heavy smoker, sustained a collapse of the lateral aspect of the posterior facet, which demonstrated osteonecrosis at revision to subtalar arthrodesis. One elderly man bore full weight immediately postoperatively and lost the reduction of the tuberosity fragment. The posterior facet remained flat and he desired no further treatment. The patients have been able to return to normal shoes with a plantigrade foot. They maintain approximately 50% of their subtalar motion. This is comparable with other modes of ORIF. There have been no deep infections or osteomyelitis. Eight subtalar arthrodeses have been performed for posttraumatic arthritis. Four lateral plates have been removed for peroneal tendon irritation. These were plates using standard screws with prominent screw heads. The advance to the low-profile locking mini calc plate without prominent screw heads may diminish the incidence of this procedure. One patient had a screw penetrate the subtalar joint. This was a technical error. His symptoms resolved after the screw was removed. Three patients have had neurological residuals due to the medial approach. Two of these cases were heel hypoesthesia. One patient who had an abductor flap at his index surgery had dysesthesia in the sphere of the lateral plantar nerve. Three patients had hypoesthesia in the sphere of the sural nerve.

When all things are considered, including patient satisfaction, there was greater than 85% "success" rate defined as a united fracture, ability to walk comfortably in standard shoes and maintain half of their subtalar motion centered on the neutral position.

Discussion

This technique has proven to be reliable in treating comminuted intraarticular calcaneal fractures. It is a modification of the principles and technique described by Ian McReynolds.[14] The modification is the addition of the anterolateral plate that connects the posterior to anterior constructs. Use of a small plate in this area in conjunction with subarticular screws outside the plate has been used.[17] The specially shaped anterolateral plate provides a larger washer and more purchase in the anterior fragment.

The fracture pattern creates four fragments and the fixation pattern stabilizes all fragments, reducing them to the "constant fragment" of the sustentaculum. This satisfies the principles of reduction and internal fixation of the calcaneus.

No large flaps are raised. The salvage procedure of subtalar or triple arthrodesis is done through the same lateral approach used for internal fixation, avoiding lifting a large flap for a second procedure.

The procedure allows direct visualization and direct reduction of both the medial and lateral columns of the calcaneus. There is no indirect reduction. The pattern of internal fixation stabilizes all of the fracture fragments. The staples or medial hindfoot plate resist redisplacement of the tuberosity while the plate and screws stabilize the posterior articular facet and the anterior lateral fragment. All fragments are reduced to the constant fragment.

When lateral X-rays are compared of the dual-incision fixation pattern with the present lateral plate fixation, there is similarity in the constructs resisting collapse. The reinforcing bar that goes obliquely across the tuberosity portion of the peripheral plates parallels and overlays the staple fixation of the dual incision construct (Figs. 59.38 and 59.39a, b). The results of this technique are comparable to those reported by other techniques.

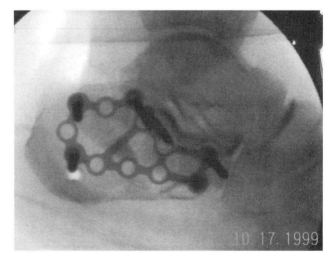

Fig. 59.38 Perimeter plate applied through a lateral incision, note the diagonal bar placed to reinforce plate

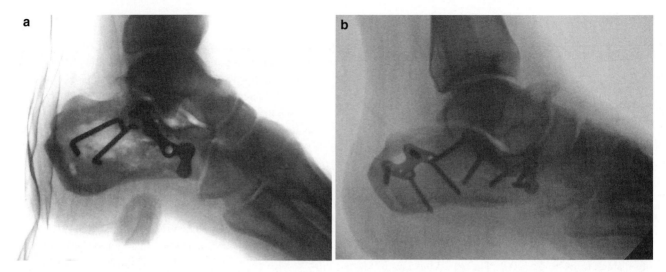

Fig. 59.39 (a) ORIF with anterolateral plate and staples. Note that the staples approximate the line and direction of oblique bar of perimeter plate. (b) ORIF with mini calc plate and medial hindfoot plate. Note that the medial plate approximates the line and direction of the oblique bar of the perimeter plate

Conclusion

The minimal dual-incision technique of open reduction and internal fixation of comminuted intraarticular calcaneal fractures is appropriate and yields satisfactory results. It should be in the foot surgeon's repertoire.

References

1. Burdeaux, B.D. Reduction of calcaneal fractures by the McReynolds medial approach technique and its experimental basis. Clin Orthop, 177:87–103, 1983
2. Carr, J.B., Hamilton, J.J., Bear, L.S. Experimental intra-articular calcaneal fractures: anatomic basis for a new classification. Foot Ankle, 10(2):81–87, 1989
3. Carr, J.B. Three dimensional CT scanning of calcaneal fractures. Orthop Trans 13: 266, 1989
4. Romash, M.M. Open reduction and internal fixation of comminuted intra articular fractures of the calcaneus using the combined medial and lateral approach. Oper Tech Ortho, 4(3):157–164, 1994
5. Sangeorzan, B.J. Open reduction and internal fixation of calcaneal fractures. In: Kitaoka, H. (ed.), Master Techniques in Orthopaedic Surgery, The Foot and Ankle. Chapter 30, Lippincott Williams and Wilkons, Philadelphia, pp. 425–447, 2002
6. Giordano, C.P., Koval, K.J. Treatment of fracture blisters: a prospective study of 53 cases. J Orthop Trauma, 9:171, 1995
7. Giordano, C.P., Koval, K.J., Zuckerman, J.D., Desai, P. Fracture blisters. Clin Orthop, 292:214, 1994
8. Atones, W. An oblique projection for roentgen examination of the talo-calcaneal joint, particularly regarding intra articular fractures of the calcaneus. Acta Radiol, 24:306, 1943
9. Broden, B. Roentgen examination of the subtaloid joint in fractures of the calcaneus. Acta Radiol, 31:85, 1949
10. Sanders, R., Dipasquale, T. Intra-operative Broden's views in the operative treatment of calcaneus fractures. Orthop Trans, 13: 26–267, 1989
11. Bohler, L. Diagnosis, pathology and treatment of fractures of the os calcis. J Bone Joint Surg, 13:75, 1931
12. Bohler, L. The Treatment of Fractures. Vol. 3, Grune and Stratton, New York, pp. 2045–2108, 1958
13. Sanders, R., Fortin, P., Di Pasquale, T., Walling, A. Operative treatment in 120 displaced intra articular calcaneal fractures: results using a prognostic computed tomography scan classification. Clin Orthop, 290:87, 1993
14. McReynolds, S. Trauma to the os calcis and heel cord. In: Jahss, M. (ed.), Disorders of the Foot and Ankle, WB Saunders, Philadelphia, p. 1497, 1984
15. Levin, L.S., Nunley, J.A. The management of soft tissue problems associated with calcaneal fractures. Clin Orthop, 290:151–156, 1993
16. Myerson, M.S., Henderson, M.R. Clinical applications of a pneumatic intermittent impulse compression device after trauma and major surgery to the foot and ankle, Foot Ankle, 14:198, 1993
17. Johnson, E.E., Gebhardt, J.S. Surgical management of calcaneal fractures using bilateral incisions and minimal internal fixation. Clin Orthop, 290:117–124, 1993

Chapter 60
Percutaneous Screw Fixation of Hallux Sesamoid Fractures

Geert I. Pagenstert, Victor Valderrabano, and Beat Hintermann

Total sesamoid excision is a powerful tool to cure recalcitrant sesamoid pain, but it has its shortcomings: excision of the lateral sesamoid led to a hallux varus, and excision of the medial sesamoid to a hallux valgus deformity in 10–20% of cases.[1–5] Excision of both sesamoids may cause cock up deformity of the hallux.[2,4,6,7] Each sesamoid is invested in the corresponding tendon sheath of the flexor hallucis brevis. The attachment of the tendon to the base of the proximal phalanx is crucial for the balance of the first metatarsophalangeal (MTP) joint. Injuries to these structures during total excision cause hallucal deviation. In addition, loss of preloading and elevation of the first metatarsal head due to sesamoid excision may lead to transfer metatarsalgia and loss of big toe push off.[8,9]

Alternative procedures have been invented to reconstruct the anatomy.[10–14] The following technique of percutaneous screw fixation of sesamoid bone fractures is one of these procedures. Moreover, the skin incisions used to approach the two sesamoid bones have been connected with adverse effects: the lateral plantar approach was reported to be associated with painful plantar scar formation, and the lateral dorsal approach with accidental harm to the intrinsic hallucal muscles and interdigital nerve neuroma. The medial approach is only useful to reach the medial sesamoid bone.[2–4,6] The percutaneous technique needs only a stap incision distal to the weight-bearing area of the sesamoid bone. Sterile strips are used for wound closure.

Indications and Contraindications

Indications for percutaneous screw fixation are a transverse sesamoid fracture, transverse nonunion, or transverse symptomatic bipartite sesamoid. Fragments have to be at least bigger than 3 mm to ensure screw fixation.

In a typical patient history, no trauma is remembered and the development of pain is insidious and chronic in character. Often these conditions are associated with endurance sports and repetitive loading of the first MTP joint as in running or dancing.[1,11,15] These symptoms may respond to activity modification alone, but generally 6–8 weeks in custom-made insoles to unburden the painful sesamoid is advised as primary treatment. However, in chronic fractures, to our experience[11,16] and in most reported cases in literature, conservative therapy is very likely to fail and further treatment will be necessary.[1,5,15]

The patient has localized pain at one sesamoid bone that exacerbates with passive dorsal extension of the hallux. To document clinical findings of unloading of the first metatarsophalangeal joint (MTP 1), pedobarography is a useful tool (Fig. 60.1).[16] On examination, conditions that stress the sesamoid complex such as cavus foot with a plantar-flexed first ray or splay foot with hallux valgus formation should be included in the surgical plan.[16]

Full weight-bearing radiographs of the whole foot and ankle are needed to asses the architecture of the foot. Special sesamoid oblique and tangential views are useful to evaluate sesamoid fracture displacement. Additional features of sesamoid pain can be visualized with magnetic resonance imaging (MRI), computed tomography (CT), and bone scan (Fig. 60.2). MRI results may show bone edema, soft tissue effusion, osteomyelitis, and tendon or ligament injuries. With the CT scan, sharp edges of sesamoid fractures can be displayed but may be absent in old fracture nonunions or bipartite sesamoids. Bone scan results adds little to find the pathology because increased uptake is unspecific.[11,12] Bone scan results are positive in asymptomatic sesamoid bones,[17] fractures, traumatized congenital bipartite bones, osteomyelitis, or tumors. Contraindications include longitudinal sesamoid fractures, comminuted fractures with multiple fragments too small for screw fixation, and infection.

Preoperative Planning

The preoperative planning for sesamoid fracture screw fixation should include treatment of the possible underlying foot

G.I. Pagenstert, V. Valderrabano, and B. Hintermann (✉)
Department of Orthopedic Surgery, University of Basel, Kantonsspital Liestal, Rheinstrasse 26, Liestal, CH-4410, Switzerland
e-mail: beat.hintermann@ksli.ch

G.R. Scuderi and A.J. Tria (eds.), *Minimally Invasive Surgery in Orthopedics*,
DOI 10.1007/978-0-387-76608-9_60, © Springer Science + Business Media, LLC 2010

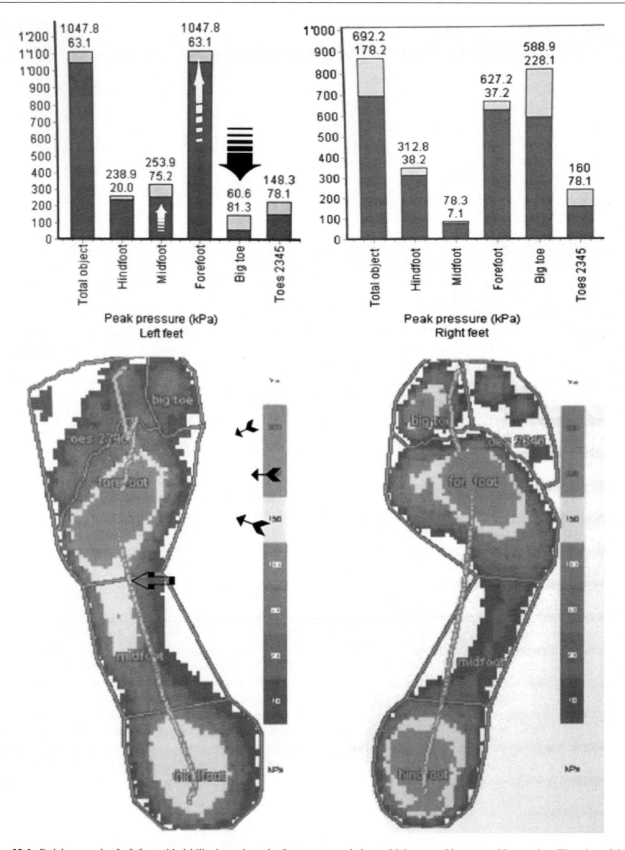

Fig. 60.1 Pedobarography. Left foot with debilitating pain at the first metatarsophalangeal joint caused by sesamoid nonunion. Elevation of the first ray has occurred with lateral drift of the central line of pressure (*arrows* on picture). Big toe push off is markedly reduced compared with the healthy contralateral side (*arrows* on chart)

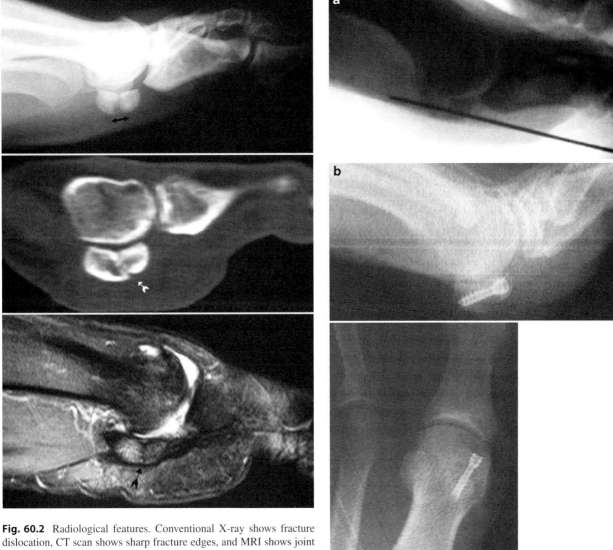

Fig. 60.2 Radiological features. Conventional X-ray shows fracture dislocation, CT scan shows sharp fracture edges, and MRI shows joint effusion, bone edema, and additional tendon and capsular injuries

deformity.[16] A metatarsus primus flexus is treated with a dorsal-extension osteotomy, a metatarsus primus varus and hallux valgus is addressed with appropriate osseus and/or soft tissue procedures. Reducing mechanical stress to the sesamoid bone osteosynthesis is thought to improve healing. However, surgical stress reduction alone may cause fracture healing even without sesamoid osteosynthesis in marked foot deformities.[16]

Technique

For percutaneous cannulated screw fixation of the sesamoid fracture, the patient is placed in the supine position. A tourniquet is not needed. A stap incision is made and a 1.5-mm K-wire is inserted to the distal pole of the sesamoid with the hallux fixed in hyperextension (Fig. 60.3). Under fluoros-

Fig. 60.3 Screw fixation. (**a**) K-wire inserted from distally; (**b**) cannulated compression screw in place

copy, the wire is guided perpendicular to the fracture line through the distal fragment. With the surgeon's thumb, the hallux is held in neutral and pressure is put on the proximal pole and the whole sesamoid bone against the metatarsal head. This procedure levels out the joint surfaces of the sesamoid fragments with the metatarsal joint surface of the metatarsal-sesamoid joint. This constant pressure is continued until the cannulated compression screw is in place to enhance the compressive forces (Fig. 60.3). The authors used 10- to 14-mm compression screw lengths (e.g., Bold-Screw, New Deal, Lyon, France). Both corticalices should be held by the screw to assure compression and fixation of the fragments. Wound closure is achieved with a sterile strip.

Complications

Improper screw placement may not deliver compression and stability to the fracture and nonunion or dislocation may occur and need sesamoid bone excision. Persistent sesamoid stress caused by unrecognized foot deformity (hallux valgus, pes cavus) may maintain sesamoid bone symptoms and may need further treatment.[16]

Postoperative Management

Full weight bearing as tolerated is allowed right after surgery at the heel in a stiff-soled shoe to prevent dorsiflexion of the first MTP joint. No suture removal or wound care is needed since the stap incision was closed by a sterile strip. At 6–8 weeks after surgery, conventional shoes and gradual return to previous activity is allowed.

Results

Blundell and colleagues[12] fixed nine sesamoid fractures in athletes with percutaneous cannulated screws and revealed excellent results. All athletes went back to their previous level of activity. No complication was reported. They concluded that percutaneous screw fixation is a safe and fast procedure. They pointed out that discerning between traumatized bipartite sesamoid and fractured sesamoid bones was not performed because treatment was the same anyway.

The authors performed percutaneous screw fixation in seven athletic patients and had excellent results with full athletic recovery. All patients were endurance athletes (running, dancing), and five were female and two were male. One lateral and six medial sesamoid bone nonunions have been treated. In two patients, the concomitant hallux valgus deformity was corrected in the same surgery and fracture compression of sesamoid screw fixation was controlled under vision.[12] Local anesthesia only was sufficient for percutaneous surgery in the most recent case. All patients went back to sports 8 weeks after surgery.

Conclusion

Percutaneous screw fixation for sesamoid bone nonunion is a safe and fast procedure that can be performed with local anesthesia. In contrast to the standard treatment of total sesamoid bone excision, the percutaneous screw fixation preserves anatomy and function of the hallux sesamoid complex.

References

1. Brodsky JW, Robinson AHN, Krause JO, and Watkins D. Excision and flexor hallucis brevis reconstruction for the painful sesamoid fractures and non-unions: surgical technique, clinical results and histo-pathological findings. J Bone Joint Surg (Br) 2000 82-B:217
2. Grace DL. Sesamoid problems. Foot Ankle Clin 2000 5:609–627
3. Inge GAL and Ferguson AB. Surgery of sesamoid bones of the great toe. Arch Surg 1933 27:466–489
4. Richardson EG. Hallucal sesamoid pain: causes and surgical treatment. J Am Acad Orthop Surg 1999 7:270–278
5. Saxena A and Krisdakumtorn T. Return to activity after sesamoidectomy in athletically active individuals. Foot Ankle Int 2003 24:415–419
6. Jahss MH. The sesamoids of the hallux. Clin Orthop Relat Res 1981 Jun;(157):88–97
7. McBryde AM, Jr. and Anderson RB. Sesamoid foot problems in the athlete. Clin Sports Med 1988 7:51–60
8. Aper RL, Saltzman CL, and Brown TD. The effect of hallux sesamoid resection on the effective moment of the flexor hallucis brevis. Foot Ankle Int 1994 15:462–470
9. Aper RL, Saltzman CL, and Brown TD. The effect of hallux sesamoid excision on the flexor hallucis longus moment arm. Clin Orthop Relat Res 1996 Apr;(325):209–217
10. Anderson RB and McBryde AM, Jr. Autogenous bone grafting of hallux sesamoid nonunions. Foot Ankle Int 1997 18:293–296
11. Biedert R and Hintermann B. Stress fractures of the medial great toe sesamoids in athletes. Foot Ankle Int 2003 24:137–141
12. Blundell CM, Nicholson P, and Blackney MW. Percutaneous screw fixation for fractures of the sesamoid bones of the hallux. J Bone Joint Surg (Br) 2002 84:1138–1141
13. Riley J and Selner M. Internal fixation of a displaced tibial sesamoid fracture. J Am Podiatr Med Assoc 2001 91:536–539
14. Rodeo SA, Warren RF, O'Brien SJ, Pavlov H, Barnes R, and Hanks GA. Diastasis of bipartite sesamoids of the first metatarsophalangeal joint. Foot Ankle 1993 14:425–434
15. Van Hal ME, Keene JS, Lange TA, and Clancy WG, Jr. Stress fractures of the great toe sesamoids. Am J Sports Med 1982 10:122–128
16. Pagenstert GI, Valderrabano V, and Hintermann B. Medial sesamoid nonunion combined with hallux valgus in athletes: a report of two cases. Foot Ankle Int 2006 27:135–140
17. Chisin R, Peyser A, and Milgrom C. Bone scintigraphy in the assessment of the hallucal sesamoids. Foot Ankle Int 1995 16:291–294

Chapter 61
Proximal Percutaneous Harvesting of the Plantaris Tendon

Geert I. Pagenstert and Beat Hintermann

For decades, in a variety of surgical specialties, the plantaris longus tendon has been used as a free autologous tendon graft.[1] The plantaris is a tendon of a rudimentary developed muscle and harvesting leaves no functional donor site morbidity. However, even foot and ankle surgeons frequently use other autografts because of difficulties finding the tendon with the established harvesting procedure at the medial calcaneus.[2,3] Enlargement of the incision, multi incisions, and painful scar formation at the level of footwear have been described.[4]

Difficulties finding the plantaris distally are explained by its inconstant insertion at the ankle joint capsule, bursa calcanei, flexor retinaculum, blending with the Achilles tendon or intermuscular septum a few centimeters above its insertion at the calcaneus.[5,6] In different reports, surgeons were able to find the tendon in only 80[7] to 88%[8] of cases, while cadaver sections and magnetic resonance imaging (MRI) or ultrasound studies have proved its prevalence in 93–98% of cases.[5,9,10] In the following discussion, we present an easy and reproductive procedure to harvest at least 30 cm of plantaris tendon over a 2-cm single incision at the medial calf.

Indications and Contraindications

In orthopedic surgery, autografts are used for reconstruction of ligaments or tendons providing mechanical function. If local tissue is absent or too weak, free grafts are indicated. The best graft tissue is located within the surgical field (no enlargement of the surgical field necessary) and provides the greatest mechanical stability, which means that it has aligned strong and elastic collagen fibers. Among autograft tissues, tendons have the highest concentration of aligned collagen fibers. However, only the plantaris tendon at the leg has no crucial function.[10] Harvesting of other tendons can be asso-

ciated with significant donor site morbidity.[11–15] A biomechanical study of Bohnsack and colleagues[16] compared tensile strength (in newtons per square millimeter) with load to failure of the peroneus longus (61 N/mm²), peroneus brevis (41 N/mm²), split peroneus brevis (52 N/mm²), split Achilles tendon (36 N/mm²), fascia lata (27 N/mm²), periostal flap (2 N/mm²), anterior talo-fibular ligament (8 N/mm²), corium (12 N/mm²), and plantaris tendon (94 N/mm²) and found that the plantaris tendon had the highest tensile strength per square millimeter.[16] Therefore, especially in the field of foot and ankle surgery, the use of the plantaris tendon is indicated.

Preoperative Planning

Magnet resonance imaging can prove existence of the plantaris tendon but should not be ordered for this purpose alone.[9,17] Ultrasound visualization is adequate.[18]

Technique

The plantaris longus tendon runs at the medial boarder of the triceps between the muscle bellies of gastrocnemius and soleus.[1,19] A 2-cm longitudinal incision 30 cm proximal to the medial malleolus is made (Fig. 61.1a). Subcutaneous blunt dissection to the fascia is performed with respect to the saphenous nerve and vein (Fig. 61.1b). Again, a 2-cm longitudinal incision is made in the fascia to enable the surgeon's finger to enter the intermuscular space (Fig. 61.1c). The only rigid tubular structure that is palpable at this location is the plantaris tendon. The tendon is developed with the finger or a nerve retractor (Fig. 61.1d). With a blunt tendon stripper, the plantaris tendon is dissected in the distal direction. The tendon stripper is advanced, keeping the tendon under tension (Fig. 61.1e). At the calcaneus level, the inner cylinder of the stripper is rotated, which cuts the tendon. The tendon is stored in a wet sponge for later use (Fig. 61.1f). Fascia is closed with interrupted sutures, and wound closure is done with a subcuticular running stitch

G.I. Pagenstert and B. Hintermann (✉)
Department of Orthopedic Surgery, University of Basel, Kantonsspital Liestal, Rheinstrasse 26, Liestal, CH, 4410, Switzerland
e-mail: beat.hintermann@ksli.ch

G.R. Scuderi and A.J. Tria (eds.), *Minimally Invasive Surgery in Orthopedics*,
DOI 10.1007/978-0-387-76608-9_61, © Springer Science + Business Media, LLC 2010

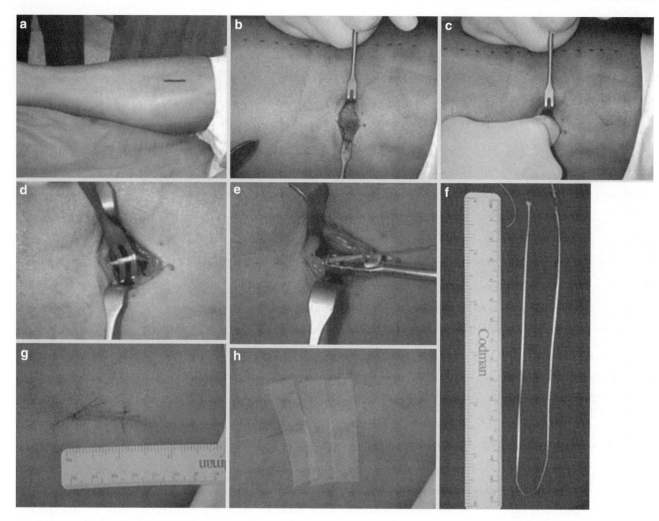

Fig. 61.1 Proximal plantaris harvesting. (**a**) Overview and skin incision to harvest the plantaris longus tendon. (**b**) Blunt dissection to the crural fascia has been made. (**c**) The only palpable tubular structure here is the plantaris tendon. (**d**) The tendon developed. (**e**) The tendon stripper is advanced distally with the tendon under tension. (**f**) The average length of the harvested tendon is 30 cm. (**g**) A small and cosmetic scar is achieved by subcuticular running suture and (**h**) sterile strips

(Fig. 61.1g). Wound tension is neutralized with sterile strips to achieve a favorable cosmetic result (Fig. 61.1h).

Complications

The authors performed proximal plantaris harvesting in more than 100 cases and had one case of mild dysesthesia at a broadened scar that did not bother the patient. No saphenous nerve or vein injury has been experienced despite anatomic nearness.

Postoperative Management

Sterile strips can reduce skin tension and broadening of the scar. After wound healing, the patient may use friction massage in case of subcutaneous adhesions.

Results

The harvesting procedure of the plantaris tendon had been controlled in the context of a clinical study that used plantaris tendon autograft for lateral ligament reconstruction of chronic ankle instability. In three (5.3%) of 56 ankle reconstructions, the plantaris tendon could not be located with the previously described harvesting procedure. In one case (1.7%), the plantaris tendon was too weak to serve as proper donor material. In 52 cases (93%), a strong 25- to 35-cm-long tendon graft was harvested.[19]

Conclusions

The proximal plantaris harvesting procedure has a higher success than has the traditional distal harvesting procedure. It is associated with no donor site morbidity or complications and may be recommended for all procedures that need strong autograft tissue, especially in the field of foot and ankle surgery.

References

1. White WL. The unique, accessible and useful plantaris tendon. Plast Reconstr Surg 25:133–141, 1960
2. Coughlin MJ, Matt V, Schenck RC, Jr. Augmented lateral ankle reconstruction using a free gracilis graft. Orthopedics 25:31–35, 2002
3. Sammarco GJ, Idusuyi OB. Reconstruction of the lateral ankle ligaments using a split peroneus brevis tendon graft. Foot Ankle Int 20:97–103, 1999
4. Weber BG. Die Verletzungen des oberen Sprunggelenks, 2nd edn, 193–196. Bern, Stuttgart, Wien: Huber, 1972
5. Daseler EH, Anson BH. The plantaris muscle. An anatomical study of 750 specimens. J Bone Joint Surg. 25:822–827, 1943
6. Harvey FJ, Chu G, Harvey PM. Surgical availability of the plantaris tendon. J Hand Surg (Am). 8:243–247, 1983
7. Weber BG, Hupfauer W. Zur Behandlung der frischen fibularen Bandruptur und der chronischen fibularen Bandinsuffizienz. Arch Orthop. Trauma Surg 65:251–257, 1969
8. Segesser B, Goesele A. [Weber fibular ligament-plasty with plantar tendon with Segesser modification]. Sportverletz Sportschaden 10:88–93, 1996
9. Saxena, A. and Bareither, D. Magnetic resonance and cadaveric findings of the incidence of plantaris tendon. Foot Ankle Int. 21:570–572, 2000
10. Tillmann B, Töndury G. Flexorengruppe der unteren Extremität. In: Leonhardt H, Tillmann B, Töndury G, Zilles K (eds.), Bewegungsapparat, pp. 584–793. Stuttgart, New York: Thieme, 1987
11. Attarian DE, McCrackin HJ, Devito DP, McElhaney JH, Garrett, WE, Jr. A biomechanical study of human lateral ankle ligaments and autogenous reconstructive grafts. Am J Sports Med 13:377–381, 1985
12. Bahr R, Pena F, Shine J, Lew WD, Tyrdal S, Engebretsen L. Biomechanics of ankle ligament reconstruction. An in vitro comparison of the Brostrom repair, Watson-Jones reconstruction, and a new anatomic reconstruction technique. Am J Sports Med 25:424–432, 1997
13. Brunner R, Gaechter A. Repair of fibular ligaments: comparison of reconstructive techniques using plantaris and peroneal tendons. Foot Ankle 11:359–367, 1991
14. Hintermann B. [Biomechanical aspects of muscle-tendon functions]. Orthopade 24:187–192, 1995
15. Hintermann B. Biomechanics of the unstable ankle joint and clinical implications. Med Sci Sports Exerc 31:S459–S469, 1999
16. Bohnsack M, SurieB, Kirsch IL, Wulker N. Biomechanical properties of commonly used autogenous transplants in the surgical treatment of chronic lateral ankle instability. Foot Ankle Int 23:661–664, 2002
17. Wening JV, Katzer A, Phillips F, Jungbluth KH, Lorke DE. [Detection of the tendon of the musculus plantaris longus - diagnostic imaging and anatomic correlate]. Unfallchirurgie 22:30–35, 1996
18. Simpson SL, Hertzog MS, Barja RH. The plantaris tendon graft: an ultrasound study. J Hand Surg (Am). 16:708–711, 1991
19. Pagenstert GI, Valderrabano V, Hintermann B. Lateral ankle ligament reconstruction with free plantaris tendon graft. Tech Foot Ankle Surg 4:104–112, 2005

Chapter 62
Percutaneous Fixation of Proximal Fifth Metatarsal Fractures

Jonathan R. Saluta and James A. Nunley

Classification

Fractures of the proximal fifth metatarsal can be divided into three general patterns: avulsion of the tuberosity (type 1), Jones fractures (type 2), and diaphyseal stress fractures (type 3).[1] Tuberosity fractures can be extraarticular or may involve the metatarsocuboid joint (Fig. 62.1). Jones fractures involve the metaphyseal-diaphyseal junction and extend transversely and medially into the 4–5 intermetatarsal joint (Figs. 62.1 and 62.2). Unlike tuberosity fractures, which reliably heal, Jones fractures have a nonunion rate between 7 and 28%.[2,3] In addition, one third of Jones fractures treated conservatively may go on to closed refracture.[4] Diaphyseal stress fractures occur distal to the 4–5 intermetatarsal joint (Fig. 62.1) and are usually associated with prodromal symptoms. Torg[5] divides diaphyseal stress fractures into three types: acute fractures with sharp margins, delayed unions with a widened fracture line and intramedullary sclerosis, and established nonunions with complete obliteration of the canal.

Treatment

For the majority of tuberosity fractures, conservative management is recommended. A rare indication for surgery would be a large articular stepoff in the metatarsocuboid joint. Depending on symptoms, patients are treated weightbearing in either a hard-soled shoe, removable boot, or cast for 3 weeks. Jones fractures are treated similarly to diaphyseal stress fractures. Nonsurgical management usually consists of nonweightbearing in a short leg cast for 6–8 weeks. However, conservative management is not as reliable in this group, and in most cases surgery is recommended. Surgical candidates include patients engaged in regular athletic activity, patients with high occupational demands, and informed patients who decline conservative treatment.

Surgical Technique

Fixation of minimally to nondisplaced fifth metatarsal base fractures is possible through a percutaneous technique. The first step is to template the fracture because choosing the proper screw is critical to the success of the surgery. Generally the largest diameter screw that will fit the canal should be used. We recommend using a 4.5-mm solid shaft screw for intramedullary canal diameters of 3.5–4.0 mm, a 5.5 screw for canal diameters of 4.1–5.0 mm, and a 6.5 screw for canal diameters of 5.1 mm or greater.[6] A commercially available screw set designed specifically for these fractures contains shaft screws of all three diameters (Fig. 62.3a, b). In addition to proper screw width, an appropriate screw length should be calculated as well. Generally a screw measuring 50% of the length of the bone is a good place to start. Because the fifth metatarsal has a plantar and lateral bow, a straight screw of greater than 60% of the overall length of the metatarsal may straighten the bow and displace the fracture.[7,8] Compression is advantageous to help heal this fracture, so if a cancellous lag screw is chosen, one must be certain that all of the threads will cross the fracture site.

Surgery is generally performed under ankle block anesthesia and in an outpatient surgical suite. The patient is positioned supine and the body shifted toward the side of the operating room table that corresponds with the affected foot. It is important that the ipsilateral knee can be flexed and the affected foot can be placed plantigrade on the edge of the table or a sterile operating room fluoroscopy unit. Proper positioning is important because it will keep the working instruments clear of the operating room table. A tourniquet is generally used to provide a bloodless field. Before an incision is made, a K wire is placed upon the lateral aspect of the foot, and fluoroscopy is used to position the pin parallel to and overlapping the proximal metatarsal shaft. This position should correspond to the target screw placement on both the anteroposterior (AP) and lateral images. Two lines are traced in ink on the skin that approximate the pin alignment in both views (Fig. 62.4).

A 2-cm longitudinal incision is made 2 cm proximal to the base of the fifth metatarsal. In our experience, displacement of the fracture commonly consists of mild angulation,

J.R. Saluta (✉) and J.A. Nunley
Department of Surgery, Division of Orthopaedic Surgery,
Duke University Medical Center, Box 2923, Durham, NC 27710, USA
e-mail: salutaj@yahoo.com

G.R. Scuderi and A.J. Tria (eds.), *Minimally Invasive Surgery in Orthopedics*,
DOI 10.1007/978-0-387-76608-9_62, © Springer Science+Business Media, LLC 2010

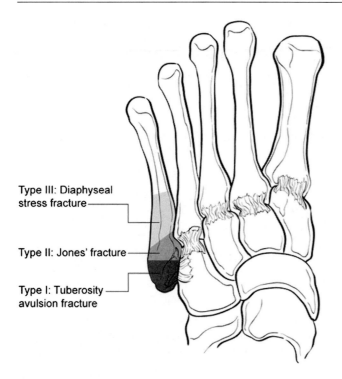

Type III: Diaphyseal stress fracture

Type II: Jones' fracture

Type I: Tuberosity avulsion fracture

Fig. 62.1 Classification of proximal metatarsal fractures

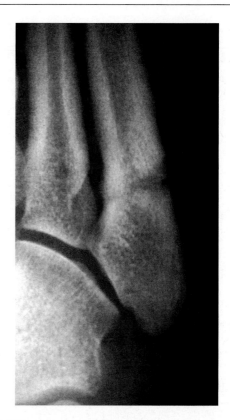

Fig. 62.2 Plain radiograph of a Jones fracture

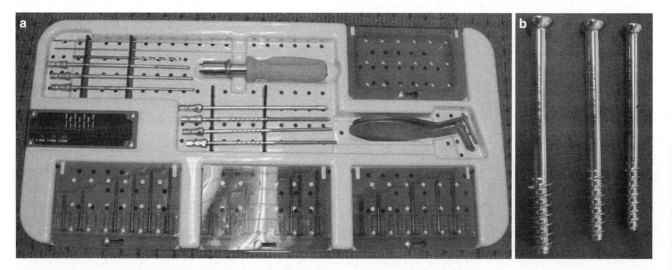

Fig. 62.3 (a) Specialty Jones set of screws and instrumentation for fixation of proximal fifth metatarsal fractures (Photo courtesy of Wright Medical). (b) 4.5-, 5.5-, and 6.5-mm screws with low-profile heads (Photo courtesy of Wright Medical)

and exposure of the fracture site is usually unnecessary. The reduction is accomplished with compression from screw insertion. An important step is to identify and protect the sural nerve and peroneus brevis tendon during screw preparation and insertion. The sural nerve is either overlying or slightly dorsal to the skin incision and can be retracted superiorly (Fig. 62.5). Anatomic studies have shown the sural nerve to lie within 5 mm of the proximal tuberosity.[9] The peroneus

brevis tendon is usually retracted inferiorly. A commonly described technique involves partially elevating the attachment of the peroneus brevis in order to gain better exposure of the entry point for the guide wire, but, in our experience, simple retraction of the tendon is adequate. A guide pin is now placed through the incision toward the "high and inside" starting point at the base of the fifth metatarsal. Fluoroscopy is used to place the tip of the pin in a center-center position

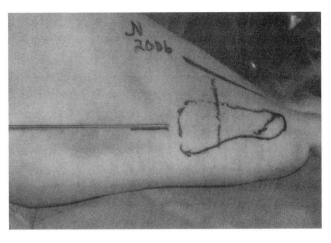

Fig. 62.4 Skin markings for guidewire placement

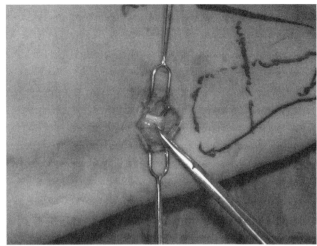

Fig. 62.5 A branch of the sural nerve

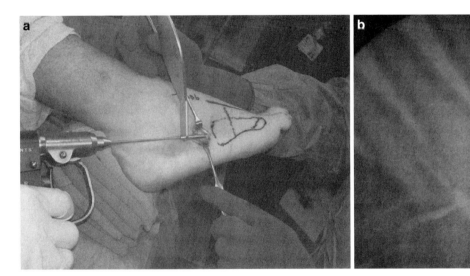

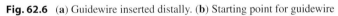

Fig. 62.6 (**a**) Guidewire inserted distally. (**b**) Starting point for guidewire

relative to the intramedullary canal on AP, lateral, and oblique views (Fig. 62.6). The medial edge of the pin should abut the cuboid. The pin is advanced two thirds of the length of the shaft through the center of the medullary canal. In order to keep the guide pin from deviating medially in the fifth metatarsal shaft, the pin should lie almost directly on the lateral calcaneal skin when being advanced.

The pin is next overdrilled with a cannulated drill under fluoroscopic guidance to avoid penetration of the fifth metatarsal cortex (Fig. 62.7). Next, the bone is carefully tapped to the proper size and length corresponding to the intended screw. Countersinking the head has not been necessary in our experience. Using a screw that is longer than the distance tapped can either distract the fracture site or explode the lateral cortex and should be avoided. The appropriate screw is finally advanced under fluoroscopy to make sure that all of the screw threads have just crossed the fracture site. The screw should compress

the fracture site, which usually results in an adequate reduction (Fig. 62.8). In our experience, drilling the canal even in sclerotic bone promotes fracture healing, which makes extensile incisions and supplemental bone grafting usually unnecessary. The incision is irrigated and closed with interrupted nylon sutures.

A technique for avoiding excessive fluoroscopy exposure during pin placement was described by Johnson.[9] His technique requires a slightly longer skin incision that exposes the plantarmost aspect of the proximal tuberosity and part of the peroneus brevis insertion. Without the use of fluoroscopy, a guide pin is placed at the starting point 1 cm dorsal to the palpable inferior margin of the tuberosity and medial to the peroneus brevis insertion (Fig. 62.9). A predetermined plantarflexion angle of 7° is marked on the skin using a goniometer (Fig. 62.10). The guide pin is advanced, overdrilled, and tapped, and the screw is inserted as previously described. A fluoroscan is used to check the final screw placement.

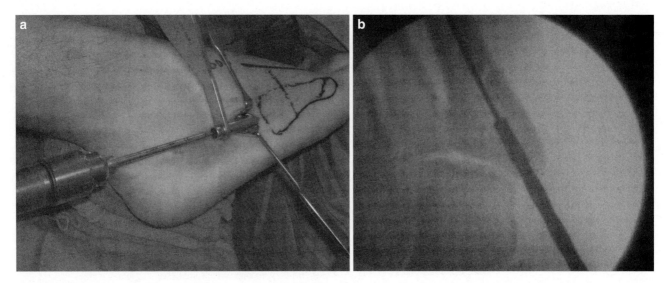

Fig. 62.7 (a) Drill inserted with protector. (b) Guidewire overdrilled

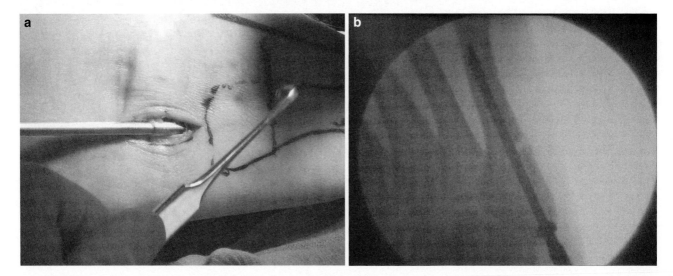

Fig. 62.8 (a) Large diameter screw inserted. (b) Screw advanced across fracture

Postoperative Management

Postoperatively, the patient is splinted and kept touchdown-weightbearing for 2 weeks. At the end of 2 weeks, the patient is allowed to begin progressive weightbearing in a removable boot and with a custom molded orthosis. By the fourth week, the orthosis is maintained, and the patient is transitioned to regular shoes with a stiff sole to reduce motion. Athletes are usually allowed to jog on a track by the fifth to sixth week, and most are back to sports by the seventh to eighth week.

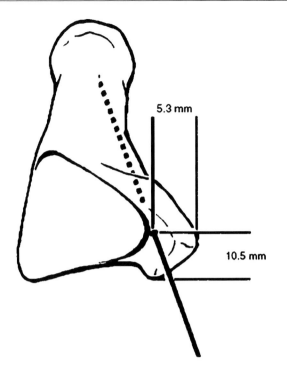

Fig. 62.9 Illustration showing the starting point in relation to the lateral and plantar portions of the fifth metatarsal tuberosity (From Johnson et al.[9] Copyright © 2004 by the American Orthopaedic Foot & Ankle Society [AOFAS], reproduced here with permission.)

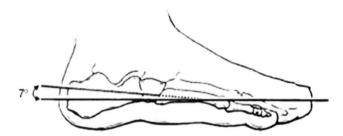

Fig. 62.10 Illustration showing the 7° plantarflexion angle with the ankle dorsiflexed to neutral. The pin would always project along the lateral aspect of the calcaneus after antegrade placement through the starting point (From Johnson et al.[9] Copyright © 2004 by the American Orthopaedic Foot & Ankle Society [AOFAS], reproduced here with permission.)

References

1. Quill G Jr. Fractures of the proximal fifth metatarsal. Orthop Clin North Am 1995;26:353–361
2. Torg J, Balduini F, Zelko R, Pavlov H, Peff T, Das M. Fractures of the base of the fifth metatarsal distal to the tuberosity: classification and guidelines for non-surgical and surgical management. J Bone Joint Surg Am 1984;66:209–214
3. Clapper M, O'Brien T, Lyons P. Fractures of the fifth metatarsal: analysis of a fracture registry. Clin Orthop Relat Res 1995;315:238–241
4. Quill G Jr. Fractures of the proximal fifth metatarsal. Orthop Clin North Am 1995;26:353–361
5. Torg J, Balduini F, Zelko R, Pavlov H, Peff T, Das M. Fractures of the base of the fifth metatarsal distal to the tuberosity: classification and guidelines for non-surgical and surgical management. J Bone Joint Surg Am 1984;66:209–214
6. Mall N, Queen R, Glisson R, Nunley JS. Patterns and risk factors of screw failure in intramedullary fixation of fifth metatarsal Jones fractures: a biomechanical study. Unpublished data, 2006
7. Horst F, Gilbert B, Glisson R, Nunley J. Torque resistance after fixation of Jones fractures with intramedullary screws. Foot Ankle Int 2004;25(12):914–919
8. Nunley J. Fractures of the base of the fifth metatarsal: the Jones fracture. Orthop Clin North Am 2001;32(1): 171–180
9. Johnson J, Labib S, Fowler, R. Intramedullary screw fixation of the fifth metatarsal: an anatomic study and improved technique. Foot Ankle Int 2004;25(4):274–277

Chapter 63
Percutaneous ORIF of Periarticular Distal Tibia Fractures

Michael P. Clare and Roy W. Sanders

Periarticular fractures of the distal tibia remain among the more challenging of fractures for the orthopedic surgeon. Traditional methods of treatment have included functional bracing, external fixation with or without limited internal fixation (hybrid fixation), intramedullary nailing, and formal open reduction internal fixation (ORIF). Cadaveric studies have previously described the somewhat tenuous vascular supply to the distal metaphysis, which, combined with inherent limitations in the surrounding soft tissue envelope, pose a risk of nonunion and have led to increasing interest in "biologic" fixation techniques.[1]

These techniques are based upon the principles of limited soft tissue stripping, maintenance of the osteogenic fracture hematoma, and preservation of vascular supply to the individual fracture fragments while restoring axial and rotational alignment, and providing sufficient stability to allow progression of motion, uncomplicated fracture healing, and eventual return to function. As such, the evolution of percutaneous plating techniques has led to the development of low-profile, precontoured implants specifically intended for subcutaneous/submuscular application in the distal tibia.

Indications and Contraindications

Percutaneous ORIF techniques are ideal for unstable distal-fourth, extraarticular fractures of the distal tibia with periarticular metaphyseal comminution or distal fracture lines precluding use of a locked intramedullary nail (OTA types 43A1-A3; 43B1).[2] Other indications include simple two-part, nondisplaced or minimally displaced intraarticular fractures (OTA type 43C1) in which the articular fragments can be anatomically reduced by an abbreviated open reduction, and the remainder completed through percutaneous means.[2]

Percutaneous ORIF is also particularly attractive in the event of open fractures, which account for up to 20% of these injuries; overlying fracture blisters, or other significant soft tissue compromise; fractures in patients who are heavy smokers (≥ 2 packs/day); and fractures in patients with diabetes mellitus, peripheral neuropathy, or other significant medical comorbidities.

We think that complex, comminuted intraarticular fractures of the tibial pilon require an anatomic articular reduction for optimum results, which thus necessitates a true open reduction and internal fixation. Percutaneous techniques in these instances are therefore contraindicated.

Surgical Technique

Depending on the extent of soft tissue injury, periarticular fractures in the distal tibia typically require temporary stabilization with a spanning external fixator, which maintains axial length and provides provisional stability until soft tissue swelling and/or fracture blisters have sufficiently resolved to allow definitive stabilization. We utilize the "wrinkle test," originally described for calcaneal fractures, as a simple means to determine soft tissue suitability for surgery.[3] The test involves gentle passive ankle dorsiflexion, paying close attention to the skin overlying the area of intended dissection; alternatively, in the presence of a prohibitive external fixator frame, the skin overlying the planned area of dissection can be gently pinched. The presence of skin wrinkles is considered a positive test, indicating that soft tissue swelling has adequately dissipated to proceed with definitive fracture stabilization.

The patient is placed supine on a radiolucent operating table with a bolster beneath the ipsilateral hip, and a pneumatic tourniquet is placed. We prefer utilizing the tourniquet for any articular reduction, as well as for open stabilization of the fibula, where necessary, in order to provide a bloodless surgical field. The percutaneous plating may then be performed with the tourniquet deflated, depending on the clinical situation. Because of the need for biplanar image intensification, standard fluoroscopy is also required. In the presence of prior external fixation, we typically remove the external fixator frame (still assembled) prior to skin preparation while

M.P. Clare and R.W. Sanders (✉)
Orthopaedic Trauma Service, Tampa General Hospital, The Florida Orthopaedic Institute, 4 Columbia Drive #710, Tampa FL, 33606, USA
e-mail: OTS1@aol.com

G.R. Scuderi and A.J. Tria (eds.), *Minimally Invasive Surgery in Orthopedics*,
DOI 10.1007/978-0-387-76608-9_63, © Springer Science+Business Media, LLC 2010

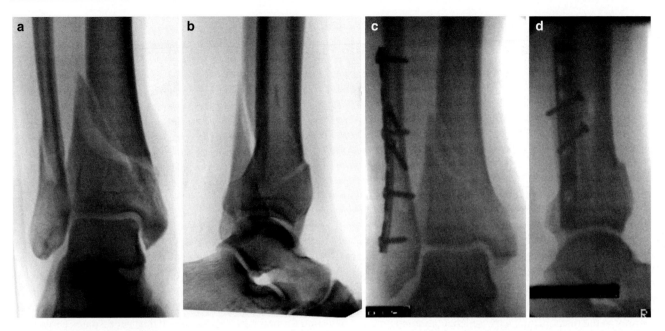

Fig. 63.1 (**a**, **b**) Preoperative radiographs of a periarticular distal tibia fracture; (**c**, **d**) intraoperative radiographs after stabilization of fibula – note the indirect reduction of the distal tibia

leaving the Schanz pins in place for assistance with indirect fracture reduction intraoperatively; the frame is then resterilized and preserved on the back table for use where needed.

In the event of an associated fibula fracture, we prefer to first stabilize the fibula to confirm axial length and rotational alignment. In most cases, and particularly with extraarticular fractures of the distal tibia, restoring fibular length and rotation will indirectly reduce the distal tibia, such that only minimal further manipulation is required with tibial stabilization (Fig. 63.1a–d).

Medial Plating of the Distal Tibia

Subcutaneous medial plating is the most common of the percutaneous stabilization techniques in the distal tibia, and is especially well suited for extraarticular distal-fourth or supramalleolar fractures (OTA types 43A1–3).[2] A small (2–3 cm) vertical incision is made in line with the medial malleolus, and the underlying saphenous nerve is identified and protected (Fig. 63.2). Alternatively, an oblique or transverse incision may be utilized. Deep dissection then continues down through the extensor retinaculum, but superficial to the underlying periosteum. The full thickness soft tissue envelope is then gently mobilized to facilitate easy passage of the plate, and a subcutaneous tunnel is then developed with a blunt periosteal elevator along the medial border of the tibia in extraperiosteal fashion.

The provisionally selected plate is placed directly on the skin overlying the medial distal tibia and assessed under fluoroscopy for adequacy of length (Fig. 63.3). The required plate length is variable depending on the fracture pattern and extent of comminution, bone quality of the patient, and screw purchase (for nonlocking implants), among other factors. As a general rule, however, four to six screw holes with two to four screws proximal to the main fracture line should provide sufficient stability. The plate is then rotationally contoured where necessary (Fig. 63.4) and gently passed in retrograde fashion under fluoroscopic guidance, specifically avoiding the saphenous nerve (Fig. 63.5). At the present time, most commercially available implants for the medial distal tibia do not have an associated outrigger for assistance with plate passage. Sagittal plane alignment of the plate relative to the tibial shaft is then confirmed fluoroscopically. A secondary incision is made at the proximal tip of the plate for manipulation where necessary until the plate is appropriately positioned.

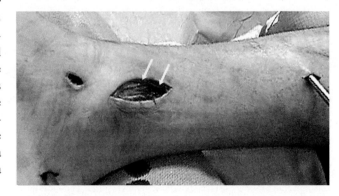

Fig. 63.2 Small medial incision for percutaneous medial plating - note the saphenous nerve (*white arrows*)

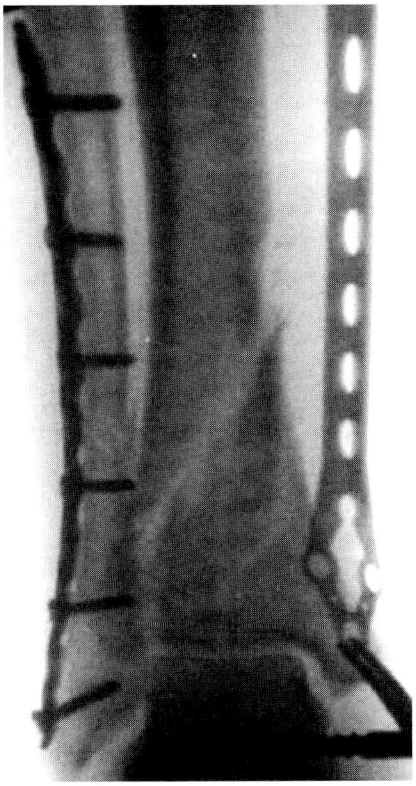

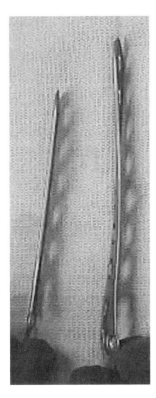

Fig. 63.3 Intraoperative radiograph with a provisionally selected plate - note the length of the plate relative to the apex of the fracture line, allowing four screw holes for the proximal fragment

Depending on the fracture pattern and extent of residual displacement, pointed reduction forceps are then used through separate stab incisions to further reduce the proximal fragment to the distal fragment(s) through the plate (Fig. 63.6a, b). In the absence of a fibula fracture, or in the event of significant residual shortening, restoration of axial length may be facilitated through a variety of indirect reduction techniques, including longitudinal traction through the previous external fixator Schanz pins, use of a femoral distractor, or an articulated tensioning device. Lag screws may be placed outside the plate through separate stab incisions to stabilize additional fracture lines where necessary.

Because of the proximity of the ankle joint, we generally prefer initially stabilizing the distal fragment to the plate, using the distal-most and proximal-most screw holes overlying the distal fragment. Typically, the distal-most screw holes are easily visualized through the small medial incision, while the more proximal screw holes are isolated under fluoroscopy and accessed through small stab incisions (Fig. 63.7). In general, three to four screws within the distal fragment should provide sufficient stability (Fig. 63.8a, b). With simple, oblique fracture patterns, lag screws may first be placed through the plate across the primary fracture line, thereby securing the distal fragment to the proximal fragment (Fig. 63.9). Additional lag screws may be placed through the plate where necessary for stabilization of vertically oriented fracture lines distally.

The proximal fragment is then secured, utilizing (as a minimum) the proximal-most and apex screw holes within the plate, respectively, which, when combined with the distal screw pattern creates an "internal external fixator" construct (Fig. 63.10a, b). Other screw holes may additionally be filled within the proximal fragment, again depending on the clinical situation, quality of screw purchase, and overall fracture and construct stability (Fig. 63.11a, b).

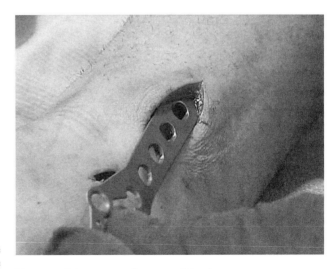

Fig. 63.5 Subcutaneous placement of the plate

Fig. 63.4 Contouring of the selected plate prior to placement - note the rotational bend through the proximal portion of the plate to match the triangular contour of the distal diaphysis

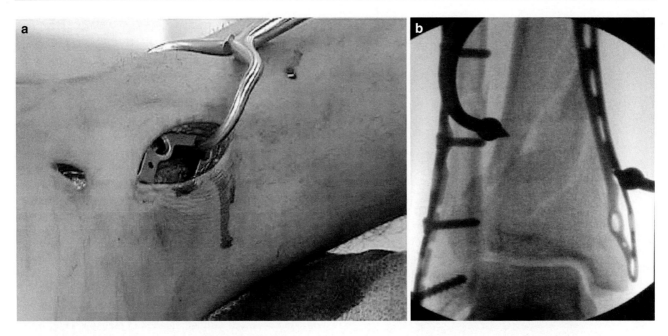

Fig. 63.6 (**a, b**) Provisional reduction of the distal tibia with a pointed reduction clamp

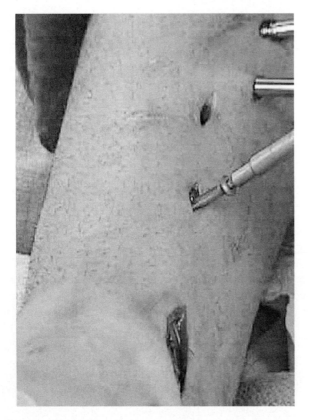

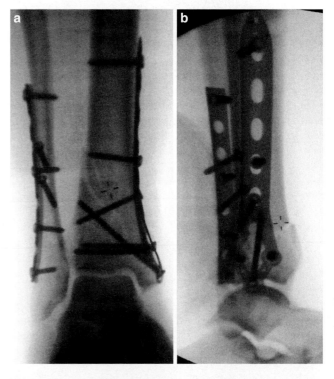

Fig. 63.8 (**a, b**) Intraoperative radiographs after definitive stabilization of a distal tibia fracture - note the three screws within the distal fragment, in addition to the cortical lag screw across the primary fracture line

Fig. 63.7 Stabilization of a proximal fragment - note the small stab incisions

Anterior/Anterolateral Plating of the Distal Tibia

Submuscular anterior or anterolateral plating is primarily used for proximal fixation in simple two-part intraarticular fractures, in which the articular fragments are reduced through an abbreviated open reduction, and with open fractures in which the traumatic laceration is extended and used for passage of the plate. In these instances, the incision or traumatic laceration itself affords visualization and mobilization

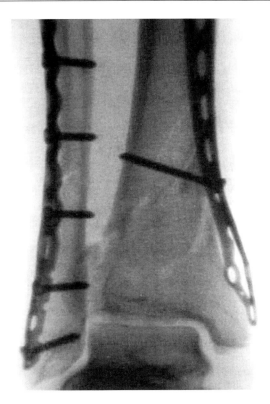

Fig. 63.9 Intraoperative radiograph demonstrating initial lag fixation (through the plate) across the primary fracture line

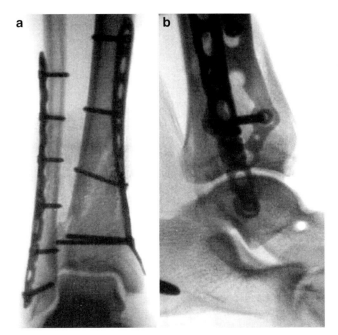

Fig. 63.10 (**a**, **b**) Intraoperative radiograph demonstrating "internal external fixator" construct

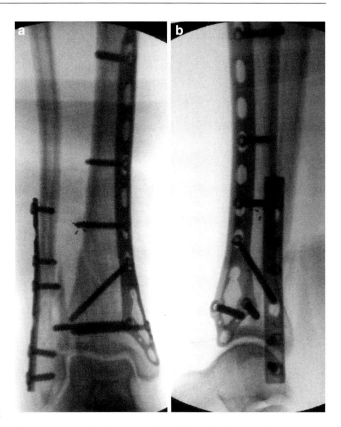

Fig. 63.11 (**a**, **b**) Intraoperative radiograph demonstrating alternate fixation pattern in an osteoporotic patient - note the longer plate and additional screws for supplemental stability

Anterior Approach

A 6-cm incision is made overlying the ankle joint in line with a point approximately one fingerbreadth lateral to the tibial crest. Deep dissection continues through the extensor retinaculum, utilizing the interval between the tibialis anterior and extensor hallucis longus tendons. Every effort is made to preserve the continuity of the tibialis anterior tendon sheath to minimize potential wound complications (Fig. 63.12). The underlying anterior tibial/dorsalis pedis artery and deep peroneal nerve, which typically course just lateral to the extensor hallucis longus tendon, are identified and protected throughout the procedure. A transverse arthrotomy is completed for full visualization of the intraarticular surface; further proximal dissection is completed in extraperiosteal fashion. The articular fragments are reduced anatomically under direct vision, provisionally stabilized with 1.6-mm Kirschner wires, and the reduction is verified fluoroscopically.

The provisionally selected anterior plate is then confirmed under fluoroscopy for adequacy of length, and passed in submuscular fashion, specifically avoiding the adjacent neurovascular bundle. A small stab incision is made at the proximal tip of the plate for manipulation where necessary until the plate is appropriately positioned. Cortical lag screws are

of the underlying neurovascular structures. The location of the intraarticular extension, as determined on computed tomographic (CT) evaluation, determines whether an anterior or anterolateral approach is used.

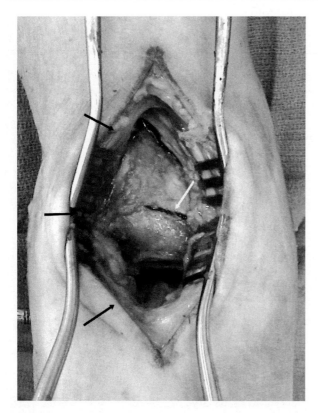

Fig. 63.12 Anterior approach - note the tibialis anterior maintained within the tendon sheath (*black arrows*) and the intraarticular fracture line (*white arrow*)

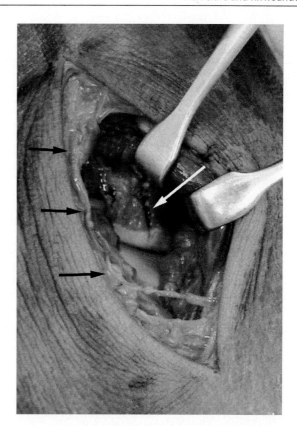

Fig. 63.13 Anterolateral approach - the peroneus tertius muscle is retracted medially. Note the superficial peroneal nerve (*black arrows*) and the intraarticular fracture line (*white arrow*)

placed through the plate distally for stabilization of a coronal plane fracture line; lag screws may alternatively be placed outside the plate for a sagittally oriented fracture line. Additional cortical screws are then placed - in general, three to four screws within the distal fragment should provide sufficient stability.

Stabilization of the proximal fragment is then completed through separate stab incisions over the respective screw holes. Because of the underlying tibialis anterior muscle, the stab incisions are made just lateral to the tibial crest to allow lateral retraction of the tibialis anterior muscle, and tend to be slightly longer than those used for medial plating.

Following stabilization and final fluoroscopic images, a deep drain is placed exiting proximally, and the extensor retinaculum is meticulously repaired. The remainder of the incision is closed in routine, layered fashion. We prefer interrupted 3–0 nylon suture for the skin layer, using the modified Allgöwer-Donati technique.

Anterolateral Approach

A 6-cm incision is made overlying the ankle joint just lateral to the extensor digitorum longus and peroneus tertius tendons.

The superficial peroneal nerve is identified and gently mobilized laterally, and deep dissection continues through the extensor retinaculum. The adjacent anterior tibial/dorsalis pedis artery and deep peroneal nerve, which typically course between the extensor hallucis longus and extensor digitorum longus tendons, are protected throughout the procedure. A transverse arthrotomy is completed for full visualization of the intraarticular surface; further proximal dissection is completed in extraperiosteal fashion (Fig. 63.13). A 4.5-mm Schanz pin may be temporarily placed in the lateral (nonarticular) talar neck for intraarticular distraction where necessary. The remainder of the procedure is completed as described for the anterior approach.

Locked Plates Versus Nonlocked Plates

The development of locked plating technology has been a major advance in the management of lower extremity fractures, and particularly in the distal tibia. The advantages of locked plating over conventional plating include increased overall construct stability, increased resistance to bending stresses, and decreased screw cutout and failure. Locked plates, however, are inherently more bulky, which may increase the risk of wound complications, as well as hardware prominence. Additionally, because of the increased stiffness of the plate, there is generally limited ability to compress comminuted metaphyseal fragments through the plate, even with initial nonlocking, cortical lag screws.

Although there are no specific guidelines as to absolute indications for locked plating, as a general rule, locked plating should be considered for fractures with significant metaphyseal comminution, whereby the locked implant bridges the comminuted segment to maintain axial length; fractures in patients with osteopenia, osteoporosis, or other significant medical comorbidities in which poor screw purchase would be otherwise anticipated.

Alternatively, a combination of locking and nonlocking screws may be utilized, creating a so-called hybrid construct. In this instance, the nonlocking screws are first placed, either in lag fashion to stabilize secondary fracture lines, or in neutral mode to reduce the plate to bone. Locking screws are used thereafter, preventing toggle and potential cutout at the bone-implant interface. In this manner, some degree of micromotion and bone elasticity is permitted, thereby allowing endosteal bony callous formation.

Postoperative Protocol

After routine wound closure, the involved limb is placed in a protective splint for 10–14 days to allow incisional healing. The patient is then converted to a venous compression stocking and fracture boot, and early progression of motion is initiated to facilitate functional limb recovery. Advancement of weightbearing is variable depending on the individual fracture pattern and overall stability of the fixation construct, and ranges from 8 to 12 weeks postoperatively.

Results and Complications

Krettek et al.[4] first described the use of percutaneous plating in the management of distal femur and proximal tibia fractures. Subsequent authors have reported percutaneous applications for fractures of the distal tibia, primarily medial plating, using a variety of implants.[5–13]

Helfet et al.[5] treated 20 complex distal tibia and pilon fractures with delayed percutaneous medial plating using precontoured ½ semitubular plates and screws, and reported no hardware failures or significant wound complications. All fractures healed and all patients in their series had good functional results.

Oh et al.[7] managed 21 extraarticular or minimal intraarticular distal tibia fractures with acute percutaneous medial plating with precontoured LC-DC plates and screws. There were no wound complications and all fractures healed without incident. Three patients had slight residual ankle stiffness, while all others regained full ankle range of motion. Similarly, Francois et al.[8] reported good results with indirect reduction and percutaneous medial plating in 10 distal tibia and plafond fractures. There were no wound complications and all fractures ultimately healed.

Khoury et al.[9] treated 24 distal tibia fractures with percutaneous medial plating using a variety of plates ranging from 3.5-mm and 4.5-mm reconstruction plates to 3.5-mm and 4.5-mm broad LC-DC plates. They too reported no deep infections and only one superficial infection, and all patients regained good ankle range of motion. All fractures healed at an average of 12 weeks postoperatively.

Collinge et al.[11] treated 17 high-energy distal tibia fractures, including 11 open injuries, with prebent 4.5-mm narrow LC-DC plates and large fragment screws. They reported three superficial wound infections, all related to external fixator pin sites, and one deep infection. All patients with closed injuries regained knee and ankle range of motion within 5° of motion of the contralateral limb, while ankle range of motion in those with open injuries averaged 10° of dorsiflexion and 20° of plantarflexion.

Percutaneous techniques are, however, technically demanding and thus strict attention to detail is necessary to prevent axial, rotational, and angular malalignment. Helfet et al.[5] had four fractures heal with significant malalignment - two with >5° of varus angulation, and two with >10° of recurvatum, although none required further surgery. Maffulli et al.[12] had seven angular malunions (7–10° of residual angular malalignment) out of 20 distal tibia fractures. Borg et al.[13] had two malunions requiring revision surgery, and Oh et al.[7] had one rotational malunion out of 21 distal tibia fractures. Khoury et al.[9] had four malunions - one with 8° of valgus angulation, one with 7° of varus angulation, and two with 4–5° of recurvatum - although none required further surgery. In both instances of coronal plane malalignment, there was significant metaphyseal comminution and a "soft" 3.5-mm reconstruction plate had been used, leading the authors to recommend use of "solid" LC-DC plates for those fractures with substantial metaphyseal comminution.

Because of the generally high-energy nature of these injuries, delayed union or nonunion may still develop despite these biologic techniques, particularly in those patients with open injuries or substantial bone loss. Collinge et al.[11] reported three delayed unions and three nonunions among their patients with open injuries, including four with significant bone loss. All six patients healed after revision surgery and bone grafting. Francois et al.[8] had two delayed unions in their series that required bone grafting and eventually healed. Borg et al.[13] had two delayed unions and two nonunions out of 21 closed distal tibia fractures.

Conclusions

Periarticular distal tibia fractures are complex, challenging fractures to effectively manage. Because of the inherently limited soft tissue envelope and vascularity in the distal tibial metaphysis, subcutaneous/submuscular plating is an attractive option for certain extraarticular and simple intraarticular fractures. These techniques allow restoration of axial, sagittal, and rotational alignment in a biologically friendly manner, thereby providing sufficient bony stability to facilitate early range of motion, uncomplicated fracture healing, and optimum return of function. Although larger, randomized series with longer-term follow-up are necessary, particularly with respect to locked implants, the current preliminary series suggest promising results with these techniques.

References

1. Borrelli J Jr, Prickett W, Song E, et al. Extraosseous blood supply of the tibia and the effects of different plating techniques: a human cadaveric study. J Orthop Trauma 2002; 16:691–95
2. Orthopaedic Trauma Association committee for coding and Classification: Fracture and dislocation compendium. J Orthop Trauma 1996; 10(Suppl 1):51–5
3. Sanders R. Intra-articular fractures of the calcaneus: present state of the art. J Orthop Trauma 1992; 6:252–65
4. Krettek C, Schandelmaier P, Tscherne H. Neue entwicklungen bei der stabilisierung dia- und metaphysarer frakturen der langen rohrenknocken. Orthopade 1997; 26:408–21
5. Helfet DL, Shonnard PY, Levine D, et al. Minimally invasive plate osteosynthesis of distal fractures of the tibia. Injury 1997; 28 (Suppl 1):SA-42–8
6. Helfet DL, Suk M. Minimally invasive percutaneous plate osteosynthesis of fractures of the distal tibia. Instr Course Lect 2004; 53:471–5
7. Oh CW, Kyung HS, Park IH, et al. Distal tibia metaphyseal fractures treated by percutaneous plate osteosynthesis. Clin Orthop Relat Res 2003; 408:286–91
8. Francois J, Vandeputte G, Verheyden F, et al. Percutaneous plate fixation of fractures of the distal tibia. Acta Orthop Belg 2004; 70:148–54
9. Khoury A, Liebergall M, London E, et al. Percutaneous plating of distal tibial fractures. Foot Ankle Int 2002; 23:818–24
10. Collinge CA, Sanders RW. Percutaneous plating in the lower extremity. J Am Acad Ortho Surg 2000; 8:211–6
11. Collinge C, Sanders R, Dipasquale T. Treatment of complex tibial periarticular fractures using percutaneous techniques. Clin Orthop Relat Res 2000; 375:69–77
12. Maffulli N, Toms AD, McMurtie A, et al. Percutaneous plating of distal tibial fractures. Int Orthop 2004; 28:159–62
13. Borg T, Larsson S, Lidsjo U. Percutaneous plating of distal tibial fractures: preliminary results in 21 patients. Injury 2004; 35:608–14

Chapter 64
Round Table Discussion of MIS of the Foot and Ankle

Mark Easley: I have invited several of the contributing authors to participate in a roundtable discussion of minimally invasive surgery (MIS) for the foot and ankle. I am pleased to share the thoughts and expertise of Juha Jaakkola, Brad Lamm, Nicola Maffulli, Martinus Richter, Robert Rozbruch, and Steve Shapiro. While all of our contributing authors provide valuable insights to MIS in their respective chapters, I anticipate that this roundtable discussion will provide the reader with an important overview of current concepts in MIS as they pertain to the management of foot and ankle disorders.

While several techniques for the management of foot and ankle pathology have traditionally been performed with limited incisions, for example fixation of fifth metatarsal fractures, the concept of minimally invasive surgery for the foot and ankle has only recently gained appreciable attention. In my opinion, the evolution of MIS for the foot and ankle lags behind that for the knee, hip, spine, shoulder, and trauma surgery. Nicola, what is your view of the apparent lag of MIS in foot and ankle surgery?

Nicola Maffulli: From the beginning, the foot and ankle has been the "Cinderella subspeciality," often drawing from the advances in other subspecialities for its development. Thus, in my mind, it is not surprising that MIS for the foot and ankle is only recently emerging. MIS techniques for the foot and ankle simply have not been devcloped for the majority of foot and ankle procedures. Moreover, similar to the timeline for advances in other subspecialities, most foot and ankle surgeons favor traditional and/or extensile exposures, leaving the development of less invasive techniques to a group of select pioneers.

Mark Easley: So, with that said, Steve, you have used several minimally invasive techniques for years with great success. While you are a dedicated academician, you are in private practice. In your mind, what are the major advantages to MIS for foot and ankle surgery?

Steve Shapiro: Besides the obvious advantage of improved cosmesis (not to be underestimated when patients recommend a surgeon to their friend), it has been my experience that MIS affords a more rapid recovery and often the advantage of more precise and focused surgery. I performed tradi-

tional approaches to the foot and ankle for years, but have not looked back since employing MIS techniques. By and large, less invasive access reliably permits a more rapid return to normal activities, without compromising functional outcome. For example, while plantar fascia release and Morton's neuroma excision are relatively minor foot and ankle procedures, traditional approaches may still lead to delayed wound healing and delayed weightbearing due to soft tissue dissection. When performed endoscopically, recovery is greatly accelerated. Furthermore, the endoscope provides a much greater detail of the pathology that, in my hands, leads to greater precision.

Mark Easley: Juha, you have adopted a minimally invasive approach to several foot and ankle procedures, some performed with the aid of arthroscopy. Where do you see advantages of arthroscopy in managing foot and ankle disorders traditionally treated with extensile exposures?

Juha Jaakkola: My experience is best explained with my approach to the surgical management of displaced, intraarticular calcaneus fractures. Traditionally I utilized an extensile exposure that affords full visualization of the lateral calcaneus and, with mobilization of the fragments, adequate visualization to achieve an anatomic reduction, albeit with considerable reliance on intraoperative fluoroscopy. Despite the extensile approach, I was rarely ever able to visualize the entire posterior calcaneal articular facet. Using the arthroscopically assisted technique, I am able, in most cases, to better visualize the articular reduction of the posterior facet than with the traditional extensile approach. In my opinion, like for acetabular fractures or other intraarticular fractures, outcome of calcaneal fractures is probably heavily dependent on a congruent articular reduction.

Mark Easley: Any downsides?

Juha Jaakkola: Well, not necessarily a downside, but timing becomes more of an issue for arthroscopically assisted management of displaced calcaneal fractures. Since the approach is limited, comprehensive mobilization of fracture fragments is not possible with the MIS technique as it is with the extensile approach. Therefore, I must perform the arthroscopically assisted technique within the first 3–4 days, much like those surgeons who use external fixation in the management of

G.R. Scuderi and A.J. Tria (eds.), *Minimally Invasive Surgery in Orthopedics*,
DOI 10.1007/978-0-387-76608-9_64, © Springer Science + Business Media, LLC 2010

displaced calcaneus fractures. Otherwise, the fracture fragments begin to bind and reduction without an extensile approach is not feasible.

Mark Easley: Should we categorize arthroscopically and endoscopically assisted surgeries as MIS?

Steve Shapiro: Absolutely! Physiologically, there is not a lot of soft tissue coverage about the foot and ankle, so often traditional approaches are not very extensive. To make the incisions even smaller, like MIS for TKA or THA, may not be plausible. Endoscopically and arthroscopically assisted techniques comprise a considerable number of procedures that define MIS of the foot and ankle.

Mark Easley: Rob, Juha mentioned external fixation. You are establishing yourself as a leader in the field of external fixation for the management of complex deformity of the foot and ankle. How does external fixation factor into MIS for foot and ankle disorders?

Robert Rozbruch: Mark, thank you for your confidence in my abilities! I am very fortunate that my institution provides me with the resources to utilize external fixation to treat foot and ankle pathology. It has been a particularly rewarding experience for me. Initially I practiced orthopedics with traditional techniques but acquired further training with several masters of external fixation. Since I have been able to apply the principles they taught me to foot and ankle deformity, I now favor external fixation over internal fixation when the indications permit. Here are some of my observations:

The use of external fixation helps promote MIS of the foot and ankle in two ways. First, the bony fixation is established through stab wounds avoiding soft tissue dissection needed for plate fixation. Second, correction of deformity is accomplished with a percutaneous osteotomy and the use of acute and/or gradual correction. This avoids the need for large exposures needed for closing wedge osteotomies and plate fixation.

Mark Easley: Any appreciable advantages in postoperative management?

Robert Rozbruch: No question. The external fixation techniques are very practical. In my hands, less exposure is less traumatic to the soft tissues and results in less postoperative pain and quicker bony healing compared with traditional extensile exposures. The use of circular external fixation is especially helpful at gaining stable fixation of the foot needed for complex ankle fusion. Moreover, the frames generally afford adequate stability to allow the patient to fully weight-bear on the operated extremity postoperatively.

Mark Easley: Brad, you also tend to favor external fixation in the management of complex foot and ankle deformity. In your practice, have principles of external fixation afforded a more minimally invasive approach compared with conventional open techniques?

Brad Lamm: Rob and I have had many occasions to share ideas, and I agree with Rob's observations. Prior to the use of external fixation in the foot and ankle, large deformities were generally corrected acutely, necessitating extensile exposures that often increased the risk for complications. With external fixation, I can now correct large deformities gradually without the need for extensile surgical exposures. As Rob mentioned, I view techniques of external fixation as minimally invasive procedures (despite the large frame construct), since the fixation (pins/wires) are placed percutaneously. When external fixation is combined with the MIS techniques of joint arthrodesis, osteotomy, and/or soft tissue releases, in my opinion, surgical outcome can be optimized and the complication rate remains low.

With respect to trauma, the combination of external fixation and MIS techniques limit soft tissue/periosteal stripping, potentially improving healing rates over conventional techniques of open reduction and internal fixation. While I recognize that percutaneous plating techniques may achieve the same goal of preserving blood supply to the fractures, external fixation confers one very important advantage! Minimally invasive plate osteosynthesis requires an anatomic reduction at the time of surgery. In contrast, while I attempt the same with external fixation, I have the luxury of making subtle adjustments postoperatively to optimize reduction and alignment, adjustments not possible with internal fixation.

Mark Easley: Some MIS techniques appear driven by technology. We are very fortunate to have a contribution by Martinus Richter, a pioneer in computer-assisted surgery (CAS) for the foot and ankle. Martinus, in your experience, what advantages does navigation provide in the evolution of MIS for the management of foot and ankle disorders?

Martinus Richter: Navigation, or more appropriately, CAS is helpful in complex three-dimensional corrections or reduction, and in closed placement of drills and/or screw positioning. I am convinced by my own experience in managing complex hindfoot and midfoot deformities that the improved accuracy afforded by CAS may lead to improved clinical outcomes compared with those reported using conventional techniques. Whereas CAS is too complex and time consuming for cases that are accurately and easily performed by the experienced surgeon, CAS provides superior guidance for procedures with limited visualization. Naturally, this advantage afforded by CAS is especially useful in MIS.

Mark Easley: Currently, the applications of CAS for the foot and ankle are few. Martinus, what developments do you anticipate for CAS in the foot and ankle, particularly with respect to MIS?

Martinus Richter: For the future, the integration of the different computerized systems will improve the handling and clinical feasibility of CAS technology. An integration of preoperative pedography, planning software, CAS, intraoperative three-dimensional imaging (ISO-C-3D™, ARCADIS™) and Intraoperative Pedography (IP) in one Integrated Computer System for Operative Procedures (ICOP) will be possible. Within this kind of ICOP, the preoperative computerized planning will be able to include preoperative radiographic, CT, MRI, and pedography data. The preoperative computerized planning result will be transferred to the CAS device. Intraoperative two-dimensional (C-arm) or three-dimensional (ISO-C-3D) imaging will allow registration-free CAS and will be matched with preoperative CT and or MRI scans. The CAS system will be guided by biomechanical assessment with IP that allows not only morphological but also biomechanical based CAS. The intraoperative three-dimensional imaging (ISO-C-3D) data and the IP-data will be matched with the data from the planning software to allow immediate improvements of reduction, correction, and or drilling/implant position in the same procedure.

While this seems terribly complex, I envision that this integration will ultimately be manageable for most foot and ankle surgeons, just like most drivers can now make use of the navigation systems in their cars. Two decades ago, many people doubted that we would have practical applications for navigation systems in our vehicles. Today most manufactures offer navigation options. While navigation is rarely used for short and easy routes, they are used effectively for long and difficult journeys. Similarly, computerized methods of improved intraoperative imaging, guidance, and biomechanical assessment will help to realize the planned operative result. We will have these systems (ISO-C-3D, CAS, IP) available in a few years, but they will not be used in the easy standard case but for difficult and complex procedures. I anticipate that even the most complex procedures may be performed with very precise, focused interventions requiring very limited exposures and soft tissue dissection. In other words, with this technology, MIS will be a reality in the management of complex foot and ankle disorders.

Mark Easley: Finally, what about CAS and MIS in managing foot and ankle trauma?

Martinus Richter: The problem with MIS in foot and ankle trauma is limited visualization. In my hands, the use of computer-based visualization, i.e., intraoperative three-dimensional imaging (ISO-C-3D™, ARCADIS™) is advantageous compared with conventional two-dimensional imaging. ISO-C-3D is most helpful in closed procedures and in providing information that is cannot be obtained with direct visualization or using a C-arm. With this technology, MIS can be effectively utilized without an increased risk of malreduction or inappropriate implant placement.

Mark Easley: Nicola, you have adopted and even developed several MIS techniques for the treatment of foot and ankle problems. I have no doubt that you are a believer in the techniques. However, would you please conclude our roundtable discussion with your views of the shortcomings of MIS in the foot and ankle.

Nicola Maffulli: Mark, I will continue to use MIS techniques for the foot and ankle and I will continue to channel some of my energies to improving and developing MIS for the foot and ankle. As I see it, there has been little or no scientific research in MIS for the foot and ankle. It is well and good to devise what appears to be a great technique, and to operate on many patients, who may be grateful to the surgeon, and surprised to find that they can return to work and normal activities in little time. However, very little has been published in peer-reviewed journals on the outcome of these procedures, and, to my knowledge, no research has compared traditional with less invasive procedures. We should channel our efforts to make sure that we do not lose sight of the fact that we wish that our patients are served well in the long term, not just that we are very clever with our saws, drills, and scalpels. I suspect that the only way in which these new techniques will become part of our armamentarium is to prove that they are indeed comparable with the traditional ones. Indications and patient selection for MIS techniques still need to be defined. Newer is not always better, and, for the time being, a technical advance is not necessarily a clinically relevant one. I look forward to prospective, randomized investigations comparing traditional and MIS techniques in the management of foot and ankle pathology necessitating surgical intervention.

Mark Easley: I thank all of you for participating in this roundtable discussion and for contributing to this section on MIS of the foot and ankle.

Section V
The Spine

Chapter 65
Minimally Invasive Spinal Surgery: Evidence-Based Review of the Literature

Max C. Lee, Kyle Fox, and Richard G. Fessler

The advances in minimally invasive spinal surgery (MISS) are unparalleled. These advances have occurred throughout the spinal axis from the occiput to the pelvis. With the progress in optics, instrumentation, and familiarity with MISS procedures, MISS can now be seen in all aspects of spine surgery.

Although MISS began as a way to assist decompressions within the lumbar spine, MISS has transitioned to address complex decompressions, tumor resections, fusions, and deformity. Decompressions include lumbar, thoracic, and cervical discs. Recurrent herniated discs, synovial cysts, and intradural and extradural tumors are within the scope of MISS. With percutaneous screws and expandable working channels, fixation is accomplished in multiple levels within the spinal axis. With thoracoscopic and transpsoas techniques, deformity can be approached within the coronal and axial plane. With bilateral extracavitary approaches, Smith-Peterson osteotomies and pedicle screw subtraction, osteotomies for deformity within the sagittal plane can also be accomplished.

Lumbar

We sought to evaluate the published literature demonstrating the advantages and complications from minimally invasive spine surgery. With respect to lumbar disc disease, MISS began with chemonucleolysis, introduced by Lyman Smith in 1964.[1] Then, percutaneous manual nucleotomy was introduced by Hijikata in 1975.[2] The first microdiscectomy was accomplished by Kravenbuhl and Yasargil in 1968.[3] This was followed with automated percutaneous lumbar discectomy and laser discectomy.[4,5] Endoscopic discectomy was first used by Schreiber and Suezawa in 1986 and improved by Mayer, Brock, and Mathews.[6–8] Then, microendoscopic discectomy (MED) was introduced by Smith, Foley, and Fessler.[9,10]

Although MISS has been associated with shorter lengths of hospitalization, decreased postoperative pain with less post-operative narcotic consumption and an earlier return to work, documentation of this has been limited. In the evaluation of video-assisted arthroscopic microdiscectomy, Hermantin et al. randomized 60 patients to either open or MISS discectomy, demonstrating equivalence in complication rates and improved outcomes with this approach within the lumbar spine.[11] In a series of 70 patients after a MED, patients demonstrated earlier ambulation, reduced blood loss, and decreased post-operative narcotic use.[12] Palmer describes 135 patients after minimally invasive lumbar discectomies. Patient satisfaction was demonstrated in 94% of these patients. Furthermore, 36% of the patients monitored returned to work within 2 weeks.[13] Similar findings were also appreciated in 17 patients undergoing MIS decompressions for far lateral discectomies[14] and in the microendoscopic approach to decompressions for lumbar stenosis via a bilateral and unilateral approach.[15,16]

Evaluating 15 patients who underwent a traditional discectomy in comparison with MED, intraoperative electromyography (EMG) activity demonstrated significantly less irritation of the nerve root and less mechanically elicited activity with both the approach and nerve root mobilization. Therefore, the smaller incision causes less tissue trauma while providing adequate exposure for visualization of the neural structures.[17] In the evaluation of 22 patients during MED or open discectomy, MED results demonstrated decreased C reactive protein (CRP) and IL-6. This decreased cytokine excretion corresponded with decreased postoperative pain with smaller incisions.[18]

This was subsequently followed with a series of outcome studies. We evaluated 150 patients who underwent the MIS procedure for treatment of a lumbar herniated disc. Based on the MacNab criteria, 77% had excellent outcomes, 17% had good outcomes, 3% had fair outcomes, and 3% had poor outcomes. The average hospitalization was 7.7 h. The average return to work was 17 days. Complications primarily included dural tears and occurred in 5% of the patients but were more frequent initially and decreased with more experience.[10] Further evaluation included a prospective study utilizing 57 patients from two centers with an average age of 81 years and with lumbar degenerative disease. The results included no major complications or deaths. Visual Analog Scale (VAS) pain scores improved from 5.7 to 2.2 for low back pain and from 5.7 to 2.3 for leg pain. Oswestry disability

M.C. Lee, K. Fox, and R.G. Fessler (✉)
Department of Neurosurgery, Feinberg School of Medicine,
Northwestern University, Chicago, IL, USA
e-mail: RFessler@nmff.org

G.R. Scuderi and A.J. Tria (eds.), *Minimally Invasive Surgery in Orthopedics*,
DOI 10.1007/978-0-387-76608-9_65, © Springer Science+Business Media, LLC 2010

index scores decreased from 48 to 27 and SF-36 Body Pain and Physical Function scores demonstrated statistical improvements with surgical intervention.[19]

In addition to MISS for herniated discs and stenosis, MISS can be utilized for recurrent herniated discs, synovial cysts, extradural tumors, and intradural tumors of the spine. We compared the MED approach with traditional open surgery in the evaluation of recurrent disc herniations and demonstrated no statistical discrepancy.[20] Recurrent disc herniation was evaluated with a retrospective study of 43 patients. The average follow-up was 31 months and, based on MacNab criteria, 81.4% had excellent or good outcomes. The average pain analog scale score was decreased from 8.72 ± 1.20 to 2.58 ± 1.55. The results were much better in patients younger than 40 years old, symptoms less than 3 months, and patients without concurrent lateral recess stenosis.[21] Seventeen patients underwent synovial cyst resection with the 18-mm METRx tubular retraction system. The average age was 64 years and the MacNab criteria was used to assess the outcomes. The average operating time was 97 min with an average blood loss of 35 mL. A result of excellent or good occurred with 94% of the patients. A dural tear complication occurred with one patient but did not violate the arachnoid membrane and required no further treatment. Lumbar spondylolisthesis occurred in 47% of the cases so the advantage of this approach prevents disruption of the ligamentous and bony structures in order to avoid destabilization of the lumbar spine with the typical benefits of MISS, including better cosmesis, less tissue trauma, and less blood loss.[22] Similar findings were demonstrated in another retrospective study following 19 patients for MISS resection of synovial cyst.[23] Six patients with an average age of 47 years underwent a unilateral approach for intradural tumor resection. There was one tumor in the cervical spine, one in the thoracic spine, and four in the lumbar spine. Each patient had successful resection. The average operative time was 247 min, with a blood loss average of 56 mL. Average hospitalization was 57 h. Five of the tumors were schwannomas and one was a myxopapillary ependymoma. In all cases, no complications occurred and postoperative magnetic resonance imaging (MRI) scan demonstrated complete resection. The conclusion was that intradural, extramedullary tumors can be safely and effectively resected with less blood loss, shorter hospitalization, and less tissue trauma compared with the open procedure if one is skilled in the MISS technique.[24]

Further advances in MISS have been demonstrated in lumbar fusions. Advances have occurred in laparoscopic anterior lumbar interbody fusion (ALIF), transforaminal lumbar interbody fusion (TLIF) with instrumentation, transsacral approaches to L5-S1, and extreme lateral approaches for ALIF. A prospective, multicenter study involved a total of 240 patients from eight centers who underwent a minimally invasive laparoscopic ALIF. The results were compared with 591 patients who underwent the standard open ALIF procedure. While there was a 10% conversion rate to an open procedure, the laparoscopic approach group demonstrated shorter hospitalization and less blood loss with no statistical difference in complication rate. The laparoscopic group also demonstrated a shorter hospitalization and reduced blood loss but longer operative time.[25] In another prospective study, 22 patients underwent a laparoscopic ALIF using recombinant human bone morphogenic protein (rhBMP)-2 rather than autogenous bone. Based on Oswestry, pain analog, and functional testing scales at 1 year postoperatively, there was 100% satisfaction with no pseudoarthrosis or complications.[26] In a comparison of this laparoscopic approach versus a transperitoneal endoscopic video-assisted procedure, minilaparotomy retroperitoneal approach or traditional retroperitoneal appr-oach for 135 patients whom underwent an ALIF, one study demonstrated the highest incidence of complications in video-assisted laparoscopic approaches - including damage to vascular structures, the sympathetic plexus, or abdominal viscera.[27]

Based on success with cadaveric studies demonstrating feasibility of percutaneous lumbar fusion via a modified micro-endoscopic microdiscectomy, the microendoscopic TLIF was performed unilaterally on 20 patients with a one-level spondylolisthesis or mechanical low back pain. Two interbody grafts were placed in each case. Bilateral percutaneous pedicle screws were placed. The results were compared with patients who underwent an open posterior lumbar interbody fusion at the same institution. The average hospitalization was 3.4 days with the MISS approach versus 5.1 days with the open approach. There were no complications with the MIS approach. Compared with the open approach, the MIS method produced less intraoperative blood loss, postoperative pain, total narcotic use, and risk of transfusion.[28] Similar findings occurred comparing 21 patients after MISS lumbar fusion with 29 patients after traditional lumbar fusion. Park and Ha demonstrated less blood loss, less postoperative pain, and shorter hospitalizations.[29] After 49 patients underwent MISS TLIF, complications included two cases of screw malposition requiring surgical revision, one graft dislodgment, and one contralateral foraminal stenosis.[30] Furthermore, 43 patients who underwent a single-level percutaneous TLIF and 10 patients who underwent a multilevel fusion were compared with 67 patients who underwent a mini-open approach using a muscle-splitting approach. Excellent and good outcomes were obtained in 87% of the 53 patients at 16 months.[31]

Another type of approach is the transsacral, percutaneous approach for fixation and fusion of the L5-S1 disc. A tunnel is created into the L5-S1 disc from this approach, permitting disc removal, bone grafting, and placement of two 9-mm-diameter titanium screws into the body of L5. There were no complications referable to screw placement, and eight of nine patients had successful fusion.[32]

Moreover, 21 patients underwent a lumbar fusion via a transpsoas approach at two different centers. Seventeen patients underwent a single-level fusion, one patient a two-level fusion, and three patients a three-level fusion via the transpsoas approach supplemented with bilateral percutaneous pedicle screws. The preoperative VAS pain score was 8.3 and was reduced by an average of 5.9 points in the 15 patients who were followed for more than 6 months and an average follow-up of 3.1 years. Postoperative paresthesias involving the thigh and groin region occurred in 30%, and 27% experienced pain in this region. However, only 10% of the patients had these symptoms for longer than 1 month.[33]

Cervical

These minimally invasive techniques have been utilized within the cervical spine. With sequential dilation of the paraspinous neck musculature, cervical decompressions may be accomplished via a tubular retractor. Four human cadavers were utilized with minimally invasive cervical foraminotomies performed on three noncontiguous levels using the microendoscopic technique versus the open technique performed on the adjacent, contralateral levels. The MED technique provided greater average vertical diameter decompression and greater percentage of facet resection.[34] Then, 25 patients with cervical root compression from foraminal stenosis or a disc herniation underwent the minimally invasive approach and were compared with 26 patients who underwent the traditional open approach. The results included the MIS approach producing less blood loss, at 138 mL versus 246 mL per level. Hospitalization was significantly decreased, at 20 h versus 68 h. Fewer narcotics were used postoperatively, at 11 equivalents versus 40 equivalents. The MISS approach had initial symptomatic improvement of 87–92% of the patients. Furthermore, patients with a primary symptom of radiculopathy and an average follow-up of 16 months and minimum follow-up of 1 year had complete resolution of their radiculopathy in 54%, improvement in 38%, and no change in 8% of cases. In comparison, the open approach had resolution in 48%, improvement in 40%, and remained unchanged in 12%. For those with the primary symptom of neck pain, 40% completely resolved, 47% improved, and 13% were unchanged. Open results were 33% complete resolution, 56% improvement, and 11% no change. With that being said, the MISS approach produced effective results comparable to both the open group and those published in literature, while demonstrating a shorter hospitalization, less blood loss, and less postoperative pain medication utilization.[35] In a retrospective study of 100 patients who underwent a cervical decompression via microendoscopic approach, 97% demonstrated good or excellent results with no serious complications.[36]

Endoscopic partial laminectomy was performed in ten patients with degenerative compressive cervical myelopathy. All of the ten patients experienced symptomatic improvement with only minimal postoperative incisional pain. The average operating time was 164 min, with an average of 45.5 mL of blood loss.[37]

These minimally invasive techniques within the cervical spine have been expanded to cervical laminoplasty and lateral mass fusions. In cadaveric specimens, the midsagittal spinal canal was increased in size by a mean of 38% and increased by 43% at the level of C5.[38] Eighteen patients were retrospectively evaluated for lateral mass fixation. All but two patients had successful screw placement. Two cases had to be converted to the standard, open procedure due to inadequate radiographic visualization of the inferior cervical spine levels. Unilateral instrumentation was performed in six cases and bilateral instrumentation in ten cases, for a total of 39 levels instrumented. No complications occurred and postoperative computed tomographic (CT) scans showed that there were no bony violations except a few cases of bicortical purchase. Complete fusion occurred without evidence of pseudoarthrosis.[39]

Thoracic

The MIS approach is suggested as a treatment for lateral disc herniations in order to avoid a thoracoscopic approach that requires entry into the ventral chest. Nine cadaveric discectomies were performed in the mid and lower thoracic regions at the T5–6 and T9–10 levels. The average operating time was 60 min. An average of 3.4 mm of the ipsilateral facet was removed, which is an average of approximately 35% of the facet complex, and canal decompression was 73.5%. This approach does give access to the majority of the canal with only a minimal amount of bony removal.[40] Seven patients with a total of nine herniated discs were surgically treated. The herniations were either soft lateral or midline herniations. Results were based on the modified Prolo scale, which showed five patients with excellent results, one with a good result, and one with a fair result. None of the cases were converted to an open approach. The average operative time was 1.7 h per level, with an average blood loss of 111 mL per level.[41]

A thoracoscopic approach can access the anterior and anterolateral aspects of the vertebrae and spinal canal. Han et al. describe 241 thoracoscopic procedures that were performed: 164 thoracic sympathectomies, 60 discectomies, 5 neurogenic tumor resections, 8 corpectomies and spinal reconstructions, 2 anterior releases, and 2 biopsies. In this study, they were able to demonstrate the efficacy of thoracoscopic spinal surgery with less morbidity than open procedures and with improved postoperative pain.[42] Then, 55 patients underwent thoracoscopy for the resection of herniated thoracic discs. Thirty-six patients presented with myelopathies and 19 with incapacitating thoracic radicular pain. These patients were compared with 15 patients who underwent a costotransversectomy. Clinical and neurological outcomes were excellent, with a mean follow-up period of 15 months.[43]

Beisse et al. describe 30 patients with thoracolumbar canal compromise who underwent endoscopic anterior spinal canal decompression, interbody reconstruction, and stabilization for fractures totaling 27 cases, and one case each for tumor, infection, and severe degenerative disc disease. Spinal canal clearance quantified on preoperative and postoperative CT scans improved from 55% to 110%. A total of 25% of patients with complete paraplegia and 65% of those with incomplete neurological deficit improved neurologically. The complication rate was 16.7% and included one reintubation, two pleural effusions, one intercostal neuralgia, and one persistent lesion of the sympathetic chain.[44] Beisse reported his data between May 1996 and May 2001 in which 371 patients with fractures of the thoracic and thoracolumbar spine (T3-L3) were treated with a thoracoscopically assisted procedure. In the first 197 patients, a conventional open anterior plating system was used. The last 174 patients were treated with the MACS-TL system (Aesculap, Tuttlingen, Germany), which was designed specifically for endoscopic placement, thereby significantly reducing operative times. Seventy-three percent of the fractures were located at the thoracolumbar junction. In 35% of patients, a stand-alone anterior thoracoscopic reconstruction was performed. In 65% of patients, a supplemental posterior pedicle-screw construct was also placed either before or after the anterior construct. The severe complication rate was low, at 1.3%, with one case each of aortic injury, splenic contusion, neurological deterioration, cerebrospinal fluid leak, and severe wound infection. Compared with a group of 30 patients treated with open thoracotomy, thoracoscopically treated patients required 42% less narcotics for pain treatment after the operation.[45]

Thoracoscopic release for scoliotic deformity has also been well described.[46] Correction of thoracic scoliosis has been described. Fifty patients with primary thoracic scoliosis were corrected with 24–45 months of follow-up data retrospectively studied. Curve correction averaged 50.2%, improving to 68.6% in the last ten cases. The hospital stays averaged 2.9 days. Picetti et al. describe their initial complications, which diminished with further experience.[47]

Conclusion

Minimally invasive spine surgery continues to evolve since its inception nearly half a century ago. MISS has proven to

be both a safe and effective alternative to the traditional approaches, allowing patients to recover faster and with less postoperative pain. Thus, the demand by the patient population for less invasive spine surgery will continue to grow.

References

1. Smith L. Chemonucleolysis. *Clin Orthop Relat Res* 1969 Nov-Dec, 67:72–80
2. Hijikata S. Percutaneous nucleotomy. A new concept technique and 12 years' experience. *Clin Orthop Relat Res* 1989 Jan, 238:9–23
3. Kravenbuhl H, Yasargil MG. Use of the microscope in surgery of the central nervous system. *Praxis* 1968, 57(7):214–7
4. Onik G, Helms CA, Ginsberg L, Hoaglund FT, Morris J. Percutaneous lumbar diskectomy using a new aspiration probe: porcine and cadaver model. *Radiology* 1985, 155(1):251–2
5. Choy DS, Ascher PW, Ranu HS, Saddekni S, Alkaitis D, Liebler W, Hughes J, Diwan S, Altman P. Percutaneous laser nucleolysis of lumbar disks. *N Engl J Med* 1987, 317(12):771–2
6. Schreiber A, Suezawa Y. Transdiscoscopic percutaneous nucleotomy in disk herniation. *Orthop Rev* 1986, 15(1):35–8
7. Mayer HM, Brock M, Berlien HP, Weber B. Percutaneous endoscopic laser discectomy (PELD). A new surgical technique for non-sequestrated lumbar discs. *Acta Neurochir Suppl (Wien)* 1992, 54:53–8
8. Mathews HH. Transforaminal endoscopic microdiscectomy. *Neurosurg Clin N Am* 1996, 7(1):59–63
9. Foley KT, Smith MM, Rambersaud YR. Microendoscopic approach to far lateral lumbar disc herniations. *Neurosurg Focus* 1999, 7(5):e5
10. Perez-Cruet MJ, Foley KT, Isaacs RE, Rice-Wyllie L, Wellington R, Smith MM, Fessler RG. Microendoscopic lumbar discectomy: technical note. *Neurosurgery* 2002, 51(5Suppl):S129–36
11. Hermantin FU, Peters T, Quartararo L, Kambin P. A prospective, randomized study comparing the results of open discectomy with those of video-assisted arthroscopic microdiscectomy. *J Bone Joint Surg* 1999, 81(7):958–65
12. Muramatsu K, Hachiya Y, Morita C. Postoperative magnetic resonance imaging of lumbar disc herniation: comparison of microendoscopic discectomy and Love's method. *Spine* 2001, 26:1599–605
13. Palmer S. Use of a tubular retractor system in microscopic lumbar discectomy: 1 year prospective results in 135 patients. *Neurosurg Focus* 2002, 13(2):E5
14. Cervellini P, De Luca GP, Mazzetto M, Colombo F. Microendoscopic discectomy (MED) for far lateral disc herniation in the lumbar spine. Technical note. *Acta Neurochir Suppl* 2005, 92:99–101
15. Guiot BH, Khoo LT, Fessler RG. A minimally invasive technique for decompression of the lumbar spine. *Spine* 2002, 27:432–8
16. Palmer S, Turner R, Palmer R. Bilateral decompression of lumbar spinal stenosis involving a unilateral approach with microscope and tubular retractor system. *J Neurosurg* 2002, 97(2 Suppl):213–7
17. Schick U, Dohnert J, Richter A, Konig A, Vitzthum H. Microendoscopic lumbar discectomy versus open surgery: an intraoperative EMG study. *Eur Spine J* 2002, 11(1):20–6
18. Huang TJ, Hsu RW, Li YY, Cheng CC. Less systemic cytokine response in patients following microendoscopic versus open lumbar discectomy. *J Orthop Res* 2005, 23(2):406–11
19. Rosen DS, O'Toole JE, Eichholz KM, Hrubes M, Huo D, Sandhu FA, Fessler RG. Minimally invasive lumbar spinal decompression in the elderly: outcomes of 50 patients aged 75 years and older. *Neurosurgery* 2007, 60(3):503–9; discussion 509–10
20. Isaacs RE, Podichetty V, Fessler RG. Microendoscopic discectomy for recurrent disc herniations. *Neurosurg Focus* 2003, 15(3):E11

21. Ahn Y, Lee SH, Park WM, Lee HY, Shin SW, Kang HY. Percutaneous endoscopic lumbar discectomy for recurrent disc herniation: surgical technique, outcome, and prognostic factors of 43 consecutive cases. *Spine* 2004, 29(16):E326–32

22. Sandhu FA, Santiago P, Fessler RG, Palmer S. Minimally invasive surgical treatment of lumbar synovial cysts. *Neurosurgery* 2004, 54(1):107–11; discussion 111–2

23. Sehati N, Khoo LT, Holly LT. Treatment of lumbar synovial cysts using minimally invasive surgical techniques. *Neurosurg Focus* 2006, 20(3):E2

24. Tredway TL, Santiago P, Hrubes MR, Song JK, Christie SD, Fessler RG. Minimally invasive resection of intradural-extramedullary spinal neoplasms. *Neurosurgery* 2006, 58(1 Suppl):ONS52–8; discussion ONS52–8

25. Regan JJ, Yuan H, McAfee PC. Laparoscopic fusion of the lumbar spine: minimally invasive spine surgery. A prospective multicenter study evaluating open and laparoscopic lumbar fusion. *Spine* 1999, 24(4):402–11

26. Kleeman TJ, Ahn UM, Talbot-Kleeman A. Laparoscopic anterior lumbar interbody fusion with rhBMP-2: a prospective study of clinical and radiographic outcomes. *Spine* 2001, 26(24):2751–6

27. Escobar E, Transfeldt E, Garvey T, et al. Video assisted versus open anterior lumbar spine fusion surgery: a comparison of four techniques and complications in 135 patients *Spine* 2003, 28; 729–32

28. Isaacs RE, Podichetty VK, Santiago P, Sandhu FA, Spears J, Kelly K, Rice L, Fessler RG. Minimally invasive microendoscopy-assisted transforaminal lumbar interbody fusion with instrumentation. *J Neurosurg Spine* 2005, 3(2):98–105

29. Park Y, Ha JW. Comparison of one level posterior lumbar interbody fusion performed with a minimally invasive approach or a traditional open approach. *Spine* 2007, 32(5):537–43

30. Schwender JD, Holly LT, Rouben DP, Foley KT. Minimally invasive transforminal lumbar interbody fusion: technical feasibility and initial results. *J Spinal Disord Tech* 2005, 18:Suppl: S1–6

31. Scheufler KM, Dohmen H, Vougioukas VI. Percutaneous transforminal lumbar interbody fusion for the treatment of degenerative lumbar instability. *Neurosurgery* 2007, 60(4) :(Operative Neurosurgery Supplement 2):203–13

32. MacMillan M, Fessler RG, Gillespy M, Montgomery WJ. Percutaneous lumbosacral fixation and fusion: anatomic study and two-year experience with a new method. *Neurosurg Clin of N Am* 1996, 7(1):99–106

33. Bergey DL, Villavicencio AT, Goldstein T, Regan JJ. Endoscopic lateral transpsoas approach to the lumbar spine. *Spine* 2004, 29(15):1681–8

34. Roh SW, Kim DH, Cardoso AC, Fessler RG. Endoscopic foraminotomy using MED system in cadaveric specimens. *Spine* 2000, 25(2):260–4

35. Fessler RG, Khoo LT. Minimally invasive cervical microendoscopic foraminotomy: an initial clinical experience. *Neurosurgery* 2002, 51(5 Suppl 2):S37–S45

36. Adamson TE. Microendoscopic posterior cervical laminoforaminotomy for unilateral radiculopathy: results of a new technique in 100 cases. *J Neurosurg* 2001, 95(1 Suppl):51–7

37. Yabuki S, Kikuchi S. Endoscopic partial laminectomy for cervical myelopathy. *J Neurosurg Spine* 2005, 2(2):170–4

38. Wang MY, Green BA, Coscarella E, et al. Minimally invasive cervical expansile laminoplasty: an initial cadaveric study. *Neurosurgery* 2003, 52:370–73

39. Wang MY, Levi A. Minimally invasive lateral mass screw fixation in the cervical spine: initial clinical experience with long-term follow-up. *Neurosurgery* 2006, 58(5):907–12

40. Isaacs RE, Podichetty VK, Sandhu FA, Santiago P, Spears JD, Aaronson O, Kelly K, Hrubes M, Fessler RG. Thoracic microendoscopic discectomy: a human cadaver study. *Spine* 2005, 30(10):1226–31

41. Perez-Cruet MJ, Kim BS, Sandhu F, Samartzis D, Fessler RG. Thoracic microendoscopic discectomy. *J Neurosurg Spine* 2004, 1(1):58–63

42. Han PP, Kenny K, Dickman CA. Thoracoscopic approaches to the thoracic spine: experience with 241 surgical procedures. *Neurosurgery* 2002, 51(5 Suppl):S88–95

43. Rosenthal D, Dickman CA. Thoracoscopic microsurgical excision of herniated thoracic discs. *J Neurosurg* 1998, 89(2):224–35

44. Beisse R, Muckley T, Schmidt MH, Hauschild M, Buhren V. Surgical technique and results of endoscopic anterior spinal canal decompression. *J Neurosurg Spine* 2005, 2(2):128–36

45. Khoo LT, Beisse R, Potulski M. Thoracoscopic-assisted treatment of thoracic and lumbar fractures: a series of 371 consecutive cases. *Neurosurgery* 2002, 51(5 Suppl):S104–17

46. Nymberg SM, Crawford AH. Video-assisted thoracoscopic releases of scoliotic anterior spines. *AORN J* 1996, 63(3):561–2, 565–9; 571–5

47. Picetti GD III, Pang D, Bueff HU. Thoracoscopic techniques for the treatment of scoliosis: early results in procedure development. *Neurosurgery* 2002, 51(4):978–84; discussion 984

Chapter 66
Endoscopic Foraminoplasty: Key to Understanding the Sources of Back Pain and Sciatica and Their Treatment

Martin Knight

Since 1990, I have been practicing aware state surgery and have regularly found that the exiting nerve is being irritated or compressed by facet joint osteophytes, the superior foraminal ligament (SFL), and or shoulder osteophytes and tethering of the exiting nerve to the billowing or inflamed disc. These features are grossly underdemonstrated by magnetic resonance imaging (MRI) and computed tomography (CT) scans. In addition, these investigative tools fail to account for neural anomalies. The key finding however is that pressure on the medial border of the irritated nerve produces back pain whilst the core of the nerve produces oft-atypical dermatomal pain and the disc wall seldom produces back pain. Consequently, endoscopic minimally invasive spine surgery involving transforaminal decompression and foraminoplasty offers a paradigm shift in the treatment of chronic lumbar spondylosis and back pain, degenerative disc disease and failed back surgery by treating the causal factors, mobilising the nerve and the dorsal root ganglion. This surgery is performed in the aware state, thus allowing accurate determination of the single most relevant foraminal level, avoiding open surgery, retaining segmental movement, and maintaining the options for the patient as new techniques such as keyhole nuclear replacement become established.

Background

Hitherto, our appreciation of the role of the foramen in the production of back pain and sciatica has relied on cadaveric anatomical and imaging studies and the results of surgical intervention on the unconscious patient and midline studies in the aware state.

M. Knight
The University of Manchester, Manchester, UK
The University of Central Lancashire, Preston, UK
The Spinal Foundation, Sunnyside, Highfield Road, Congleton, Cheshire CW12 3AQ, UK
e-mail: mknight@spinal-foundation.org

The posterolateral approach conducted with the patient under intravenous analgesia (aware state) allows the foramen to be examined endoscopically and palpated with patient feedback. This has revealed a number of unexpected pain sources and mechanisms that required evaluation that is more detailed.

This chapter describes the incidence of expected and unrecognised anatomical structures and pain sources encountered during endoscopy and included the SFL, shoulder osteophytes, disc pads, and safe working zone inflammation. The pain evoked directly from each structure, when addressed from the posterolateral approach, had not been previously described. Currently, the nerve is considered to respond homogeneously, but selective probing revealed clinically significant variations in response. The role of LRS in pain production has focused upon compromised foraminal volume occasioned by loss of disc height, facet joint hypertrophy, or venous engorgement. The role of facet joint, ligamentous and osteophytic tethering, and impaction upon the exiting nerve appears underestimated.

Material and Methods

Study Construct

The study was designed prospectively to determine the pathologies present in the foramen and the distribution of symptoms evoked directly from painful sources.

Methodology

Cohort Selection

The patient group consisted of 127 consecutive patients with two-level degenerative disc disease treated by aware state posterolateral endoscopic lumbar foraminotomy (ELF) between January 1997 and January 1998.

Inclusion and Exclusion Criteria

Patients with MRI scan-proven two-level disc disease and a combination of back, buttock, or leg pain present for over a year, resistant to 3 months or more of muscle balance physiotherapy were included. These patients were substratified for compressive radiculopathy, non-compressive radiculopathy, and failed back surgery (FBS). Inclusion criteria, which were employed for the feedback studies, are presented here:

- Chronic lumbar spondylosis
- Compressive radiculopathy with sensory or motor impairment
- Disc protrusion, extrusion, or sequestration with non-compressive radiculopathy
- Lateral recess and foraminal stenosis with non-compressive radiculopathy
- Failed Back Surgery syndrome with compressive radiculopathy
- Failed Back Surgery syndrome with non-compressive radiculopathy

Exclusion criteria, which were employed for the spinal probing and discography (SP and D) study, are presented here:

- Multilevel (>two-level MRI scan proven) degenerative disc disease
- Concordant or overlapping symptoms evoked at adjacent levels
- Spondylolytic spondylolisthesis
- Facet joint cysts
- Cauda equina syndrome
- Painless motor deficits
- Tumours

Definitions

Compressive radiculopathy denotes a subject with objective evidence of impaired sensory or motor function of dermatomal or myotomal distribution. Non-compressive radiculopathy describes a patient with referred pain into the limb without objective evidence of sensory or motor impairment, aggravated at least in part by manipulation of a spinal segment or by knee extension in the upright sitting position or decubitus straight leg raising in the absence of local or systemic neuropathy.

If the MRI scan identified loss of foraminal space, loss of perineural fat, and a foraminal dimension of <5 mm, then patients were deemed to have LRS.

Outpatient Data Acquisition

Pre-operative and post-operative questionnaires included full details of history and symptoms, a pain manikin, visual analog pain scale (VAP) and Oswestry disability index (ODI) scores. Patients were evaluated at 6 and 12 weeks after surgery unless clinical symptoms required closer supervision. During the first 6 weeks, patients completed a pain diary three times a day, relating back, buttock, and leg pain levels to activity levels.

Clinical Evaluation

Full clinical, neurological, and postural analyses were performed together with radiographic studies at initial assessment. If the pain intensity remained unacceptable, after 3 months of compliant MPB, then patients were referred for an MRI scan. Gadolinium enhancement was added where prior spinal surgery had been involved or perineural scarring was suspected.

Surgical Protocol

SP and D were performed at levels that clinically reproduced the site of back pain or peripheral radiation or were shown to evidence clinically relevant pathology on radiological or imaging investigations. Concordant symptom reproduction indicated the foraminal level for ELF but discordant or indistinguishable levels indicated the need for differential discography (ΔD).

Spinal Probing

The nurse, sitting beside the patient, records the distribution of discomfort produced by probing the lateral facet wall, and the degree to which this reproduces the predominant presenting symptoms (PPS) is noted on the per-operative Pain Distribution and Reproduction (PDR) record.

The patient may score the severity of the perceived pain as on the VAP scale. This is an imperfect measure because the response depends upon the pressure exerted and the level of circulating analgesia. The PDR record is important when analysing the outcome of ΔD or definitive surgery when there are multiple levels of disc degeneration contributing to symptoms.

The anterior border of the facet joint and the interval between the facet joint and disc are next probed to elicit the presence of specific PPS arising from structures tethered to the joint and from adjacent structures referred to under SP and D.

A correct approach has been secured once the pliant disc wall is felt. The cannula alone or the cannula with the round-ended trocar is used to probe the disc wall in at least three positions. Annular symptoms are being evoked where peripheral radicular symptoms are avoided. Annular symptoms may consist of back and paravertebral gutter pain with radiation to the buttock, sacrum, groin, and thighs down to the level of the knee, as appropriate to the interrogated level. This response may fade with repetition. An irritated disc wall can produce peripheral symptoms radiating to the distal thigh from the lower two lumbar discs. Elicitation of more peripheral pain should be assumed to be radicular in origin and due to compression of a displaced nerve root until proved otherwise under direct endoscopic vision.

When the nerve is medially displaced, the probe should be withdrawn and a more shallow approach utilised to reach the disc wall, often commencing on the posterior inferior vertebral wall sweeping superiorly onto the annulus. If this fails, then probing will have to be replaced by endoscopic inspection. Once the disc wall has been reached, then the nerve may be swept gently laterally to achieve the ideal point of entry. Retention of the shallow alignment without correction will lead to an unwanted medial, shallow, and possibly annular placement of the discography needle or laser probe. This carries the risk of imperfect and misleading discography and jeopardy to neural structures. Similarly, too inclined an approach may produce a lateral annular placement with imperfect discography and runs the risk of visceral injury. The distribution of discomfort produced by facet joint margin probing, facet joint/disc interval probing, and annular probing is recorded in the PDR record and entered into the database.

Discography

Entry into the disc is effected through the SWZ with either the standard needle or the thin straight or curved needle as dictated by the available disc height and the presence of olisthesis and the obliquity of the approach. The needle point should be placed in the middle of the disc equidistant from the endplates and the annular margins. Omnipaque® 240 (Nycomed Ltd, Romsey, Hampshire, England) or an equivalent viscosity radio-opaque dye is inserted under guidance from serial X-ray shots, providing the patient is not allergic to Halogens. The purpose of the discography is to demonstrate the distribution of the dye and hence the areas of maximal degeneration. The dye also demonstrates the integrity and thickness of the posterior wall, posterior annular collections, and subligamentous and transligamentous leaks. The point of collection or discharge is further defined on the

anteroposterior (AP) projection because this may demonstrate "horns" of degeneration "pointing" to the foramen.

Much has been made of discography pressures, but as these vary within loci of the disc, this was found to be of indefinite diagnostic targeting value. Pressurised discography carries the risk of enlargement of a disc protrusion or extrusion and should be used with caution. Reliance should be placed upon probing for pain reproduction with added information arising from gentle discography or from the pain caused during leakage.

Discography also provides the acceptance volume of the disc. This is the amount of dye that the disc accepts prior to spring back into the syringe. This provides an indication of the volume of disc material that has been broken down and has leached from the disc and the degree of disc degeneration therein.

The normal acceptance volume is 0.5 ml up to the age of 20 years, 1.0 ml at 30 years, 2.0 ml at 40 years, and 2.5 ml at 50 years, after which the increase in acceptance volume in healthy discs tends to plateau. The volume accepted by the disc space beyond these amounts at a given age is an indication of the void occasioned by disc material loss arising from disc degeneration. The pattern of dye distribution, symptom reproduction, leakage, acceptance volume, and outline of the posterior annulus is recorded in the PDR record and entered into the database.

Once discography is complete, the guide wire replaces the needle and either LDD or ELF can be effected, depending upon the pathology and the inclusion criteria. Alternatively, if probing and discography findings are equivocal, then a ΔD should be effected.

Endoscopic Approach

Once the index level has been targeted by segmental probing and radiopaque discography, indigo carmine marker dye is inserted into the disc to distinguish annulus from scar and disc pad. Once the discography needle has been replaced with the solid guidewire, the standard cannula and dilator are railroaded to the foramen using an oscillating rotating action. Additional local anaesthetic may be needed to secure comfort at the rib margin or iliac crest margin. When two-dimensional X-ray results confirm that the dilator has been placed in the foramen, the standard cannula is replaced with the "cut away" slotted cannula, which can more easily be introduced without the curved edges snagging tissues during insertion. The cannula is attached to the suction friction lock water seal, the 00 or 200 endoscope is inserted over the guide wire, and the position of the guide wire in relation to the exiting nerve root and the facet joint is ascertained. With experience, the guide wire is removed once the cannula is in situ.

Camera and Drape Setup

The 00 endoscope is selected early in the learning curve. The camera is attached via a sterile tubular drape (Mildrape camera drape, Surgical Innovations Ltd., Leeds, England) that is secured with an additional supplied adhesive thong. The camera is locked on the objective eyepiece of the endoscope and the objective is rotated to orientate the picture.

Endoscope Choice and Setup

The endoscopes are shaped elliptically to match the configuration of the foramen. The system consists of a small-bore 00 and 200 elliptical endoscope and a large-bore 200 elliptical endoscope. In the initial learning stages, the small-bore 00 endoscope is to be recommended. The 200 endoscope improves visualisation across the midline of the epidural space, improves epidural visualisation medial to the proximal and distal pedicles, and improves visualisation of the posterior annulus during intradiscal surgery. With experience and orientation established, the 200 endoscope becomes the more versatile instrument and it can be used throughout the procedure.

Positive suction drainage is linked to the drain tap on the cannula. The endoscope is designed to be attached to two 3-l bags of saline on the side taps. These are elevated to between approximately 1 and 2 m above the height of the endoscope.

Bleeding in the operative working zone is controlled by the balance of gravity-fed inflow and the rate of suction and irrigation dictated by the drainage tap. The use of the laser to seal bleeding points should be carried out meticulously throughout the procedure. Cooling the inflow fluid and the use of adrenaline in the irrigant are not usually necessary. Excessive inflow pressure should be avoided because it increases tissue fluid extravasation and may cause pressure effects upon the dura with consequent effects on cerebral and neural blood flow.

Oblique endoscope taps are provided for back flushing of the working channels if they become blocked or for use of additional straight firing laser probes, ultrasonic or radiofrequency probes.

The large-bore elliptical endoscope is utilised after adequate clearance of the foramen and definition and mobilisation of the nerves has been achieved. The function of this endoscope is to transmit larger instrumentation such as reamers or punches. To ensure the safe use of such equipment, vital structures such as the nerve must be sufficiently mobilised to ensure their safeguard.

Because the large-bore endoscope has only one irrigation channel, suction should be applied to the cannula with irrigation applied to the irrigation channel of the endoscope and the laser probe. When using the reamer, reversal of connections with fluid applied to the cannula and suction applied to the reamer may be the optimal configuration, especially when working in tight corners. The powered reamer may be exchanged for large-bore punches or osteotomes.

ELF Lasing Technique

The side-firing laser probe has individual irrigation led from a 1-l bag of saline attached by a giving set with a Luer lock and three-way tap. This allows continuous flow during use and irrigation over the mirror and side fire window with preservation thereof. The focus of the beam is tested prior to insertion against a white swab using the guide or pilot beam.

The Omnipulse Max (Trimedyne Inc., Irvine, CA, USA) laser generator is set at DP1 for the initial clearance stage (Table 66.1). The single pulse mode is less effective for bone ablation and, in this mode, higher wattages need to be used to achieve the same effect and the patient feels greater thermoacoustic discomfort from each impact.

The position of cannula, endoscope, and probe is checked in the AP and lateral planes radiographically before commencing. Clearance of the soft tissues commences seeking to define the bone margin of the facet joint. Once the soft tissues have been defined, facet joint undercutting may be started. Bone ablation is best effected at a setting of DP3–DP5. The total energy used ranges from 40 to 150,000 J.

Care should be maintained to avoid energy flashback from reflective structures such as bone because the rebounding energy will damage the side-firing window. Maintaining an appropriate distance from the target and approaching while observing the ablation effect avoids flashback. Hemostasis is achieved by either reducing the energy levels or increasing the distance between the probe and the target.

Power Osteotome Utilisation

A power-driven oscillating osteotome (MDS, Zurich, Switzerland) can be inserted down the 00 and 200 endoscopes for the removal of facet joint overhang and osteophytes. Under

Table 66.1 Laser settings used in endoscopic laser foraminoplasty.

Setting and double pulse (DP)	Power (W)	Pulses per second	Maximum duration (s)	Energy (joules per pulse)
DP1	12	12	6	0.500
DP2	20	18	20	0.556
DP3	30	18	20	0.833
DP4	40	18	20	1.111
DP5	50	18	20	1.389

direct vision, the osteotome consists of a longitudinal hand piece into which can be inserted straight and curved osteotomes with straight working edges. The tips have marks at 1-mm intervals to guide the surgeon regarding the depth of entry of the osteotome blade into the bone.

The power generator should be set at 0.1 Bar and single shots initially. As the surgeon becomes familiar with the technique, then the setting can be upgraded to repetitive shots and the power increased to 2–4 Bar.

The osteotome can be used to clear the deepest reaches of the foraminal isthmus where laser clearance may be impeded by the presence of the transiting nerve passing across the deep/epidural face of the foramen and often lying obscured by the lower border of the medial facet. The laser can be used to trim and seal the bone surface subsequently.

The osteotome can be used to remove larger segments of bone from the foraminal entrance by joining up the indentations made by the osteotome until the section of bone becomes loose. The segment can be mobilised by gentle twisting of the osteotome in the cleavage created. The fragment is then removed by punches either through the small- or large-bore endoscope or through the cannula with the endoscope removed.

Manual Instruments

Instruments are available for use through the large- and small-bore endoscopes described.

Powered Reamer

The powered reamer consists of an electric hand piece into which the reamers are slotted. The speed and direction of rotation or oscillation is controlled by a foot piece. The standard reamers consist of burrs with a distal guard to allow bone resection and undercutting of the foramen. Powered eccentric reamers are available for specific applications such as endplate reaming in preparation for endoscopic fusion.

Flexible Endoscopes

Flexible fibreoptic endoscopes are available with a working channel for a forward-firing laser fibre for inspection and clearance in the epidural and intradiscal space.

Extraforaminal Zone. The initial view in the extraforaminal region is dictated by the underlying pathology. In a case of prior surgery with advanced settlement, short pedicles and perineural scarring, the first view is likely to be a wall of scar with evidently tender structures trapped within (Fig. 66.1).

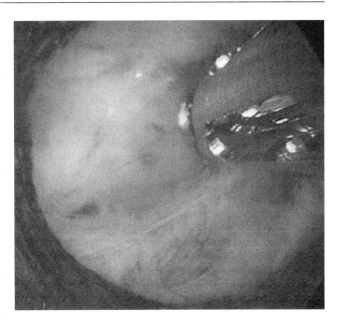

Fig. 66.1 Extraforaminal initial endoscopic clearance

This contrasts with an unadulterated surgical field in a patient with a large protrusion and reasonable disc height and normal pedicle lengths. In this situation, the exiting nerve will be readily visible together with readily definable foraminal margins containing a disc protrusion occluding the foramen.

The surgeon aims for the bone margin of the foramen and clears the anterior margin and lateral surfaces of the facet joint. The borders from the superior pedicle, the facet joint margin, and the external surface of the inferior pedicle are cleared. In the area of the inferior pedicle, the exiting nerve root can be found and identified more easily because it may be less incarcerated at this point.

The side-firing laser is suited to the clearance of scar because of the discrete depth of laser ablation and the concurrent self-sealing effect. Irrigated lasing maintains a clear field of view and appears to deter subsequent scarring.

The scar and infolded ligamentum flavum (LF) found anterior to the facet joint capsule and in the superior and inferior notches are gradually removed until the exiting nerve root is freed from the bone of the ascending facet joint, the superior notch, the disc, and the inferior notch boundaries.

The intertransversus muscle may be seen passing from the superior transverse process and overlaps the lateral border of the exiting nerve root, especially where there is scoliosis. The nerve root may be adherent to this muscle. The view of the lateral border and the limits of the nerve may be obscured by this structure. The medial muscle fibres may need to be divided and the adherent border dissected from the nerve to mobilise the nerve and gain line of sight.

Lateral osteophytes may form an overhanging claw incarcerating the exiting nerve or more commonly may displace the nerve dorsally and medially into the extraforaminal zone and foramen. The soft tissues need to be removed from the bone. Subsequently, the overhanging or underlying osteophytes need to be resected from the posterior and anterior aspects of the nerve. These frequently occur at the lateral margin of the vertebral body and the nerve may be inflamed and narrowed along this discrete section.

Foraminal Stage. The foraminal zone consists of a quadrangular space as shown in Fig. 66.2. The superior and inferior notches function as sumps to accommodate the exiting nerve in extension and flexion, respectively, and ipsilateral and contralateral rotation, respectively.

These notches become obscured by hypervascular soft tissues and the SFL in the superior notch or by the disc inferiorly. The middle notch becomes narrowed by facet joint hypertrophy, LF infolding, and shoulder osteophytes with further compromise due to the tethering of the nerve to the ascending facet or disc.

Figure 66.3 shows the laser probe tip with the window pointing towards the facet joint margin. The nerve has been partially cleared but further tethering scar needs to be removed. The cannula and endoscope position in the foramen is demonstrated in the lateral X-ray insert. The nerve is freed of incarcerating scar or tethering bands. The laser probe is then directed at the facet joint margin to undercut the facet to allow access to the epidural space.

The right-angle probe or dissector may be insinuated anterior to the facet and swept along the medial surface of the facet joint in order to mobilise the traversing nerve root that is often tethered to the medial aspect of the facet joint. In cases of settlement or facet joint hypertrophy or extensive scarring, the power reamer or osteotome may be used once the nerves have been displaced to a point of safety.

The external surface of the facet joint may be addressed with the power osteotome once it has been cleared by lasing. A curved line is marked out on the bone. The cut of the osteotome is directed as horizontally as needed and deepened at each point along this line to form a continuous fissure. The action of the osteotome is observed directly and the depth of cut monitored from the millimetre gauge marks on the osteotome blade and on the AP X-ray view. Penetration is ceased when the epidural space is entered or at the first evidence of neural discomfort from the patient. Until experience is gained, it is safer to angle the osteotome towards the annulus at the midpedicular line. With experience, a more horizontal direction may be used but penetration beyond the medial pedicular line should be avoided. The osteotome cuts are amalgamated until the fissure is widened and the bone fragment becomes loose. The fragment is mobilised by gently rotating the osteotome blade in the bone fissure (Fig. 66.4).

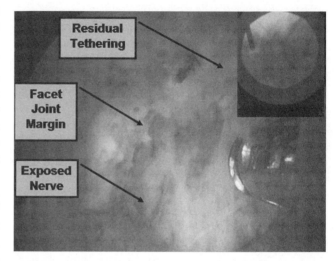

Fig. 66.3 Right-hand side approach to the L4/5 foramen with inset lateral X-ray

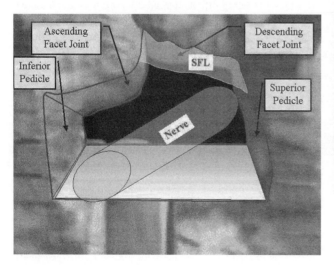

Fig. 66.2 The quadrangular space

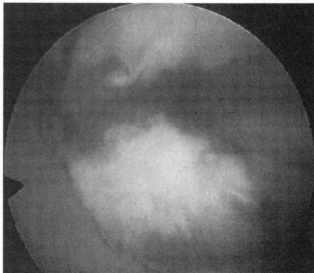

Fig. 66.4 Powered osteotome mobilising a fragment of the facet joint rim

The fragment may be removed through the large-bore endoscope or the endoscope may be removed and the fragments grasped by forward bone graspers and withdrawn through the approach cannula. The raw bone surface is then sealed with the laser to control oozing. This process will provide more space in which to manoeuvre the endoscope. If the cavity of the foramen remains too small, the process can be repeated or additional power reamers and punches may be used. This clearance allows the medial border of the oft flattened and medially displaced nerve root to be clearly visualised and the foramen to be effectively undercut and decompressed.

Further exploration of the superior notch and clearance of the impinging SFL is then undertaken, using the laser probe to ablate scar, tethering, the SFL, and local facet margin osteophytes until the "functional" axilla is exposed and cleared. Clearance may be supplemented by use of the powered guarded burr and bone punches.

The SFL originates from the ascending facet joint and attaches to the base of the transverse process (Fig. 66.5). This often binds onto the exiting nerve root, a feature often declared by the presence of marked local injection and hyperaemia of the nerve at this point. Under these circumstances, the SFL needs to be resected and the nerve mobilised. Attention is then directed to clearance of the nerve root axilla and thereafter the inferior notch to expose the disc.

At this stage, the nerve root may be mobilised along the medial and lateral border of the nerve. The laser probe or the angled dissector may be used to free gradually the anterior surface of the nerve from the bone and disc. The nerve may evidence discrete areas of redness and inflammation. Examination of these areas may reveal a shoulder osteophyte lying anterior to the nerve if the redness is coincident with the vertebral body margin or a leaking annular tear if coincident with the annulus. Under these circumstances, the shoul-

der osteophyte should be ablated by lasing, powered reaming, or forward-cutting punches. Mobilising the nerve until it is clear of the tear and entering the disc at the point of the tear and removing degenerate disc material from the margins of the tear and clearing degenerate intradiscal tissues and nucleus pulposus should effectively address the radial tear.

A thick sheet of sensitive hypervascular tissue often masks the annulus, termed the "Disc Pad". This needs to be cleared to define the margins of the disc wall. The disc pad may be adherent to the dura or to the local nerves.

In the superior notch, hypervascular sensitive tissues may bind the posterior aspect of the vertebra to the adjacent nerve and occasionally to the facet joint capsule and form a firm tender mass in the superior part of the SWZ. This should be mobilised and ablated until the functional axilla is mobilised. Removal of this tissue, swollen veins, and the fibrous impediment may play a significant part in relieving neural claudicant symptoms. Clearance still leaves a venous complex around the nerve and balances concern regarding excessive venous ablation jeopardising the vascular supply locally or within the dura. The dorsal ganglion may be bound to the superior pedicle and the superior notch and may require mobilisation.

In cases of LRS, the exposed superior notch is commonly the site of facet joint osteophytes attached to the exiting nerve. These need to be mobilised from the nerve and resected especially when the nerve is reddened at this point. This is effected by laser ablation and power burrs.

The nerve, once mobilised, should be displaced and restored to the correct pathway. Inspection of the nerve may reveal particular adherence at the level of the vertebral margin. The nerve needs to be rolled laterally to expose a shoulder osteophyte. This is often covered by a fibrous cap. This offers a plane for dissection and neural mobilisation. With the nerve displaced and protected by the "cut away" cannula, the shoulder osteophyte may be removed by side-fire laser ablation and forward bone-cutting punches with laser haemostasis.

Intradiscal Zone. After the disc surface has been cleared of the attendant disc pad by laser ablation and manual punches, the annular knife is passed through the endoscope and placed upon the disc wall. The position is checked by bi-dimensional radiography to ensure an ideal placement of the annular entry point, equidistant between the endplates at the mid-pedicular line.

In cases of advanced disc degeneration, the knife may be replaced by the laser probe or alternative ablative or thermoplastic instruments in the entry point and rotated until the entry portal is enlarged to allow easy egress of gases generated during lasing or intradiscal clearance (Fig. 66.6).

In cases of larger disc protrusion or degeneration, the endoscope may be removed and trephines used to open the disc wall. The discal contents may be removed by manual punches

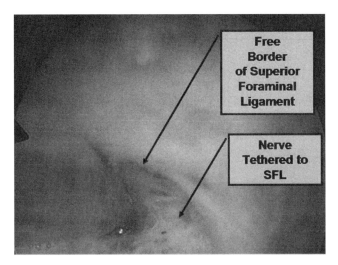

Fig. 66.5 The L4/5 superior foraminal ligament

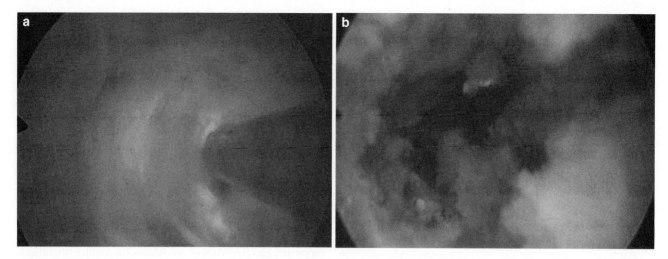

Fig. 66.6 (**a**) Endoscopic views of a large disc protrusion and (**b**) an intradiscal view

passed through the cannula under X-ray control. Removal should be confined to disc material staining darkly with indigo carmine. The paler the staining, the healthier the disc wall, and the more likely that it should be retained. When degeneration is widespread, the endoscope is removed and forward-cutting, back-cutting, and dynamically angled punches are inserted to remove freely degenerate disc material.

The powered reamers can be inserted in the disc space for additional clearance. The endoscope is replaced with the 200 endoscope to facilitate visualisation of the posterior annulus, the recesses of the disc, and the endplates. The side-firing laser probe is used to complete removal of residual degenerate intradiscal tissue and to allow thermoplastic shrinkage of the posterior wall from within the annulus (thermoplastic annealing).

Transforaminal Zone. The 200 endoscope is withdrawn from the intradiscal space and passed through the isthmus of the foramen. Sufficient foraminal enlargement and resection of the ascending facet joint should have been completed prior to discectomy. The laser can be used to enlarge the foramen where it binds on the endoscope and limits exploration. The 200 angle allows the dura to be visualised, together with improved inspection of the medial aspect of the facet joint. Medial overhanging bone can be freed from the transiting nerve by the use of the angled probe, the spatula, or the distal end of the side-firing irrigated laser probe itself. Once the transiting nerve is mobilised and displaced, then the curtain of remaining bone can be removed by lasing or by upcutting punches.

Rotation of the endoscope allows examination of the inner aspects of respective pedicles and the dorsum of the disc. In this way, the dorsal protrusion of the disc can be visualised and shrunk by additional external thermoplastic annealing of the collagen in the disc wall. In the case of an extrusion or sequestra, lasing and flexible grasping forceps may be used to remove the disrupted disc material; haemostasis is achieved by lasing the bleeding vessels. Dorsal osteophytes can be cleared and freed from the dura by direct visualised lasing.

In patients without prior surgery, the dura pulsates once suction is open. After prior surgery, the dura may be adherent to the posterior longitudinal ligament (PLL) and the disc and may have to be dissected free by a combination of spatula dissection and lasing. This is achieved by using side-fire lasing parallel to the dural margin or angled anteriorly, thus avoiding perforation.

Far Lateral Zone. For far lateral disc protrusions and lateral osteophytes, the medial and lateral borders of the nerve are identified and mobilised by neurolysis from the disc protrusion and or lateral osteophytes. The protrusion may be anterior to the nerve or protruding both from the medial or lateral aspect of the nerve. The nerve is often adherent to the disc wall and must be mobilised before the protrusion can be defined and removed. The protrusion is then entered by incision with the endoscopy knife. The laser probe widens the entry portal. Clearance is effected by laser ablation and manual clearance as outlined above. The osteophytes are resected by gradual endoscopic laser ablation, side-arm manual punches and powered tools.

The osteophyte is usually covered with a fibrotic layer and the nerve can be mobilised using this plane. Once the nerve is fully mobilised, then the laser probe can be used to retract the nerve and, by aiming at 90° away from the nerve, the osteophyte can be ablated progressively and safely.

Operative Data Acquisition

During our surgeries, assistants versed in the collection of this data over the preceding 4 years recorded the patients' responses. The distribution of evoked sensations was recorded on a data sheet describing the response during the transit through the paravertebral musculature, during lateral facet joint surface, foraminal interval, and annular probing.

Care was taken to avoid reproduction of radicular pain evoked below the knee. If there was overlap in evoked symptoms during probing or discography at adjacent levels, then patients underwent ΔD.

During discography, the distribution, pattern, acceptance volume, and leakage of radio-opaque dye were noted, together with the distribution of endstage pain during discography pressurisation.

During the procedure, the presence of SFL impingement, superior notch osteophytosis, dorsal vertebral and shoulder osteophytosis, facet joint nerve tethering and impaction, facet joint cysts, pars interarticularis tethering, safe working zone and notch engorgement, LF infolding, disc pad irritation, PLL irritation, intertransverse ligament and muscle entrapment, inferior external pedicular tethering, annular irritation and nerve tethering, annular tears, lateral osteophytosis, paravertebral bone graft tethering, post-fusion discitis, instrumentation neural tethering, perineural and dural scarring, and irritation were recorded. The distribution of pain emanating from these sites and from the medial border and core of the nerve were recorded during the probing of the nerve with a 2-mm right-angled probe.

Indices

The VAP and ODI scores were noted before and after surgery. The outcome was measured by observing the percentage change in scores as shown in the formula in which an index of ^{3}90% was deemed an excellent result, ^{3}50% deemed good, and ^{3}20% deemed improved, whilst <20% was deemed poor and negative values were deemed a worse result.

Follow-Up

Patients were discharged the same day or morning after surgery. The muscle balance physiotherapy regime was re-commenced on the first day after surgery, amplified with neural mobilisation drills, and continued on a monitored self-help basis for 3 months. Patients were reviewed at 6 and 12 weeks after surgery with their pain diaries, follow-up questionnaires, and pain manikins. A postal review was performed 2 years after surgery to ascertain whether the patient had required additional surgical intervention.

Group Data

Pre-operative diagnosis and demographics are presented in Tables 66.2 and 66.3. All patients had back, buttock, or leg pain with or without sciatica syndrome. Twenty-seven of 127 patients required a ΔD. All underwent a hospital stay of less than 24 h. Fifty-six patients had obtained opinions from one or more spinal or orthopaedic surgeons or neurosurgeons prior to referral and had been deemed unsuitable for open surgery. These patients included 39 patients with prior failed open conventional lumbar spinal surgery.

Table 66.2 Pre-operative diagnosis

Pre-operative diagnosis	Number
Compressive radiculopathy	32
Non-compressive radiculopathy	68
Lateral recess stenosis	42
Predominant back/buttock pain	59
Perineural scarring (MRI confirmed)	32
Advanced settlement (>75% loss of disc height on MRI scan)	30
Prior discectomies, decompressions or revisions	34
Prior fusions or revision fusions	18

Table 66.3 Patient demographic data for pain sources and risk studies

Demographics - aware-state feedback studies	
Period of recruitment	January 1997 and January 1998
Number of patients - total cohort	127
Number of patients - total cohort minus 27 patients excluded for differential discography	100
Men	47
Women	53
Cohort integrity at 3-month follow-up	100%
Cohort integrity at 2-year postal review	98%
Mean age	52 years (range, 29–88 years; SD 12.9)
Mean duration of symptoms	6.8 years (range, 4–27 years; SD 2.4)
Prior open surgery ($N = 39$)	
One prior operation	29
Two prior operations	7
Three prior operations	3
Patients with failed laser disc decompression	0
Levels operated	
T12-L4	3
L4–L5	46
L5–S1	51
Pre-operative Oswestry Disability Index (100 patients)	46.2 (SD 11.3)
Work accidents	12
Litigation and compensation cases	9
Patients on morphine sulphate	8
Patients with residential prior pain management courses	41
Patients with multiple prior opinions	56
Patients with diabetes mellitus	2

Results

Pain Provocative Sites

During our surgeries, the patients' responses were recorded by assistants versed in the collection of this data during the preceding 4 years. Each response during spinal probing, discography, and endoscopy was correlated to the following structures, deemed pain provocative sites.

Ascending Facet Joint Tethering

Facet joint and nerve need to be resected and the facet joint undercut to remove this dynamic impaction. Such dynamic impaction may be the mechanism underlying many instances of so-called instability. Figure 66.7 represents a right-sided view of the foramen. In Fig. 66.7a, the nerve is tethered to the SFL, indicated by black shadowed arrows. In Fig. 66.7b, the SFL is seen pressing upon the exiting nerve. The nerve is reddened as shown by the red arrow at this point of impaction and tethering. In Fig. 66.7c, the grey shadowed arrows demonstrate the area of scar resection and the exposure of a contained osteophyte is indicated by the black arrow.

Superior Foraminal Ligament Tethering and Impingement

The SFL passes from the ascending facet to the base of the transverse process. As settlement occurs, this ligament bears down on the exiting nerve and the exiting nerve may become tethered causing local hyperaemia and irritation of the nerve at that point. This irritation is further aggravated by occasional calcification of the ligament. Perineural scarring replaces tethering with dense, more rigid tissue, causing greater entrapment. The section of inflammation is usually discretely limited to the zone of entrapment. While normal radicular symptoms may be elicited from quiescent sections of the same nerve, the inflamed nerve may produce atypical dysaesthesiae.

Superior Notch Osteophytosis

As the SFL is resected, superior notch osteophytes may be displayed adherent to the exiting nerve, producing further local inflammation. These osteophytes arise from the descending (inferior) facet joint margin and from the apex of the ascending (superior) facet joint.

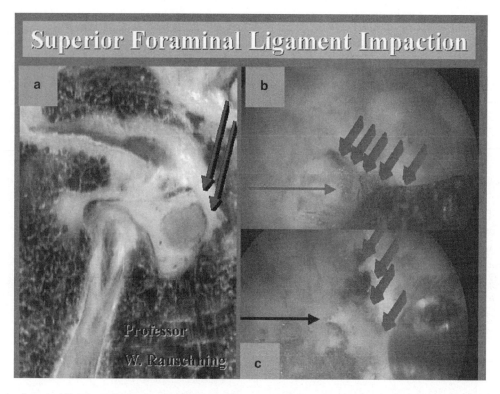

Fig. 66.7 Superior foraminal ligament tethering and impingement (Courtesy of Wolfgang Rauschning MD, PhD, The Swedish Medical Research Council, Stockholm; Department of Orthopaedic Surgery, University Hospital, Uppsala, Sweden.)

Dorsal and Shoulder Osteophytes

A soft tissue cap, which increases the compressive effect on adjacent tissues, covers these osteophytes. Tethering between the osteophyte fibrous cap and the nerve, the dura, or tenting of the PLL worsens this effect. Shoulder osteophytes can be found as a peripheral extension of dorsal osteophytes or as individual laterally placed entities. Usually the dorsal osteophyte arises from the upper vertebral body margin and produces midline or medial foraminal tethering, inflammation, and displacement of the nerve pathway. This tethering or displacement is especially noticeable during flexion.

Figure 66.8 demonstrates the presence of a shoulder osteophyte partially resected medially and the nerve root mobilised and displaced laterally. Shoulder osteophytes may arise from the superior or inferior vertebral margin in the foramen or lateral foramen lying anterior to the nerve and tethering it. These are often hidden from view unless an active search is made on the medial or anterior (deep) surface of the nerve. These appear to lie in the pathway of the abutting impacting ascending facet joint and may indeed arise because of such impaction. The endoscopy cannula can be used to mobilise and retract the nerve. Once the nerve is separated from the fibrous cap of the osteophyte, the underlying osteophyte can be ablated.

Safe Working Zone and Notch Engorgement

Hypervascular tissue consisting of scar, hypervascular veins, and arterioles can be found in the superior and inferior notch and in the safe working zone. This tissue can become engorged, producing stenotic and claudicant symptoms and may itself be directly tender when inflamed.

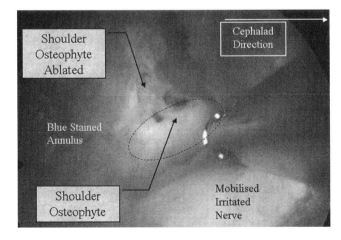

Fig. 66.8 Shoulder osteophytosis tethering

Ligamentum Flavum Infolding

The LF infolds as disc height is reduced. The infolding crowds the exiting nerve root in the superior notch and in the inferior notch if the nerve has been displaced medially. On occasions, the LF may be found to blend with the posterior disc pad and PLL. Resection of the LF at these sites serves to decompress the exiting and traversing nerve roots and mobilise them from local tethering. The procedure should be combined with anterior mobilisation of the nerve at the index level to achieve full mobilisation. The LF may blend with the foraminal ligament that passes from the superior notch, blends with the capsule, and extends to the inferior notch but, of itself, does not appear to cause compression.

Figure 66.9 represents a right-sided view of the foramen. In (a), the annulus is tethered to the ascending facet joint, indicated by black shadowed arrows. In (b), the ascending facet joint has been partially resected and is seen pressing upon the annulus at C. The nerve has been mobilised and displaced laterally. Exposure of the apex of the ascending facet joint can be seen in (a) along with superior displacement of the tethered nerve root.

Annular Facet Joint Tethering and Impaction

In cases of extensive degeneration, loss of disc height, and concomitant osteophytosis, the ascending facet joint may impinge upon the annulus and associated osteophytes. This impedes access to the epidural space. Importantly, this results in displacement of the nerve into the superior notch with crowding of vascular tissues. Associated tethering restricts nerve mobility, allowing it to be impacted by the ascending facet joint, whose apex is now exposed by the overriding of the facet joint.

Figure 66.10 represents a right-sided view of the foramen. In (a), the annulus evidences a minor foraminal bulge but is associated with tethering to the exiting nerve, indicated by black shadowed arrows. In (b), the annulus is stained blue as indicated by a blue shadowed arrow. The exiting nerve has been rolled laterally to expose the tethering of the nerve to the underlying annulus indicated by the black shadowed arrows. This section of the nerve root is seen to be locally irritated.

Annulus

The annulus may extrude or protrude into the foramen, lateral foraminal zone, or posterolateral or central epidural zones. Discectomy or resection of the central or posterolateral bulging

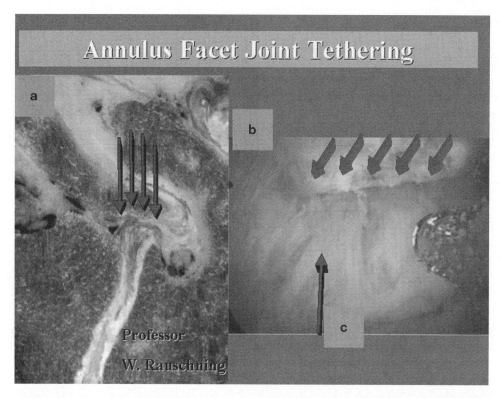

Fig. 66.9 Annulus facet joint tethering and impingement. This image is copied from a microtome picture prepared by and with the permission of Professor Rauschning

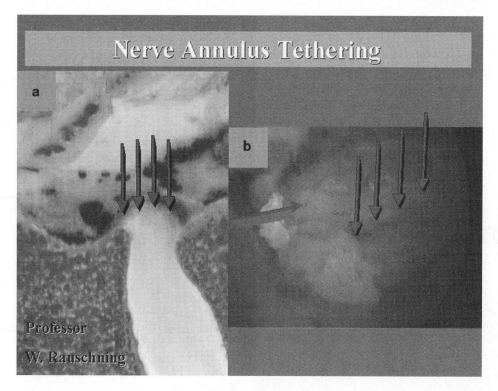

Fig. 66.10 Nerve annulus tethering. This image is copied from a microtome picture prepared by and with the permission of Professor Rauschning

disc may be appropriate and concur with expected clinical findings. However, protrusions in the lateral foramen may impact upon the exiting nerve and produce unexpected clinical signs, especially where the annulus is tethered to the nerve. The disc protrusion in this area may be surprisingly small and discrete yet produce significant impact upon the nerve, especially where the nerve is tethered to the disc wall. Under these circumstances, the disc protrusion may be imperceptible on the MRI scan.

In situations of degenerate disc height loss, the wall of the disc may be seen to be playing only a limited role in the pathogenesis of symptoms and, under these circumstances, the wall of the disc may be shrunk thermo-plastically with the laser rather than removed and damaged further. The emphasis of treatment needs to focus upon the clearance of the foramen and enlargement of foraminal boundaries in these circumstances. In more than three quarters of cases, intradiscal clearance may be performed without pain.

In cases where the MRI scan does not show a disc bulge, yet concordant pain is reproduced at a given level, endoscopy often shows a discrete weakness and bulging of the annulus at the posterolateral corner of the disc and adjacent to the nerve. The effect of the bulge is amplified where the nerve is adherent to the disc at this point.

Annular Tears

The annulus may be the site of intradiscal tears that may breach the annulus either under the PLL (subligamentous) or through the PLL (transligamentous), occasioning symptoms according to the point of liberation and direction of breakdown products. The most symptomatic are those ejecting breakdown products directly onto the nerve in the foramen. Their effect is amplified where the nerve is tethered adjacent to the exit portal of the tear. The reaction to the leakage may be to lay down perineural scarring, causing further adherence of the nerve to the disc thus impeding movement of the nerve away from the point of leakage during flexion or rotation. The fibrous response may cause encapsulation of the leakage, resulting in containment and concentration of the breakdown products around the nerve. These effects enhance

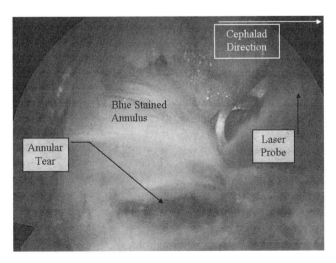

Fig. 66.11 Endoscopic view of a leaking radial tear

the symptoms and are found in patients with long-term pre-operative symptoms.

Opening of the radial tear orifice and removal of debris, often holding the tear open, should complement clearance of the perineural scarring and mobilisation of the nerve (Fig. 66.11). The course of the tear is often serpiginous, so the route of the tear cannot be fully explored. Therefore, the nucleus should be explored and the degenerate material removed manually and by laser ablation. The wall of the disc is then treated by thermoplastic annealing thus contracting the walls of the tear.

Disc Pad

On the posterior aspect of the disc, a pad of tissue may be found that is thick and contains multiple blood vessels and nerves that may be locally tender in contradistinction to the annulus itself which, if not injected, is often pain-free to concurrent probing. Removal of the pad may produce immediate relief of local back pain. This may occur in the absence of a posterior collection of dye in the annulus or a leak. However, it is more common to find this in association with annular collections or leaks.

Posterior Longitudinal Ligament Irritation

The PLL may be inflamed and locally tender but this is usually found in this state when adjacent tissues such as the disc are inflamed. Local neurolysis and ablation of adjacent inflamed tissues can resolve the inflammation. Probing of the inflamed PLL will produce pain arising in territories normally expected to be subtended by both the index and adjacent levels.

Figure 66.12 represents a right-sided view of foraminal sources of pain. In (**a**), the normally silver annulus evidences injection and proved to be locally tender. In (**b**), the disc can be seen stained blue. Dorsal to the annulus are tissues that are hyperaemic and lying as a disc pad on the dorsum of the disc. These tissues appeared irritated and proved to be locally tender. The underlying annulus was asymptomatic. In (**c**), a shoulder osteophyte has been exposed by lateral displacement and mobilisation of the nerve root. The laser probe points at the bony osteophyte whose fibrous cap has been resected. The side-firing laser probe was used to ablate the osteophyte, and the nerve was allowed to roll back free of local impingement by the osteophyte. In (**d**), the SWZ on the dorsum of the vertebral body has been exposed and the tissues were found to be tender, hyperaemic, and were injected. On this occasion, there was a leaking radial tear in the annulus at the base of the safe working zone. The adjacent section of the nerve root was locally irritated.

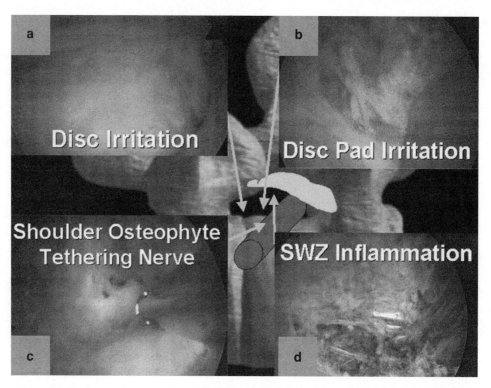

Fig. 66.12 A collage of pain sources

Intertransverse Ligament and Muscle Entrapment

The intertransverse ligament and muscle pass on the lateral aspect of the exiting nerve. In the degenerate state, the nerve may be tethered on the medial aspect to the intertransverse ligament and muscle, causing local inflammation. Degenerative loss of disc height may aggravate this dorsolateral crowding of the exiting nerve, limiting the excursion of the nerve and impeding escape from the impacting ascending facet. Endoscopic neurolysis and modest division of the medial limits of the ligament and muscle relieves the lateral constraint and assists access and mobilisation of the nerve root.

Inferior External Pedicular Tethering

The exiting nerve may be tethered to the external surface of the inferior pedicle, especially after previous surgery and prior posterolateral bone grafted fusion. Local endoscopic neurolysis allows mobilisation of the nerve root from the pedicle and resection of dorsally encroaching hypertrophic tethering bone graft.

Lateral Osteophytosis

Lateral osteophytes displace the exiting nerve root dorsally and into the inferior notch, amplifying compression by the redundant annulus at that point. In addition, the lateral osteophytes cause displacement of the nerve into the middle section of the foramen thus placing the nerve in the path of the impacting facet joint. Partial resection of the osteophytes where they displace the nerve is valuable as part of general undercutting and enlargement of the foramen.

Paravertebral Bone Graft Tethering

After instrumented and non-instrumented fusion, paravertebral bone graft causes tethering to exiting nerve roots with profound entrapment, often in the presence of a secure and technically correct fusion. Wide neurolysis on the anterior surface of the graft results in nerve root mobilisation and amelioration of symptoms resulting from extraforaminal entrapment.

Post-fusion and Aseptic Discitis

Post-fusion discitis and aseptic discitis are manifest endoscopically as a highly injected and tender annulus. This irritation appears to be relieved by manual and laser discectomy under endoscopic control. If clinical or MRI evidence of infection exists, then a fine cannula can be placed intradiscally to insert antibiotics until intravenous conversion is appropriate. In cases of aseptic discitis, removal of the inflamed disc contents serves to significantly reduce the back pain and possibly to accelerate resolution.

Instrumentation and Neural Tethering

Pedicle screw instrumentation can produce neural tethering either by direct impingement of the metalwork or by tethering of the nerve to misplaced metalwork or microfractures of adjacent pedicles. The former, when identified, can be treated by endoscopic mobilisation of the nerve and removal of the metalwork. The latter can be treated by mobilisation of the nerve only.

Perineural Tethering and Nerve Irritation

Perineural tethering may arise because of direct irritation from a disc protrusion, extrusion, or post-traumatic bleed aggravated by facet joint impaction or the release of breakdown products. The nerve may be reddened because an impacting facet joint with osteophytes or inflamed engorged hypervascular tissues in the notch may entrap it. Displacement of the nerve by scarring, lateral small knuckles of disc protrusion, and shoulder osteophytes may aggravate the displacement, tethering, mechanical irritation, or inflammation. Annular tears, by direct release of intradiscal breakdown products onto the nerve, cause irritation associated with perineural scarring.

Neural Response to Probing

The core of the exiting or traversing nerve root will produce normal radicular signs with compression. However, the irritated reddened nerve will often produce dysaesthesiae of unexpected distribution. Despite this, adjacent non-irritated sections of the same nerve core may produce symptoms in expected territories. The medial border of the nerve however produces back pain and atypical symptoms of proximal referred pain accounting for beneficial reduction in such

symptoms after clearance and reduction of dynamic impaction upon the medial border of the nerve. Endoscopy reveals that it is the medial border of the nerve that is most vulnerable to impaction by the ascending facet joint (Tables 66.4 and 66.5).

Radial tears cause symptoms during discography seemingly related to the products liberated by discography and the direction in which they flow and the tissues upon which they impinge (Tables 66.6 and 66.7).

Table 66.4 Incidence of endoscopically determined pain sources

Pain sources	Number
Superior foraminal ligament impingement	53
Superior foraminal ligament tethering	48
Superior notch osteophytosis	34
Ascending facet joint impaction	74
Ascending facet joint - nerve tethering	58
Quiescent annulus	66
Tender annulus or pain during intradiscal manipulation	34
Foraminal nerve - disc tethering	62
Disc pad inflammation	15
Safe working zone inflammation	11
Unexpected foraminal bulge	32
Shoulder osteophytosis - nerve tethering	20
Lateral osteophytosis posteromedial nerve displacement	09
External inferior pedicle tethering	17
Post-fusion inflamed annulus	06
Posterolateral graft - nerve tethering	04
Post-fusion instrumentation - nerve tethering	02

Table 66.5 Pattern of pain evoked during endoscopic foraminal nerve palpation

Neural responses	L5 exiting at L5/S1	L4 exiting at L4/5
Nerve medial border	Local back pain	Local back pain
	Pain at L5/S1 facet joint	Pain at L4/5 facet joint
	L5/S1 paravertebral pain	L4/5 paravertebral pain
	Lateral buttock pain	Medial buttock pain
	Lateral groin	Iliac crest pain
Core of nerve	L5 radicular distribution	L4 radicular distribution
	S1 distribution to lateral malleolus	L5 distribution to medial malleolus
Inflamed nerve	Global dysaesthesia	Global dysaesthesia

Table 66.6 Distribution patterns of pain evoked by radial leaks during discography

Radial leaks	Pain distribution
Midline leak	Local segmental back pain, ascending or descending axial pain
Posteromedial leak	Local segmental back pain and transiting nerve irritation
Foraminal leak	20 nerve irritation, see Table 66.7
Lateral leak	Back pain, paravertebral pain, descending exited nerve pain

Table 66.7 Incidence of anatomical structures and their relation to pain production

Anatomical structure	Number detected	Number painful	Pain distribution
Medial border of the nerve	100	100	Back pain at the index level
Core of the nerve	100	100	Referred pain, often proximal dermatomal, often not conforming to dermatomal patterns
Superior foraminal ligament	88	0	None
Superior foraminal ligament impingement	53	100	Secondary nerve root referred pain
Superior notch osteophytes	34	0	None
Superior notch osteophyte impingement	34	100	Secondary nerve root referred pain
Superior foraminal ligament - nerve tethering	48	100	Secondary nerve root referred pain
Ligamentum flavum (infolded)	82	0	
Posterior foraminal ligament - separated from ligamentum flavum	47	2	Local backache
Facet joint capsule - separated from posterior foraminal ligament	18	4	Local backache
Ascending facet joint - nerve tethering (incidence)	100		
Ascending facet joint - nerve tethering - inflamed	58		Secondary nerve root referred pain
Ascending facet joint impaction	74	74	Secondary nerve root referred pain
Disc pad (irritated)	15	15	Backache + axial radiation
Disc pad (no inflammation)	25	2	Mild backache
Posterior longitudinal ligament irritation without disc pad inflammation	9	5	Backache + axial radiation
Safe working zone (no inflammation)	23	3	Mild discomfort
Safe working zone (irritated)	11	11	Local backache
Superior notch engorgement	32	0	
Quiescent annulus	66	0	
Annular irritation	29	29	Back pain
Intradiscal pain on manipulation	5	5	Back pain
Foraminal annulus - nerve tethering	62	59	Secondary nerve root referred pain
Unexpected foraminal bulge	32		See annular irritation
Annular tears	37		Secondary nerve root referred pain
Dorsal vertebral osteophytic nerve tethering			Transiting nerve distribution
Shoulder osteophytic nerve tethering	20	20	Secondary nerve root referred pain
Lateral osteophytic nerve - tethering with medial displacement	9	7	Secondary nerve root referred pain
Intertransverse ligament and muscle - nerve entrapment	3	2	Secondary nerve root referred pain
Inferior external pedicular tethering	17	9	Secondary nerve root referred pain
Paravertebral bone graft nerve tethering	4	4	Exiting nerve irritation
Post-fusion disc inflammation	8	6	Local back pain
Fusion instrumentation - nerve tethering	2	2	Exiting nerve irritation
Peridural scarring with irritation	8	2	Mild backache
Perineural scarring with irritation	63	60	Secondary nerve root referred pain

Discussion

The use of the lumbar posterolateral approach in patients in the aware or semiconscious state affords the opportunity to examine structures in the extraforaminal zone, the foramen, the anterior epidural space, the annulus, and the interstices of the disc. It has allowed the mapping of pain arising directly from these structures and analysis of the effect of their impingement upon the exiting nerve.

Neural Responses

The medial border of the nerve produces pain in a local distribution, predominantly evoking back pain with radiation around the facet joint, into the paravertebral muscle or buttock.

The distribution differs at each segmental level. The core of the nerve, by contrast, evokes pain of a distribution that mimics various combinations of the given and adjacent segmental level dermatomes. When the nerve exhibits obvious visual signs of irritation, the symptoms evoked by pressure are more global and often involve the whole limb.

In Fig. 66.13a, the core of the nerve has been decompressed of the impacting facet joint. The nerve is partially covered by mobilised epidural fat. In (**b**), the nerve has been laterally displaced. Endoscopy allows discrete areas of the nerve to be gently probed and the elicited response recorded.

Facet Joint Mimicry

Symptoms evoked from the medial border of the nerve mimic those thus far attributed to the facet joint. These findings

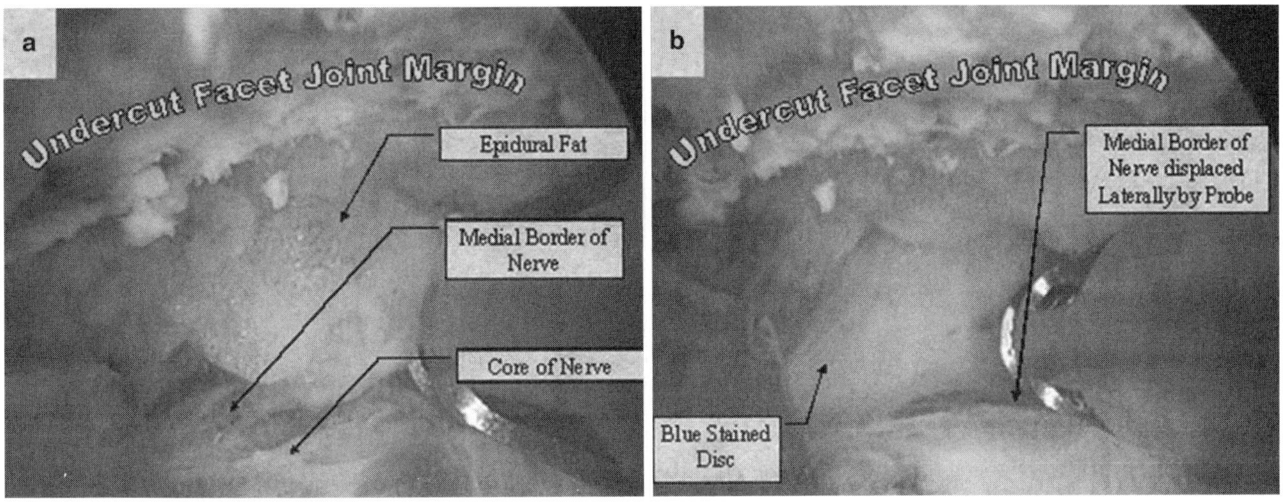

Fig. 66.13 Endoscopic view of exiting nerve before and after displacement

suggest that the benefit arising from facet joint steroid injections may be a reflection of the effect of the steroid upon the nerve tethered anteriorly. The corollary is that where facet joint injections offer temporary relief, endoscopic mobilisation of the nerve and removal of local nerve root impaction may offer longer-term resolution of symptoms.

Neural Displacement and Impaction

Medial displacement of the nerve is noted frequently, arising because of adhesion to the facet joint, epidural scarring, or lateral or shoulder osteophytosis. This displacement results in unavoidable impaction by the SFL, contained osteophytes, or the ascending facet joint.

Foraminal Annular Bulging and Tethering

Small bulges in the foramen may go undetected on non-weight-bearing MRI scans. Endoscopically, these bulges may be manifest as little more than an area of weakness in the annular wall. This can be seen to bulge preferentially during extension of the lumbar spine during the procedure. The effect of the bulge is amplified where the nerve is tethered to the disc, where it causes direct distortion of the trapped nerve. The bulge also causes a disproportionate effect where the nerve is trapped to the facet joint proximally and to the external border of the inferior pedicle distally.

Shoulder Osteophytes

The presence of a concomitant shoulder osteophyte adds further local tethering but with marked local irritation and neural sensitivity at the point of impact.

Facet Joint Impaction and Instability

The nerve is frequently noted adherent to the ascending facet joint and the SFL. Where there is loss of disc turgor, micromovements may occur, allowing these structures to impact upon the exiting nerve with consequent irritation and propensity to evoke pain. As loss of disc height occurs, overriding of the ascending facet joint increases in patients with capsular strain. Predisposition to overriding may be linked to the orientation of the facet joints. Overriding exposes the apex of the ascending facet joint and increases the impaction upon the nerve root, especially where the disc is triangular and preferentially extends during extension. The effect is enhanced where the nerve is tethered to the facet joint or medially displaced into the path of the facet joint by perineural scarring. This process of impaction provides an explanation of the causation of symptoms so often termed *instability*.

Annular Response

Intriguingly, less than a quarter of the patients reported pain when the annulus was directly probed or the interstices of the disc or the endplate were manipulated. This contrasts to the generally held precept that back pain arises from discogenic pain or endplate margin irritation or annular irritation promoted by instability.

Perineural Scarring

Post-operative perineural scarring aggravates tethering between the nerve and the ascending facet joint, SFL, or the annulus. By spreading into the SWZ, it may distort the pathway of the nerve medially. The scarring may involve the anterior and lateral aspects of the dura, causing irritation of the descending nerve. The scarring may extend dorsally and contralaterally, but ELF only allows limited exploration of these zones. Endoscopy reveals that post-operative perineural scarring can spread through the foramen, often replacing local tethering with thick stiff scar with great entrapment of the nerve. This is associated in most cases with irritation of the nerve and sensitivity to pain. The area of nerve irritation is often discrete and confined to the area of scarring. Distal or proximal sections of the nerve may be swollen but be of normal colour and sensitivity to probing.

Shortcomings of MRI Scans

The presence of these pathologies may account for the shortcomings in sensitivity and specificity of MRI scans because unloaded scans may be unable to detect many small foraminal bulges and tethering of the nerve to the ascending facet joint and the SFL. Awareness of shoulder osteophytes may allow these to be detected on MRI scans on occasions, thus increasing diagnostic accuracy.

MRI Scan Underestimation of Irritated Epidural and Foraminal Tissues

MRI scans underestimate the degree of scarring encountered endoscopically, especially where this is inspected more than 3 years after the onset of attributed symptoms. The clinical effect of foraminal scarring is underestimated by the MRI scan results, seemingly because the volume of the foramen is small and definition between the enclosed structures and bone margins is compromised by their coaption. It also arises particularly in patients with mature scarring, where gadolinium enhancement is subdued, especially as the sectional length of nerve irritation in cases of impaction or post-operative perineural scarring is usually discrete and short. MRI scans fail to detect the irritation found in the SWZ, PLL, or in the disc pad.

Conclusions

Abnormal micro-movements combined with tethering and malalignment of the nerve are associated with discrete areas of nerve irritation resulting from impaction by the ascending facet joint, SFL, foraminal annulus, and shoulder osteophytes. Less frequently, irritation of the annulus and the disc interstices may contribute to the production of back pain.

Indifferent outcomes after technically satisfactory conventional nerve root decompression or fusion may reflect a failure to treat these unrecognised foraminal pathologies.

Lateral peridural scarring may be dense but not associated with such mechanically provoking tethering and irritation as that which constrains the nerve in the foramen. Clinically significant sections of scarring appear to be related to areas of concomitant foraminal narrowing and tethering. This offers the opportunity that minimalist techniques addressing the foramen may effect symptom amelioration without the need for the wider exposure required by conventional techniques. The posterolateral approach increases the foraminal volume more effectively than medial decompression.

The foramen is a space, the volume of which is dictated by the congenital construct of the pedicles and impingement resulting from facet joint hypertrophy, overriding and osteophytosis, ligamentous impaction from the SFL, infolding LF, redundant disc, and dorsal and shoulder osteophytes (Fig. 66.14). The nerve may become tethered to these structures and medially displaced into the pathway of the ascending facet. Such tethering is aggravated by short perineural fibrosis.

The foramen and contents are subject to flexion, extension, and rotatory motion. These are distorted by loss of disc turgor, retrolisthesis, and anterior olisthesis. The nerve is subjected to combinations of traction and impaction within the same foramen. The nerve itself can produce back pain when the medial border is irritated, and a mixture of conventional dermatomal patterns arise from the core.

Failure to appreciate and treat these mechanisms and pathological entities may account for persisting symptoms after midline surgery. Their presence raises the possibility of effective diagnosis by probing the foraminal structures and effective remedy of back pain and referred pain by their discrete and precise treatment.

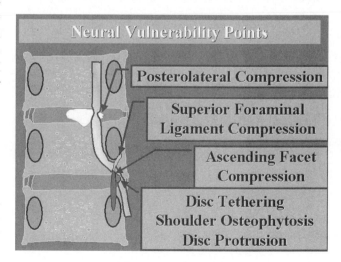

Fig. 66.14 Diagrammatic synopsis of foraminal pain sources highlighted by endoscopy

The provocative effect of these foraminal pathologies calls into question the conventional precept that a posterolateral disc protrusion at the level above the exiting nerve root foramen is causal of particular dermatomal symptoms. This is particularly likely to result in misdiagnosis in cases of multilevel degeneration. The clinical relevance of these factors and the diagnostic benefits of SP and D and ΔD will be evaluated in future publications.

Chapter 67
Minimally Invasive Thoracic Microendoscopic Discectomy

Kurt M. Eichholz, John E. O'Toole, Griffin R. Myers, and Richard G. Fessler

Thoracic disc herniations present the spine surgeon with a distinctive set of challenges with regard to patient selection, surgical anatomy, and potential complications. The reported incidences of thoracic disc herniations range from 1 in 1,000 to 1 in 1,000,000[1-3] and are decreased in comparison with those of their cervical and lumbar counterparts; this is likely a result of the increased rigidity of the thoracic cage, which results in a reduction in the flexion, extension, and rotation of the thoracic spine.[4,5] Notwithstanding this decreased incidence and the even smaller number of patients who ultimately require surgical intervention, patients with thoracic disc herniations may present with a wide variety of symptoms. Furthermore, a multitude of surgical approaches have been developed to treat these patients, including posterior (laminectomy), posterolateral (costotransversectomy, transfacet pedicles-sparing discectomy, transpedicular discectomy, and transversoartropediculectomy), lateral (extracavitary, rachiotomy), transthoracic (transpleural, extrapleural, and transsternal), and thoracoscopic approaches. This wide spectrum of therapeutic options, coupled with the relatively low incidence of operable pathologies, is a testament to the difficulty a spine surgeon faces when attempting to treat patients with thoracic disc herniations.

Obviously each of these surgical approaches has its characteristic advantages and disadvantages. Anterior and lateral approaches, for example, allow for maximal access to the intervertebral disc and vertebral body while introducing additional risk to the thoracic contents. Conversely, posterior approaches, while inherently safer with respect to the thoracic organs, demand larger incisions and the removal of larger amounts of bone, which can result in significant blood loss, paraspinal pain, and potential mechanical instability. Whatever the chosen approach, the surgical treatment of a thoracic disc herniation risks a variety of complications. The thoracic cord does not carry as significant a risk of spinal root injury when compared with the cervical or lumbar regions; however, the thoracic spine, especially the more rostral portion, is a vascular watershed region, which leaves it susceptible to ischemic injury. In the worst cases, damage to this tenuous vascular supply can result in paraplegia.

Given this multitude of suboptimal therapeutic options and their corresponding risks, a new approach to the surgical repair of thoracic disc herniations has been developed. The thoracic microendoscopic discectomy (TMED) is a modification of the lumbar microendoscopic technique that has been used with great success in treatment of numerous pathologies of the lumbar spine, including stenosis,[6] disc herniations,[7] and instability.[8,9] The TMED procedure allows the surgeon to repair thoracic herniations via a minimally invasive posterior approach and has been shown to result in significant decreases in blood loss, hospital stay, postoperative pain, and recovery time. This chapter will explore the indications and patient selection criteria for TMED, the details of the surgical technique, and its risks and benefits in treatment of thoracic disc herniations.

Indications and Patient Selection

As with all surgical interventions, patient selection is of prime importance. In the case of thoracic disc herniations, a detailed history is required, with special attention paid to recent traumas, infections, or signs of malignancy. Additionally, a complete physical exam must be performed, with emphasis on focal sensory deficits in the thoracic region. Lateral herniations are expected to cause pain that radiates laterally around the thorax, and central herniations are expected to result in myelopathy with spastic paraparesis of the lower extremities. However, in practice, symptomatology may vary; for example, herpes zoster can mimic this radiculopathy, as can metastatic lesions.

Indeed, a review of the literature suggests that thoracic disc herniations may present with wide variation. Eleraky described three patients with presenting symptoms resembling those of cardiac disease: an intense, stabbing back pain that radiated to the lateral chest wall. After negative results from cardiac workups, magnetic resonance imaging (MRI)

K.M. Eichholz, J.E. O'Toole, G.R. Myers, and R.G. Fessler (✉)
Department of Neurosurgery, Feinberg School of Medicine,
Northwestern University, 303 East Chicago Avenue, ChicagoIL,
60611-3008, USA
e-mail: RFessler@nmff.org

results demonstrated significant thoracic disc herniations.[10] Georges described a patient with colicky pain not unlike that of renal stones, which was later proven a result of a calcified T11–12 disc herniation.[11] Other authors have cited unilateral paresis of the abdominal wall musculature.[12] Neurogenic claudication, most commonly attributable to lumbar stenosis, has also been described as a presenting symptom of thoracic herniations.[13,14] Xiong reported the case of a woman with abdominopelvic pain whose gynecologic studies demonstrated endomyometritis; after an unsuccessful course of nonsteroidal anti-inflammatory drugs and narcotics, the patient underwent a T9–10 laminectomy and discectomy with dramatic improvement.[15] One patient, described by Bunning, suffered recurrent dislocation of his total hip prosthesis due to spasticity caused by a thoracic disc herniation and its resultant myelopathy.[16] An acute herniation was reported to present with a sudden, flaccid paraplegia,[17] while a chronic incidence caused symptoms during a 10-year period with the rotatory movement provoked by a golf swing.[18] Thoracic disc herniations have been reported in association with Scheuermann's disease[19,20] and as a result of chiropractic manipulation.[21] Furthermore, up to 37% of asymptomatic patients have been shown to have significant thoracic disc herniations.[22–26]

As a result of these varied presentations and the high incidence in asymptomatic patients, the surgeon must correlate the patient's history and physical examination findings with the corresponding radiographic details in making the diagnosis of thoracic disc herniation. Examples of such radiographic findings are given in Figs. 67.1 and 67.2, which demonstrate sagittal and axial T2-weighted MRI images of a patient with a symptomatic disc herniation at T6–7.

Surgical Intervention

Thoracic disc herniations have been treated with numerous surgical approaches yielding variable success. Posterior approaches, while familiar, lack the ability of the surgeon to retract the thecal sac below the conus, as these approaches do in the lumbar region. Moreover, the thoracic spinal cord is highly susceptible to injury with only minimal retraction. This fact precludes direct lateral approaches to the thoracic spine, because they do not allow for access to the central portions of the intervertebral disc. Posterolateral approaches, including the costotransversectomy and the transpedicular approach, require removal of supporting bone structure from the vertebral column, and, while this approach allows safer access to more centrally located disc herniations, the amount of bone that must be removed may be a cause of significant postoperative pain and morbidity. Lateral and anterior approaches necessarily allow greater access to the disc with

minimal risk to the spinal cord, though it comes at the expense of increased risk to the vital structures of the thoracic cavity. Transthoracic approaches have been reported to cause disabling intercostal neuralgia in 50% of patients and atelectasis and pulmonary dysfunction in 33%, although studies have shown improvements to 16% and 7%, respec-

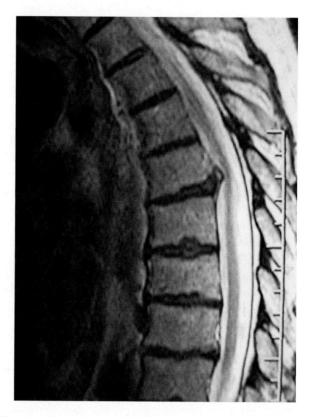

Fig. 67.1 Sagittal T2-weighted MRI of a patient with a T6–7 disk herniation

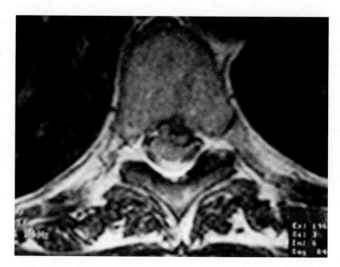

Fig. 67.2 Axial T2-weighted MRI of a patient with a T6–7 disk herniation

tively, when a thoracoscopic approach is taken. Additional complications to these anterior approaches include pleural effusion, pulmonary contusion, hemothorax, and chylothorax.[27–29]

Surgical Technique

The surgical technique for TMED is a modification of the same microendoscopic technique that is used successfully in the lumbar spine.[7] The procedure is conducted using general anesthesia with the patient positioned prone on a radiolucent Wilson frame mounted on a Jackson table. The Jackson table is preferred in this case to facilitate use of the C-arm fluoroscope when necessary. The patient's arms are positioned above the patient with care to avoid extension beyond 90°. Continuous somatosensory evoked potential monitoring is utilized during the procedure, and the endoscope and fluoroscope monitors are positioned opposite the surgeon to facilitate visualization. Localization of the appropriate operative spinal level is of critical importance; to ensure accuracy, the authors utilize lateral and anterior-posterior fluoroscopy to twice count the spinal level from either the occiput or the sacrum.

Once the appropriate spinal level has been identified, a superficial skin incision is made 3–4 cm lateral to the midline. In larger patients, a more lateral approach may be prudent to reduce manipulation of the spinal cord during disc removal. A K-wire is introduced at the superior aspect of the caudal transverse process at the spinal level of interest, and a series of tubular muscle dilators are then placed over the K-wire under fluoroscopic guidance. A tubular retractor is placed over the final dilator and attached to a table-mounted flexible arm. Next, a rigid endoscope with a 30° lens is attached to the tubular retractor; this endoscope is oriented in such a manner that the medial anatomy appears at the top of the monitor, and the lateral anatomy at the bottom. This orients the rostrocaudal axis and allows the surgeon parallel visualization of the endoscope monitor and the operative field. It is imperative that the surgeon maintains proper visual orientation throughout the procedure, because failure to do so may lead to inadvertent entry into the spinal canal. Figure 67.3 contains an endoscopic view with the proper rostrocaudal orientation of the exposed disc space.

With the endoscope suitably placed, the muscle and soft tissue overlying the field is extracted with an insulated monopolar electrocautery. This exposure yields the proximal transverse process and lateral facet, and, as before, the placement of the dilator in the mediolateral axis based upon patient body habitus is essential in minimizing manipulation of the spinal cord. Using a long, tapered high-speed drill, the rostral aspect of the inferior transverse process and lateral facet are removed. This maneuver reveals the pedicle of the caudal

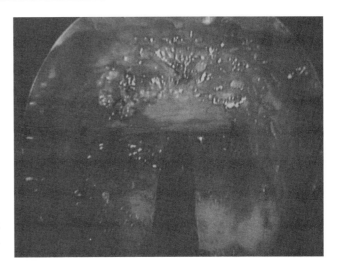

Fig. 67.3 Intraoperative endoscopic visualization of surgical field during a right-sided approach for a T6–7 microendoscopic discectomy. The spinal cord is labeled. For endoscopic orientation: *R* rostal; *C* caudal; *L* lateral; *M* medial

vertebral body, which is followed ventrally to the level of the disc space. At this point, the superior aspect of this pedicle may be removed with the drill to facilitate entry into the disc space.

Once the disc space has been exposed, the annulus is incised using an annulotomy knife. The herniated disc fragment is then removed using a combination of curettes and pituitary rongeurs. The oblique lateromedial trajectory of the retractor, in combination with the 30° angle of the endoscope, allows for direct access to the intervertebral disc space without manipulation of the spinal cord or other neural elements. Using this technique, lateral disc herniations can be removed under direct visualization. Conversely, medial disc herniations require the use of a downgoing curette or Woodson elevator to direct the fragment into the disc space; this allows it to be safely removed from the lateral annulotomy, again without manipulation of the spinal cord.

Once the herniated portion of the disc is removed, the operative field is copiously irrigated, and thorough hemostasis is achieved. The retractor is removed, and the thoracodorsal fascia is closed with a suture. Interrupted subcutaneous sutures are placed, and the skin is closed with adhesive glue.

Discussion

As with any surgical intervention, the potential for complication exists. This potential in endoscopic procedures is considered to be a result of the surgeons' relative lack of familiarity with the minimally invasive techniques, because most complications occur during the initial steep phase of the learning curve. Most neurosurgeons performing spinal procedures lack experience with endoscopic techniques, which demands unique hand-eye coordination. The surgeon must adapt to the use of longer instruments, which provide significantly less tactile feedback, and the two-dimensional endoscopic monitor lacks the depth of field offered by most surgical microscopes. These factors, along with the technical skill required, present the potential for complication. One potential complication of note is dural violation. Using the minimally invasive technique, notably including the muscle-splitting retractors, the incidence of pseudomeningocele is significantly lower than when performing open surgery.[30] However, when it does occur in the thoracic region, dural violation is more likely to result in neural injury.

Other less invasive posterolateral approaches have been proposed to repair thoracic disc herniations. Stillerman et al.[31] described the transfacet pedicle-sparing approach, which utilizes a 4-cm incision to remove the medial facet complex in which an open rigid endoscope may be used to assist in the discectomy. This approach avoids the need for a chest tube and has a reduced incidence of pulmonary complication. Stillerman later advocated for the pedicle-sparing approach over a transpedicular approach due to the decreased destruction of bone and soft tissue and the resultant improvement in postoperative back pain. Jho followed suit in describing an endoscopic transpedicular approach to thoracic herniations that utilizes a 2-cm incision to allow for stripping of the muscle from the lamina and face with a periosteal elevator. A drill is then used to remove the lateral lamina, medial facet, and one third of the pedicle; a 70° endoscope can be used to facilitate in the discectomy.[32] The TMED described here utilizes a more lateral trajectory and a 30° endoscope, which allows for improved visualization without compromising the surgeon's orientation.

TMED is a safe and effective surgical approach to treatment of thoracic disc herniations. This procedure grants surgical access via a minimally invasive, muscle-splitting posterolateral approach that avoids risk to the thoracic contents. TMED offers exposure and visualization equal to that of similar open techniques, such as costotransversectomy and the transpedicular approach, while minimizing the morbidity resulting from their associated muscle dissection.

Microendoscopic discectomy has proven effective in the lumbar spine with shorter length of stay, less postoperative pain, decreased blood loss, and shorter recovery time. These same advantages can be expected in the thoracic spine given appropriate patient selection and proper surgical technique.

References

1. Arce CA, Dohrmann GJ. Thoracic disc herniation. Improved diagnosis with computed tomographic scanning and a review of the literature. *Surg Neurol*. 1985;23(4):356–361

2. Brown CW, Deffer PA Jr, Akmakjian J, Donaldson DH, Brugman JL. The natural history of thoracic disc herniation. *Spine*. 1992;17(6 Suppl):S97–S102

3. Stillerman CB, Chen TC, Couldwell WT, et al. Transfacet pedicle-sparing approach. In: Benzel EC, Stillerman CB (eds), *The Thoracic Spine*. St. Louis: Quality Medical, 1999, pp. 338–345

4. Adams MA, Hutton WC. Prolapsed intervertebral disc. A hyperflexion injury 1981 Volvo Award in Basic Science. *Spine*. 1982;7(3):184–191

5. White AA, Panjabi MM. *Clinical Biomechanics of the Spine*. Philadelphia: Lippincott, 1990

6. Khoo LT, Fessler RG. Microendoscopic decompressive laminotomy for the treatment of lumbar stenosis. *Neurosurgery*. 2002;51(5 Suppl):S146–S154

7. Perez-Cruet MJ, Foley KT, Isaacs RE, et al. Microendoscopic lumbar discectomy: technical note. *Neurosurgery*. 2002;51(5 Suppl):S129–S136

8. Fessler RG. Minimally invasive percutaneous posterior lumbar interbody fusion. *Neurosurgery*. 2003;52(6):1512

9. Isaacs RE, Podichetty VK, Santiago P, et al. Minimally invasive microendoscopy-assisted transforaminal lumbar interbody fusion with instrumentation. *J Neurosurg Spine*. 2005;3(2):98–105

10. Eleraky MA, Apostolides PJ, Dickman CA, Sonntag VK. Herniated thoracic discs mimic cardiac disease: three case reports. *Acta Neurochir (Wien)*. 1998;140(7):643–646

11. Georges C, Toledano C, Zagdanski AM, et al. Thoracic disk herniation mimicking renal crisis. *Eur J Intern Med*. 2004;15(1):59–61

12. Meyer F, Feldmann H, Toppich H, Celiker A. [Unilateral paralysis of the abdominal wall musculature caused by thoracic intervertebral disk displacement]. *Zentralbl Neurochir*. 1991;52(3):137–139. [German]

13. Hufnagel A, Zierski J, Agnoli L, Schutz HJ. [Spinal claudication caused by thoracic intervertebral disk displacement]. *Nervenarzt*. 1988;59(7):419–421. [German]

14. Morgenlander JC, Massey EW. Neurogenic claudication with positionally dependent weakness from a thoracic disk herniation. *Neurology*. 1989;39(8):1133–1134

15. Xiong Y, Lachmann E, Marini S, Nagler W. Thoracic disk herniation presenting as abdominal and pelvic pain: a case report. *Arch Phys Med Rehabil*. 2001;82(8):1142–1144

16. Bunning RD, Witten CM. Thoracic disk herniation and recurrent dislocation of total hip prosthesis. *South Med J*. 1992;85(4):416–418

17. Hamilton MG, Thomas HG. Intradural herniation of a thoracic disc presenting as flaccid paraplegia: case report. *Neurosurgery*. 1990;27(3):482–484

18. Jamieson DR, Ballantyne JP. Unique presentation of a prolapsed thoracic disk: Lhermitte's symptom in a golf player. *Neurology*. 1995;45(6):1219–1221

19. Kapetanos GA, Hantzidis PT, Anagnostidis KS, Kirkos JM. Thoracic cord compression caused by disk herniation in Scheuermann's disease: a case report and review of the literature. *Eur Spine J*. 19 2006:1–6

20. Lesoin F, Leys D, Rousseaux M, et al. Thoracic disk herniation and Scheuermann's disease. *Eur Neurol*. 1987;26(3):145–152

21. Lanska DJ, Lanska MJ, Fenstermaker R, Selman W, Mapstone T. Thoracic disk herniation associated with chiropractic spinal manipulation. *Arch Neurol*. 1987;44(10):996–997

22. Carson J, Gumpert J, Jefferson A. Diagnosis and treatment of thoracic intervertebral disc protrusions. *J Neurol Neurosurg Psychiatry*. 1971;34(1):68–77

23. Love JG, Schorn VG. Thoracic-disk protrusions. *JAMA*. 1965;191:627–631

24. Russell T. Thoracic intervertebral disc protrusion: experience of 67 cases and review of the literature. *Br J Neurosurg*. 1989;3(2):153–160

25. Wood KB, Blair JM, Aepple DM, et al. The natural history of asymptomatic thoracic disc herniations. *Spine*. 1997;22(5): 525–529; discussion 529–530
26. Wood KB, Garvey TA, Gundry C, Heithoff KB. Magnetic resonance imaging of the thoracic spine. Evaluation of asymptomatic individuals. *J Bone Joint Surg Am*. 1995;77(11):1631–1638
27. Bohlman HH, Zdeblick TA. Anterior excision of herniated thoracic discs. *J Bone Joint Surg Am*. 1988;70(7):1038–1047
28. Faciszewski T, Winter RB, Lonstein JE, Denis F, Johnson L. The surgical and medical perioperative complications of anterior spinal fusion surgery in the thoracic and lumbar spine in adults. A review of 1223 procedures. *Spine*. 1995;20(14):1592–1599
29. Fessler RG, Sturgill M. Review: complications of surgery for thoracic disc disease. *Surg Neurol*. 1998;49(6):609–618
30. Perez-Cruet MJ, Smith M, Foley K. Microendoscopic lumbar discectomy. In: Perez-Cruet MJ, Fessler, RG (eds), *Outpatient Spinal Surgery*. St. Louis: Quality Medical Publishing, Inc., 2002, pp. 171–183
31. Stillerman CB, Chen TC, Day JD, Couldwell WT, Weiss MH. The transfacet pedicle-sparing approach for thoracic disc removal: cadaveric morphometric analysis and preliminary clinical experience. *J Neurosurg*. 1995;83(6):971–976
32. Jho HD. Endoscopic transpedicular thoracic discectomy. *J Neurosurg*. 1999;91(2 Suppl):151–156

Chapter 68
Minimally Invasive Cervical Foraminotomy and Decompression of Stenosis

John E. O'Toole, Kurt M. Eichholz, and Richard G. Fessler

Many types of degenerative cervical spine disease can be treated with well-established posterior decompressive procedures.[1–4] Even as anterior cervical procedures have gained prominence, posterior cervical laminoforaminotomy still provides symptomatic relief in 92–97% of patients with radiculopathy from foraminal stenosis or lateral herniated discs.[3, 5] Similarly, posterior cervical decompression for cervical stenosis achieves neurological improvement in 62.5–83% of myelopathic patients undergoing either laminectomy or laminoplasty.[4, 6–8] Moreover, these operations avoid the complications attendant to anterior approaches to the cervical spine, namely, esophageal injury, vascular injury, recurrent laryngeal nerve paralysis, dysphagia, and accelerated degeneration of adjacent motion segments after fusion.[9–11]

However, open posterior approaches to the cervical spine require extensive subperiosteal stripping of the paraspinal musculature that leads to postoperative pain, spasm, and dysfunction and can be persistently disabling in 18–60% of patients.[4, 9, 12, 13] Furthermore, preoperative loss of lordosis combined with long-segment decompression increases the risk for postoperative sagittal plane deformity,[14–17] a complication that frequently prompts instrumented arthrodesis at the time of laminectomy. Employing these extensive posterior fusion techniques increases operative time, surgical risks, and blood loss; exacerbates early postoperative pain; and potentially contributes to adjacent level degeneration.

The fundamental tenet of minimal access techniques is reduction of approach-related morbidity. To that end, the advent of muscle-splitting tubular retractor systems and improvements in endoscopic technology and associated instruments have allowed for the application of minimally invasive techniques to posterior cervical decompressive procedures.[13, 18] The microendoscopic cervical foraminotomy/discectomy (CMEF/D) was first described in a cadaver model and demonstrated the ability to achieve equivalent bone removal and nerve root exposure when directly compared with open technique.[19, 20] The reports of CMEF/D used

clinically[9, 13, 21] have demonstrated that efficacy is equivalent to open cases (87–97% rate of symptom relief) but that blood loss, length of stay, and postoperative pain medication usage are all reduced in CMEF/D cases. We have recently reviewed clinical outcomes after CMEF/D using validated outcome instruments in a prospective cohort of 30 patients (unpublished data). In these patients, mean Visual Analog Scale (VAS) scores decreased from 2.0 to 0.6 for headache, 5.0 to 2.1 for neck pain, and 4.8 to 1.9 for arm pain. Mean Neck Disability Index scores improved from 37.7 to 20.8, and mean Short Form-36 scores showed statistically significant improvements for bodily pain, physical function, and role physical subscales. The mean operative blood loss was 80 mL, and the mean hospital stay for the cohort was 10 h. When added to the collected literature to date, this data establish CMEF/D as a safe, effective, minimally invasive outpatient procedure for the treatment of isolated cervical radiculopathy.

The feasibility of minimal access multilevel laminectomy and laminoplasty techniques was also first demonstrated in cadaver models.[22, 23] In separate studies, both techniques demonstrated a 43% expansion of the cross-sectional area of the spinal canal.[16, 22, 23] Clinical application of minimally invasive posterior cervical decompression for stenosis, however, has not been studied as extensively as CMEF/D. The use of minimally invasive cervical laminoplasty has been reported in four patients as technically safe and feasible with a mean improvement of 1.25 points on the Nurick Scale postoperatively.[22] The authors of the minimally invasive laminoplasty studies have noted technical difficulties associated with elevating the lamina and inserting bone grafts.

Cervical microendoscopic decompression of stenosis (CMEDS), on the other hand, is based on more familiar techniques that have already been applied to lumbar stenosis.[24] By preserving much of the normal osteoligamentous anatomy of the cervical spine, the CMEDS procedure reduces the risk for post-laminectomy kyphosis as well as problems associated with the post-laminectomy membrane.[4, 16] Yabuki et al.[25] published their series of ten patients operated upon for cervical spondylotic myelopathy utilizing the endoscopic METRx system (Medtronic Sofamor Danek, Memphis, TN). Using bilateral dilations and laminotomies to remove dorsal bony

J.E. O'Toole (✉), K.M. Eichholz, and R.G. Fessler
Department of Neurosurgery, Rush University Medical Center, 1725 West Harrison Street, Suite 970, Chicago, IL, 60612, USA
e-mail: john_otoole@rush.edu

G.R. Scuderi and A.J. Tria (eds.), *Minimally Invasive Surgery in Orthopedics*,
DOI 10.1007/978-0-387-76608-9_68, © Springer Science+Business Media, LLC 2010

and ligamentous compression, they treated up to two levels of stenosis and reported a mean operative time of 164 min, a mean blood loss of 45 mL, and mean posterior neck VAS scores of 2.8 on postoperative day 1 and 0.8 on postoperative day 3.[25] Although no control group was presented, the authors anecdotally thought that the decrease in postoperative neck pain compared with open procedures was dramatic. At a mean of 15 months of follow-up, patients had a mean improvement in their Japanese Orthopedic Association score of 2.5 points. They had no complications, postoperative instability, or need for reoperation.[25]

In an effort to preserve the contralateral bony and ligamentous structures and perform only one muscle dilation, we have adopted the *unilateral* approach to CMEDS as described below. Perez-Cruet and the senior author (RGF) have previously reported on five patients undergoing CMEDS at one, two, or three levels.[16] All patients demonstrated improvement in their myelopathy and returned to work with the only complication being one unintended durotomy that sealed spontaneously.

Indications

CMEF/D is indicated for radiculopathy due to lateral disc herniations or foraminal stenosis (single or multilevel) (Fig. 68.1), persistent or recurrent root symptoms after anterior cervical discectomy and fusion, and cervical disc disease in patients for whom anterior approaches are relatively contraindicated (anterior neck infection, tracheostomy, prior

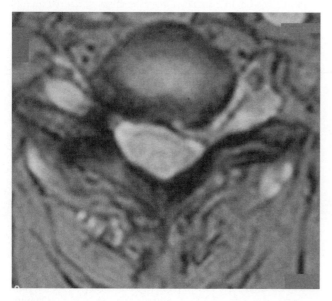

Fig. 68.1 Axial T2-weighted cervical spine MRI results demonstrate a laterally herniated disc to the left with resultant effacement of the lateral thecal sac and compression of the exiting nerve root

irradiation, or previous radical neck surgery for neoplasm).[13] CMEDS is indicated for central spondylotic stenosis (e.g., ligamentum flavum or facet hypertrophy) in patients presenting with myelopathy or myeloradiculopathy. The neurological symptoms should correlate with radiographic findings.

Contraindications to these procedures include pure axial neck pain without neurological symptoms, gross cervical instability, symptomatic central disc herniation, excessive burden of ventral disease (e.g., diffuse ossification of the posterior longitudinal ligament [OPLL]) or a kyphotic deformity that would make posterior decompression ineffective, or an inability to tolerate general anesthesia.

Preoperative Evaluation

The preoperative radiographic evaluation follows a detailed history and physical examination and should include magnetic resonance imaging (MRI) or post-myelographic computed tomography (CT) scans, and anteroposterior (AP), lateral, and dynamic cervical radiographs. Preoperative electromyography (EMG) and nerve conduction studies may also assist in the neurological localization of specific radiculopathy.

Equipment

The CMEF/D and CMEDS techniques described below require the following specific equipment: (1) Mayfield or other head fixation device compatible with the sitting position; (2) tubular retractor system with compatible endoscope; (3) endoscopic camera system with appropriate monitor; (4) endoscopic spinal instruments (including microcurettes and 1- and 2-mm rongeurs); and (5) intraoperative fluoroscopy.

Setup

General endotracheal anesthesia is induced with fiberoptic intubation employed in patients with chronic spinal cord compression. Somatosensory evoked potentials (SSEP) and myotomal EMG are monitored throughout the case. An arterial line is often helpful to maintain normotension with the patient in the sitting position in order to avoid spinal cord hypoperfusion. A precordial Doppler may be used to monitor for air embolism, although this has not presented a problem to date likely due to the fact that, given the small exposure, the risk of air embolism is very low. Foley catheterization is generally not needed. Routine perioperative antibiotics are administered as is an intravenous corticosteroid at the surgeon's discretion. Paralytic agents are minimized after induction to allow for physical intraoperative feedback of nerve root irritation. The table is then turned 180° relative to the anesthesia station. The patient is placed in Mayfield three-point head fixation, and the table progressively flexed and put into Trendelenburg to bring the patient into a semisitting position such that head is flexed but not rotated and the posterior neck is perpendicular to the floor (Fig. 68.2). The sitting position confers the advantages of decreased blood pooling in the operative field, decreased blood loss, decreased operative times, and gravity-dependent positioning of the shoulders for better lateral fluoroscopic images.[9, 13] The Mayfield is secured to a table-mounted cross-bar, and the patient's arms are folded across the lap or chest depending upon body habitus. The legs, hands, and arms are well padded, particularly over the cubital tunnel to prevent positional ulnar neuropathy. The fluoroscopic and endoscopic monitors are placed next to the head of the patient opposite the side of approach so that the surgeon can look directly at the monitors while standing behind the patient and operating through the tubular retractor at a comfortable height. The base of the fluoroscopic C-arm is placed on the side ipsilateral to the surgical approach. The C-arm

may be arranged beneath (Fig. 68.2), above, or in front of the patient, depending upon the design specifics of the C-arm and operating table, and whether or not AP images will be needed during the case. The neck is checked a final time to ensure the position allows adequate jugular venous drainage and airway patency.

Technique Description

This section outlines the technique for posterior CMEF/D[5, 9, 13, 18] and CMEDS.[16, 22, 25] The procedures described here utilize the METRx retractor and endoscope system (Medtronic Sofamor Danek, Memphis, TN); however, the principles are the same regardless of the retractor system used.

Prior to draping, an initial fluoroscopic image is acquired to confirm adequate visualization and to plan the initial entry point. The posterior neck is shaved, scrubbed, prepared, and draped in the usual manner. It is helpful to use adhesive lined drapes and/or an antibacterial adhesive layer such as Ioban (3M Health Care, St. Paul, MN) to maintain the orientation and position of the drapes during the procedure. Suction tubing, cautery lines, and endoscope light source and camera cables are typically draped over the top or side of the field and secured against the drapes. The operative level(s) is once again confirmed on lateral fluoroscopy while a long K-wire or Steinman pin is held over the lateral side of the patient's neck. A 1.8-cm longitudinal incision is marked out approximately 1.5 cm off the midline on the operative side, and this is injected with local anesthesia. For two-level procedures, the incision should be placed midway between the targeted levels. For bilateral procedures, a midline skin incision can be used and the skin retracted to each side for independent dilations. After an initial stab incision, the K-wire is advanced slowly though the musculature under fluoroscopic guidance and docked at the inferomedial edge of the rostral lateral mass of the level of interest (Fig. 68.3). It is critical to engage bone and not penetrate the interlaminar space where the laterally thinned ligamentum flavum may not protect against iatrogenic dural or spinal cord injury. At this point, the incision is completed approximately 1 cm above and below the K-wire entry point and the wire is removed. The axial forces that are applied during muscle dilation in the lumbar spine are more hazardous in the cervical spine. Therefore, the cervical fascia is incised equal to the length of the incision using monopolar cautery or scissors so that muscle dilation can proceed in a safe and controlled fashion. The K-wire is replaced under fluoroscopy again, and the tubular muscle dilators are serially inserted. Alternatively, once the fascia is incised, the first dilator may be placed without the repeated use of the K-wire. After dilation, the final 16- or 18-mm tubular METRx retractor is placed over the dilators and fixed

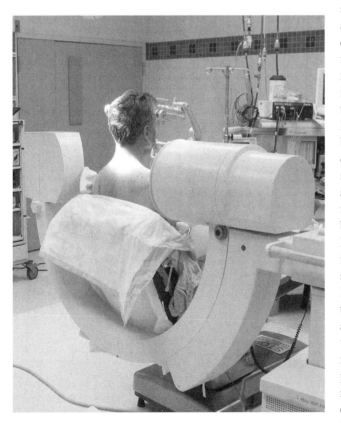

Fig. 68.2 Operative positioning of a patient in Mayfield head fixation for CMEF/D or CMEDS with the intraoperative fluoroscope C-arm beneath the patient

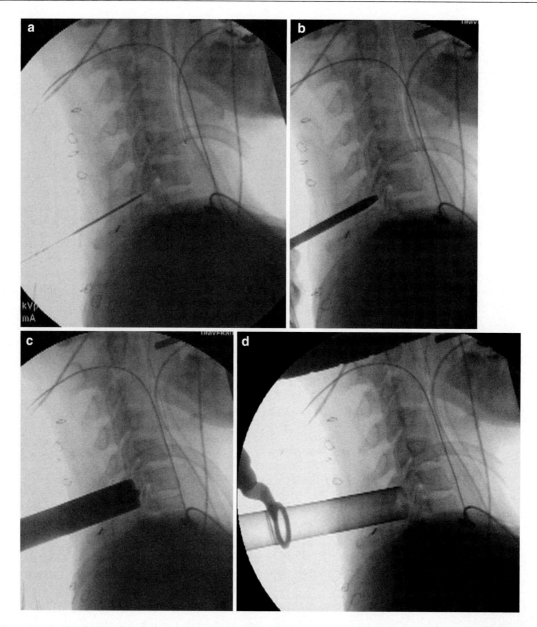

Fig. 68.3 Intraoperative lateral fluoroscopic images demonstrating the process of muscle dilation. (**a**) A K-wire is docked on the laminofacet junction over the intervertebral foramen of interest (C6–7 in this case). (**b**) The first two muscle dilators are inserted serially. (**c**) Progression to the largest dilator is complete. (**d**) An 18-mm tubular retractor is fixed into place and dilators are removed

into place over the laminofacet junction with a table-mounted flexible retractor arm, and the dilators are removed (Fig. 68.3). The 25° angled glass rod endoscope is attached to the camera, white balanced, and treated with an anti-fog solution prior to insertion and attachment to the tube via a cylindrical plastic friction-couple (Fig. 68.4).

Monopolar cautery and pituitary rongeurs are used to clear the remaining soft tissue off of the lateral mass and lamina of interest, taking care to start the dissection over solid bone laterally (Fig. 68.5a). A small up-angled curette is used to gently detach the ligamentum flavum from the undersurface of the inferior edge of the lamina and a Kerrison punch with a small footplate is used to begin the laminotomy.

At this point, the CMEF/D and CMEDS diverge in their course. We describe the technique for CMEF/D first, followed by CMEDS.

CMEF/D Technique

The subsequent steps of the operation differ little from the open procedure. Depending upon the degree of facet hypertrophy, the Kerrison may be used to complete most of the laminotomy and early foraminotomy or the drill may be required early in the course of bone removal. The use of a fine

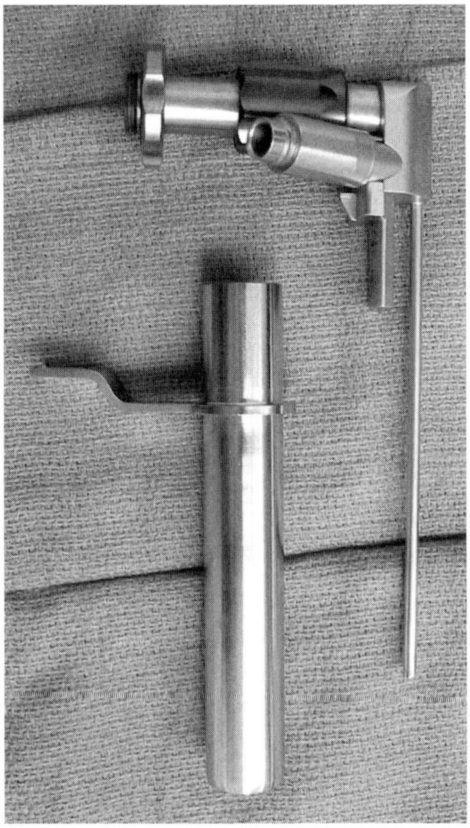

Fig. 68.4 Photograph of the METRx tubular retractor and rigid 25° glass rod endoscope

cutting bit and adjustable guard sleeve greatly facilitates the use of the drill around critical nervous structures. The ligamentum flavum can be removed medially after the laminotomy to identify the lateral edge of the dura and the proximal portion of the nerve root (Fig. 68.5b). The dorsal bony resection should follow the nerve root into the foramen by removal of part of the medial facet. It is crucial to preserve at least 50% of the facet to maintain biomechanical integrity[26] This amount of resection permits adequate exposure of the root in the foramen. At this point, the venous plexus overlying the nerve root should be carefully coagulated with bipolar cautery and incised. Fortunately, the use of the sitting position makes blood pooling and obscuring of the operative field less of a concern. With the root well visualized, a fine angled dissector can be used to palpate ventral to the nerve root for osteophytes or disc fragments. Should an osteophyte be present, a down-angled curette may be used to tamp the material further ventrally into the disc space or fragment it for subsequent removal. In the case of a soft disc herniation, a nerve hook may be passed ventrally and inferiorly to the root to gently tease the fragment away from the nerve for ultimate removal with a pituitary rongeur. In either case, additional drilling of the superomedial quadrant of the caudal pedicle allows greater access to the ventral pathology and obviates the need for excessive nerve root retraction superiorly. The foramen is inspected one final time for any further signs of compression, and the field is irrigated with antibiotic-impregnated solution. Hemostasis is achieved with bipolar cautery, bone wax, and

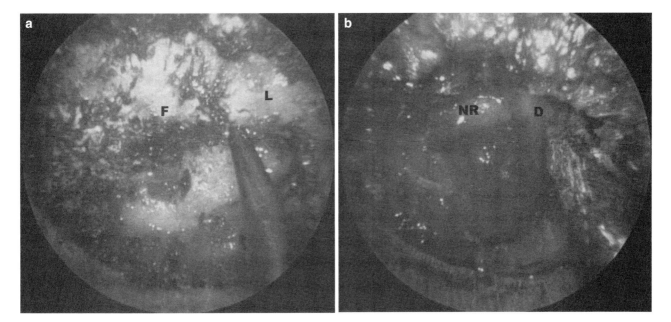

Fig. 68.5 Intraoperative endoscopic photographs during left-sided CMEF. In both photos, rostral is to the *top* and medial is to the *right*. (**a**) Initial exposure reveals the lateral edge of lamina (*L*) joining the medial facet (*F*) with a fine up-going curette inserted under the caudal edge of the lamino-facet junction. (**b**) After foraminotomy, the lateral edge of the dura (*D*) and decompressed nerve root (*NR*) in the proximal foramen are revealed

any of a variety of commercially available operative hemostatic agents. A methylprednisolone-soaked pledget may be placed over the root to reduce postoperative inflammation. Closure and postoperative care proceed as described below.

CMEDS Technique

After completion of the ipsilateral laminotomy, the ligamentum flavum is left in place to protect the dura. The tube is then angled approximately 45° off the midline such that the endoscope and tube are oriented to visualize the contralateral side. A plane between the ligament and undersurface of the spinous process is gently dissected with a fine curette. The undersurface of the spinous process and contralateral lamina are progressively drilled until reaching the contralateral facet. This initial decompression allows greater working space within which to remove hypertrophied ligament while avoiding downward pressure on the dura and spinal cord. Dissection and removal of the ligament with curettes and Kerrison rongeurs may now proceed safely. Any compressive elements of the contralateral facet or the superior edge of the caudal lamina may also be drilled off or removed with Kerrison rongeurs at this time because their impact on the dura is more apparent with the ligament removed. After gently confirming decompression over to the contralateral foramen with a fine probe, the tube is returned to its original position to complete the ipsilateral removal of ligament and bone. This should then reveal completely decompressed and pulsatile dura (Fig. 68.6). If indicated, ipsilateral foraminotomy as described above may be performed at this time as well. The field is irrigated with antibiotic-impregnated solution and hemostasis is achieved with bipolar cautery, bone wax, and hemostatic agents. Fig. 68.7 demonstrates a representative case of single level C4–5

stenosis treated with CMEDS. The typical extent of bony decompression is seen on postoperative CT (Fig. 68.7c).

Closure and Postoperative Care

The tube is removed, and local anesthetic is injected into the fascia and muscles surrounding the incision. The wound is closed using one or two absorbable stitches for the fascia,

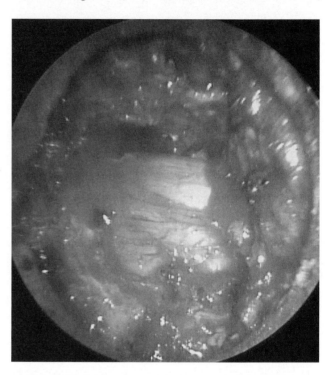

Fig. 68.6 Intraoperative endoscopic photograph during a right-sided approach for CMEDS. The dura is seen to be completely decompressed in this image after removal of offending bone and ligament. Rostral is to the *right* and lateral is to the *bottom*

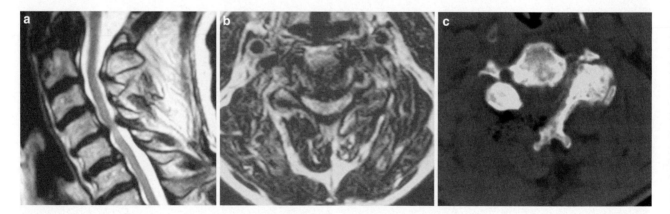

Fig. 68.7 An 80-year-old man presented with chronic myelopathy from cervical stenosis and underwent right-sided approach for C4–5 MEDS. (**a**) Sagittal T2-weighted MRI results demonstrate focal C4–5 spondylotic stenosis with signal change in the spinal cord. (**b**) Axial T2-weighted MRI reveals severe focal compression at C4–5. (**c**) Postoperative axial CT image shows typical extent of bony resection required to achieve adequate decompression of the spinal cord. Note the preservation of the dorsal spinous process and contralateral lamina and facet. Also note the minimal impact on paraspinal soft tissues on the approach side (postoperative air is seen on approach side and at the site of the laminotomy)

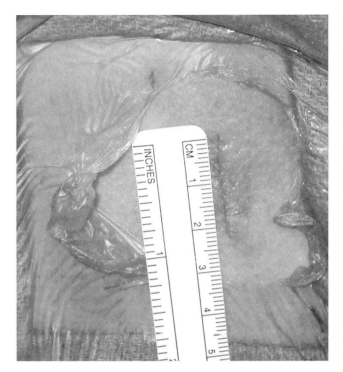

Fig. 68.8 CMEF/D or CMEDS incision after closure is only 2 cm in length

CA). Using this approach, overnight bedrest is usually sufficient to seal the defect. For larger dural tears that cannot be primarily closed, 2–3 days of lumbar CSF drainage may prevent a leak. Ultimately, the small opening and relative lack of dead space after minimally invasive procedures has made the incidence of postoperative pseudomeningoceles and CSF-cutaneous fistulae negligible.

Potential neurological complications include radicular injury from manipulation within the tight foramen or direct mechanical spinal cord injury during dilation or decompression. Vertebral artery injury can be avoided by early detection of dark venous bleeding from the venous plexus surrounding the artery that may arise from accidental dilation lateral to the facet or during overly aggressive dissection laterally in the foramen. This type of bleeding can typically be controlled by packing with Gelfoam or another hemostatic product. As mentioned previously, despite the use of the semisitting position, air embolism has not presented a problem to date. Delayed complications such as recurrent disease or postoperative instability also have not yet been observed in our use of these techniques thus far.

Conclusion

Posterior CMEF/D and CMEDS offer the benefits of decreases in blood loss, length of stay, postoperative pain, and muscle spasm; preservation of motion segments; and decreased risk of iatrogenic sagittal plan deformity, but still deliver efficacy equivalent to their open counterparts.[9] Ultimately, it is the reduction in immediate and delayed morbidity combined with safe and effective decompression that makes these minimally invasive approaches to cervical degenerative disease so appealing. Their use will and should continue to expand as more surgeons become familiar with microendoscopic techniques.

two or three inverted stitches for the subcutaneous layer, and a running subcuticular stitch and Dermabond for the skin (Fig. 68.8). No dressing need be applied. The patient is returned to a supine position and the Mayfield is removed. After awaking from general anesthesia, the patient is brought to the postanesthesia care unit and mobilized as early as possible. No collar is necessary. If medically stable, patients are typically discharged home after 2–3 h, although in some cases we have chosen to observe our CMEDS patients overnight. Discharge medications generally include an opioid/acetaminophen combination pain reliever and a muscle relaxant. Nonsteroidal anti-inflammatory agents are also commonly used.

Complications

Typical complication rates from posterior cervical decompressive procedures range from 2 to 9% and are mostly attributable to infection and cerebrospinal fluid (CSF) leak.[9] We have not had any infections in our series to date, and our unintended durotomy rate has dropped from 8% in the initial series of patients[9] to approximately 1% more recently. Direct suture repair of durotomy is difficult through the narrow diameter tubes. Therefore, one technique for handling small defects is to simply cover the durotomy with muscle, fat, Gelfoam, or dural substitute followed by fibrin glue or synthetic sealant such as Coseal (Baxter Healthcare, Glendale,

References

1. Aldrich F. Posterolateral microdisectomy for cervical monoradiculopathy caused by posterolateral soft cervical disc sequestration. *J Neurosurg.* 1990;72(3):370–377
2. Crandall PH, Batzdorf U. Cervical spondylotic myelopathy. *J Neurosurg.* 1966;25(1):57–66
3. Henderson CM, Hennessy RG, Shuey HM Jr, Shackelford EG. Posterior-lateral foraminotomy as an exclusive operative technique for cervical radiculopathy: a review of 846 consecutively operated cases. *Neurosurgery.* 1983;13(5):504–512
4. Ratliff JK, Cooper PR. Cervical laminoplasty: a critical review. *J Neurosurg.* 2003;98(3 Suppl):230–238
5. Khoo LT, Perez-Cruet MJ, Laich DT, Fessler RG. Posterior cervical microendoscopic foraminotomy. In: Perez-Cruet MJ, Fessler RG (eds). *Outpatient Spinal Surgery.* St. Louis: Quality Medical Publishing, Inc., 2006, pp. 71–93

6. Kumar VG, Rea GL, Mervis LJ, McGregor JM. Cervical spondylotic myelopathy: functional and radiographic long-term outcome after laminectomy and posterior fusion. *Neurosurgery.* 1999;44(4):771–777; discussion 777–778

7. Wang MY, Green BA. Laminoplasty for the treatment of failed anterior cervical spine surgery. *Neurosurg Focus.* 15 2003;15(3):E7

8. Wang MY, Shah S, Green BA. Clinical outcomes following cervical laminoplasty for 204 patients with cervical spondylotic myelopathy. *Surg Neurol.* 2004;62(6):487–492; discussion 492–483

9. Fessler RG, Khoo LT. Minimally invasive cervical microendoscopic foraminotomy: an initial clinical experience. *Neurosurgery.* 2002;51(5 Suppl):S37–S45

10. Hilibrand AS, Robbins M. Adjacent segment degeneration and adjacent segment disease: the consequences of spinal fusion? *Spine J.* 2004;4(6 Suppl):190S–194S

11. Ishihara H, Kanamori M, Kawaguchi Y, Nakamura H, Kimura T. Adjacent segment disease after anterior cervical interbody fusion. *Spine J.* 2004;4(6):624–628

12. Hosono N, Yonenobu K, Ono K. Neck and shoulder pain after laminoplasty. A noticeable complication. *Spine.* 1996;21(17):1969–1973

13. Siddiqui A, Yonemura KS. Posterior cervical microendoscopic diskectomy and laminoforaminotomy. In: Kim DH, Fessler RG, Regan JJ (eds). *Endoscopic Spine Surgery and Instrumentation: Percutaneous Procedures.* New York: Thieme, 2005, pp. 66–73

14. Albert TJ, Vacarro A. Postlaminectomy kyphosis. *Spine.* 1998; 23(24):2738–2745

15. Kaptain GJ, Simmons NE, Replogle RE, Pobereskin L. Incidence and outcome of kyphotic deformity following laminectomy for cervical spondylotic myelopathy. *J Neurosurg.* 2000;93(2 Suppl):199–204

16. Perez-Cruet MJ, Samartzis D, Fessler RG. Microendoscopic cervical laminectomy. In: Perez-Cruet MJ, Khoo LT, Fessler RG (eds). *An Anatomic Approach to Minimally Invasive Spine Surgery.* St. Louis: Quality Medical Publishing, Inc., 2006, pp. 16-11–16-17

17. Yonenobu K, Okada K, Fuji T, Fujiwara K, Yamashita K, Ono K. Causes of neurologic deterioration following surgical treatment of cervical myelopathy. *Spine.* 1986;11(8):818–823

18. Khoo LT, Bresnahan L, Fessler RG. Cervical endoscopic foraminotomy. In: Fessler RG, Sekhar L (eds). Atlas of Neurosurgical Techniques: Spine and Peripheral Nerves, vol. 1. New York: Thieme, 2006, pp. 785–792

19. Burke TG, Caputy A. Microendoscopic posterior cervical foraminotomy: a cadaveric model and clinical application for cervical radiculopathy. *J Neurosurg.* 2000;93(1 Suppl):126–129

20. Roh SW, Kim DH, Cardoso AC, Fessler RG. Endoscopic foraminotomy using MED system in cadaveric specimens. *Spine.* 2000;25(2):260–264

21. Adamson TE. Microendoscopic posterior cervical laminoforaminotomy for unilateral radiculopathy: results of a new technique in 100 cases. *J Neurosurg.* 2001;95(1 Suppl):51–57

22. Perez-Cruet MJ, Wang MY, Samartzis D. Microendoscopic cervical laminectomy and laminoplasty. In: Kim DH, Fessler RG, Regan JJ (eds). *Endoscopic Spine Surgery and Instrumentation: Percutaneous Procedures.* New York: Thieme, 2005, pp. 74–87

23. Wang MY, Green BA, Coscarella E, Baskaya MK, Levi AD, Guest JD. Minimally invasive cervical expansile laminoplasty: an initial cadaveric study. *Neurosurgery.* 2003;52(2):370–373; discussion 373

24. Khoo LT, Fessler RG. Microendoscopic decompressive laminotomy for the treatment of lumbar stenosis. *Neurosurgery.* 2002;51(5 Suppl):S146–S154

25. Yabuki S, Kikuchi S. Endoscopic partial laminectomy for cervical myelopathy. *J Neurosurg Spine.* 2005;2(2):170–174

26. Raynor RB, Pugh J, Shapiro I. Cervical facetectomy and its effect on spine strength. *J Neurosurg.* 1985;63(2):278–282

Chapter 69
Minimally Invasive Transforaminal Lumbar Interbody Fusion

Alfred T. Ogden and Richard G. Fessler

During the past 75 years, surgical technique, spinal instruments and instrumentation, and molecular biology have advanced the notion of lumbar interbody fusion from what Mercer[1] described, in 1936, as perhaps "technically impossible" to a routine operation with a high rate of success. Pedicle screw augmentation of the posterior lateral interbody fusion (PLIF) described by Cloward[2] made possible a decompressive operation and arthrodesis with "360°" of stabilization from a single posterior approach. The transforaminal lumbar interbody fusion (TLIF) described by Harms and Rolinger[3] in 1982 offered the same biomechanical result as the PLIF but has gained more widespread popularity because it requires less manipulation of neural structures during graft placement. Although both the PLIF and TLIF are viable using minimally invasive techniques, the minimally invasive TLIF (miTLIF) has become the dominant minimally invasive lumbar fusion procedure.

Retrospective surgical series have reported high rates of efficacy for both open PLIF and open TLIF in terms of fusion rates and clinical outcome for a variety of indications.[4–12] These results have been supported by the majority of Class I data.[13–18] Although debate continues over whether the theoretical advantages of an instrumented 360° fusion have translated into a clinical benefit over noninstrumented fusions or posterior lateral onlay fusions (PLF),[19,20] posterior interbody grafting and percutaneous pedicle screw placement has enabled the development of minimally invasive lumbar fusion procedures that would not otherwise be possible.

The miTLIF is superior to open lumbar fusion in terms of perioperative morbidity, and two outcome studies indicate that minimally invasive fusion is at least as efficacious as open lumbar fusion at 1–2 years.[21–26] The routine use of recombinant human bone morphogenetic protein (rhBMP) has likely contributed to this success and has led investigators to question the need for bilateral pedicle screw fixation. This chapter discusses the indications for the miTLIF and its current state of evolution. The procedure as performed by the authors is described in detail.

A.T. Ogden and R.G. Fessler (✉)
Department of Neurological Surgery, Northwestern Memorial
Hospital, Chicago, IL, USA

General Indications

The indications for lumbar fusion are varied and somewhat controversial. Lumbar fusion has been offered as the preferred treatment for a broad range of lumbar pathologies including lumbar disc herniation,[27] spinal stenosis,[27–29] spondylolisthesis with or without segmental instability from multiple etiologies,[3,6,8,11,12,19,30–34] failed back syndrome,[35–37] recurrent disc herniation,[38–41] and degenerative disc disease with mechanical back pain.[5,14,42,43] Methods of lumbar fusion are varied as well and include anterior procedures anterior lumbar interbody fusion (ALIF), extreme/direct lateral interbody fusion (XLIF/DLIF), the posterior interbody fusions (PLIF and TLIF), interspinous fusions, and PLF. These techniques can be supplemented with a variety of fixation methods, including pedicle screws, facet screws, and vertebral body screw systems. Given the range of possible indications and techniques, it is not surprising that opinions differ regarding when to offer patients a lumbar fusion and how to pursue it technically. No particular method has proved to be definitively superior to another and, to a degree, choice of method is influenced by specific pathology on a case-by-case basis; nevertheless, the miTLIF offers many general advantages. These include 360° fixation, an interbody graft, direct and indirect decompression of neural elements, and the possibility of reduction of spondylolisthesis - all through a single minimally invasive approach.

Evidence-Based Data

It is impossible to understand the specific indications for miTLIF without summarizing the debate over the efficacy of lumbar fusion in general. Only in the last several years have randomized prospectively collected data regarding lumbar fusions become available, with validated, quantifiable outcome measures that enable reasonable study-to-study comparisons. In the United States, the Oswestry Disability Index (ODI) and SF-36 physical component score (PCS) form have emerged as the gold standards for evaluations of treatments of disabling chronic diseases. The US Food and Drug Administration (FDA) has set a decrease of 15 points in the ODI with maintenance or improvement in the SF-36 as a clear, clinically meaningful treatment response.[44,45]

Evidence-based assessments of lumbar fusion have focused on a handful of studies that can be placed into two general groups: (1) randomized, prospective clinical trials from Europe comparing open lumbar fusion with conservative therapy and (2) the control arms of prospectively collected data from FDA investigational device exemption (IDE) studies from the United States in trials of artificial lumbar discs. Two large prospective randomized trials from Europe, comparing open lumbar fusion with conservative management in the treatment of discogenic back pain have demonstrated conflicting results. One large Swedish study[14] showed a fairly clear clinical benefit from surgery - although below the FDA cutoff (ΔODI surgery = 11.6), whereas another large study from England[46] showed a negligible benefit from surgery. Two other smaller studies from Norway[47,48] that failed to show a benefit from lumbar fusion for discogenic back pain[48] and back pain after previous discectomy[47] have been criticized for being so underpowered as to render their results meaningless.[45,49] Another study from Sweden examined outcomes from lumbar fusion compared with conservative management in the treatment of isthmic spondylolisthesis and showed a clear benefit from surgery as measured by a Disability Rating Index (DRI) > 19.[50] The mixed results from these trials have led some to question the pervasiveness of lumbar fusion, particularly as a treatment modality for discogenic back pain.

Advocates of lumbar fusion point toward data collected in the United States in FDA trials of lumbar artificial discs as additional evidence of the efficacy of lumbar fusion.[15,16] These show ΔODIs of approximately 20 for patients undergoing lumbar fusion for a variety of indications and significant improvements in SF-36 scores[13,18] - well above the FDA cutoff. Cost-benefit analysis of this data demonstrates similar or better ratios for operations such as hip replacement, knee replacement, and coronary artery bypass grafting.[16] Critics counter that IDE data, although robust in its manner of collection, lack a nonsurgical arm, rendering it less valid than the European studies.[45] More recently, the results from the degenerative spondylolisthesis arm of the SPORT trial were published, revealing a clear benefit from surgery over conservative management in the "as-treated" analysis.[17]

Minimally Invasive TLIF: Advantages and Outcomes

Compared with open lumbar fusion, the miTLIF has consistently shown reduced blood loss, lower transfusion rates, decreased postoperative narcotic use, and shorter length of stay than open fusions[23,26,51,52] and even "mini-open" techniques.[25] The routine use of rhBMP has largely obviated the need to harvest second site autografts. Some investigators have cautioned a steep learning curve to minimally invasive fusion, citing a higher complication rate,[52] but this has not been the authors' experience nor the experience of other investigators. Experience to date indicates that infection rates from minimally invasive fusions are lower than for open procedures.[69] Thus, the miTLIF already addresses many of the criticisms of lumbar fusion (graft site morbidity, significant infection rate) and continues to evolve.

Whether miTLIF can improve long-term outcomes of spinal fusion patients remains to be seen. Milder postoperative pain after miTLIF is considered to stem in large part from a reduction in retraction-induced muscle ischemia and subperiosteal muscle dissection. Pathological changes in paraspinal musculature after open spine surgery have been well documented and have been associated with poor outcomes.[53-58] Minimally invasive techniques for lumbar fusion greatly reduce the amount of pressure seen by the paraspinal musculature during surgery, and this more gentle manipulation correlates with reduced muscle edema on postoperative magnetic resonance imaging (MRI) scans,[59] lower postoperative serum muscle protein levels, and decreased measurements of serum inflammatory markers.[60] To date, validated pain and disability indices show minimally invasive fusion to be at least as effective as open lumbar fusion after 1–2 years of follow-up.[26,52,61] If iatrogenic muscle injury is indeed a major limitation to favorable outcomes after open procedures, then minimally invasive techniques could increase the overall efficacy of lumbar fusion. Whether the procedure can deliver such an improvement over open fusion beyond the perioperative period can only be answered by further study.

Current Practices

It is our practice to offer a miTLIF to our spondylolisthesis patients (grades 1 and 2 only) with demonstrable instability on dynamic radiographs (Fig. 69.1). These patients are clear beneficiaries of lumbar fusion. We will offer a miTLIF to patients with degenerative disc/facet disease and mechanical back pain as well, but only after a careful selection process. Patients first must demonstrate unremitting back pain for at least 6 months that significantly affects quality of life and has not responded to a reasonable course of conservative management, including a 6-week course of physical therapy and an aggressive pain management program. There must be evidence of severe degenerative changes at one level, or two adjacent levels, out of proportion to other levels and/or reproducible symptoms on provocative testing, such as a discogram. Additionally, upright X-ray results are reviewed. If

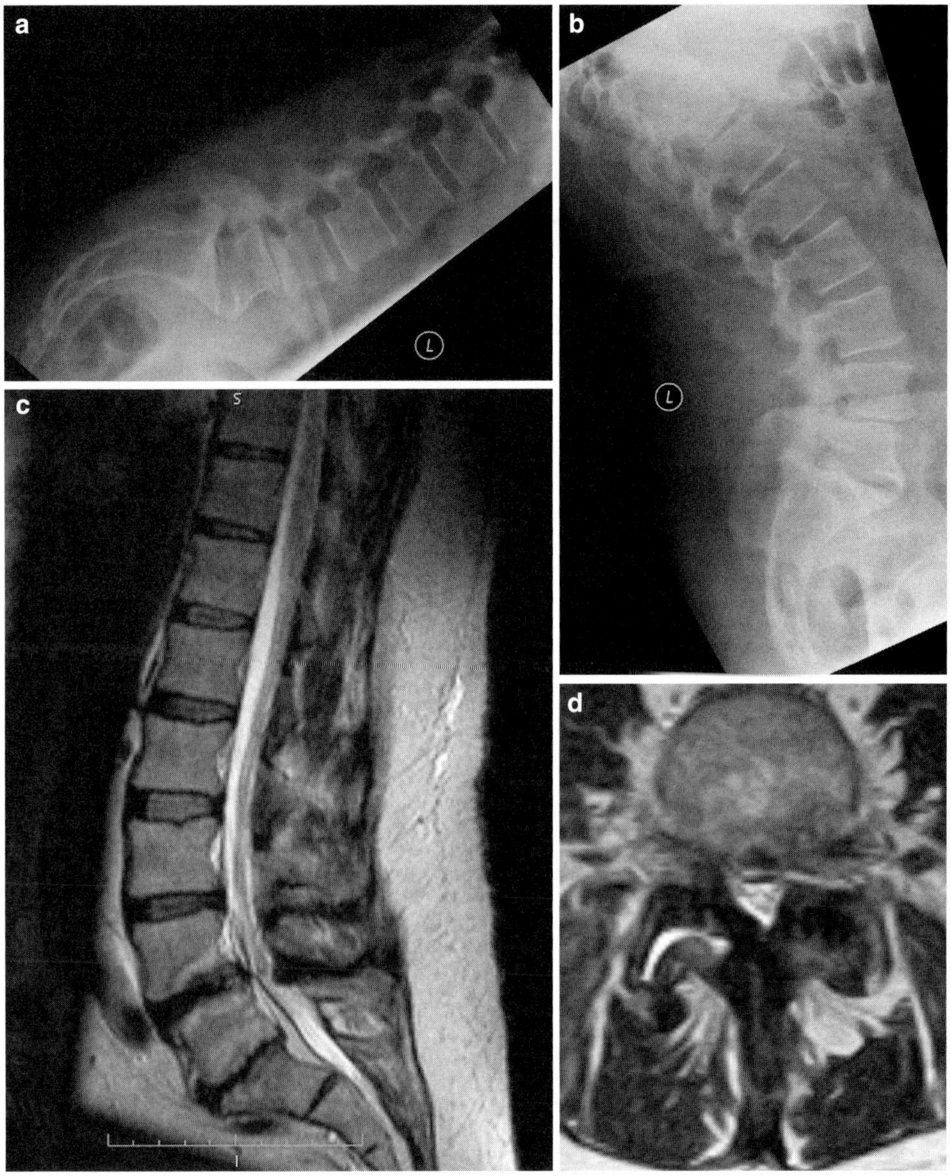

Fig. 69.1 Preoperative imaging. Radiographic studies of a 61-year-old man with chronic low back pain and a left L5 radiculopathy. Plain X-ray results demonstrated a grad.e I spondylolisthesis of L4 on L5 with instability on flexion (**a**) and extension (**b**) views. An MRI revealed severe disc degeneration (**c**) and stenosis (**d**)

necessary, upright scoliosis "long cassette" films are obtained to assess deformity. Patients with significant coronal imbalance, sagittal imbalance, or location of the pain generator at the apex of a curve may be better served by procedures that more thoroughly address their deformity issues. We generally do not recommend fusion for recurrent disc herniations or massive disc herniations, preferring microendoscopic discectomy as an initial procedure. These patients may ultimately require a fusion, but, by employing minimally invasive techniques, this may be postponed, perhaps indefinitely.

Surgical Procedure

Equipment

The miTLIF requires the following equipment: C-arm fluoroscopy, a tubular retraction system, a laminectomy tray with modified instruments for working through a tubular retractor, a high-speed drill, tools for endplate preparation, an interbody graft, and a percutaneous pedicle screw system. Currently, we place all our instrumentation using fluoroscopy, although image guidance systems are improving and will likely gain in popularity. We use an expandable tubular retractor (Fig. 69.2a) (X-Tube, Medtronic Sofamor Danek, Memphis, TN), which has a diameter of 26 mm proximally at the skin entry but can be expanded in situ to a final working diameter of 44 mm distally. This feature is particularly helpful for two-level fusions. Use of an endoscope is optional; we generally use loupe magnification with a headlight. The decompression is performed with standard laminectomy instruments that are lengthened and bayoneted for working through a tubular retractor. The tools for readying the disc space for graft placement consist of distractors (7–14 mm), rotating cutters, endplate scrapers, and a chisel. Many options exist for interbody graft material. We have had good results when using either allograft bone or cages, but our current practice is to use a PEEK cage with autograft collected during facetectomy and recombinant human bone morphogenic protein (rhBMP)-2 (Infuse, Medtronic Sofamor Danek). Placement of percutaneous screws requires an 11-gauge bone biopsy needle (Jamshidi, CardinalHealth), a Kocher clamp, K-wires, a drill, fluoroscopy, and a percutaneous pedicle screw system. We use the Sextant system (Fig. 69.2b, c) (Medtronic Sofamor Danek).

Operating Room Set-up and Positioning

The operating table is placed in the center of the room, with anesthesia at the patient's head and the fluoroscopy monitor at the patient's feet. The C-arm base is placed on the opposite side from where the TLIF is to be performed. The operating room technician and equipment tables are kept behind the surgeon on the operative side and a Mayo stand is situated over the feet to pass instruments in active use.

After induction and intubation, a Foley catheter is placed and neurophysiological monitoring with free-running electromyography (EMG) capabilities is set up. After intubation, the anesthetist should avoid the use of relaxants and nitrous

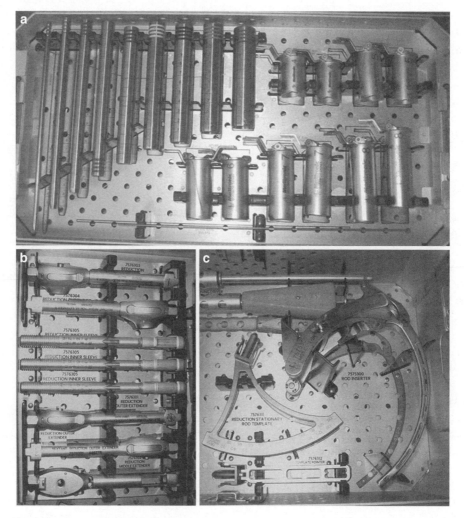

Fig. 69.2 Equipment. Trays holding the X-Tube dilating retractor system (**a**) and the Sextant percutaneous screw system screw extenders (**b**) and rod inserter (**c**)

oxide, which may interfere with EMG recordings. A single dose of appropriate antibiotic is administered. Sequential compression devices are placed on the legs and the patient is positioned on the operating table. The patient is positioned prone on a Wilson frame and Jackson table. All arm joints are bent to <90 and placed along side the patient's head. The knees, axilla, elbows, and wrists are carefully padded. The legs are elevated with pillows to reduce stretch on the sciatic nerve. The face is placed in a padded mask that has a mirrored surface (Prone View, Dupaco, Oceanside, CA) to ensure visualization of the eyes and the endotracheal tube throughout the procedure. An occlusive barrier is placed at the top of the gluteal cleft, and the skin is prepped and draped in standard fashion. The C-arm is brought in for a lateral view of the affected level and draped into the field.

Surgical Technique

Localization and Exposure

Localization of the appropriate level is performed with fluoroscopy and a K-wire. Once marked, a stab incision is made 3 cm from midline, and the K-wire is inserted until it rests on bone. Ideally, the point should be on the facet complex of the affected level, orthogonal to the disc space (Fig. 69.3a). If the localization is satisfactory, the skin incision is extended to a final length of 2.5–3 cm, with the K-wire bisecting the incision. Sequential dilators from the tubular access system are passed to expand the soft tissue in a stepwise fashion (Fig. 69.3b). Fluoroscopy is used to confirm positioning. After insertion of the final dilator, a depth measurement is made and a working channel of appropriate length is introduced. The ideal final position of the working channel is over the facet, perpendicular to the disc space, and spanning the pedicles to be instrumented (Fig. 69.3c). Inevitably, some residual muscle and soft tissue remains after dilation and this is cleared from the lamina and facet with monopolar cautery in preparation for the decompression (Fig. 69.3d).

Laminotomy/Facetectomy

A straight curette is used to define the interlaminar space, a plane is developed between the ligamentum flavum and bone with an angled curette, and the level is confirmed with fluoroscopy (Fig. 69.3e). A laminotomy is performed with Kerrison rongeurs, revealing the ligamentum flavum and defining the lateral extent of the spinal canal (Fig. 69.3f). The inferior articular process of the rostral level is removed with osteotomes guided by fluoroscopy (Fig. 69.3g, h), exposing the superior articular process of the caudal level

(Fig. 69.3i). All bone is saved for later use in the interbody fusion. The decompression should extend from pedicle to pedicle in a rostral-caudal direction. Fluoroscopy can be used as needed to assess position and evaluate the extent of decompression. Laterally, a near-total or total facetectomy is done to provide adequate space for graft placement; however, the portion of facet directly over the pedicle distal to the disc space should be preserved to provide an adequate platform for pedicle screw starting points. The ligamentum flavum is removed. If necessary, the working channel can be angled medially for a contralateral decompression, as described elsewhere.[62] Epidural veins are coagulated with bipolar cautery and divided if necessary. The lateral edge of the dura, the nerve root, and the disc space should be clearly visualized (Fig. 69.3j).

Interbody Fusion

A 15-blade scalpel is used to cut the annulus, and the initial discectomy proceeds using curettes and pituitary rongeurs. A wedge chisel may be needed to access the disc space (Fig. 69.3k). A down-angled curette is helpful to ensure that subligamentous disc fragments and the contralateral disc are properly removed. Next, the rotating cutter is introduced parallel with the disc space and twisted to prepare the vertebral body endplates (Fig. 69.3l). The endplates are scraped, and debris is removed with a pituitary rongeur. A chisel or Kerrison can be used to expand the annulotomy or to remove osteophytes. The endplates are now ready for graft placement (Fig. 69.3m). Templates are then inserted to expand and to measure the interbody space for the appropriately sized graft. Before placing the PEEK cage, we first lay a rhBMP-2-soaked sponge along the anterior annulus, followed by a generous amount of autograft. Another rhBMP-2-soaked sponge and more autograft is placed in the cage and inserted obliquely, such that it is centered in the disc space. Fluoroscopy is used to confirm graft position (Fig. 69.3n) and the inserter is unscrewed from the graft (Fig. 69.3o). Hemostasis is achieved using standard techniques, and the working channel is withdrawn slowly in order to permit periodic cauterization.

Pedicle Screw Fixation

The miTLIF relies on anteroposterior (AP) and lateral fluoroscopy for pedicle screw placement. After rotation of the C-arm for a true AP view in parallel to the disc space, starting points for screws are marked over the center of the pedicle. A bone biopsy needle is passed through the soft tissue and docked onto the entry point. We try to orient the needle directly in line with the pedicle, such that the needle will

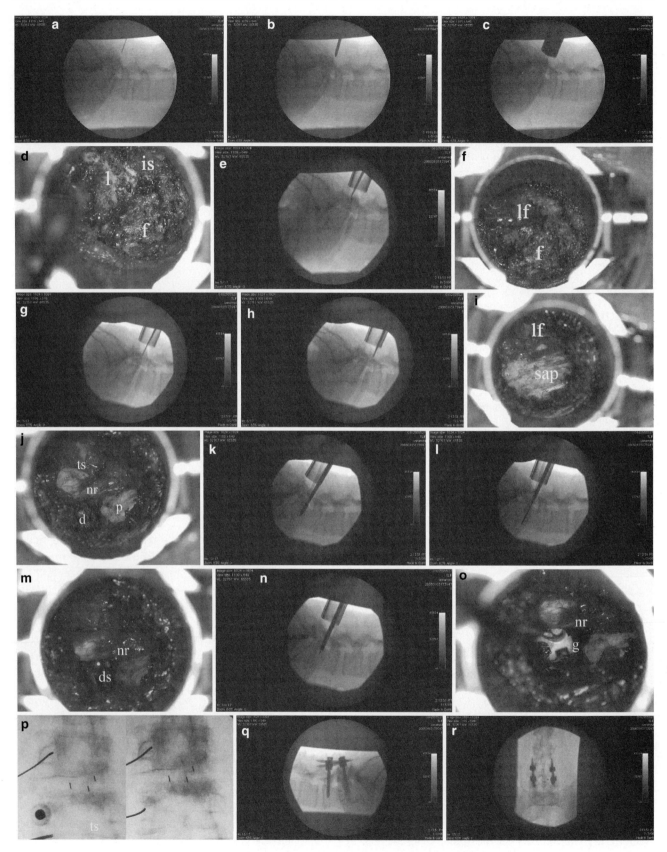

Fig. 69.3 Operative procedure: L4–5 TLIF. A K-wire is inserted through a stab incision and docked on the facet orthogonal to the disc space (**a**). Sequential dilators expand the opening to accommodate a 28-mm working port (**b, c**). After removal of a thin layer of residual soft tissue, the superficial osseous structures overlying the disc space are revealed (**d**); *f* facet; *l* lamina; *is* interlaminar space. The plane between the lamina and the interlaminar ligaments is developed with an angled curette and the level is confirmed (**e**). A laminotomy is performed, exposing the ligamentum

Conclusions

Through minimally invasive techniques, an interbody fusion with anterior and posterior stabilization can be achieved with similar or greater efficacy and significantly reduced perioperative morbidity compared with open techniques. The miT-LIF is the preferred procedure to this end. The best outcomes are achieved after careful patient selection for a variety of indications, including segmental instability and discogenic back pain. Current research is focused on further reduction of the procedure's invasiveness through the evaluation of unilateral vs. bilateral pedicle fixation and the use and development of image guidance and robotic systems.

References

1. Mercer R. Spondylolisthesis with a description of a new method of operative treatment and notes of ten cases. *Edinb Med J* 1936;43: 545–572
2. Cloward RB. The treatment of ruptured lumbar intervertebral discs by vertebral body fusion. I. Indications, operative technique, after care. *J Neurosurg* 1953;10:154–168
3. Harms J, Rolinger H. [A one-stager procedure in operative treatment of spondylolistheses: dorsal traction-reposition and anterior fusion (author's transl)]. *Z Orthop Ihre Grenzgeb* 1982;120:343–347
4. Chastain CA, Eck JC, Hodges SD, et al. Transforaminal lumbar interbody fusion: a retrospective study of long-term pain relief and fusion outcomes. *Orthopedics* 2007;30:389–392
5. Gill K, Blumenthal SL. Posterior lumbar interbody fusion. A 2-year follow-up of 238 patients. *Acta Orthop Scand Suppl* 1993;251: 108–110
6. Hackenberg L, Halm H, Bullmann V, et al. Transforaminal lumbar interbody fusion: a safe technique with satisfactory three to five year results. *Eur Spine J* 2005;14:551–558
7. Haid RW Jr, Branch CL Jr, Alexander JT, et al. Posterior lumbar interbody fusion using recombinant human bone morphogenetic protein type 2 with cylindrical interbody cages. *Spine J* 2004;4:527–538; discussion 38–39
8. Lauber S, Schulte TL, Liljenqvist U, et al. Clinical and radiologic 2–4-year results of transforaminal lumbar interbody fusion in degenerative and isthmic spondylolisthesis grades 1 and 2. *Spine* 2006;31:1693–1698
9. Okuda S, Miyauchi A, Oda T, et al. Surgical complications of posterior lumbar interbody fusion with total facetectomy in 251 patients. *J Neurosurg Spine* 2006;4:304–309
10. Okuda S, Oda T, Miyauchi A, et al. Surgical outcomes of posterior lumbar interbody fusion in elderly patients. *J Bone Joint Surg Am* 2006;88:2714–2720
11. Potter BK, Freedman BA, Verwiebe EG, et al. Transforaminal lumbar interbody fusion: clinical and radiographic results and complications in 100 consecutive patients. *J Spinal Disord Tech* 2005;18:337–346
12. Rosenberg WS, Mummaneni PV. Transforaminal lumbar interbody fusion: technique, complications, and early results. *Neurosurgery* 2001;48:569–575
13. Blumenthal S, McAfee PC, Guyer RD, et al. A prospective, randomized, multicenter Food and Drug Administration investigational device exemptions study of lumbar total disc replacement with the CHARITE artificial disc versus lumbar fusion: part I: evaluation of clinical outcomes. *Spine* 2005;30:1565–1575; discussion E387-E391
14. Fritzell P, Hagg O, Wessberg P, et al. 2001 Volvo Award Winner in Clinical Studies: Lumbar fusion versus nonsurgical treatment for chronic low back pain: a multicenter randomized controlled trial from the Swedish Lumbar Spine Study Group. *Spine* 2001;26:2521–2532; discussion 32–34
15. Glassman S, Gornet MF, Branch C, et al. MOS short form 36 and Oswestry Disability Index outcomes in lumbar fusion: a multicenter experience. *Spine J* 2006;6:21–26
16. Polly DW Jr, Glassman SD, Schwender JD, et al. SF-36 PCS benefit-cost ratio of lumbar fusion comparison to other surgical interventions: a thought experiment. *Spine* 2007;32:S20–S26
17. Weinstein JN, Lurie JD, Tosteson TD, et al. Surgical versus nonsurgical treatment for lumbar degenerative spondylolisthesis. *N Engl J Med* 2007;356:2257–2270
18. Zigler J, Delamarter R, Spivak JM, et al. Results of the prospective, randomized, multicenter Food and Drug Administration investigational device exemption study of the ProDisc-L total disc replacement versus circumferential fusion for the treatment of 1-level degenerative disc disease. *Spine* 2007;32:1155–1162; discussion 63
19. Ekman P, Moller H, Tullberg T, et al. Posterior lumbar interbody fusion versus posterolateral fusion in adult isthmic spondylolisthesis. *Spine* 2007;32:2178–2183
20. Videbaek TS, Christensen FB, Soegaard R, et al. Circumferential fusion improves outcome in comparison with instrumented posterolateral fusion: long-term results of a randomized clinical trial. *Spine* 2006;31:2875–2880
21. Fessler RG. Minimally invasive percutaneous posterior lumbar interbody fusion. *Neurosurgery* 2003;52:1512
22. Foley KT, Holly LT, Schwender JD. Minimally invasive lumbar fusion. *Spine* 2003;28:S26–S35
23. Holly LT, Schwender JD, Rouben DP, et al. Minimally invasive transforaminal lumbar interbody fusion: indications, technique, and complications. *Neurosurg Focus* 2006;20:E6
24. Kim KT, Lee SH, Lee YH, et al. Clinical outcomes of 3 fusion methods through the posterior approach in the lumbar spine. *Spine* 2006;31:1351–1357; discussion 8
25. Scheufler KM, Dohmen H, Vougioukas VI. Percutaneous transforaminal lumbar interbody fusion for the treatment of degenerative lumbar instability. *Neurosurgery* 2007;60:203–212; discussion 12–13
26. Schwender JD, Holly LT, Rouben DP, et al. Minimally invasive transforaminal lumbar interbody fusion (TLIF): technical feasibility and initial results. *J Spinal Disord Tech* 2005;18(Suppl):S1–S6

Fig. 69.3 (continued) xflavum (**f**); *lf* ligamentum flavum; *f* facet. Using osteotomes under fluoroscopic guidance (**g, h**), the left inferior articular process of L4 is removed, revealing the left superior articular process of L5 (**i**); *sap* superior articular process. The ligamentum flavum is removed, along with the facet overlying the disc space and nerve root. The thecal sac (*ts*), nerve root (*nr*), disc (*d*), and pedicle (*p*) are identified and the epidural vessels over the disc space are cauterized and divided (**j**). A wedge chisel is used to enter the disc space (**k**) and a discectomy is performed using a variety of instruments (**l, m**); *ds* disc space; *nr* nerve root. After endplate preparation and packing of the disc space with rhBMP-2 and local bone, the interbody graft is placed under fluoroscopic guidance (**n, o**); *g* graft; *nr* nerve root. The working channel is removed and pedicles screws are placed percutaneously. A hollow biopsy needle is used guide trajectories using the "bull's eye" technique, and pedicles are cannulated using guide wires (**p**). A cannulated tap and screws permits percutaneous pedicle screw placement and rods are swung into position through separated incisions using the Sextant system. Intraoperative X-rays confirm satisfactory construct position (**q, r**)

27. Cloward RB. Posterior lumbar interbody fusion updated. *Clin Orthop Relat Res* 1985;Mar(193):16–19

28. Hutter CG. Spinal stenosis and posterior lumbar interbody fusion. *Clin Orthop Relat Res* 1985;Mar(193):103–114

29. Trouillier H, Birkenmaier C, Rauch A, et al. Posterior lumbar interbody fusion (PLIF) with cages and local bone graft in the treatment of spinal stenosis. *Acta Orthop Belg* 2006;72:460–466

30. Ekman P, Moller H, Hedlund R. The long-term effect of posterolateral fusion in adult isthmic spondylolisthesis: a randomized controlled study. *Spine J* 2005;5:36–44

31. Miyakoshi N, Abe E, Shimada Y, et al. Outcome of one-level posterior lumbar interbody fusion for spondylolisthesis and postoperative intervertebral disc degeneration adjacent to the fusion. *Spine* 2000;25:1837–1842

32. Molinari RW, Sloboda JF, Arrington EC. Low-grade isthmic spondylolisthesis treated with instrumented posterior lumbar interbody fusion in U.S. servicemen. *J Spinal Disord Tech* 2005;18(Suppl):S24–S29

33. Moller H, Hedlund R. Instrumented and noninstrumented posterolateral fusion in adult spondylolisthesis - a prospective randomized study: part 2. *Spine* 2000;25:1716–1721

34. Thomsen K, Christensen FB, Eiskjaer SP, et al. 1997 Volvo Award winner in clinical studies. The effect of pedicle screw instrumentation on functional outcome and fusion rates in posterolateral lumbar spinal fusion: a prospective, randomized clinical study. *Spine* 1997;22:2813–2822

35. Duggal N, Mendiondo I, Pares HR, et al. Anterior lumbar interbody fusion for treatment of failed back surgery syndrome: an outcome analysis. *Neurosurgery* 2004;54:636–643; discussion 43–44

36. Markwalder TM, Battaglia M. Failed back surgery syndrome. Part II: Surgical techniques, implant choice, and operative results in 171 patients with instability of the lumbar spine. *Acta Neurochir (Wien)* 1993;123:129–134

37. Skaf G, Bouclaous C, Alaraj A, et al. Clinical outcome of surgical treatment of failed back surgery syndrome. *Surg Neurol* 2005;64:483–488; discussion 8–9

38. Chitnavis B, Barbagallo G, Selway R, et al. Posterior lumbar interbody fusion for revision disc surgery: review of 50 cases in which carbon fiber cages were implanted. *J Neurosurg* 2001;95:190–195

39. Choi JY, Choi YW, Sung KH. Anterior lumbar interbody fusion in patients with a previous discectomy: minimum 2-year follow-up. *J Spinal Disord Tech* 2005;18:347–352

40. Lee SH, Kang BU, Jeon SH, et al. Revision surgery of the lumbar spine: anterior lumbar interbody fusion followed by percutaneous pedicle screw fixation. *J Neurosurg Spine* 2006;5:228–233

41. Vishteh AG, Dickman CA. Anterior lumbar microdiscectomy and interbody fusion for the treatment of recurrent disc herniation. *Neurosurgery* 2001;48:334–337

42. Folman Y, Lee SH, Silvera JR, et al. Posterior lumbar interbody fusion for degenerative disc disease using a minimally invasive B-twin expandable spinal spacer: a multicenter study. *J Spinal Disord Tech* 2003;16:455–460

43. Leufven C, Nordwall A. Management of chronic disabling low back pain with 360 degrees fusion. Results from pain provocation test and concurrent posterior lumbar interbody fusion, posterolateral fusion, and pedicle screw instrumentation in patients with chronic disabling low back pain. *Spine* 1999;24:2042–2045

44. Dimar JR, Glassman SD, Burkus KJ, et al. Clinical outcomes and fusion success at 2 years of single-level instrumented posterolateral fusions with recombinant human bone morphogenetic protein-2/compression resistant matrix versus iliac crest bone graft. *Spine* 2006;31:2534–2539; discussion 40

45. Mirza SK, Deyo RA. Systematic review of randomized trials comparing lumbar fusion surgery to nonoperative care for treatment of chronic back pain. *Spine* 2007;32:816–823

46. Fairbank J, Frost H, Wilson-MacDonald J, et al. Randomised controlled trial to compare surgical stabilisation of the lumbar spine with an intensive rehabilitation programme for patients with chronic low back pain: the MRC spine stabilisation trial. *BMJ* 2005;330:1233

47. Brox JI, Reikeras O, Nygaard O, et al. Lumbar instrumented fusion compared with cognitive intervention and exercises in patients with chronic back pain after previous surgery for disc herniation: a prospective randomized controlled study. *Pain* 2006;122:145–155

48. Brox JI, Sorensen R, Friis A, et al. Randomized clinical trial of lumbar instrumented fusion and cognitive intervention and exercises in patients with chronic low back pain and disc degeneration. *Spine* 2003;28:1913–1921

49. Hagg O, Fritzell P. Re: Brox JI, Sorensen R, Friis A, et al. Randomized clinical trial of lumbar instrumented fusion and cognitive intervention and exercises in patients with chronic low back pain and disc degeneration. Spine. 2003; 28:1913–1921. *Spine* 2004;29:1160–1161

50. Moller H, Hedlund R. Surgery versus conservative management in adult isthmic spondylolisthesis - a prospective randomized study: part 1. *Spine* 2000;25:1711–1715

51. Isaacs RE, Podichetty VK, Santiago P, et al. Minimally invasive microendoscopy-assisted transforaminal lumbar interbody fusion with instrumentation. *J Neurosurg Spine* 2005;3:98–105

52. Park Y, Ha JW. Comparison of one-level posterior lumbar interbody fusion performed with a minimally invasive approach or a traditional open approach. *Spine* 2007;32:537–543

53. Gejo R, Matsui H, Kawaguchi Y, et al. Serial changes in trunk muscle performance after posterior lumbar surgery. *Spine* 1999;24:1023–1028

54. Kawaguchi Y, Matsui H, Tsuji H. Back muscle injury after posterior lumbar spine surgery. A histologic and enzymatic analysis. *Spine* 1996;21:941–944

55. Kawaguchi Y, Matsui H, Tsuji H. Back muscle injury after posterior lumbar spine surgery. Part 2: Histologic and histochemical analyses in humans. *Spine* 1994;19:2598–2602

56. Kawaguchi Y, Matsui H, Tsuji H. Changes in serum creatine phosphokinase MM isoenzyme after lumbar spine surgery. *Spine* 1997;22:1018–1023

57. Mayer TG, Vanharanta H, Gatchel RJ, et al. Comparison of CT scan muscle measurements and isokinetic trunk strength in postoperative patients. *Spine* 1989;14:33–36

58. Sihvonen T, Herno A, Paljarvi L, et al. Local denervation atrophy of paraspinal muscles in postoperative failed back syndrome. *Spine* 1993;18:575–581

59. Stevens KJ, Spenciner DB, Griffiths KL, et al. Comparison of minimally invasive and conventional open posterolateral lumbar fusion using magnetic resonance imaging and retraction pressure studies. *J Spinal Disord Tech* 2006;19:77–86

60. Kim KT, Lee SH, Suk KS, et al. The quantitative analysis of tissue injury markers after mini-open lumbar fusion. *Spine* 2006;31:712–716

61. Jang JS, Lee SH. Minimally invasive transforaminal lumbar interbody fusion with ipsilateral pedicle screw and contralateral facet screw fixation. *J Neurosurg Spine* 2005;3:218–223

62. Khoo LT, Fessler RG. Microendoscopic decompressive laminotomy for the treatment of lumbar stenosis. *Neurosurgery* 2002;51:S146–S154

63. Beringer WF, Mobasser JP. Unilateral pedicle screw instrumentation for minimally invasive transforaminal lumbar interbody fusion. *Neurosurg Focus* 2006;20:E4

64. Deutsch H, Musacchio MJ Jr. Minimally invasive transforaminal lumbar interbody fusion with unilateral pedicle screw fixation. *Neurosurg Focus* 2006;20:E10

65. Holly LT, Foley KT. Three-dimensional fluoroscopy-guided percutaneous thoracolumbar pedicle screw placement. Technical note. *J Neurosurg* 2003;99:324–329

66. Grutzner PA, Beutler T, Wendl K, et al. [Intraoperative three-dimensional navigation for pedicle screw placement]. *Chirurg* 2004;75:967–975

67. Villavicencio AT, Burneikiene S, Bulsara KR, et al. Utility of computerized isocentric fluoroscopy for minimally invasive spinal surgical techniques. *J Spinal Disord Tech* 2005; 18:369–375

68. Shoham M, Lieberman IH, Benzel EC, et al. Robotic assisted spinal surgery - from concept to clinical practice. *Comput Aided Surg* 2007;12:105–115

69. O. Toole, J.E., Eichholy, J.M., Fossler, G.G. Surgicalsite infection notes after minimally invasive surgey. Zournal of Neuosurgery in press

Chapter 70
Minimally Invasive Treatment of Spinal Deformity

Christopher M. Zarro and Baron S. Lonner

There has been a rapid evolution in the operative management of spinal deformity during the past century. While much has changed in the surgical theater, the goals of treatment have remained the same; to achieve balanced curve correction, obtain solid arthrodesis, prevent future deformity, improve and/or prevent back pain, and avoid cardiopulmonary compromise.[1] In the first half of the 20th century, the standard of care was posterior arthrodesis followed by prolonged bed rest and casting.[2] In the late 1950s, Harrington introduced instrumentation to achieve improved curve correction, lower pseudarthrosis rates, and allow early patient mobilization. Harrington utilized a nonsegmental system to distract across the concave side of a curvature and, in doing so, elongated the spine.[3] The coronal plane correction achieved was desirable but the sagittal plane distraction forces resulted in a loss of lumbar lordosis and flat back syndrome in many patients.[4]

In the early 1980s, segmental spinal instrumentation was introduced by Luque. This consisted of two longitudinal contoured rods fixed to the spine via multiple sublaminar wires. The mechanism of curve correction in the Luque system involved predominantly translation. This resulted in correction of the coronal plane deformity while preserving the sagittal plane contour and improving fixation.[5] While an improvement over the Harrington system in some respects, passage of sublaminar wires in the spinal canal resulted in an increased risk of neurologic injury. During the next 20 years, the concept of segmental instrumentation was further developed and improved upon. Cotrel and Dubousset introduced bilateral segmental hook fixation with dual rods. Cotrel-Dubousset instrumentation allowed selective distraction and compression at different levels, improving correction and construct rigidity and maximizing the number of preserved motion segments. The improved construct rigidity allowed immediate patient mobilization without an orthosis.[6] In the 1990s, multisegmental instrumentation expanded to include the use of pedicle screws in the lumbar and, later, the thoracic spine. Suk popularized the use of pedicle screws at all levels of the thoracic spine, resulting in improved curve correction and construct stability.[7]

As posterior surgical techniques were developed during the past century, a simultaneous evolution occurred in anterior surgical approaches for deformity correction. In 1960, Hodgson and Stock described an anterior approach for resection and fusion of vertebral tuberculosis.[8] Dwyer, in 1969, introduced a cable and screw system to treat thoracolumbar scoliosis via a short segment anterior arthrodesis. Coronal plane correction was achieved, but the procedure was complicated by high rates of implant failure, pseudarthrosis, and kyphotic deformity.[9,10] In an effort to lessen these complications, Zielke introduced a threaded rod instead of a cable in 1976, but maintaining lordosis was still noted to be a problem without anterior structural support.[11,12] Current techniques involve an anterior structural graft or mesh cage and rigid dual rod systems such as those described by Kaneda in 1996 with or without interbody structural grafting.[13]

A major advantage of anterior fusion procedures is the ability to utilize shorter constructs in the thoracolumbar spine thereby saving distal motion segments. Hall recommended fusion of one vertebral level above and one level below the curve apex when fusion is performed anteriorly. If the apex is at a disc, then arthrodesis should include two levels above and two levels below.[14] The more commonly used alternative to this so called short-segment fusion, is an arthrodesis including the Cobb end vertebrae of the curvature. Although fusion levels may be spared with anterior arthrodesis, there is concern about the impact of the anterior approach on pulmonary function. In an effort to allay some of these concerns, Regan and Picetti introduced video-assisted thoracoscopic spine surgery for thoracic deformity in the early 1990s.[15] Advantages of thoracoscopy over traditional open thoracic approaches include reduced postoperative pain, less pulmonary morbidity, less intraoperative blood loss, shorter hospital stay, better intraoperative visualization, and improved cosmesis.[16] The major disadvantages of the approach are the technical demands of the procedure and significant learning curve. Early on in a surgeon's training with the procedure, one can utilize a mini open thoracoscopic-assisted procedure until the surgeon becomes more adept at procedures done entirely through the scope. These minimally invasive alternatives to an open thoracotomy can be employed for anterior releases, anterior fusions with corrective instrumentation and various growth modulation

C.M. Zarro and B.S. Lonner (✉)
NYU Hospital for Joint Diseases,
820 2nd Avenue, Suite 7A, New York, NY 10017
e-mail: blonner@nyc.rr.com

G.R. Scuderi and A.J. Tria (eds.), *Minimally Invasive Surgery in Orthopedics*,
DOI 10.1007/978-0-387-76608-9_70, © Springer Science+Business Media, LLC 2010

techniques including stapling, and other tethers. The focus of this chapter is on these minimally invasive surgical techniques, their applications, and potential complications.

Video-Assisted Thoracoscopic Spine Surgery

During the past 15 years, thoracoscopy has become a valuable tool in the surgical treatment of spinal deformity. The large open space of the chest cavity makes the thorax an ideal location for less invasive endoscopic techniques.[17] Thoracoscopic surgery minimizes the morbidity of the anterior approach while retaining several of its advantages. Advantages of anterior thoracic fusion and instrumentation include fusion of fewer motion segments, less blood loss, and better restoration of sagittal contour compared with the posterior approach. These advantages come at a price when performing an open thoracotomy, which results in decreased pulmonary function and shoulder girdle strength.[18] Landreneau and others have found that there is less postoperative pain, a more rapid recovery, shorter hospital stay, improved cosmesis, less impact on pulmonary and shoulder girdle function, and less blood loss when comparing thoracoscopy with an open thoracotomy.[19,20] Additionally, intraoperative visualization is improved due to the use of multiple ports, angled scopes, magnification, and illumination. The disadvantages of the procedure as noted by Newton and Lonner are the steep learning curve and the expense of the new equipment required.[20]

Anterior release and fusion is indicated for the treatment of rigid scoliosis and kyphosis, scoliosis in patients at risk for crankshaft due to continued anterior column growth, after posterior arthrodesis in skeletally immature patients with an open triradiate cartilage, and patients at increased risk for pseudarthrosis from stand-alone posterior procedures such as patients with neurofibromatosis. The absolute indications for thoracoscopy as a means of obtaining anterior release and/or fusion are not established. However, Al-Sayyad and Wolf report the following indications: (1) rigid idiopathic scoliosis with curves of 75° that do not correct to less than 50° on side-bending radiographs; (2) to prevent crankshaft in immature children with greater than 50° curves; (3) patients with kyphotic deformities that do not correct to less than 50° on hyperextension radiographs; (4) progressive congenital deformities within the thorax requiring anterior epiphysiodesis; (5) patients with neuromuscular deformities and an "at risk" pulmonary status; (6) severe rib hump deformity not corrected by spinal instrumentation; (7) patients with neurofibromatosis who have intrathoracic tumors in addition to spinal deformity; (8) pseudarthrosis after anterior intervertebral fusion; (9) excision of the first rib for thoracic outlet syndrome; (10) rib and intercostal nerve tumors; and (11) instrumentation of thoracic spinal deformity above the diaphragm. These indications continue to evolve as stand-alone posterior procedures

have become more powerful with the use of thoracic pedicle screws. Growth-modulation procedures will likely be an indication for thoracoscopic surgery in increasing numbers in the future. Contraindications include patients who are unable to tolerate single-lung ventilation, those who have had previous ipsilateral thoracic procedures or pleural infections resulting in pleural adhesions, those with severe or acute respiratory insufficiency, and those with high airway pressures with positive pressure ventilation.[21]

Technique for Anterior Release

The authors' preferred technique involves positioning the patient prone on the Jackson frame after obtaining single-lung ventilation using a double-lumen endotracheal tube or bronchial blocker. A sterile prep of both the back and right chest is performed. The thoracoscopic portals (usually three) are placed in a linear fashion along the posterior axillary line (Fig. 70.1). The initial portal is made at the seventh or eighth intercostal space to avoid diaphragmatic injury upon entry into the chest, and a 45° scope is introduced. Visibility may be enhanced by utilizing carbon dioxide insufflation at 8 mmHg of pressure, which allows the use of a standard endotracheal tube. If rib graft is to be obtained, 6- to 8-cm segments of rib can be obtained through the incision for the portal without the need to extend the incision. After the placement of the first portal, additional portals are placed under direct visualization of the chest wall, using the scope to avoid injury to the diaphragm, lung, or other structures within the thoracic cavity. The ribs are counted to identify the levels to be released and/or fused, depending on the preoperative plan. The first rib hides deep to the pulsating

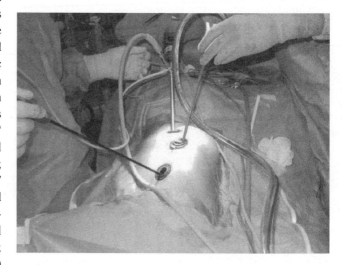

Fig. 70.1 Correct portal placement. Three portals are utilized: one for the camera, one for a suction device, and the third working portal for passage of instruments. This patient is positioned in the left lateral decubitus position

subclavian artery. Typically, three portals are used, which house the thoracoscope, a suction device, and the working instrument. Subsequently, pleural incision is performed with a harmonic scalpel (Fig. 70.2). The pleura is then bluntly dissected to expose the anterior longitudinal ligament (ALL) and contralateral annulus of the discs to be excised. After coagulating and incising the segmental vessels over the levels to be operated on, the ALL and annulus are incised and Cobb elevators are employed to separate the disc and endplate from the vertebral body. The disc material is then removed with long-handle endoscopic curettes, pituitary rongeurs, and Kerrison punches back to the posterior annulus (Fig. 70.3). A long-handle rasp is used for final endplate preparation. This sequence is repeated at all levels as determined by the preoperative plan. Rib autograft then may be placed for

fusion. A chest tube is placed through the caudal portal. It is left in place postoperatively until the output is less than 50 mL per 8-h shift.

Thoracoscopic Anterior Instrumentation

In the 1950s and through the 1980s, long fusions to the lower lumbar spine were common. The current trend, using guidelines set forth in the Lenke classification system, is to avoid fusion into the lumbar spine in patients who have primary structural thoracic curves.[22] Curve correction is comparable between anterior and posterior surgery, although by limiting the fusion to the proximal end vertebra and the distal end vertebra of the structural curve, anterior instrumentation has been shown to save up to 2.5 distal fusion levels. An additional benefit is improvement in sagittal plane correction while avoiding spinal extensor muscle disruption.[23] Adaptations to the instrumentation used in traditional open thoracotomies have enabled surgeons to use anterior instrumentation thoracoscopically (Fig. 70.4). The ideal candidate for thoracoscopic fusion and instrumentation at the authors' institution is a patient with a single structural thoracic curve (Lenke 1), of a magnitude between 40 and 70°, with less than 40° of kyphosis that corrects by a minimum of 50% on bending radiographs. Contraindications include patients with greater than 40° of kyphosis, those with severe lung disease, and those unable or unwilling to wear a brace postoperatively.

There are many technical pearls to consider during thoracoscopic instrumentation to ensure patient safety and successful fusion. As with open procedures, segmental bicortical fixation is desirable at all vertebral levels included within the fusion. However, a unicortical screw design allows for similar screw purchase without bicortical fixation. Screw insertion requires

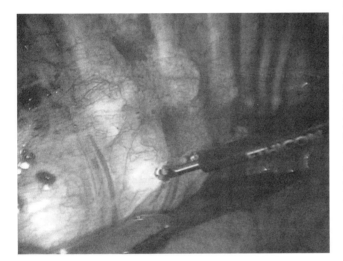

Fig. 70.2 An intraoperative view using the thoracoscope. The segmental vessels are seen traversing along the vertebral body; the harmonic scalpel is used to expose the disc space

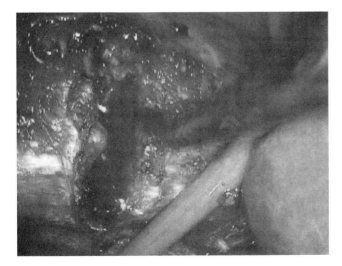

Fig. 70.3 The use of a pituitary rongeur through a working cannula to perform the discectomy is shown

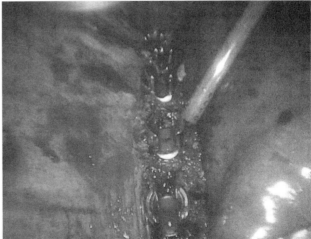

Fig. 70.4 Screw placement in the vertebral bodies using a thoracoscopic approach

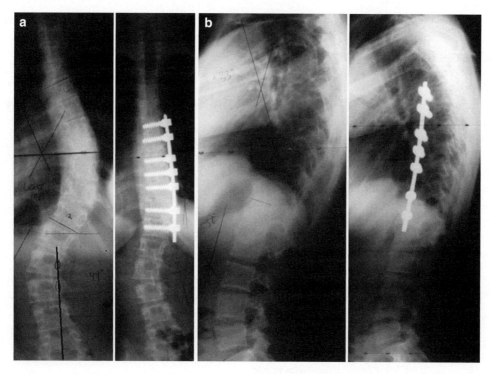

Fig. 70.5 (**a**) The preoperative and postoperative anteroposterior (AP) radiograph and (**b**) a preoperative and postoperative lateral radiograph of a patient who underwent a thoracoscopic anterior fusion

careful portal placement, which is planned under fluoroscopic guidance. The working portals should be placed in the posterior axillary line for a direct lateral view of the spine. The starting point for the screws is just anterior to the rib head and in the midportion of the vertebral body. At more proximal levels, gaining access to the starting position may necessitate rib head excision. Screw placement requires ligation of the ipsilateral segmental vessels. As with open procedures, careful discectomy, endplate preparation, and bone grafting, using autologous rib or iliac crest, are the key to obtaining a solid fusion (Fig. 70.5).

Outcomes

Thoracoscopic spine surgery is a relatively new technique and, as such, long-term follow-up data is lacking. However, several studies do report on the immediate postoperative and 2-year outcomes compared with traditional open anterior approaches as well as with posterior approaches. Lonner et al. evaluated outcomes utilizing the Scoliosis Research Society questionnaire (SRS-22) regarding quality of life and reported better results in 28 patients who underwent thoracoscopic anterior fusion and instrumentation compared with 23 patients who underwent posterior surgery with all hook or hook-screw hybrid constructs.[24] Landreneau et al. reported less postoperative pain and a statistically significant shorter length of stay in patients treated with thoracoscopy as

compared with open thoracotomy in thoracic surgery patients.[19] Newton's 2003 case series compared pulmonary function testing in two groups of patients; the first underwent thoracoscopic anterior instrumented fusion and the second underwent open anterior instrumentation. Pulmonary function testing for the thoracoscopic group demonstrated a return of forced vital capacity (FVC) and forced expiratory volume in 1 s (FEV1) by 6 months. He also reported a significantly larger decline in FVC at 3 months in the thoracotomy group. In that same study, the effect of the approach on shoulder abduction strength was compared at three time points; preoperatively, the day of discharge, and 6 weeks postoperatively. There was a trend suggesting a more rapid return of strength in the thoracoscopic group at the 6-week time point.[20] Wall et al. evaluated the adequacy of surgical release between open and thoracoscopic techniques in an animal model and found no statistically significant difference between the groups.[25] Lonner et al. also showed there to be no significant difference in the percentage of curve correction obtained between patients who underwent thoracoscopic fusion (58% correction) and those who had posterior procedures (55.5% correction). In the same study, the average fusion levels required in the thoracoscopic group were 5.8, compared with 9.3 in the posterior group; blood loss was 359 and 537 ml, respectively. It is important to note that there was a significant difference in operative time, with the thoracoscopic group taking 366 min compared with 192 min for the posterior group.[24] Lonner et al. recently presented data on 17 patients treated by thoracoscopic anterior instrumentation compared with a matched (age, sex, curve type, and magnitude) group of 17 patients treated by posterior fusion with all pedicle screw constructs. Although percent corrections were statistically equivalent (57% vs. 64%) they trended toward being greater for the all-pedicle screw group. The number of pedicle screw anchors utilized are greater today than for the patients reported so that the differences are likely to be greater. No differences were found between the two groups in SRS-22 outcomes.[26] Further development of thoracoscopic instrumentation is required to improve corrections and maintenance of correction. Newton studied the operative time, and found that as the frequency of cases increased to greater than 30, the operative time per disc excised decreased from 29 to 22 min.[27]

Fusionless Scoliosis Treatment

The natural history of scoliosis is dependent on the curve severity, curve pattern, and skeletal maturity of the patient. Patients who present with large curves and significant growth potential are likely to have curve progression. Sixty-eight percent of patients presenting with curves measuring 20–29° and Risser grade 0–1 will have curve progression.[28] Indications for bracing include curves between 30 and 40° on initial presentation, or curves greater than 20° that exhibit progression skeletally immature patients.[17] The success of brace wear is dose-dependent, with better results reported for so-called full-time bracing vs. part-time bracing.[29] This results in a high rate of noncompliance among adolescents.[30,31] Furthermore, bracing does not typically result in curve correction, rather, its goal is to halt curve progression and it is effective approximately 70% of the time.[32]

Fusionless techniques using minimally invasive approaches to the anterior thoracic spine have been developed in an effort to obtain curve correction and avoid brace wear. These techniques are often referred to as anterior thoracoscopic vertebral stapling, convex tethering, mechanical growth modulation, or internal bracing. Utilizing the Hueter Volkman principle, these techniques inhibit progression and may correct scoliotic deformities while preserving growth, motion, and function of the spine and do not rely on patient compliance for efficacy.[33] Additionally, they may prevent adjacent segment degeneration seen with more traditional fusion technology. A number of centers are evaluating these concepts. Braun et al. created scoliosis in a goat model and used a ligament tether and bone anchors on the curve convexity to show modest correction and stabilization of curves less than 70°.[33] Early applications of vertebral stapling had disappointing results and were complicated by staple dislodgement or failure.[34] Betz et al. reported that the initial stainless steel staples used were prone to dislodge because their tines were placed parallel to the vertebral body endplates, making them unable to withstand the motion that occurs in the spine. To address

this concern, he employs a proportionally sized Nitinol staple (Medtronic Sofamor Danek, Memphis TN) to fit the size of the patient and thereby cross the disc space to gain purchase into the adjacent vertebral bodies. Nitinol is a shape memory metal alloy composed of 50% nickel and 50% titanium that, when cooled, has straight prongs, but, at body temperature, clamps into a "C" shape for secure fixation into bone. His early results in 21 patients showed a cessation of curve progression or curve correction for the majority of those with initial curves less than 30°, there were three minor complications and no major complications. The procedure was performed with thoracoscopic assistance placing staples at all vertebrae within the measured Cobb curve.[35]

Although there is evidence of success for these techniques in the literature, absolute indications are unclear. Questions remain regarding when an operative intervention should be applied to patients who are currently treated nonoperatively with observation or bracing. Perhaps advances in genetics may shed light on which patients will progress, and when and what type of treatment should be initiated.[36]

Complications

Complications related to thoracoscopic anterior spinal release and fusion for deformity are relatively few and can be related to surgical technique, patient positioning, and anesthesia. They include the need for conversion to an open thoracotomy for the inability to control bleeding, recurrent pleural effusions requiring chest tube reinsertion, chylothorax, intercostal neuralgia, lung parenchymal injury, and superficial wound infection.[36,37] The major disadvantage of thoracoscopic approaches to the spine for anterior instrumentation is the learning curve and prolonged operative time compared with traditional open techniques. This learning curve exists not only for the surgeon but for the anesthesiologist as well, because the anesthesiologist must become adept at obtaining and maintaining single-lung ventilation.[38,39] In 2002, Sucato published a case report of a patient who sustained bilateral pneumothoraces, pneumomediastinum, pneumoperitoneum, and subcutaneous emphysema as a result of tracheal and bronchial tears caused by an inappropriately sized double-lumen tube.[37] The requirement for single-lung ventilation and prolonged positioning in the lateral decubitus position may result in prolonged postoperative atelectasis, pneumonia, and mucous plugs.[39]

For the patient undergoing an anterior release followed by a posterior fusion, prone positioning for the thoracoscopic release has advantages over lateral positioning by avoiding the need for repositioning and reprepping. More importantly, it alleviates the pressure on the dependent lung caused by the body weight and mediastinum, and the tendency for congestion and mucous plugging on the down-side lung. It makes retraction of the lung less difficult because the lung falls anteriorly due to gravity, and it may avoid single-lung ventilation if bilateral ventilation can be performed at lower tidal volumes.[40] Carbon dioxide insufflation is another option that permits bilateral ventilation while maintaining satis-factory visualization (Tim Oswald, personal communication, Atlanta, GA).

The learning curve for the surgeon involves mastering hand eye coordination, becoming facile with long instruments where tactile feedback may be less than with standard tools, and interpreting two-dimensional images of three-dimensional structures on video screens. In order to avoid complications, a surgeon considering thoracoscopic spinal surgery should first be comfortable with the anatomy of the anterior approach. The surgeon should attend didactic and hands-on courses, train in a cadaver or animal laboratory, and ensure that the surgeon has adequate surgical volume to justify the learning curve, a minimum of 15 cases per year. Lonner found that a significant improvement in the learning curve was noted after 28 cases, as noted by a decrease in operative time, pseudarthrosis, and implant breakage.[39] A further suggestion may be to perform the procedure as a mini open thoracotomy with thoracoscopic assistance. In 2002, Hasharino et al. described a thoracoscopically assisted mini open thoracotomy to perform anterior releases in 15 patients with either rigid scoliotic curves or kyphosis greater than 90°. The procedure was performed with the patient in the lateral decubitus position through a 5- to 7-cm incision over the apical vertebra. The study showed the mini open procedure is efficient, easy to learn, effective, and may be more cosmetically appealing than its traditional open counterpart.[41] In an effort to hasten progression of the learning curve, efficiency can be improved by maintaining a consistent operating room team.

Conclusion

Minimally invasive techniques for spinal deformity will have an increasing role in the future. The application of growth-modulation approaches such as stapling and tethers hold promise to result in curve correction without the need for fusion. Further studies are needed to evaluate the long-term outcomes of these techniques and their future applications.

References

1. Hibbs RA, Risser JC, Ferguson AB. Scoliosis treated by the fusion operation: an end-result study of three hundred and sixty cases. J Bone Joint Surg 1931;13:91–104
2. Cobb J. Spine arthrodesis in the treatment of scoliosis. Bull Hosp Joint Dis 1958;29:187–209
3. Harrington P. Treatment of scoliosis: correction and internal fixation by spine instrumentation. J Bone Joint Surg 1962;44:591–610
4. Bridwell K. Spinal instrumentation in the management of adolescent scoliosis. Clin Orthop Relat Res 1997 Feb;(335): 64–72
5. Luque E. Segmental spinal instrumentation for correction of scoliosis. Clin Orthop Relat Res 1982 Mar;(163):192–198
6. Cotrel Y, Dubousset J. A new technique for segmental spinal osteosynthesis using the posterior approach. Rev Chir Orthop Reparatrice Appar Mot 1984;70(6):489–494
7. Suk S, Lee C, Jeong S. Segmental pedicle screw fixation in the treatment of thoracic idiopathic scoliosis. Spine 1995; 20: 1399–1405
8. Hodgson A, Stock F. Anterior fusion for the treatment of tuberculosis of the spine: the operative findings and results of treatment in the first on hundred cases. J Bone Joint Surg 1960;42:295–304
9. Dwyer A, Newton N, Sherwood A. An anterior approach to scoliosis. A preliminary report. Clin Orthop Relat Res 1969 Jan-Feb;(62): 192–202
10. Lonner B. Emerging minimally invasive technologies for the management of scoliosis. Orthop Clin North Am 2007;38:431–440
11. Zielke K, Pellin B. New instruments and implants for supplementation of Harrington system. Z Orthop Ihre Grengeb 1976;114: 5347–5359
12. Lowe T, Peters J. Anterior spinal fusion with Zielke instrumentation for idiopathic scoliosis: a frontal and sagittal curve analysis in 36 patients. Spine 1993;18:423–426
13. Kaneda K, Shono Y, Satoh S, et al. New anterior instrumentation for the management of thoracolumbar and lumbar scoliosis. Application of Kaneda two rod system. Spine 1996;22:1358–1368
14. Bernstein R, Hall J. Solid rod short segment anterior fusion in thoracolumbar scoliosis. J Pediatr Orthop B 1998;7:124–131
15. Mack M, Regan J, Bobechko W, et al. Application of thoracoscopy for diseases of the sine. Ann Thorac Surg 1993;56:736–738
16. Newton P, Shea K, Granlund K. Defining the pediatric spinal thoracoscopy learning curve: sixty five consecutive cases. Spine 2000; 25:1028–1035
17. Herkowitz H. Rothman-Simeone The Spine, 5th edn. Elsevier, Philadelphia, 2006
18. Vedantam R, Lenke L, Bridwell K, et al. A prospective evaluation of pulmonary function in patients with adolescent idiopathic scoliosis relative to the surgical approach used for spinal arthrodesis. Spine 2000;25:82–90
19. Landreneau R, Hazelrigg S, Mack M. Postoperative pain related morbidity: video assisted thoracoscopy versus thoracotomy. Ann Thorac Surg 1993;56:1285–1289
20. Newton P, Marks M, Faro F, et al. Use of video-assisted thoracoscopic surgery to reduce perioperative morbidity in scoliosis surgery. Spine 2003;28(20):S249–S254
21. Al-Sayyad M, Crawford A, Wolf R. Early experience with video assisted thoracoscopic surgery: our first 70 cases. Spine 2004;29(17): 1945–1951
22. Lenke L, Betz R, Harms J, et al. Adolescent idiopathic scoliosis: a new classification to determine extent of spinal arthrodesis. J Bone Joint Surg 2001;83:1169–1181
23. Betz R, Shufflebarger H. Anterior versus posterior instrumentation for the correction of thoracic idiopathic scoliosis. Spine 2001;26: 1095–1100
24. Lonner B, Kondrachor D, Siddiqi F, et al. Thoracoscopic spinal fusion compared with posterior spinal fusion for the treatment of thoracic adolescent idiopathic scoliosis. J Bone Joint Surg 2006; 88:1022–1034
25. Wall E, Bylski-Austrow D, Shelton F, et al. Endoscopic discectomy increases thoracic spine flexibility as effectively as open discectomy: a mechanical study in a porcine model. Spine 1998;23:9–16
26. Lonner BS, Auerbach JD, Estreicher M, et al. Video-Assisted Thoracoscopic Spinal Fusion Compared with Thoracic Pedicle Screws for Thoracic Adolescent Idiopathic Scoliosis. J Bone Joint Surg 2009;91:398–408

27. Newton P, Cardelia J, Farnsworth C, et al. A biomechanical comparison of thoracoscopic and open anterior spinal release in a goat model. Spine 1998;23(5):530–535

28. Lonstein J, Carlson J. The prediction of curve progression in untreated idiopathic curve progression during growth. J Bone Joint Surg 1984;66:1061–1071

29. Allington N, Bowen J. Adolescent idiopathic scoliosis: treatment with the Wilmington brace: a comparison of full time and part time use. J Bone Joint Surg 1996;78A:1056–1062

30. Clayson D, Luz-Alterman S, Cataletto M, et al. Long term psychological sequelae of surgically versus nonsurgically treated scoliosis. Spine 1987;12:983–986

31. Noonan K, Dolan L, Jacobson W, et al. Long term psychosocial characteristics of patients treated for idiopathic scoliosis. J Pediatr Orthop 1997;17:712–717

32. Nachemson A, Peterson L. Effectiveness of treatment with a brace in girls who have adolescent idiopathic scoliosis. J Bone Joint Surg 1995;77:815–822

33. Braun J, Akyuz E, Udall H, et al. Three dimensional analysis of 2 fusionless scoliosis treatments: a flexible ligament tether versus a rigid shape memory alloy staple. Spine 2006;31(3):262–268

34. Smith A, Von Lakum H, Wylie R. An operation for stapling vertebral bodies in congenital scoliosis. J Bone Joint Surg 1954;36A:342–348

35. Betz R, Kim J, D'Andrea, et al. An innovative technique of vertebral body stapling for the treatment of patients with adolescent idiopathic scoliosis: a feasibility, safety and utility study. Spine 2003;28(205):S255–S265

36. Thompson G, Lenke L, Akbarnia B, et al. Early onset scoliosis: future directions. J Bone Joint Surg 2007;89A:163–166

37. Sucato D, Girgis M. Bilateral pneumothoraces, pneumomediastinum, pneumoperitoneum and subcutaneous emphysema following intubation with a double lumen endotracheal tube for thoracoscopic anterior spinal release and fusion in a patient with idiopathic scoliosis. J Spinal Disord Tech 2002;15(2):133–138

38. Perez-Cruet M, Fessler R, Perin N. Review: complications of minimally invasive spinal surgery. Neurosurgery 2002;51(2):S26–S36

39. Dieter R, Kuzycz G. Complications and contraindications of thoracoscopy. Int Surg 1997;82:232–239

40. Sucato D, Elerson E. A comparison of the prone and lateral position for performing a thoracoscopic anterior release and fusion for pediatric spinal deformity. Spine 2003;28(18):2176–2180

41. Hasharino A, Errico T, Lonner B, et al. Mini open thoracotomy, thoracoscopically assisted, for anterior thoracic spine release. J Bone Joint Surg Br 2002;84(Suppl III):297–298

Chapter 71
Percutaneous Vertebral Augmentation: Vertebroplasty and Kyphoplasty

Richard L. Lebow, John E. O'Toole, Richard G. Fessler, and Kurt M. Eichholz

Vertebroplasty and balloon kyphoplasty are two percutaneous surgical options for the treatment of osteoporotic vertebral compression fractures (VCF) that have become increasingly utilized since their development in the mid 1980s. These well-described techniques can also address VCF caused by metastatic lesions, multiple myeloma, and hemangiomas. Physicians from several disciplines including neurosurgery, orthopedic surgery, and radiology now perform vertebroplasty and balloon kyphoplasty as a routine part of their practice. The surgical goals of vertebroplasty are to stabilize the fractured vertebral body and provide relief from pain. Pain is thought to be alleviated from bonding and strengthening the fractured vertebral body, as well as from the thermal reaction that occurs during the curing of the polymethylmethacrylate (PMMA) cement. Balloon kyphoplasty has similar goals, but also aims at partially correcting the deformity by restoring the vertebral body height. However, controversy does exist over whether the pain is relieved from fracture stabilization, the PMMA thermal reaction, or from the restoration of vertebral height. Recent developments have included using an arc osteotome, which is placed through a percutaneous transpedicular approach, for cavity creation prior to filling the defect with PMMA cement. This chapter summarizes the indications, techniques, and complications for both the vertebroplasty with and without cavity creation.

Indications

Vertebroplasty was initially described by Galibert et al. in 1987 as a percutaneous technique to treat vertebral angiomas.[1] Since that time, the treatment indication for vertebroplasty has expanded to include osteoporotic compression fractures, metastatic spinal lesions, and traumatic vertebral body fractures.[2]

Affecting more than 24 million Americans, osteoporosis is a systemic metabolic bone disorder characterized by low bone density and the progressive microarchitectural deterioration of bone tissue leading to increased bone fragility and thus an increased risk of fracture.[3] Vertebral fractures are the most common type of osteoporotic fracture and are a significant cause of morbidity and mortality in the elderly population in the United States.[4] The incidence of osteoporotic vertebral fractures is difficult to accurately quantify given that only approximately 30% come to medical attention.[5] The risk of developing VCF has been shown to increase with age. Slightly less than 25% of women over the age of 50 years are afflicted by osteoporotic bone fractures.[6] This number increases only slightly into the seventies, after which there is an abrupt rise into the 40–50% range for female octogenarians.[5,7] However, this is not solely a women's disease, as a review by Olszynski et al. demonstrated that VCF occur in approximately 40% of men surviving into their eighth decade.[8] Osteoporosis has a significant socioeconomic impact, as the estimated cost of osteoporotic bone fractures within the United States in 1995 was approximately $746 million.[3] Considering the increasing life expectancy in the United States, as well as the growth in the senior citizen population, the "baby boomer generations" ages, the prevalence and economic impact of this disease will continue to magnify in the near future. Other factors that increase the risk of developing VCF include rheumatoid arthritis, cirrhosis, renal insufficiency, menopause, prolonged immobilization or immobility, chronic steroid therapy, diabetes mellitus, and malnutrition.[9]

Metastatic spinal lesions that cause compression fractures have also been treated with vertebroplasty. Metastatic disease commonly affects the spine and is symptomatic in more than a third of patients afflicted with cancer.[10,11] Spinal metastases are the presenting symptom in approximately 10% of cases.[12] The majority of primary lesions are breast, lung, and prostate, which account for approximately 60% of cases, while gastrointestinal and renal malignancies are each responsible for 5% of cases.[13] Metastases are typically osteolytic processes, and result in subsequent weakness and fracture of the vertebral bodies. Symptomatically, these lesions result in debilitating pain, deformity, and neurologic compromise.[10,11,13] These sequelae have a detrimental impact on the quality of life for patients who already have systematic neoplastic disease. Vertebroplasty has become a useful treatment for symptomatic

R.L. Lebow, J.E. O'Toole, R.G. Fessler (✉), and K. Eichholz
Department of Neurosurgery, Feinberg School of Medicine,
Northwestern University, 303 East Chicago Avenue, Chicago, IL,
60611-3008, USA
e-mail: RFessler@nmff.org

relief for spinal metastatic disease[14–17] as well as multiple myeloma,[18] has been used to treat malignant compression fractures with epidural involvement,[19] and has been combined with radiotherapy.[20]

Vertebroplasty has also been employed in the treatment of burst fractures,[2] although this should be done with trepidation. Detailed analysis of radiographic images is essential to ensure that injection of cement does not cause further retropulsion of loose bone fragments into the canal. It has been shown that balloon vertebroplasty may be used safely in cases where damage to the longitudinal ligaments is expected.[21] In the setting of vertebral burst fracture, careful consideration must be made in the decision to perform cavity creation, and with what method (balloon or arc osteotome).

Natural History and Conservative Management

Osteoporosis-induced VCF can be a self-perpetuating cycle. Ross et al. examined how bone mass density and the presence of VCF were predictive of the development of future fractures.[22] After a mean follow-up of 4.7 years, they concluded that patients who had a bone mass less than two standard deviations from the mean has a fivefold increased risk of developing VCF. This increased risk was the same for patients with average bone density and a prior single VCF. However, in the presence of two or more VCF, this risk is magnified to 12-fold. In the rare setting of a patient with a bone mass in the 33rd percentile and two or more fractures, the risk of future fractures is increased by 75-fold compared with women with bone density above the 67th percentile and no prior history of VCF. Although this population is at high risk for the development of multiple fractures, only approximately two thirds of patients with acute symptomatic fractures improve despite the management initiated.[23]

Traditional conservative treatment includes oral analgesic therapy and bed rest. However, bed rest may accelerate bone loss and increases the risk of developing deep venous thromboses.[24] The pain caused by vertebral fractures may last for months and prove to be severely debilitating. Unfortunately, the use of analgesic medical therapy occasionally results in narcotic dependence. In a predominantly elderly population, this can alter mood and mental status, thus compounding the patient's condition.[25] Chronic pain, sleep deprivation, depression, decreased mobility, and loss of independence are all sequelae of VCF.[26,27] In addition, both thoracic and lumbar compression fractures can lead to a decrease in lung capacity.[28]

Alternatively, physical therapy and use of a hardshell brace that appropriately immobilizes the affected segment may decrease the risks of complications due to bed rest. As noted above, the majority of patients improve regardless of the treatment prescribed, usually within 4–6 weeks. Several additional medical treatments have been studied with mixed results. Bisphosphonates, calcitonin, parathyroid hormone, or raloxifene have been shown to reduce subsequent fracture rates, whereas the results for calcitriol, etidronate, fluoride, and pamidronate have been mixed and inconclusive.[29] In comparing conservative treatment with vertebroplasty, Diamond et al. conducted a prospective, nonrandomized trial of osteoporotic patients with acute VCF.[30] It was shown that vertebroplasty provided a rapid and significant reduction in pain and an improvement in physical activity scores compared with medical treatment and it was concluded that vertebroplasty is a viable treatment option.

Patient Evaluation and Selection

It is important to obtain a thorough medical history with specific attention to risk factors for VCF as well surgical candidacy. Evaluation continues with a detailed neurological examination documenting any motor or sensory changes, and paying attention to any existing radiculopathies. Preoperative investigations should include routine laboratory work and coagulation studies. In addition, if malignancy is suspected, an appropriate work-up is indicated, including the determination of a tissue diagnosis, if possible. Radiologic evaluation includes anteroposterior (AP) and lateral radiographs of the spine as well as a thin-cut, reconstructed computed tomography (CT) scan. The CT scan is scrutinized to evaluate the integrity of the posterior cortex, which may suggest an increased risk of cement extrusion into the spinal canal during the procedure, as well as the size of the pedicles, should a transpedicular route be considered. In patients with signs of myelopathy, it is essential to obtain an magnetic resonance imaging (MRI) or postmyelogram CT scan (if MRI is contraindicated) to evaluate for evidence of cord compression. The presence of bone marrow or endplate edema has been shown to be a positive prognostic sign for patients undergoing vertebroplasty.[31] Alvarez et al. also showed that signal changes in the vertebral body on MRI scan as well as 70% or greater collapse of the vertebral body are both highly predictive of positive outcome.[32]

The primary indication for vertebroplasty is failure of conservative management of a vertebral fracture in which patients continue to have pain that affects their mobility and activities of daily living. It is important in determining if vertebroplasty is indicated to ensure that the pain be localized and attributable to the fracture level. There is no evidence available in the medical literature to guide the duration of conservative therapy before it is deemed a failure. Typically, patients are selected whose duration of pain from fracture is greater than 6 weeks, but less than 1 year. Others have reported successfully treating painful fractures of 2-year duration.[33] While complete relief of pain is less likely in older fractures,[34,35] Irani reported symptomatic improvement in fractures up to 5 years old.[36] Guidelines and reviews have been published to aid in the selection of patients, although the decision to undergo surgery is made by the treating surgeon.[37,38] Painful osteoporotic and osteolytic fractures without myelopathy constitute the vast majority of cases in most practices. Contraindications for vertebroplasty include severe wedge deformity with loss of greater than 90% of vertebral height (vertebra plana), comminuted burst fracture, spinal canal compromise >20%, epidural tumor extension, myelopathy, inability to lie prone, uncorrected coagulopathy, inability to localize source of pain, allergy to cement or radio-opaque dye, and infection (local or systemic). There has been considerable debate into the merits of prophylactic verte-broplasty in selected patients;[37,38] however, it is the practice of the senior authors to only include symptomatic patients, because many patients never develop clinical symptoms. It is also prudent to have the facilities and capability to perform emergent decompressive surgery should extravasation of bone cement into the spinal canal occur, resulting in spinal cord compromise.

Kyphoplasty is a modification of the vertebroplasty technique that was developed in the late 1990s.[39,40] This technique attempts to restore vertebral body height with the introduction of cement into a lower-pressure cavity. The use of a balloon creates a cavity for placement of the cement, and may result in a lower incidence of cement extravasation.[41] Verlaan showed a reduced incidence of endplate fractures in balloon vertebroplasty.[42] In addition, recent developments have included the use of an arc osteotome, which creates a cavity for cement placement without attempting to restore vertebral body height. The indications for these procedures mirror those for vertebroplasty; however, with the goal of fracture reduction, the age of the fracture affects the success rate, although the exact timing has yet to be determined.[38,43] In addition, technical considerations require a minimum of 8 mm of residual vertebral height to introduce the materials.[38]

Vertebroplasty Technique

After obtaining appropriate medical clearance and written, informed consent, the patient is brought to either an interventional radiology suite or operating room (Fig. 71.1). Although in many centers both a radiologist and a surgeon are present, in other centers, the procedure is performed with only the surgeon present. The procedure may be performed under general anesthetic or under local anesthetic with mild sedation. Which type of anesthetic should be determined based on the patients general medical condition, comorbidities, and in conjunction with the anesthesiologist. While the patient may be monitored for neurological dysfunction if the procedure is

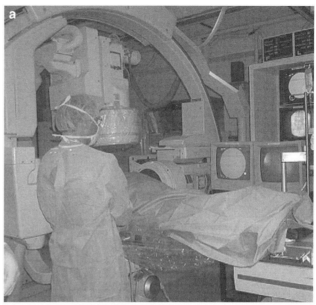

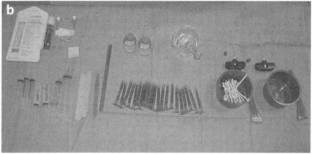

Fig. 71.1 Patient positioning and angiography suite setup (**a**) with biplanar fluoroscopy is shown. Basic surgical supplies needed to perform percutaneous vertebroplasty are pictured (**b**)

performed under local anesthetic, this method is typically uncomfortable for the patient. General anesthetic may be used safely, with frequent use of intraoperative fluoroscopy to prevent cement extravasation. The patient is placed in the prone position with their arms above their head and adequately padded for comfort and to prevent compressive peripheral neuropathies. A wide area of skin overlying the level of interest is then prepped and draped in strict sterile fashion to minimize the chance of a postoperative infection.

Once the patient is satisfactorily positioned, the fracture site is identified using biplanar fluoroscopy. Although some authors have advocated CT scanning to facilitate needle placement,[33,44] it is our experience that CT guidance is necessary only in a few rare instances when anatomical constraints prohibit easy identification of an appropriate trajectory and placement of the needle. A mark is placed on the skin overlying the pedicle of interest. The skin is infiltrated with a buffered anesthetic solution containing 0.5 or 0.25% Marcaine, 1:200,000 epinephrine (Abbot Labs, Chicago, IL), and Na bicarbonate (American Pharmaceutical Partners, Los Angeles, CA) down to the level of the periosteum over the pedicle.

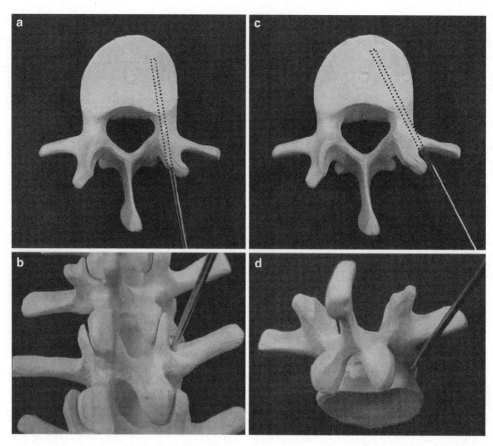

Fig. 71.2 Model illustrations depicting the entry points and needle trajectories for both the transpedicular (**a** and **b**) and parapedicular (**c** and **d**) approaches

Currently, there is a wide selection of needles and cement from several vendors that can be used for percutaneous vertebroplasty. In addition, there is no standardized technique for needle placement. The senior authors use either a transpedicular or a parapedicular approach (Fig. 71.2). Biplanar fluoroscopy is used to confirm the appropriate trajectory regardless of which approach is used (Fig. 71.3). A 2-mm stab incision is created with a #11 scalpel blade lateral to the midline at the point previously marked to identify the pedicle. A #11 Jamshidi needle with the trocar in place is introduced. In the transpedicular approach (Fig. 71.4), the needle is advanced until it docks onto the pedicle. The preferred entry point is at the upper and outer quadrant of the pedicle, because perforation at this location has few consequences compared with the inferomedial quadrant, which places the exiting nerve root at risk. In this "bull's eye" approach, the needle forms the center, while the cortex of the pedicle is the outer ring. The location and trajectory are again confirmed with fluoroscopy, and the needle is advanced into the vertebral body. An identical procedure is then repeated for the contralateral pedicle.

When utilizing the parapedicular approach (Fig. 71.5), only a unilateral cannulization is necessary because the more lateral approach allows for a more centrally directed needle. The Jamshidi needle is docked on the transverse process and advanced immediately caudal to the transverse process. The appropriate entry point is at the lateral vertebral body on the AP projection and at, or immediately ventral to, the posterior cortex on the lateral fluoroscopic image. The biplanar fluoroscopic images are used to help guide the needle trajectory, keeping the needle tip equidistant from the vertebral body on both AP and lateral views. Once the vertebral body in encountered, the needle is advanced toward the center of the body. While there is a theoretical increased risk of pneumothorax and bleeding with this approach,[45] it has been our experience that the complication rates are similar between the two approaches.

Regardless of which approach is used, the target of the needle tip should be in the anterior half of the vertebral body on the lateral views and the medial third in the AP views. The bevel of the needle can be directed in the most optimal direction for cement placement for each given patient. Given the frequency of fluoroscopic image acquisition, a clamp may be used to stabilize the needle during imaging to minimize the exposure of the operator's hand. Intraosseous venography had been advocated in some centers, particularly within the United States, prior to injection of cement.[46–48] However, as more centers have increased their experience with this technique, it has become apparent that there is no

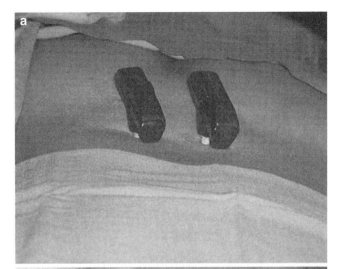

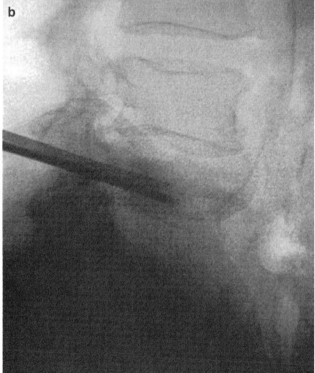

Fig. 71.3 Percutaneous access to both pedicles with 11-gauge biopsy needles is depicted (**a**); radiographic confirmation of adequate placement of the needles is obtained on lateral fluoroscopy (**b**)

increase in safety afforded by venography.[49–51] In most centers, venography is typically no longer used prior to cement injection. To avoid the introduction of air during the injections, the needle is filled with sterile saline after adequate placement has been confirmed.

There are a number of cement products and suppliers available and the choice is left to the surgeon performing the procedure based on their experience and training. The increased application of percutaneous vertebroplasty has led to advances in the mixing and administration devices so that one can achieve a uniform, consistent product and minimize exposure to vapors. PMMA is provided in two separate components, a methylmethacrylate polymer in powder form and a liquid methylmethacrylate monomer. When combined, an exothermic polymerization reaction occurs and the resulting compound progresses from a liquid to solid state. The ideal time for injection is when the consistency of the polymer approximates that of toothpaste. The timing will vary depending upon the specific product used. Most commercially available products come with an aliquot of a radio-opaque marker, which is combined with the PMMA to facilitate visualization during the injection process. If not available, sterile barium sulfate powder can be added to the methylmethacrylate polymer and mixed thoroughly with the compound. The thickened PMMA solution is poured into a 10-cc syringe or one of the many commercial delivery devices available. Some vertebroplasty application devices require placement of a guidewire through the Jamshidi needle, removal of the Jamshidi needle, and placement of a larger working cannula. The delivery device is then attached to the hub of the Jamshidi needle or working cannula and, under intermittent fluoroscopic monitoring, the PMMA is injected slowly under a consistent pressure (Fig. 71.5). In general, it is typically possible to inject 5–10 cc of PMMA into each treated vertebral body; the thoracic spine accepts less volume than the lumbar spine due to their relative sizes. Extravasation of cement beyond the confines of the vertebral body is an indication to stop the injection. It is not clear what volume of cement is necessary to reliably produce pain relief, nor is it known by what mechanism the pain relief is achieved. Possible proposed mechanisms include mechanical stabilization of the fracture site[45] and neural thermal necrosis secondary to the heat generated during the curing process.[52]

Once the operator is satisfied with the injection, the inner cannula is replaced and the needle removed is removed with a twisting motion. Closure of the wound is usually unnecessary. Occasional bleeding is controlled with direct pressure. Patients are kept recumbent for 2 h and are then allowed to sit and ambulate with assistance. A postoperative CT scan of the region treated to assess the degree of vertebral body filling and to rule out any occult spinal cord compression and X-rays are obtained as a baseline for lateral comparison. Patients are then discharged home on nonsteroidal anti-inflammatory drugs (NSAIDS) and muscle relaxants later the same day. Ambulation is encouraged and participation in routine activities of daily living is emphasized.

Kyphoplasty Technique

Kyphoplasty is a procedure whereby a cavity is created in the vertebral body for cement injection with an inflatable bone tamp or balloon. The procedure attempts to restore the vertebral

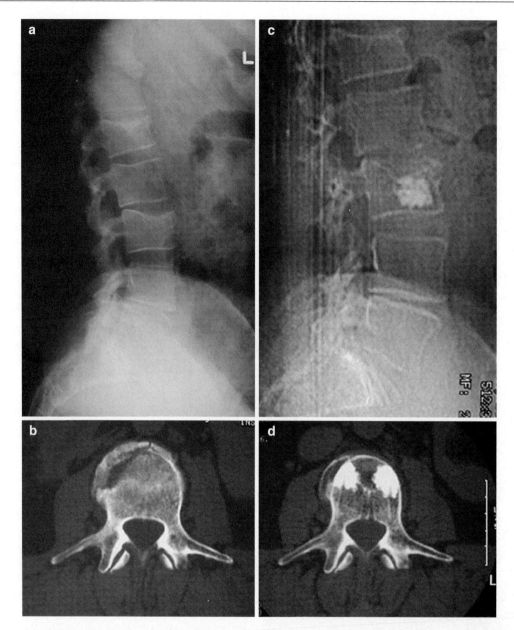

Fig. 71.4 Illustration of the transpedicular approach. A 46-year-old man suffered a traumatic compression fractures at L1 and L3. He complained of chronic back pain for several months after the injury, which was localizable to the L3 level. Lateral lumbosacral X-ray (**a**) and axial CT scan (**b**) demonstrate the L3 fracture. He underwent vertebrop lasty with bipedicular injection of PMMA. Lateral X-ray (**c**) and axial CT scan (**d**) show good placement of cement in the anterior third of the vertebral body

body back to its original height. In doing so, it is thought that a low-pressure cavity is created within the bone that may then be filled with cement.[40,53] However, restoration of vertebral body height does not correlate with pain relief or improvement in quality of life.[54,55] Expansion of the vertebral body is followed radiographically by placing contrast medium in the balloon. Alternatively, an arc osteotome may be used to create a cavity. However, this form of cavity creation does not result in restoration of vertebral body height.

The kyphoplasty procedure was first described by Garfin et al.[40] The bone tamp is placed using either the transpedicular or parapedicular approach. This is accomplished with the aid of a guide pin and biplanar fluoroscopy. Once cannulation of the vertebral body has occurred, an obturator is passed over the guidewire and inserted into the vertebral body. A working cannula is then passed over the obturator until the cannula tip is in the posterior portion of the vertebral body. The inflatable tamp is passed through a corridor created by drilling along the cannula path. Once in place, the device is inflated under fluoroscopic guidance to a pressure of no more than 220 psi. An inline pressure gauge allows for constant pressure monitoring within the balloon. Once a sufficiently sized cavity has been created and an appropriate reduction has been obtained, the PMMA cement is prepared. At this point, smaller cannulas

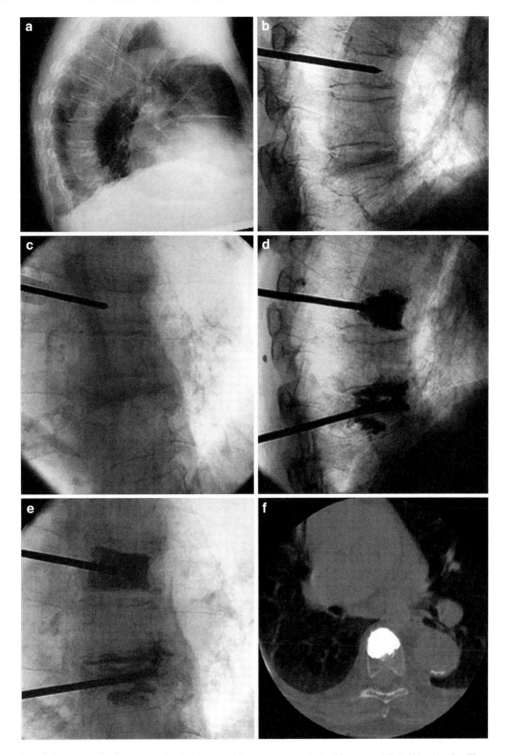

Fig. 71.5 Illustration of the parapedicular approach. A 64-year-old woman presented with a complaint of back pain. There was no history of trauma or malignancy. Compression fractures of T8 and T10 were identified and both were thought to be symptomatic. Lateral thoracic X-ray (**a**) demonstrates the fractures. Lateral (**b**) and AP (**c**) images confirm the cannulation of T8. Lateral (**d**) and AP (**e**) images after injection of T8 and during injection of T10. Postoperative CT scan demonstrates good filling of the anterior portion of the T8 vertebral body (**f**)

filled with cement are inserted into the working cannula. The cement-filled cannula is inserted into the working cannula, with subsequent passage into the vertebral body. A plunger-like effect is obtained by using a stainless steel stylet to extrude the cement into its target location. Filling the cavity with cement continues under lateral fluoroscopic guidance and ceases when the mantle of cement reaches approximately two thirds of the way to the posterior cortex of the vertebral body.

When utilizing an arc osteotome system such as the Arcuate XP system (Medtronic Sofamor Danek, Memphis, TN), vertebral body access is obtained as described above through either the parapedicular or transpedicular approach. A guidewire is then placed through the Jamshidi needle, and the Jamshidi needle is removed. A working channel with a port in the lateral aspect of the anterior aspect of the channel is then placed into the vertebral body. A flexible metal arc osteotome is then placed, and deployed through the port. The surgeon will feel variable resistance depending on the degree of osteoporosis present. The port is turned to allow deployment of the osteotome superiorly, medially, and inferiorly, allowing creation of a cavity. Once the cavity is created, the osteotome is removed, an inner cannula is placed that occludes the side port, and PMMA is injected through the tip of the working channel. Closure proceeds as described above.

Complications

The overall complication rates for vertebroplasty and kyphoplasty are in the range of 1–2% for osteoporotic fractures and 5–10% for metastatic lesions.[37,45] The most common complication after vertebroplasty is a transient increase in pain at the injected level. This is readily treated with NSAIDs and typically resolves within 48–72 h.[45] Acute radiculopathy has been reported to occur in up to 5% of cases. The symptoms are often transient and a short course of steroids may be of benefit, however, in some cases surgical decompression is necessary. The relatively higher complication rate in malignancy is now well recognized and documented.[37] Chiras et al. reported on a series of vertebroplasty cases and documented a complication rate of 1.3% in osteoporotic compression fractures, while higher complication rates were noted with more destructive bone lesions such as hemangiomas (2.5%) and vertebral malignancies (10%).[56] Cement leakage is a common problem, particularly in lytic lesions,[45] and has been reported in up to 30–70% of cases; fortunately, most of these occurrences are asymptomatic.[57] Some have reported cement leakage necessitating surgical intervention, with surgical findings consistent with thermal injury due to the exothermic reaction of the PMMA.[58] Other reported complications include fractures of the rib or pedicle, pneumothorax, spinal cord compression, and infection. There have been reports of embolic complications such as pulmonary embolism,[13,59-64] embolization of cement into the vena cava and pulmonary arteries[65] and into the renal vasculature,[66,67] and death[47,68] occurring during or shortly after vertebroplasty. The cause of these events has not been delineated, however, it has been postulated that cement with low viscosity and a large number of levels treated concurrently may play a role.[45] Other rare but reported complications include acute pericarditis,[69] osteomyelitis treated successfully with antibiotics[70]

and necessitating subsequent corpectomy,[71,72] cardiac perforation,[73] and fat and bone marrow embolization.[74]

Fracture of adjacent vertebral levels after vertebroplasty has been known to occur. The cause is most likely multifactorial and may include the diffuse nature of the osteoporotic disease, relief of pain with a subsequent return to higher level of physical activity, and increased strength in vertebrae that are subject to increased loads from kyphotic deformity. In 2005, Syed performed a retrospective analysis of 253 female patients who were treated with vertebroplasty. Of these patients, 21.7% experienced a new symptomatic VCF within 1 year.[75] Tanigawa showed that one third of patients who underwent vertebroplasty had a new compression fracture, half of which occurred at the adjacent level within 3 months of the procedure.[76] Kim et al. reported an increased incidence of new compression fractures after percutaneous vertebroplasty when treatment was performed at the thoracolumbar junction, and when a greater degree of height was restored.[77] Lin et al. reviewed their series of patients treated with vertebroplasty for compression fractures, concluding that cement leakage into adjacent disc spaces was related to an increased rate of adjacent level fracture.[78] Gradual increase in activity and continued use of orthotic devices (for 6 weeks after vertebroplasty), may help prevent adjacent level fracture in those at high risk.

There have been no reported complications related to balloon tamps during kyphoplasty procedures.[40,53] Several complications related in some way to needle insertion have been documented. During Phase 1 testing of an inflatable bone tamp, Lieberman et al. found that kyphoplasty was a safe procedure, with no significant complications related to their device. Cement extravasation was the most common problem occurring in 8.6% of their patients.[53] There were no clinical sequelae resulting from cement extravasation. Furthermore, the authors were encouraged that rates of cement extravasation during their kyphoplasty procedure were lower than those of published vertebroplasty series, which may indicate that cavity creation may prevent cement extravasation.

The exposure to ionizing radiation must be considered for both the patient and the treating team. Mehdizade et al. evaluated the radiation dose received by operators in a series of 11 cases.[79] They noted significant radiation dosage measurements, particularly on the operator's hands. Kruger and Faciszewski made a similar observation, however they were able to demonstrate that proper shielding and limiting the radiation used significantly reduced the measured exposure.[80]

Outcomes

Currently, there are no randomized, controlled trials comparing the outcomes of vertebroplasty and kyphoplasty with each other, or with conventional medical therapies. Most of the data available is derived from retrospective studies, although there have been a few reports on prospective, observational cohorts.

Vertebroplasty has been shown to reduce pain in 90–95% of patients suffering osteoporotic vertebral fractures.[45,57,81] Additionally, improvements in mobility and in activities of daily living occur. Also of note, patients who have undergone percutaneous vertebroplasty have a tendency to decrease their use of narcotic pain medications. Furthermore, the reduction in pain is rapid, usually within 48–72 h.[43] The analgesic effect has been shown to persist in a cohort of patients followed prospectively for a minimum of 5 years.[82] The success rate is slightly less in patients with metastatic disease, with approximately 65–80% reporting significant improvement in pain scores.[45,83]

In 2001, Lieberman et al. reported the results of a Phase 1 clinical trial examining the efficacy of kyphoplasty in osteoporotic fractures.[53] They reported that, in 70% of levels operated, a mean restoration of 47% of the lost vertebral body height was achieved. In addition, the patients demonstrated a significant improvement in measures of pain, activity, and energy. Similar results have been reported in patients with multiple myeloma.[84]

Conclusions

Percutaneous vertebroplasty and kyphoplasty provide minimally invasive options for the management of osteoporotic and osteolytic vertebral body compression fractures. These techniques provide substantial pain relief and support without having to sacrifice mobility, and have been shown to have an acceptable complication rate. These procedures allow stabilization of VCF through a short procedure, and also allow rapid mobilization of the patient. However, clinical trials need to be done comparing these various approaches for the different indications to which they are applied. In this way, surgeons will have better information upon which to base the decision to choose vertebroplasty or kyphoplasty. In addition, cost effectiveness of any new treatment should be evaluated and scrutinized. Currently, the cost of kyphoplasty is significantly greater than vertebroplasty. To justify the additional cost, kyphoplasty must be shown to be safer and/or to provide added clinical benefit such as greater stability, better pain relief, or reduced operating time. Most published studies demonstrate equivalent results in stability and pain relief, as well as complication rates, though some have suggested lower rates of cement extravasation. In addition, both procedures utilize a similar technique and are roughly equivalent in technical difficulty to perform. Therefore, at this time, it seems reasonable to question the cost/benefit ratio of the kyphoplasty procedure when compared with vertebroplasty.

Regardless, vertebral augmentation techniques such as vertebroplasty and kyphoplasty provide pain relief and improvement in quality of life in the highly selected patient.[85–87] Complications can be avoided with careful surgical technique, and good outcomes can be achieved with proper patient selection.

References

1. Galibert P, Deramond H, Rosat P, Le Gars D. [Preliminary note on the treatment of vertebral angioma by percutaneous acrylic vertebroplasty]. Neurochirurgie 1987;33(2):166–168
2. Chen JF, Wu CT, Lee ST. Percutaneous vertebroplasty for the treatment of burst fractures. Case report. J Neurosurg Spine 2004;1(2): 228–231
3. Ray NF, Chan JK, Thamer M, Melton LJ III. Medical expenditures for the treatment of osteoporotic fractures in the United States in 1995: report from the National Osteoporosis Foundation. J Bone Miner Res 1997;12(1):24–35
4. Kado DM, Browner WS, Palermo L, Nevitt MC, Genant HK, Cummings SR. Vertebral fractures and mortality in older women: a prospective study. Study of Osteoporotic Fractures Research Group. Arch Intern Med 1999;159(11):1215–1220
5. Cooper C, Atkinson EJ, O'Fallon WM, Melton LJ III. Incidence of clinically diagnosed vertebral fractures: a population-based study in Rochester, Minnesota, 1985–1989. J Bone Miner Res 1992;7(2): 221–227
6. Lyles KW. Management of patients with vertebral compression fractures. Pharmacotherapy 1999;19(1 Pt 2):21S–24S
7. Melton LJ III. Epidemiology worldwide. Endocrinol Metab Clin North Am 2003;32(1):1–13, v
8. Olszynski WP, Shawn Davison K, Adachi JD, et al. Osteoporosis in men: epidemiology, diagnosis, prevention, and treatment. Clin Ther 2004;26(1):15–28
9. Rao RD, Singrakhia MD. Painful osteoporotic vertebral fracture. Pathogenesis, evaluation, and roles of vertebroplasty and kyphoplasty in its management. J Bone Joint Surg Am 2003;85-A(10):2010–2022
10. Fourney DR, Schomer DF, Nader R, et al. Percutaneous vertebroplasty and kyphoplasty for painful vertebral body fractures in cancer patients. J Neurosurg 2003;98(1 Suppl):21–30
11. Wise JJ, Fischgrund JS, Herkowitz HN, Montgomery D, Kurz LT. Complication, survival rates, and risk factors of surgery for metastatic disease of the spine. Spine 1999;24(18):1943–1951
12. Greenlee RT, Murray T, Bolden S, Wingo PA. Cancer statistics, 2000. CA Cancer J Clin 2000;50(1):7–33
13. Aebi M. Spinal metastasis in the elderly. Eur Spine J 2003;12 (Suppl 2):S202–S213
14. Burton AW, Reddy SK, Shah HN, Tremont-Lukats I, Mendel E. Percutaneous vertebroplasty - a technique to treat refractory spinal pain in the setting of advanced metastatic cancer: a case series. J Pain Symptom Manage 2005;30(1):87–95
15. Chow E, Holden L, Danjoux C, et al. Successful salvage using percutaneous vertebroplasty in cancer patients with painful spinal metastases or osteoporotic compression fractures. Radiother Oncol 2004;70(3):265–267
16. Masala S, Lunardi P, Fiori R, et al. Vertebroplasty and kyphoplasty in the treatment of malignant vertebral fractures. J Chemother 2004;16(Suppl 5):30–33
17. Yamada K, Matsumoto Y, Kita M, Yamamoto K, Kobayashi T, Takanaka T. Long-term pain relief effects in four patients undergoing percutaneous vertebroplasty for metastatic vertebral tumor. J Anesth 2004;18(4):292–295

18. Diamond TH, Hartwell T, Clarke W, Manoharan A. Percutaneous vertebroplasty for acute vertebral body fracture and deformity in multiple myeloma: a short report. Br J Haematol 2004;124(4): 485–487

19. Shimony JS, Gilula LA, Zeller AJ, Brown DB. Percutaneous vertebroplasty for malignant compression fractures with epidural involvement. Radiology 2004;232(3):846–853

20. Jang JS, Lee SH. Efficacy of percutaneous vertebroplasty combined with radiotherapy in osteolytic metastatic spinal tumors. J Neurosurg Spine 2005;2(3):243–248

21. Verlaan JJ, van de Kraats EB, Oner FC, van Walsum T, Niessen WJ, Dhert WJ. Bone displacement and the role of longitudinal ligaments during balloon vertebroplasty in traumatic thoracolumbar fractures. Spine 2005;30(16):1832–1839

22. Ross PD, Davis JW, Epstein RS, Wasnich RD. Pre-existing fractures and bone mass predict vertebral fracture incidence in women. Ann Intern Med 1991;114(11):919–923

23. Lieberman I. Vertebral augmentation for osteoporotic and osteolytic vertebral compression fractures: vertebroplasty and kyphoplasty. In: Haid RW Jr, Subach BR, Rodts GE Jr (eds.), Advances in Spinal Stabilization, vol. 16. pp. 240–250. Basel: Karger, 2003

24. Uhthoff HK, Jaworski ZF. Bone loss in response to long-term immobilisation. J Bone Joint Surg Br 1978;60-B(3):420–429

25. Silverman SL. The clinical consequences of vertebral compression fracture. Bone 1992;13(Suppl 2):S27–S31

26. Cook DJ, Guyatt GH, Adachi JD, et al. Quality of life issues in women with vertebral fractures due to osteoporosis. Arthritis Rheum 1993;36(6):750–756

27. Gold DT. The clinical impact of vertebral fractures: quality of life in women with osteoporosis. Bone 1996;18(3 Suppl):185S–189S

28. Schlaich C, Minne HW, Bruckner T, et al. Reduced pulmonary function in patients with spinal osteoporotic fractures. Osteoporos Int 1998;8(3):261–267

29. Lippuner K. Medical treatment of vertebral osteoporosis. Eur Spine J 2003;12(Suppl 2):S132–S141

30. Diamond TH, Champion B, Clark WA. Management of acute osteoporotic vertebral fractures: a nonrandomized trial comparing percutaneous vertebroplasty with conservative therapy. Am J Med 2003;114(4):257–265

31. Tanigawa N, Komemushi A, Kariya S, et al. Percutaneous vertebroplasty: relationship between vertebral body bone marrow edema pattern on MR images and initial clinical response. Radiology 2006;239:195–200

32. Alvarez L, Perez-Higueras A, Granizo JJ, de Miguel I, Quinones D, Rossi RE. Predictors of outcomes of percutaneous vertebroplasty for osteoporotic vertebral fractures. Spine 2005;30(1):87–92

33. Barr JD, Barr MS, Lemley TJ, McCann RM. Percutaneous vertebroplasty for pain relief and spinal stabilization. Spine 2000;25(8): 923–928

34. Brown DB, Gilula LA, Sehgal M, Shimony JS. Treatment of chronic symptomatic vertebral compression fractures with percutaneous vertebroplasty. AJR Am J Roentgenol 2004;182(2):319–322

35. Brown DB, Glaiberman CB, Gilula LA, Shimony JS. Correlation between preprocedural MRI findings and clinical outcomes in the treatment of chronic symptomatic vertebral compression fractures with percutaneous vertebroplasty. AJR Am J Roentgenol 2005;184(6):1951–1955

36. Irani FG, Morales JP, Sabharwal T, Dourado R, Gangi A, Adam A. Successful treatment of a chronic post-traumatic 5-year-old osteoporotic vertebral compression fracture by percutaneous vertebroplasty. Br J Radiol 2005;78(927):261–364

37. McGraw JK, Cardella J, Barr JD, et al. Society of Interventional Radiology quality improvement guidelines for percutaneous vertebroplasty. J Vasc Interv Radiol 2003;14(7):827–831

38. Stallmeyer MJ, Zoarski GH, Obuchowski AM. Optimizing patient selection in percutaneous vertebroplasty. J Vasc Interv Radiol 2003; 14(6):683–696

39. Garfin SR, Lin G., Lieberman I. Retrospective analysis of the outcomes of balloon kyphoplasty to treat vertebral body compression fracture (VCF) refractory to medical management. Eur Spine J 2001;10(Suppl 1):S7

40. Garfin SR, Yuan HA, Reiley MA. New technologies in spine: kyphoplasty and vertebroplasty for the treatment of painful osteoporotic compression fractures. Spine 2001;26(14):1511–1515

41. Togawa D, Kovacic JJ, Bauer TW, Reinhardt MK, Brodke DS, Lieberman IH. Radiographic and histologic findings of vertebral augmentation using polymethylmethacrylate in the primate spine: percutaneous vertebroplasty versus kyphoplasty. Spine 2006;31(1): E4–E10

42. Verlaan JJ, van de Kraats EB, Oner FC, van Walsum T, Niessen WJ, Dhert WJ. The reduction of endplate fractures during balloon vertebroplasty: a detailed radiological analysis of the treatment of burst fractures using pedicle screws, balloon vertebroplasty, and calcium phosphate cement. Spine 2005;30(16):1840–1845

43. Phillips FM. Minimally invasive treatments of osteoporotic vertebral compression fractures. Spine 2003;28(15 Suppl):S45–S53

44. Gangi A, Kastler BA, Dietemann JL. Percutaneous vertebroplasty guided by a combination of CT and fluoroscopy. AJNR Am J Neuroradiol 1994;15(1):83–86

45. Mathis JM, Wong W. Percutaneous vertebroplasty: technical considerations. J Vasc Interv Radiol 2003;14(8):953–960

46. Do HM. Intraosseous venography during percutaneous vertebroplasty: is it needed? AJNR Am J Neuroradiol 2002;23(4):508–509

47. Jensen ME, Evans AJ, Mathis JM, Kallmes DF, Cloft HJ, Dion JE. Percutaneous polymethylmethacrylate vertebroplasty in the treatment of osteoporotic vertebral body compression fractures: technical aspects. AJNR Am J Neuroradiol 1997;18(10):1897–1904

48. McGraw JK, Heatwole EV, Strnad BT, Silber JS, Patzilk SB, Boorstein JM. Predictive value of intraosseous venography before percutaneous vertebroplasty. J Vasc Interv Radiol 2002;13(2 Pt 1): 149–153

49. Gaughen JR Jr, Jensen ME, Schweickert PA, Kaufmann TJ, Marx WF, Kallmes DF. Relevance of antecedent venography in percutaneous vertebroplasty for the treatment of osteoporotic compression fractures. AJNR Am J Neuroradiol 2002;23(4):594–600

50. Vasconcelos C, Gailloud P, Beauchamp NJ, Heck DV, Murphy KJ. Is percutaneous vertebroplasty without pretreatment venography safe? Evaluation of 205 consecutives procedures. AJNR Am J Neuroradiol 2002;23(6):913–917

51. Wong W, Mathis J. Is intraosseous venography a significant safety measure in performance of vertebroplasty? J Vasc Interv Radiol 2002;13(2 Pt 1):137–138

52. Belkoff SM, Molloy S. Temperature measurement during polymerization of polymethylmethacrylate cement used for vertebroplasty. Spine 2003;28(14):1555–1559

53. Lieberman IH, Dudeney S, Reinhardt MK, Bell G. Initial outcome and efficacy of "kyphoplasty" in the treatment of painful osteoporotic vertebral compression fractures. Spine 2001;26(14):1631–1638

54. Dublin AB, Hartman J, Latchaw RE, Hald JK, Reid MH. The vertebral body fracture in osteoporosis: restoration of height using percutaneous vertebroplasty. AJNR Am J Neuroradiol 2005;26(3): 489–492

55. McKiernan F, Faciszewski T, Jensen R. Does vertebral height restoration achieved at vertebroplasty matter? J Vasc Interv Radiol 2005;16(7):973–979

56. Chiras J, Depriester C, Weill A, Sola-Martinez MT, Deramond H. [Percutaneous vertebral surgery. Technics and indications]. J Neuroradiol 1997;24(1):45–59

57. Cortet B, Cotten A, Boutry N, et al. Percutaneous vertebroplasty in the treatment of osteoporotic vertebral compression fractures: an open prospective study. J Rheumatol 1999;26(10):2222–2228

58. Teng MM, Cheng H, Ho DM, Chang CY. Intraspinal leakage of bone cement after vertebroplasty: a report of 3 cases. AJNR Am J Neuroradiol 2006;27(1):224–229

59. Choe du H, Marom EM, Ahrar K, Truong MT, Madewell JE. Pulmonary embolism of polymethyl methacrylate during percutaneous vertebroplasty and kyphoplasty. AJR Am J Roentgenol 2004;183(4):1097–1102

60. Monticelli F, Meyer HJ, Tutsch-Bauer E. Fatal pulmonary cement embolism following percutaneous vertebroplasty (PVP). Forensic Sci Int 2005;149(1):35–38

61. Pott L, Wippermann B, Hussein S, Gunther T, Brusch U, Fremerey R. [PMMA pulmonary embolism and post interventional associated fractures after percutaneous vertebroplasty]. Orthopade 2005;34(7): 698–700, 702

62. Righini M, Sekoranja L, Le Gal G, Favre I, Bounameaux H, Janssens JP. Pulmonary cement embolism after vertebroplasty. Thromb Haemost 2006;95(2):388–389

63. Yoo KY, Jeong SW, Yoon W, Lee J. Acute respiratory distress syndrome associated with pulmonary cement embolism following percutaneous vertebroplasty with polymethylmethacrylate. Spine 2004;29(14):E294–E297

64. Padovani B, Kasriel O, Brunner P, Peretti-Viton P. Pulmonary embolism caused by acrylic cement: a rare complication of percutaneous vertebroplasty. AJNR Am J Neuroradiol 1999;20(3):375–377

65. Baumann A, Tauss J, Baumann G, Tomka M, Hessinger M, Tiesenhausen K. Cement embolization into the vena cava and pulmonal arteries after vertebroplasty: interdisciplinary management. Eur J Vasc Endovasc Surg 2005;31(5):558–561

66. Chung SE, Lee SH, Kim TH, Yoo KH, Jo BJ. Renal cement embolism during percutaneous vertebroplasty. Eur Spine J 2006;15 (Suppl 5):590–594

67. Freitag M, Gottschalk A, Schuster M, Wenk W, Wiesner L, Standl TG. Pulmonary embolism caused by polymethylmethacrylate during percutaneous vertebroplasty in orthopaedic surgery. Acta Anaesthesiol Scand 2006;50(2):248–251

68. Childers JC Jr. Cardiovascular collapse and death during vertebroplasty. Radiology 2003;228(3):902; author reply 902–903

69. Park JH, Choo SJ, Park SW. Images in cardiovascular medicine. Acute pericarditis caused by acrylic bone cement after percutaneous vertebroplasty. Circulation 2005;111(6):e98

70. Schmid KE, Boszczyk BM, Bierschneider M, Zarfl A, Robert B, Jaksche H. Spondylitis following vertebroplasty: a case report. Eur Spine J 2005;14(9):895–899

71. Walker DH, Mummaneni P, Rodts GE Jr. Infected vertebroplasty. Report of two cases and review of the literature. Neurosurg Focus 2004;17(6):E6

72. Yu SW, Chen WJ, Lin WC, Chen YJ, Tu YK. Serious pyogenic spondylitis following vertebroplasty - a case report. Spine 2004; 29(10):E209–E211

73. Kim SY, Seo JB, Do KH, Lee JS, Song KS, Lim TH. Cardiac perforation caused by acrylic cement: a rare complication of percutaneous vertebroplasty. AJR Am J Roentgenol 2005;185(5):1245–1247

74. Syed MI, Jan S, Patel NA, Shaikh A, Marsh RA, Stewart RV. Fatal fat embolism after vertebroplasty: identification of the high-risk patient. AJNR Am J Neuroradiol 2006;27(2):343–345

75. Syed MI, Patel NA, Jan S, Harron MS, Morar K, Shaikh A. New symptomatic vertebral compression fractures within a year following vertebroplasty in osteoporotic women. AJNR Am J Neuroradiol 2005;26(6):1601–1604

76. Tanigawa N, Komemushi A, Kariya S, Kojima H, Shomura Y, Sawada S. Radiological follow-up of new compression fractures following percutaneous vertebroplasty. Cardiovasc Intervent Radiol 2006;29(1):92–96

77. Kim SH, Kang HS, Choi JA, Ahn JM. Risk factors of new compression fractures in adjacent vertebrae after percutaneous vertebroplasty. Acta Radiol 2004;45(4):440–445

78. Lin EP, Ekholm S, Hiwatashi A, Westesson PL. Vertebroplasty: cement leakage into the disc increases the risk of new fracture of adjacent vertebral body. AJNR Am J Neuroradiol 2004;25(2):175–180

79. Mehdizade A, Lovblad KO, Wilhelm KE, et al. Radiation dose in vertebroplasty. Neuroradiology 2004;46(3):243–245

80. Kruger R, Faciszewski T. Radiation dose reduction to medical staff during vertebroplasty: a review of techniques and methods to mitigate occupational dose. Spine 2003;28(14):1608–1613

81. Deramond H, Depriester C, Galibert P, Le Gars D. Percutaneous vertebroplasty with polymethylmethacrylate. Technique, indications, and results. Radiol Clin North Am 1998;36(3):533–546

82. Perez-Higueras A, Alvarez L, Rossi RE, Quinones D, Al-Assir I. Percutaneous vertebroplasty: long-term clinical and radiological outcome. Neuroradiology 2002;44(11):950–954

83. Cortet B, Cotten A, Boutry N, et al. Percutaneous vertebroplasty in patients with osteolytic metastases or multiple myeloma. Rev Rhum Engl Ed 1997;64(3):177–183

84. Dudeney S, Lieberman IH, Reinhardt MK, Hussein M. Kyphoplasty in the treatment of osteolytic vertebral compression fractures as a result of multiple myeloma. J Clin Oncol 2002;20(9):2382–2387

85. Kumar K, Verma AK, Wilson J, LaFontaine A. Vertebroplasty in osteoporotic spine fractures: a quality of life assessment. Can J Neurol Sci 2005;32(4):487–495

86. McKiernan F, Faciszewski T, Jensen R. Quality of life following vertebroplasty. J Bone Joint Surg Am 2004;86-A(12):2600–2606

87. Winking M, Stahl JP, Oertel M, Schnettler R, Boker DK. Treatment of pain from osteoporotic vertebral collapse by percutaneous PMMA vertebroplasty. Acta Neurochir (Wien) 2004;146(5): 469–476

Chapter 72
Round Table Discussion of a MIS Spine Surgery Case

History

The patient is a 23-year-old woman, who was doing well until she was thrown from her horse. Since then she has had excruciating low back pain, radiating into her buttocks, the lateral aspect of her thighs, and into her lateral calves bilaterally. Neurologic examination is normal. She has no other medical comorbidities. This pain has been going on for 1 year and has not responded to pain medication, physical therapy, bracing, epidural steroids, and chiropractic manipulations with anything other than partial, temporary relief. She wishes to proceed with some type of surgery.

Richard Fessler: What is your thought process in evaluating her? What would you recommend?

Mick Perez-Cruet: This is a classic case of Grade I spondylolisthesis. Certainly this condition may have and probably was preexisting before the accident, the accident just brought on the symptoms that she is currently experiencing. I usually try a course of rehabilitation and targeted L4,5 epidural steroids. However, if significant instability exists, which I suspect is the case, these treatments are usually only temporary at best. Therefore, I think this patient would benefit from surgical intervention. I would offer her a minimally invasive fusion and instrumentation and reduction.

The current instrumentation available has really facilitated this procedure. I would preform a transforaminal lumbar interbody fusion (TLIF), using a peak TLIF shaped cage device, followed by percutaneous instrumentation and reduction using the Pathfinder system (I am very familiar with the nuances of this system). Alternatively, the Sextant would work as they also have a new reduction device, although I have not used it yet.

One of the questions in the case is whether she is in need of a minimally invasive decompression as well. She does not seem overly tight and usually the interbody placement with reduction will sufficiently open the canal as well as restore foraminal height. Alternatively, as we are involved in an Optimesh investigational device exemption (IDE) investigation, she would make an excellent candidate for this interbody device as well.

Some of the complications that I discuss with the patient prior to surgery are the following: risks of anesthesia including and not limited to coma, stroke, paralysis, and death. The risk of the surgical procedure would include injury to a nerve root with motor and or sensory deficit; and dural tear, and I would explain the repair process to the patient; injury to abdominal viscera including the need for an anterior approach to repair bowel or major blood vessel injury; failure of fusion and or instrumentation and need for additional surgery; and no improvement or worsening symptoms.

We have a program called "Back to Back" in which spine patients undergoing similar procedures can talk to other patients; this really lets them know what to expect and often calms them and answers many of their questions.

Lastly, I like to show patients images of the procedure and of course review their radiographs with them. I find that visual aids are usually remembered better than the spoken explanation.

John O'Toole: The presence of what sounds like bilateral L5 radiculopathy probably necessitates a decompression of the lateral recesses and her L4–5 isthmic spondylolisthesis requires arthrodesis/fixation. I would favor the fairly standard MIS TLIF but with bilateral decompression and bilateral instrumentation with reduction screws of some sort.

Fred Ogden: I agree that a minimally invasive TLIF (miTLIF) is the way to go. Given her age and activity level, one would have liked to try a direct pars repair; however, even if she reduces on the table, such an approach would likely fail given the incompetence of the intervertebral disc. The issue of whether an indirect decompression of the contralateral nerve root through obliteration of movement, reduction of spondylolisthesis, and restoration of disc height is sufficient or a bilateral direct decompression is warranted as well is a judgment call.

Justin Smith: I agree that miTLIF is certainly a reasonable management approach and would enable foraminal decompression if this is thought to be necessary. However, in this case, the compression appears to be secondary to the spondylolisthesis and some loss of disc height. I would favor a lateral approach, such as a direct lateral interbody fusion (DLIF) or extreme lateral interbody fusion (XLIF), in order to restore disc height and provide indirect decompression. The lateral approach would minimize disruption of the posterior elements, and, if adequate reduction is achieved, a lateral plate could be used for stabilization, thereby saving the patient from needing L4–5 pedicle screw instrumentation. If adequate reduction is not achieved with the lateral procedure, minimally invasive posterior L4–5 fusion could then be performed with reduction screws.

Section VI
Computer Navigation

Chapter 73
Computer-Assisted Orthopedic Surgery (CAOS): Pros and Cons

James B. Stiehl

Computer-assisted orthopedic surgery (CAOS) has recently evolved as an important technical application that has offered substantial improvements over conventional instrumented methods. The possibility of using computers in total joint replacement surgery is not a recent discovery, as Bargar and Paul introduced the first successful robotic application for total hips in 1987.[1] Their system was a development effort with IBM, which had identified a considerable research program to apply robotics to medicine. Perhaps the most significant discovery at the time was to refine digital software algorithms to the level of "pixel accuracy" (20–30 mm). This was required for the machining of custom total hip femoral implants that were implanted at that time. The next years of evolution occurred in Europe, where computer algorithms were advanced to allow intraoperative registration, removing the need for preoperative fiducial placement. DiGioia and Jaramaz developed the first computed tomography (CT) system that could be applied for navigation of the acetabular component.[2] Actually, this approach was a step backward because the complex robot was not needed. Imageless total knee applications were an even simpler method because preoperative images were no longer needed.

From a purely scientific point of view, the proof of these systems for increasing surgical precision and presumed benefit has been straightforward. The literature that I will outline clearly indicates the benefit of computer-assisted techniques over conventional instrumentation. Even in imageless total hip applications with lesser accuracy, computer-assisted surgery (CAS) provides a statistical improvement over conventional techniques from most studies. In this chapter, I offer a broad overview of the current state of the art. As with minimally invasive surgery (MIS), there are a group of early advocates who may offer a more enthusiastic viewpoint. As demonstrated, I will describe my current experience and research, which would question some of the claims regarding electromagnetic applications and imageless total hip

applications, for example. However, this technology is a moving target, and improvements are being developed as we speak.

Literature Review

Total Knee Arthroplasty

Numerous authors have investigated outcomes after total knee arthroplasty (TKA), finding that malalignment of greater than 3° resulted in a significantly higher potential for mechanical loosening and implant failure. Petersen and Engh investigated the radiographic results of 50 patients who underwent primary TKA with conventional methods, noting a 26% failure to achieve alignment within the optimum of 3° of varus or valgus.[3] Berend et al. investigated tibial component failure mechanisms, noting that malalignment of the tibial component in more than 3° of varus increased the odds of failure.[4]

Computer-assisted alignment devices were developed to improve the positioning of implants during TKA. These systems include image-based and image-free navigation systems. Image-based systems use preoperative CT scans or operative fluoroscopic images to assist in implant positioning. Image-free navigation systems use information obtained in the operating suite with the aid of infrared probes (Fig. 73.1). Early data on the use of these systems appear positive with improved mechanical alignment, frontal and sagittal femoral axis alignment, and frontal tibial axis alignment. Furthermore, no studies have demonstrated increased complications compared with hand-guided techniques. Yau et al. compared the combined intraobserver error for image-free acquisition of reference landmarks during TKA, finding that the maximum combined error for the coronal plane mechanical axis alignment was 1.32°.[5] Bathis et al. compared an image-free navigation system with a conventional method using an intramedullary femoral guide and an extramedullary tibial guide. They reported the postoperative mechanical

J.B. Stiehl (✉)
Department of Orthopaedic Surgery, Medical College of Wisconsin, MilwaukeeWI, USA
e-mail: jbstiehl@me.com

G.R. Scuderi and A.J. Tria (eds.), *Minimally Invasive Surgery in Orthopedics*,
DOI 10.1007/978-0-387-76608-9_73, © Springer Science+Business Media, LLC 2010

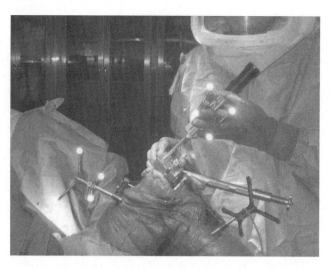

Fig. 73.1 Computer navigation in total knee arthroplasty using optical line-of-sight tracking, reflective balls on tracker, and LEDs on tracker

Table 73.1 Recent publications comparing navigated with manual or conventional methods of determination of the mechanical axis compared to CAS.

References	N	Navigated (%)	Manual (%)	% Difference
Haaker et al. (2005)	100	96	75	21
Sparmann et al.[7]	120	98	78	20
Victor and Hoste[9]	50	100	74	27
Jenny[15]	235	97	74	23
Jenny et al. (2001)	50	94	78	16
Kim et al. (2005)	69, 78	78	58	20
Perlick et al. (2004)	40	93	75	18
Song et al. (2005)	47, 50	96	76	20
Bathis et al. (2004)	160	96	78	18
Perlick et al. (2004)	50	92	72	20
Hart et al. (2003)	60	88	70	18
Oberst et al. (2006)	13	100	62	39
Anderson et al. (2005)	116, 51	95	84	11
		94	73 (P < 0.001)	20

alignment to be within 3° varus or valgus in 96% of the navigation cases vs. 78% in the conventional group.[6] Sparmann et al. determined an image-free navigation system to produce a significant improvement in mechanical alignment, frontal and sagittal femoral alignment, and the frontal tibial alignment (P < 0.0001) compared with a hand-guided technique. The postoperative mechanical alignment was within 3° varus or valgus in 87% of the conventional group vs. 100% of the navigation group.[7]

Table 73.1 lists a number of recent studies that compare the use of imageless computer-assisted navigation with conventional methods for TKA. All studies are able to demonstrate a statistically significant improvement in terms of placing the final mechanical alignment of the knee within 3° of the ideal mechanical axis. Furthermore, we note that 94% of the overall cases reach this level of precision with computer navigation compared with 73% where conventional methods are used, and the difference does not change as the number of cases are accumulated from the various series.

There are other image acquisition and tracking methods beyond the current standard imageless total knee systems and these would include CT, fluoroscopy, and electromagnetic tracking. Bathis et al. compared CT with imageless referencing methods in TKA, finding that 92% of CT vs. 97% with imageless referencing methods produced TKA mechanical axis alignment <3°.[8] Victor and Hoste used a fluoroscopic image acquisition in a randomized study with TKA to find 100% of navigated knees to have a mechanical alignment within ±2° while 73% of conventional TKAs were within ±2°.[9] Lionberger et al. compared electromagnetic trackers vs. optical line-of-site trackers in a prospective study using an imageless referenced TKA system, finding that 93% of cases with electromagnetic trackers had an alignment of

<3° from the mechanical axis compared with 90% of cases where optical trackers were used.[10]

Because of the recent popularity of electromagnetic trackers, a short discussion of accuracy issues is warranted. Lionberger et al. has studied the various facets of electromagnetic technologies, pointing out the important weaknesses of signal distortion from any conductive material and degradation of the signal by any ferrous or magnetic material. While software optimization has been developed with system lockout for various form of signal degradation, this has not been comprehensive enough to include materials such as copper or brass. In these examples, an error may be registered before the system can detect abnormality. The working space for an electromagnetic coil is roughly a 30-cm cube. That means the tracking device or coil must remain within this limited space, and be held relatively rigid or still for appropriate signal acquisition. We have studied these factors in a simulated operating room setting for TKA, finding comparable accuracy with the standard optical line-of-sight system, with the caveat that unexplained "outliers" still occurred during testing (Fig. 73.2). We would caution that this technology, while promising, has not reached the industrial grade of precision present with most standard optical line-of-sight systems.

Blood loss has been shown to be significantly reduced with the use of computer navigation and avoidance of intramedullary rods. Kalairajah et al. were able to reduce the mean blood loss from 1,747 to 1,351 mL by using the pin-placed trackers instead of intramedullary guided femur and tibia jigs, which was a significant difference in 60 patients.[11] Kalairajah et al. performed a transcranial Doppler study on 14 patients, finding that all patients who had undergone intramedullary instrumentation of the femur and tibia with

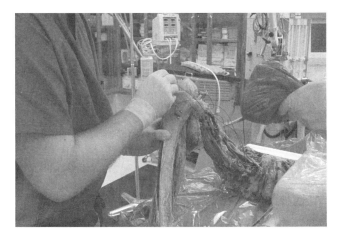

Fig. 73.2 Experimental registration using electromagnetic trackers for total knee arthroplasty

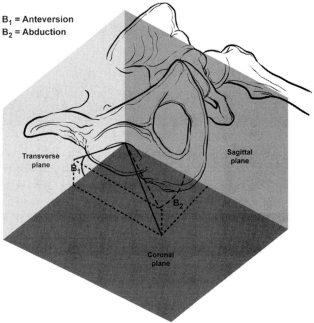

B_1 = Anteversion
B_2 = Abduction

Fig. 73.3 Pelvic coordinate system used for standard measurement of cup inclination and anteversion with anterior pelvic plane

conventional TKA had documented intracranial microemboli compared with only 50% of those who had undergone procedures where only intracortical tracking pins had been placed.[12]

Unicondylar knee arthroplasty is a procedure that also may benefit from CAS. Cobb et al. used a computer-navigated robotic system to insert Oxford unicondylar knee implants, finding that, with CAS, all patients had the final implant placement within 2° of the planned position compared with 40% using conventional instruments.[13] Cossey et al. demonstrated that CAS-directed mechanical alignment for unicondylar arthroplasty was optimal in all cases while the conventional aligned cases had 4 of 15 cases where the axis was placed in the lateral joint compartment from mild overcorrection.[14] Jenny clearly demonstrated the improvement of unicondylar arthroplasty using navigation, both for a standard and a minimally invasive approach.[15] Keene et al. compared the results of conventional and CAS navigated unicondylar arthroplasties performed in bilateral cases, finding that 87% of navigated cases were within 2° of planned alignment compared with 60% of conventional cases.[16]

Total Hip Arthroplasty

DiGioia et al. first described the use of CT for preoperative image acquisition subsequently utilized in the navigated surgical procedure.[17] This was done originally for acetabular component insertion. The other significant innovation was the description of the anterior pelvic plane as the baseline anatomical reference for measuring the position of the cup (Fig. 73.3). Several reports describe the accuracy of the cup placement in relation to the transverse axial plane to be 1°/1

mm. Haaker et al. compared the results of free-hand conventional instrumentation vs. CT navigation using postoperative CT for final evaluation in 98 patients. The target acetabular component position was 45° inclination and 20° anteversion. After CAS, average cup position was 43° abduction (95% confidence interval [CI]: 0.97) and 22.2° anteversion (95% CI: 1.72). For freehand, average cup position was 45.7° abduction (95% CI: 9.1°) and 28.5° anteversion (95% CI: 10.2°). The F ratio was 5.56 for abduction and 3.67 for anteversion ($P < 0.0001$).[18]

Imageless applications have been developed to eliminate the complexity and expense required for using CT. Kalteis et al. found that imageless referencing was comparable to CT navigation in a randomized and controlled trial.[19] Using the Lewinnek criteria of radiologic cup positioning to avoid dislocation of 40° inclination and 15° anteversion, 17% of CT navigated patients were outside the ±10° limits compared with 7% imageless navigation.[20] In that study, a "flip technique" was used for imageless referencing in the supine position and then repositioning to the lateral position. Nogler et al. attempted with cadavers to show an improvement over conventional acetabular cup positioning.[21] While a clear advantage was evident, the error was up to 8°, with a high standard deviation of 4.5° with the imageless method. Wixson et al. utilized CAS in patients who had undergone minimally invasive posterior hip approaches for cup placement. At surgery, the mean values for inclination and anteversion in the CAS group were 42.38 ± 1.88° (range 38–47°) and 20.78 ± 2.58° (range 13–29°), respectively. They studied cup anteversion, finding that 30% of navigated cups were within a narrow range of 17–23° compared with only 6% of a manual control group.

While imageless methods of referencing have been advocated for total hip navigation, several authors have questioned the accuracy and precision of this approach. Stiehl et al. used several cadaver studies to evaluate cup positioning after imageless referencing[22] (Fig. 73.4). Using the

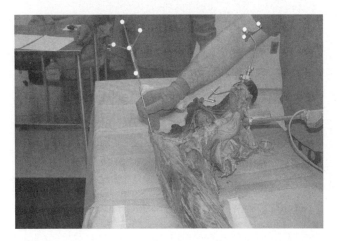

Fig. 73.4 Experimental registration of imageless total hip computer navigation system touch point marking the anterior superior iliac spine

imageless optical tracking referencing surgical navigation, mean acetabular inclination was 43.59° (standard deviation [SD] = 3.56°) and anteversion was 17.03° (SD = 1.01°). Their conclusion was that determination of cup inclination lacked precision, based on the relatively large standard deviation and range that was found. This was related in part to the relatively large area for touch point matching the anterior superior iliac spines. Another issue is the error created by the subcutaneous fat layer between skin and the bone landmarks, which has been determined to add 0.5° error for each millimeter of thickness.

Fluoroscopic referencing has been attempted as well for total hip arthroplasty, but suffers from similar precision issues (Fig. 73.5). Most importantly, the field of vision of most standard fluoroscopy C-arms is limited to approximately 9 in. This makes image acquisition difficult, particularly if the patient is on the operating table. Stiehl et al. found that visualizing and referencing the pubic symphysis was problematic using fluoroscopy, leading to poor precision with cup anteversion[23] (Fig. 73.6). Cup inclination, on the other hand, was relatively accurate. Grutzner et al. has demonstrated significant improvements when fluoroscopy was combined with percutaneous touch pointing methods for determination of the anterior pelvic plane, perhaps rendering a more suitable system.[24]

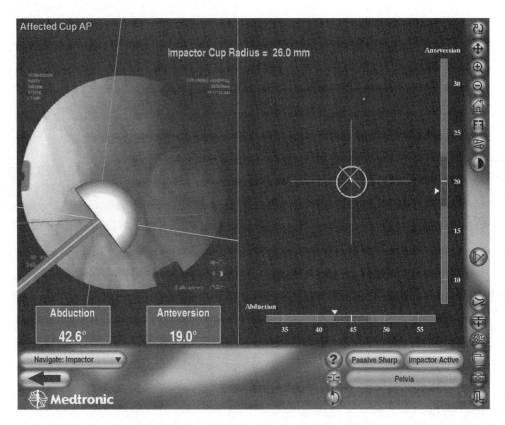

Fig. 73.5 Screen portrayal of fluoroscopic navigation of acetabular component, note projected inclination of 42° and anteversion of 19°

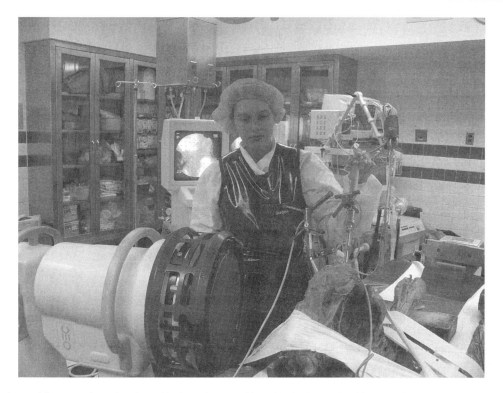

Fig. 73.6   Experimental fluoroscopic registration with the cadaver positioned in the lateral decubitus position

Pros

Total Knee Arthroplasty

Navigating a TKA has become my standard practice, beginning in September 2003, with now more than 250 cases completed. My hospital purchased the Medtronic Treon Stealth system, which uses optical cameras but has a variety of instruments and tracker options. The original "Universal Total Knee" software system was simple with excellent screen graphics and continues to be my software of choice. After experiencing several other examples, I think that any system to be of value for the surgeon must not add more than 5–15 min to the surgical procedure. From experience, I have developed a medial placement of the dynamic reference base (DRB) placing pins in the medial femoral transepicondylar axis and in the medial tibial shaft (Fig. 73.7). The idea is to have the frames located in the sagittal plane on the medial side of the leg, so that they are out of the way for all instrument placements, yet allowing easy access to the camera that is placed beyond the contralateral leg. Reference point matching is the critical step, and the most important points are the anterior femoral cortex (because I use an anterior cortical reference for the anterior-posterior cuts), femoral center, tibial center, and the distal malleoli (Fig. 73.8). In fact, the precision of any navigation system relies on how accurately these points are referenced. The

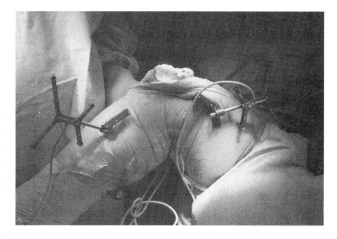

Fig. 73.7   Placement of LED trackers in the sagittal plane with femoral transepicondylar percutaneous position and medial tibial shaft percutaneous placement of dynamic reference bases

points of the procedure for which I rely almost solely on the computer are the initial ligament balancing, which is done in extension, tibial cut, distal femoral cut, anterior femoral cut, and gap measurements. With experience, one learns to rely on the computer for these measurements and will override positions suggested by conventional instruments.

A clinical study was done on my first 86 total knee cases comparing the final computer alignment readings with standing anteroposterior (AP) radiographs of the lower extremity, finding that 95% were within ±2° of the mechanical axis cen-

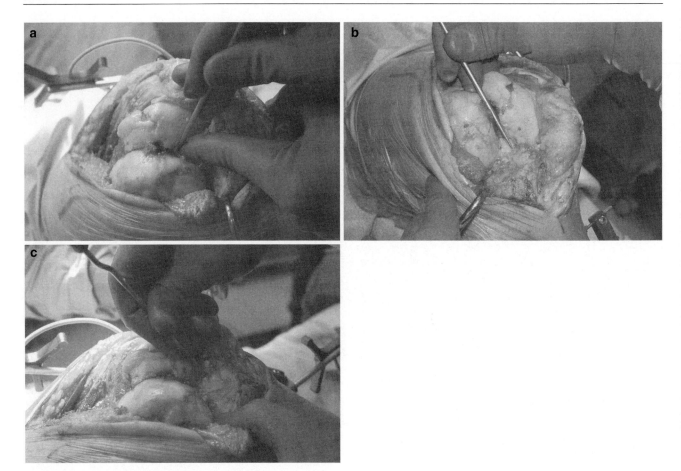

Fig. 73.8 (**a**) Touch point referencing of the femoral center, which is the bisection of the transepicondylar line and the anterior/posterior axis (Whiteside) line in total knee arthroplasty. (**b**) Touch point referencing of the femoral anterior/posterior axis, which also coincides with the tibial shaft axis in total knee arthroplasty. (**c**) Touch point referencing of the tibial center, which is the bisection of the transtibial axis

ter line. I found that other measurements, including the transepicondylar axis, Whiteside's AP axis, and the tibial rotational axes were too variable and of limited value in absolute terms. Joint line position reflected a resection amount within 1–2 mm of the healthy joint surface but required some judgment. Particular problems are best resolved with computer navigation. For example, any varus deformity greater than 10° from the mechanical axis requires a ligament release that can be assessed by the computer (Fig. 73.9). I have learned that prior to surgical navigation, I was not fully releasing most of these knees. Stripping of the superficial collateral ligament is fairly extensive, going down 7–10 cm, and a "pop" of the medial ligament is needed to get the anatomical alignment. Similar findings are noted with valgus knee, where release will usually require a complete release of the iliotibial tract insertion, lateral capsule, and occasionally the femoral origin of the lateral collateral ligament. Old fracture deformities are best resolved with navigation (Fig. 73.10). Because femoral alignment is conventionally done with intramedullary instrumentation, bone blocks of the femoral canal usually require computer navigation for accurate assessment. Ligament-balancing

measurements have become an important part of my techniques, and I strive for 1–2 mm laxity in full extension and less than 3 mm in flexion. This is done with gentle varus/valgus stresses throughout the range of motion. There are no practical instruments for assessing ligament balance currently available.

I have navigated ten failed total knees during revision TKA and found significant information in each case that subsequently guided the surgical technique. Several revisions have been done to correct chronic instability found after MIS "quadriceps-sparing" approaches. The typical problem is a residual varus deformity of 5–7°, which leaves the knee tight on the medial side in extension but lax on the lateral side in extension and on both sides in flexion. I have used the computer to correct the original deformity and then to appropriately balance the gaps, allowing for a simple exchange of a thicker polyethylene insert. The computer can also be used to define abnormal tibial and femoral component rotation that can be found with cases requiring revision for patella subluxation or dislocation.

Computer navigation has been an excellent intraoperative method to assess the precision and efficacy of newer MIS instruments (Fig. 73.11). I have found most of these

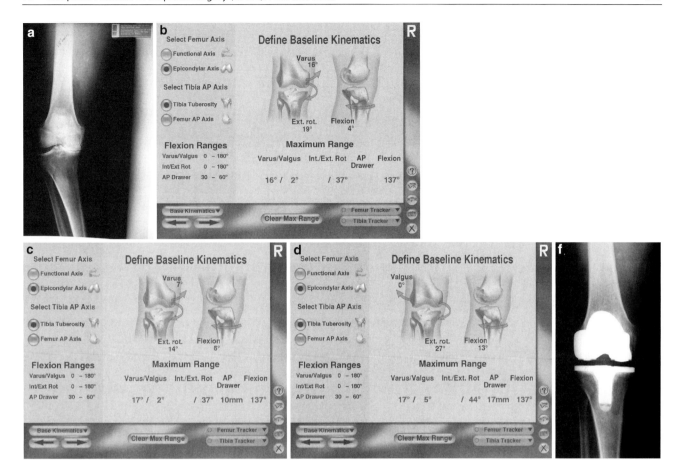

Fig. 73.9 (**a**) A 69-year-old man with a varus deformity that measures 16° from the mechanical axis. (**b**) Baseline screen shot on a computer demonstrates a 16° varus deformity. (**c**) Typical release with extensive stripping of the superficial medial collateral ligament and judged to be "adequate" by clinical experience is shown to be still in 7° of varus. (**d**) Further release to the point of "pop" of the superficial medial collateral ligament allows not for correction of 0° to the mechanical axis. (**e**) Postoperative AP standing radiograph shows correction with femorotibial axis of 6°

instruments to have a "toggle" or "wiggle" that easily translates into a 2-mm error. When performing MIS procedures, I heavily rely on the computer for all cuts, ligament release, and final measurements.

Total Hip Arthroplasty

The potential for satisfactory surgical navigation in total hip arthroplasty is very different from that in total knees. There is a suitable method for surgical navigation in total hips that has an accuracy approximating 1 mm/1°, but this requires the use of preoperative CT. Several studies have validated this fact. To date, there are no similar validations of imageless or fluoroscopic image acquisition techniques. Secondly, the primary applications for total hip arthroplasty have been for cup placement. Several new systems now offer the potential of determining femoral offset, femoral canal version, and leg length assessment. Most lack published scientific validation.

Cons

Total Knee Arthroplasty

The problems with computer navigation can be defined by two factors, increased cost and surgical time. Most early adopters have an advantage for costs because the benefits of the method can be marketed, increasing surgical case load. This was clearly my situation, and I noted that patients were clamoring for the new technology. That stated, a typical capital system will cost the hospital $200,000, with the need of a maintenance contract of $20,000–$40,000 for software upgrades and other problems. This technology is in constant evolution requiring frequent adjustments. Surgical time is an important consideration and I would note that several current systems are cumbersome and time consuming. I have cut out all of the extra steps, doing only those things that I think are "value added" for my system. A typical case is lengthened only 7–10 min over the conventional approach.

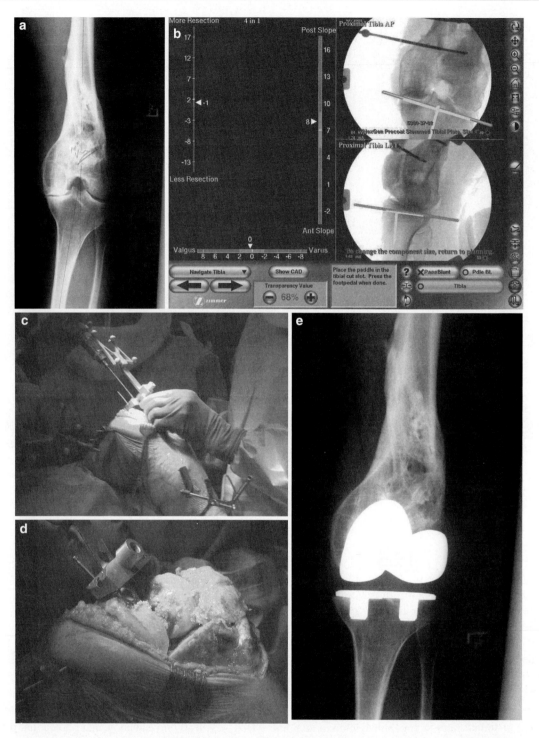

Fig. 73.10 (a) Difficult total reconstruction in an old distal femoral fracture deformity. (b) Navigation of tibial cut shows planned cut to be 8° posterior slope, 1 mm of medial tibial plateau, and 0° to the mechanical axis. (c) Freehand navigation of the distal femoral cutting guide into the desired resection level and correct angle for the coronal and sagittal planes. (d) The distal femoral cut is made based on the freehand navigated position of the cut guide. (e) The final radiograph shows the "perfect" position of the distal femoral cut, with a final mechanical axis measurement of 1° varus

For the community surgeon with lower surgical volume, purchasing a capital system may not be an option. Several companies now offer laptop systems that utilize innovative tracking methods such as the Zimmer Axiem electromagnetic system. The hospital rents the system on a per-case basis that closely approximates the cost of the typical capital system. Small electromagnetic trackers may be placed within the wound, avoiding the need for percutaneous pin placement. The disadvantage is the fact that any ferrous material, including instruments, operating table, etc. can degrade the

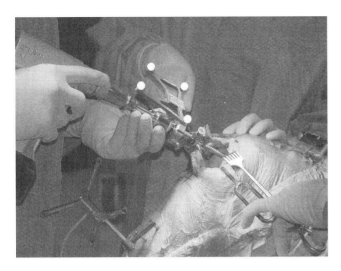

Fig. 73.11 Navigation of minimally invasive surgical distal femoral cut guide into the appropriate position

accuracy of the system. In addition, an assistant must carefully position the magnetic coils to limit motion and to effectively collect the signal from the trackers. These problems limit the accuracy and efficacy of this technology.

A third factor that could be equated with costs is the expense of the "learning curve." This could require the surgeon and their staff to attend a surgical skill course to learn computer navigation. I personally spent several hours in the anatomy lab learning my system before performing live surgery. However, much effort has been made to create appropriate product literature to limit this process.

Total Hip Arthroplasty

Cost can be identified as the major drawback with total hip navigation and this carries all the problems noted above for total knees. The other serious reservation is time, and my experience with both the fluoroscopic and imageless systems has been that they are very time consuming. The current imageless applications require either a "flip technique" where the patient is moved from the supine to the lateral decubitus position, or a touch point matching method with the patient positioned in the lateral position. The point matching may be superficial or through percutaneous punctures. The "flip technique," although easy to perform, adds at least 15–20 min as a separate procedure. The reference base plate must be placed into position with percutaneous pins, the trackers must be attached with the quick release, and the optical camera positioned. After referencing, the tracker is removed, the patient is repositioned into lateral decubitus, and the pelvis and leg are prepped and draped for the formal total hip replacement. I have utilized fluoroscopic referencing for the lateral approach and virtually abandoned

this approach. The field of view of the standard fluoroscopic C-arm is limited, making image acquisition challenging and time consuming. I think that these limitations will be resolved with new emerging technologies, such as intraoperative CT, that should allow for automated referencing and have a much larger field of view. Finally, any of these methods that use percutaneous pin placement expose the patient to pin site infection, bone fracture, neuroma formation, or sensitive scar formation, although there are no reported cases to date of these problems.

Conclusions

CAS for total knee and hip arthroplasty has offered substantial improvements in the precision of the operative technique that should provide long-term benefits to the patient. In addition, the gains for minimally invasive surgery, although not proven, could be logically assumed. Optical systems for tracking are highly accurate and robust for this application. Electromagnetic tracking offers promise, although current systems are not presently as accurate. Total knee applications have evolved easily to an efficient imageless referencing protocol. Total hip applications remain cumbersome, and non CT-based systems lack the important precision that is needed. Significant improves loom on the horizon.

References

1. Bargar WL, Bauer A, Boerner M. (1998) Primary and revision total hip replacement using ROBODOC. Clin Orthop Relat Res Sep;(354):82–91
2. Jaramaz B, DiGioia AM III, Blackwell M, Nikou C. (1998) Computer assisted measurement of cup placement in total hip replacement. Clin Orthop Relat Res Sep;(354):70–81
3. Petersen T, Engh G. (1988) Radiographic assessment of knee alignment after total knee arthroplasty. J Arthroplasty 3:67–72
4. Berend M, Ritter M, Meding J, et al. (2004) Tibial component failure mechanisms in total knee arthroplasty. Clin Orthop Relat Res Nov;(428):26–34
5. Yau WP, Leung A, Chiu KY, Tang WM, Ng TP. (2005) Intraobserver errors in obtaining visually selected anatomic landmarks during registration process in nonimage based navigation-assisted total knee arthroplasty. J Arthroplasty 20:591–599
6. Bathis H, Perlick L, Tingart M, et al. (2004) Alignment in total knee arthroplasty. J Bone Joint Surg Br 86:682–687
7. Sparmann M, Wolke B, Czupalla H, et al. (2003) Positioning of total knee arthroplasty with and without navigation support. J Bone Joint Surg Br 85:830–835
8. Bathis H, Perlick L, Tingart M, et al. (2004) Radiological results of image-based and non-image-based computer-assisted total knee arthroplasty. Int Orthop 28:87–90
9. Victor J, Hoste D. (2004) Image-based computer-assisted total knee arthroplasty leads to lower variability in coronal alignment. Clin Orthop Relat Res Nov;(428):131–139

10. Lionberger, DR. (2006) The attraction of electromagnetic computer navigation in orthopaedic surgery. In *Navigation and Minimally Invasive Surgery*, JB Stiehl, A Digioia, W Konermann, R Haaker (eds). Springer, Heidelberg

11. Kalairajah Y, Simpson P, Cossey AJ, Verrall GM, Spriggins AJ. (2005) Blood loss after total knee arthroplasty, effects of computer assisted surgery. J Bone Joint Surg Br 87:1480–1482

12. Kalairajah Y, Cossey AJ, Verall GM, Ludbrook G, Spriggins AJ. (2005) Are systemic emboli reduced in computer assisted surgery. J Bone Joint Surg Br 88:198–202

13. Cobb J, Henckel J, Gomes P, et al. (2006) Hands on robotic unicompartmental knee replacement. J Bone Joint Surg Br 88:188–197

14. Cossey AJ, Spriggins AJ. (2005) The use of computer-assisted surgical navigation to prevent malalignment in unicompartmental knee arthroplasty. J Arthroplasty 20:29–33

15. Jenny J-Y. (2005) Navigated unicompartmental knee replacement. Orthopaedics 28:1263–1267

16. Keene G, Simpson D, Kalairag Y. (2006) Limb alignment in computer assisted minimally-invasive unicompartmental knee replacement. J Bone Joint Surg Br 88:44–48

17. DiGioia AM, Jaramaz B, Plakseychuk AY, et al. (2002) Comparison of a mechanical acetabular alignment guide with computer placement of the socket. J Arthroplasty 17:359–364

18. Haaker R, Tiedjen K, Ottersbach A, Stiehl JB, Rubenthaler F, Shockheim M. (2007) Comparison of freehand versus computer assisted acetabular cup implantation. J Arthroplasty 22(2): 151–159

19. Kalteis T, Handel M, Bathis H, Perlick L, Tingart M, Grifka J. (2006) Imageless navigation for insertion of the acetabular component in total hip arthroplasty. J Bone Joint Surg Br 88:163–167

20. Lewinnek GE, Lewis JL, Tarr R, et al. (1978) Dislocations after total hip-replacement arthroplasties. J Bone Joint Surg Am 60:217–220

21. Nogler M, Kessler O, Prassl A, et al. (2004) Reduced variability of acetabular cup positioning with use of an imageless navigation system. Clin Orthop Relat Res Sep(426):159–163

22. Stiehl JB, Heck DA. (2006) Validation of imageless total hip navigation. In *Navigation and Minimally Invasive Surgery in Orthopaedics*, JB Stiehl, A Digioia, W Konermann, R Haacker. (eds). Springer, Heidelberg

23. Stiehl JB, Heck DA, Jarmaz B, Amiot L-P. Comparison of fluoroscopic and imageless referencing in navigation of total hip arthroplasty. J Comput Assist Surg in press

24. Grutzner PA, Zheng G, Langlotz U, et al. (2004) C-arm based navigation in total hip arthroplasty - background and clinical experience. Injury 35(Suppl 1):A90

Chapter 74
Computer-Guided Total Hip Arthroplasty

James B. Stiehl

Computed-assisted orthopedic surgery (CAOS) has been recently defined as the ability to use sophisticated computer algorithms to allow the surgeon to determine three-dimensional (3D) placement of total hip implants in situ.[1] A rapid ongoing evolution of technical advances has allowed the ability to move from cumbersome systems requiring a preoperative computed tomography (CT) scan of the patient's hip joint to more elegant systems that use image-free registration or the simple use of fluoroscopy at the time of surgery. In total hip replacement, several reports have cited the accuracy with which implants can be placed using computer-aided robotic devices or surgical navigation.

From a historical perspective, ROBODOC was the first modern attempt to use computers to place implants in bones; in this example, a cementless metal femoral stem in the proximal femoral canal. The goal was to improve the precision of implant placement, and to eliminate errors from a variety of sources including inaccurate plain radiographic templating, morphological anatomical variation, and problems related to the insertion of the implants. The ROBODOC system was conceived in 1986 by Bargar and Paul, and developed over the next several years with grants from IBM. That team developed proprietary software for the CT imaging to obtain an accuracy of one pixel for the raw data, which then allowed them to create CT 3D reconstructions for choosing the implant sizes and planning the robotic surgical intervention. Originally, the fiducial markers for the robotic system were placed during a separate operative procedure and the marker was used to specifically orient the robotic tool into the inner canal of the proximal femur. This changed with the ability to register the unique anatomy of the patient intraoperatively. With improvements in software, the system could be referenced by using a digitizing probe for the key areas of the proximal femur, and small incisions were used about the midshaft of the femur for distal referencing. Currently, referencing may be done using a highly sophisticated combination of local touch point referencing and image overlay. The ROBODOC system is amenable to very small incisions that are limited in length only by the size of the implants.[2,3]

In the early 1990s, other possibilities arose for computer navigation and, although *active* or robotic navigation held promise, *passive* navigation developed with the possibility of remotely tracking the instruments and anatomy (Fig. 74.1). The idea here was to reference the target object, which in this case would be the human acetabulum and then track the instruments passively in space. For navigation about the hip, CT scanning was first used to acquire a digital representation of the structure of the pelvis and femur.[4] Optoelectronic tracking was developed because that system was readily available from other industrial processes. Furthermore, the inputs were not affected by the surgical environment, as were other methods such as electromagnetic trackers and ultrasound. A negative feature, however, is the need for unobstructed view of the camera and the markers.

In order to determine the exact spatial orientation of the patient or any surgical instrument, at least three noncollinear points on a fixed body (dynamic reference base [DRB]) must be recognized by a camera system, which then inputs data into the computer for virtual referencing. The referencing protocol collects all components, including the patient's anatomy and all registered surgical instruments. The DRBs may be active, consisting of light emitting diodes (LEDs), in which two or three charge-coupled devices (CCD) of the camera system pick up the light signal; or passive, in which reflector balls are placed on the DRB and reflect infrared light originating from a light source on the camera. By differentiating the sphere arrangements on the DRBs, the computer could then detect the specific DRB, such as the marker on the pelvis or a reaming instrument.

Registration is the process by which the computer recognizes the various 3D objects that it must *virtually* characterize. For all DRBs, the process is simply finding the appropriately defined DRB with the camera and registering it with the computer. For instruments and implants, the exact dimensions and orientation of the referencing source are encrypted into the software. For the patient, the goal is to reference or *match* the anatomy

J. Stiehl (✉)
Department of Orthopaedic Surgery, Medical College of Wisconsin, Milwaukee, WI, USA
e-mail: jbstiehl@me.com

* Adapted from Stiehl JB, Computer-guided total hip arthroplasty, in Scuderi G, Tria A, Berger R (eds), MIS in Orthopedics, New York, Springer, 2006, with kind permission of Springer Science + Business Media.

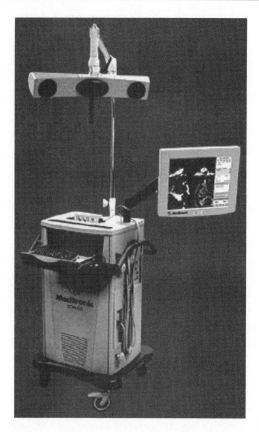

Fig. 74.1 The computer navigation system consists of a camera, DRBs on the patient, the computer platform, and the method of image acquisition, in this case, fluoroscopy

of the patient into the computer model. Two methods exist for performing this step. Paired-point matching takes prominent anatomical points that have been predetermined on the CT scan and then intraoperatively using a space digitizer (pointer probe) that identifies or matches the same landmark. Surface registration is a secondary referencing method in which a small number of points may be digitized into the system to describe a surface contour such as the dome of the acetabulum. An additional step is verification, which is cross-referencing additional points on the anatomy with the virtual object on the computer. From this information, the surgeon may judge the operational accuracy of the system.

The advantage of the CT scan for referencing is that it provides a 3D data set for creating the virtual model in the computer. However, acquisition of the CT scan adds additional logistical and financial factors to the process. The CT scan must be obtained preoperatively and must be digital in format for use on the computer. Additional time will be required by the surgical team to manipulate the data, pick the primary referencing points, templating, etc. In addition, there are certain examples such as in navigated fracture reduction, in which the bone topology of the CT is intentionally altered during the surgical procedure. Other options exist such as acquiring the images with two-dimensional (2D) fluoroscopy or using a direct surgeon-defined anatomical approach. Fluoroscopy

requires specific calibration to maintain the desired accuracy of the imaging technique. It is known that the earth's magnetic forces significantly distort the image acquired from the fluoroscope camera and this must be accounted for. In practice, a calibrated grid with markers of known size and spatial relationship are combined with the image to create an accurate virtual portrayal on the computer. The images are then acquired with the patient's DRB in position to obtain the virtual model that allows navigation of the fluoroscopic image.[5]

The surgeon-defined anatomy approach requires the surgeon to create the virtual model by digitizing the various points of the anatomy with a navigated probe. This is particularly applicable to open total knee replacement, where most of the important landmarks are visible and readily identified. A novel kinematic approach has evolved for determining the hip center location in which the center of rotation of the hip joint is determined by simply rotating the lower extremity in a large circular motion. The computer automatically finds the smallest point of movement, which in this case should be the center of the femoral head, if the pelvis is held absolutely rigid. The mechanical axis of the lower extremity is defined by point matching the center of the distal femur, the center of the proximal tibia, and a factored point between the ankle malleoli for the most distal center. Certain proprietary software applications have added surface matching to this direct method to supplement anatomical features.

The applications to minimally invasive surgery will evolve from a unique combination of the previously noted techniques. For example, the two-incision hip approach, which already uses fluoroscopy for identifying the anatomy, will now have a virtual fluoroscopy image on the computer for navigating both the acetabulum and the femur. Direct anatomical landmarks may be point match referenced on such areas as the anterior superior iliac spine, which is readily accessible. For the other landmarks, such as the pubic symphysis, indirect referencing may be done by obtaining calibrated fluoroscopic images in two planes. For the total knee arthroplasty, a similar combination of direct and fluoroscopic referencing will be done. While one may easily identify the lower extremity centers for the total knee minimally invasive quadriceps-sparing technique, accessory landmarks such as the distal femoral epicondyles may not be readily obtained. Future applications include newer technologies such as electromagnetic sensors that can be made into miniature DRBs and the use of more sophisticated imaging systems such as ultrasound, 3D C-arms, and the use of intraoperative CT scanners.

Acetabular Component Navigation

Optimal acetabular component orientation in total hip arthroplasty is a complex 3D problem with failure leading to increased wear and instability. Recent publications have demonstrated a connection between the positioning of the prosthesis and the frequency of dislocation.[6–8] Lewinnek et al. noted an increase of the hip dislocation rate from 1.5% to 6.1% if a safe range of 15 ± 10° radiographic anteversion or 40 ± 10° acetabular abduction were exceeded.[9] Recent computer simulations have studied range of motion and concluded that the greatest range of motion was noted with acetabular anteversion of 20–25°, acetabular abduction of 45°, and femoral stem anteversion of 15°.[10,11]

The positioning of the acetabular component during surgery is dependent on the orientation of the bony acetabulum and position of the patient's pelvis on the operating table. McCollum et al. have stated that patient positioning is not always reproducible in the lateral decubitus position and often leads to pelvic malalignment with resultant improper cup alignment. Pelvic flexion and adduction are virtually unavoidable in this position, placing greater demands on the surgical technique for satisfactory outcome.[12] Therefore, improvement in cup implantation occurs if either the pelvis position can be standardized or a method of correctly localizing the anatomical orientation of the acetabulum can be created.

Computed Tomography for Acetabular Navigation

I describe the method of computer-assisted navigation recently used in a group of patients in whom CT was the source of image referencing. In patients undergoing computer-assisted navigation of the acetabular components, a preoperative anal-ysis and planning was required (Figs. 74.2 and 74.3). The digital CT study was loaded into the Surgigate (Medivision, Oberdorf, Switzerland) software program and

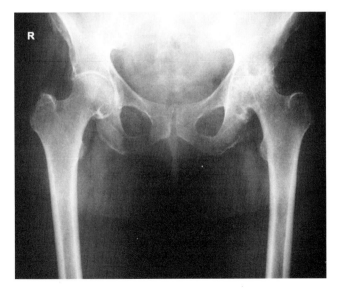

Fig. 74.2 Anterior pelvic radiograph of a preoperative patient with severe degenerative arthritis of the left hip

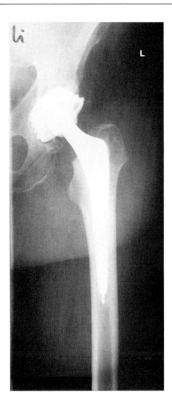

Fig. 74.3 Postoperative anterior-posterior radiograph of the left hip revealing a screw-in cup and pressfit femoral stem

the 3D model was then created. The femoral head was extracted from the image and the sagittal plane of view was drawn over the acetabular inlet. This then allowed visualization of the acetabulum in three planes and the 3D model of the pelvis (Fig. 74.4). The frontal plane reference was created, which was the landmarking reference subsequently used at the time of surgery. This reference consisted of the plane formed by the points of the anterior superior iliac spines and the pubic symphysis. In most patients, this plane is parallel to the long axis of the patient and is perpendicular to the floor. The Surgigate software automatically creates all images in the sagittal, frontal, and axial planes with a 90° reference to the frontal plane reference (Fig. 74.5). With the 3D model, at least three additional points of reference were identified to be used at the time of surgery. These included the points in the acetabular dome, the acetabular floor, and the cotyloid notch on the lateral wall of the quadrilateral plate. The final step allowed positioning of a virtual acetabular component into the pelvis at the chosen position of 45° acetabular abduction and 20° acetabular anteversion. Additionally, the surgeon has the ability in this planning step to deepen or medialize the cup position and preferentially position the cup more anteriorly or posteriorly. Final cup position was demonstrated in three planes and also on the 3D pelvic model that had the femoral head extracted (see Fig. 74.4).

The intraoperative computer-assisted navigation system consisted of an infrared camera (Optotrack 3020, Northern

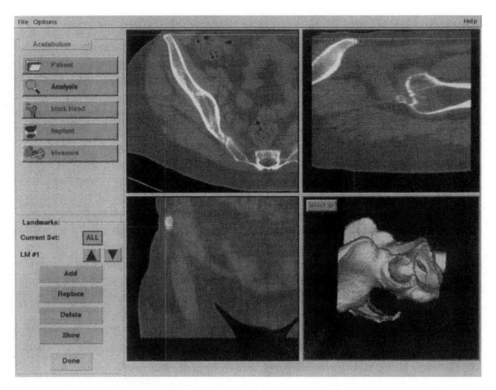

Fig. 74.4 Computer screen *analysis* image after acquisition of the CT study, noting the position of the ipsilateral anterior superior iliac spine for registration. The point is shown with sagittal, axial, and frontal plane views with a composite 3D model of the pelvis

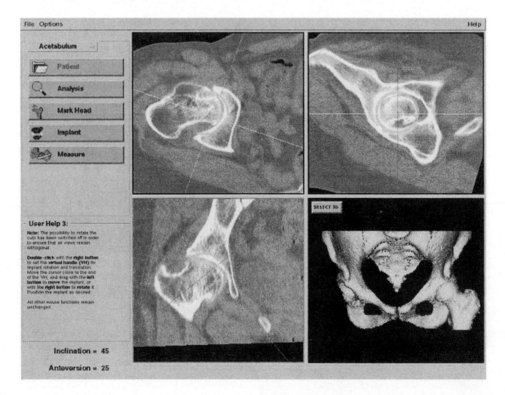

Fig. 74.5 In this preoperative planning step, the cup implant in size, design, and position is added to the 3D model of the pelvic bone. The position is defined by the anteversion (25°), the inclination (45°), and the depth of the implant

Digital, Waterloo, Canada) on an overhead boom and the Surgigate system including the video with monitor, and Unix Ultra 10 workstation with appropriate Surgigate software.

The conventional instruments for the implantation of hip endoprostheses was equipped with infrared transducers or LEDs. With these optoelectronic markers, the position of all instruments were tracked in space by the optical camera and transmitted to the computer system. A special pointer was used to indicate landmarks defined in preoperative planning phase and now used for referencing those points in the patient's acetabulum. The pointer was also used to initiate certain computer functions by activating or taping designated areas on a virtual keyboard. In addition, a DRB, an instrument equipped with infrared transducers, was securely fastened to the pelvic skeleton of the patient. This was done by using a Steinman pin attached approximately 2 cm cranial of the acetabular rim or, alternatively, fixed to the anterior superior iliac spine, depending on the surgical exposure. Fixation of the DRB must be absolutely rigid because this reference allows the computer system to track the patient's movements on the operation table.

The intraoperative navigation can be divided in two major steps, registration and surgical implantation. First, the instruments and the reference base need to be checked for positional error, which is typically less than 0.5 mm. After this step, pair point matching was done, which identifies and registers the same landmarks as determined during the preoperative planning phase. Subsequently, surface matching was done, in which a cloud of points consisting of at least 12 separate points were placed on the pelvis of the patient. Preferred areas were the anterior superior iliac spines, acetabular dome, and lateral ilium surrounding the

lip of the acetabulum. With this registration process, the Surgigate software attempted to find a *best fit* between the demonstrated points and the 3D pelvic model generated in the preoperative planning phase. The computer then generated a *quality index*, which defined the precision of which the patient's pelvis could be matched to that of the virtual pelvis. The manufacturer of the system required a maximum quality index value of 10 after the pair point matching and 2 after the surface point matching. The final step in registration was a verification step during which the software sought the best solution to "align the virtual and the actual pelvis." The surgeon identified a known point on the pelvis and this point must precisely match the point identified on the virtual pelvic model.

At this point, the surgeon was then capable of navigating both the milling process and the subsequent cup implantation. Both of the instruments used for this process, including the reamer and the cup inserter, were instrumented with an LED, which allowed for precise positioning in the acetabulum. The surgeon used visual cues and numerical positional data displayed on the computer screen to determine exact reamer and cup position compared with the preoperative planning position. For all patients with acetabular navigation in this study, we recorded the final cup position as indicated on the screen at the conclusion of the procedure (Fig. 74.6).

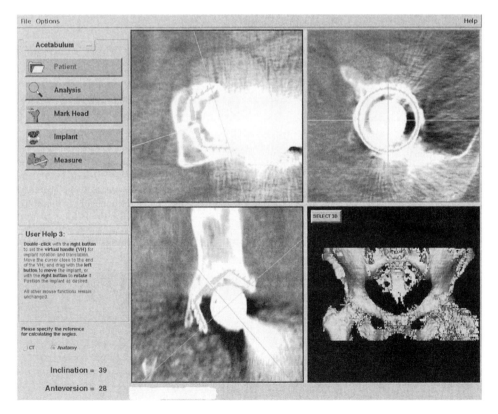

Fig. 74.6 Computer screen view demonstrates three postoperative views through the center of the acetabulum from the CT scans, including the sagittal, axial, and frontal views followed by a 3D model of the pelvis. Note the calculated acetabular inclination of 39° and anteversion of 28°

Postoperative Assessment Using CT Computer Analysis

Analysis of all postoperative CT study results was done using the Surgigate Data Analysis software module (Medivision, Oberdorf, Switzerland; now Praxim, Grenoble, France), which allowed for accurate interpretation of implanted acetabular components. Computer hardware used was an Ultra 10 Sun Microsystems workstation (Sun Microsystems, Schwerzenbach, Switzerland). This was a multistep process requiring each CT scan to be loaded into the Surgigate software module. The computer then created a 3D model of the pelvis. From this model, the frontal plane was defined by touch pointing the appropriate landmarks, which include the bilateral anterior superior iliac spines and the bilateral pubic tubercles, as noted previously. This then defined the reference base of subsequent measurements of acetabular component position. The scans demonstrating the implanted cups were brought into view using the computer touch screen. Using a library of computer-aided design models of each specific acetabular component, the appropriately sized and positioned virtual images were then overlaid to the implanted devices (Fig. 74.6). After DiGioia et al., operative acetabular abduction and anteversion was described for each implanted device. Specifically, the acetabular abduction was defined as the angle between the projection of the opening plane of the cup in the coronal plane and the sagittal plane; and the anteversion angle was defined as the angle between the projection of the opening plane of the cup in the frontal plane and the sagittal plane.[13,14]

Clinical Experience with CT Navigation

A control group of 69 patients underwent CT scanning for preoperative planning for surgical navigation of the contralateral total hip replacement after a previously placed conventional total hip replacement.[15] Each CT scan was taken through the pelvis with 3-mm slices, using a digital format. The cohort of the conventional implanted group was aged 63.4 years (46.5–76.8 years). There were 43 women and 26 men. Forty-one pressfit cups and 28 screw-in cups were implanted. All patients had reached at least 12 months follow-up at the time radiographic study. The acetabular implant position was assessed in the conventionally placed implants in this group. A second group of 98 patients underwent total hip replacement using the computer-assisted navigation system where the acetabular component had been inserted using computer guided indices. In the computer-assisted cup implantation cohort, we found an average age of 66.9 years (42.4–81.0 years). Sixty-three women and 35 men underwent this operation. The implanted prostheses included 64 screw-in cups, 26 pressfit cups, and 8 cemented cups. The primary diagnosis

was osteoarthritis in 86% of cases, with the remaining cases being other including inflammatory arthritis and dysplasia.

From analysis of the postoperative CT scans, the average acetabular abduction for computer navigation was 43.03° (standard deviation [SD]: 4.59; 95% confidence interval [CI]: 0.97; range: 30–58°); and, for acetabular anteversion, the average was 22.22° (SD: 7.39; 95% CI: 1.72; range: 5–38°). For the freehand group, the average acetabular abduction was 45.74° (SD: 9.09; 95% CI: 2.63°; range 26–64°). The average acetabular anteversion was 28.51° (SD: 10.25; 95% CI: 3.80°; range 9–53°). The average last saved Surgigate computer-navigated acetabular abduction was 43.1° (95% CI: 0.87°; range 42.22–43.98°) and the acetabular anteversion was 22.4° (95% CI: 1.48°; range 20.94–23.92°). Using the F test for comparing the difference in the amount of variation between the two surgical methods, the ratio was 5.56 for abduction ($p < 0.0001$) and 3.67 for anteversion ($p < 0.0001$), indicating that the variation could not be attributed to chance for either variable and that computer navigation is significantly more accurate than free-hand conventional methods. The F ratio for the last Surgigate computer-navigated acetabular abduction position compared with the CT control was 0.30 and that for acetabular anteversion was 1.55, not reaching statistical significance.

Comparing both groups with the anteversion "safe zone" described by Fontes et al., we found that 28% of the freehand cups were placed outside of 11–35° anteversion; 4.7% were placed with less than 11° of anteversion and 23.4% have been implanted with an anteversion exceeding 35°. In the computer-navigated group, 7% were outside the parameters of 11–35° anteversion; 4.7% of the cups were implanted with less anteversion than 11°; and 2.5% exceeded 35° of anteversion.

Fluoroscopic Computer-Assisted Navigation

The use of fluoroscopy has been a more recent evolution of CAOS and represents the diversification of other methods used in neurosurgery and ear-nose-throat applications.[16,17] As mentioned previously, the technique requires accurate referencing of the fluoroscopic grid, which transfers the images to the computer for point matching and subsequent navigation. I have gained experience with fluoroscopic navigation using the Stealth Universal Hip Application (Medtronic ST, Denver, CO) and describe its use in both the acetabulum and the femur.

Technique of Acetabular Navigation

Fluoroscopic navigation of the pelvis requires that an unobstructed image be acquired in two different planes. This means that the camera must see both the DRB and the grid of the

C-arm during the image acquisition. I have used the Jackson operative imaging table for this purpose, which allows the patient to be placed in either the supine or lateral decubitus position. Once the grid has been acquired by the computer, the following images must be acquired for cup navigation: (1) contralateral anterior superior iliac spine in two views; (2) affected acetabulum in two views; and (3) pubic tubercle in two views. I have found several modifications helpful for obtaining the contralateral anterior superior iliac spine images, which may be the "downside" with the lateral decubitus minimally invasive lateral approach. First, a simple clamp wrapped in foam tape for insulation may be place directly adjacent to the ASIS by palpation. The patient is then prepped and draped, and a DRB is applied to the anterolateral wing of the ilium (Fig. 74.7). The fluoroscope C-arm is then brought over the area, and tilted 15–20° oblique to the frontal plane (Fig. 74.8). This brings the ASIS into relief compared with the remaining pelvis and with the marker, allows easy identification of the outline of the pelvic ilium, even in obese patients where abdominal contents overlie the image (Fig. 74.9). With the C-arm at the same tilt, the affected cup can then be imaged in the oblique view, and the presence of the pins from the DRB in the superior corner confirm the correct side. The image may be moved parallel to the frontal reference plane and the pubic tubercle lateral may be obtained (Figs. 74.10 and 74.11). This structure is a bit inferior to the acetabulum and is roughly on a transverse line just above the lesser trochanter and below the infracotyloid tubercle.

It will be anterior to the acetabulum by roughly 5 cm. The next structure is the anterior-posterior view of the pubic tubercle, which is very easily defined by fluoroscopy. In the lateral decubitus position, the C-arm is parallel to the floor (Figs. 74.12 and 74.13). The C-arm is tilted 15–20° oblique to the floor and the final images are made, which is the anterior-posterior affected cup view and the anterior-posterior ASIS view (Fig. 74.14). Again, the foam-covered clamp enables finding the later structure. The affected side ASIS may be acquired by touch pointing the anatomical structure in the field.

Referencing the fluoroscopic images that have been acquired is done by touching or mouse pointing the appropriate anatomic structures on the computer screen. This includes the center of the acetabulum or femoral head, the pubic tubercle, and the contralateral side ASIS. One interesting point is that the easily identified reference points, such as the *downside* lateral ASIS and anterior-posterior pubic tubercle provide a reference line on the other associated view for which the same structure must exist. Thusly, the anterior-posterior downside ASIS position, which is difficult to interpret, can be more easily identified. For the Stealth system, a final check is to determine if all of the reference lines match appropriately with the axes of the extremity.

When referencing is completed, the final step before actual navigation is to reference the DRBs attached to the reamers and the cup impactor (Fig. 74.15). Navigation then proceeds with the appropriate steps in the operative procedure.

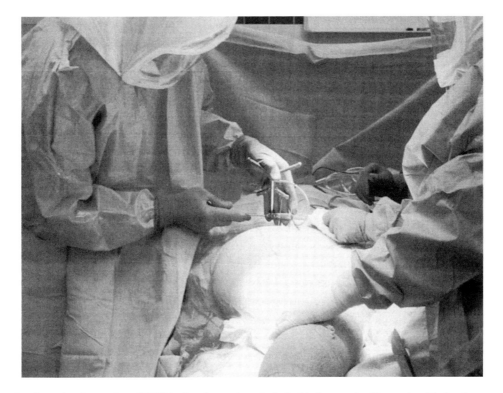

Fig. 74.7 The active dynamic reference base (DRB) is placed on a pin pod attached to the superior iliac crest and facing the camera system at the head of the operating table

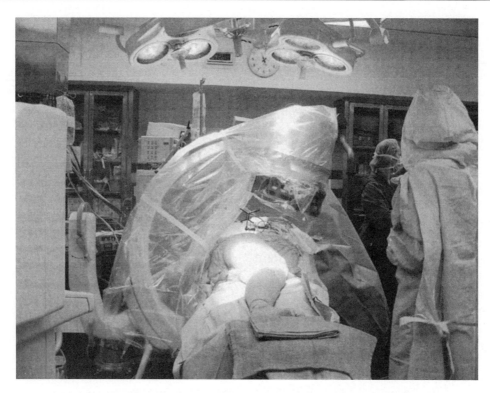

Fig. 74.8 Imaging the *downside* anterior superior iliac spine by tilting the C-arm approximately 20° oblique to the vertical to bring the ASIS into relief

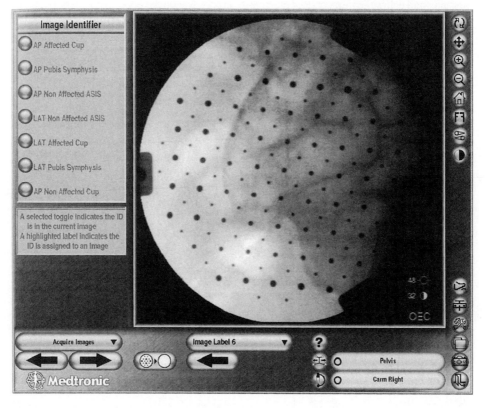

Fig. 74.9 Acquired image of the *downside* anterior superior iliac spine

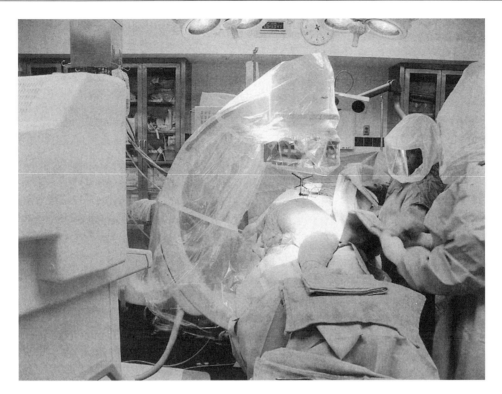

Fig. 74.10 Imaging the pubic tubercle from the lateral view of the pelvis with the C-arm vertical to the floor

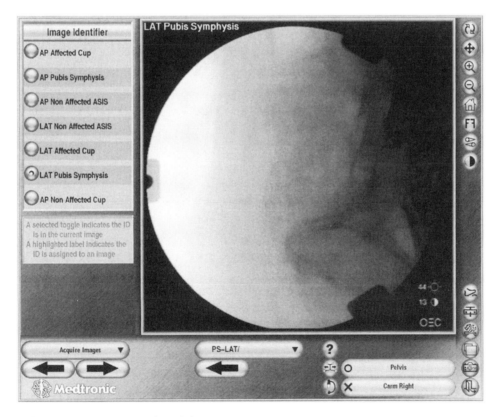

Fig. 74.11 Acquired image of the pubic tubercle lateral view

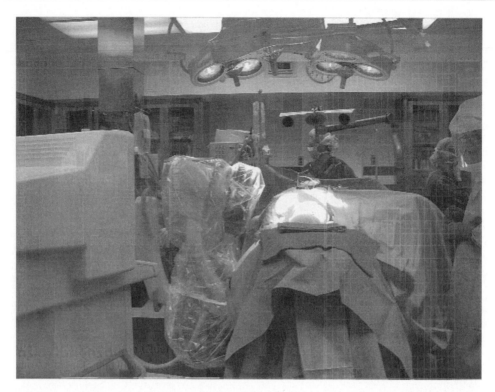

Fig. 74.12 Imaging the anterior-posterior view of the *downside* anterior superior iliac spine and the frontal view of the pubic tubercle

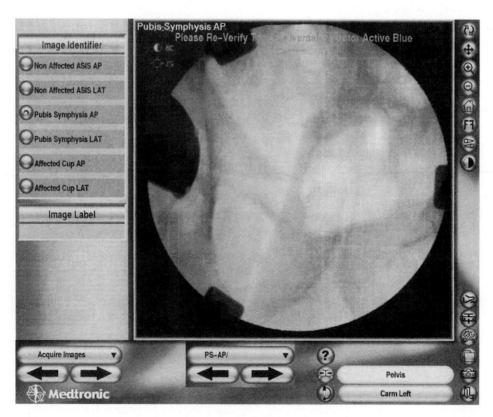

Fig. 74.13 Acquired image of the pubic tubercle on the anterior-posterior view

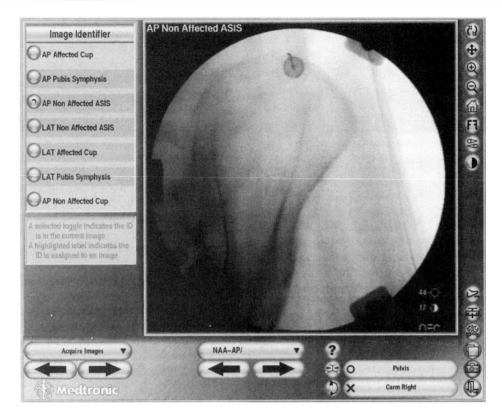

Fig. 74.14 Acquired image of the *downside* anterior superior iliac spine on the anterior-posterior view

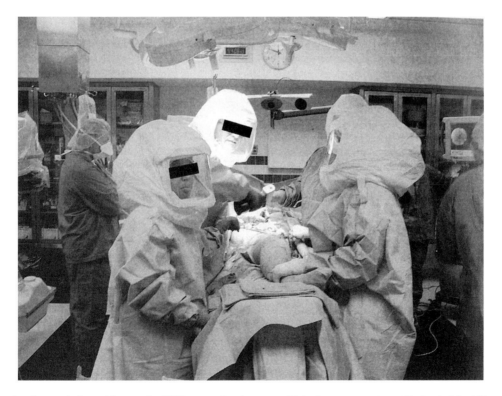

Fig. 74.15 Reaming the acetabulum with an *active* DRB mounted to the reamer. Note the camera system at the head of the table and the computer screen in *upper right hand corner*

As noted previously, the optimal position determined for cup positioning is 45° abduction and 20° anteversion. The reamer and cup inserter are instrumented with an appropriate DRB. Both reaming and final cup insertion can be virtually observed on the computer, and the operator can carefully match the instruments with the screen calibration targets and numbers (Figs. 74.16 and 74.17). I have found the cup insertion usually parallels my "experience" with this effort, but surprisingly little motion of the insertion handle can make a big difference. Postoperative radiographs are difficult to interpret because the frontal pelvic reference frame is not always appropriately positioned.

Discussion

Acetabular component placement in total hip arthroplasty can be difficult, with optimal placement required to prevent chronic instability, exaggerated wear, and implant migration. Recent investigators have sought to define the radiographic analysis of cup position in the clinical setting, prosthetic issues such as range of motion and component impingement, and technical issues at the time of surgery, such as body position and how to place the prosthesis in the desired location. Computer-assisted navigation represents a new technology that can be used to deal with all of these problems.[18–24]

The spatial orientation of the natural acetabulum and prosthetic components placed at surgery is a complex 3D problem and most authors have attempted to describe a 2D radiographic answer. Murray has provided the most complete insight into this problem by defining geometrically exactly what these solutions represent (Fig. 74.18). For simple comparison, the acetabular abduction is defined as the angle formed to the transverse plane of the patient when the superior

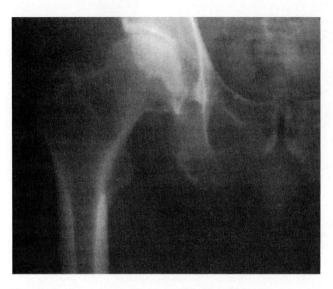

Fig. 74.16 Anterior-posterior view of the affected hip

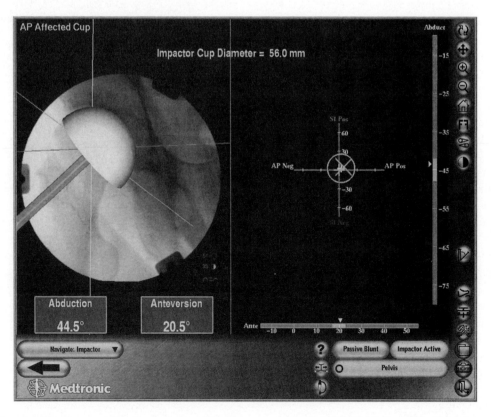

Fig. 74.17 Final cup position documented on the computer, with a 56-mm cup inserted at 44° abduction and 20° anteversion

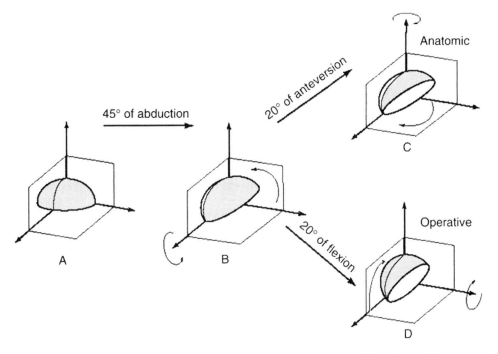

Fig. 74.18 Concept of acetabular abduction and anteversion with the various measurement possibilities. (From DiGioia et al.,[14] by permission of Elsevier, Inc.)

cup is tilted toward the longitudinal axis of the patient, or, in the anatomical specimen, a line drawn from the superior lip down to the inferior cotyloid notch on the anterior-posterior radiograph. The more complex issue is how to determine the acetabular anteversion or flexion, and three possibilities are possible based on how the cup is measured. Operative anteversion occurs when the acetabular component is flexed in the coronal plane of the patient, essentially rotating about a line through the acetabulum, which is perpendicular to the longitudinal axis of the patient. This is the maneuver accomplished by most freehand surgical guides and is the planar measurement made by determining the angulation of the cup in the frontal plane compared with the sagittal plane by looking at the coronal section CT scan. Radiographic anteversion occurs when the anterior cup lip is rotated superiorly around the oblique transverse axis of the acetabulum, which lies in the coronal plane of the patient. This measurement was typically used on cemented cups of known dimension that had wire radio-opaque markers. Anatomical anteversion is the position that occurs when the abducted acetabulum position is internally rotated around the longitudinal axis of the patient. This measurement has been used to assess acetabular anatomical position in dysplasia. Murray has concluded that the operative anteversion is the most practical and should be used to describe cup position in total hip arthroplasty.[25] For the computer application, DiGioia et al. have concluded that the operative acetabular abduction and anteversion measurements are the most straightforward, reducing the conclusions to strict planar 2D terms.[13,14] We used this method for our

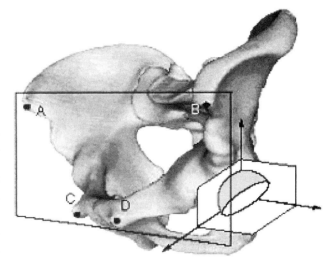

Fig. 74.19 Frontal pelvic reference frame marking the anterior superior iliac spine and the pubic promontory. (From DiGioia et al.,[14] by permission of Elsevier, Inc.)

abduction and anteversion measurements and have found no other variations in recent publications concerning computer navigation.

Lewinnek et al. were first to describe the concept of the anterior pelvic plane, which is defined as a coronal slice passing through bilateral anterior superior iliac spines and the bilateral anterior pubic tubercles[9] (Fig. 74.19). In the normal standing position, this plane is usually parallel to the longitudinal axis of the patient. McCollum et al. have shown

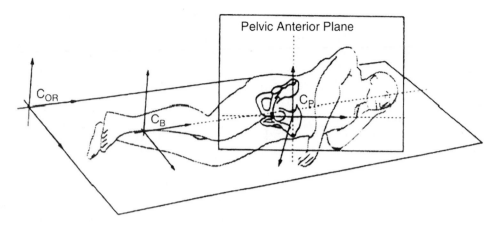

Fig. 74.20 Tripod used to establish the pelvic reference frame parallel to the table for a patient undergoing radiography in the supine position

that this plane may altered, especially if patients are placed in the lateral decubitus position, or there is hip flexion reducing the normal lumbar lordosis.[12] Lewinnek et al. employed a crude device with three legs and a bubble level applied to the pelvic crests and pubis to make certain that the pelvic plane was parallel to the plane of the table prior to taking their anterior-posterior radiographs of the pelvis for anteversion measurement[9] (Fig. 74.20). An important step in the registration procedure for computer-assisted navigation is to define the anterior pelvic plane using the same references generating a standardized pelvic position.

Numerous investigators have questioned the accuracy of standard radiographic methods for measuring cup position. For radiographic views, the X-ray beam must be carefully directed in a standardized fashion centered over the pelvis, and the pelvis must be level with the beam perpendicular to the pelvic frontal plane in each case. However, Ackland et al. stated that an error of as much as 5° could be introduced if the X-ray was centered over the symphysis pubis and not the hip joint itself.[26] Pelvic rotation certainly is an important consideration, and Thorén et al. demonstrated a 2.5° alteration of cup anteversion for 5° of pelvic rotation.[27] Herrlin et al. found that 5° of pelvic flexion or extension could introduce a maximum error of 8° in acetabular anteversion.[28] CT assessments done with computer navigation, on the other hand, have been described as the gold standard for measuring cup abduction and anteversion, with an accuracy of approximately 1–2° based on current methodologies.

Optimal acetabular component orientation has been a subject of much debate, but most recent investigations conclude that the approximate position of 45° abduction or inclination and 20° radiographic anteversion is the ideal target. Obviously, retrospective studies such as those of Lewinnek et al. and Fontes et al. define a "safe" envelope or range about which hip stability after arthroplasty is much greater.[9,29] However, Barrack et al. have used a complex 3D computer analysis to refine the optimization to the above parameters and have shown that certain positions such as cup abduction below 25° or cup anteversion below 0° are clearly unsatisfactory for positions such as sitting or stooping.[10] Acetabular stability and impingement relates not only to component position but also to prosthetic design dimensions and related femoral stem positioning. The average cup position after navigation in our study was acetabular inclination of 43° and cup anteversion of 22°, closely approximating the best position in the majority of cases.

DiGioia et al. used a computer-assisted navigation system similar to the method we used to study the problems of mechanical alignment in the conventional operative setting with the lateral decubitus position and with the use of typical freehand alignment guides.[30] They found that the mean pelvic position was close to the desired anterior pelvic plane prior to dislocation, but, after dislocation, the pelvis tilted anteriorly, causing a shift of the mean anteversion of the pelvis to 18°. Of 74 cups, 58 were placed outside the desired anteversion of 20 ± 10°, while only one cup was outside of the desired abduction of 45 ± 10°. In another study, they were able to determine that postoperative radiographs produced variable and inaccurate results compared with their precise intraoperative computer-generated measurements.

The use of computer-assisted navigation will be an important asset for surgeons attempting to improve total hip implant insertion. This will be especially true for minimally invasive approaches, which offer great challenge if the typical landmarks are obscured. The computer offers a virtual image of the pelvis and femur, which is then used for accurate placement of the implants. The current accuracy of most computer navigation systems is within 1 mm or 1°. That being said, the true accuracy relates more to the skill of the surgeon in carefully identifying the appropriate landmarks and carefully inserting a stable DRB. A *stacking* or magnification of errors may occur if simple mistakes are made at several steps. For that reason, both system validation and observer validation is important to maintain system reliability. I presented a recent study where CT was used for reference image acquisition. Interestingly, neither the company developing the system for that study, Medivision, nor the CT technique utilized are currently being sold. I currently favor the use of fluoroscopic referencing using the Medronic ST Stealth station, because the referencing can be done real time and in a few minutes. Studies are currently in process to validate the clinical in vivo results. In conclusion, recent studies have proven the efficacy of the surgical technique at least to accomplish given surgical goals. Clinical validation and efficacy will require ongoing studies.

References

1. Knolte LP, Langlotz F. (2003) Basics of computer-assisted orthopaedic surgery (CAOS). In Stiehl JB, Konermann WH, Haaker RG, (eds) *Navigations and Robotics in Total Joint and Spinal Surgery*, Springer, Berlin Heidelberg New York Tokyo

2. Bargar WL, Bauer A, Bomer M. (1998) Primary and revision total hip replacement using ROBODOC. Clin Orthop Relat Res Sep;(354):82–91

3. Bargar WL. (2003) Robotic surgery and current development with the ROBODOC system. In Stiehl JB, Konermann WH, Haaker RG, (eds) *Navigations and Robotics in Total Joint and Spinal Surgery*, Springer, Berlin Heidelberg New York Tokyo

4. Weise M, Schmidt K, Willburger RE. (2003) Clinical experience with CT-based Vectorvision system. In Stiehl JB, Konermann WH, Haaker RG, (eds) *Navigations and Robotics in Total Joint and Spinal Surgery*, Springer, Berlin Heidelberg New York Tokyo

5. Hagena FW, Kettrukat M, Christ RM, Hackbart M. (2003) Fluoroscopy-based navigation in Genesis II total knee arthroplasty with the Medtronic "Viking" system. In Stiehl JB, Konermann WH, Haaker RG, (eds) *Navigations and Robotics in Total Joint and Spinal Surgery*, Springer, Berlin Heidelberg New York Tokyo

6. Giurea A, Zehetgruber H, Funovics P, Grampp S, Karamat L, Gottsauner-Wolf F. (2001) Risk factors for dislocation in cementless hip arthroplasty - a statistical analysis. Z Orthop Ihre Grenzgeb 139:194–199

7. Kennedy JG, Rogers WB, Soffe KE, Sullivan RJ, Griffen DG, Sheehan LJ. (1998) Effect of acetabular component orientation on recurrent dislocation, pelvic osteolysis, polyethylene wear and component migration. J Arthroplasty 13:530–534

8. Bader RJ, Steinhauser E, Willmann G, Gradinger R. (2001) The effects of implant position, design, and wear on the range of motion after total hip arthroplasty. Hip Int 11:80–90

9. Lewinnek GE, Lewis JL, Tarr R, Compere CL, Zimmermann JR. (1978) Dislocations after total hip replacement arthroplasties. J Bone Joint Surg Am 60:217–221

10. Barrack RL, Lavernia C, Ries M, Thornberry R, Tozakoglou E. (2001) Virtual reality computer animation of the effect of component position and design on stability after total hip arthroplasty. Orthop Clin North Am 32:569–577

11. Seki M, Yuasa N, Ohkuni K. (1998) Analysis of optimal range of socket orientations in total hip arthroplasty with use of computer-aided design simulation. J Orthop Res 16:513–517

12. McCollum DE, Gray WJ. (1990) Dislocation after total hip replacement. Clin Orthop Relat Res Dec;(261):159–170

13. DiGioia AM, Jamaraz B, Blackwell M, Simon DA, Morgan F, Moody JE, Nikou C, Colgan BD, Aston CA, LaBarca RS, Kischell E, Kanade T. (1998) Image guided navigation system to measure intraoperatively acetabular implant alignment. Clin Orthop Relat Res Oct;(355):8–22

14. Di Gioia AM, Jamaraz B, Nikou C, LaBarca RS, Moody JE, Colgan S. (2000) Surgical navigation for total hip replacement with the use of HipNav. Oper Tech Orthop 10:3–8

15. Haaker R, Tiedjen K, Ottersbach A, Stiehl JB, Rubenthaler F, Shockheim M. (2004) Comparison of freehand versus computer assisted acetabular cup implantation. J Bone Joint Surg Br [Submitted]

16. Hofstetter R, Slomczykowski M, Bourquin Y, Nolte LP. (1997) Fluoroscopy based surgical navigation. In Lemke HU, Vannier MW, Inamura K, (eds) *Computer Asssited Radiology and Surgery*, Elsevier Science B.V., Amsterdam, pp 956–960

17. Hofstetter R, Slomczykowski M, Sati M, Nolte LP. (1999) Fluoroscopy as an imaging means for computer-assisted surgical navigation. Comput Aided Surg 4:65–76

18. Hassan DM, Johnston GHF, Dust WNC, Watson G, Dolovich AT. (1998) Accuracy of intraoperative assessment of acetabular prosthesis placement. J Arthroplasty 13:80–84

19. Bernsmann K, Langlotz U, Ansari B, Wiese M. (2000) Computer-assistierte navigierte Pfannenplatzierung in der Hüftendoprothetik Anwenderstudie im klinischen Routinealltag. Z Orthop Ihre Grenzgeb 138:515–521

20. Bernsmann K, Langlotz U, Ansari B, Wiese M. (2001) Computerassistierte navigierte Platzierung von verschiedenen Pfannentypen in der Hüftendoprothetik - eine randomisierte kontrollierte Studie. Z Orthop Ihre Grenzgeb 139:512–517

21. Jarmaz B, DiGioa AM, Blackwell M, Nikou C. (1998) Computer assisted measurement of cup placement in total hip replacement. Clin Orthop Relat Res Sep;(354):70–81

22. Jolles BM, Genoud P. (2001) Accuracy of computer-assisted placement in total hip arthroplasty. Int Congr Ser 1230:314–318

23. Leenders T, Vandervelde D, Nahiew G, Nuyts R. (2002) Reduction in variability of acetabular cup abduction using computed assisted surgery: prospective and randomized study. Comput Aided Surg 7:99–106

24. Mian SW, Truchly G, Pflum FA. (1992) Computed tomography measurement of acetabular cup anteversion and retroversion in total hip arthroplasty. Clin Orthop Relat Res Mar;(276):206–209

25. Murray DW. (1993) The definition and measurement of acetabular orientation. J Bone Joint Surg Br 75:228–232

26. Ackland MK, Bourne WB, Uhthoff HK. (1986) Anteversion of the acetabular cup. J Bone Joint Surg Br 68:409–413

27. Thoren B, Sahlstedt. (1990) Influence of pelvic position on radiographic measurements of the prosthetic acetabular component. Acta Radiol 31:133–136

28. Herrlin K, Pettersson H, Selvik G. (1998) Comparison of two- and three-dimensional methods for assessment of orientation of the total hip prosthesis. Acta Radiol 29:357–361

29. Fontes D, Benoit J, Lortat-Jacob A, Didry R. (1991) Luxation of total hip endoprosthesis. Statistical validation of a modelization of 52 cases. Rev Chir Orthop Reparatrice Appar Mot 77:163–170

30. DiGioa AM, Jaramaz B, Plakseychuk AY, Moody JE, Nikou C, LaBarca RS, Levison TJ, Picard F. (2002) Comparison of a mechanical acetabular alignment guide with computer placement of the socket. J Arthroplasty 17:359–364

Chapter 75
Computer Navigation with Posterior MIS Total Hip Arthroplasty

Aamer Malik, Zhinian Wan, and Lawrence D. Dorr

The majority of literature on computer-assisted surgery of the hip shows how navigation assists the surgeon in more accurate component placement as compared with techniques that use mechanical guides or are freehand.[1–5] Our work has been with imageless navigation technology, which allows real-time intraoperative knowledge of the quantitative direction and depth of reaming; adjustment during reaming for variations in the bony anatomy to allow for correct cup coverage with optimal inclination; and adjustment of the anteversion of a cup to a desired combined anteversion through knowledge of the fixed femoral anteversion.[6]

We have validated the results of the imageless computer navigation by comparison with postoperative computed tomography (CT) scans, which are considered the gold standard. We also compared the precision of the computer with postoperative radiographs and with the surgeons' estimates of cup position.

Methods

Institutional Review Board approval and proper informed consent for prospective review of data was obtained from 60 consecutive patients with 66 total hip replacements performed between July 2005 and March 2006. The Navitrack Imageless Computer Hip System (Orthosoft, Montreal, Canada) was used for each of these hip replacements. Data was collected during the operation. The operation for total hip replacement used was the posterior minimally invasive incision.[6,7] The preoperative diagnosis for surgery was primary osteoarthritis in 56 cases (85%), congenital hip dysplasia in 7 cases (11%), rheumatoid arthritis in 2 cases (3%), and idiopathic necrosis of the femoral head in 1 case (1%). The demographics of the patients studied are listed in Table 75.1.

A. Malik, Z. Wan, and L.D. Dorr (✉)
Dorr Arthritis Institute, 637 S. Lucas Ave, 5th Fl, Los Angeles, CA, 90017, USA
e-mail: Patriciajpaul@yahoo.com

Posterior MIS Technique

The operative technique for the total hip replacement was the posterior minimally invasive surgery (MIS) operation, which was performed by one experienced hip surgeon (LDD).[7–9] Components used were the porous coated Converge cup (Zimmer, Warsaw, IN) and Anatomic Porous Replacement (APR) stem (Zimmer), which were implanted cementless.

Computer Registration

For tracking, we used baseplates secured on the pelvis and femur with three threaded 1/8″ pins to bone. An optical tracker was attached to the baseplate. The anterior pelvic plane (APP) was registered with the patient in the supine position by percutaneous (puncturing the skin and ensuring firm bony contact) digitization of both anterosuperior iliac spines and the pubis near the tubercles (Fig. 75.1). The femoral baseplate was attached to the anterior lateral femur 8 cm cephalad from the superior pole of the patella and anterior to the anterior edge of the iliotibial band. The patient was then turned to the lateral position for the operation. The longitudinal axis of the patient was registered by using the posterior body supports - the Flip technique (Fig. 75.2). The pelvic tilt with the patient in the lateral position was calculated by computer software relative to the APP. The acetabular component position was displayed on the screen as adjusted inclination and anteversion, being adjusted for the pelvic tilt. This adjustment changed the inclination and anteversion from the anatomic plane to the radiographic plane as defined by Murray.[10] The longitudinal plane of the leg was registered from the two femoral condyles and ankle malleoli.

Posterior Approach

The incision is made over the posterior 1/3 of the trochanter, and extends proximally from the level of the vastus tubercle for 8–10 cm cephalad (Fig. 75.3). The first incision into hip tissue is done in the gluteus maximus muscle, which is incised

G.R. Scuderi and A.J. Tria (eds.), *Minimally Invasive Surgery in Orthopedics*,
DOI 10.1007/978-0-387-76608-9_75, © Springer Science+Business Media, LLC 2010

for 6–8 cm along the posterior border of the greater trochanter. The second is through the small external rotators and the posterior capsule with the leg in 90° of internal rotation. It is made as a single flap from just proximal to the quadratus femoris muscle through the piriformis tendon, including 1–2 cm of the gluteus minimus muscle, which lies under the piriformis tendon. Thereafter, the hip is dislocated and the corresponding templated neck is cut for restoration of leg length made (Fig. 75.4). The third incision is of the inferior medial capsule, which is incised from the anterior femur to the acetabulum through the transverse acetabular ligament.

Femoral Preparation

The preparation of the femur was performed first so that the anteversion of the femur was known prior to the preparation and implantation of the acetabulum. The femur is presented through the wound by the positioning of special long-handled retractors (Zimmer) as shown in Fig. 75.5. Femoral

Table 75.1 Demographics of 60 patients with 66 total hip replacements performed between July 2005 and March 2006

Patients (hips)	60 (66)
Age (years)	64 (33–89)
Sex (M/F)	40 (60%)/26 (40%)
Height (in.)	68.4 (54–78)
Weight (pounds)	186.1 (100–300)
Body mass index (BMI)	27.6 (17–40)

preparation was done by reaming and broaching. The intramedullary canal of the femur was registered by inserting the tool into the opened intramedullary canal and registering five points of the intramedullary canal into the software. The software could then determine the position of the implants in the femoral bone by calculating the intramedullary canal relative to the plane of the leg. The anteversion of the broach

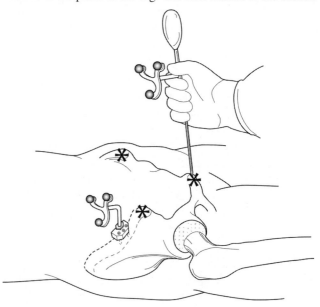

Fig. 75.1 The pelvic base antenna is pinned to the iliac crest. The two anterosuperior iliac spines and symphysis pubis are touched by the pointer guide. Percutaneous incisions are made to ensure that the guide obtains bony contact through the skin

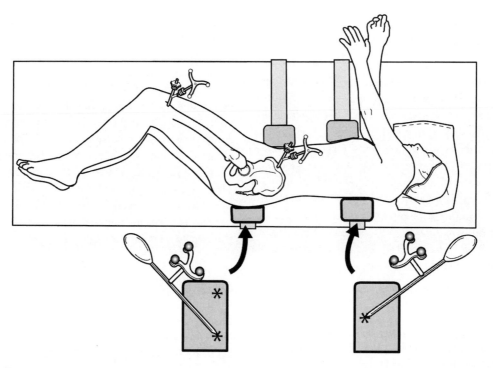

Fig. 75.2 In the flip technique, once the patient is changed to a lateral decubitus position, a triangle is formed using the posterior supports of the pelvis and chest to register the longitudinal axis of the body. Pelvic tilt in the lateral position relative to the longitudinal axis is also obtained

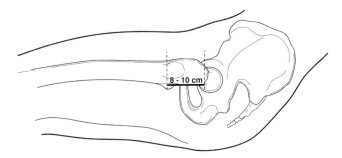

Fig. 75.3 Schematic representation of cut 1. The incision must be made along the posterior border of the greater trochanter. The average length of the incision is 8–10 cm

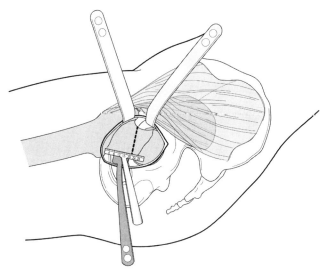

Fig. 75.4 The neck cut that has been templated preoperatively is validated for hip and leg length measurement. A ruler is used to measure the cut from the distal edge of the femoral head because the lesser trochanter is not visible because the quadratus is not incised

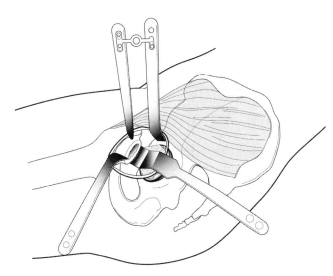

Fig. 75.5 Femoral exposure: the femur is presented through the wound posteriorly with the aid of the special long retractors. The anterior retractors separate the greater trochanter and the gluteus medius tendon. The posterior retractor inferiorly is placed retracting the quadratus muscle and the superior jaws retractor is under the anterior femoral neck

(and subsequently the stem) was computed as it was implanted into the bone (Fig. 75.6). Knowledge of the femoral anteversion permits customized placement of the cup to provide a combined anteversion of stem and cup of 35 ± 5°.[11] This technique of initially preparing the femur and determining femoral anteversion with subsequent cup implantation and positioning is a paradigm shift in the performance of the total hip replacement operation.

Acetabular Preparation

Once again, specialized long-handled retractors are placed to obtain correct exposure of the acetabulum (Fig. 75.7). Three registrations of the acetabulum are done prior to acetabular preparation: (1) center of rotation (COR) and diameter of the bony acetabulum; the acetabulum is digitized 16 times to obtain these values; (2) three to four points on the cortical bone on the cotyloid notch to digitize the medial wall; and (3) inclination and anteversion of the native acetabulum is registered by touching the periphery of the acetabular bone 6 times, which is displayed on the computer screen as both anatomic and adjusted values. The surgeon can control the depth of reaming in both the medial and superior directions while visualizing the change in the COR position on the computer screen. This is important because it allows the surgeon to obtain the correct depth that permits adequate coverage of the cup with an inclination between 35 and 45°; and it gives the surgeon the ability to keep the COR within 1 cm of the original native COR.

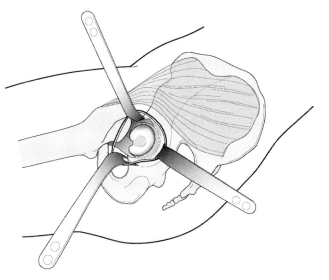

Fig. 75.6 Acetabular exposure: the snake retractor is placed anteriorly on the ilium through an incision made on the anterosuperior acetabulum and retracts the greater trochanter anteriorly. The anterior-superior acetabular wall is thus visualized. The number 7 inferior retractor is placed with its tip on the cotyloid notch and the paddle on the ischium. The number 4 retractor is placed posterosuperiorly and the whole acetabulum can be visualized

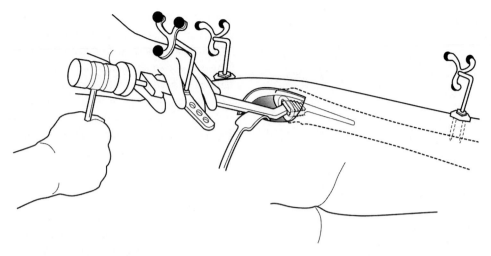

Fig. 75.7 The broach is inserted into the femur and the light-emitting diode (LED) on the broach handle allows the computer to recognize the broaches position in the intramedullary canal. The anteversion of the femur is thus obtained from this broach so that the combined anteversion can be obtained for acetabular cup placement

Table 75.2 Accuracy of computer navigation for acetabulum

	CT inclination	Navitrack inclination	CT anteversion	Navitrack anteversion
N hips	14	14	14	14
Mean value (°)	41.8 ± 4.6	41.2 ± 4.7	24.4 ± 6.3	22.8 ± 8.9
Precision (°)	3.6		4.4	
Mean of differences (bias) (°)	0.64		0.5	
Intraclass correlation coefficient	0.88		0.97	

N hips = the number of hips studied

Postoperative CT Scans

Postoperatively, 14 patients had a CT scan of their pelvis for comparison of the inclination and anteversion of the cup on the CT scan to that measured by computer navigation. The CT scan value was considered the true value and the accuracy of the computer navigation value was determined by comparison with this CT scan true value. We defined the absolute difference of values of more than 5° between the CT scan and the computer navigator to be an outlier.

The computed axial tomography scans were obtained in the Radiology department (MX8000, Phillips, Highland Heights, OH). The CT data was analyzed by the hip plan module of the CT-based Navitrack System (Navitrack Computed Tomography Based Hip Application, Orthosoft, Montreal, Canada). By means of this software, a virtual three-dimensional model of the patient's pelvis, as well as the implanted cup, were reconstructed using the CT data. The APP was used to establish an anatomic coordinate reference system. A virtual cup was positioned over the reconstructed cup to match its position and orientation. The software then calculated the resulting standardized computer radiographic anteversion and inclination values based on Murray's equations.[10]

Radiographic Measurements

Six-week postoperative anterior-posterior radiographs were taken with the patient supine and the beam centered over the symphysis pubis. These radiographs were measured using a digitized program with cup inclination by the method of Callaghan et al.,[12] and anteversion by a method previously described by us.[13] By our method, a correction factor of 4° was added to the anteversion measurement obtained on the AP pelvis radiograph. Precision of the radiographs was calculated by comparison of the radiographic measurements with the final cup position by computer navigation. Computer navigation was known to be accurate within 1° (Table 75.2), so the precision of the radiographs was a consequence of greater measurement errors associated with the radiographic technique.[14] We defined the absolute difference of values of more than 5° for inclination and/or anteversion between the computer navigator and postoperative X-rays to be an outlier.

Surgeon's Estimates

The computer navigation technique is valuable to the surgeon only if it is better than the surgeon in precision of cup placement. We measured the ability of both an experienced surgeon and surgeons in fellowship training to correctly judge the cup position of inclination and anteversion. The trial acetabular cup was placed into the acetabulum using the mechanical holder with a tracking guide and the computer screen was blinded to the surgeons. The cup holder was removed and the two surgeons estimated the position of the cup within the acetabular bone. These estimates were then compared with the adjusted numbers for inclination and anteversion displayed on the computer screen. The mean precision found for computer values allowed us to use it as the true value (Table 75.2). We defined the absolute difference of values of more than 5° for inclination and/or anteversion between the computer navigator and surgeons estimates to be an outlier. The percentage of outliers for inclination and anteversion were then determined.

Statistics

The statistical analysis was performed with SPSS software (SPSS Inc., Chicago, IL). The Kolmogorov-Smirnov test for normal distribution was used before further statistical analysis was conducted. For analysis of measurements, the means and standard deviations were calculated. One-way analysis of variance (ANOVA) was used to determine statistical difference in measurements between anteroposterior pelvic tilt. The repeatability between femoral anteversion of computer navigation and CT scan results was calculated using intraclass correlation coefficient by the reliability analysis. The bias and precision were calculated according to the American Society for Testing and Materials (ASTM) definitions. A p value of less than or equal to 0.05 was considered significant.

Results

The accuracy and precision of computer measurements for inclination and anteversion compared with postoperative CT scans were excellent and are shown in Table 75.2. We defined the absolute difference of values of more than 5° between the CT scan and the computer navigator to be an outlier, and found no outliers for inclination nor for anteversion with computer navigation.

The mean values of the surgeons' estimates and of postoperative X-rays for inclination and anteversion, are compared with those of computer navigation in Table 75.3. The

precision of the radiographic measurements and the surgeons' estimates for inclination and anteversion are listed in Table 75.4. There was a statistically significant difference between computer values and experienced doctors for anteversion ($p = 0.009$) and inexperienced doctors for inclination ($p = 0.007$) and anteversion ($p = 0.011$).

Experienced surgeons had 27% outliers for inclination and 35% for anteversion; less experienced surgeons had 49% outliers for inclination and 46% for anteversion. Experienced surgeons are more precise than less experienced surgeons for inclination ($p = 0.004$), but there is no statistical difference for anteversion ($p = 0.852$).

The precision measurements mean that a surgeon can be as much as 11–15° wrong in the position of inclination that he/she thinks the position of inclination or anteversion of the cup is in. Therefore, even though the surgeon has a mean inclination and anteversion very near that determined by the computer, the data shows that anywhere from 30 to 50% of the time the surgeon is wrong by 5° or more and can be wrong by as much as 15°.

Table 75.3 Computer, surgeon, and radiographic measurements: means and standard deviations

	Mean ± SD, in degrees (range)
Computer navigation-adjusted inclination	40.3 ± 3.8 (31–59)
Computer navigation-adjusted anteversion	25.9 ± 5.4 (3–39)
X-ray inclination	44.4 ± 4.9 (35–58)
X-ray anteversion	23.6 ± 5.2 (9–33)
Experienced surgeons inclination	40.6 ± 3.9 (33–50)
Experienced surgeons anteversion	23.2 ± 4.7 (14–35)
Less experienced surgeon's inclination	42.7 ± 5.1 (25–54)
Less experienced surgeon's anteversion	23.0 ± 5.7 (5–36)

Numbers are in degrees. Adjusted numbers are not adjusted for tilt. Radiographic measurements are included to compare with computer numbers

Table 75.4 Computer measurements compared with surgeon and radiographic measurements: precision and bias

	Precision (degrees)	Bias (degrees)	P value
X-ray inclination	9.1	3.9	0.000
X-ray anteversion	11.5	2.1	0.006
Experienced surgeon's inclination	11.4	0.4	0.56
Experienced surgeon's anteversion	12.3	2.1	0.009
Less experienced surgeon's inclination	14.6	2.6	0.007
Less experienced surgeon's anteversion	13.6	2.2	0.011

Precision is the reproducibility of results of surgeons and X-rays compared with the computer navigator

Bias is the error compared with the computer

Statistical significance is achieved when $P £ 0.05$

There was also a statistically significant difference between computer values and postoperative X-ray values for inclination (p = 0.000) and anteversion (p = 0.006). Radiographic outliers were 22 (33%) of 66 for inclination and 19 of (29%) 66 for anteversion. Our results for the X-rays compared with the computer show that they are wrong by more than 5° approximately 33% of the time for inclination and 29% for anteversion, with the most inaccurate reading of up to 20°.

Pelvic Tilt

The influence of tilt on inclination and anteversion is shown in Table 75.5, which has a comparison of the adjusted and unadjusted measurements. Unadjusted measurements are statistically related to pelvic tilt, whereas, when the anteversion is adjusted for tilt, the values are the same.

Discussion

Posterior single-incision MIS total hip replacement is a safe and effective operation that benefits patients.[7,8,15–18] Clinical data has demonstrated the favorable outcomes with the posterior MIS operation technique and show that it achieves the goal of better function early for patients.[7] The posterior MIS total hip replacement is a more difficult operation to perform than a traditional incision and requires specialized training and instruments. It can be easily learned by those surgeons who perform a traditional posterior approach by gradually reducing the length of the incision and using the instruments we have described[9] (as manufactured by Zimmer).

Until recently, the ability to reproducibly position a cup to any target numbers had depended greatly on a surgeon's experience and intuition. However, even the accuracy of experienced surgeons varies at different surgeries, and it is impossible to say that at every surgery the desired cup posi-

tion can be obtained.[1,2,4,5] Studies have shown that the use of mechanical guides based on the body axis for alignment are inferior to the computer with its knowledge of tilt and position of the acetabulum in space in relation to the APP.[2,5,15]

When associated with minimally invasive surgery, computer navigation can reduce errors in cup placement and help restore the COR, despite the decreased vision with smaller incisions. The ability of the surgeon to have real-time information of the components' position significantly increases the accuracy of implantation.[8,16] Our mean bias (system error) with the computer was within 1° of postoperative CT scans. The precision (reproducibility) of the computer values was always within 5° of the measured component position, whereas surgeons' precisions varied from 11 to 15° and resulted in outliers of cup position beyond 5° in 27–49% of cases for inclination and/or anteversion.

A second advantage of computer navigation is to customize the cup position rather than target it. By preparing the femur first and knowing the anteversion of the femoral component, the cup can be anteverted the correct degrees to provide a combined anteversion of 35 ± 5°. The inclination can be customized by controlling the depth of reaming to maintain the COR within 10 mm of the original bony acetabular COR and yet permit inclination to be 35–40° with correct coverage of the cup.

In this study, we learned that femoral component anteversion is not the 10–15° that laboratory studies have used (Table 75.6).[19] Indeed, up to 30% of the femoral stems in this

Table 75.6 Accuracy of computer navigation for femoral anteversion

Statistics	CT anteversion	Navitrack anteversion
N hips	9	9
Mean value (°)	9 ± 6.2	6.8 ± 4.5
t Test	P = 0.07	
Mean of differences (bias)	2.2	
95% CI of differences	−0.23 to 4.67	
Intraclass correlation coefficient	0.906	

N hips = the number of hips studied
95% CI is the confidence interval

Table 75.5 Influence of anterior-posterior pelvic tilt on inclination and anteversion

Computer measurement	Posterior tilt 10–20°	Posterior tilt 1–9°	Anterior tilt 0–9°	Anterior tilt 10–20°	P value
Computer inclination[a]	36.7 ± 1.4	38.7 ± 2.8	42.4 ± 5.5	45.0 ± 2.8	0.001
Computer-adjusted inclination	40.3 ± 1.6	40.0 ± 2.7	41.2 ± 5.5	40.0 ± 1.4	0.752
Computer anteversion[a]	18.5 ± 1.7	22.0 ± 5.6	27.8 ± 5.5	39.0 ± 4.2	0.000
Computed-adjusted anteversion	28.2 ± 2.1	25.5 ± 5.4	25.2 ± 6.1	31.0 ± 2.8	0.337

Numbers in degrees. The anteroposterior tilt of the pelvis is divided into four categories according to the number of degrees of tilt. The effect of adjustment by pelvic tilt is shown by the difference in unadjusted computer inclination and anteversion values compared with the similarity of adjusted inclination and adjusted anteversion values

[a] The number of degrees of anterior-posterior pelvic tilt is statistically related to these measurements

study were relatively retroverted. With noncemented components, the mean femoral anteversion was 7° and was greater by 4° in women than men, which confirmed the cadaver study of Maruyama et al.[20] Furthermore, the anteversion of the noncemented femoral component was fixed and therefore not a variable that the surgeon could control. This fact makes it important to customize the cup for each patient's anatomy. This paradigm shift permits the acetabular anteversion to be adapted in accordance with the femoral anteversion to provide a combined anteversion of approximately 35°. To customize the cup, rather than use target numbers, requires femoral preparation prior to acetabular preparation.

More than 25 years have passed since Lewinnek et al. described the safe zone for acetabular component positioning as 30–50° for inclination and 5–25° for anteversion.[21] We propose that the safe zone for inclination should be narrowed to 35–45° and for anteversion changed to 20–30° for patients operated in the posterior position. Surgeons who operate on patients with an anterior approach often state that a cup position of 10–15° anteversion is optimal.[22] However, we suspect that surgeons who operate with the anterior approach, and particularly with the patient in the supine position, visualize the cup position by the anatomic plane and not the radiographic plane. Surgeons who operate through the posterior approach with the patient in the lateral position visualize the cup more with the radiographic plane. This may account for differences in the numbers quoted by surgeons. If we take impingement or wear as endpoints, it does not seem reasonable that different numbers should be used for different surgical approaches.

The inclination of the cup should not exceed 45° to optimize the wear of the articulation surface.[23] The ideal inclination is a horizontal abduction of approximately 35°. The advantage of this position is optimum coverage of the femoral head when compared with a position of 45°, and a greater range of motion (ROM) with less impingement when compared with a position of 25°.[24,25] We found that the position of 35° can be obtained if the COR is reamed approximately 4–5 mm superior and at least 6 mm medial (on average). Our experience would suggest that an inclination of 35–40° is more important for minimizing wear than is maintenance of the COR within 5–10 mm of the original COR. Therefore, we are willing to move the COR as much as 10 mm from the original COR to allow adequate coverage of the cup and provide an inclination between 35 and 40°. In this group of patients, the mean superior displacement of the COR was 1.56 ± 3.3 mm and medialization was 5.19 ± 5.4 mm, which is well within accepted limits of reconstruction of the COR.[26]

Navigation is a great source of data for correlating component position with impingement, to thereby reduce its prevalence. We found that lateralized cup positions had a much higher prevalence of impingement of the metal neck on the metal shell. Cups with a mean 3.2 ± 3.5 mm of medialization had greater impingement ($p = 0.03$) vs. those cups medialized on average 5.8 ± 4.9 mm.

There is one technique that we have learned that is necessary in hips with a low anteversion of the femoral stem. When the hip is in maximum flexion and internal rotation, these hips can impinge against the ilium, and specifically the anterior-inferior iliac spine. In hips with low anteversion of the femoral stem, the anterior-superior capsule should be excised and a portion of the anterior-inferior spine should be removed. We remove this bone with a power burr. By clearing this anterior-superior iliac space, the femoral bone will not impinge against the ilium in the flexion internal rotation position. This is especially important if a small femoral head is used, such as a 28- or 32-mm head. With larger femoral heads, the radius is greater and this is less likely to occur, but it can still occur and we still clear this area even when we use a large femoral head. By using this technique, it also allows the avoidance of dislocation precautions for these patients because impingement has been prevented.

The benefit to patients of the avoidance of outliers and customization of the cup to femoral anatomy is better mating of the femoral head into the cup. The more medial (and the less vertical) the vector of load is into the cup, the lower the linear rate of wear will be. Secondly, the more horizontal the cup (35–40° instead of 45–50°), with a combined anteversion closer to 35°, the better the coverage of the femoral head is for promoting hip stability. When these positions can be achieved every time at surgery (and, with computer navigation, the surgeon can avoid all outliers) then the durability of the operation can be projected to have been optimized. When these component positions are combined with correct soft tissue balance (hip length and offset) and excellent head-neck ratios, dislocation will become rare.

Precision measurements confirmed prior observations that that radiographs are not as accurate as the computer. The imprecision of 10° is caused by variable flexion of the pelvis on the X-ray table, the rotation of radiographs, and the variations from the direction of the X-ray beams.[5,14,27] The most basic element that orthopedic surgeons have relied on for postoperative control of most orthopedic procedures, the X-ray, is not as reliable as we surgeons have thought, and the computer is superior to them.

Our results show that computer navigation affords a more precise (reproducible) acetabular component reconstruction, with less bias (error) than that offered by even the most experienced surgeons. We have seen from our CT scan study that the computer is a tool that surgeons can rely on during surgery. It has permitted us to explore new techniques such as customizing hip reconstructions to accommodate a patient's individual anatomy and reducing impingement by medialization. Outcomes of this more accurate hip reconstruction for decreased complication rates and requirements for revision are being observed by us in our patient population.

References

1. Nogler M, Kessler O, Prassl A, et al. Reduced variability of acetabular cup positioning with use of an imageless navigation system. Clin Orthop Relat Res2004 Sep;(426):159–163
2. Leenders T, Vandevelde D, Mahieu G, Nuyts R. Reduction in variability of acetabular cup abduction using computer assisted surgery: a prospective and randomized study. Comput Aided Surg 2002;7(2):99–106
3. Kalteis T, Handel M, Herold T, Perlick L, Baethis H, Grifka J. Greater accuracy in positioning of the acetabular cup by using an image-free navigation system. Int Orthop 2005;29(5):272–276
4. Jolles BM, Genoud P, Hoffmeyer P. Computer-assisted cup placement techniques in total hip arthroplasty improve accuracy of placement. Clin Orthop Relat Res 2004 Sep;(426):174–179
5. DiGioia AM, Jaramaz B, Blackwell M, et al. The Otto Aufranc Award. Image guided navigation system to measure intraoperatively acetabular implant alignment. Clin Orthop Relat Res 1998 Oct;(355):8–22
6. Dorr LD, Hishiki Y, Wan Z, Newton D, Yun A. Development of imageless computer navigation for acetabular component position in total hip replacement. Iowa Orthop J 2005;25:1–9
7. Inaba Y, Dorr LD, Wan Z, Sirianni L, Boutary M. Operative and patient care techniques for posterior mini-incision total hip arthroplasty. Clin Orthop Relat Res 2005 Dec;(441):104–114
8. Berry DJ, Berger RA, Callaghan JJ, et al. Minimally invasive total hip arthroplasty. Development, early results, and a critical analysis. Presented at the Annual Meeting of the American Orthopaedic Association, Charleston, South Carolina, USA, June 14, 2003. J Bone Joint Surg Am 2003;85-A(11):2235–2246
9. Dorr LD. *Hip Arthroplasty Minimally Invasive Techniques and Computer Navigation*. Saunders Elsevier, Philadelphia, PA; 2006
10. Murray DW. The definition and measurement of acetabular orientation. J Bone Joint Surg Br 1993;75(2):228–232
11. Widmer KH, Zurfluh B. Compliant positioning of total hip components for optimal range of motion. J Orthop Res 2004;22(4):815–821
12. Callaghan JJ, Salvati EA, Pellicci PM, Wilson PD Jr, Ranawat CS. Results of revision for mechanical failure after cemented total hip replacement, 1979 to 1982. A two to five-year follow-up. J Bone Joint Surg Am 1985;67(7):1074–1085
13. Wan Z, Dorr LD. Natural history of femoral focal osteolysis with proximal ingrowth smooth stem implant. J Arthroplasty 1996; 11(6):718–725
14. Tannast M, Langlotz U, Siebenrock KA, Wiese M, Bernsmann K, Langlotz F. Anatomic referencing of cup orientation in total hip arthroplasty. Clin Orthop Relat Res 2005 Jul;(436): 144–150
15. Wixson RL, MacDonald MA. Total hip arthroplasty through a minimal posterior approach using imageless computer-assisted hip navigation. J Arthroplasty 2005;20(7 Suppl 3):51–56
16. Ogonda L, Wilson R, Archbold P, et al. A minimal-incision technique in total hip arthroplasty does not improve early postoperative outcomes. A prospective, randomized, controlled trial. J Bone Joint Surg Am 2005;87(4):701–710
17. Chimento GF, Pavone V, Sharrock N, Kahn B, Cahill J, Sculco TP. Minimally invasive total hip arthroplasty: a prospective randomized study. J Arthroplasty 2005;20(2):139–144
18. Berger RA, Duwelius PJ. The two-incision minimally invasive total hip arthroplasty: technique and results. Orthop Clin North Am 2004;35(2):163–172
19. Barrack RL, Lavernia C, Ries M, Thornberry R, Tozakoglou E. Virtual reality computer animation of the effect of component position and design on stability after total hip arthroplasty. Orthop Clin North Am 2001;32(4):569–577, vii
20. Maruyama M, Feinberg JR, Capello WN, D'Antonio JA. The Frank Stinchfield Award: morphologic features of the acetabulum and femur: anteversion angle and implant positioning. Clin Orthop Relat Res 2001 Dec;(393):52–65
21. Lewinnek GE, Lewis JL, Tarr R, Compere CL, Zimmerman JR. Dislocations after total hip-replacement arthroplasties. J Bone Joint Surg Am 1978;60(2):217–220
22. Siguier T, Siguier M, Brumpt B. Mini-incision anterior approach does not increase dislocation rate: a study of 1037 total hip replacements. Clin Orthop Relat Res 2004 Sep;(426):164–173
23. Kennedy JG, Rogers WB, Soffe KE, Sullivan RJ, Griffen DG, Sheehan LJ. Effect of acetabular component orientation on recurrent dislocation, pelvic osteolysis, polyethylene wear, and component migration. J Arthroplasty 1998;13(5):530–534
24. D'Lima DD, Urquhart AG, Buehler KO, Walker RH, Colwell CW Jr. The effect of the orientation of the acetabular and femoral components on the range of motion of the hip at different head-neck ratios. J Bone Joint Surg Am 2000;82(3):315–321
25. Robinson RP, Simonian PT, Gradisar IM, Ching RP. Joint motion and surface contact area related to component position in total hip arthroplasty. J Bone Joint Surg Br 1997;79(1):140–146
26. Karachalios T, Hartofilakidis G, Zacharakis N, Tsekoura M. A 12- to 18-year radiographic follow-up study of Charnley low-friction arthroplasty. The role of the center of rotation. Clin Orthop Relat Res 1993 Nov;(296):140–147
27. Amiot LP, Poulin F. Computed tomography-based navigation for hip, knee, and spine surgery. Clin Orthop Relat Res 2004 Apr;(421): 77–86

Chapter 76
Minimally Invasive Total Knee Arthroplasty with Image-Free Navigation

S. David Stulberg

Computer-assisted surgery (CAS) is beginning to emerge as one of the most important technologies in orthopedic surgery. Many of the initial applications of this technology have focused on adult reconstructive surgery of the knee. The value of CAS in total knee arthroplasty (TKA) has been established in many studies. Minimally invasive surgical (MIS) techniques for performing TKA are also receiving extensive and intensive attention. The goals of this chapter are to (1) present the rationale for the use of image-free CAS in knee surgery, (2) explain the rationale for combining CAS with MIS techniques, (3) describe the basic components of an image-free navigation system, (4) illustrate a typical CAS MIS technique, and (5) present the initial results using this technique.

Rationale for the Use of Computer-Assisted Surgery in Knee Reconstruction

A successful surgical reconstruction of the knee requires proper patient selection, appropriate perioperative management, correct implant selection, and accurate surgical technique. The consequences of performing a knee reconstruction inaccurately have been well documented for total knee arthroplasties, unicondylar arthroplasties, anterior cruciate ligament reconstructions, and high tibial osteotomies.[1-35]

Although mechanical instrumentation has significantly increased the accuracy and reliability with which knee reconstructions are performed,[36] errors in implant and limb alignment continue to occur, even when the procedures are performed by experienced surgeons. The accuracy with which these procedures are performed using manual instrumentation is dependent on the knowledge and experience of the surgeon and the frequency with which the surgeon performs the procedures.

Computer-assisted surgical techniques have been developed to address the inherent limitations of mechanical instrumentation.[37-72] The goals of integrating CAS with knee reconstruction techniques are to increase the accuracy of these procedures and reduce the proportion of alignment outliers that occur when these procedures are performed.

Errors in the alignment of bone resection can occur at numerous points during the performance of a knee reconstruction.[73, 74] The placement of the cutting blocks or ligament alignment jigs may be inaccurate. The attachment of these tools to bone may produce an error in their placement. The actual performance of the cut or drilling of the hole may be inaccurate (e.g., the saw blade may deflect). The final insertion of the implant may be inaccurate. Mechanical instrumentation does not provide a method for checking the accuracy of each of these steps of a knee reconstructive procedure. Integrating CAS with knee reconstruction allows the surgeon a means of placing cutting blocks accurately and measuring the accuracy with which each step of the procedure is performed. During the performance of an MIS TKA, visualization of each step of the procedure is difficult. Therefore, the ability to measure each step of the TKA procedure using CAS may be particularly important for MIS TKA.[73-75]

The goal of knee reconstructive procedures is to align limbs and implants correctly. Restoration of appropriate kinematic relationships and ligamentous stability to the knee is also sought.[76-78] Mechanical instrumentation cannot measure the precision with which knee kinematics and ligament stability is restored. CAS techniques make it possible to determine the presurgical kinematic relationships and ligamentous stability of the knee and help guide the surgeon to restore the desired kinematic relationships and ligamentous balance.

Rationale for Combining MIS and CAS TKA Techniques

The rationale for an MIS TKA is that an accurate and properly executed TKA can be carried out safely using a surgical technique that may decrease the morbidity, accelerate the recovery, and improve the outcome of the surgical procedure.

S.D. Stulberg (✉)
Department of Orthopaedic Surgery, Feinberg School of Medicine, Northwestern University, Chicago, IL, USA
e-mail: Jointsurg@northwestern.edu

G.R. Scuderi and A.J. Tria (eds.), *Minimally Invasive Surgery in Orthopedics*,
DOI 10.1007/978-0-387-76608-9_76, © Springer Science+Business Media, LLC 2010

MIS TKA exposures provide reduced visualization of critical surgical anatomy. This has led to the development of a number of modifications in the usual TKA procedure. The concept of a "mobile window" (visualization of a portion of the entire surgical field at any given time) has been described. Special retractors to enhance visualization have been developed. Instruments that are unique to less invasive surgery have been designed. A variety of exposures of the knee joint, including the subvastus, mid-vastus, and tri-vector, have been described in an attempt to optimize the goals of MIS TKA. In addition, the need for "assistants' choreography" (precise, atraumatic exposure by experienced personnel) has been emphasized.

The consequences of the reduced visualization associated with minimally invasive total knee exposures include: (1) implant malposition; (2) fracture of the femur, tibia, or patella; (3) neurovascular injuries; (4) compromised wound healing; and (5) prolonged operative time.

Computer-assisted techniques were developed to overcome the inherent limitations of manual instrumentation. The initial reports of performing TKAs with computer-assisted techniques using conventional, extensile surgical exposures indicate that increased accuracy of limb and implant alignment and reduced incidence of alignment outliers occurs.[38, 67, 68, 77, 79–105] Therefore, the rationale for combining computer-assisted and MIS techniques is that the reduction in perioperative morbidity and the improvement in early postoperative function that are achieved with less invasive exposures can be realized while retaining the accuracy of implant and limb alignment that can be achieved with computer techniques, even when crucial surgical anatomic landmarks are not visible.

The introduction of less invasive total knee surgical techniques has required the development of instruments and cutting guides that are compatible with smaller incisions and less extensile exposures. If computer-assisted techniques are to be applied to less invasive total knee procedures, the hardware, software, and navigation instruments must also be reconfigured for these reduced exposures. As the computer technologies are adapted to less invasive knee procedures, it is essential that they are: (1) safe; (2) accurate; (3) efficient; (4) cost effective; and (5) compatible with less invasive surgical sequences and tools. It is critical that the accuracy and safety associated with the use of computer-assisted technologies for total knee replacements performed using conventional exposures be retained when this technology is applied to less invasive knee replacement exposures. The accurate registration of critical anatomic landmarks must not be compromised when small incisions are used. Trackers and miniaturized navigated cutting blocks must remain securely fixed to bone during the performance of the less invasive procedures.

Hardware and Software Requirements for Surgical Navigation

A detailed description of the hardware and software needed to perform computer-assisted reconstructive knee surgery is beyond the scope of this chapter. However, it is important that knee surgeons understand the basic components of a computer-assisted orthopedic system so that they can use the system correctly, safely, and efficiently, and so that they can make intelligent choices regarding the appropriateness of various systems for their surgical needs.

The hardware devices common to CAS systems are: (1) imaging devices; (2) computers and the peripherals and interfaces to allow them to function in the operating room; and (3) localizers and trackers (Fig. 76.1a, b).

The imaging devices that are currently available for use with computer-assisted orthopedic surgery systems include computed tomography (CT), magnetic resonance imaging (MRI), and fluoroscopy.[42, 58, 62, 64, 79, 93–95, 106, 107] These devices are used to acquire anatomical information on which a presurgical or intraoperative surgical plan is made. This plan becomes the basis for placing cutting tools intraoperatively and for establishing the alignment and stability of the knee. Although potentially extremely useful for knee reconstruction surgery, especially for robotic or customized surgery, imaging devices as currently employed with CAS knee systems have been perceived by surgeons as requiring additional and cumbersome steps to well-established knee procedures without providing significant benefits. Consequently, image-free computer-assisted systems have emerged as the most desired form of CAS for knee reconstruction.

A CAS knee navigation system can be thought of as an aiming device that enables real-time visualization of surgical action with an image of the operated structures. In order for this navigation to occur, it is necessary that the position and orientation of an instrument be visualized with respect to the anatomical structures to which it is attached. Therefore, contactless systems are used to communicate between the extremity and the computer system. Information can be transmitted using infrared light, electromagnetic fields, or ultrasound. Each method has its advantages and drawbacks. All of these methods allow several objects (e.g., two bones) to be viewed simultaneously.

The function of software in CAS systems is to integrate medical images and mathematical algorithms with surgical tools and surgical techniques.[41, 42, 44] A relatively small number of software components underlie most CAS image-free systems. These components include registration, navigation, procedure guidance, and safety.

Image-free CAS knee systems use as their preoperative plan concepts of limb and implant alignment that are currently used

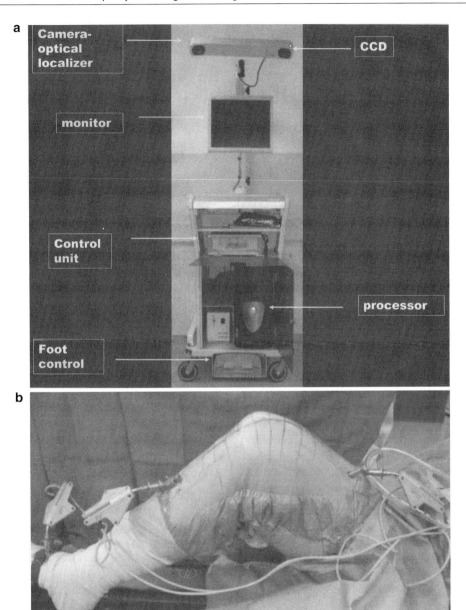

Fig. 76.1 (**a**) A typical image-free computer-assisted hardware system consisting of an optical tracker with charge-coupled devices (CCDs; the "cameras"), a computer monitor, control unit and processor, and a foot control system for communication between surgeon and the system. (**b**) Active trackers (also called rigid bodies or fiducials) attached to bicortical screws rigidly fixed to the femur and tibia

with manual instrumentation (e.g., restoration of the mechanical axis). In order to accomplish this plan, anatomic and kinematic information about a patient must be transmitted to the software on the computer and geometrically transformed using registration algorithms. Because bones are rigid and assumed unlikely to deform during the procedure, the algorithms used are termed *rigid*. These algorithms also require that the trackers attached to bones do not move during the procedure. Fiducial-based registration is a type of rigid registration. Therefore, the objects to which the LEDs are attached may be referred to as fiducials, trackers, or rigid bodies. Fiducial registration requires that at least three sets of markers be implanted into each bone or

attached to each tool to determine the object's position and orientation. Therefore, each tracker must have at least three LEDs or reflecting spheres. Some CAS knee systems currently use shaped-based registration as an alternative to fiducial-based registration. These systems measure the shape of the bone surface intraoperatively and match the acquired shape to a surface model created from medical images and stored in the computer. The registration process for image-free knee navigation systems requires that information be acquired using kinematic techniques (e.g., circumducting the leg to determine the center of the femoral head) and/or surface registration techniques (e.g., touching bone landmarks with a probe).

Once the software takes anatomic and kinematic input from the extremity and geometrically transforms it, the surgeon is presented with a user interface that depicts, in sequence, the steps of the knee procedure. One of the most important objectives of software development in CAS knee surgery is to depict procedure sequences that are familiar to surgeons and with which they have become comfortable using manual instrumentation.

Example of an Image-Free, Minimally Invasive CAS Surgical Technique for TKA

Computer-assisted surgical technologies require that surgeons incorporate new tools into surgical routines with which they are experienced and comfortable. In fact, the most successful application of CAS occurs when surgeons are very familiar with all aspects of the procedure in which CAS is used. Although the details of the CAS application for one knee procedure (e.g., TKA) vary from those of another knee procedure (e.g., anterior cruciate ligament [ACL] reconstruction), the basic principles and intraoperative steps are very similar for all of them. The TKA image-free navigation application is currently the most rapidly developing and most widely used CAS knee reconstruction technique. A brief description of a typical CAS MIS TKA will be described.[69, 70, 107, 108]

Image-free CAS techniques do not require any special preoperative planning. The methods surgeons normally use to determine desired frontal and sagittal limb and implant alignment and implant sizes can be used to guide the intraoperative use of the CAS system. Mechanical alignment and CAS techniques use similar approaches for patient positioning and surgical exposure. Leg holders and pneumatic tourniquets that are routinely used with mechanical instrumentation can also be used with CAS.

The initial step in a TKA using CAS is the placement of the screws or pins in the distal femur and proximal tibia to which are attached the trackers (Fig. 76.1b). These are placed outside of the skin incision in a position that avoids injury to neurovascular structures and allows clear visualization of the trackers by the camera. Once the skin incision is made and the distal femur and proximal tibia are exposed, the anatomic landmarks critical for CAS-guided navigation are located. The center of the femoral head is determined using a kinematic registration technique (Fig. 76.2a, b). The hip is circumducted in a path guided by the visual cues displayed on the computer screen. The centers of the knee and ankle joint can be established using kinematic (Fig. 76.2c–f) or surface (Fig. 76.3a–i) registration techniques or a combination of both. The other anatomic landmarks located with a CAS probe are: (1) the distal femur (Fig. 76.3d, e); (2) the posterior condylar line (Fig. 76.3d, e); (3) the anterior femoral

cortex (Fig. 76.3f); (4) the epicondylar axis; and (5) the medial and lateral tibial articular surfaces (Fig. 76.3g–i). The presurgical frontal and sagittal alignment, medial-lateral laxity in flexion and extension, and range of motion can then be measured and recorded (Fig. 76.4).

Both ligament balancing techniques (similar to those first described by Insall[13]) and anatomic approaches[12] can be used with CAS MIS TKA techniques. As with mechanically based techniques, the CAS anatomic procedures can begin with either the femoral or tibial preparation. In the example illustrated, the anatomic approach is used and the distal femur is resected first. A distal femoral cutting block with an attached tracker is placed on the anterior cortex of the femur. The proximal-distal, varus-valgus, and flexion-extension position of this block are guided by the CAS system (Fig. 76.5a, b). The CAS determination of femoral implant size and anterior-posterior placement can be made using either anterior or posterior referencing techniques. The rotation of the femoral component using CAS can be established using the posterior condylar line, the epicondylar line, or the patellar groove (Whitesides' line). A single navigation tool can be used to establish all of these femoral alignment and sizing objectives (Fig. 76.6a, b). The tibial cutting block, to which a tracker is attached, is placed in the desired position of varus-valgus and flexion-extension and at the desired resection level guided by the CAS system (Fig. 76.7a, b).

Once the femoral and tibial resections are completed, a trial reduction is carried out. The polyethylene insert that best balances the knee in flexion and extension is selected. The navigation system is used to measure the final alignment of the extremity, the amount of medial-lateral laxity in extension and flexion, and the final range of motion. The system can be used to guide the release of tight soft tissues medially, laterally, and posteriorly if this is necessary to establish a balanced, well-aligned knee. After the actual implants are inserted, the navigation system is used to measure the final frontal and sagittal alignment of the extremity, the final medial-lateral stability, and the final range of motion (Fig. 76.8).

Clinical Results of CAS MIS for Total Knee Arthroplasty

A prospective study was carried out to compare the effectiveness of CAS MIS TKA with manually performed MIS TKA.

Methods

Seventy-eight consecutive MIS TKA were performed by a single surgeon with extensive prior experience in both manual and CAS MIS TKA. Of the 78 TKA, 40 were performed

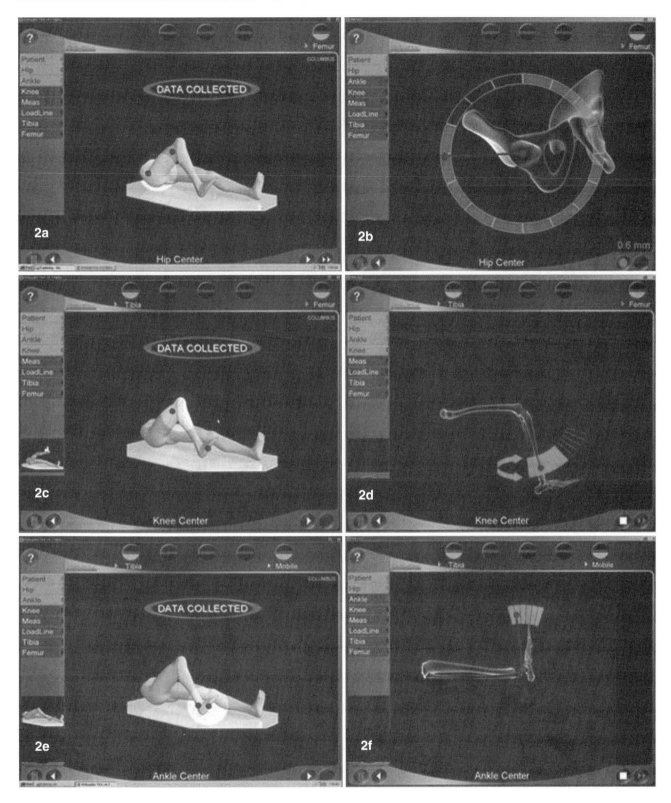

Fig. 76.2 Computer interfaces illustrating motion necessary to acquire adequate kinematic information to establish location of center of the (**a**, **b**) hip joint; (**c**, **d**) knee joint; and (**f**, **g**) ankle joint

with MIS manual instruments and 38 with CAS MIS instruments. The groups were identical with regard to age, sex, body mass index (BMI), diagnosis, surgical technique, implants, and perioperative management. Preoperative and postoperative clinical examinations at 4 weeks, 6 months, and 1 year were performed by a physician blinded to the surgical techniques.

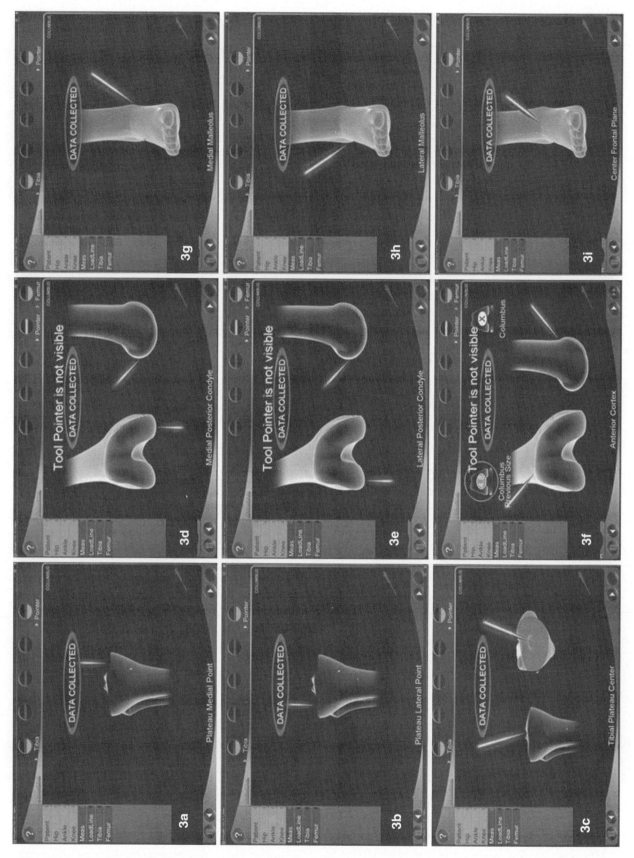

Fig. 76.3 Computer interfaces illustrating the position of the surface registration pointer necessary to acquire: (**a–c**) tibial medial and lateral articular surfaces and tibial mid-point; (**d–e**) the location of distal femoral articular surfaces and posterior condylar line; (**f**) the location of anterior femoral cortex; and (**g–i**) the location of center of ankle joint

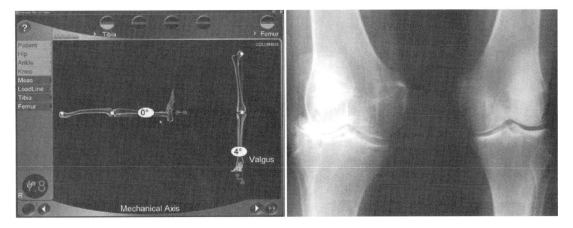

Fig. 76.4 Presurgical alignment depicted on the computer screen correlates with the alignment seen on the standing preoperative X-ray

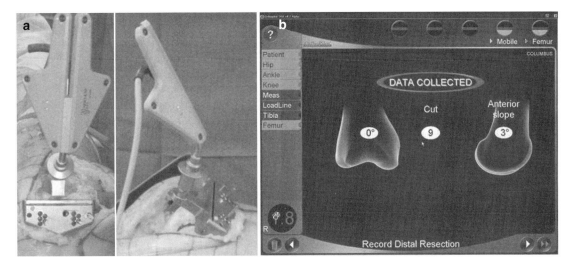

Fig. 76.5 Resection of a distal femur. (**a**) Frontal and sagittal position of a distal femoral cutting block with attached tracker. (**b**) Computer interface indicating the position of the distal femoral cutting block with regard to the frontal (0°) and sagittal (3° anterior slope) mechanical alignment and depth of resection (9 mm)

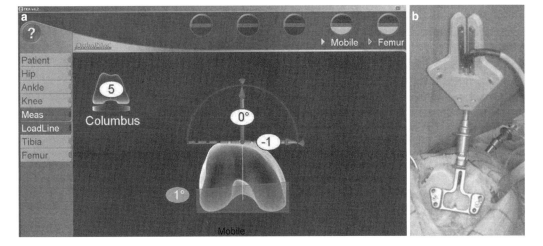

Fig. 76.6 Establishing position of four in one femoral cutting block. (**a**) Computer interface indicating rotation (0° relative to Whitesides' line) of the cutting block and anterior-posterior position of (in this case, the number 5) femoral component (1 mm above anterior cortex). (**b**) Navigation tool with attached tracker to establish rotation and anterior-posterior position of four in one femoral cutting block

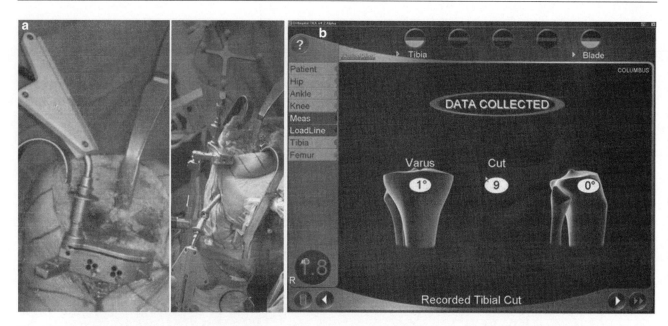

Fig. 76.7 Resection of a proximal tibia. (**a**) Frontal and sagittal position of a proximal tibial cutting block with attached tracker. (**b**) Computer interface indicating the position of the proximal tibial cutting block with regard to frontal (1° varus) and sagittal (0°) mechanical alignment and depth of resection from the least-involved tibial surface (9 mm)

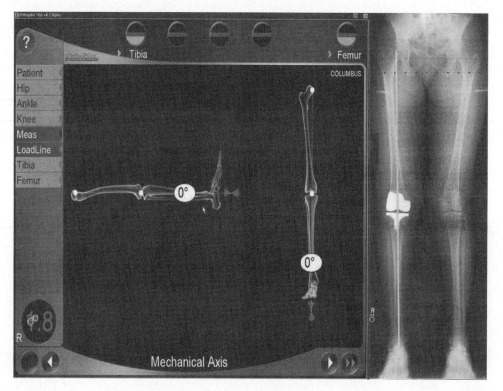

Fig. 76.8 Final frontal and sagittal alignment depicted on the computer screen correlates with the postoperative standing long X-ray

Preoperative and postoperative radiographic measurements of the anterior-posterior mechanical axis and the sagittal tibial and femoral axes were evaluated by an observer blinded to the surgical technique. The Knee Society scoring system was used to assess clinical and functional outcomes relating to measures of range of motion, pain, knee stability, patient mobility, and movement independence (Table 76.1). Aesculap's Columbus cruciate-retaining, condylar implants

Table 76.1 Demographic data

	Unilateral manual	Unilateral CAS	Total
Number of patients	40	38	78
Age, in years (range)	64.0 (25.1–87.5)	65.7 (48.0–86.1)	64.8 (25.1–87.5)
Sex (% male)	43%	37%	40%
Diagnosis (% osteoarthritis)	100	100	100
BMI average (range)	31.5 (19.6–54.8)	33.9 (23.9–44.2)	32.7 (19.6–54.8)
Preoperative mechanical axis alignment (range); varus (+); valgus (−)	5.2 (−27 to 22)	8.9 (−12 to 20)	6.8 (−27 to 22)
Preoperative knee score (range)	48.1 (17–77)	44.5 (22–79)	46.3 (17–79)
Preoperative function score (range)	56.7 (35–80)	50.4 (30–80)	53.6 (30–80)
Preoperative range of motion (range)	113.7 (70–140)	112.1 (70–140)	112.9 (70–140)
Preoperative pain calculation (range)	12.8 (0–30)	12.0 (0–45)	12.4 (0–45)

were used in each patient. The Aesculap's OrthoPilot image-free navigation system was used for computer-assisted TKA. The study was approved by the Institutional Review Board of Northwestern University. The accuracy of the MIS manual instruments used by the surgeon at the beginning of his CAS experience has been previously reported.[69]

Results

Clinical and functional scores were not significantly different between MIS CAS TKA and manual MIS TKA patients at 1 and 6 months postoperatively (Table 76.2). The average change in clinical and functional scores from preoperative to 1 and 6 months postoperative was also similar. Pain calculations were slightly higher (less pain) for CAS patients at 1 month postoperatively; however, no difference was noted at 6 months. Range of motion was not significantly different at 1 and 6 months postoperatively. The number of units of blood transfused was slightly greater for CAS patients and tourniquet time was on average, 27 min longer for CAS compared with manual TKA (Table 76.2). Mechanical axis, sagittal femoral axis, and sagittal tibial axis radiographic results were not significantly different (Table 76.3).

Discussion

Unlike the senior author's initial experience working with CAS,[71, 103] this study found no statistically significant radiographic alignment differences between TKAs performed using CAS and manual techniques. This suggests either that external factors such as advancements in implants and mechanical alignment systems have resulted in manual TKA being performed more accurately, or that an improvement in the manual TKA technique has been realized through more than 4 years of extensive CAS utilization by the senior author. The MIS manual instruments used in this study were developed from alignment information obtained using image-free navigation techniques.[37, 69, 73] Although modifications in manual instrumentation can improve the accuracy with which MIS TKA can be performed, there are still have inherent limitations in the ability of this instrumentation to accurately determine the location of crucial alignment landmarks.[37, 45] Moreover, intraoperative measurements of the accuracy with which each step of a MIS TKA is performed can not be made with manual instrumentation. Many studies have demonstrated superior radiographic alignment outcomes with CAS as compared with manual TKA. Therefore, the changes in the MIS mechanical alignment system do not seem sufficient to explain the equivalent alignment results obtained in this study.

This study suggests that it is also the intraoperative feedback and training effects realized through extensive use of a navigation system that has enabled the radiographic measures of manual MIS TKA to parallel those of CAS MIS TKA. It is possible for refinements in alignment perception, improvements in intraoperative judgment, and advances in technique to evolve to the point that no significant differences in radiographic alignment are apparent between CAS and manual TKA.

Clinical and patient-perceived functional results were not significantly different for CAS and manual TKA in this study. Outcome measures such as one's level of pain, range of motion, knee stability, mobility, and movement independence, which are measures of greatest importance to the TKA patient, were not significantly different in early follow-up. Thus, even if standard radiographs are not sensitive enough to detect subtle differences in alignment, these differences are not significant enough to influence short-term clinical and functional results. It is important to note the limitations of this study in terms of its duration. The long-term success of TKA is highly dependent on proper limb and implant alignment, thus, it is possible that alignment differences that were too minor to be exposed via standard radiograph in the short-term may become more readily apparent in long-term patient follow-up.

Table 76.2 Selected variable results

	Unilateral manual			Unilateral CAS			Total		
	Average	Range	SD	Average	Range	SD	Average	Range	SD
Knee score[a] (preoperative)	48.1	(17, 77)	15.0	44.6	(22, 79)	13.7	46.3	(17, 79)	14.4
Knee score (1 month postoperative)	69.1	(40, 100)	14.3	75.4	(45, 98)	13.5	72.2	(40, 100)	14.1
Knee score (6 months postoperative)	84.6	(23, 100)	18.3	83.4	(32, 100)	18.5	84.0	(23, 100)	18.2
Function score[a] (preoperative)	56.7	(35, 80)	17.8	50.4	(30, 80)	12.2	53.6	(30, 80)	12.6
Function score (1 month postoperative)	48.9	(20, 100)	17.8	50.3	(20, 90)	14.9	49.6	(20, 100)	16.3
Function score (6 months postoperative)	62.0	(45, 90)	15.7	64.0	(30, 100)	19.4	62.9	(30, 100)	20.0
ROM (preoperative)	113.7	(70, 140)	15.7	112.1	(70, 140)	15.0	112.9	(70, 140)	15.3
ROM (1 month postoperative)	103.2	(65, 135)	13.5	105.1	(80, 125)	10.2	104.1	(65, 135)	11.9
ROM (6 months postoperative)	116.0	(100, 135)	8.7	117.0	(105, 135)	8.1	116.4	(100, 135)	8.4
Pain calculation[b] (preoperative)	12.8	(0, 30)	9.1	12.0	(0, 45)	9.7	12.4	(0, 45)	9.3
Pain calculation (1 month postoperative)	25.6	(10, 50)	12.5	29.3	(0, 50)	12.9	27.4	(0, 50)	12.8
Pain calculation (6 months postoperative)	39.5	(20, 50)	10.7	36.5	(0, 50)	15.6	38.1	(0, 50)	13.1
Units of blood transfused	0.4	(0, 4)	0.76	0.6	(0, 3)	0.82	0.48	(0, 4)	1.1
Tourniquet time (min)	72.9	(47, 110)	13.7	99.6	(60, 131)	16.3	85.1	(47, 147)	19.3
Mechanical axis (postoperative X-ray): Varus (+); Valgus (−)	−0.24	(−6, 8)	3.5	2.1	(−3, 7)	2.7	0.80	(−6, 8)	3.1
Femoral angle (postoperative)	2.6	(−6, 9)	3.2	2.2	(−2, 7)	2.2	2.5	(−6, 9)	2.6
Tibial angle (postoperative)	88.1	(83, 91)	1.7	88.0	(83, 92)	1.9	88.0	(83, 92)	1.8

[a]Best assessment = 100

[b]Maximum pain = 0; no pain = 50

SD, standard deviation; ROM, range of motion

Table 76.3 Variable change between preoperative, and 1- and 6-month follow-up

	Unilateral manual			Unilateral CAS			Total		
	Average	Range	SD	Average	Range	SD	Average	Range	SD
Knee score change; preoperative -1 month postoperative	20.9	(−18, 64)	21.3	30.8	(−15, 71)	20.6	25.8	(−18, 71)	21.4
Knee score change; preoperative - 6 months postoperative	36.7	(−26, 76)	26.0	36.9	(−6, 73)	25.7	36.8	(−26, 76)	25.5
Function score change; preoperative - 1 month postoperative	−4.4	(−40, 65)	21.0	−2.0	(−35, 55)	22.3	−3.2	(−40, 65)	21.4
Function score change; preoperative - 6 months postoperative	4.6	(−20, 35)	14.5	12.7	(−20, 30)	13.5	8.7	(−20, 35)	14.3
Range of motion change; preoperative - 1 month postoperative	−10.5	(−57, 38)	16.7	−4.7	(−48, 100)	24.4	−7.7	(−57, 100)	20.8
Range of motion change; preoperative - 6 months postoperative	3.3	(−15, 30)	11.6	8.1	(−87, 100)	36.1	5.5	(−87, 100)	25.7
Pain calculation change; preoperative - 1 month postoperative	12.8	(−20, 45)	13.7	17.4	(−25, 45)	15.2	15.1	(−25, 45)	14.6
Pain calculation change; preoperative - 6 months postoperative	25.5	(0, 50)	15.2	21.5	(−10, 50)	17.9	23.6	(−10, 50)	16.4

Summary

The widespread interest in minimally invasive arthroplasty surgery is focusing surgeons' attention on the importance of retaining accurate implant and limb alignment as exposure of surgical anatomy is reduced.[75] Techniques using nonfrontal resection planes (e.g., the "quadrant sparing" medial approach) are making clear how the position of an implant in one plane critically affects its position in all other planes.[74] CAS systems have the potential for greatly facilitating the evolution of MIS knee surgery. However, the CAS hardware and software must be configured to support safely, accurately, and efficiently the MIS systems that are being developed.

References

1. Aglietti P, Buzzi R. Posteriorly stabilized total-condylar knee replacement. J Bone Joint Surg 1988; 70-B(2): 211–216
2. Ayers DC, Dennis DA, Johanson NA, et al. Common complications of total knee arthroplasty. J Bone J Surg 1997; 2(79A): 278–311
3. Bargren JH, Blaha JD, Freeman MAR. Alignment in total knee arthroplasty: correlated biomechanical and clinical observations. Clin Orthop Relat Res 1983 Mar;(173): 178–183
4. Berger RA, Crosset LS, Jacobs JJ. Malrotation causing patellofemoral complications after total knee arthroplasty. Clin Orthop Relat Res 1998 Nov;(356): 144–153
5. Cartier P, Sanouillier JL, Frelsamer RP. Unicompartmental knee arthroplasty surgery. 10-year minimum follow-up period. J Arthroplasty 1996; 11: 782–788
6. Dorr LD, Boiardo RA. Technical considerations in total knee arthroplasty. Clin Orthop Relat Res 1986 Apr;(205): 5–11
7. Ecker ML, Lotke PA, Windsor RE, et al. Long-term results after total condylar knee arthroplasty. Significance of radiolucent lines. Clin Orthop Relat Res 1987 Mar;(216): 151–158
8. Fehring TK, Odum S, Griffin WL, Mason JB, Naduad M. Early failures in total knee arthroplasty. Clin Orthop Relat Res 2001 Nov;(392): 315–318
9. Feng EL, Stulberg SD, Wixson RL. Progressive subluxation and polyethylene wear in total knee replacements with flat articular surfaces. Clin Orthop Relat Res 1994 Feb;(299): 60–71
10. Goodfellow JW, O'Connor JJ. Clinical results of the Oxford knee. Clin Orthop Relat Res 1986 Apr;(205): 21–24
11. Hsu HP, Garg A, Walker PS, Spector M, Ewald FC. Effect on knee component alignment on tibial load distribution with clinical correlation. Clin Orthop Relat Res 1989 Nov;(248): 135–144
12. Insall JW. Surgical approaches to the knee. In Insall JN (ed), *Surgery of the Knee*, Churchill Livingston, New York, 1984, pp. 41–54
13. Insall JN, Binzzir R, Soudry M, Mestriner LA. Total knee arthroplasty. Clin Orthop Relat Res 1985 Jan-Feb;(192): 13–22
14. Insall JN, Ranawat CS, Aglietti P, Shine J. A comparison of four models of total knee-replacement prosthesis. J Bone Joint Surg 1976; 58A: 754–765
15. Jeffcote B, Shakespeare D. Varus/valgus alignment of the tibial component in total knee arthroplasty. Knee 2003; 10(3): 243–247
16. Jeffery RS, Morris RW, Denham RA. Coronal alignment after total knee replacement. J Bone Joint Surg 1991; 73B: 709–714
17. Jiang CC, Insall JN. Effect of rotation on the axial alignment of the femur. Clin Orthop Relat Res 1989 Nov;(248): 50–56
18. Laskin RS. Alignment of the total knee components. Orthopedics 1984; 7: 62
19. Laskin RS. Total condylar knee replacement in patients who have rheumatoid arthritis. A ten year follow-up study. J Bone Joint Surg 1990; 72A: 529–535
20. Laskin RS, Turtel A. The use of an intramedullary tibial alignment guide in total knee replacement arthroplasty. Am J Knee Surg 1989; 2: 123
21. Nuno-Siebrecht N, Tanzer M, Bobyn JD. Potential errors in axial alignment using intramedullary instrumentation for total knee arthroplasty. J Arthroplasty 2000; 15: 228–230
22. Oswald MH, Jacob RP, Schneider E, Hoogewoud H. Radiological analysis of normal axial alignment of femur and tibia in view of total knee arthroplasty. J Arthroplasty 1993; 8: 419–426
23. Petersen TL, Engh GA. Radiographic assessment of knee alignment after total knee arthroplasty. J Arthroplasty 1988; 3: 67–72

24. Piazza SJ, Delp SL, Stulberg, SD, Stern SJ. Posterior tilting of the tibial component decreases femoral rollback in posterior-substituting knee replacement. J Orthop Res 1998; 16: 264–270

25. Ranawat CS, Boachie-Adjei O. Survivorship analysis and results of total condylar knee arthroplasty. Clin Orthop Relat Res 1988 Jan;(226): 6–13

26. Rand JA, Coventry MB. Ten-year evaluation of geometric total knee arthroplasty. Clin Orthop Relat Res 1988 Jul;(232): 168–173

27. Ritter MA, Faris PM, Keating EM, Meding JB. Postoperative alignment of total knee replacement. Its effect on survival. Clin Orthop Relat Res 1994 Feb;(299): 153–156

28. Ritter M, Merbst WA, Keating EM, Faris PM. Radiolucency at the bone-cement interface in total knee replacement. J Bone Joint Surg 1991; 76A: 60–65

29. Sharkey PF, Hozack WJ, Rothman RH, et al. Why are total knee arthroplasties failing today? Clin Orthop Relat Res 2002 Nov;(404): 7–13

30. Stern SH, Insall JN. Posterior stabilized prosthesis: results after follow-up of 9–12 years. J Bone Joint Surg 1992; 74A: 980–986

31. Teter KE, Bergman D, Colwell CW. Accuracy of intramedullary versus extramedullary tibial alignment cutting systems in total knee arthroplasty. Clin Orthop Relat Res 1995 Dec;(321): 106–110

32. Tew M, Waugh W. Tibiofemoral alignment and the results of knee replacement. J Bone Joint Surg 1985; 67B: 551–556

33. Townley CD. The anatomic total knee: instrumentation and alignment technique. The Knee: papers of the First Scientific Meeting of the Knee Society. Baltimore University Press, Baltimore, MD, 1985, pp. 39–54

34. Vince KIG, Insall JN, Kelly MA. The total condylar prosthesis. 10 to 12 year results of a cemented knee replacement. J Bone Joint Surg 1989; 71B: 93–797

35. Wasielewski RC, Galante JO, Leighty R, Natarajan RN, Rosenberg AG. Wear patterns on retrieved polyethylene tibial inserts and their relationship to technical considerations during total knee arthroplasty. Clin Orthop Relat Res 1994 Feb;(299): 31–43

36. Hungerford DS, Kenna RV. Preliminary experience with a total knee prosthesis with porous coating used without cement. Clin Orthop Relat Res 1983 Jun;(176):95–107

37. Currie J, Varshney A, Stulberg SD, Adams A, Woods O. The reliability of anatomic landmarks for determining femoral implant = rotation in TKA surgery: implications for CAOS TKA. Presented at the Annual Meeting of Mid-America Orthopaedic Association, Amelia Island, FL, 2005

38. Delp SL, Stulberg SD, Davies B, Picard F, Leitner F. Computer assisted knee replacement. Clin Orthop Relat Res 1998 Sep; (354): 49–56

39. Eichorn H.-J. Image-free navigation in ACL replacement with the OrthoPilot System. In Steihl JB, Konermann WH, Haaker RG (eds), Navigation and Robotics in Total Joint and Spine Surgery, Springer, Berlin, 2004, pp. 387–396

40. Ellis RE, Rudan JF, Harrison, MM. Computer-assisted high tibial osteotomies. In DiGioia AM, Jaramaz B, Picard R, Nolte PL (eds), Computer and Robotic Assisted Knee and Hip Surgery, Oxford University Press, Oxford, 2004, pp. 197–212

41. Fadda M, Bertelli D, Martelli S, et al. Computer assisted planning for total knee arthroplasty. Proceedings of the First Joint Conference on Computer Vision, Virtual Reality and Robotics in Medicine and Medial Robotics and Computer Assisted Surgery, Grenoble, France. Springer, Berlin, 1997, pp. 619–628

42. Froemel M, Portheine F, Ebner M, Radermacher K. Computer assisted template based navigation for total knee replacement. North American Program on Computer Assisted Orthopaedic Surgery, 6–8 July 2001, Pittsburgh, PA

43. Garbini JL, Kaiura RG, Sidles JA, Larson RV, Matsen FA. Robotic instrumentation in total knee arthroplasty. 33rd Annual Meeting, Orthopaedic Research Society, 19–22 January 1987, San Francisco, CA

44. Garg A, Walker PS. Prediction of total knee motion using a three-dimensional computer graphics model. J Biochem 1990; 23: 45–58

45. Jenny JY, Boeri C. Low reproducibility of the intra-operative measurement of the transepicondylar axis during total knee replacement. Acta Orthop Scand 2004; 75(1): 74–77

46. Julliard R, Lavallee S, Dessenne V. Computer assisted anterior cruciate ligament reconstruction of the anterior cruciate ligament. Clin Orthop Relat Res 1998 Sep;(354): 57–64

47. Julliard R, Plaweski S, Lavallee S. ACL surgetics: an efficient computer-assisted technique for ACL reconstruction. In Steihl JB, Konermann WH, Haaker RG (eds), Navigation and Robotics in Total Joint and Spine Surgery, Springer, Berlin, 2004, pp. 405–411

48. Kaiura RG. Robot assisted total knee arthroplasty investigation of the feasibility and accuracy of the robotic process. Master's Thesis, Mechanical Engineering, University of Washington, Seattle, WA, 1986

49. Kienzle TC, Stulberg SD, Peshkin M, et al. A computer-assisted total knee replacement surgical system using a calibrated robot. Orthopaedics. In Taylor RH, et al. (eds), Computer Integrated Surgery. MIT Press, Cambridge, MA 1996, pp. 409–416

50. Kinzel V, Scaddan M, Bradley B, Shakespeare D. Varus/valgus alignment of the femur in total knee arthroplasty. Can accuracy be improved by pre-operative CT scanning? Knee 2004; 11(3): 197–201

51. Klos TVS, Habets RJE, Banks AZ, Banks SA, Devilee RJJ, Cook FF. Computer assistance in arthroscopic anterior cruciate ligament reconstruction. In DiGioia AM, Jaramaz B, Picard R, Nolte PL (eds), Computer and Robotic Assisted Knee and Hip Surgery, Oxford University Press, Oxford, 2004, pp. 229–234

52. Krackow K, Serpe L, Phillips MJ, et al. A new technique for determining proper mechanical axis alignment during total knee arthroplasty. Orthopedics 1999; 22(7): 698–701

53. Kuntz M, Sati M, Nolte LP, et al. Computer assisted total knee arthroplasty. International symposium on CAOS: 2000, February 17–19, Davos, Switzerland

54. Leitner F, Picard F, Minfelde R, et al. Computer-assisted knee surgical total replacement. First Joint Conference of CVRMed and MRCAS, Grenoble, France. Springer, Berlin, 1997, pp. 629–638

55. Leitner F, Picard F, Minfelde R, et al. Computer assisted knee surgical total replacement. Proceedings of the First Joint Conference on Computer Vision, Virtual Reality and Robotics in Medicine and Medical Robotics and Computer Assisted Surgery, Grenoble, France.. Springer, Berlin, 1997, pp. 630–638

56. Martelli M, Marcacci M, Nofrini L, LA Palombara F, Malvisi A, Iacono F, Vendruscolo P, Pierantoni M. Computer- and robot-assisted total knee replacement: analysis of a new surgical procedure. Ann Biomed Eng 2000; 28(9): 1146–1153

57. Matsen FA, Garbini JL, Sidles JA. Robotic assistance in orthopaedic surgery. A proof of principle using distal femoral arthroplasty. Clin Orthop Relat Res 1993 Nov;(296): 178–186

58. Nizard R. Computer assisted surgery for total knee arthroplasty. Acta Orthop Belg 2002; 68(3): 215–230. [Review]

59. Noble PC, Sugano N, Johnston JD, Thompson MT, Conditt MA, Engh CA Sr, Mathis KB. Computer simulation: how can it help the surgeon optimize implant position? Clin Orthop Relat Res 2003 Dec;(417): 242–252. [Review]

60. Peterman J, Kober R, Heinze R, Frolich JJ, Heeckt PF, Gotzen L. Computer-assisted planning and robot assisted surgery in anterior cruciate ligament reconstruction. Oper Techn Orthop 2000; 10: 50–55

61. Picard F, Leitner F, Raoult O, Saragaglia D. Computer assisted knee replacement. Location of a rotational center of the knee. Total knee arthroplasty. International Symposium on CAOS, February 2000

62. Picard F, Moody JE, DiGioia AM, Jaramaz B, Plakseychuk AY, Sell D. Knee reconstructive surgery: preoperative model system. In DiGioia AM, Jaramaz B, Picard R, Nolte PL (eds), Computer and Robotic Assisted Knee and Hip Surgery, Oxford University Press, Oxford, 2004, pp. 139–156

63. Picard F, Moody JE, DiGioia AM, Martinek V, Fu FH, Rytel MJ, Nikou C, LaVarca RS, Jaramaz B. ACL reconstruction-preoperative model system. In DiGioia AM, Jaramaz B, Picard R, Nolte PL (eds), *Computer and Robotic Assisted Knee and Hip Surgery*, Oxford University Press, Oxford, 2004, pp. 213–228

64. Radermacher K, Staudte HW, Rau G. Computer assisted orthopaedic surgery with image-based individual templates. Clin Orthop Relat Res 1998 Sep;(354): 28–38

65. Saragaglia D, Picard F. Computer-assisted implantation of total knee endoprosthesis with no pre-operative imaging: the kinematic model. In Steihl JB, Konermann WH, Haaker RG (eds), *Navigation and Robotics in Total Joint and Spine Surgery*, Springer, Berlin, 2004, pp. 226–233

66. Sati M, Staubli HU, Bourquin Y, Kunz M, Nolte LP. CRA hip and knee reconstructive surgery: ligament reconstructions in the knee-intra-operative model system (non-image based). In DiGioia AM, Jaramaz B, Picard R, Nolte PL (eds), *Computer and Robotic Assisted Knee and Hip Surgery*, Oxford University Press, Oxford, 2004, pp. 235–256

67. Siebert W, Mai S, Kober R, Heeckt PF. Technique and first clinical results of robot-assisted total knee replacement. Knee 2002; 9(3): 173–180

68. Stulberg SD, Eichorn J, Saragaglia D, Jenny J-Y. The rationale for and initial experience with a knee suite of computer assisted surgical applications. Third International CAOS Meeting, June, 2003, Marbella, Spain

69. Stulberg SD, Picard F, Saragaglia D. Computer assisted total knee arthroplasty. Operative techniques. Orthopaedics 2000; 10(1): 25–39

70. Stulberg SD, Saragaglia D, Miehlke R. Total knee replacement: navigation technique intra-operative model system. In DiGioia AM, Jaramaz B, Picard R, Nolte PL (eds), *Computer and Robotic Assisted Knee and Hip Surgery*, Oxford University Press, Oxford, 2004, pp. 157–178

71. Stulberg SD, Sarin V, Loan P. X-ray vs. computer assisted measurement techniques to determine pre and post-operative limb alignment in TKR surgery. Proceedings of the Fourth Annual American CAOS meeting, July 2001, Pittsburgh, PA

72. Tibbles L, Lewis C, Reisine S, Rippey R, Donald M. Computer assisted instruction for preoperative and postoperative patient education in joint replacement surgery. Comput Nurs 1992; 10(5): 208–212

73. Koyonos L, Granieri M, Stulberg SD. At what steps in performance of a TKA do errors occur when manual instrumentation is Used. Presented at the Annual Meeting of American Academy of Orthopaedic Surgeons, 2005, Washington, DC

74. Stulberg SD, Koyonos L, McClusker S, Granieri M. Factors affecting the accuracy of minimally invasive TKA. Presented at the Annual Meeting of American Academy of Orthopaedic Surgeons, 2005, Washington, DC

75. Tria AJ Jr. Minimally invasive total knee arthroplasty: the importance of instrumentation. Orthop Clin North Am 2004; 35(2): 227–234

76. Briard JL, Stindel E, Plaweski S, et al. CT free navigation with the LCS surgetics station: a new way of balancing the soft tissues in TKA based on bone morphing. In Steihl JB, Konermann WH, Haaker RG (eds), *Navigation and Robotics in Total Joint and Spine Surgery*, Springer, Berlin, 2004, pp. 274–280

77. Konermann WH, Kistner S. CT-free navigation including soft-tissue balancing: LCS-TKA and vector vision systems. In Steihl JB, Konermann WH, Haaker RG (eds), *Navigation and Robotics in Total Joint and Spine Surgery*, Springer, Berlin, 2004, pp. 256–265

78. Strauss JM, Ruther W. Navigation and soft tissue balancing of LCS total knee arthroplasty. In Steihl JB, Konermann WH, Haaker RG (eds), *Navigation and Robotics in Total Joint and Spine Surgery*, Springer, Berlin, 2004, pp. 266–273

79. Bathis H, Perlick L, Tingart M, Luring C, Perlick C, Grifka J.Radiological results of image-based and non-image-based computer-assisted total knee arthroplasty. Int Orthop 2004; 28(2): 87–90

80. Bohler M, Messner M, Glos W, Riegler ML. Computer navigated implantation of total knee prostheses: a radiological study. Acta Chir Aust 2000; 33(Suppl): 63

81. Clemens U, Konermann WH, Kohler S, Kiefer H, Jenny JY, Miehlke RK. Computer-assisted navigation with the OrthoPilot System using the search evolution TKA prosthesis. In Steihl JB, Konermann WH, Haaker RG (eds), *Navigation and Robotics in Total Joint and Spine Surgery*, Springer, Berlin, 2004, pp. 236–241

82. Jenny JY, Boeri C. Computer-assisted total knee prosthesis implantation without preoperative imaging. A comparison with classical instrumentation. Presented at the Fourth Annual North American Program on Computer Assisted Orthopaedic Surgery, 2000, Pittsburgh, PA

83. Jenny JY, Boeri C. Implantation d'une prothese totale de genou assistee par ordinateur. Etude comparative cas-temoin avec une instrumentaiton traditionnelle. Rev Chir Orthop 2001; 87: 645–652

84. Jenny JY, Boeri C. Navigated implantation of total knee prostheses: a comparison with conventional techniques. Z Orthop Ihre Grenzgeb 2001; 139: 117–119

85. Jenny JY, Boeri C. Unicompartmental knee prosthesis. A case-control comparative study of two types of instrumentation with a five year follow-up. J Arthroplasty 2002; 17: 1016–1020

86. Jenny JY, Boeri C. Unicompartmental knee prosthesis implantation with a non-image based navigation system. In DiGioia AM, Jaramaz B, Picard R, Nolte PL (eds), *Computer and Robotic Assisted Knee and Hip Surgery*, Oxford University Press, Oxford, 2004, pp. 179–188

87. Konermann WH, Sauer MA. Postoperative alignment of conventional and navigated total knee arthroplasty. In Steihl JB, Konermann WH, Haaker RG (eds), *Navigation and Robotics in Total Joint and Spine Surgery*, Springer, Berlin, 2004, pp. 219–225

88. Lampe F, Hille E. Navigated implantation of the Columbus total knee arthroplasty with the OrthoPilot System: Version 4.0. In Steihl JB, Konermann WH, Haaker RG (eds), *Navigation and Robotics in Total Joint and Spine Surgery*, Springer, Berlin, 2004, pp. 248–253

89. Mattes T, Puhl W. Navigation in TKA with the Navitrack System. In Steihl JB, Konermann WH, Haaker RG (eds), *Navigation and Robotics in Total Joint and Spine Surgery*, Springer, Berlin, 2004, pp. 293–300

90. Miehlke RK, Clemens U, Jens J-H, Kershally S. Navigation in knee arthroplasty: preliminary clinical experience and prospective comparative study in comparison with conventional technique. Z Orthop Ihre Grenzgeb 2001; 139: 1109–1129

91. Miehlke RK, Clemens U, Kershally S. Computer integrated instrumentation in knee arthroplasty: a comparative study of conventional and computerized technique. Fourth Annual North American Program on Computer Assisted Orthopaedic Surgery, Pittsburgh, PA, 2000, pp. 93–96

92. Nishihara S, Sugano N, Ikai M, Sasama T, Tamura Y, Tamura S, Yoshikawa H, Ochi T. Accuracy evaluation of a shape-based registration method for a computer navigation system for total knee arthroplasty. J Knee Surg 2003; 16(2): 98–105

93. Perlick L, Bathis H, Luring C, Tingart M, Grifka J. CT based and CT-free navigation with the brainLAB vector vision system in total knee arthroplasty. In Steihl JB, Konermann WH, Haaker RG (eds), *Navigation and Robotics in Total Joint and Spine Surgery*, Springer, Berlin, 2004, pp. 304–310

94. Perlick L, Bathis H, Tingart M, Perlick C, Grifka J. Navigation in total-knee arthroplasty: CT-based implantation compared with the conventional technique. Acta Orthop Scand 2004; 75(4): 464–470

95. Perlick L, Bathis H, Tingart M, Kalteis T, Grifka J. [Usability of an image based navigation system in reconstruction of leg alignment in total knee arthroplasty - results of a prospective study] Biomed Tech (Berl) 2003; 48(12): 339–343. [German]

96. Picard F. Leitner F, Raoult O, Saragaglia D, Cinquin P. Clinical evaluation of computer assisted total knee arthroplasty. Second Annual North American Program on Computer Assisted Orthopaedic Surgery, Pittsburgh, PA, 1998, pp. 239–249.

97. Saragaglia D, Picard F, Chaussard C, et al. Computer-assisted knee arthroplasty: comparison with a conventional procedure: results of 50 cases in a prospective randomized study. Rev Chir Orthop Reparatrice Appar Mot 2001; 87: 215–220

98. Saragagaglia D, Picard F, Chaussard D, Montbarbon E, Leitner F, Cinquin P. Computer assisted total knee arthroplasty: comparison with a conventional procedure. Results of 50 cases prospective randomized study. Presented at the First Annual Meeting of Computer Assisted Orthopaedic Surgery, Davos, Switzerland, 2001

99. Sparmann M, Wolke B. Knee endoprosthesis navigation with the Stryker System. In Steihl JB, Konermann WH, Haaker RG (eds), *Navigation and Robotics in Total Joint and Spine Surgery*, Springer, Berlin, 2004, pp. 319–323

100. Sparmann M, Wolke B. [Value of navigation and robot-guided surgery in total knee arthroplasty]. Orthopade 2003; 32(6): 498–505. [German]

101. Stockl B, Nogler M, Rosiek R, Fischer M, Krismer M, Kessler O. Navigation improves accuracy of rotational alignment in total knee arthroplasty. Clin Orthop Relat Res 2004 Sep;(426): 180–186

102. Stulberg SD. CAS-TKA reduces the occurrence of functional outliers. Presented at the Annual Meeting of Mid-America Orthopaedic Association, Amelia Island, FL, 2005

103. Stulberg SD, Loan P, Sarin V. Computer-assisted navigation in total knee replacement: results of an initial experience in thirty-five patients. J Bone Joint Surg 2002; 84-A(Suppl 2): 90–98.

104. Wiese M, Rosenthal A. Bernsmann K. Clinical experience using the SurgiGATE System. In Steihl JB, Konermann WH, Haaker RG (eds), *Navigation and Robotics in Total Joint and Spine Surgery*, Springer, Berlin, 2004, pp. 400–404

105. Wixson RL. Extra-medullary computer assisted total knee replacement: towards lesser invasive surgery. In Steihl JB, Konermann WH, Haaker RG (eds), *Navigation and Robotics in Total Joint and Spine Surgery*, Springer, Berlin, 2004, pp. 311–318

106. Bathis H, Perlick L, Luring C, Kalteis T, Grifka J. [CT-based and CT-free navigation in knee prosthesis implantation. Results of a prospective study] Unfallchirurg 2003; 106(11): 935–940. [German]

107. Insall J, Scott N, Surgery of the knee, Chapter 95. Elsevier, Philadelphia, 2006, pp. 1675–1688

108. Mahfouz MR, Hoff WA, Komistek RD, Dennis DA. A robust method for registration of three-dimensional knee implant models to two-dimensional fluoroscopy images. IEEE Trans Med Imaging 2003; 22(12): 1561–1574

Chapter 77
The Utility of Robotics in Total Knee Arthroplasty

Mohanjit Kochhar and Giles R. Scuderi

In the last decade, instrumentation for total knee arthroplasty (TKA) has improved the accuracy, reproducibility, and reliability of the procedure. In recent years, minimally invasive surgery (MIS) TKA introduced instrumentation that was reduced in size to fit within the smaller operative field. As the operative field becomes reduced in size, the impact and influence of technology becomes proportionately larger.[1] The introduction of computer navigation with MIS is an attempt to improve the surgeon's visibility in a reduced operative field. The intended goal is to improve the position of the resection guides and ultimately the position of the final components, in essence, providing improved visualization in the limited field. This new technology is an enhancement tool or enabler in MIS TKA because, after registration of the anatomic landmarks, the instruments are dynamically tracked with real-time feedback on the angle and depth of the femoral and tibial resection. Currently, there are two types of computer-navigated systems for TKA: imaged-guided and imageless systems. Image-guided systems rely on data from preoperative radiographs or computed tomography (CT) scans that are registered into the computer system. Imageless navigation systems eliminate the need for preoperative imaging and rely on the registration of intraoperative landmarks, and then compare the registered data with a library of anatomic specimens recorded within the computer databank. The next distinctive feature is the mode of instrument tracking, which can be either by optical line of sight with a series of arrays that are detected by an infrared camera, or an electromagnetic (EM) system that utilizes trackers that are attached to the bone and an EM field generator. Each computer navigation system has their proponents. Either way, advocates of computer-navigated surgery have reported in clinical studies that navigation has shown an improvement in the accuracy of component position within 3° of the desired position over conventional instrumentation.[2,3] The computer relies on the

registration of anatomic landmarks and interprets this data to create a three-dimensional (3D) virtual model of the knee. Refinements in the process of collecting the landmark data will create a more accurate virtual model and guidance system. The ideal system should be simple to use, accurate, and reliable without interfering with the operative field and should serve as an enabler in the limited operative field, reliably reporting the knee alignment and intraoperative kinematics.[4]

Although it may be appealing to rely on computer navigation to perform a TKA, it is not artificial intelligence and does not make any of the surgical decisions. The procedure still is surgeon directed, and navigation should serve as a tool of confirmation with the potential for improvements in surgical accuracy and reproducibility. Computer navigation is the first step in introducing advanced technologies into the operating room. The accuracy and safety of conventional instrumentation in TKA have always been dependent on the surgeon's judgment, experience, ability to integrate images, ability to utilize preoperative radiographs, knowledge of anatomic landmarks, knowledge of knee kinematics, and hand-eye coordination. Recent advances in medical imaging, computer vision, and robotics have provided enabling technologies. Synergistic use of computers and robotic technology, which are designed to develop interactive patient-specific procedures, optimize the accurate performance of the surgery.[5] The successful use of this technology requires that it not replace the surgeon, but support the surgeon with enhanced feedback, integration of information, and visual dexterity. The surgeon needs to clearly understand the goals, applications, and limitations of such a system.[6]

TKA is ideally suited for the application of robotic surgery. The ability to isolate and rigidly fix the femur and tibia in known positions allows robotic devices to be securely fixed to the bone or within the desired plan of resection.[7] The bone is treated as a fixed object, simplifying the computer control of the robotic system. In developing the ideal robotic system, the technology must be safe; accurate; compatible with the operative field in size and shape, and be able to be sterilized; and must show measurable benefits, such as reduced operative time, reduced surgical trauma, and

M. Kochhar and G.R. Scuderi (✉)
Insall Scott Kelly Institute, 210 East 64th Street, 4th Floor, New York, NY, 10021, USA
e-mail: gscuderi@iskinstitute.com

G.R. Scuderi and A.J. Tria (eds.), *Minimally Invasive Surgery in Orthopedics*,
DOI 10.1007/978-0-387-76608-9_77, © Springer Science+Business Media, LLC 2010

improved clinical outcomes.[8] Advocates think that this is attainable and that robotic-assisted TKA can achieve levels of accuracy, precision, and safety not accomplished by computer-assisted surgery.[7]

The robotic systems rely on the creation of a 3D virtual model of the knee joint, which is formed from the identification of fixed anatomic landmarks. With all systems, the knee is rigidly secured in the same position with a leg-holding device throughout the referencing stage, as well as during the procedure to ensure accuracy. This establishes a relationship between the robot, the patient, and the surgical field. Using this information and the created virtual model of the knee, the robot enables the surgeon to perform the guided surgery within a defined operative field. Commercially available robotic systems can be categorized as either passive or active devices. This classification is dependent on the control the surgeon has on the robot. With a passive system, the surgeon and robot interact and communicate during the procedure. While there is surgeon apprehension about active robots and automated surgery, passive systems that are in development may relieve the negative impression of robotics, the perception of increased risk, and potentially improve the surgeon's accuracy. A passive robotic system maintains surgeon control, which one does not want to relinquish, throughout the procedure. The surgeon selects the anatomic landmarks, which establishes the coordinate system that creates the virtual 3D model of the knee that guides the instrumentation. Surgeon input is preserved with confirmation of the implant size, the angle of resection, component rotation, and depth of resection. All of these factors can be adjusted prior to final positioning of the automated cutting guide. Once the cutting guide is guided into place, the surgeon resects the femur and tibia, as the surgeon would routinely do with standard instruments. Further concepts in development will provide intraoperative quantifiable information on soft tissue balancing, alignment, range of motion, and kinematics.

Passive robotic systems can be either with a haptic robot or a nonhaptic robot. With a haptic robot, a preoperative plan, established by the input of fixed bone landmarks, determines the boundaries of the surgical area. The tactile feedback with the cutting tool allows the surgeon to feel the boundaries of the bone resection and prevents movement outside of the planned operative field. Examples of this are the ACROBOT (Acrobot Co. LTD, United Kingdom) and the Haptic Guidance System (HGS) (MAKO Surgical Corp., Ft. Lauderdale, FL), which constrain the range of movement of the surgical tool held by a robotic arm. HGS is a haptic surgeon-assisted robotic system that allows the surgeon to accurately plan the implant size, and optimize the position and orientation of the implant relative to a CT scan acquired preoperatively. The system eliminates the need for cutting guides that are used in conventional knee arthroplasty. During the bone resection, the HGS system with its proprietary software continuously provides the surgeon with visual, tactile, and auditory guidance.[9]

The nonhaptic robot assists the surgeon in accurately positioning the cutting guides based upon a preoperative plan and the recorded anatomic landmarks. The surgeon then performs the bone resection through the positioned cutting guide. There is no tactile feel to the resection, and the surgeon performs the resection through the cutting guide, as the surgeon would do with standard instrumentation. BRIGIT (Zimmer, Warsaw, IN) is a system in development that is an example of a passive robot. It is a multifunctional tool that serves as a passive assistant through an automated arm that positions and holds the resection guide according to the surgeon's surgical plan. The surgeon performs each step in the planned femoral and tibial resection for the desired knee implant as the robotic arm with the multifunctional cutting guide is positioned in place for each bone resection. The orientation and depth of resection is determined by the system software and confirmed by the surgeon. The bone resection is performed with a conventional saw. There is no tactile guidance during the bone preparation. The advantage of the robotic multifunctional cutting guide is that it eliminates the vast majority of instruments needed to perform the procedure, and the multifunctional cutting guide does not have to be pinned in place. It is locked in the plane of resection by the system during bone resection.

In contrast to a passive system, an active system follows a complete preoperative plan, which is carried out without surgeon intervention. After registration of the anatomic landmarks, the automated cutting tool resects the femur and the tibia. Examples of an active system are CASPAR (Universal Robot Systems, Germany) and ROBODOC (Integrated Surgical Supplies LTD, Sacramento, CA), which direct a milling device automatically according to preoperative planning.[10] These systems use preoperative CT images as part of the preoperative templating, including the angle and depth of bone resection, and the size of the components. After intraoperative registration of the anatomic landmarks, the computer matches this data with the CT scan and a virtual model of the knee is created. The surgeon then guides the robotic cutting tool to the desired location and the robot then prepares the bone autonomously. Upon completion of the bone preparation, the surgeon completes the TKA by balancing the soft tissues and implanting the components.

Robotic surgery is helping us take the next step into the operating room of the future. The role of robots in the operating room has the potential to increase as technology improves and appropriate applications are defined.[1] Joint replacement arthroplasty may benefit the most due to the need for high precision in placing instruments, aligning the limb, and implanting components. In addition, this technology will reduce the number of instruments needed for the procedure, improving efficiency. As technology advances, robots may be commonplace in the operating room and potentially transform the way TKA is done in the future. This is important because there has been an exponential rise in the number of TKA performed annually. With baby boomers coming of age, the rise in the number of people with arthritis and reported success of TKA in improving the quality of life, the number of TKA performed annually is rising. A recent report by Kurtz predicted that the number of primary TKA performed annually will increase to 3.48 million by 2030.[11] This demand on surgeon and the hospital system will need improvements in technology in order to treat more patients and maintain the quality of care. Robotic surgery is new innovative technology and it will remain to be seen whether history will look on its development as a profound improvement in surgical technique or a bump on the road to something more important.

References

1. Scuderi GR. Smart tools and total knee arthroplasty. Am J Orthop 36(95)Supplement: 8–10, 2007
2. Alan RK, Shin MS, Tria AJ. Initial experience with electromagnetic navigation in total knee arthroplasty: a radiographic comparative study. J Knee Surg 20(2): 152–157, 2007
3. Stiehl JB. Computer navigation in primary total knee arthroplasty. J Knee Surg 20(2): 158–164, 2007
4. Scuderi GR. Computer navigation in total knee arthroplasty. Where are we and where are we heading. Am J Knee Surg 20(2): 151, 2007
5. DiGioia AM, Jaramaz B, Colgan BD. Computer assisted orthopedic surgery. Image guided and robotic assistive technologies. Clin Orthop Relat Res 354: 8–16, 1998
6. Specht LM, Koval KJ. Robotics and computer assisted orthopedic surgery. Bull Hosp Jt Dis 60: 168–172, 2001
7. Adili A. Robotic assisted orthopedic surgery. Semin Laparosc Surg 11(2): 89–98, 2004
8. Hurst KS, Phillips R, Viant WJ, etal. Review of orthopedic manipulator arms. Stud Health Technol Inform 50: 202–208, 1998
9. Roche M. Changing the way surgeons plan and execute minimally invasive unicompartmental knee surgery. Orthopedic Product News July/August 2006
10. Surgano N. Computer assisted orthopedic surgery. J Orthop Sci 8(3): 442–448, 2003
11. Kurtz S, Ong K, Lau E etal. Projection of primary and revision hip and knee arthroplasty in the United States 2005–2030. J Bone Joint Surg 89A: 780–785, 2007

Chapter 78
Electromagnetic Navigation in Total Knee Arthroplasty

Rodney K. Alan and Alfred J. Tria

Accurate limb alignment in total knee arthroplasty (TKA) is an essential part of the reconstructive procedure. Good alignment has been shown to correlate with improved outcomes. Malalignment of components greater than 3–4° may be associated with early failure.[1–7] The goal of computer-assisted TKA is to improve alignment. Theoretically, improved alignment should decrease the incidence of failure due to surgical technique.

Traditionally, intramedullary and extramedullary guides have been used to facilitate accurate bone cuts in TKA. Intramedullary alignment guides have been shown to have a high level of accuracy for the femur, but are less accurate for the tibia because the intramedullary canal does not always allow easy insertion of the reference rods.[8–14] Intramedullary guides align the limb relative to the anatomic axis. When using intramedullary guides, most surgeons cut the distal femur between 4 and 7° of anatomic valgus. Unlike conventional TKA, navigated TKA references the mechanical axis. With navigated TKA, the mechanical axis is more likely to show less variation postoperatively.[4,15–25] Slotted cutting guides have also been used to help to control the saw blade to increase bone cutting accuracy.[26] With the advent of computer-assisted surgery, slotted cutting guides can be positioned by navigation. This technique has been used effectively to improve the accuracy of alignment relative to the mechanical axis. Multiple studies have shown that postoperative alignment is improved using computer-assisted navigation when compared with performing TKA with conventional alignment guides.[4,15–25,27] Based on these studies, computer-assisted navigation in TKA may lead to improved outcomes.

Two types of navigation systems are available for TKA: image-assisted navigation and image-free navigation. Image-assisted techniques require radiographic studies to complete the procedure. Preoperative computed tomography (CT) scans or intraoperative fluoroscopic images are used by the computer as a reference for the anatomy. Image-assisted navigation increases the amount of time and planning required for performing navigated TKA and also exposes the patient to radiation.

Many navigation systems have transitioned into image-free techniques. The advantage of image-free navigation is the elimination of preoperative or intraoperative imaging. Image-free navigation requires kinematic localization of the hip center in order to identify the alignment of the limb.

Optical (or line-of-sight) navigation systems are available as image assisted and image free. With line-of-sight navigation, placement of optical tracking units (arrays) is detected by an infrared camera. All of the current studies on computer-assisted navigation in TKA use the line-of-site technique.[4,15–25]

Electromagnetic (EM) navigation is different from optical navigation. With EM technology, small dynamic referencing frames (DRF) are attached to the femur and the tibia within the operative exposure (Fig. 78.1), and a small handheld electromagnetic emitter is used to track the DRFs (Fig. 78.2).

Advantages and Disadvantages of EM Navigation

EM navigation does not require a line-of-sight. The emitter sets up a field around the DRFs and the instruments. The computer can see the devices in the field and relate them to known anatomic landmarks identified by the surgeon. The emitter eliminates the need for the camera and the difficulties of lining the camera up with the reflective spheres of the arrays. The line-of-sight arrays required percutaneous pin fixation to the underlying femur and tibia. This exposes the knee to possible stress fracture through the pin holes and can lead to persistent drainage with the possibility of associated infection. The DRFs take the place of the arrays and are attached to the bone with small cortical screws.

Metal interference is a major problem with EM navigation. In the clinical setting, if there is too much interference, there is no image on the computer screen. It is possible that minor interference will still allow tracking but decrease the accuracy of the measurements.[28] The DRFs must be placed in a protected area in the knee so that no instruments change the

R.K. Alan and A.J. Tria (✉)
Institute for Advanced Orthopaedic Study, The Orthopaedic Center of New Jersey, 1527 State Highway 27, Suite 1300, Somerset, NJ 08873, USA
e-mail: Atriajrmd@aol.com

G.R. Scuderi and A.J. Tria (eds.), *Minimally Invasive Surgery in Orthopedics*, DOI 10.1007/978-0-387-76608-9_78, © Springer Science+Business Media, LLC 2010

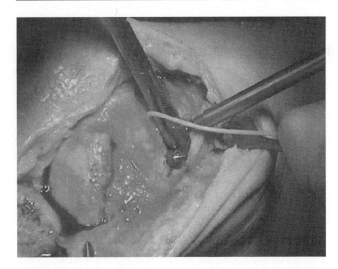

Fig. 78.1 The femoral DRF is attached to the medial metaphyseal bone

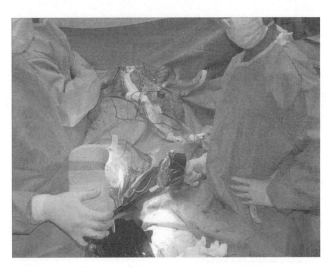

Fig. 78.2 The emitter is handheld with a sterile cover over it

position of the sensing devices. The DRFs presently have wires that are attached to the computer, and these wires sometimes interfere with the surgical exposure. If the wire is cut, the DRF must be replaced and all of the land marking must be repeated.

Patients with cardiac pacemakers should not have EM navigation unless their pacemaker has been approved for use with EM navigation. The vendor who provides the device also provides a list of approved cardiac pacemakers that do not preclude EM navigation.

The kinematic hip center registration does require motion of the hip on the ipsilateral side to the TKA. The most recent software for EM navigation requires approximately 15° of abduction and adduction and 10° of combined internal and external rotation to localize the hip center. Thus, if the hip is fused, the EM navigation will not be possible. The emitter should be placed in a firm holding base for the kinematic

centering of the hip because slight motion delays the process and sometimes invalidates the result. During the remainder of the operative procedure, the emitter can be handheld.

Technique

EM navigation can be used with any surgical approach for TKA. The technique does not require any change in the preparation of the case or in the surgical draping. All of the steps for EM navigation are carried out during the surgical procedure within the operative field. EM navigation requires the computer, the emitter, some retractors with decreased iron content, and the disposables. The disposables are sterile and include a registration stylus, a paddle probe, one DRF for the femur, one DRF for the tibia, and small screws for securing the referencing frames. The emitter and disposables should be connected prior to making the incision.

The DRFs are positioned and secured on the femur and the tibia after making the initial approach to the knee. Extensive soft tissue releases should be avoided until the initial alignment is recorded with the navigation. The placement of the DRFs is important because any motion of the referencing frames will diminish the accuracy of navigation. The referencing frames should be placed away from the areas of the bone that may be disturbed by the saw blade or broaches or instruments. The femoral referencing frame should be placed on the medial aspect of the femur at least 2 cm above the joint line, and the tibial referencing frame should be placed on the medial aspect of the tibia at least 1.5 cm below the joint line. The instruments are closest to the femoral DRF during the anterior resection of the femoral cortex. The tibial DRF is at greatest risk during the intramedullary broaching for the tibial stem.

After placing the DRFs, kinematic registration of the hip center can be completed. The EM field should be large enough so that the DRFs will remain in the field for approximately 15° of abduction and adduction and 10° of combined internal and external rotation of the limb. It is essential that there is no motion in the emitter or the pelvis during localization of the hip center. An emitter holder attached to the operating room table expedites the process (Fig. 78.3). The land marking of the knee is completed using the disposable pointer probe.

Throughout the remainder of the operative procedure, the navigation can be used to make the primary cuts or to check the cuts after they are completed with traditional instrumentation. It is best to use a mixture of both approaches until the surgeon is familiar with the technique. The EM monitoring can be used for the femoral rotation and the alignment in the coronal and sagittal planes. The tibial cut can also be monitored in the coronal and sagittal planes but the software is not currently able to evaluate the axial rotation of the component.

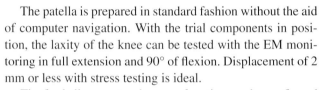

Fig. 78.3 The emitter holder attaches to the operating table and holds the device stable for navigation of the hip center (Innovative Medical Products, Plainville, CT, USA)

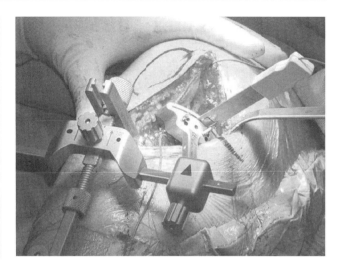

Fig. 78.4 The EM paddle is placed into the cutting slot of the extramedullary tibial guide for direct referencing of the cut

The patella is prepared in standard fashion without the aid of computer navigation. With the trial components in position, the laxity of the knee can be tested with the EM monitoring in full extension and 90° of flexion. Displacement of 2 mm or less with stress testing is ideal.

The final alignment and range of motion can be confirmed after the final components are inserted. The DRFs are disposable, but the authors have used the referencing frame in the contralateral knee on bilateral procedures without any difficulty.

Materials and Methods

After obtaining institutional review board (IRB) approval, 60 consecutive patients who underwent TKA with EM navigation were reviewed. The navigation was used to measure the preoperative and postoperative alignment, and to confirm the cuts during the procedure. A standard intramedullary femoral alignment guide was used to make the distal femoral resection, and a modified extramedullary alignment guide was used to resect the proximal tibia (Fig. 78.4). After each bone resection, the paddle was used to measure the alignment of the cut (Fig. 78.5).

Preoperative and postoperative X-rays were used to measure the coronal plane alignment of the knee and the alignment of the tibial component. All X-rays were taken with the same technique. The knee was in full extension with the patella directed perpendicular to the X-ray beam.[29]

The radiographic alignment of the knee was compared with the EM navigated alignment of the knee, using 6° of anatomic valgus as neutral for radiographs, and a mechanical axis of zero as neutral for EM navigation. Paired differences between

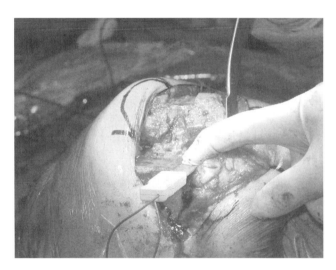

Fig. 78.5 The EM paddle is placed onto the cut surface of the tibia to recheck the cut

X-ray and EM measures of alignment were generated to determine the relationship between radiographic alignment measured on a 14 × 17-in. cassettes and EM-navigated alignment.

A separate analysis with another consecutive series of 20 patients was completed using preoperative and postoperative mechanical axis radiographs. Paired differences were analyzed to assess the relationship between mechanical axis radiographs and EM navigation.

Results

In the initial experience, EM navigation was abandoned in three operative procedures. On one occasion, the technical problem was solved by replacing the emitter. In another case, one of the DRFs was slightly loose and the computer began generating abnormal data. A wire was incidentally cut during one procedure.

When compared with anatomical alignment measured on short radiographs, the alignment measured by EM was within 3° of the predicted preoperative alignment in 63% (33/52) of cases. The alignment measured by EM was within 3° of the predicted postoperative alignment in 67% (38/57) of cases. The alignment of the tibial component measured by EM was within 3° of the predicted postoperative X-ray alignment in 87% (48/55) of cases.

When compared with mechanical axis radiographic alignment, the alignment measured by EM was within 3° of the predicted preoperative alignment in 90% (18/20) of cases. The postoperative alignment was within 3° in 90% (18/20) of cases; and the tibial component position was within 3° in 95% (19/20) of cases.

Discussion

Improvement of alignment during TKA and avoiding the potential concerns of optical navigation systems prompted the authors to investigate EM navigation. The technique is not difficult and can be adapted in a step-wise fashion until the surgeon becomes proficient with the system. Although the referencing frame and the wires are in the operative exposure, careful technique can eliminate the concern for cutting them during the procedure. The average tourniquet time was 69 min for the entire operative procedure in the author's initial experience with EM navigation. There were no surgical delays due to interruption in camera line-of-sight and no difficulties with debris interfering with arrays. There were no major complications. In three cases where the computer malfunctioned or the DRF was disturbed, the surgeries were completed with standard instrumentation.

The relationship between radiographic alignment and EM alignment was evaluated to determine the accuracy of EM navigation. Although there is some inherent variability in X-ray measurements,[30,31] it is currently the standard for evaluating limb alignment after TKA.[8–14] The maximum difference between the alignment demonstrated by EM navigation and alignment measured by mechanical axis radiographs was 4.2°. The mean differences are within 3° in 89% of cases. Two degrees may be the limit of what can be measured by X-rays;[32] therefore, EM navigation appears to be accurate.

When compared with anatomical alignment measured on short X-rays, the maximum difference can be as high as 9° when neutral is considered to be 6° of anatomic valgus. Many surgeons continue to use short X-rays to evaluate the results of TKA. Extraarticular deformity such as bowing is commonly not seen on short radiographs.[33] This causes the anatomic alignment to vary relative to the mechanical alignment. Six degrees of anatomic valgus is not neutral in all patients.[34] Surgeons who use navigation and rely on short radiographs only should be aware of the variability of the anatomical axis after navigated TKA.

The assumption of some articles regarding navigation is that the alignment determined by the computer is absolutely accurate.[35] This assumption is not entirely correct and the operating surgeon must be aware of the limitations of any system that is used for operative support. All systems that rely on kinematic hip center determination may have some error in assessing alignment. Victor and Hoste reported a mean deviation between the kinematic and radiographic hip center of 1.6 mm with a range of 0–5 mm.[25] They also suggested that other systems may have even more variability. Anatomical landmark registration is also a source for computer error. It is sometimes difficult to accurately identify all of the anatomic landmarks that are necessary for navigation.[36] Motion in the referencing frames adversely effects computer measurement of alignment and anatomic variation makes it difficult for any one software program to calculate the alignment correctly on every occasion. Finally, navigated alignment is determined with the knee joint in the non-weight-bearing position on the operating room table with the patella subluxated laterally and with a portion of the deep medial collateral ligament released as a part of the surgical approach. The radiographs are taken with the knee in the weight-bearing position and without any opening or laxity of the capsule. These factors can contribute to differences in alignment when measured by navigation and X-rays.

Conclusions

EM navigation for TKA can be adopted for clinical use with a short learning curve. The system appears to be accurate within 1 or 2°, comparable to optical navigation. The pitfalls of metallic interference and DRF motion are not difficult to surmount. Navigation is, in general, a supportive tool that can improve the accuracy of TKA but it must also be monitored throughout the operative procedure.

References

1. Bargren JH, Blaha JD, Freeman MA. Alignment in total knee arthroplasty. Correlated biomechanical and clinical observations. Clin Orthop Relat Res 1983 Mar;(173):178–83
2. Hvid I, Nielsen S. Total condylar knee arthroplasty. Prosthetic component positioning and radiolucent lines. Acta Orthop Scand 1984 Apr;55(2):160–5
3. Jeffery RS, Morris RW, Denham RA. Coronal alignment after total knee replacement. J Bone Joint Surg Br 1991 Sep;73(5):709–14

4. Kim SJ, MacDonald M, Hernandez J, Wixson RL. Computer assisted navigation in total knee arthroplasty: improved coronal alignment. J Arthroplasty 2005 Oct;20(7 Suppl 3):123–31

5. Lotke PA, Ecker ML. Influence of positioning of prosthesis in total knee replacement. J Bone Joint Surg Am 1977 Jan;59(1):77–9

6. Ritter MA, Faris PM, Keating EM, Meding JB. Postoperative alignment of total knee replacement. Its effect on survival. Clin Orthop Relat Res 1994 Feb;(299):153–6

7. Wasielewski RC, Galante JO, Leighty RM, Natarajan RN, Rosenberg AG. Wear patterns on retrieved polyethylene tibial inserts and their relationship to technical considerations during total knee arthroplasty. Clin Orthop Relat Res 1994 Feb;(299):31–43

8. Bono JV, Roger DJ, Laskin RS, Peterson MG, Paulsen CA. Tibial intramedullary alignment in total knee arthroplasty. Am J Knee Surg 1995 Winter;8(1):7–11

9. Cates HE, Ritter MA, Keating EM, Faris PM. Intramedullary versus extramedullary femoral alignment systems in total knee replacement. Clin Orthop Relat Res 1993 Jan;(286):32–9

10. Dennis DA, Channer M, Susman MH, Stringer EA. Intramedullary versus extramedullary tibial alignment systems in total knee arthroplasty. J Arthroplasty 1993 Feb;8(1):43–7

11. Evans PD, Marshall PD, McDonnell B, Richards J, Evans EJ. Radiologic study of the accuracy of a tibial intramedullary cutting guide for knee arthroplasty. J Arthroplasty 1995 Feb;10(1):43–6

12. Ishii Y, Ohmori G, Bechtold JE, Gustilo RB. Extramedullary versus intramedullary alignment guides in total knee arthroplasty. Clin Orthop Relat Res 1995 Sep;(318):167–75

13. Reed SC, Gollish J. The accuracy of femoral intramedullary guides in total knee arthroplasty. J Arthroplasty 1997 Sep;12(6):677–82

14. Teter KE, Bregman D, Colwell CW Jr. The efficacy of intramedullary femoral alignment in total knee replacement. Clin Orthop Relat Res 1995 Dec;(321):117–21

15 Anderson KC, Buehler KC, Markel DC. Computer assisted navigation in total knee arthroplasty: comparison with conventional methods. J Arthroplasty 2005 Oct;20(7 Suppl 3):132–8

16. Bathis H, Perlick L, Tingart M, Luring C, Perlick C, Grifka J. Radiological results of image-based and non-image-based computer-assisted total knee arthroplasty. Int Orthop 2004 Apr;28(2):87–90. Epub 2004 Jan 17

17. Bathis H, Perlick L, Tingart M, Luring C, Zurakowski D, Grifka J. Alignment in total knee arthroplasty. A comparison of computer-assisted surgery with the conventional technique. J Bone Joint Surg Br 2004 Jul;86(5):682–7

18. Bolognesi M, Hofmann A. Computer navigation versus standard instrumentation for TKA: a single-surgeon experience. Clin Orthop Relat Res 2005 Nov;440:162–9

19. Chauhan SK, Scott RG, Breidahl W, Beaver RJ. Computer-assisted knee arthroplasty versus a conventional jig-based technique. A randomized, prospective trial. J Bone Joint Surg Br 2004 Apr;86(3):372–7

20. Decking R, Markmann Y, Fuchs J, Puhl W, Scharf HP. Leg axis after computer-navigated total knee arthroplasty: a prospective randomized trial comparing computer-navigated and manual implantation. J Arthroplasty 2005 Apr;20(3):282–8

21. Hankemeier S, Hufner T, Wang G, Kendoff D, Zheng G, Richter M, Gosling T, Nolte L, Krettek C. Navigated intraoperative analysis of lower limb alignment. Arch Orthop Trauma Surg 2005 Aug;12:1–5

22. Matsumoto T, Tsumura N, Kurosaka M, Muratsu H, Kuroda R, Ishimoto K, Tsujimoto K, Shiba R, Yoshiya S. Prosthetic alignment and sizing in computer-assisted total knee arthroplasty. Int Orthop. 2004 Oct;28(5):282–5. Epub 2004 Aug 14

23. Perlick L, Bathis H, Tingart M, Perlick C, Grifka J. Navigation in total-knee arthroplasty: CT-based implantation compared with the conventional technique. Acta Orthop Scand 2004 Aug;75(4):464–70

24. Sparmann M, Wolke B, Czupalla H, Banzer D, Zink A. Positioning of total knee arthroplasty with and without navigation support. A prospective, randomized study. J Bone Joint Surg Br 2003 Aug;85(6):830–5

25. Victor J, Hoste D. Image-based computer-assisted total knee arthroplasty leads to lower variability in coronal alignment. Clin Orthop Relat Res 2004 Nov;(428):131–9

26. Plaskos C, Hodgson AJ, Inkpen K, McGraw RW. Bone cutting errors in total knee arthroplasty. J Arthroplasty 2002 Sep;17(6):698–705

27. Stockl B, Nogler M, Rosiek R, Fischer M, Krismer M, Kessler O. Navigation improves accuracy of rotational alignment in total knee arthroplasty. Clin Orthop Relat Res 2004 Sep;(426):180–6

28. Stiehl JB. Comparison of imageless and electromagnetic referencing protocols in total knee arthroplasty. Presented at the closed meeting of The Knee Society, September, 2006

29. Hall-Rollins J. Lower limb. In: Bontrager KL (ed.) Textbook of Radiographic Positioning and Related Anatomy. St. Louis, MO: Mosby; 2001, p. 231

30. Lonner JH, Laird MT, Stuchin SA. Effect of rotation and knee flexion on radiographic alignment in total knee arthroplasties. Clin Orthop Relat Res 1996 Oct;(331):102–6

31. Swanson KE, Stocks GW, Warren PD, Hazel MR, Janssen HF. Does axial limb rotation affect the alignment measurements in deformed limbs? Clin Orthop Relat Res 2000 Feb;(371):246–52

32. Laskin RS. Alignment of total knee components. Orthopedics 1984;7:62–72

33. Petersen TL, Engh GA. Radiographic assessment of knee alignment after total knee arthroplasty. J Arthroplasty 1988;3(1):67–72

34. Hsu RW, Himeno S, Coventry MB, Chao EY. Normal axial alignment of the lower extremity and load-bearing distribution at the knee. Clin Orthop Relat Res 1990 Jun;(255):215–27

35. Stulberg D. How accurate is current TKR instrumentation? Clin Orthop Relat Res 2003 Nov;(416):177–84

36. Robinson M, Eckhoff DG, Reinig KD, Bagur MM, Bach JM. Variability of landmark identification in total knee arthroplasty. Clin Orthop Relat Res 2006 Jan;442:57–62

Chapter 79
Computer Navigation in the Foot and Ankle Surgery

Martinus Richter

Foot and ankle surgery at the end of the 20th century was characterized by the use of sophisticated computerized preoperative and postoperative diagnostic and planning procedures.[1-3] However, intraoperative computerized tools that assist the surgeon during his or her struggle for the planned optimal operative result are missing. This results in an intraoperative "black box" without optimal visualization, guidance, and biomechanical assessment.[2] The future will be characterized by breaking up this intraoperative "black box." We will have more intraoperative tools to achieve the planned result.[2,3] Intraoperative three-dimensional (3D) imaging (ISO-C-3D), computer-assisted surgery (CAS), and intraoperative pedography (IP) are three possible innovations to realize the planned procedure intraoperatively.[3] These devices might be especially helpful for minimally invasive surgery.

These novel methods are in clinical use at our institution for further development. This chapter especially analyzes the feasibility and potential clinical benefit of navigation for foot and ankle surgery. Because ISO-C-3D and IP are two other innovations that are closely connected to navigation, these two methods are also described.

Intraoperative Three-Dimensional Imaging

In foot and ankle trauma care, malposition of extraosseous or intraarticular screws and gaps or steps in joint lines frequently remain undiscovered when using intraoperative fluoroscopy, and are only recognized on postoperative computed tomography (CT) scans.[4] Earlier preclinical studies showed that evaluation of reduction and implant position with a new C-arm-based 3D imaging device (ISO-C-3D) is better than with plain films or a C-arm alone and comparable to CT scans.[5-9]

ISO-C-3D (Siemens AG, Germany) is a motorized C-arm that provides fluoroscopic images during a 190° orbital rotation computing a 119-mm data cube (Fig. 79.1a). From these 3D data sets, two-dimensional (2D) and multiplanar reconstructions can be obtained on the screen of the device without delay (Fig. 79.1b). For scanning, the situs is draped with a sterile plastic bag that is pulled over the legs and the table.

Study Results

A prospective consecutive clinical study was performed in a level one trauma center.[10] The aim of the study was to evaluate the feasibility and benefit of the intraoperative use of the ISO-C-3D for foot and ankle trauma care in this special environment. The hypothesis was that the ISO-C-3D could detect failures of reduction or implant position that had not been detected with a conventional C-arm in a considerable percentage of cases.

Patients with foot and ankle trauma or reconstruction surgery who were treated in the Trauma Department of the Hannover Medical School between July 1, 2003 and June 30, 2005 were considered for inclusion in the study. Before the use of the device, the reduction and implant position had to judged to be correct by the surgeon using a conventional C-arm. The patients were placed either on a special metal-free carbon table or on a standard table. Time spent, changes after use of the ISO-C-3D, and surgeons' ratings (visual analog scale [VAS], 0–10 points) were recorded. The surgeons' ratings for image quality for the carbon table and the standard table were compared (t test, significance level 0.05). The surgeons' ratings for image quality for the carbon table and the standard table were compared (t test, significance level 0.05).

One hundred and one patients/cases (no bilateral ISO-C-3D use) were included (Fractures: pilon, $n = 15$; Weber-C ankles, $n = 12$; isolated dorsal Volkmann, $n = 3$; talus, $n = 7$; calcaneus, $n = 32$; navicular, $n = 2$; cuboid, $n = 2$; Lisfranc fracture-dislocation, $n = 8$; ankle/hindfoot arthrodesis with or without correction, $n = 4/16$). Carbon table was use in 80 cases (79%) and a standard table in 21 cases (21%). The operation was interrupted for 430 s on average (range, 300–700 s); 100 s on average for preparation, 120 s on average for the ISO-C-3D scan, and 210 s on average for evaluation of the images by the surgeon. In 39% (39 of 101) of the cases,

M. Richter (✉)
II Chirurgische Klinik, Unfallchirurgie, Orthopädie und Fußchirurgie, Klinikum Coburg, Ketschendorfer Str. 33, 96450 Coburg, Germany
e-mail: martinus.richter@klinikum-coburg.de

G.R. Scuderi and A.J. Tria (eds.), *Minimally Invasive Surgery in Orthopedics*,
DOI 10.1007/978-0-387-76608-9_79, © Springer Science+Business Media, LLC 2010

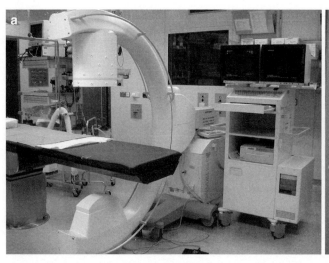
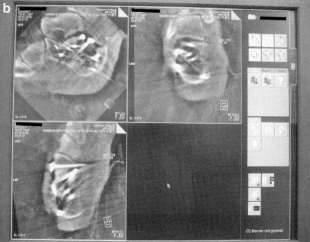

Fig. 79.1 Intraoperative three-dimensional (3D) imaging (ISO-C-3D). ISO-C-3D device in the operating room and carbon fracture table (**a**). Monitor view of an ISO-C-3D device showing multiplanar reformations of a calcaneus after open reduction and internal fixation with a plate and screws (**b**). *Top left* parasagittal reformation; *top right* coronal reformation; *bottom left* axial/horizontal reformation. The reformation planes can be chosen by the surgeon in any orientation compared with a CT scan

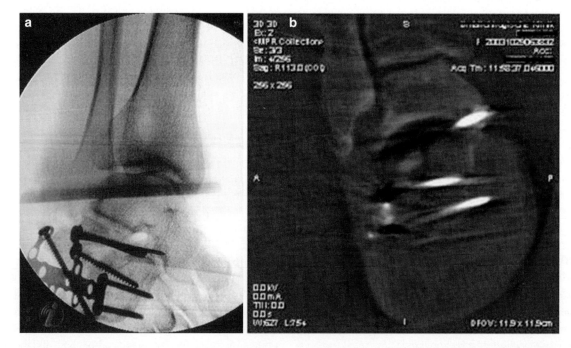

Fig. 79.2 Intraoperative 3D imaging (ISO-C-3D). Calcaneus fracture after open reduction and internal fixation with plate and screws. After evaluation with a C-arm including Broden's view (**a**), a correct reduction and implant position was confirmed by the surgeon. The ISO-C-3D scan showed a screw penetrating the posterior facet medially (**b**), and the screw position was corrected during the same procedure

the reduction ($n = 16$, 16%) and/or implant position ($n = 30$, 30%) was corrected after ISO-C-3D scan during the same procedure. The ratings of the eight surgeons involved were 9.2 (range, 5.2–10) for feasibility, 9.5 (range, 6.1–10) for accuracy, and 8.2 (range, 4.5–10) for clinical benefit. The image quality was rated 9.1 (range, 8.0–10) for the carbon tables, and 8.7 (range, 7.0–10) for the standard tables (difference rating carbon table vs. standard table, t test, $p > 0.05$).

The image quality was rated 9.1 (range, 8.0–10) for the carbon tables, and 8.7 (range, 7.0–10) for the standard tables (difference rating carbon table vs. standard table, t test, not significant). Fig. 79.2 shows a clinical example.

In this study, in almost 40% of cases, reduction and/or implant position was corrected after ISO-C-3D scan at the same procedure. The radiation contamination is comparable to a standard CT scan and corresponds to 39 s fluoroscopy time with a modern digital C-arm. The image quality with a carbon table is not better than with a standard table. Consequently, the use of a carbon table is not necessary for ISO-C-3D scan at the foot region.

In conclusion, the intraoperative 3D visualization with the ISO-C-3D can provide important information in foot and ankle trauma care that cannot be obtained from plain films or C-arm alone.[11] The use is not considerably time consuming. The ISO-C-3D is extremely useful in evaluating reduction and/or implant position intraoperatively and can replace a postoperative CT scan.

Computer-Assisted Surgery

CT-Based Computer-Assisted Surgery

The accuracy of the reduction in hindfoot and midfoot fractures and fracture-dislocations correlates with the clinical result.[12–20] The same is true for the correction of hindfoot and midfoot.[19,21–29] However, an accurate correction or reduction with the conventional C-arm-based procedure is challenging.[19,30,31] CT-based CAS has become a valuable tool for the correction and reduction in other body regions.[32–53] Especially a more exact reduction could be achieved.[32,34,38–40,43–47,49,52,54–5] [7] CT-based CAS may also be useful for the correction of hindfoot and midfoot deformities and for the reduction in hindfoot or midfoot fractures and fracture-dislocations, although it has not been used in the foot region so far.[58]

Study Results

The purpose of an experimental study at our institution was to compare CT-based CAS assisted correction of hindfoot and midfoot deformities with C-arm-based correction.[59] Sawbone (Pacific Research Laboratories, Vashon, WA, USA) specimen models "Large Left Foot/Ankle," "Large Left Foot/Ankle with Equinus Deformity," "Large Left Foot/Ankle with Calcaneus Malunion," and "Large Left Foot/Ankle with Equinovarus Deformity" were used. A CT scan of each deformity specimen model ($n = 3$) was performed. The goal of the correction was to transform the shape of the pathology specimen models into the shape of the normal specimen model. Two methods were used for the correction: (a) conventional C-arm-based correction and (b) CAS-based (CT based, Surgigate™, Medivision, Oberdorf, Switzerland & Northern Digital Inc., Waterloo, Ontario, Canada) correction. Five specimens of each deformity model were corrected with each method. Standardized osteotomies were performed before the correction when necessary (in models with calcaneus malunion and equinovarus). The surgeon's direct view to the

specimens was disabled by drapes. During the correction procedure, the visualization of the specimen was exclusively provided by the image of the C-arm or the CAS device. Retention was performed with 1.8-mm titanium K-wires. The following parameters were registered: time needed for entire procedure and different steps of the procedure, time of fluoroscopy, foot length, length and height of the longitudinal arch, calcaneus inclination, hindfoot angle for all models ($n = 30$), and additionally Boehler's angle and the calcaneus length for the "calcaneus malunion" specimen models ($n = 10$). The shape of the corrected specimens was graded as normal, nearly normal, abnormal, or severely abnormal. The parameters of the two correction method groups (CAS vs. C-arm) were statistically compared (t test, c^2 test). According to the specimen measurements, the differences between the corrected specimen models and the normal specimen model were also compared.

The shape was graded as normal in all specimens ($n = 15$) in the CAS group, and in eight of the specimens in the C-arm group (other grades in C-arm group: nearly normal, $n = 6$; abnormal, $n = 1$; c^2 test, $p = 0.05$). The time needed for the procedure was longer in the CAS group, and the fluoroscopy time was shorter in the CAS group than in the C-arm group (mean values and range shown, t test utilized):

– Time for the entire procedure, CAS, 782 s (range, 450–1,020 s), C-arm, 410 s (range, 210–600 s), $p < 0.001$
– Fluoroscopy time, CAS, 0 s, C-arm, 11 s (range, 8–19 s), $p < 0.001$

In three cases in the CAS group, the system crashed and was restarted (the times for the entire procedure in these cases were 1,000, 1,010, and 1,020 s).

The measurement *differences* between the corrected specimens and the normal specimen model were as follows (mean values and standard deviation shown, t test utilized): foot length, CAS, -1.7 ± 1.9 mm, C-arm, -4.1 ± 3.8 mm, $p = 0.03$; length of longitudinal arch, CAS, -0.9 ± 0.9 mm, C-arm, -5.6 ± 4.9 mm, $p = 0.001$; height of longitudinal arch, CAS, -0.1 ± 0.5 mm, C-arm, 1.7 ± 4.3 mm, $p = 0.14$; calcaneus inclination, CAS, $0.1 \pm 1.4°$, C-arm, $2.7 \pm 4.8°$, $p = 0.05$; calcaneus length, CAS, -0.5 ± 0.4 mm, C-arm, -2.8 ± 1.3 mm, $p = 0.005$; Boehler's angle, CAS, $0.4 \pm 1.1°$, C-arm, $4.1 \pm 8.6°$, $p = 0.37$.

When further analyzing the correction in the different pathology specimen models, the highest differences (lowest t values) between the CAS group and the C-arm group were observed in "calcaneus malunion" specimen model, followed by the "equinus deformity" and the "equinovarus deformity" specimen models.

In conclusion, in an experimental setting, CT-based CAS provided higher accuracy for the correction of hindfoot and midfoot deformities than C-arm-based correction.[59]

The reasons for the double time needed with CT-based CAS in comparison with the C-arm-based method are the requirements of the data transfer of the DICOM data of the preoperative CT scan to the CAS device and especially the very time consuming matching process during the registration procedure. The main problems with the matching are based on the difficult bony architecture of the foot with 28 bones and more than 30 joints. Due to these anatomic conditions, the foot does not regularly maintain its complete integrity and position during the preoperative CT and the registration. This makes the registration in the foot much more difficult than in other body regions like the spine or the pelvis with lesser and larger bones and joints.[36,38,47,58,60]

In the clinical application of CT-based CAS at the foot, the problems with the registration will still increase, although the soft tissue coverage is favorable thin. When the registration was finally finished, the CT-based CAS as used in our study was more accurate and even easier and faster than the conventional C-arm, but the problems with the registration will prevent broad clinical use. Fortunately, while this experimental study was planned and performed, two CAS methods without registration were introduced, the C-arm-based CAS and the ISO-3-D-based CAS. These CAS methods without registration are especially interesting for the foot region. Clinical studies must show whether these registration-free methods can achieve high accuracy like CT-based CAS in real operations, and if this leads to better clinical results.

ISO-C-3D-Based Computer-Assisted Surgery

In our institution, ISO-C-3D-based CAS was co-developed and first used for retrograde drillings in osteochondral defects of the talus.[61] The goal in osteochondral defects of the talus in stages I and II, according to Berndt and Harty, is revascularization of the lesion.[62] A debridement of the chondral part is required if symptomatic.[63,64] This debridement is limited to loose cartilage or cartilage with poor quality.[63–65]

Subchondral drilling of the lesion allows revascularization. Retrograde drilling leaves the chondral surface intact and is therefore advantageous compared with antegrade drilling.[66] Arthroscopically guided drilling is limited to those lesions that could be arthroscopically identified.[65] In the remaining cases, open procedures are justified.[67] Based on these principles, CT-based CAS-guided retrograde drilling of osteochondral lesions has been described with promising results as a new technique.[66,68] CT- and fluoroscopy-based navigation systems in current use are limited in their flexibility.[59,61] The drawbacks of fluoroscopy are lack of 3D imaging intraoperatively. CT-based navigation still requires intraoperative cumbersome registration, extra preoperative planning, and imaging with further technical resources.

In addition to the current method of arthroscopic evaluation and treatment, we also introduce an alternative technique of using ISO-C-3D-based CAS-guided retrograde drilling of lesions.

Study Results

All patients with symptomatic osteochondrosis dissecans stadium I and II, according to Berndt and Harty, of the talus between June 1, 2003 and July 31, 2003 were included in a follow-up study. Exclusion criteria were a higher stadium or if the device was not available for the study because it was also being used for procedures other than foot and ankle. The patients were treated with ISO-C-3D-based navigated retrograde drilling. Time spent, accuracy, problems, and surgeons' rating (VAS, 0–10 points) were recorded and analyzed. The accuracy of the drillings were assessed by the intraoperative 3D imaging device (ISO-C-3D™). Clinical and radiological follow-ups were performed using the following scores: VAS foot and ankle (VAS FA) and SF36 (standardized on a possible 100-point maximum scale for better comparison with the VAS FA).

Technical Background

An ISO-C-3D (description above, Fig. 79.1) is connected to a navigation system (Surgigate™, Medivision, Oberdorf, Switzerland & Northern Digital Inc.). After fixation of a dynamic reference basis (DRB) to the bone (Fig. 79.3a), an ISO-C-3D scan follows (Fig. 79.4b). The data are transferred to the navigation system. The starting point and end point, and direction and length of the drilling is planned on the screen of the navigation system using the standard software. A trajectory for the drilling is placed in the virtual bone on the screen. The drilling is performed with a modified navigated electrical power drilling machine (Powerdrive, Synthes Inc., Bochum, Germany, Fig. 79.3a, b). The direction and length of the drilling is shown on the monitor of the navigation device. Standard fluoroscopy is not needed during the entire procedure.

Ten patients ($n = 6$ at lateral talar shoulder; $n = 4$ at medial talar shoulder) were treated with ISO-C-3D-based CAS-guided retrograde drilling. The time needed for preparation, including the placement of the DRB, scanning time, and preparation of the trajectories was 580 s (range, 500–750 s). All drillings were in the correct positions (deviation from planned position less than 2° and 2 mm). No surgery-related complication, in particular, no infection occured. The surgeons' ratings were: feasibility, VAS 9 (range, 7.3–10); accuracy 8.5 (range, 5.8–10); and clinical benefit 8.5 (range, 5.7–10). The time of follow-up was 18 months (range, 12–28 months). Nine patients could be included in the follow-up study. One patient required OATS after initial clinical improvement, and had to be excluded. The VAS FA was 92 (range, 86–98), and

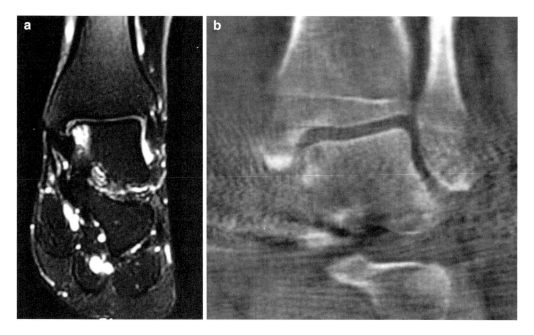

Fig. 79.3 ISO-C-3D based computer-assisted surgery (CAS). ISO-C-3D-based CAS-guided retrograde drilling in osteochondrosis dissecans tali. MRI image (**a**) and ISO-C-3D image from data transferred to the navigation system (**b**) of an osteochondrosis dissecans tali (Hepple/Winson stadium II)

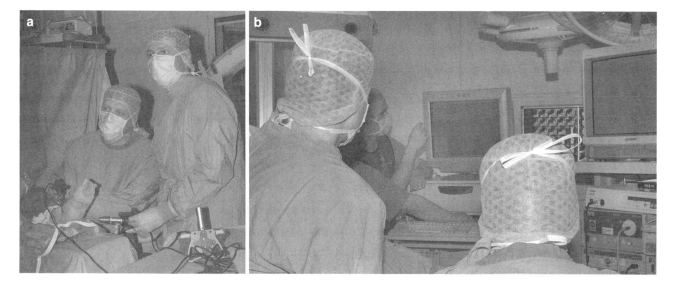

Fig. 79.4 ISO-C-3D-based computer-assisted surgery (CAS). ISO-C-3D-based CAS-guided retrograde drilling in osteochondrosis dissecans tali. Retrograde drilling with starting point at the lateral talar process (**a**) and visualization on the screen of the CAS device in real time (**b**)

the SF36 was 89 (range, 79–97). The different score categories averaged as follows:

– Pain: VAS FA, 85 (range, 69–100); SF36, 87 (range, 80–100)
– Function: VAS FA, 94 (range, 88–99); SF36, 96 (range, 83–100)
– Other complaints: VAS FA, 96 (range, 87–99); SF36, 85 (range, 67–93)

The ISO-C-3D-based CAS worked without problems in the described cases. However, the handling of the system is very complex. During the developing process, the systems was very trouble-prone due to computer control failures.

The introduced system was reliable and in frequent use at our department for surgical procedures in different body regions. The advantages of the introduced technique are an actual and almost real-time ISO-C-3D for the use of navigation without the need for anatomical registration and an immediate intraoperative control of surgical treatment.[2] Our results reveal that ISO-C-3D-based CAS-guided retrograde drilling is an alternative to arthroscopically guided or open drilling for osteochondral lesions of the talus. To date, we use the same ISO-C-3D, but a different navigation device that is easier to use (VectorVision™, BrainLAB Inc., Kirchheim-Heimstetten, Germany; for description, see below). The tremendous device costs for the ISO-C-3D-based CAS will prevent standard use for retrograde drilling in osteochondral lesions of the talus alone, despite the advantages. However, the ISO-C-3D-based CAS is also useful for other body regions such as the spine and pelvis. Furthermore, the ISO-C-3D alone is a valuable tool for intraoperative 3D visualization, as described above. Radiation protection for the patient and personnel is another essential topic. The radiation of an ISO-C-3D-based CAS-guided drilling procedure is, of course, higher compared with arthroscopically based drilling. However, the ISO-C-3D-based CAS procedures produce less radiation than all conventional C-arm-based procedures and CT-based CAS.

C-Arm-Based Computer-Assisted Surgery

As described above, CAS is considered to be useful for the correction of hindfoot and midfoot deformities and for the reduction in hindfoot or midfoot fractures and fracture-dislocations.[59] CT-based CAS provided high accuracy in an experimental setting, but the very cumbersome obligatory registration process prevented clinical use.[59] A registration-free C-arm-based CAS-guided correction was fortunately developed and studied at our institution.

Study Results

Patients with posttraumatic deformities of the ankle or subtalar joint with deformity (malalignment) were included in a prospective clinical follow-up study. C-arm-based CAS-guided arthrodeses with correction of the deformity were performed. Time spent, accuracy, problems, surgeons' rating (VAS, 0–10 points), and follow-up (VAS FA, American Orthopaedic Foot and Ankle Society Hindfoot Score [AOFAS], SF36) were analyzed. The accuracy of the corrections was assessed by a new C-arm-based 3D imaging device (ISO-C-3D).

Technical Background

A navigation system with wireless DRBs was used (VectorVision™, BrainLAB Inc.). The system was connected with a modified C-arm (Exposcope™, Instrumentarium Imaging Ziehm Inc., Nuremberg, Germany; Fig. 79.5a). One DRB was fixed to each of the two bones or fragments that had been planned for correction in relation to each other.

With the C-arm, anteroposterior and lateral digital radiographic images were obtained, and the data were transferred to the navigation device. Then the correction was performed. During the correction, the angle motion and translational motion between the bones or fragments in all degrees of freedom were displayed on the screen of the navigation system (Fig. 79.5a). Furthermore, virtual radiographs with the moving bones or fragments were displayed on the screen. The C-arm was not used during the correction process. After correction, retention was performed with 2.0-mm K-wires. Then the accuracy of the correction was checked with C-arm and intraoperative 3D imaging with ISO-C-3D (Siemens Inc., Germany). Finally, screw fixation followed. The insertion of the screws was also C-arm-based CAS guided (data not shown).

Twelve patients were included (ankle correction arthrodesis, $n = 3$; subtalar correction arthrodesis, $n = 6$; combined ankle/subtalar joint correction arthrodesis, $n = 2$; Lisfranc correction arthrodesis, $n = 1$). The time needed for preparation, scanning time, and preparation on the screen for the correction was 500 s (range, 400–900 s). The correction process took 45 s (range, 30–60 s). All planned angles and translations were exactly achieved as planned before (deviation from planned correction less than ±2° for angles or ±2 mm for translations). Three surgeons were involved. Feasibility by VAS was 9.5 (range, 9–10); accuracy was 9.8 (range, 9.5–10); and clinical benefit was 9 (range, 8–10). Ten (83%) patients completed follow-up after 14 months (range, 6–27 months). All arthrodeses were fused at follow-up. The corrected angles and translations at follow-up (analyzed on radiographs) did not differ significantly from those measured intraoperatively (see above; t test, $p > 0.05$). The VAS FA averaged 47 (range, 25–81); the AOFAS Hindfoot Score, 57 (range, 40–64); and the SF36, 54 (range, 34–80). The different score categories averaged as follows: pain: VAS FA 47 (range, 14–85), SF36 46 (range, 11–93); function: VAS FA 41 (range, 14–85), SF36 45 (range, 8–85); and other complaints: VAS FA 52 (range, 19–83), SF36 70 (range, 55–84).

The feasibility of the introduced method was favorable. The time spent was less than 10 min for preparation. The correction process is very fast and extremely accurate, especially regarding the problems with the conventional C-arm-based correction. In our experience, the correction without CAS guidance needs more time because the necessary frequent C-arm controlling. Furthermore, it is much more difficult, not only because of the difficult visualization, but also because the very demanding correction process with 3D motion of two different fragments in relation to each other.

In conclusion, C-arm-based CAS-guided correction of posttraumatic deformities of the ankle and hindfoot region is feasible and provides very high accuracy and a faster correction process.[2,69] The significance of the introduced method is high in these cases because the improved accuracy may lead to an improved clinical outcome.[19,21–29,58]

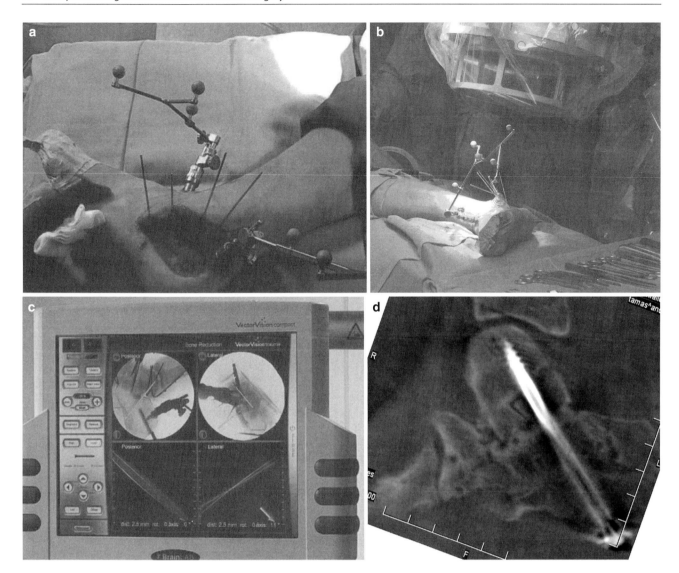

Fig. 79.5 C-arm-based computer-assisted surgery (CAS). C-arm-based CAS-guided correction of hindfoot deformity after malunited calcaneus fracture with flattening of the longitudinal arch and the Boehler's angle (0°), and hindfoot varus (10°). A correction arthrodesis of the subtalar joint with elevation of the longitudinal arch (planned Boehler's angle 30°) and correction of the varus was indicated. (**a**) The DRBs were fixed to the talar neck and to the posterior process of the calcaneus. Image acquisition and verification had been performed. (**b**) Image acquisition. (**c**) Monitor view during the navigation process. (**d**) Intraoperative imaging with ISO-C-3D (Siemens, Germany) after correction and screw fixation with bone blocks in the subtalar joint. The achieved supposed Boehler's angle was 30°. For the measurement of the Boehler's angle, the formerly posterior edge of the posterior facet was defined as the point located at the middle, i.e., the half height of the posterior rim of the posterior bone block

Intraoperative Pedography

For any kind of reduction or correction at the foot and ankle, an immediate biomechanical assessment of the reduction result would be desirable.[19,21–29] This is especially true for a CAS-guided reduction or correction, which is supposed to be more accurate than a conventional reduction.[2,61] The reduction or correction control is normally performed with a C-arm or an ISO-C-3D, if available.[2,10,59] Analyzing the position of the bones radiographically allows conclusions about the biomechanics of the foot.[19,70] However, pedography is considered to be more effective for the analysis of the biome-chanics of the foot.[71] So far, pedography for biomechanical assessment was only available during clinical follow-up.[2] An IP would be useful for immediate intraoperative biome-chanical assessment.[2]

Study Results

A new device was developed to perform IP. A feasibility study was first performed.[72] Then a study for validation followed to compare the introduced method with standard dynamic pedography.[73] Finally, a prospective consecutive randomized multicenter study is in progress to analyze the clinical benefit of IP.

For an intraoperative introduction of standardized forces to the foot sole, a device named Kraftsimulator Intraoperative Pedographie (KIOP, manufactured by the Workshop of the Hannover Medical School, Hannover, Germany; registered design no. 202004007755.8 by the German Patent Office, Munich, Germany, Figs. 79.6a, b and 79.7) was developed. The pedographic measurement is performed with a custom-made mat with capacitive sensors (PLIANCE™, Novel Inc., Munich, Germany). The system allows real-time pedography and comparison with the contralateral side. The measurements were performed in the neutral ankle position. In this neutral ankle position, the influence of the missing muscle action in the anesthetized patient is considered to be minimal because the electromyelogram (EMG) in awake standing individuals with a comparable ankle position is silent.[74–76]

Validation Study

The validation was performed in two steps:

Step 1 was a comparison of standard dynamic pedography (three trials, walking, third step; and three trials, mid stance force pattern), static in the standing position (three trials), and pedography with KIOP in healthy volunteers (three trials; total force, 400 N). For dynamic pedography and pedography in the standing position, a standard platform (EMED™, Novel Inc.) was used.

Step 2 was a comparison of pedography in the standing position, pedography with KIOP in non-anesthetized and anesthetized patients (three trials; total force, 400 N). Patients with operative procedures performed at the knee or distal to the knee were excluded. Only patients with general or spinal anesthesia were included.

Additionally, a qualitative analysis was performed for both steps (Fig. 79.8a, b). The analysis was focused on the force distribution and not on the force values. The relation of the forces of different regions; the hindfoot, midfoot, and forefoot (first metatarsal, second to fourth metatarsal, fifth metatarsal), and medial vs. lateral were compared. The different measurement and qualitative analyses were compared (*t* test, one-way analysis of variance [ANOVA]).

The results of the validation process were as follows. In step 1, 30 individuals were included (age, 26.1 ± 8.6 years; sex, male:female = 24:6). In step 2, 30 individuals were included (age, 55.3 ± 30.3 years; sex, male:female = 24:6). No statistically significant differences were found in either

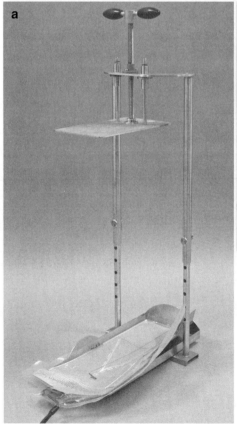
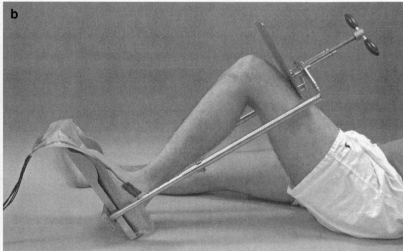

Fig. 79.6 Intraoperative pedography (IP). The newly developed device for intraoperative force introduction (KIOP) (**a**). The custom-made mat for force registration (PLIANCE™, Novel, Inc.) is covered intraoperatively with a sterile plastic bag and is placed on the KIOP, as also shown in Fig. 79.7. The size of the mat is 16 × 32 cm. The mat includes 32 × 32 sensors with a sensor size of 0.5 × 1 cm. Fig. 79.7 shows a scheme of the modus for IP

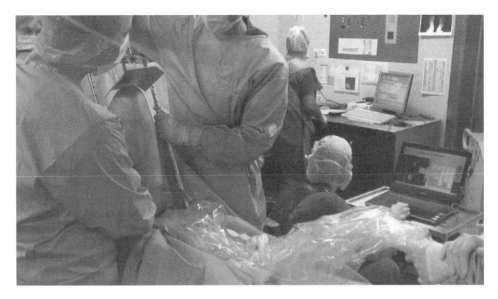

Fig. 79.7 Intraoperative pedography (IP). IP during a correction arthrodesis at the talonavicular joint (performed during a feasibility prestudy); 400 N comparable to half body weight was applied. The force measurements were displayed in real time on the screen of the pedography system. During the IP, KIOP is entirely sterile and the force measurement mat (PLIANCE™, Novel Inc.) is covered by a sterile plastic bag

step between the methods, nor between the methods of step 1 and 2 (*t* test and ANOVA, *p* > 0.05).Clinical Prospective Study

Sixteen patients were included until March 15, 2006 (ankle correction arthrodesis, *n* = 2; subtalar joint correction arthrodesis, *n* = 4; correction arthrodesis midfoot, *n* = 4; correction forefoot, *n* = 4; Lisfranc fracture-dislocation). Nine patients were randomized for the use of IP, whereas four patients had no intraoperative measurement. The mean preoperative scores were as follows: AOFAS, 51.6 ± 22.6; VAS FA, 45.2 ± 14.4; and SF36, 47.3 ± 21.4. No score differences between the two groups occurred (*t* test, *p* > 0.05). The mean interruption of operative procedure for the IP was 323 ± 32 s. In four (44%) of the nine patients, changes were made after IP during the same operative procedure (correction modified, *n* = 3; screw tightened, *n* = 1). The follow-up has not been completed so far.

In conclusion, IP is feasible and valid because no statistical significant differences were found between the measurements of the introduced method for IP in anesthetized individuals and the standard dynamic and static pedography. In the future, dynamic IP with registration of the entire foot sole is planned for an even more sophisticated biomechanical assessment.[2,72,73] During clinical use, in 50% of the cases, a modification of the surgical correction was made after IP in the same surgical procedure. A follow-up of these patients has to be completed to show whether these changes improve the clinical outcome. In any case, IP was able to detect insufficient biomechanical behavior of the foot and it may lead to modifications in the same procedure, instead of after pedography in the office weeks or months later.[2,72,73]

What Do We Need When?

The perfect surgeon who does not make any mistakes without any guidance does not need any of the introduced systems. However, the surgical staff involved in foot and ankle surgery consists of experienced surgeons as well as interns, residents, and fellows in training. In times of increasing legal pressure regarding working hours, the acquisition of surgical experience is harder. Tools for improved intraoperative imaging (ISO-C-3D), guidance (CAS), or biomechanical assessment (IP) may help the surgeon in training to achieve the planned result with less experience.[3]

Iso-c-3d

ISO-C-3D is most helpful in closed procedures and/or when axial reformations provide information that is not possible to obtain with a C-arm or with direct visualization.[10] Weber-C fractures and calcaneus fractures are examples for these special situations. The ISO-C-3D is less helpful when easy visualization with a C-arm or under direct vision is possible, as, for example, in Weber-B fractures during open reduction and internal fixation.

Computer-Assisted Surgery

CAS is helpful in complex 3D corrections or reduction, and in closed placement of drillings and/or screw positioning.[2,59]

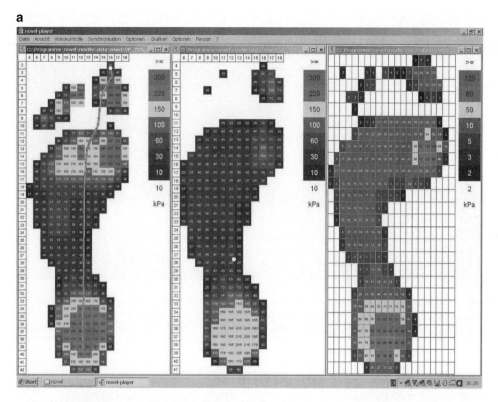

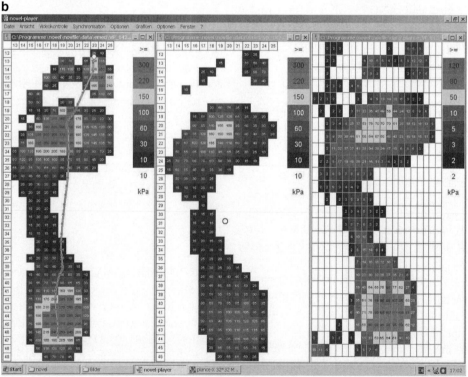

Fig. 79.8 Intraoperative pedography (IP). Images from the qualitative analysis of the validation process of IP. (a) Step 1: awake volunteer - *left* pedography with KIOP; *middle* static pedography in standing position; *right* standard dynamic pedography. For dynamic pedography and pedog-raphy in the standing position, a standard platform (EMED Novel Inc.) was used. (b) Step 2: non-anesthetized/anesthetized patient - *left* pedography in the standing position; *middle* pedography with KIOP in a non-anesthetized individual; *right* IP in an anesthetized individual

The significance of the introduced CAS methods is high in those cases because the improved accuracy may lead to an improved clinical outcome like complex corrections in the hindfoot and midfoot deformities.[19,21–29] CAS is too complex and time consuming for cases that are accurately and easily performed by the experienced surgeon.

Intraoperative Pedography

IP will be useful for cases in which biomechanical assessment may lead to an immediate improvement of the achieved surgical result.[2,72,73] The same cases that are currently analyzed with clinical preoperative or postoperative pedography will potentially profit from IP. The surgeon's experience is also crucial for the use of IP, because experienced surgeons who do not use pedography in their office may also not use it intraoperatively. IP as introduced was made possible by the newly developed device for intraoperative force introduction (KIOP).

Integrated Computer System for Operative Procedures

For the future, the integration of the different computerized systems will improve the handling and clinical feasibility. An integration of preoperative pedography, planning software, CAS, ISO-C-3D, and IP in one integrated computer system for operative procedures (ICOP) will be favorable. Within this kind of ICOP, the preoperative computerized planning will be able to include preoperative radiographic, CT, magnetic resonance imaging (MRI), and pedography data. The preoperative computerized planning result will be transferred to the CAS device. Intraoperative 2D (C-arm) or 3D (ISO-C-3D) imaging will allow registration-free CAS and will be matched with preoperative CT and or MRI images. The CAS-system will be guided by biomechanical assessment with IP that allows not only morphological but also biomechanical-based CAS. The ISO-C-3D data and the IP data will be matched with the data from the planning software to allow immediate improvements of reduction, correction, and or drilling/implant position in the same procedure.[3]

In conclusion, in the future, computerized methods for improved intraoperative imaging, guidance, and biomechanical assessment will help to realize the planned operative result.[3]

The development will be similar to navigation systems in the car. Two decades ago, many people doubted that we need these systems. Today almost everybody has a system, but, of course, no one uses them for short and easy routes; rather, they are used for long and difficult journeys. Similarly, we will have these systems (ISO-C-3D, CAS, IP) available in a few years, but they will not be used in the easy standard case but for difficult and complex procedures. The costs of these systems are high, but the increased outcome will decrease the overall costs for the medical system.[3]

Acknowledgments   The author thanks Christian Krettek, MD, FRACS, Director or Trauma, Stefan Zech, MD, Jens Geerling, MD, Michael Frink, MD, Tobias Huefner, MD, Daniel Kendoff, MD, Musa Citak, MD, Nicolas Vanin, Patricia Droste, Claudia Schultz-Blum, Alke Bretzke, Carolina Böse, Angelika Heinrich, and Vital Karch, Trauma Department, Hannover Medical School, Hannover Germany for their valuable contribution in carrying out the surgical procedures and the handling of the introduced technical devices.

References

1. Dahlen C, Zwipp H. [Computer-assisted surgical planning. 3-D software for the PC]. Unfallchirurg 2001; 104(6):466–479.
2. Richter M. Foot and Ankle Surgery: Today and in the Future. In: 5th Congress of the European Foot and Ankle Society (EFAS), Montpellier, 29 April–01 May 2004, Abstracts, 2004.
3. Richter M. Computer based systems in foot and ankle surgery at the beginning of the 21st century. Fuss Sprungg 2006; 4(1):59–71.
4. Euler E, Wirth S, Linsenmaier U, Mutschler W, Pfeifer KJ, Hebecker A. [Comparative study of the quality of C-arm based 3D imaging of the talus]. Unfallchirurg 2001; 104(9):839–846.
5. Kotsianos D, Rock C, Euler E, Wirth S, Linsenmaier U, Brandl R et al. [3-D imaging with a mobile surgical image enhancement equipment (ISO-C-3D). Initial examples of fracture diagnosis of peripheral joints in comparison with spiral CT and conventional radiography]. Unfallchirurg 2001; 104(9):834–838.
6. Kotsianos D, Rock C, Wirth S, Linsenmaier U, Brandl R, Fischer T et al. [Detection of tibial condylar fractures using 3D imaging with a mobile image amplifier (Siemens ISO-C-3D): comparison with plain films and spiral CT]. Rofo Fortschr Geb Rontgenstr Neuen Bildgeb Verfahr 2002; 174(1):82–87.
7. Kotsianos D, Wirth S, Fischer T, Euler E, Rock C, Linsenmaier U et al. 3D imaging with an isocentric mobile C-arm comparison of image quality with spiral CT. Eur Radiol 2004; 14(9):1590–1595.
8. Rock C, Kotsianos D, Linsenmaier U, Fischer T, Brandl R, Vill F et al. [Studies on image quality, high contrast resolution and dose for the axial skeleton and limbs with a new, dedicated CT system (ISO-C-3 D)]. Rofo Fortschr Geb Rontgenstr Neuen Bildgeb Verfahr 2002; 174(2):170–176.
9. Rock C, Linsenmaier U, Brandl R, Kotsianos D, Wirth S, Kaltschmidt R et al. [Introduction of a new mobile C-arm/CT combination equipment (ISO-C-3D). Initial results of 3-D sectional imaging]. Unfallchirurg 2001; 104(9):827–833.
10. Richter M, Geerling J, Zech S, Goesling T, Krettek C. Intraoperative three-dimensional imaging with a motorized mobile C-arm (SIREMOBIL ISO-C-3D) in foot and ankle trauma care: a preliminary report. J Orthop Trauma 2005; 19(4):259–266.
11. Richter M, Geerling J, Kendoff D, Hufner T, Krettek C. Intraoperative 3-D Imaging with a Mobile Image Amplifier (ISO-C 3D) in Foot and Ankle Trauma Care. In: American Orthopaedic Foot and Ankle Society, 19th Annual Summer Meeting, Final Program 78, 2003.
12. Adelaar RS. The treatment of complex fractures of the talus. Orthop Clin North Am 1989; 20(4):691–707.
13. Amon K. Luxationsfraktur der kuneonavikularen Gelenklinie. Klinik, Pathomechanismus und Therapiekonzept einer sehr seltenen Fussverletzung. Unfallchirurg 1990; 93(9):431–434.

14. Brutscher R. Frakturen und Luxationen des Mittel- und Vorfusses. Orthopäde 1991; 20(1):67–75.

15. Hansen STJ. Functional reconstruction of the foot and ankle. Philadelphia, PA: Lippincott Williams & Wilkins, 2000.

16. Hildebrand KA, Buckley RE, Mohtadi NG, Faris P. Functional outcome measures after displaced intra-articular calcaneal fractures. J Bone Joint Surg Br 1996; 78(1):119–123.

17. Richter M, Wippermann B, Krettek C, Schratt E, Hufner T, Thermann H. Fractures and fracture dislocations of the midfoot - occurrence, causes and long-term results. Foot Ankle Int 2001; 22(5):392–398.

18. Suren EG, Zwipp H. Luxationsfrakturen im Chopart- und Lisfranc-Gelenk. Unfallchirurg 1989; 92(3):130–139.

19. Zwipp H. Chirurgie des Fusses, 1st edn. Berlin Heidelberg New York: Springer, 1994.

20. Zwipp H, Dahlen C, Randt T, Gavlik JM. Komplextrauma des Fusses. Orthopäde 1997; 26(12):1046–1056.

21. Adelaar RS, Kyles MK. Surgical correction of resistant talipes equinovarus: observations and analysis - preliminary report. Foot Ankle 1981; 2(3):126–137.

22. Coetzee JC, Hansen ST. Surgical management of severe deformity resulting from posterior tibial tendon dysfunction. Foot Ankle Int 2001; 22(12):944–949.

23. Koczewski P, Shadi M, Napiontek M. Foot lengthening using the Ilizarov device: the transverse tarsal joint resection versus osteotomy. J Pediatr Orthop B 2002; 11(1):68–72.

24. Marti RK, de Heus JA, Roolker W, Poolman RW, Besselaar PP. Subtalar arthrodesis with correction of deformity after fractures of the os calcis. J Bone Joint Surg Br 1999; 81(4):611–616.

25. Mosier-LaClair S, Pomeroy G, Manoli A. Operative treatment of the difficult stage 2 adult acquired flatfoot deformity. Foot Ankle Clin 2001; 6(1):95–119.

26. Sammarco GJ, Conti SF. Surgical treatment of neuroarthropathic foot deformity. Foot Ankle Int 1998; 19(2):102–109.

27. Stephens HM, Walling AK, Solmen JD, Tankson CJ. Subtalar repositional arthrodesis for adult acquired flatfoot. Clin Orthop Relat Res 1999 Aug; (365):69–73.

28. Toolan BC, Sangeorzan BJ, Hansen ST Jr. Complex reconstruction for the treatment of dorsolateral peritalar subluxation of the foot. Early results after distraction arthrodesis of the calcaneocuboid joint in conjunction with stabilization of, and transfer of the flexor digitorum longus tendon to, the midfoot to treat acquired pes planovalgus in adults. J Bone Joint Surg Am 1999; 81(11):1545–1560.

29. Wei SY, Sullivan RJ, Davidson RS. Talo-navicular arthrodesis for residual midfoot deformities of a previously corrected clubfoot. Foot Ankle Int 2000; 21(6):482–485.

30. Bailey EJ, Waggoner SM, Albert MJ, Hutton WC. Intraarticular calcaneus fractures: a biomechanical comparison or two fixation methods. J Orthop Trauma 1997; 11(1):34–37.

31. Trnka HJ, Easley ME, Lam PW, Anderson CD, Schon LC, Myerson MS. Subtalar distraction bone block arthrodesis. J Bone Joint Surg Br 2001; 83(6):849–854.

32. Bargar WL, Bauer A, Borner M. Primary and revision total hip replacement using the Robodoc system. Clin Orthop Relat Res 1998 Sep; (354):82–91.

33. Claes J, Koekelkoren E, Wuyts FL, Claes GM, Van Den HL, Van De Heyning PH. Accuracy of computer navigation in ear, nose, throat surgery: the influence of matching strategy. Arch Otolaryngol Head Neck Surg 2000; 126(12):1462–1466.

34. Delp SL, Stulberg SD, Davies B, Picard F, Leitner F. Computer assisted knee replacement. Clin Orthop Relat Res 1998 Sep; (354):49–56.

35. DiGioia AM III, Jaramaz B, Colgan BD. Computer assisted orthopaedic surgery. Image guided and robotic assistive technologies. Clin Orthop Relat Res 1998 Sep; (354):8–16.

36. DiGioia AM III, Jaramaz B, Plakseychuk AY, Moody JE Jr, Nikou C, Labarca RS et al. Comparison of a mechanical acetabular alignment guide with computer placement of the socket. J Arthroplasty 2002; 17(3):359–364.

37. Hassfeld S, Muhling J. Navigation in maxillofacial and craniofacial surgery. Comput Aided Surg 1998; 3(4):183–187.

38. Jaramaz B, DiGioia AM III, Blackwell M, Nikou C. Computer assisted measurement of cup placement in total hip replacement. Clin Orthop Relat Res 1998 Sep; (354):70–81.

39. Kamimura M, Ebara S, Itoh H, Tateiwa Y, Kinoshita T, Takaoka K. Accurate pedicle screw insertion under the control of a computer-assisted image guiding system: laboratory test and clinical study. J Orthop Sci 1999; 4(3):197–206.

40. Kato A, Yoshimine T, Hayakawa TM et al. [Computer assisted neurosurgery: development of a frameless and armless navigation system (CNS navigator)]. No Shinkei Geka 1991; 19(2):137–142.

41. Kerschbaumer F. ["Numerical imaging, operation planning, simulation, navigation, robotics". Do the means determine the end? (editorial)]. Orthopade 2000; 29(7):597–598.

42. Klos TV, Banks SA, Habets RJ, Cook FF. Sagittal plane imaging parameters for computer-assisted fluoroscopic anterior cruciate ligament reconstruction. Comput Aided Surg 2000; 5(1):28–34.

43. Klos TV, Habets RJ, Banks AZ, Banks SA, Devilee RJ, Cook FF. Computer assistance in arthroscopic anterior cruciate ligament reconstruction. Clin Orthop Relat Res 1998 Sep; (354):65–69.

44. Laine T, Lund T, Ylikoski M, Lohikoski J, Schlenzka D. Accuracy of pedicle screw insertion with and without computer assistance: a randomised controlled clinical study in 100 consecutive patients. Eur Spine J 2000; 9(3):235–240.

45. Langlotz F, Bachler R, Berlemann U, Nolte LP, Ganz R. Computer assistance for pelvic osteotomies. Clin Orthop Relat Res 1998 Sep; (354):92–102.

46. Merloz P, Tonetti J, Cinquin P, Lavallee S, Troccaz J, Pittet L. [Computer-assisted surgery: automated screw placement in the vertebral pedicle]. Chirurgie 1998; 123(5):482–490.

47. Merloz P, Tonetti J, Pittet L, Coulomb M, Lavallee S, Troccaz J et al. Computer-assisted spine surgery. Comput Aided Surg 1998; 3(6):297–305.

48. Ploder O, Wagner A, Enislidis G, Ewers R. [Computer-assisted intraoperative visualization of dental implants. Augmented reality in medicine]. Radiologe 1995; 35(9):569–572.

49. Radermacher K, Portheine F, Anton M, Zimolong A, Kaspers G, Rau G et al. Computer assisted orthopaedic surgery with image based individual templates. Clin Orthop Relat Res 1998 Sep; (354):28–38.

50. Schlenzka D, Laine T, Lund T. Computer-assisted spine surgery. Eur Spine J 2000; 9(Suppl 1):S57–S64.

51. Tonetti J, Carrat L, Blendea S, Merloz P, Troccaz J, Lavallee S et al. Clinical results of percutaneous pelvic surgery. Computer assisted surgery using ultrasound compared to standard fluoroscopy. Comput Aided Surg 2001; 6(4):204–211.

52. Tonetti J, Carrat L, Lavallee S, Pittet L, Merloz P, Chirossel JP. Percutaneous iliosacral screw placement using image guided techniques. Clin Orthop Relat Res 1998 Sep; (354):103–110.

53. Weihe S, Wehmoller M, Schliephake H, Hassfeld S, Tschakaloff A, Raczkowsky J et al. Synthesis of CAD/CAM, robotics and biomaterial implant fabrication: single-step reconstruction in computer aided frontotemporal bone resection. Int J Oral Maxillofac Surg 2000; 29(5):384–388.

54. Birkfellner W, Huber K, Larson A, Hanson D, Diemling M, Homolka P et al. A modular software system for computer-aided surgery and its first application in oral implantology. IEEE Trans Med Imaging 2000; 19(6):616–620.

55. Schiffers N, Schkommodau E, Portheine F, Radermacher K, Staudte HW. [Planning and performance of orthopedic surgery with the help of individual templates]. Orthopade 2000; 29(7):636–640.

56. Schlenzka D, Laine T, Lund T. [Computer-assisted spine surgery: principles, technique, results and perspectives]. Orthopade 2000; 29(7):658–669.

57. Thoma W, Schreiber S, Hovy L. [Computer-assisted implant positioning in knee endoprosthetics. Kinematic analysis for optimization of surgical technique]. Orthopade 2000; 29(7):614–626.

58. Bechtold JE, Powless SH. The application of computer graphics in foot and ankle surgical planning and reconstruction. Clin Podiatr Med Surg 1993; 10(3):551–562.

59. Richter M. Experimental comparison between computer assisted surgery (CAS) based and C-Arm based correction of hind- and midfoot deformities. Osteo Trauma Care 2003; 11:29–34.

60. Foley KT, Smith MM. Image-guided spine surgery. Neurosurg Clin N Am 1996; 7(2):171–186.

61. Richter M, Geerling J, Zech S, Krettek C. ISO-C-3D based computer assisted surgery (CAS) guided retrograde drilling in a osteochondrosis dissecans of the talus: a case report. Foot 2005; 15(2):107–113.

62. Berndt AL., Harty M. Transchondral fractures (osteochondritis dissecans) of the talus. Am J Orthop 1959; 41-A:988–1020.

63. Alexander AH, Lichtman DM. Surgical treatment of transchondral talar-dome fractures (osteochondritis dissecans). Long-term follow-up. J Bone Joint Surg Am 1980; 62(4):646–652.

64. Tol JL, Struijs PA, Bossuyt PM, Verhagen RA, van Dijk CN. Treatment strategies in osteochondral defects of the talar dome: a systematic review. Foot Ankle Int 2000; 21(2):119–126.

65. Taranow WS, Bisignani GA, Towers JD, Conti SF. Retrograde drilling of osteochondral lesions of the medial talar dome. Foot Ankle Int 1999; 20(8):474–480.

66. Fink C, Rosenberger RE, Bale RJ, Rieger M, Hackl W, Benedetto KP et al. Computer-assisted retrograde drilling of osteochondral lesions of the talus. Orthopade 2001; 30(1):59–65.

67. Seil R, Rupp S, Pape D, Dienst M, Kohn D. [Approach to open treatment of osteochondral lesions of the talus]. Orthopade 2001; 30(1):47–52.

68. Rosenberger RE, Bale RJ, Fink C, Rieger M, Reichkendler M, Hackl W et al. [Computer-assisted drilling of the lower extremity. Technique and indications]. Unfallchirurg 2002; 105(4):353–358.

69. Richter M, Geerling J, Frink M, Zech S, Knobloch K, Dammann F et al. Computer assisted surgery based (CAS) based correction of posttraumatic ankle and hindfoot deformities - preliminary results. Foot Ankle Surg 2006; 12:113–119.

70. Zwipp H. Biomechanik der Sprunggelenke. Unfallchirurg 1989; 92(3):98–102.

71. Rosenbaum D, Becker HP, Sterk J, Gerngross H, Claes L. Functional evaluation of the 10-year outcome after modified Evans repair for chronic ankle instability. Foot Ankle Int 1997; 18(12):765–771.

72. Richter M, Frink M, Zech S, Droste P, Knobloch K, Krettek C. Technique for intraoperative use of pedography. Tech Foot Ankle 2006; 5(2):88–100.

73. Richter M, Frink M, Zech S, Vanin N, Geerling J, Droste P et al. Intraoperative pedography - a new validated method for intraoperative biomechanical assessment. Foot Ankle Int 2006; 27(10):833–842.

74. Duranti R, Galletti R, Pantaleo T. Electromyographic observations in patients with foot pain syndromes. Am J Phys Med 1985; 64(6):295–304.

75. Kawakami O, Sudoh H, Watanabe S. Effects of linear movements on upright standing position. Environ Med 1996; 40(2):193–196.

76. Trepman E, Gellman RE, Solomon R, Murthy KR, Micheli LJ, De Luca CJ. Electromyographic analysis of standing posture and demi-plie in ballet and modern dancers. Med Sci Sports Exerc 1994; 26(6):771–782.

Chapter 80
Robotics in Total Knee Arthroplasty

Werner Siebert, Sabine Mai, and Peter F. Heeckt

Total knee arthroplasty (TKA) has become the standard procedure in the management of degenerative joint disease after conservative therapy options have been exhausted. However, despite conscientious planning and carefully performed procedures, surgeons are often unsatisfied with implant alignment. Various authors described significant axial or rotational malalignment, and mediolateral and ventrodorsal tilt.[1-4] Seemingly small displacements of 2.5 mm potentially alter the range of motion by as much as 20°.[5] None of the contemporary improvements in implant design and instrumentation has alleviated these problems.

This led to the development of various robotic systems for improved precision in surgery. Robots are able to accurately position and move tools, thereby reducing human error. These systems rely on preoperative imaging, registration, and planning. The first clinical use was reported 1985 in the field of neurosurgery.[6] Orthopedic surgeons started using robotic devices around 1992 for total hip arthroplasty.[7] The active surgical robot CASPAR® (Computer-Assisted Surgical Planning and Robotics) was adapted for total hip and knee arthroplasty and for anterior cruciate ligament repair.[8] The first robot-assisted knee replacement with this system was performed in March of 2000 in the Orthopedic Center Kassel. A total of 108 consecutive cases were operated on at this institution and followed-up for at least 5 years in a prospective study.[9]

Surgical Technique

Robot-assisted TKA consists of the placement of fiducial markers, computed tomographic (CT) scanning, preoperative planning, and surgery.

W. Siebert (✉), S. Mai, and P.F. Heeckt
Vitos Orthopaedic Center Kassel, Wilhelmshoeher Allee 345,
34131 Kassel, Germany
e-mail: werner.siebert@vitos-okk.de

Placement of Fiducial Markers

To facilitate orientation, the robot requires placement of a femoral and a tibial pin that serve as fiducial markers for each bone (Fig. 80.1). The robot uses these pins for spatial orientation and performs geometric calculations based on their location.

CT Scanning and Preoperative Planning

A helical CT scan is obtained immediately after the pins have been placed. Particular attention is paid to the areas of the femoral head, the pins, the knee, and the ankle. The CT data are then transferred into the PC-based planning station. The technical quality of the scan is automatically checked and the pin position is verified. The surgeon identifies specific anatomical landmarks. The anatomical and mechanical axes of the femur and tibia are then calculated in the frontal and sagittal planes. The joint line, epicondylar twist, torsion of the tibia, as well as the relationship of the dorsal part of the tibia and the condylar line serve as additional important parameters. All angles and possible geometric translations are displayed on the video screen at the end of the planning procedure (Fig. 80.2).

The system allows the user to select and position a specific implant in different sizes. Unintentional notching can easily be avoided. With computer-assisted planning, the strong interdependence of all parameters, including the mechanical axes, becomes quite evident. Implant fit can be accurately assessed by scrolling through the scan. The system informs the user about the expected change in "extension" and "flexion gaps" and the resulting ligament tension. After positioning the implants, it is important to specify the milling areas in order to avoid redundant cutting and to protect the surrounding soft tissue. As a last step, the system prints out an overview of the final plan. All data are stored on a PC card and transferred to the robot control unit immediately before surgery.

G.R. Scuderi and A.J. Tria (eds.), *Minimally Invasive Surgery in Orthopedics*,
DOI 10.1007/978-0-387-76608-9_80, © Springer Science+Business Media, LLC 2010

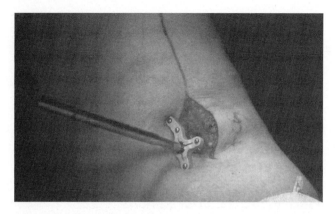

Fig. 80.1 Fastening of the special CT cross on the tibial pin (From Konermann W, Haaker R (eds.), Navigation und Robotic in der Gelenk- und Wirbelsäulenchirurgie. Berlin, Springer, 2003, with kind permission of Springer Science + Business Media, Inc.)

Robot-Assisted Surgery

A conventional median incision with parapatellar approach to the knee joint is used. The knee joint is secured by a trans-femoral and transtibial self-cutting screw to a specially designed frame. This rigid frame is also used for fixation of self-holding soft tissue retractors. In order to control for unwanted micro-movements of the leg during robotic surgery, rigid bodies with light-emitting diodes (LEDs) are firmly attached to the frame. The LED signal is constantly monitored by an infrared camera system, which will automatically shut off the robot in the event of excessive motion (Fig. 80.3). After registration of the fiducial markers, robotic milling is started by the surgeon. The cutting tool is equipped with internal water cooling and irrigation. A splash guard helps to keep the operative field and LEDs dry and clean (Fig. 80.4). Milling heads are changed during the procedure depending on the type of cut to be made. Varying with the size of the

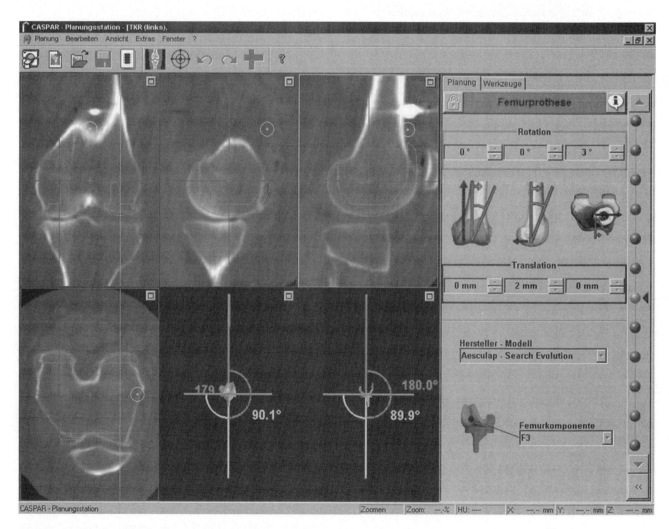

Fig. 80.2 Original screen-shot from the planning station showing the PC-based planning of the femoral component and the resulting mechanical leg axis (From Konermann W, Haaker R (eds.), Navigation und Robotic in der Gelenk- und Wirbelsäulenchirurgie. Berlin, Springer, 2003, with kind permission of Springer Science + Business Media, Inc.)

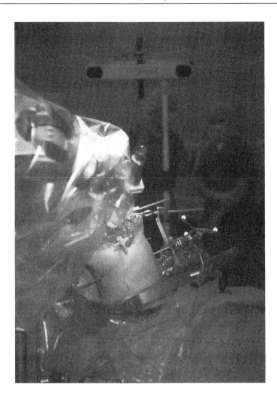

Fig. 80.3 View of the working robot. Unwanted motion is detected by an infrared camera system as seen in the background and corresponding rigid bodies fixed to the frame in the foreground (From Konermann W, Haaker R (eds.), Navigation und Robotic in der Gelenk- und Wirbelsäulenchirurgie. Berlin, Springer, 2003, with kind permission of Springer Science + Business Media, Inc.)

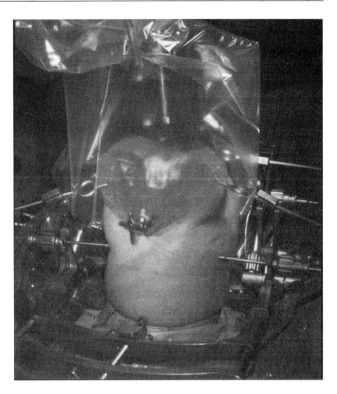

Fig. 80.4 Knee securely fixed with cutting tool and splash guard in place right before femoral milling action commences. The tibial registration cross is still in place at the distal end of the incision (From Konermann W, Haaker R (eds.), Navigation und Robotic in der Gelenk- und Wirbelsäulenchirurgie. Berlin, Springer, 2003, with kind permission of Springer Science + Business Media, Inc.)

implant and bone density, the entire milling procedure takes approximately 18 min. If required, it is possible to revert to conventional manual technique at any point during surgery.

The resulting bone surfaces are accurately shaped and smooth (Fig. 80.5). After the fixation frame and pins are removed, soft tissues are balanced and the components of the implant are inserted. In this study, we started with the cemented LC Search Evolution knee system (Aesculap, Tuttlingen, Germany) in the robotic group because this was the first knee implant system geometry that was loaded into the planning software.

Patients and Methods

A total of 108 knees were operated on using the robot system CASPAR. The following cruciate-retaining implant designs were used: 70 Search Evolution (Aesculap), 31 PFC Sigma® (DePuy Orthopedics, Inc., Warsaw, IN), and 7 Genesis (Smith & Nephew, Memphis, TN). Of these, 55 were implanted with both components being cemented (Figs. 80.6a, b and 80.7a, b), 46 implants were hybrids (tibia cemented, femur cementless), and 7 were completely cement-

less (Fig. 80.8). The average age of the patients (74 women, 34 men) was 66 years (range, 37–87 years). Patients were clinically evaluated before and after surgery according to the Knee Society Score.[10] All patients were followed up at intervals of 3, 6, 12, 24, and 60 months after surgery. No patients were lost to follow-up.

Before and 2 weeks after surgery, standing long-leg anteroposterior roentgenograms were taken of all patients to control for correct alignment. The mechanical leg axis was measured on these X-ray films and directly compared with the preoperative plan. Data were statistically analyzed by using a two-tailed Student's t-test. Statistical significance was assumed at a p value smaller than 0.01.

Results

General Observations and Complications

Operating time for the 108 robotic cases averaged 137 min (80–200 min). At discharge, all patients had 90° or greater of flexion. No major adverse events, directly related to the

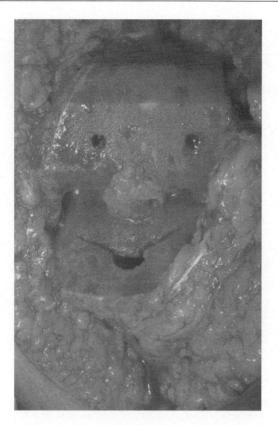

Fig. 80.5 Final tibial and femoral bone surfaces with preserved posterior cruciate ligament (From Konermann W, Haaker R (eds.), Navigation und Robotic in der Gelenk- und Wirbelsäulenchirurgie. Berlin, Springer, 2003, with kind permission of Springer Science + Business Media, Inc.)

CASPAR system, have been noted. A minor complication occurred in one patient. Due to a defective registration marker, the femoral milling process could not be completed as planned. Full correction was achieved by converting to a manual technique. Three patients had superficial infections at one of the sites where the fiducial marker pins had been fixed to the bone. All infections resolved under conservative management.

Postoperative Tibiofemoral Alignment

In the computerized preoperative planning procedure, the mechanical axis was routinely corrected to a tibiofemoral angle of 0°. The overall mean difference between the preoperative plan and postoperative result for tibiofemoral alignment was 0.8°, with a standard deviation of 1.0° and a range from 0 to 3°. In addition, the joint line with respect to the position of the femoral and tibial components was in good alignment. In 2004, Decking, with postoperative CT scans, proved the accuracy of this system in all planes, frontal, sagittal, and transverse.[11] The mean tibiofemoral angle in a comparable manual group (NexGen CR Prosthesis, Zimmer, Inc., Warsaw, IN) was 2.6° with a standard deviation of 2.2° and a range from 0 to 7°. Eighteen patients (35%) had a deviation >3°, with a maximum of 7°. The exact distribution of varus

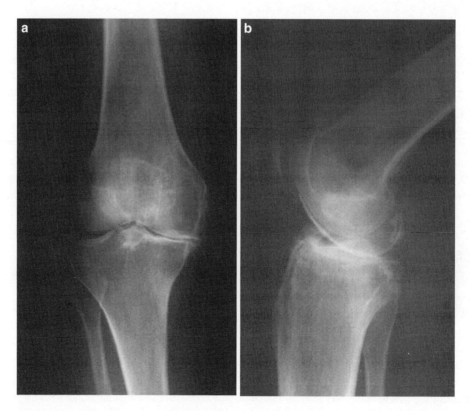

Fig. 80.6 (**a, b**) Anteroposterior and lateral X-rays of a patient with medial gonarthrosis before robotic TKA (From Siebert et al.,[9] with permission of Elsevier, Inc.)

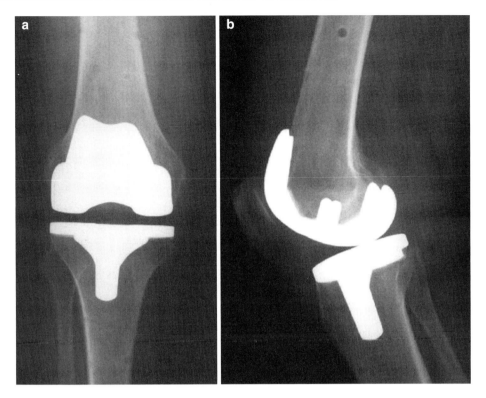

Fig. 80.7 (**a**, **b**) Anteroposterior and lateral X-rays of the same patient after robotic TKA (Search Evolution, Aesculap, Tuttlingen, Germany) (From Siebert et al.,[9] with permission of Elsevier, Inc.)

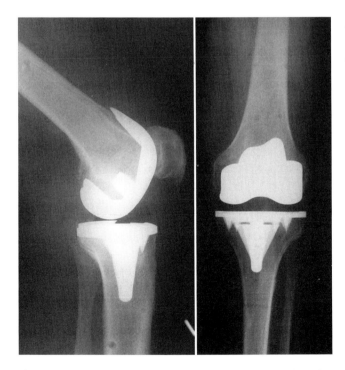

Fig. 80.8 Anteroposterior and lateral X-rays of the same patient after robotic TKA (Genesis, Smith & Nephew, Memphis, TN) (From Siebert et al.,[9] with permission of Elsevier, Inc.)

and valgus deviations of the mechanical axis is shown in Fig. 80.9. The difference in tibiofemoral alignment was highly significant at $p < 0.0001$.

Knee Society Score

The Knee Society Score is divided into the Knee score and the Function score. In each score, the patient can achieve a maximum of 100 points. The difference between the preoperative score and the scores at 12, 24, and 60 months after surgery was significant (Table 80.1). Unfortunately, comorbidity may influence the surgical results, therefore, some patients, especially older patients, rarely achieve the full score and continue loosing functional capabilities as evidenced by slightly lower values at 24 and 60 months postoperatively (Table 80.2).

Discussion

Various experimental active and semi-active robotic systems have been developed to improve the accuracy of implant alignment.[12] To our knowledge, this is the only clinical report of robotic TKA in a large series of consecutive patients with a 5-year follow-up.

Our results clearly demonstrate that, after a short learning period, an active robotic system allows the surgeon to execute the preoperative plan with unparalleled accuracy with a mean error below 1° and achieve optimum to very good results regarding tibiofemoral alignment in more than 95% of cases

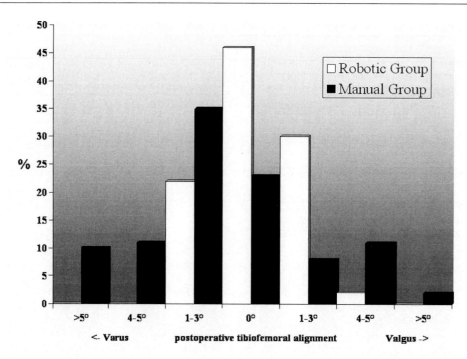

Fig. 80.9 Postoperative tibiofemoral angles of patients after manual and robotic TKA. Measured values show a much broader variation of varus or valgus angles after manual TKA compared with robotic technique ($p < 0.0001$) (From Siebert et al.,[9] with permission of Elsevier, Inc.)

Table 80.1 Comparison of knee score preoperative and after 60 months is highly significant in robot-assisted TKA

Knee score	Preoperative	12 months	24 months	60 months
Mean	38.60	87.73	91.59	90.49
Standard deviation	16.36	13.17	11.66	12.09
Number	108	105	96	85

Table 80.2 Comparison of function score preoperatively and after 60 months is highly significant in robot-assisted TKA

Function score	Preoperative	12 months	24 months	60 months
Mean	53.15	81.62	86.72	84.51
Standard deviation	16.04	17.63	17.97	18.39
Number	108	105	96	85

Table 80.3 Advantages of robot-assisted surgery

- Exact preoperative planning and transfer to the robot
- High precision and safety
- Better mechanical axis
- Reduced bone loss
- Exact milling process
- Precision of implantation is less dependent on experience and skill of the surgeon

as compared with approximately 65% with manual technique. Aglietti and coworkers reported that the majority of conventionally operated patients end up with a mean valgus angle of 9.6°, ranging from 2° to 16°.[13] Correct tibiofemoral alignment seems to be particularly important because it is generally agreed that axial deviation and imprecise implantation may

lead to early loosening of implant components.[14–17] An axial deviation of more than 3° or Maquet's line not passing through the middle third of the implant is considered the most frequent cause of early TKA failure.[18–21] The results of alignment after robotic TKA are not only superior to the results with conventional technique, but also to the results of computer-assisted, navigated TKA. Miehlke and coworkers found that 63% of patients had an acceptable tibiofemoral alignment within the 2° varus/valgus range after navigated TKA. More than 4° of deviation with a maximum error of 7° were observed in almost 7% of the navigated cases.[22] This indicates that although computer-assisted navigation yields superior results to manual technique, it is still inferior to the robotic technique regarding orientation of the prosthetic components. In contrast to the CASPAR system, navigation systems for TKA still depend on intramedullary and extramedullary guides, which might be an important cause for potential errors in axial alignment.[23] Another benefit of the robotic technique might be the accurate planning of the milling track and the type of cutting used. This should result in a reduced risk for injury of ligaments, vessels, and nerves, which are undoubtedly endangered by manually directed oscillating saws. The osseous insertion of the posterior cruciate ligament, for instance, can always be preserved. Implants fit more exactly because the milled surfaces are always precisely flat; a matter of particular importance when cementless systems are used. Finally, the amount of removed bony substance can be minimized, which could facilitate later revision surgery.

There are certain advantages and disadvantages in robot-assisted surgery, as shown in Tables 80.3 and 80.4.

Table 80.4 Disadvantages of robot-assisted surgery.

- Additional cost
- Increased planning time
- Longer operation time
- Soft tissue balancing depending on experience of surgeon
- Additional pins
- Rigid fixation of leg
- Additional CT

Robotic systems hold great promise in assisting surgeons to perform difficult procedures with a high degree of accuracy and repeatability. Preoperative plans can reliably be translated into clinical reality with the help of a robotic device. The CASPAR system fulfilled these requirements, but had major drawbacks, such as added costs, need for additional surgery, and CT imaging, as well as increased time for preoperative planning and surgery. Being a modified industrial robot that is, e.g., used for computer chip production in clean room environments, the CASPAR system represented quite a cumbersome piece of capital equipment, which, for many hospitals, is difficult to purchase and maintain. Despite excellent clinical results, in particular, in the area of knee arthroplasty, the CASPAR robot did not become a commercial success and the manufacturer stopped production and sales in 2001. Other robotic systems are currently being clinically investigated. Passive robotic systems that leave more control to the surgeon but limit the surgeon's path and range of milling and cutting seem to be ideal candidates for future clinical use, especially when combined with real-time computer navigation.[24–26]

References

1. Aglietti P, Buzzi R. Posteriorly stabilised total-condylar knee replacement. J Bone Joint Surg 70B: 211, 1988
2. Jeffery RS, Morris RW, Denham RA. Coronal alignment after total knee replacement. J Bone Joint Surg 73B: 709, 1991
3. Petersen TL, Engh GA. Radiographic assessment of knee alignment after total knee arthroplasty. J Arthroplasty 3: 67, 1988
4. Tew M, Waugh W. Tibiofemoral alignment and the results of knee replacement. J Bone Joint Surg 67B: 551, 1985
5. Garg A, Walker PS. Prediction of total knee motion using a three-dimensional computer graphics model. J Biochem 23: 45, 1990
6. Kwoh YS, Hou J, Jonckheere EA, Hayati S. A robot with improved absolute positioning accuracy for CT guided stereotactic brain surgery. IEEE Trans Biomed Eng 35(2): 153–160, 1998
7. Börner M, Bauer A, Lahmer A. Rechnerunterstützter Robotereinsatz in der Hüftendoprothetik. Orthopäde 26: 251–257, 1997
8. Petermann J, Kober R, Heinze, R, Frölich JJ, Heeckt PF, Gotzen L. Computer-assisted planning and robot-assisted surgery in anterior cruciate ligament reconstruction. Oper Tech Orthop 10: 50, 2000
9. Siebert W, Mai S, Kober R, Heeckt PF. Technique and first clinical results of robot-assisted total knee replacement. Knee 9: 173–180, 2002
10. Insall JN, Dorr LD, Scott R, Scott WN. Rationale of the knee society clinical rating system. Clin Orthop Relat Res 248: 13, 1989
11. Decking J, Theis C, Achenbach T, Roth E, Nafe B, Eckhardt A. Robotic total knee arthroplasty: the accuracy of CT-based component placement. Acta Orthop Scand 75: 573–579, 2004
12. Howe RD, Matsuoka Y. Robotics for surgery. Annu Rev Biomed Eng 1: 211, 1999
13. Aglietti P, Buzzi R, Gaudenzi A. Patellofemoral functional results and complications with the posterior stabilized total condylar knee prosthesis. J Arthroplasty 3: 17, 1988
14. Ecker ML, Lotke PA, Sindsor RE, Cella JP. Long-term results after total condylar knee arthroplasty. Significance of radiolucent lines. Clin Orthop Relat Res 216: 151, 1987
15. Feng EL, Stuhlberg SD, Wixon RL. Progressive subluxation and polyethylene wear in total knee replacements with flat articular surfaces. Clin Orthop Relat Res 299: 60, 1994
16. Laskin RS. Total condylar knee replacement in patients who have rheumatoid arthritis. A ten year follow-up study. J Bone Joint Surg 72A: 529, 1990
17. Ritter M, Merbst WA, Keating EM, Faris PM. Radiolucency at the bone-cement interface in total knee replacement. J Bone Joint Surg 76A: 60, 1991
18. Goodfellow JW, O'Connor JJ. Clinical results of the Oxford knee. Clin Orthop Relat Res 205: 21, 1986
19. Insall JN, Ranawat CS, Aglietti P, Shine J. A comparison of four models of total knee-replacement prosthesis. J Bone Joint Surg 58A: 754, 1976
20. Insall JN, Binzzir R, Soudry M, Mestriner LA. Total knee arthroplasty. Clin Orthop Relat Res 192: 13, 1985
21. Ranawat CS, Adjei OB. Survivorship analysis and results of total condylar knee arthroplasty. Clin Orthop Relat Res 323: 168, 1988
22. Miehlke RK, Clemens U, Kershally S. Computer integrated instrumentation in knee arthroplasty – a comparative study of conventional and computerized technique. Presented at the Fourth Annual North American Program on Computer Assisted Orthopaedic Surgery, Pittsburgh, PA, June 2000
23. Nuño-Siebrecht N, Tanzer M, Bobyn JD. Potential errors in axial alignment using intramedullary instrumentation for total knee arthroplasty. J Arthroplasty 15: 228, 2000
24. Shi F, Zhang J, Liu Y, Zhao Z. A hand-eye robotic model for total knee replacement surgery. Med Image Comput Comput Assist Inverv Int Conf Med Image Comput Comput Assist Interv.8(Pt2): 122–30, 2005
25. Adili A. Robot assisted orthopedic surgery. Semin Laparosc Surg 11(2): 89, 2004
26. Jakopec M, Harris SJ, Rodriguez y Baena F, Gomes P, Cobb J, Davies BL. The first clinical application of a « hands on » robotic knee surgery system. Comput Aided Surg 6(6): 329, 2001

Index

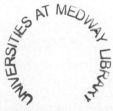Printed in the United States of America